THE
HISTORY OF
CARDIOLOGY

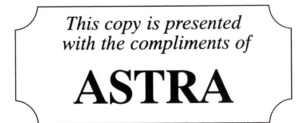

*This copy is presented
with the compliments of*

ASTRA

To my wife Dorothy
without whose forbearance and support
this work would not have been possible

THE
HISTORY OF
CARDIOLOGY

Louis J. Acierno, M.D., F.A.C.C., F.A.C.P.
Professor, Cardiopulmonary Sciences
University of Central Florida

The Parthenon Publishing Group
International Publishers in Medicine, Science & Technology

LONDON   *CASTERTON*   NEW YORK

British Library Cataloguing-in-Publication Data
Acierno, L. J.
   History of Cardiology
   I. Title
   616.1009

   ISBN   1-85070-339-6

Library of Congress Cataloging-in-Publication Data
Acierno, Louis J., 1920–
   A history of cardiology/L. J. Acierno.
        p.   cm.
   Includes bibliographical references and index.
   ISBN 1-85070-339-6
   1. Cardiology--History.   I. Title
   [DNLM: 1. Cardiology – History. WG 11.1
   A181h 1993]
   RC666.5. A24 1993
   616. 1'2'009 – dc20
   DNLM/DLC
   for Library of Congress   93–22688
                                         CIP

Published in the UK and Europe by
The Parthenon Publishing Group Limited
Casterton Hall, Carnforth
Lancs. LA6 2LA

Published in North America by
The Parthenon Publishing Group Inc.
One Blue Hill Plaza, PO Box 1564
Pearl River, New York 10965, USA

Copyright © 1994 Parthenon Publishing Group Ltd

First published 1994

Composed by Ryburn Typesetting, Keele University
Printed and bound by The Bath Press, Avon

Contents

Introduction

The high level of diagnostic and therapeutic sophistication in the management of cardiovascular disease today has truly been one of the most outstanding achievements of mankind. This level of excellence did not emerge *de novo*. As in all human endeavors, it rests upon concepts established in the past and contributed by researchers from various countries throughout the world, but especially from those of the western civilization. Furthermore, no matter how novel each new concept or technique may appear to be, it is, in reality, but an extension or refinement of an earlier contribution.

Although many of us tend to deprecate the technological mantle that surrounds the practice of cardiology in this enlightened twentieth century, it is, nevertheless, important to emphasize the distinct benefits that have accrued because of this technological orientation. Without it, cardiology would still be a primitive discipline. Utilized wisely and coupled with the maturity of thought formulated by our predecessors, technological advancements have been the solid rock upon which all modern 'miracles' are being performed today. An often quoted statement in medicine is that progress has been made by placing ourselves on the shoulders of the giants that preceded us. The truism of this statement becomes even more evident as we trace the roots of all current knowledge. Cardiology is what it is today simply because of the monumental contributions of the great minds throughout the centuries.

There have been many admirable publications concerning the history of cardiology. Another text would add really little of value other than updating the developments that constitute the core of modern cardiological practice. On the other hand, an approach utilizing a matrix consisting of anatomical, pathological, physiological, and patho-physiological components constitutes the *raison d'etre* of this book.

A history of cardiology in terms of these components would then have two objectives. It could serve as a vehicle for understanding the modern concepts that govern the current practice of cardiology, and provide, at the same time, the means for incorporating each new concept into the present state of knowledge. The sequel to such an approach would result in an in-depth under-standing of the various diagnostic tools used today and provide simultaneously a rational basis for the various current therapeutic modalities.

The realization of the internationalism of medical thought and activity is another ancillary benefit. This, coupled with the acquisition and presentation of detailed and intimate portraits of the personalities involved (with varied national and ethnic backgrounds), should present us with unlimited opportunities for cultural enrichment.

No single nation can claim total contribution towards cardiovascular knowledge. At the same time, no single individual can claim complete originality or independence of thought. In fact, the very fabric of medicine itself is tightly interwoven with the threads of internationalism so that a knowledge of the significant historical developments of cardiology will nullify any ethnic prejudice or chauvinism that may be harbored initially.

The intricacies involved, the complexity and vastness of the subject matter, and the abstruse nature of the various scientific disciplines that have played a role in the evolution of cardiovascular knowledge, present a challenge to anyone who attempts to convey the historical information at the level of the general reader. The reader may be an individual truly curious about the historical developments in cardiology but who lacks the scientific background to unravel the maze of medical jargon. The reader can be a student in the field of nursing and allied health, or a student enrolled in a discipline far removed from the biological sciences. Finally, the reader can be that individual who needs to understand the complexities of modern cardiological practice in order to cope with his own illness. A knowledge of the evolution of current concepts in cardiology would help that patient in sorting out and appreciating the various diagnostic and therapeutic options available today. In any case, the motivation to read a book of this kind would be a sincere desire to learn more about the men and ideas responsible for the present day management of cardiovascular disturbances.

This is the audience for whom these words are intended. In an attempt to accomplish this, I have striven to present the material in as lucid a manner as possible. Whenever a new idea or technical term is introduced, I have couched it in phraseology that should be understood without an intensive background in the biological or associated sciences.

The study of history can be likened to the journey of a ship through many seas, stopping at various ports of call through the centuries and adding, with each stop, another bit of cargo to its store of knowledge. There are times during this journey when the ship appears to have no rudder, meandering aimlessly or moving in tangential directions, only to resume once more its forward thrust. Time and again, it appears to be overloaded with superfluous cargo and sinking under the weight of erroneous information only to return once more on a true course under the hands of a new and aggressive captain. At the same time, the realization of the importance of each member of the crew becomes increasingly evident in the light of each individual's contribution to the total sum of knowledge. There are times when the captain merely collates these efforts. There are times, however, where the captain is so brilliant and forceful that it is he and he alone who is responsible for the forward motion of the ship and who causes it to make great strides. This is history, whether it applies to social and geopolitical changes or scientific advances. This has certainly been the history of cardiology.

The most difficult task in the preparation of this work was to determine how the information was to be presented. A mere concatenation of events would not have sufficed. Should the text consist of flashbacks starting with current diagnostic and therapeutic techniques? Would it be better to formulate the approach on the basis of disease categories, as in a standard textbook of cardiology?

It appeared to me that the most logical approach would be one that preserved the sequential nature of each contribution within the matrix as

originally described. This would allow for the proper interfacing between the various components of the matrix and the diagnostic and therapeutic advances as they occurred.

In adhering to this rather simplistic criterion, it was felt that the goal could be realized by utilizing a format consisting of the following categories: (1) the anatomy of the heart and blood vessels; (2) structural abnormalities of the heart and blood vessels; (3) functional mechanisms of the heart and blood vessels; and (4) functional disturbances of the heart and blood vessels. This would then lead us into the presentation of the evolutionary changes and diagnostic techniques, beginning with physical diagnosis and ending with current invasive and non-invasive procedures. Finally, it would allow us to trace the development of the various therapeutic modalities utilizing preventive, interventional, and pharmaceutical approaches.

The most difficult part of the task was the research of the literature. This required the utilization of both primary and secondary sources. Many of the older primary sources were available only at specific libraries. I visited the National Library of Medicine in Bethesda, Maryland, the libraries at Cambridge and Oxford Universities and the University of Bologna. Primary bibliographic material was made available to me also by the Wellcome Institute, the Royal Society of Medicine and the Royal College of Physicians. I also utilized the facilities of our own libraries at the University of Central Florida and Florida Hospital of Orlando.

The spelling of names varies depending on the translator and ethnic source. The reader will notice some names spelled differently in different chapters. This too was dependent upon the source of the material.

The work was made possible through the unstinting help of the staff at all of the above institutions. My thanks alone could never repay them. I must thank in particular the following who were singularly helpful in my task. Dr John Parascandola, Chief of the Division of the History of Medicine at the National Library of Medicine was a delight to meet, an able scholar, and above all a constant source of help and encouragement in this endeavor. His associates in the photo archives went out of their way to help in procuring many of the illustrations. They are Jan Lazarus and Lucy Keister. Barbara Breckner and Pat Vaughan of the Florida Hospital Library staff were always ready to procure for me still another reference whenever I asked, and I am indebted to them for their cooperation. Among my colleagues at the University of Central Florida I must acknowledge with gratitude the efforts of L. Timothy Worrell, who helped me in so many ways, and Dan Crittenden for the proofreading of the manuscript. I must also acknowledge the efforts on the part of our departmental secretary, Toni Painter, who, despite a heavy load from other members of the faculty, found the time to obtain permissions for the reproduction of the illustrations. My heartfelt thanks go to Mary Busbee for her painstaking care in transcribing onto the printed page my handwritten manuscript. Finally, I must acknowledge with the utmost appreciation the editorial assistance of the Parthenon Publishing Group for their meticulous attention to detail, conducted under the able guidance of Jean Wright and Julia Tissington.

Whatever errors are present are mine and mine alone.

Section 1

Anatomy of the heart and blood vessels

1   Earliest concepts (theory and myths)

Although this historical survey of the anatomy of the heart and blood vessels will focus primarily on the structural elements, it must be borne in mind that structure in and of itself is meaningless unless it can be correlated with the function that the structure must provide. This is a fundamental principle of nature and should always be kept in focus. Many of the errors spawned throughout the ages are due to loss of this correlation. Function without structure cannot exist and structure has no meaning unless it serves its functional purpose[1]. It is for this reason that statements about function are often made in this survey.

The earliest myths concerning the anatomical makeup of the heart and vessels date back to primitive man and rest upon beliefs rather than observation. Moreover, these beliefs had a mystical flavor and were religious in origin defying and rejecting, as it were, any attempts at rational analysis. Theocracy ruled supreme and when it did not, authoritarianism took its place. It was only much later when the scientific discipline of observation and experimentation became entrenched that authoritarianism was swept away. This took place at the expense of much human misery, spilled blood, humiliation and denigration of great minds and continues today despite the so-called intellectual liberation of the last two centuries.

Anatomical descriptions of the heart can be found as far back as the Bible. These biblical references to the anatomy of the heart as well as later references from the Talmud are summarized by F. Rosner in his book, *Medicine in the Bible and the Talmud*[2]. He states that there are two Hebrew words for heart. They are *lev* and *levav*. Both words or their variations appear at least 827 times in the Bible, and most of the time these words are used in a descriptive or figurative sense. The word *lev* or its Aramaic equivalent, *libba*, is found also in the Talmud but, in addition to the heart, it may have other meanings such as stomach, chest, breast or mind. Rosner cites many examples of these various meanings. He also states that the Talmud serves as a primary source of preoccupation with the anatomy of the heart. Chambers and great vessels are recognized but not valves. The following quotation from his text documents these anatomical references: 'The Mishnah recognized (*Hullin 3:1*) that if the heart [of an animal] was pierced as far as the cavity thereof, the animal cannot survive and is declared *terefah* (unfit for ritual slaughtering and consumption). R. Zera raised the question: Does it mean as far as the small cavity or as far as the large cavity? (*Hullin 45b*)'. Apparently, small cavity seems to mean the right and large cavity the left part of the heart, not a differentiation of atrium and ventricle as we now know it. Moses Maimonides, in his *Mishneh Torah*, reiterates the fatal outcome of a pierced heart, but also describes left and right chambers of the heart as follows:

> If the heart is pierced as far as the chambers thereof, whether as far as the large chamber on the left or the small one on the right, the animal is *terefah*. If only the flesh of the heart is pierced, but the perforation does not penetrate inside the chamber, it is permitted. The aorta, that is, the large artery which leads from the heart to the lung, is like the heart: if it is perforated to the smallest extent into its cavity, it is *terefah*. [*Hilhot Shehitah 6:5*]

The code of Jewish law of Joseph Karo states that the heart has three chambers (*Shulhan Arukh, Yoreh Deah 40:1*). It remained for more recent anatomists to correctly describe the four chambers of the mammalian heart. There is also no mention of heart valves in the Talmud and the major commentaries thereon. The piercing of an animal's heart, and the possible use to which such a nonviable animal may be put, is discussed in other parts of the Talmud (*Abodah Zarah 29b, Sefer Torah 1:2, Soferim 1:2*).

The aorta is also described in the Talmud as follows:

As to the aorta [lit, the artery of the heart], Rab says the slightest perforation therein [will render the animal *terefah*] and Samuel says [it is *terefah* only if] the greater portion [of its circumference was severed] … Amemar said in the name of R. Nahman: There are three main vessels, one leads to the heart [aorta], one leads to the lungs [pulmonary artery], and one leads to the liver [inferior vena cava?] [*Hullin 45b*]

The two carotid arteries are described by Maimonides in his *Commentary on the Mishnah (Hullin 1:1)*, where he calls them the pulsating vessels on the side of the neck.

In pre-hellenic times there are only the vaguest allusions to anatomical detail. The first references to structure, and quite superficial at that, are to be found in a collection of writings that were discovered in the ruins of Ashurbanipal, a palace in Nineveh[1]. Among these writings are included the code of Hammurabi which provides a very good insight into the practice of medicine during the Babyl-Assyrian era[3].

Against a background of magic, religious beliefs, idolatry and satanism, the Babylonian practitioners of this epoch had a very confused conception of cardiovascular anatomy[3]. First of all, they made no distinction between arteries and veins although they did refer to arterial blood as blood of the day and venous blood as blood of the night. There was not the slightest idea concerning the physiological implications of the anatomy of these blood vessels and their contents.

It was no better during the succeeding civilization in Egypt. Here again, theology interfered with objective observation. It is true that the Egyptians were experts at embalming. This practice was raised to a high art primarily because the Egyptians believed that under no circumstances was the body to fall prey to animals for, in so doing, the body would lose its former spirit and could never be reunited. Since worms were considered animals, mummification was developed to prevent the desecration of the body by these scavengers. Despite the level of sophistication that their embalming methods reached, the Egyptians failed to acquire any significant knowledge of human anatomy during the process. Figure 1 is an engraving by Pomet showing Egyptian mummies, corpse, pyramid, and embalming process.

The most important and enlightening sources regarding the Egyptians' grasp of cardiovascular anatomy are to be found in three papyri. These are named after their discoverers and are known as: The Edwin Smith Surgical Papyrus, The Ebers Papyrus and the Brugsch Papyrus. The word papyrus refers to a paper-like material derived from the stem of the paper reed, *Cyperus papyrus*, a plant cultivated in ancient times in the Nile Delta region of Egypt. The invention of the alphabet along with the discovery of the papyrus as a vehicle for the preservation of the written word accelerated the diffusion and transmission of knowledge to an unbelievable degree, abolishing forever the pitfalls and constraints of oral passage of information and its clay and stone substitutes.

Edwin Smith acquired the papyrus named after him in Thebes in 1862. It remained as an obscure item among the archives of the New York Historical Society to which it had been bequeathed by Smith's daughter until 1920 at which time J. H. Breasted of the Oriental Institute of the University of Chicago translated and deciphered it at the request of the society[4]. The author of this document is unknown though the name of Imhotep, the earliest known physician, has been advanced as being responsible for it. It is a very old document perhaps dating as far back as 3000 BC. In it the heart is described as being the center of a system of blood vessels extending peripherally to various parts of the body without reference to what they are distributing. A direct correlation is made between the pulse and the heart, but again, there is no insight into the true mechanism of the circulation though the pulse is said to be influenced by the force and action of the heart[5].

The second papyrus was also discovered in Thebes; this time by George Ebers. He apparently acquired it in 1872 from an inhabitant of that city, who, in turn, probably procured it from a grave robber. Neither the location of the grave nor the mummy that occupied it are known. This document is probably at least 1500 years younger that the Edwin Smith papyrus. It too describes the heart as being the center of a system of vessels supplying the various parts of the body. Many more vessels are listed than in the Smith document. Again, the anatomical descriptions are meager and erroneous. The Ebers papyrus does state that the heart is located on the left side unless displaced by disease. The manuscript is now at the University of Leipzig having been originally translated into

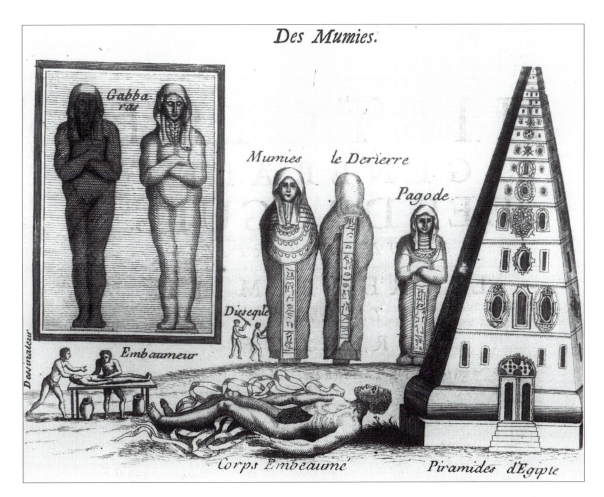

Figure 1 Embalming: showing Egyptian mummies, corpse, pyramids, and embalming process. *Photo Source National Library of Medicine. Literary Source Pomet: Histoire generale des drogues, Paris, 1694. Courtesy of National Library of Medicine*

German by H. Joachim[6–8]. A page from the Ebers papyrus is depicted in Figure 2.

The Brugsch papyrus also describes the heart in similar terms as in the Ebers Papyrus[9]. In addition, there is a superficial description of the anatomy of the veins. This papyrus is also known as the Greater Berlin Papyrus. Its author is unknown with Castiglioni dating its origin, however, within the reign of Casti, the fifth king of the first dynasty[10]. Willius and Dry[11] ascribe the following quotation regarding its discovery to a Mr. Passalacqua in his catalogue of books[12]:

It was carefully covered up in a vase of baked clay, along with the small manuscript 1,559 in similar hieratic writing, and bearing a date and cartouches; this vase was discovered alone amongst the ruins, at a depth of about ten feet, near the pyramids of Sakarah at Memphis.

These authors also state the possibility that Galen may have referred to this papyrus in his writings.

The true evolution of anatomical knowledge, general as well as cardiovascular, can be described as being fueled during five major epochs of western civilization. These would include those eras dominated by the Greeks, Alexandrians and Romans and those two periods of time referred to as the Middle Ages and the Renaissance. During each era, certain great personalities stand out as we shall see.

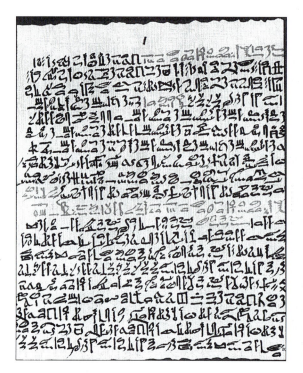

Figure 2 Ebers papyrus. *Photo Source National Library of Medicine. Literary Source Wreszinski, Walter: Atlas zur Altaegyptischen Kulturgeschichte, J.C. Henrichs Buchhandlung, Leipzig, 1914–1946. Courtesy of National Library of Medicine*

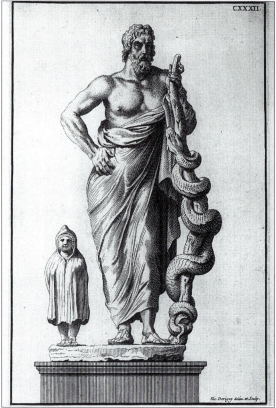

Figure 3 Aesculapius. *Photo Source National Library of Medicine. Literary Source Ni. Dorigny delin. et Sculp. Courtesy of National Library of Medicine*

Although Greek culture relied heavily on Egyptian and Babylonian sources, the independent mind of the Greek in time divorced itself from this background and established new practices while clinging to the rituals of old. This was particularly evident in their approach to disease. It meant the gradual establishment of the art of healing that was stripped of sacerdotal monopoly while still paying lip service to pagan deities that were part of the panoply of healing gods. The most important of these healers was Aesculapius, the god of medicine, and supposedly, the son of Apollo (see Figure 3) [13,14].

A whole cult of healing grew up around Aesculapius. Temples were built in his name. They were called Asclepions and the priests staffing these temples were called Asclepiads. A facade of an Asclepion is shown in Figure 4. These medical priests persisted for centuries. Their beliefs and concepts were influenced a great deal not only by their predecessors but also by the teachings of the numerous philosophers that continually sprung up in ancient Greece like so many weeds. Eventually the sacerdotalism surrounding these practitioners was discarded along with the custom of attending to the sick within the walls of the Asclepions. Gradually, the term Asclepiad began to acquire a new meaning, indicating a physician belonging to a family of physicians that had produced well-known physicians for many generations.

Perhaps the greatest of these Asclepiads, or at least the best known, is Hippocrates, reputed to be a descendant of Aesculapius himself. Hippocrates was born on the island of Cos, Greece, in 460 BC and died in 377 BC. Details of his life are rather scanty, but it is known that he traveled widely in Greece and Asia Minor practicing medicine and teaching. Plato, a contemporary, referred to Hippocrates as a famous Asclepiad with a philosophical approach to medicine. Aristotle also

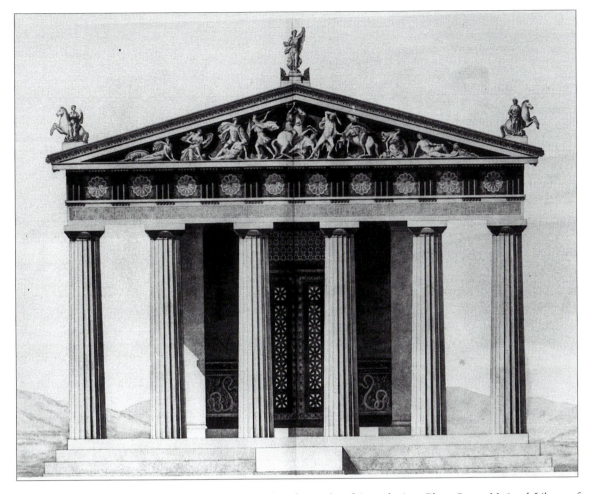

Figure 4 Medicine – Greek and Roman: Facade of Temple of Aesculapius. *Photo Source National Library of Medicine. Literary Source Lechat: Epidaure, restauration et description. Paris, 1895. Courtesy of National Library of Medicine*

alluded to Hippocrates as the great physician and commented on his small stature[15]. A Roman bust of Hippocrates is depicted in Figure 5.

Although a considerable body of medical literature existed before him, the writings of Hippocrates and those of his followers supersede all the previous ones because of the totality of their approach to various aspects of medical practice. The works are quite variable in length, style and orientation. Out of the original 70 in number, only 60 are still extant. Some of the works are philosophical rather than medical. Some were written for physicians, others for their assistants or students, and still others for laymen. The whole compendium of treatises is known as the Hippocratic Collection (Corpus Hippocraticum)[16].

Only those parts that deal specifically with cardiovascular anatomy are of particular importance to us. These anatomical descriptions are woefully inaccurate, and represent, for the most part, a hodge-podge of misinformation, myths and beliefs passed from one author to another, distorted or embellished by all to finally emerge as unchallenged and unproven statements of fact which they definitely are not. The valves of the heart, the ventricles and the great vessels are described with little attention to detail or pathological alterations. The heart is described as a firm thick mass so richly supplied with fluid that it does not suffer harm or manifest pain[17]. How untrue! However, he did identify four cavities. The left ventricle was described as being rougher

7

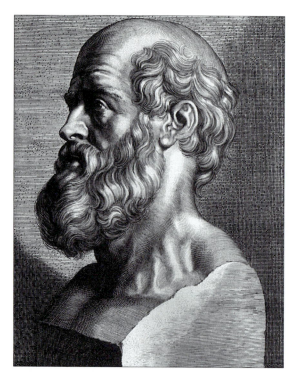

Figure 5 Hippocrates. *Photo Source National Library of Medicine. Literary Source P.P. Rubens delineauit. P. Pontius Sculp. Courtesy of National Library of Medicine*

than the right due to its being filled with untempered heat[18]. He did prove that the aortic valve could only open one way by showing that no leakage occurred back into the ventricle when water was poured into the aorta above the valve. Because of its shape, the aortic valve was called the sigmoid valve. The pulmonary valve was also called sigmoid since its shape was similar to that of the aortic. The pericardium was described as a smooth mantle surrounding the heart and containing a small amount of fluid resembling urine[19].

Several other personalities of the Hippocratic era should be mentioned for their contributions to the field of cardiovascular anatomy. These are Polybus (fl. 375 BC), the son-in-law of Hippocrates; Diocles of Corystus (fl. 400 BC); and Aristotle (384 –322 BC)[20]. Diocles is alleged to have been responsible for distinguishing the aorta from the vena cava but without having offered any insight into their relationship with the rest of the vascular system. Aristotle, on the other hand, attempted to

establish a relationship by describing two large vessels placed ventral to the spinal column, the smaller of which he termed the aorta, which he located to the left of the column while the larger was placed to the right of the column. He claimed they arose from the heart, which he located quite accurately, but he became confused by the vena cava and pulmonary artery[21]. Aristotle also was somewhat confused about the gross anatomy of the heart. He did not notice the valves and he made no distinction between arteries and veins. He described the heart as having only three cavities. Bonnabeau advances the opinion that this marked error was due to the fact that he killed his animals prior to dissection by strangulation and proceeded with his dissection with the heart remaining *in situ*[22]. Since in doing so both the right atrium and ventricle were engorged with blood, these two chambers appeared as one cavity.

During the Alexandrian period all forms of science were fostered. Among these disciplines were anatomy and physiology with dissection being carried out on condemned criminals[23]. Erasistratus (310–250 BC) and Herophilus (335–280 BC) stand out in this era as the two strongest contributors of anatomical knowledge. Herophilus described the pulmonary artery, calling it the arterious vein. Esteem for Herophilus as an anatomist continued for centuries. Fallopius, many centuries later, evaluated him in the following words: 'Quando Galenum refutat Herophilium censeo ipsum refutare Evangelium'. (When Galen refutes Herophilus I feel that he refutes the Gospel itself)[24]. He labeled the pulmonary artery as the arterial vein because though it carried venous blood, it had the thickness of an artery. Like the Greeks, the Alexandrians erroneously believed that the blood vessels emanating from the heart contained air (the Greek's pneuma). Artery is derived from the Greek word for air, *area*. Thus, the arterial vein, though it had the thickness of an artery, carried blood instead of air. Herophilus also showed that the auricles were really cardiac structures rather than venous. Erasistratus investigated the tricuspid and mitral valves along with their chordae tendinae, calling them respectively the tricuspid and sigmoid. He must also be credited with having anticipated Malpighi's discovery of the capillary system by postulating on theoretical grounds alone a system of communicating invisible orifices between the arteries and veins[25]. Again, both men perpetuated the erroneous notion that the arteries were filled with air.

We will meet Erasistratus again in his role as a physiologist, which is what he essentially was.

Information regarding the Roman period of anatomical contributions is available to us mostly from *De Medicina*, a treatise written by Aurelius Celsus (25 BC–AD 50) at the beginning of the Christian era. It is of interest to note that Celsus, a Roman aristocrat belonging to the patrician family of Cornelii, though deeply interested in medicine, was not a physician at all. Celsus wrote the treatise primarily for the edification of his fellow Roman landlords, who, distrustful of the Greek physicians, insisted that they themselves ministered to the medical needs of their servants, slaves and tenants. Figure 6 is a likeness of Celsus. *De Medicina* was actually part of a monumental encyclopedia dealing with philosophy, rhetoric, military art, law, agriculture and medicine. The treatise on medicine is the only portion that has survived, and it contains one of the first accounts of heart disease. It had enjoyed a greater acclaim posthumously than during his lifetime, being largely ignored by his contemporaries. It is now considered one of the greatest medical classics of antiquity. It became one of the most important medical reference works of the Renaissance following its discovery by Pope Nicholas V, and with the invention of the printing press the impetus for its wide dissemination was assured[26]. This work of Aurelius Celsus must be regarded as the first significant treatise on medicine since the Hippocratic Collection, and despite its imprecise expressions, it has become an important primary source for the latinized nomenclature of anatomy[27,28]. Pliny's natural history also shares this distinction[29].

Another avid student of anatomy and physiology during the early Christian era was Aretaeus of Cappadoccia (2nd–3rd century). Unlike Celsus, Aretaeus was a physician. He studied medicine in Alexandria but practiced in Rome as well. Although he was advanced by some historians as the greatest physician after Hippocrates, very few currently subscribe to this view. Aretaeus wrote two treatises and we are indebted to F. Adams for their translation into English[30]. Although his contributions to cardiovascular anatomy are nil, he is of interest because he pointed out the correlation that exists between cardiac and pulmonary activities, though he erroneously maintained that the heart stimulated respiratory function.

Galen, probably the best known figure in the history of medicine, also enacted his role during the

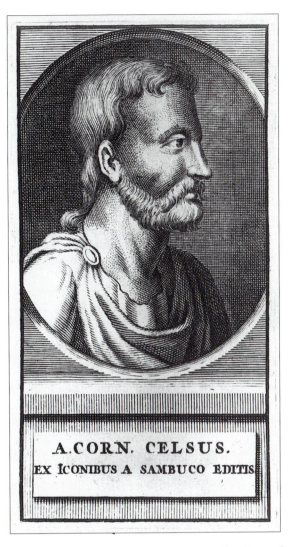

A.CORN. CELSUS.
EX ICONIBUS A SAMBUCO EDITIS

Figure 6 Celsus. *Photo Source National Library of Medicine. Literary Source Photo Archives. Courtesy of National Library of Medicine*

2nd century. Claudius Galen was born in Pergamis, Mysia (modern Bergama in Turkey) in AD 129 and died c.AD 199[31]. He too placed a great deal of stress on the value of anatomy, though, since dissection of the human body was illegal in his day, his anatomical descriptions were derived from pigs and apes, especially the barbary ape. Only 83 of his more than 200 works have come down to us. Galen was chief physician of the gladiators and this is probably why his forte was musculoskeletal anatomy. He had rather formidable features as seen in Figure 7.

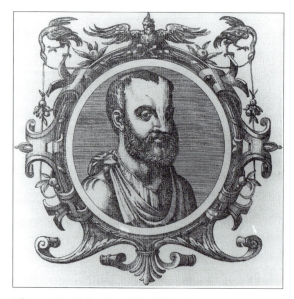

Figure 7 Galen (AD 130–200). *Photo Source National Library of Medicine. Literary Source Photo Archives. Courtesy of National Library of Medicine*

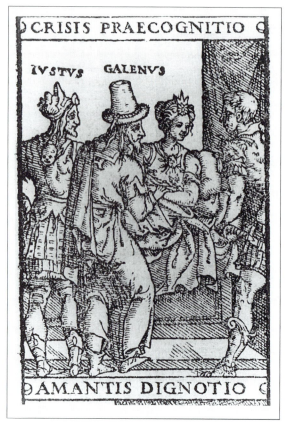

Figure 8 Galen treating a woman in love. *Photo Source National Library of Medicine. Literary Source Photo Archives. Courtesy of National Library of Medicine*

After Hippocrates, it is Galen who appears to be the foremost of Greek physicians. His monolithic contributions came to be regarded as the Bible of Medicine. Galen was not only an anatomist and experimental physiologist but a highly successful practitioner as well (Figure 8). He was somewhat anachronistic in that, while attempting to seek the truth by experimentation and dissection, he still believed in many of the mystical notions of his predecessors. Though he contributed greatly towards medical practice, his influence extended over too long a period of time, so that ultimately he had a retarding influence on the scientific development of medicine. It was not until thirteen hundred years after his death with the waning of his influence that medicine really began to progress[32].

Galen's contributions to cardiovascular anatomy are at best meager and quite erroneous. He thought that all the vessels which were connected with the heart were arteries while those connected with the liver were veins. Galen's concept of the cardiovascular system is depicted in Figure 9. He also subscribed to the view that the interventricular septum was riddled with invisible pores which allowed the blood to pass from the right ventricle to the left ventricle. In contradistinction to these erroneous views, Galen contributed by experi-

mentation and observation some very important facts regarding the pulse and heart. For example, he proved that the heart had the intrinsic ability to beat after being excised, indicating its independence of anatomical control by the brain or spinal cord. This bit of information can certainly help to explain how transplanted hearts can continue to function without being tethered to the recipients' nervous systems. Galen's views on the pulse are presented in Section 5, while his views on circulation are discussed in detail in Section 3. Figure 10 is a vignette showing Galen using a pig in an anatomical demonstration.

With Galen's death, further development of general anatomical knowledge remained at a standstill. The transmission of medical knowledge, such as it was, came to rely more and more on his written teachings and those of Hippocrates; being

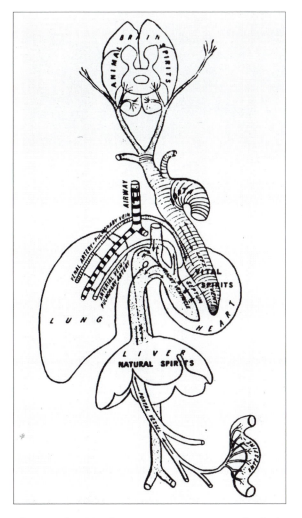

Figure 9 Circulatory system as conceived in ancient times. *Photo Source National Library of Medicine. Literary Source Photo Archives. Courtesy of National Library of Medicine*

transmitted from generation to generation by the preceptor system. For centuries, Byzantine physicians were important in preserving this inherited body of knowledge, collating it, and passing it on to their preceptees. This practice persisted until the Arabians began to make their own contributions through their translations of the Greek texts. As in all translations, it was inevitable that personal opinions and errors would creep in and considerable confusion created by failure to substitute the exact word in the translation for the original. Translations alone, without concomitant independent investi-

gation, resulted in increasingly greater reliance on authority so that Galen's influence became even more pervasive. Anatomical knowledge could not progress under these conditions.

It was during this time that the initial beginnings of the university system came into being. From the humble beginnings of a master and his pupils, gathered together in a single room bereft of comfort, larger groups gradually evolved consisting of students and several masters, pooling their resources but studying several disciplines. A group of this sort was initially called studium or studium generale. It was not until the 14th century that the word university was first applied to designate this type of teaching arrangement; the analogy being guild or corporation since this was the original meaning of the stem word universitas.

The most reputable and important prototype of a university was the somewhat loosely formed school of medicine that was established in Salerno and which came to be called Civitas Hippocratica. Its origins are shrouded in obscurity but with most scholars agreeing that it could rightfully be called the first Christian European Medical School.

Salerno is a seaport situated on the Western coast of southern Italy just at the end of that beautiful serpentine littoral road known as the Amalfi Drive. Its salubrious climate made it an ideal health resort, guaranteeing, as it were, the continued growth and popularity of its medical school. Royal favor and an edict by Emperor Frederick II in 1224 regulating educational prerequisites for the practice of surgery further assured its existence as a center of learning until the founding of the Neapolitan school.

An immensely popular poem entitled *Regimen Sanitatis Salernitanum* attests to the fame of the Salernitan school throughout most of the Middle Ages. This poem, originally written in Latin, was translated into many European tongues and outlines the Salernitan rules for hygiene and medical treatment. An English translation was made available in 1920[33].

Still under the influence of Hippocrates, Galen and other authoritarian sources, anatomical knowledge at Salerno, however, continued to remain stagnant. Only one dissection a year was carried out, and this was on a pig with anatomy being taught for the most part from the ancient texts or later from texts written by Salernitan teachers that were, in reality, compilations and rearrangements of older manuscrips[34].

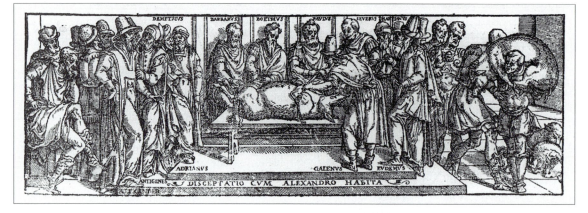

Figure 10 Vignette from title page showing Galen using a pig in an anatomical demonstration. *Photo Source National Library of Medicine. Literary Source Photo Archives. Courtesy of National Library of Medicine*

It was during this era, the early part of the Middle Ages, that our Islamic heritage manifested itself. Among the many important Muslim physicians, there were four that contributed greatly towards the advancement of cardiovascular anatomy and, concomitantly, towards the physiology of the heart and vessels. Their works span the years between AD 948 and AD 1200. They are Ali Husain Gilani (AD 948), Ibn Cena (AD 980), Abul Sahl Masihi (AD 1027), and Alanddin Qarshi Ibn an-Nafis (AD 1200)[35]. It is quite difficult at times to trace these individuals since there may be several variations in the spelling of their names. For example, Cena is also written as Sn and at the same time he is also known to us as Avicenna.

Avicenna is the most widely known of the four. He wrote a five volume tome entitled *Canon of Medicine (Al-Qanun fil-Tibb)*. It was used at many medical schools, even at Montpellier as late as 1650. Avicenna has been called the prince of physicians. He was a Persian. His writings were not restricted to medical topics but also involved geology and chemistry. Avicenna apparently also practiced physical therapy. Figure 11 depicts him massaging a man's back for possibly a muscle or bone disorder. Willius and Dry relate how Avicenna became ill with colic while discharging his duties as a military surgeon[36]. His symptoms suggest the possibility that they were the initial manifestations of a chronic colitis and reinforce the age-old adage that the doctor who has himself for a patient has a fool for a doctor. Avicenna had eight enemas given to him on the first day of his bout with colic, weakening him

severely and, still more so, when the dysentery became recurrent with continued administration of more enemas and opium. Avicenna apparently died from this ailment at the age of 57.

Avicenna described the anatomy of the heart believing, erroneously, that it had three ventricles. He also postulated the existence of anastomoses between the arteries and the veins in the extremities to keep the blood moving. This certainly seems to indicate some realization of the anatomical basis for the circulation. An interatrial communication during infancy was also suggested by him[36].

Prior to Avicenna, Gilani described the cusps of the cardiac valves stating that there were eleven in all[36]. He also described how the aortic root arose from the outflow tract of the left ventricle and how the aortic valve resembles the Greek letter Sigma when open, and a triangle when closed. Current echocardiographic descriptions refer to the cusps of the closed aortic valve as resembling the letter Y or the symbol of the Mercedes automobile, while in the open state the three cusps assume a triangular configuration.

Masihi, a contemporary of Avicenna, provided further insight into the structure and function of the heart valves. He taught that the vena cava opened into the right ventricle and that the pulmonary artery arose from the right ventricle carrying unoxygenated blood into the lungs. He referred to unoxygenated blood as smoking vapor. He further described the manner in which the aortic cusps opened allowing for unidirectional flow only, so that the special air (oxygenated blood)

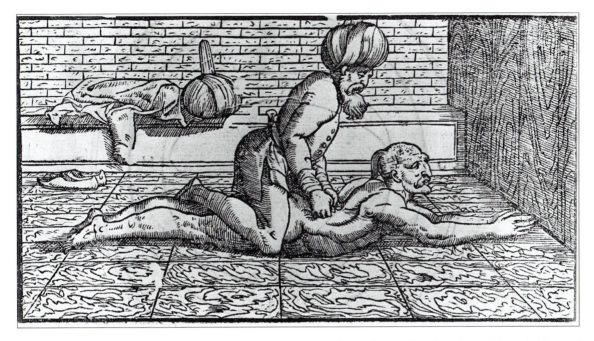

Figure 11 Avicenna massaging a man's back (for muscle or bone disorder?). *Photo Source National Library of Medicine. Literary Source Avicenna. Avicennae Arabum medicorum principis...Venice, 1595. Courtesy of National Library of Medicine*

could be ejected into the aorta for ultimate distribution throughout the body. These are rather prescient observations, certainly antedating the definitive observations of William Harvey, and underscoring, once more, the continuous linkage of current knowledge with the views of previous investigators (see Section 3).

The existence of the lesser or pulmonary circulation was also recognized during this era. Ibn-an Nafis disputed Avicenna's teachings and advanced in their stead the belief that the pulmonary artery was the conduit for transporting the blood into the pores of the lungs where it became purified with air (oxygen) and then was transported to the left ventricle via the pulmonary veins[37]. This account of the pulmonary circulation was not to be recognized in Europe for at least another three hundred years[38].

The description of the pulmonary circulation as well as a discussion of the general physiologic principles of respiration are all to be found in Ibn an-Nafis' *Commentary on the anatomy in the Canon of Ibn Sn* (*Shash Tashrih al-Qanun li-bn Sn*)[39]. He restated that the heart had two ventricles instead of the three that Avicenna claimed. Moreover, he also

recorded the existence of the coronary circulation stating that the heart was nourished by its vessels. The existence of Galen's interventricular pores was also refuted by him (stating in his commentary that the interventricular septum was a solid structure with no evidence of passage between the two ventricles). Figure 12 is from the manuscript on the anatomy of the body by Tashrih al-badan. It is a human figure showing the labeled components of the circulatory system.

Ghalioungui's comments on Ibn-an-Nafis are worthy of repetition. I quote,

> ... The riddle of Ibn-an-Nafis is whether he performed dissections. Otherwise, in spite of his denials, how could he assert that the blood runs from the right ventricle to the left ventricle through the lungs and not through the septal pores that Galen imagined? How could he deny the existence of three ventricles asserted by Aristotle and Avicenna? How could he oppose the view that the heart is nourished by a sediment left by the blood in the right ventricle, and declare that the heart obtains its nourishment from the blood that runs in its substance[40].

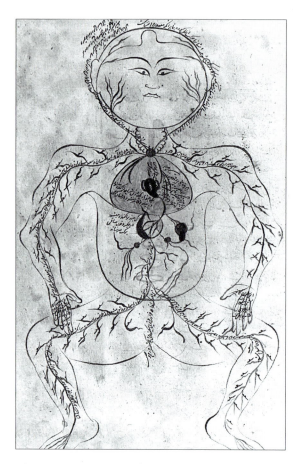

Figure 12 Human figure with organs of the circulatory system shown and labeled. *Photo Source National Library of Medicine. Literary Source Tashrih al-badan (Anatomy of the body). MSS. p. Courtesy of National Library of Medicine*

Human dissection did not reappear until the latter part of the middle ages when it became an important teaching tool at the University of Bologna sometime in the early 13th century. The initial impetus was given by Taddeo Alderotti (Thaddeus of Florence, 1223–1303) but it did not become firmly entrenched as an integral part of the curriculum until the tenure of Mondino de Luzzi. Mondinus was a student of Alderotti and received his doctorate from the university of Bologna. He lived between 1270 and 1326, spending all of his professional life at the University of Bologna where he occupied the chair of anatomy. Mondinus would lecture while dissecting the cadaver in front of his students or demonstrate anatomical specimens

prepared for him by two prosectors of exceptional skill, one of whom was a woman, Alessandra Gilliani[41]. His book was the first original text on practical anatomy in the Middle Ages. It was in reality a dissecting manual of human anatomy discarding completely the ape or pig. The book survived Mondinus for at least two centuries[42].

Although his anatomical description of the heart was quite accurate, especially the details regarding the valves, his correlation of structure with function was not, he being still unable to remove completely the shackles of Galenism. Despite this, the earliest European rumblings against Galen's anatomical description of the heart must be attributed to Mondino de Luzzi. His questioning of the existence of pores in the interventricular septum as postulated by Galen was a remarkable piece of effrontery for the times. The authority of Galen was so formidable that for more than a millennium the dictum was: If there proved to be no holes in the septum, it clearly followed that nature must have undergone changes since Galen[43]. The irrevocable authoritarian stamp of this statement becomes more fully appreciated when one realizes that it was made many years before Darwin advanced his theory of evolution. Figure 13 is an engraving showing Mondino de Luzzi lecturing while his prosector dissects.

Further advances in the study of cardiac anatomy were made at about the same time by Henri de Mondeville (c.1260–1320). Also a radical with an independent bent of mind, he held three chairs at Montpellier (anatomy, surgery and medicine). He, too, was skeptical of Galen's infallibility, declaring that God did not exhaust all his creative power in making Galen[44]. Montpellier was a center of medical learning that had become the premier medical school as Salerno's influence and reputation began to decline.

Henri de Mondeville was primarily a surgeon and it was in his treatise on surgery that he described the anatomy of the heart in a meticulous fashion. He described the heart as containing two cavities or ventricles with a small cavity between them. This could have been the fossa ovalis. The appendages above the ventricles, also with cavities, he called auricles. He regarded the auricles as reservoirs for the blood and air needed to nourish the heart[45]. Despite his strong anatomical foundation, he still adhered to the Galenic concepts of pneuma and spirits (see Section 3).

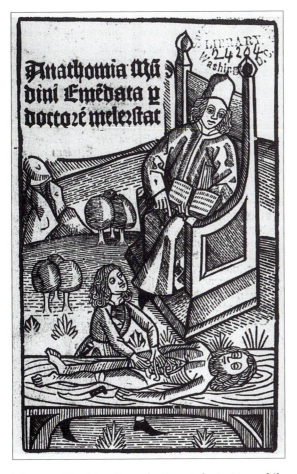

Figure 13 Mondino de Luzzi lecturing while prosector dissects. *Photo Source National Library of Medicine. Literary Source Photo Archives. Courtesy of National Library of Medicine*

REFERENCES

1. Mettler, C.C. (1947). *History of Medicine*, p. 3. (Philadelphia, The Blackiston Co.)

2. Rosner, F. *Medicine in the Bible and the Talmud*. pp. 77–85. (New York: Yeshiva Univ. Press)

3. Harper, R.F. (1904). *The Code of Hammurabi, King of Babylon about 2500 BC*. (Chicago)

4. Breasted, J.H. (1930). *The Edwin Smith Surgical Papyrus*. Published in facsimile and hieroglyphic transliteration with commentary in two volumes. Vol. 1. (Chicago: The University of Chicago Press)

5. Hamburger, W.W. (1939). The earliest known reference to the heart and circulation; the Edwin Smith surgical papyrus, circa 3000 BC, *Am. Heart J.*, **17**, 259–274

6. Joachim, H. (1875). *Papyros Ebers: Das hermetische Buch ueber die Arzneimittel der alten Aegypten in hieratischen Schrift*. 2 vols. (Leipzig). Also quoted by Finlayson, James

7. Joachim, H. (1890). *Das alteste Buch ueber Heilkunde aus dem Aegyptischen zum erstenmal vollstndig bersetzt*. (Berlin). Also quoted by Finlayson, James

8. Finlayson, J. (1893). Ancient Egyptian medicine (a bibliographical demonstration in the library of the faculty of physicians and surgeons, Glasgow, January 12th, 1893.) *Br. Med. J.*, **1**, 748–52 (Apr. 8); 1014–16 (May 13); 1061–4 (May 20)

9. Brugsch, H. (1963). *Recueil de Monuments Egyptiens*, pt 2

10. Castiglioni, A. (1941). *A History of Medicine* (Translated by E. B. Krumbhaar), p. 49. (New York: Alfred A. Knopf)

11. Willius, F.A. and Dry, T.J. (1948). *A History of the Heart and the Circulation*, p. 18. (Philadelphia: W.B. Saunders Co)

12. Passalacqua: (1826). *Catalogue raisonné et historique*, No. 1, 558, p. 207

13. Walton, A. (1894). *The Cult of Aesculapius*. (New York: Cornell)

14. Combrie, J.D. (1910). *Pre-Hippocratic Medicine*. (London)

15. Hippocrates: (1974). *Encyclopaedia Britannica*, 15th edn., vol. 8, p. 942

16. Adams, F. (1849). *The Genuine Works of Hippocrates*, 2 vols. (London)

17. Herrick, J.B. (1942). *A Short History of Cardiology*, p. 8. (Springfield, Ill.: Charles C. Thomas)

18. Bonnabeau, R.C. (1983). The school of Alexandria and the vascular system. *Minn. Med.*, pp. 100–1

19. Boyd, L.J. and Elias, H. (1955). Contributions to diseases of the heart and pericardium, I. Historical introduction. *Bull. New York Med. Coll.*, **18**, 1–37

20. Mettler, C.C. (1947). *Op. cit.*, p. 15

21. Mettler, C.C. (1947). *Op. cit.*, p. 16

22. Bonnabeau, R.C. (1983). *Op. cit.*, p. 100

23. Spencer, W.G. (1935–38). *Celsus, De Medicina*, vol. 1, p. 15. (Cambridge)

24. Ghalioungui, P. (1984) Four landmarks of

Egyptian cardiology. *J. R. Soc. Phys. London*, **18**, 182–6

25. Spencer, W.G., *Op. cit.*, p. 16
26. Celsus, A. (1974). *Encyclopaedia Britannica, Micropaedia*, 15th edn., p. 674
27. Spencer, W.G., *Op. cit.*
28. Bostoch, J. and Riley, H.T. (1856). *The Natural History of Pliny*, vol. 5, p. 374. (London)
29. Bostoch, J. and Riley, H.T. *Op. cit.*, vol. 5, p. 376
30. Adams, F. (1856). *The Extant Works of Aretaeus the Cappadocian.* (London)
31. Galen, C. (1974). *Encyclopaedia Britannica*, 15th edn., vol. 7, p. 849
32. Herrick, J.B. (1942). *Op. cit.*, pp. 6–22
33. Harrington, Sir J. (1920). *The School of Salernum (Regimen Sanitatis Salernitatum), The English Version.* (New York: Paul B. Hoeber)
34. Pucinotti, F. (1850–60). *Storia della Medicina*, vol. 1, 317. (Leghorn)
35. Ilyas, M. (1985). Cardiovascular medicine, Islamic heritage: concepts and contributions. *J.P.M.A.*, 290–2
36. Willius, F.A. and Dry, T.J. (1948). *Op. cit.*, p. 20
37. Bicton, E.D. (1935). The Williams Soler Medal Essay, *Bull. Hist. Med.*
38. Elgwood, G. (1951). *Medical History of Persia*, p. 335
39. Meyerhof, M. (1935). Ibn-an-Nafis (XIIIth cent.) and his theory of the lesser circulation, *Isis*, **23**, 100–20
40. Ghalioungui, P. (1984). *Op. cit.*, p. 185
41. Walsh, J. (1920). *Medieval Medicine*, p. 164. (London)
42. Singer, C. (1925). *The Evolution of Anatomy.* (London: Kegan Paul, Trench, Trubner)
43. Snellen, H.A. (1984). *History of Cardiology*, p. 21. (Rotterdam: Donker Academic Publications)
44. Herrick, J.B. (1942). *Op. cit.*, p. 11
45. Nicaisse, E. (1893). *Chirurgie de Maître Henri de Mondeville*, pp. 61–2. (Paris)

2   Accurate description by dissection

During the 14th century, teachers at Bologna were, in actuality, appointed by the students. The statutes of the university at that time mandated that teachers of anatomy maintain this appointment by dissecting corpses brought to them for anatomical study. Body snatching for this purpose became rather commonplace by students and riff-raff as well. In addition, bodies of executed criminals were turned over to the university for such purposes and for postmortem examinations. This practice was not legal but officially condoned by lack of disciplinary action on the part of the authorities.

As the Renaissance approached, it provided an even more inviting ambience for the furtherance of anatomical knowledge. As more favorable laws were enacted, and as the impact of the intellectuals of the era became more evident, human dissection, as an integral part of anatomical research, became increasingly frequent and fruitful. A most important impetus to human dissection was provided by the Bull of Sixtus IV which removed all official restraints by the Roman Catholic Church. The structural foundations for the physiologic discoveries of the 17th century were being laid during this exciting time of western civilization. The department of anatomy became the center of interest in many of the universities of northern Italy and Europe attracting not only students and physicians, but lay people as well. In fact, a carnival atmosphere prevailed at times with food and drink available in rooms adjoining the amphitheater of dissection. The interior of an anatomical theater is shown in Figure 1. A dissection is taking place by candlelight.

It is during this period that the true beginnings of cardiovascular anatomy are to be found, and among the various outstanding personalities involved, the name of Vesalius must be assigned first place. The publication of Vesalius' text in 1543 entitled *De Humani Corporis Fabrica* constitutes a momentous achievement because it presented anatomy as a true scientific discipline, shattering

once and for all Galen's authoritarian grip on anatomy, and also because it became the nidus for the development of physiology and morbid anatomy, two branches of medical science that, as we shall see later, were very important for the advancement of cardiologic knowledge. The title page of this landmark work is illustrated in Figure 2.

Before delving further into the contributions of Vesalius, credit must also be given to Leonardo Da Vinci, a true Renaissance man, who, arguably, was perhaps the greatest genius that ever lived. Born illegitimately to a peasant woman and a lawyer, Leonardo's interests were not confined to art but were rather wide in range and included mathematics, engineering and aerodynamics among so many other fields. Perhaps, Leonardo's greatest defect was his failure to complete many of his projects. This is probably due to the fact that he was primarily a conceptualist and once he realized the validity of a concept, the remainder of the project could no longer hold his interest.

Da Vinci's anatomical drawings antedate those in Vesalius' text by some thirty years. His interest in anatomy was initially aroused by Marc Antonio Della Torre, a young anatomist of this period. Young Della Torre had requisitioned Leonardo Da Vinci to povide the illustrations for a new text in anatomy based on the former's dissection. This work was never completed because of Della Torre's death, but Da Vinci, with his interest aroused, continued with his own dissections and sketches. This multigifted man produced most of his anatomical drawings from a functional point of view as an aid to his artistic endeavors, but he also portrayed in a very accurate manner the valves, muscle and coronary vasculature of the heart. He was able also to show that no air entered the heart from the lungs by way of the arteria venalis (pulmonary vein)[1].

Unfortunately, no one knew of Leonardo's work since it was never published. The importance and accuracy of his work came to light long after his

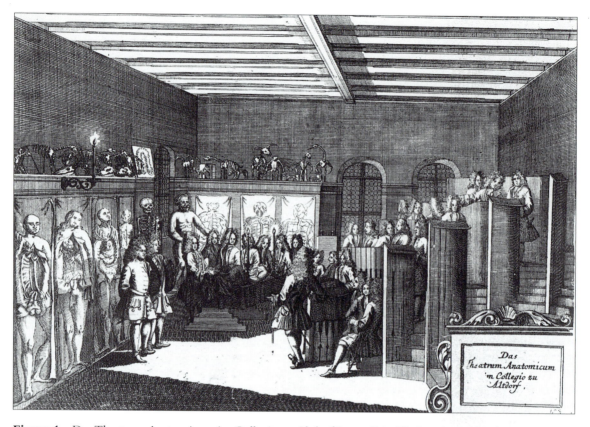

Figure 1 Das Theatrum Anatomicum im Collegio zu Altdorf (engr. [16 – ?]). Interior of the theatre, founded ca. 1650, with dissection taking place by candlelight. Anatomical charts on walls. *Photo Source National Library of Medicine. Literary Source Altdorf, Ger. Universitat. Medizinische Facultat. Courtesy of National Library of Medicine*

death when William Hunter in 1784 called attention to Da Vinci's anatomical drawings[2]. Blumenbach also participated in the recovery of these drawings. The entire collection was first published between 1898–1916 after having been collated from the holdings of the Royal Library at Windsor, the Ambrosian Library at Milan and the Institut de France. These renderings, long hidden and unnoticed, were further camouflaged by Leonardo's mirror, hand-written notes. Figure 3 is a photograph of Leonardo's drawing of the heart and Figure 4 is a self-portrait of the artist himself.

Some of Da Vinci's remarks on the heart as culled from the Windsor collection are worthy of quotation: 'The heart … is a vessel made of thick muscle, kept alive and nourished by artery and vein as the other muscles are'. (Anat. Ms. B, fol, 33v). 'The heart is a muscle of pre-eminent power over other muscles'. (Ms. G, fol IV). He distinguished

the ventricles which he called lower ventricles, from the other chambers which he called upper ventricles, and from the auricular appendages which he called ears (Quad. Anat. I, fol. 3r). He called the pericardial sac, the cassula (capsule) of the heart, and commented on the fluid it contained, which, according to him, was more plentiful in the corpse than in life. (Anat. Ms. B. fol. 17r, p.114). He described the coronary arteries as arising from the two external openings of the left ventricle (Quad. Anat II, fol. 3v).

One of the drawings depicts the papillary muscles and the trabeculae carnae of the ventricular walls. They are described as follows:

Between the cords (cordae) and threads of the muscles of the right ventricle there are interwoven a quantity of minute threads; and these wind themselves around the most minute

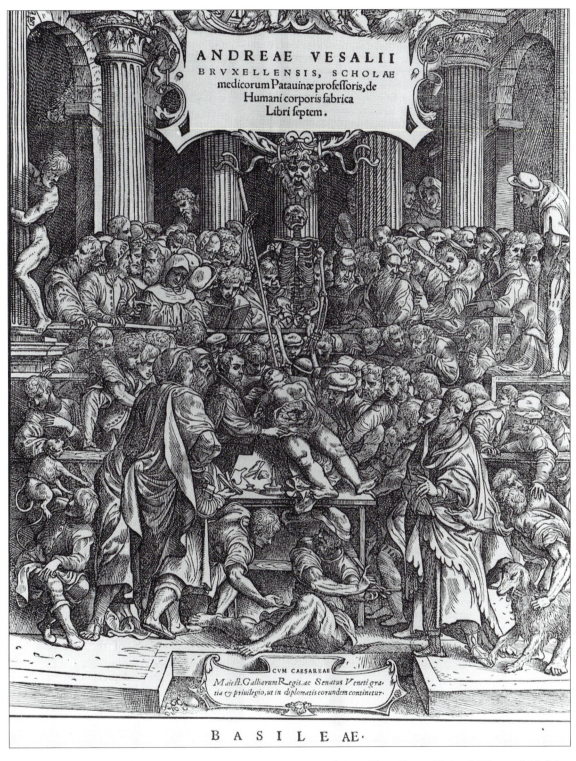

Figure 2 Title page from Vesalius: De Humani Corporis Fabrica. *Photo Source National Library of Medicine.*
Literary Source Facsimile Edition. Courtesy of National Library of Medicine

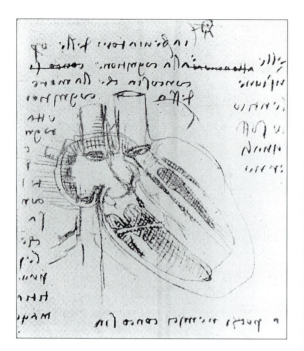

Figure 3 Reproduction of Leonardo da Vinci's drawing of the heart. *Photo Source University of Central Florida Library. Literary Source Quad.d'Anatomia, published by O.C.L. Vangensten, A. Fonahn, and H. Hopstock. Christiana, 1911–1916, Vol. 11, Folio 4 Recto. Courtesy of University of Central Florida Library*

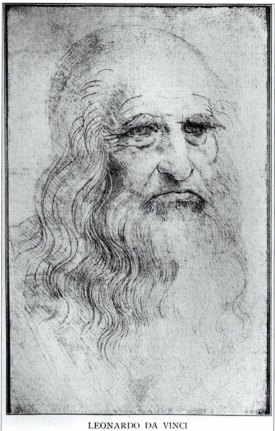

LEONARDO DA VINCI

Figure 4 Self portrait of Leonardo da Vinci. *Photo Source National Library of Medicine. Literary Source Photo Archives. Courtesy of National Library of Medicine*

and imperceptible nerves (tendons) and weave themselves with them. And these muscles are in themselves very capable of expansion and contraction, and they are situated within the fury of the rush of the blood, which passes in and out among the minute cords (tendinous prolongations) of the muscles before they are converted into the panniculi (membranes of the uscioli) (cusps of the valves) (Quad. Anat. IV, fol 13r).

For further insight into Leonardo's precise descriptions and terminology, reference should be made to Favaro's publication[3].

We now return to Vesalius. He was born in Brussels in 1514 and died in 1564. Andreas Vesalius is the latinized form of Andre Wesel. He studied for a time under Sylvius in Paris, but rapidly became disenchanted with his teacher and returned to Louvain where he had pursued his earlier studies and now completed them to earn his Bachelor of

Medicine degree. He then attended the University of Padua which at that time had a strong reputation for anatomical dissection, received his M.D. degree from this institution and was immediately appointed a lecturer in surgery with the responsibility of giving anatomical demonstrations[4].

His life can be divided into three phases: an early academic and research oriented phase; an interlude of twenty years of academic-free indolence and a third phase characterized by a return to academia and research. It was during his first phase at the young age of 29 that his fame was made with the publication of his tome *De Humani Corporis Fabrica Libri Septem*. During the second phase he was court physician to Charles V and later to his son, Philip II. During this time it appears he had no interest at all in academic pursuits but rather enjoyed the perquisites that came with the role of court physician. His return to his first love, anatomy, was prompted by the publication of a text written by Fallopio, a former student of his who had become professor of anatomy at Padua[5].

The Fabrica, as this outstanding work of Vesalius is generally called, is actually an outgrowth of an atlas-compendium consisting of seven books. It was illustrated by an outstanding artist, Jan Calcar, a student of Titian. The third book in the collection is devoted to the vascular system while the sixth book deals primarily with the heart and briefly with the lungs. Unfortunately, the least satisfactory of the seven books is the one dealing with the vascular system. Although the anatomical description of the heart is quite good, it is not exceptional and is again marred by Galenic misconceptions regarding function. *The Fabrica* owes much of its elegance to the organizational clarity of the author, the excellent wood block engravings of the drawings, and to the unsurpassed printing facilities at Basel, Switzerland. It was truly a labor of love with Vesalius even supervising personally the actual printing in Basel. It is because of this work that Vesalius has been aptly called the founder of descriptive anatomy. A woodcut of Vesalius attributed to Jan Calcar is illustrated in Figure 5, and a lithograph of Vesalius before a dissecting table with a cadaver is seen in Figure 6.

Vesalius' book went through two editions. Incidentally, it was the invention of the printing press that helped accelerate the publication and widespread dissemination of many scientific works, including this one, during the turbulently active epoch known as the Renaissance. In his first edition, he questioned somewhat hesitantly the existence of the interventricular septal pores with these remarks: 'We are driven to wonder at the handiwork of the Almighty, by means of which blood sweats from the right into the left ventricle through passages which escape the human vision'. It was in his second edition that he unabashedly refutes Galen's mythical pores. 'I do not, therefore, see how even the smallest particle can be transferred from the right to the left ventricle through it'[6].

As a matter of fact, Vesalius' view of Galen was in marked contrast to that held by Jacobus Sylvius, a leading authority at the time, and as mentioned before, a former teacher. It was during his formative years as a young student that Vesalius became disenchanted with Sylvius. This break

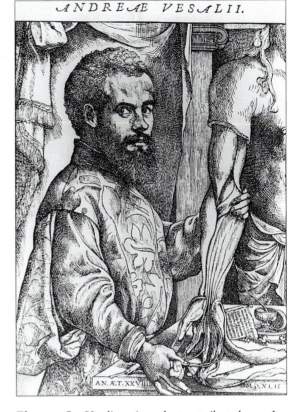

Figure 5 Vesalius (woodcut attributed to Jan Kalcar). *Photo Source National Library of Medicine. Literary Source Photo Archives. Courtesy of National Library of Medicine*

developed into a constant feud between former teacher and renowned pupil, fueled over the years by recurrent acrimonious debates, and with each one vying with the other for the lion's share of new pupils. Sylvius never relinquished the belief that Galen was infallible, that Galen's *De usu partium* was divine, and that any knowledge past Galen was impossible[7].

It is interesting to note that this former teacher of Vesalius, also known as Jacques Dubois Sylvius, never had a formal education until after he had attracted quite a large student following with his private instructions. This popularity engendered quite a bit of envious controversy among his formally accredited colleagues. Finally, at the age of 53, Sylvius attempted to neutralize this opposition by obtaining the Bachelor's degree in Medicine from the University of Montpellier[8].

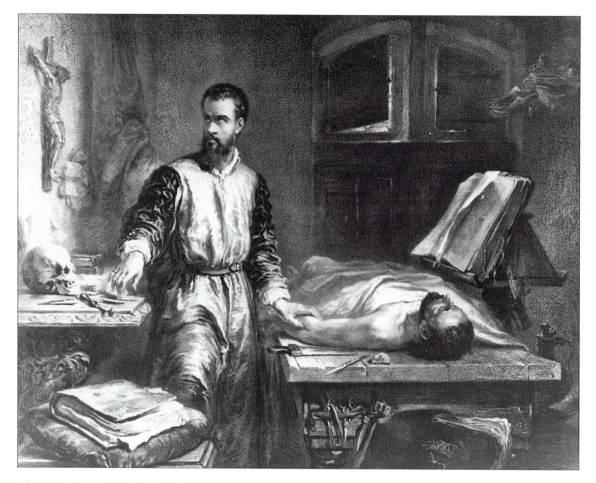

Figure 6 Lithograph of Vesalius before a dissecting table with a cadaver. *Photo Source National Library of Medicine. Literary Source Photo Archives. Courtesy of National Library of Medicine*

Despite Sylvius' fanatical adherence to Galen's errors, he did contribute somewhat to the anatomical knowledge of the cardiovascular system. Although Eustachio is given credit for initially describing the valve that bears his name between the inferior vena cava and the right atrium, it appears that this honor should probably go to Sylvius instead[8]. Sylvius also helped standardize anatomic nomenclature by utilizing classical names as much as possible, and eliminating the many Arabic and hybrid expressions that accumulated over the years.

This momentary digression from Vesalius to Sylvius cannot be ended without reiterating Baker's description of how Sylvius became a symbol of mockery in his old age, completely overshadowed by the fame and respect enjoyed by his former student, Vesalius. In fact, ultimately, Sylvius was completely rejected by his students and his apparently avaricious nature accompanied him to his grave by a cruel inscription on his tomb dripping with sarcasm:

> In this grave lies old Sylvius, during his day
> He never gave aught without getting full pay;
> And though dead as a Herring, so naught could be worse,
> He is vexed he cant charge you for reading this verse[9].

Returning again to Vesalius, although the noted anatomist utilized human cadavers in his dissections, many of his anatomical descriptions combined the structures of animal anatomy, especially that of the barbary ape. One has but to look at the illustrations of the bones and muscles in his *De Fabrica* to become aware of this. Vesalius did not restrict his dissections to cadavers alone. He often resorted to vivisection utilizing live animals as a means of correlating function with structure. The following excerpt from Chapter XIX, Book VII of his *De Fabrica* attests to this: What May Be Learned By Dissection of The Dead and What of The Living

> Just as the dissection of the dead teaches well the number, position and shape of each part, and most accurately the nature and composition of its material substance, thus also the dissection of a living animal clearly demonstrates at once the function itself, at another time it shows very clearly the reasons for the existence of the parts. Therefore, even though students deservedly first come to be skilled in the study of dead animals, afterward when about to investigate the action and use of the parts of the body they must become acquainted with the living animal.
>
> On the other hand since very many small parts of the body are endowed with different uses and functions, it is fitting that no one doubt that dissections of the living present also many contradictions.

This particular passage can be found in Logan Clendening's *Source Book of Medical History*[10].

Vesalius was also quite observant and accurate in his description of the gross anatomy of the pericardium. To wit: 'The entire heart is covered with a certain membraneous involucrum, to which it is joined at no point. This involucrum is much more ample than the heart and is moistened by an aqueous humor …'[11].

De Fabrica continued to be printed long after Vesalius died. Its latest printing was in 1782. Many of Vesalius' original figures were copied and plagiarized. Two of the most notorious plagiarizers were Ambrose Pare and Helkiah Cooke. Singer recounts how Cooke added insult to injury by accusing Vesalius of having slighted Galen[12].

Vesalius epitomizes the well-known aphorism: Honest labor bears a lovely face. Even as a youngster his interest in anatomy was keen, as manifested by his constant dissection of animals. His life's work, *De Fabrica*, was the result of an intense, dedicated, undeviating labor compressed into five short years and establishing permanently his exalted position as an esteemed anatomist. He approached anatomy in terms of function.

Notice how the skeleton is positioned from a functional point of view in Figure 7. His training was galenic but his mind was that of a skilled observer and explorer bent on reforming old concepts and methods. The frontispiece of his book (Figure 2) is a vivid indication of how popular and well-attended his lectures were. It also depicts Vesalius as the actual dissector. This was one of the basic reforms that Vesalius instituted while holding the professorship at Padua. He did away with both demonstrators and ostensors. A typical product of the Renaissance, Vesalius was an artist, humanist and naturalist, and should be included among the giants of medicine.

There were many other contemporaries of Vesalius but the majority do not figure strongly in the advancement of cardiovascular anatomy. The few that are worthy of mention in this regard are Aranzi, Botallo, Fallopio, Eustachio, Cesalpino, Fabrizio, Serveto, Berengario, Colombo and Canano.

Guido Cesare Aranzi (1530–89), also known as Aranzio, was a student of Vesalius at Padua but received his doctorate at Bologna, at which institution he stayed as professor of medicine and surgery until his death. He was an avid student and is noted particularly for describing the anatomical differences between the hearts of the adult and the fetus. He pointed out the closure of the ductus arteriosus and foramen ovale in the post-natal period. The cartilaginous nodules of the semilunar valves are named after him since he was the first to describe them. Another eponym is the Arantius ligament since it was he that noted that during intra-uterine life, it was the communicating channel between the umbilical and portal veins. It should be noted that many other anatomists including Galen were also aware of the existence of the foramen ovale and ductus arteriosus[13]. Among them is Leonardo Botallo who is honored by the eponym, Botallo's ligament, the remnant of the ductus arteriosus.

Eustachio (1520–74) was also a bitter contemporary opponent of Vesalius. He held the chair of anatomy at the Collegia della Sapienza at Rome. His only contribution to cardiac anatomy was the discovery of the valve in the right atrium that carries his name and which is a remnant of the valve over the inferior vena cava, being situated at its junction with the right atrium. Born to be buried in obscurity by the vast majority of medical students, this structure is important to echocardiographers

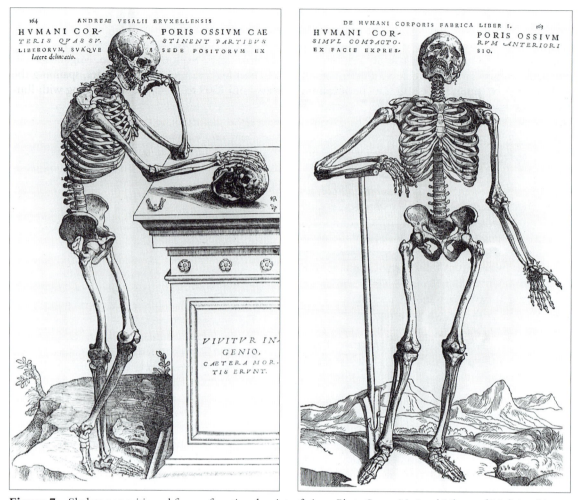

Figure 7 Skeletons positioned from a functional point of view. *Photo Source National Library of Medicine. Literary Source Vesalius A, Kalkar JS: Tabulae Anatomica, P.D. Bernardi, Venice, 1538. Courtesy of National Library of Medicine*

since it is a normal structure that can be confused with cardiac tumors on those occasions when it is visualized.

Gabriele Fallopio (Fallopius 1523–62) was born at Modena. He too was a student of Vesalius, and ironically he was the author of the text that rekindled his former teacher's interest in anatomy. Fallopius was an accurate and careful dissector correcting many of the errors found in *De Fabrica*. He gave careful descriptions of the jugular and vertebral veins, and the intracranial branchings of the carotid arteries. Most of his anatomical contributions were, however, outside of the cardiovascular system. His most outstanding work was *Medici mutinensis*

observationes. In it he described the coronary vessels as well as a nerve plexus in the heart.

There are two important bearers of the name Fabricius. One is Fabrizio d'Acquapendente and the other is the surgeon Fabricius Hildanus. Fabrizio d'Acquapendente (1537–1619) carried on the anatomical tradition at Padua by studying anatomy under Fallopio and continuing to demonstrate with actual dissections while serving there as professor of surgery. His fame became so great that a huge amphitheater was specially built in his honor by the Venetian authorities to supplant a large one that he himself had had constructed at his own expense. It was his treatise on the valves of the veins that is thought to have provided the nidus for Harvey's interest and experimentation into the physiology of the circulation.

Despite the fact that he was a careful and dependable observer, he too resorted to speculation as illustrated by his remarks on the pericardium with respect to how it is nourished. He felt that the clear fluid of the chick egg nourished the cold parts while the yolk provided the nutrition for the hot parts. Extrapolating this belief to the pericardium, he wrote as follows:

> Now, of course, the entire substance of an animal is composed of two elements, hot and cold; for all sanguinous and red parts ... are hot; but on the contrary, white and bloodless parts are cold, such as ... all membranous structures like the stomach, the intestines, the uterus, the pericardium, and whatever other parts may be...[14].

Andrea Cesalpino emerges as probably one of the most important anatomists of this era simply because of the contentious controversy surrounding his place in the annals of medical history. Cesalpino was born probably in 1519 at Arezzo in Tuscany and served as professor of Medicine at Pisa as well as physician to Pope Clement VIII. Arcieri[15] goes to great lengths in an attempt to establish Cesalpino rather than Harvey as the true discoverer of the circulation. Arcieri advances as evidence for this position precise references to Cesalpino's detailed dissections, and observations on the motions of the heart and vessels. Needless to say, this belief though reinforced by other Italian historians is bitterly contested by the British. As we shall see later, the British feel that Harvey should be awarded priority simply because his conclusions were based on experimentation, a valid scientific approach.

Be that as it may, the observations recorded in his works appear to indicate that Cesalpino had a very comprehensive view and accurate appreciation of the circulatory system in general. Cesalpino wrote two texts: *Quaestionum peripateticarum* in 1571, and *Quaestionum medicarum* in 1593. In them, he delineates the difference in structure and function between the pulmonary artery and vein, and postulates the existence of communicating channels between the smallest ramifications of the pulmonary artery and vein as well as between the systemic arteries and veins. He did establish by observations rather than conjecture, as above,

the presence of communications between the inferior vena cava and the portal veins.

A rather pathetic figure of this period is the Spaniard from Villaneuva de Sigena, Miguel Serveto (Michael Servetus). His life was brief, spanning the years from 1509 to 1553. He stands along with Ibn-an-Nafis as an early describer of the pulmonary circulation. Servetus was primarily a theologian and this description was part of a religious treatise entitled *Restituto Christianismi*. It is to be found in the fifth book of the text that brought down upon Servetus the wrath of John Calvin and which eventually caused Servetus to be burned at the stake. In this book, he describes both the nature of the Holy Spirit and the pulmonary circulation. Ibn-an-Nafis described the pulmonary circulation three centuries earlier, but knowledge was more easily disseminated during the time of Servetus, and this, coupled with a stronger historical interest in Servetus because of his pathetic martyrdom on the pyre, may account for the relative lack of appreciation with respect to the contribution of Ibn-an-Nafis.

To add to the ever proliferating list of priorities, Matteo Colombo of Cremona is also credited as being the discoverer of the pulmonary circulation. Colombo had been the prosector of Vesalius at Padua. Krumbhaar quotes a passage from Colombo's *De Re Anatomica* describing in a rather arrogant and peer-disparaging manner this anatomist's view of the pulmonary circulation[16]. Colombo also practiced vivisection, demonstrating in this manner that the pulmonary veins contained blood rather than air and vapors. Despite this accurately noteworthy description, he erred in believing that the veins carried nutritive substances throughout the body and that the liver, rather than the heart, was the center of the cardiovascular system, this being a heritage of Galen's teachings.

Jacopo Berengario da Carpi, listed among the contemporaries of Vesalius, was another in the long line of Bolognese anatomists that figured so prominently during this phase of scientific anatomical discoveries. Berengario is also referred to as Berenger and Berengarius. He was one of the first to utilize copper engravings for his anatomical illustrations. He published an isogogue in 1592 and in it he described the cardiac valves[17]. An isogogue is an introductory text, a form of publication used by many scholars of this era. Berengario noted the oblique position of the heart, described the pericardium, cardiac cavities and the aorta.

He carefully described the carotid arteries and their ramifications outlining these as well as other arteries by injecting them with tepid water, disdaining the usage of tinted liquids. He mistook the anterior spinal artery, however, for a nerve[18]. Four views of the heart in various stages of dissection, as sketched by Berengario, are seen in Figure 8.

According to Castiglioni, it was Canano rather than Vesalius who first demonstrated the valves of the veins[19]. Giovanni Battista Canano was a great anatomist in his own right who, as a contemporary of Vesalius, was overshadowed, as other anatomists of this era, by the great Vesalius. Again, regarding the difficulty of assigning priorities, the valves of the veins were also described by a French anatomist, Charles Etienne, a pupil of Sylvius. He referred to them as apophyses membranarum[20]. Etienne is also known as Carolus Stephanus, a member of a family prominent in the field of printing.

Before proceeding with the next century it should be noted that three important works were produced in France during the 16th century that exercised a great deal of influence on modern anatomical terminology including that dealing with cardiac structure[21]. These were the index to the works of Galen by Antonio Musa Brassavola, an Italian living and working in France; a philological dictionary of medical terms by Henri Etienne, a nephew of the anatomist Charles Etienne; and a dictionary of the same genre by Jean De Gorris.

The 17th century saw the emergence of concise accounts of new discoveries and observations in the various journals that were being published as part of the transactions of newly-formed learned societies. This was a new departure from the previous practice of publishing a whole text so that the author could air his views regarding a particular subject. Knowledge was more easily disseminated now with improved methods of printing, copper-plate engraving, newer techniques regarding the preparation of anatomical specimens, and further diminution of ecclesiastical restraints against human dissection, though the last was somewhat erratic and not uniformly applied throughout Europe. The American influence was yet to emerge since the western hemisphere was still a colony striving to conquer the savagery of its environment as well as its own savagery. However, although medical scholarship was still virtually non-existent throughout both North and South America, the indigenous plants of the hemisphere began to give up some of their secrets so that such remedies as quinine, jalop and ipecac began to arrive in Europe.

Anatomy was still the important foundation of medical knowledge in Italy and interest in it was now widespread throughout Europe. Dissection was being practiced with greater freedom and frequency. Grave robbing became more and more common to meet the increasing demand of dissectors. Grave robbing was not a new phenomenon though; it was practiced with regularity in the early 16th century as the woodcut in Figure 9 indicates. Figure 10 is a caricature of an anatomist overtaken by the watch indicating that body snatching in England continued well into the 18th century. It shows Dr. William Hunter running from the scene as he and an accomplice are overtaken by a policeman (?) while stealing a cadaver (that of Miss Waats).

It was during the latter part of the 17th century that the anatomy of the lymphatics was first delineated, thus forging another link in the anatomy of the circulatory system. It was also during this era that injection and corrosion techniques were being developed and refined for the preservation and study of the blood vessels and lymphatics. Foremost among the innovators of these techniques was Frederick Ruysch of Amsterdam who injected wax into anatomical specimens. He perfected this method to such a high degree that it allowed him to describe in minute detail the vessels and structure of the lungs as well as the vascular network of the skin. Most of his observations, though made in the 17th century, were published, however, between the years 1701–15 in a 10 volume Thesarius of anatomy noted for its humorous and artistic illustrations[22].

Anatomical knowledge of the lymphatic system evolved through the combined efforts of several men working independently of each other, though not in all cases, oblivious of the others' work. At times, a discovery was the result of serendipity. Among the earliest investigators was Gasparo Aselli followed by several others from England and different parts of the continent. These were Pauli, Meutel, Vesling, Pecquet, Joyliffe, Rudbeck and Bartholin; a veritable league of nations and again reflective of the international flavor of cardiological discoveries.

Gasparo Aselli was professor of anatomy at Pisa[23]. He discovered the lacteal vessels while dissecting a dog that had just eaten a fatty meal. This was in 1622 and in his treatise on the matter,

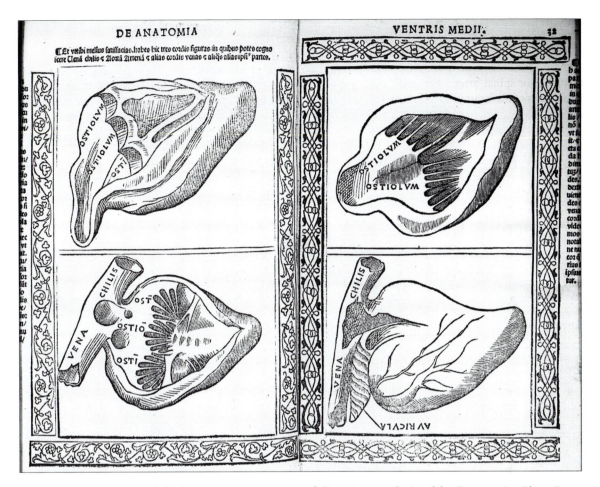

Figure 8 Four views of the heart in various stages of dissection, as depicted by Berengario. *Photo Source National Library of Medicine. Literary Source Photo Archives. Courtesy of National Library of Medicine*

he erroneously described them as emptying into the liver rather than the thoracic duct. Aselli's work also enjoys the unique position of being the first book dealing with anatomy that was illustrated with colored plates. Two years were to pass before Jacques Meutel described the thoracic duct, a feat of rediscovery since it had been originally described by Eustachius. A Parisian physician by the name of Jean Pecquet described how the lymph in dogs was carried from the intestines to the thoracic duct from whence it drained into that part of the venous system formed by the junction between the left jugular and subclavian veins[24]. Further details of the lymphatic network were then supplied by three men: Joyliffe from England, Rudbeck from Sweden and Thomas Bartholin

from Denmark. Bartholin confirmed in man what Pecquet described in the dog, and then carried on over the years a lively debate with Pecquet concerning priorities of discovery and accuracy of description[25]. Olaf Rudbeck, independently and concurrently, recognized and described the lymphatics of the viscera utilizing cattle. He also dissected the subepicardial lymphatics tracing them to their connection with the mediastinal lymph nodes[26]. It was not until 1653 that he became aware of Bartholin's work. Joyliffe, in turn, became aware of Rudbeck's work several months later, and in due time, also became involved in controversy with Bartholin[26]. Each member of this triangle of glory seekers was not hesitant in aiming at each other repeated fusillades of verbal onslaughts with

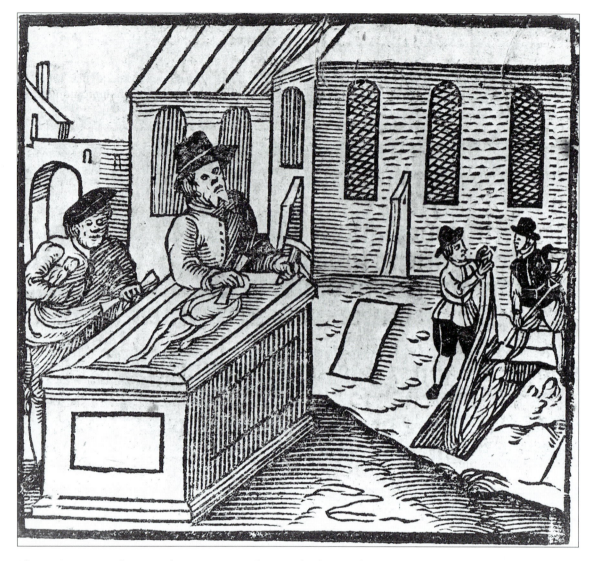

Figure 9 Man in foreground examining a cadaver; in background two men are robbing a grave. *Photo Source National Library of Medicine. Literary Source Damhouder, Joost (1506–1581): Practycke in criminele saecken. Rotterdam, 1628. Courtesy of National Library of Medicine*

exaggerated claims of their own findings and denigrating remarks concerning their opponents. Nuck did not become involved in this controversy but in 1691 he too became interested in the subepicardial lymphatics and outlined them by injecting mercury[27].

Another great anatomist of this era was Niels Stensen, who, after studying under Thomas Bartholin, spent some time at Amsterdam. Stenson's major interest was the structure of glands but this did not prevent him from becoming embroiled in a major controversy of the time as to whether or not the heart was a muscular organ. Miller recounts how Stenson was quite convinced of the muscular nature of the heart[28]. Stenson expressed his conviction that the heart was purely and exclusively a muscular organ in his *De musculis and glandulis observationum specimen*[29]. This was later reconfirmed by Lower in 1669[30] in his treatise *Tractatus de Corde*. Lower described the spiral course of the myocardial fibers as well as the cardiac valves and the coronary vessels. He also utilized the

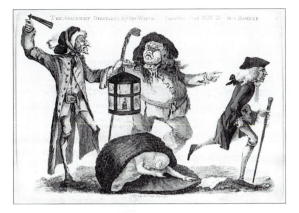

Figure 10 The Anatomist overtaken by the Watch … Carrying off Miss Waats in a hamper. *Photo Source National Library of Medicine. Literary Source Color etching by William Austin. Courtesy of National Library of Medicine*

injection technique in his study of the coronary vessels, outlining with this method the anastomoses among these vessels.

Despite the exacting anatomical contributions of this era, the blind proponents of galenic errors continued to remain in force in scattered centers of learning. Jean Riolan (1577–1657) is notorious for being one of these diehards of galenic traditions. We shall hear more of him later when we discuss his fierce opposition to Harvey's concepts. He is mentioned at this time because despite his accurate description of the internal carotid arteries he stated that the vital spirit of Galen was distilled from their small communicating branches to be emptied into the ventricles of the brain where it was converted into animal spirit and then transported by the nerves to various parts of the body. This was refuted by a younger contemporary, Johann Jakob Wepfer[31]. Jean Riolan served as Royal Professor of Anatomy and Botany in Paris, having been appointed to the chair by Louis XIII. He figures prominently as a loud voice, persistently opposing the numerous contributions made during the century by the many innovative experimenters and observers who dared defy the teachings of Galen with scientific proof. He clung to the very end in support of Galen's errors but truth will prevail so that by the final days of the 17th century, Galen's influence had been virtually nullified, despite all attempts to the contrary.

Joseph Guichard Duverney of France is another anatomist who merits attention. His lifetime spanned the latter part of the 17th century and the first 30 years of the 18th. He is credited with being the first to demonstrate that the cerebral sinuses (of the brain) were actually venous reservoirs and that they ultimately drained into the jugular veins. He also traced the ultimate communication of the veins of the spinal cord with the azygos system.

Raymond Vieussens' life also straddled the 17th and 18th centuries. He should be remembered in the history of cardiology primarily because in his treatise on the heart he attempted to correlate structure with function[32–34]. He called the muscular fibers of the heart conduits charni, mistakenly believing that they were conduits emanating from the coronary arteries and emptying into the veins. Vieussens' isthmus or ring is actually the annulus ovalis. We shall return to this earnest student of anatomy again in his role as clinician and physiologist.

Probably the most outstanding among the many anatomists of the 17th century is the name of Marcello Malpighi. His contributions have affected the entire field of medicine but our interest in him at this point lies primarily in his landmark work concerning the capillaries. This was the link that firmly secured the anatomical foundation for circulatory physiology; the channels that connect the arterial with the venous side of the heart, both at the pulmonary and peripheral levels. Figure 11 is an engraving of a sketch by Malpighi on the lungs and lung capillaries of a frog, the latter seen through a microscope.

Marcello Malpighi was born in 1628, in Crevalcore, just outside Bologna, Italy. He earned a doctorate in both philosophy and medicine at the University of Bologna, though the granting of the degree was initially opposed by the University authorities presumably because he was not a native of Bologna. His teaching career and anatomical studies began at Bologna but the hostile environment at Bologna caused Malpighi to transfer his activities in an intermittent fashion between Pisa and Bologna, then Messina and Bologna. It was at Pisa that Malpighi began a friendship with Giovanni Borelli that was to last a lifetime. While teaching and practicing medicine at these three institutions, Malpighi assiduously continued his investigations with the newly invented microscope. It was during his tenure at Messina that Malpighi's studies began to be published in the Philosophical Transactions of the Royal Society of London. Malpighi had been

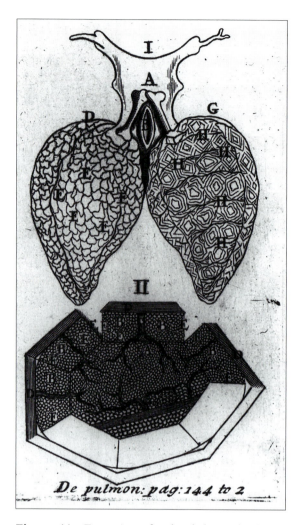

De pulmon: pag:144 to 2

Figure 11 Engraving of a sketch by Malpighi on the lungs and lung capillaries of a frog, the latter seen through a microscope. *Photo Source National Library of Medicine. Literary Source Photo Archives. Courtesy of National Library of Medicine*

granted honorary membership in the Royal Society, and for the remainder of his academic career, the Transactions of the Royal Society constituted the vehicle for Malpighi's publications.

Despite his modesty and gentleness, the immense scope and impact of Malpighi's microscopic studies engendered a great deal of envy, jealousy and criticism on the part of his contemporaries. This opposition reached a boiling point in his 56th year when Malpighi's villa was burned, his papers, notes and manuscripts destroyed and his laboratory equipment reduced to pieces.

This shattering experience was soothed somewhat by his appointment, several years later, as archiater to Pope Innocent XII. Further honors were soon after heaped upon him redeeming somewhat the vilification that he suffered and endured for so many years[35].

Malpighi used the microscope for almost 40 years establishing the groundwork for future students of botany, embryology, human anatomy and pathology. He can rightfully be called the first histologist. Insofar as cardiology is concerned, his greatest achievement was the establishment by direct observation of an anatomical linkage between arteries and veins, a monumental achievement since it solidified Harvey's views on the circulation. Malpighi's discovery of the capillaries was first made known in two letters that he wrote to his intimate friend Giovanni Borelli[36]. This was in 1661. In these letters the ramifications of the bronchial tree into alveoli are described along with the rete mirabili of Malpighi (the terminal branches of the pulmonary artery).

The following is a translation by M. Foster of Malpighi's description of the capillaries in the frog's lungs as well as in those of the tortoise[37]:

For, while the heart is still beating, two movements contrary in direction though accomplished with difficulty are observed in the vessels so that the circulation of the blood is clearly laid bare; and indeed the same may be even more happily recognized in the mesentery and in other larger veins contained in the abdomen. And thus by this impulse the blood is showered down in minute streams through the arteries, after the fashion of a flood, into the several cells, one or other conspicuous branch passing right through or leaving off there, and the blood, thus repeatedly divided, loses its red colour, and, carried round in a sinuous manner, is poured out on all sides until it approaches the walls, and the angles and the absorbing branches of the veins.

The power of the eye could not be carried further in the opened living animal; hence I might have believed that the blood itself escaped into an empty space and was gathered up again by a gaping vessel and by the structure of the walls. But an objection to this view was afforded by the movement of the blood being tortuous and scattered in different directions and by its

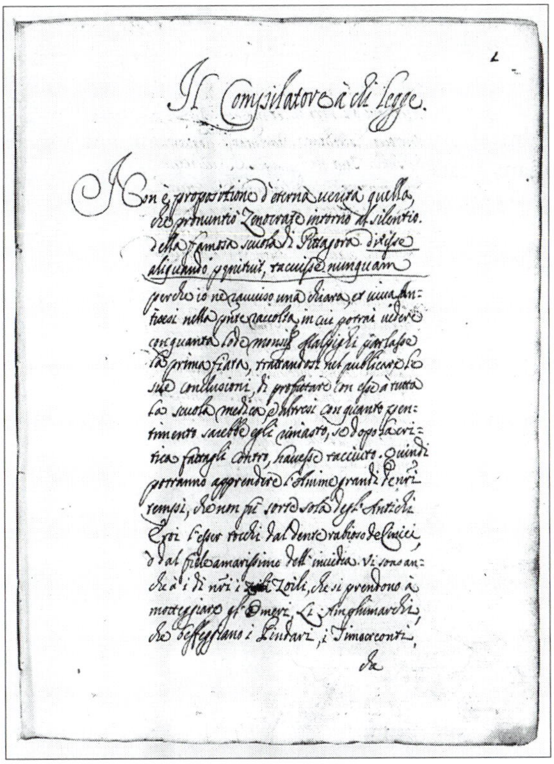

Il Compilatore à chi legge.

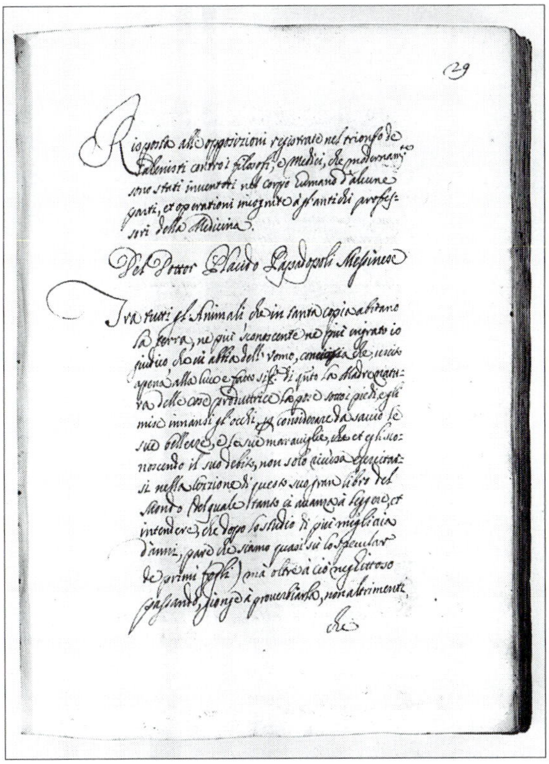

Del Dottor Placido Papadopoli Messinese

Figure 12 Marcello Malpighi, Raccolta di 46 conclusioni mediche. *Photo Source Wellcome Institute Library. Literary Source Marcello Malpighi, Raccolta da 46 conclusioni mediche, s.l., [Italy?], n.d.,[c. 1695] WIHM Western MS 3412, fol 1. By courtesy of the Wellcome Trustees*

being united again in a determinate part. My doubt was changed into certainty by the dried lung of the frog which to a very marked extent had preserved the redness of the blood in very minute tracts (which were afterwards found to be vessels) where by the help of our more perfect glass there met the eye no longer scattered points resembling the skin which is called Sagrino, but vessels joined together in a ring-like fashion. And such is the wandering about of these vessels, as they proceed on this side from the vein and on the other side from the artery that the vessels no longer maintain a straight direction, but there appears a network made up of the continuations of the two vessels. This network not only occupies the whole area but extends to the walls, and is attached to the outgoing vessel, as I could more abundantly and yet with greater difficulty see in the oblong lung of the tortoise, which is equally membranous and transparent. Hence it was clear to the senses that the blood flowed away along tortuous vessels and was not poured into spaces, but was always contained within tubules, and that its dispersion is due to the multiple winding of the vessels. Nor is it a new thing in Nature to join to each other the terminal mouths of vessels, since the same obtains in the intestines and other parts; and, indeed, what seems more wonderful, she joins together by a conspicuous anastomosis the upper and lower terminations of veins as the most learned Fallopius has very well observed.

In order, however, that you may more easily grasp what I have just stated, and follow it with your own eyes, ligature with a thread at the spot where it joins the heart, the protruded and turgid lung of a frog whose body has been laid open, doing this while a copious supply of blood is flowing through the whole of it.

This even when dried will preserve its vessels turgid with blood. And this you will see exceedingly well if you examine it with a microscope of a single lens against the horizontal sun.

In 1985, W.E. Knowles Middleton published an unknown letter written by Malpighi to his life-long friend, Borelli, that fills a gap in the correspondence between the two men about Malpighi's work on the lungs. The following translation as quoted from his article underscores the unique relationship that existed between these men, and the veneration and esteem that Malpighi had for Borelli[38]:

Most illustrious and excellent Sir, my reverend master: While I was writing out the enclosed letter I received a courteous one from you[a], from which I understand the motives that again urge you not to write an epistle[b], and also the reasons that you add for me to moderate my first ideas with a second epistle; and although in my last letter[c] I showed myself unwilling to do this, now as you will see I am very ready to do it, and I am more than ordinarily indebted to you for instructing and defending me with such great kindness.

This week, and not before, I have been able to obtain frogs, and while I investigated the substance of the lungs with a microscope in the sun or by a light, I found with great labor what is inserted in the epistle[d]. I do not believe that this has been observed by others, and it seems to me that it is of great consequence. You will be so good as to consider the enclosed, and to take your pen and correct it, cutting it down or adding to it where you please, if indeed you judge that it can be published as the second epistle. Do not show so much respect for me, but behave firmly and speak freely, because I am ever your grateful scholar. You could show it to Their Highnesses[e] if you think it deserves to be brought to light.

In the last few days, for the first time, I have had the good luck to see a uterine placenta, which has at its end the distinct little lobes of the same shape as are observed in the lungs, rather than cartilaginous particles, as Signor Fracassati[f] has called them in dissecting it several times. The superstition in this city does not allow me to see one except once every Holy Year[g], in the presence of the relatives.

If you need to make the experiments of the first epistle, note that in the lungs of dogs the little lobes are very obscure, though in others they are clearly observed.

About the comet, some of the people have seen it. Signor Cassini[h] is at Ferrara, and in the meanwhile I do not know whether it has been observed by anyone in the Profession. Signor Fracassati greets you, and if he should get the money for his business begs you for your attention[i], while I, awaiting your reply with anxiety, remain with Signor Mariani[j] etc.

If people need to observe the lungs of the frog, let them look for microscopes of very fine quality, and do it in the sun, and with patience, or otherwise they will not see anything more. There seems nothing else for me to say, while I sign myself from Bologna, 16 March 1661,

Of your most illustrious and excellent self the most devoted and obliged servant
Marcello Malpighi

a. Probably the letter 11 March 1661 (Adelmann, ed., *Correspondence of Malpighi*, 1: letter 39, pp. 76–79).
b. Malpighi had suggested that Borelli write a letter to amplify and criticize his results.
c. Letter of 22 February 1661 (Adelmann, ed., *Correspondence of Malpighi*, 1: letter 36, pp. 69–71).
d. i.e., the letter that became the second part of *De pulmonibus*.
e. The Grand Duke Ferdinand II and his brother Prince Leopold, both patrons of scientific research.
f. Carlo Fracassati (d. 1672) was a colleague at Bologna. He later moved to Pisa.
g. i.e., once in a blue moon.
h. Giovanni Domenico Cassini (1625–1712), professor of astronomy at Bologna; one of the leading astronomers of his time. In 1669 he became the first director of the new Paris Observatory.
i. This phrase is obscure.
j. Mario Mariani (d. 1709), the son of Malpighi's teacher, Andrea Mariani (1593–ca. 1661).

Malpighi died of a massive cerebral hemorrhage; the necropsy being conducted by one of his most outstanding pupils, and an outstanding anatomist in his own right, Giorgio Baglivi. The details of the autopsy are to be found in *The Practice of Physick*, published in London in 1694[39].

Although Baglivi's life spanned both the 17th and 18th centuries, most of his contributions occurred in the last decade of the 17th century. He occupied the anatomy chair at Rome at a very early age. His most famous work, *De praxi medica*, was published when he was only 28 years old. Unfortunately, his promising career remained largely unfulfilled with death occurring prematurely at the age of 38[40].

Perhaps his most outstanding characteristic was his correlation of structure with function and his ability to utilize descriptive analogies in this regard. For example, he likened the heart and blood vessels to a pump and hydraulic system[41]. He was the first to distinguish the differences between smooth and striated muscle. Later on we shall note his important contributions to cardiovascular physiology, pathology and the clinical syndrome of heart failure.

The 18th century saw great changes in Europe involving political, economic, geographical and intellectual parameters. The turbulent activity of the Renaissance had spent itself but this in no way affected further contributions in the field of medicine though at a much slower pace. The 18th century was a time more of consolidation than advancement *per se*. Other nations besides Italy and France emerged as bright stars in the intellectual firmament. The schools of anatomy that flourished with such high esteem in Italy and France were now being challenged by newly established schools in Scotland, England, Holland and Germany. Even the fledgling North American colony began to flex its medical muscles with the establishment of several medical schools. These were the University of Pennsylvania which evolved from the medical school of the College of Philadelphia, Columbia University which began as Kings College, and soon thereafter, Harvard University and Dartmouth Medical School. Thus, the reawakening of interest and enthusiasm in knowledge that characterized the Renaissance continued to motivate and fuel, in a global manner, the scholars of this century. A relatively dark spot in all of this was France. The reigns of Louis XIV and Louis XVI had a somewhat retarding influence on intellectual activity in France. The French Revolution worsened the situation so that by the end of the century, medical progress in France was at a complete standstill. Medical facilities were dissolved. Medical practitioners were scarce and the medical profession itself was in shambles. France had to wait for Napoleon to resume its leadership role in medicine. But, despite all this, France still managed to produce some important scholars during the 18th century.

The Italian schools continued to maintain their traditional leadership but had to share this role with other European countries. There were many worthy successors to Vesalius and Malpighi and among those that played a prominent role in cardiology were Scarpa, Morgagni and Spallanzani.

Morgagni and Spallanzani, however, were not interested in normal anatomy. Their contributions will be detailed in that part of the text devoted to their fields of interest, namely, morbid anatomy for Morgagni and physiology for Spallanzani. Valsalva and Santorini were also great anatomists of the era but their contributions were not in cardiovascular anatomy. The Dutch school numbered the following important investigators in cardiac anatomy: Albinus of Frankfort-on-the-Oder and Albrecht von Haller. De Senac and Felix Vicq d'Azyr constitute the leaders in France while the Scottish school spawned primarily the Monro dynasty consisting of three generations of anatomists spanning a period of 126 years. England had great anatomists in such men as the Hunter brothers, Hewson and Cruikshank. Significant contributions in descriptive anatomy began to appear from Germany in the hands of the Meckel family, Soemmering, Vater, Lieberkuhn, and Thebesius to mention but a few. But, these men with the exception of Thebesius did not contribute anything of significance to cardiovascular anatomy.

This international melange of anatomists in the 18th century was complemented by only a brief and sporadic output from the Americans. Their minuscule output may have been due to the marked degree of resistance to dissection that prevailed among the laity in America at the time. Indeed, this abhorrence towards dissection manifested itself in the infamous doctors riot that occurred in New York City in 1788. This incident involved an unruly mob that gathered in protest against the dissecting activity of certain doctors. The mob, incensed and urged on by certain factions, finally became completely out of control and caused much damage both to persons and property. Paradoxically, this riot did have one beneficial effect in that it caused the legislature to pass a law allowing for the discretionary dissection of executed criminals. At any rate, the 18th century cannot be counted as having seen any advances in cardiovascular anatomy from America. The tremendous impact on cardiology that America was to make was yet to come.

Let us view now some of this century's personalities and their contributions. In this survey, Antonio Scarpa, among the 18th century Italian anatomists, is the only one who played a major role in cardiovascular anatomy. He was born in 1747 and died in 1832. His mentor was Morgagni, and Scarpa, while still a student, was so deeply devoted to his teacher that he continued to maintain what appeared to be a father–son relationship with the aging and enfeebled Morgagni. Scarpa went on to become professor of anatomy and clinical surgery at Modena, and then later at Pavia. He was both an artistic and anatomical genius. The first accurate delineation of the nerves of the heart are to be found in the beautifully illustrated *Tabulae neurologicae ad illustrandam historiam anatomicam cardiacorum nervorum, noni nervorum cerebri, glossopharyngaei et pharyngaei ex octavo cerebri*. Many of the illustrations were done by himself following, as it were, in Leonardo Da Vinci's footsteps. Scarpa was fortunate though in having as his assistant a master engraver by the name of Faustino Anderloni. Mann recounts how Scarpa's admiration for the ability of his master engraver did not prevent him from locking the engraver in his room until the work at hand was finished[42].

Jean-Baptiste de Senac is noted for his comprehensive textbook dealing with the anatomy, physiology, and diseases of the heart. It was the first textbook of its kind and contained many original observations on the muscular make-up of the heart. It too was accompanied by outstanding illustrations[43]. The book entitled *Traite de la structure du coeur, de son action, et de ses maladies* was published in 1749. Its systematic and exhaustive treatment of the subject made it an authoritative text for many years. A second and revised edition was published by Portal in 1783, 34 years after the first edition and 8 years after the death of Senac[44]. Senac's contributions to cardiology were not confined to his description of the structure of the heart alone. As we shall see later, his text provided many important insights into the physiology of the heart, morbid anatomy and congenital heart disease with painstaking anatomical and clinical correlation.

Felix Vicq D'Azyr was quite active, during his short life, as a private lecturer in anatomy and as permanent secretary of the Royal Society of Medicine which he helped to establish. He is mentioned here because of his important text on comparative anatomy and his book dealing with the nervous system. The former work helped define the differences in cardiac structure among mammals, especially man and apes, while his text on the neural system helped delineate the innervation of the heart[45,46].

All three generations of the Monro family of anatomists served at the University of Edinburgh.

The father, son and grandson were all named Alexander. The first Alexander (1697–1767) is now referred to, for obvious reasons, as Monro Primus. His father was a Scottish army-surgeon who helped establish the school of medicine at Edinburgh. A remarkably motivated man, the father was the persistent guiding force in the preparation of Primus, from the age of three, for a life devoted to medicine. Primus was able to realize all of his father's ambitions. He proved to be a very prolific writer and passed this trait on to his son, Monro Secundus. The least inspirational of all was the last of the dynasty, Monro Tertius. It is said that Tertius was a desultory lecturer, reading verbatim his grandfather's notes. Although none of the three Monros were on the cutting edge of anatomical discoveries in cardiology, both Primus and Secundus exerted an indirect influence by virtue of their prestige and inspirational teaching that attracted many students to the University of Edinburgh not only from England but from the North American colonies as well.

Bernhard Siegfried Albinus is remembered as one of the greatest anatomical illustrators of the 18th century. His atlases are notable for the detail and accuracy with which they depict the veins and arteries of the intestines[47]. Albrecht von Haller was a student of Albinus, who in time outstripped his teacher, to become recognized as the master physiologist of the 18th century. He became an anatomist in an effort to overcome the many shortcomings of anatomical illustrations available to him when attempting to illustrate the physiological concepts of his other teacher, the renowned Boerhave of Leyden. On the basis of personal observations gleaned from approximately 400 dissections, von Haller published a collection of these anatomical studies in seven volumes entitled *Disputationes anatomicae selectae*[48,49]. In one of these volumes, his treatment of the anatomy of blood vessels is regarded as particularly good. Haller also described quite accurately the musculature of the heart, the pericardium and the valvular elements of the veins. Haller played a far greater role in physiology, and his contributions in this area will be dealt with later.

There were two Hunter brothers, William and John. William was the older of the two and much more articulate than John (probably because John had a very poor educational background in the humanities). Despite this deficiency, John became quite a proficient anatomist by virtue of his technical ability in dissection. During the early part of the 18th century several private schools of anatomy were founded in England as an aftermath of the dissolution of the barber-surgeons trade unions and aided by a legislative act allowing dissection of executed criminals. William was the founder of one of these schools (Figures 13 and 14). It was called the Great Windmill Street School and contained, in addition to its anatomic theater, a museum. In time, the museum, because of William's constant addition of specimens, became quite valuable in terms of financial worth. His brother John also had a consuming interest in his own museum, and at the time of his death, it contained about 13,000 specimens. John achieved greater renown than his brother William, and we shall speak of him again in the chapter dealing with coronary artery disease. Both brothers discovered the independence of the fetal and maternal circulations. The foundation of placental anatomy rests upon this discovery[50–52].

William Hewson and William Cruikshank were both students of the Hunter brothers. Hewson is credited with giving the first complete account of the comparative anatomy of the lymphatic system. Cruikshank was also interested in the lymphatics and he gave a detailed account of this system in his treatise entitled *The Anatomy of the Absorbing Vessels of the Human Body*[53].

The analogue to the Monros was the Prussian family of Meckel. This dynasty also spanned three generations. It started with Johann Friedrich (1724–74) followed by his son Philipp (1756–1803) and ended with Philipp's son, also called Johann Friedrich (1781–1833). Although all great anatomists, they did not contribute in any significant manner to cardiovascular anatomy. The grandfather, Johann, was aware of the relationship between the veins and lymphatics but did not offer any original descriptions in this field. This family deserves to be mentioned in any history of cardiology simply because, like the Monros, they exerted an indirect influence through their teachings in the general field of anatomy.

Adam Christian Thebesius of Germany (1686–1732) is better known to cardiologists since he described the venae minimae cordis now known as the veins of Thebesius, the orifices of these veins (Thebesius foramina), and the valve of the coronary vein now referred to by the eponym, Thebesius valve[54].

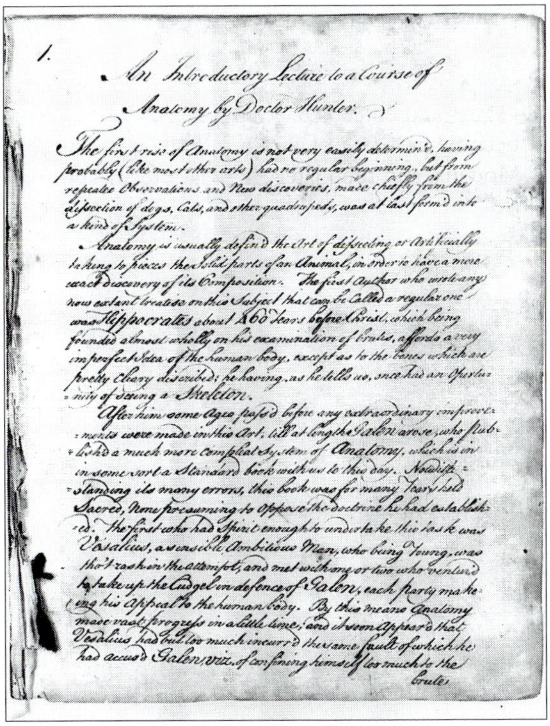
1.

An Introductory Lecture to a Course of Anatomy by Doctor Hunter.

The first rise of Anatomy is not very easily determin'd, having probably (like most other arts) had no regular beginning, but from repeated Observations and New discoveries, made chiefly from the dissection of dogs, Cats, and other quadrupeds, was at last form'd into a kind of System.

Anatomy is usually defin'd the Art of dissecting or Artificially taking to pieces the solid parts of an Animal, in order to have a more exact discovery of its Composition. The first Author who wrote any now extant treatise on this Subject that can be Called a regular one was Hippocrates about 460 Years before Christ, which being founded almost wholly on his examination of brutes, affords a very imperfect Idea of the human body, except as to the bones which are pretty Cleary described; he having, as he tells us, once had an Opportu-nity of seeing a Skeleton.

After him some Ages pass'd before any extraordinary improve-ments were made in this Art, till at length Galen arose, who pub-lish'd a much more compleat System of Anatomy, which is in some sort a Standard book with us to this day. Notwith-standing its many errors, this book was for many Years held Sacred, None presuming to Oppose the doctrine he had establish-ed. The first who had Spirit enough to undertake this task was Vesalius, a sensible Ambitious Man, who being Young, was tho't rash in the attempt, and met with one or two who ventur'd to take up the Cudgel in defence of Galen, each party make-ing his Appeal to the human body. By this means Anatomy made vast progress in a little time, and it soon Appear'd that Vesalius had but too much incurr'd the same fault of which he had accus'd Galen, viz. of confining himself too much to the brutes

Figure 13 William Hunter, Lectures on Anatomy. *Photo Source Wellcome Institute Library. Literary Source William Hunter, Lectures on Anatomy, London, n.d.[c. 1755] WIHM Western MS 2965, fol 1. By courtesy of the Wellcome Trustees*

The study of anatomy during the 19th century again was carried on mostly by European and to a lesser extent by American investigators. Anatomy continued to remain a vital part of physiology and with ever increasing new techniques becoming available, microscopic anatomy began to make a great deal of headway. We shall see in the section dealing with electrophysiology, how important histologic descriptions of the heart muscle were in establishing fundamental concepts of cardiac rhythm from initiation of impulse to its propagation throughout the heart. The cellular basis of cardiac function whether it be contractility or rhythm became firmly established as a result of these histologic studies.

Significant advances in microscopic anatomy, however, had to wait until the latter part of the 19th century. It was not until then that, because of refinement in methods, consistently high quality preparations, relatively free of

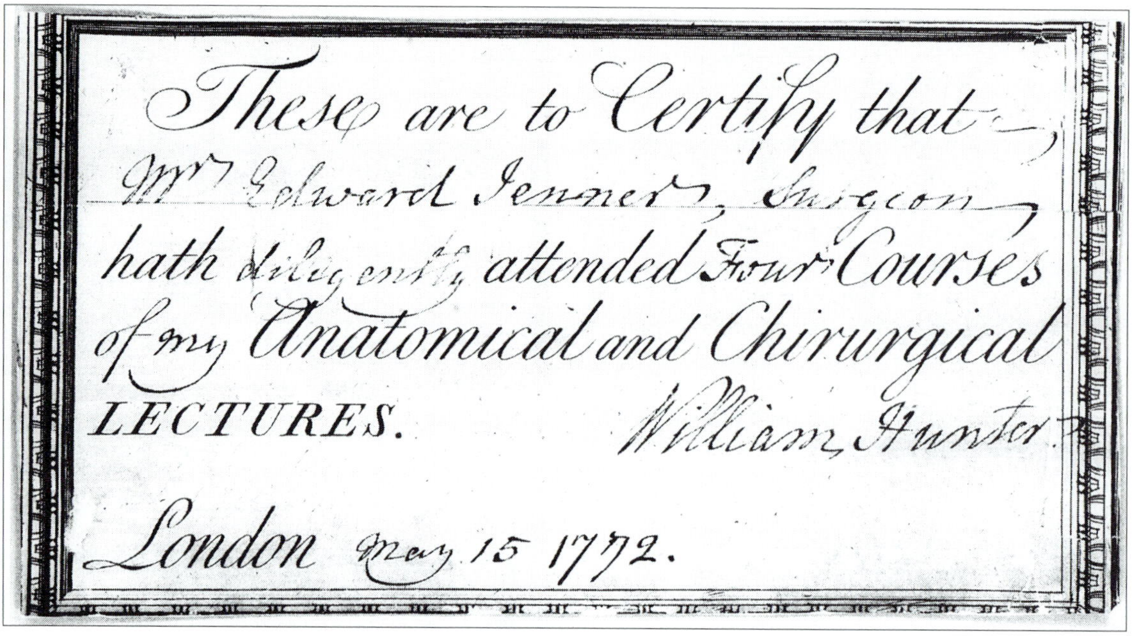
These are to Certify that
Mr Edward Jenner, Surgeon
hath diligently attended Four Courses
of my Anatomical and Chirurgical
LECTURES. William Hunter.
London May 15 1772.

Figure 14 Edward Jenner's certificate of attendance at lectures by William Hunter, London, 1772. *Photo Source Wellcome Institute Library. Literary Source WIHM Western MS 5231/1. By courtesy of the Wellcome Trustees*

distortion, were possible. Before that time, tissue specimens were prepared in a rather crude manner. Stains were few and erratic. Embedding agents for histologic study were unknown. Animal tissues could be studied only by tearing them apart with needles. Serial sectioning was impossible except with botanical tissue since only plants (being more rigid) could be sliced in this fashion, and then only in a crude manner by using a razor for this purpose. Really effective serial sections were not possible until the advent of high quality reliable microtomes. This plus the introduction of a wide variety of staining agents, good cheap glassware and improvements in the microscope were necessary before histology began to bear fruit.

Germany seemed to provide the lion's share of the great anatomists during this century. Among them were Müller, Schwann, Schleiden, Stilling, Henle, Schultze, von Koelliker, Burdach and His. Other countries including America gave us Purkinje, Bell, Hyrtl, Wistar, Dorsey, Horner, Warren, Oliver Wendell Holmes, Mall, Ramsay, Golgi, von Baer, and many others, too numerous to mention.

To Stilling belongs the credit for rendering animal tissue more rigid for slicing by freezing[55]. Purkinje was one of the first to use the microtome and canadian balsam. He was to elaborate on the histology of the conducting tissue that His first described but with a far more efficient and reliable microtome. Jacob Henle is remembered today mostly for the microscopic loop of cells in the kidneys which is the pharmacological site for many of the currently popular diuretics. He also contributed to our knowledge of the histology of the smaller arteries by noting the presence of smooth muscle in the middle layer. Henle had a long and fruitful life. He was successively professor of anatomy at Zurich, Heidelberg, and then Göttingen where he remained until his death in 1885.

One of the foremost microscopists of the 19th century was Rudolph von Koelliker. He too had a long and active career, working and remarkably productive until the age of 85 when he resigned at Würzburg after having held the chair for 55 years. He wrote two texts on microscopic anatomy, one of which was a handbook[56,57]. They are both classics and remained important sources of histology references for many years. In them, he elaborated still further on Henle's description of the muscular layer of the blood vessels.

By the end of the 19th century, histologic knowledge of the heart was quite well advanced. Photomicrography was introduced during this era but ultrastructure of the cardiovascular system

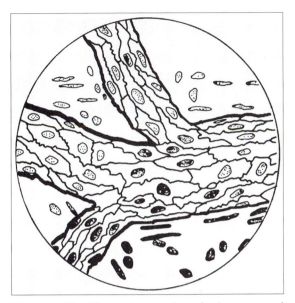

Figure 15 Photomicrograph of the external epithelium of a frog's skin. *Photo Source University of Central Florida. Literary Source Varcho, S.: J.J. Woodward (1870) on the histology and photomicrography of minute blood vessels. American Journal of Cardiology, 30:542–546,1972. With permission*

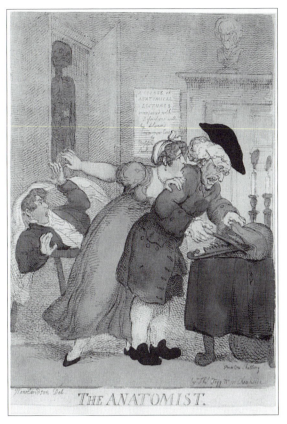

Figure 16 The Anatomist *Photo Source National Library of Medicine. Literary Source Rowlandson del. [Pub.] by Thos. Tegg, no. 111 Cheapside. Courtesy of National Library of Medicine*

would not be explored until well into the 20th century with the invention of the electron microscope. J. J. Woodward was a leading expert in photomicrography. He utilized this technique, achieving magnifications of 400 diameters in his studies at the newly established Army Medical Museum[58]. His work documented the existence of the morphologic substrate that was necessary for the phenomenon of diapedesis of leukocytes in the inflammatory process. Diapedesis had originally been proposed by Waller and was later expanded upon by Conheim. Woodward's photomicrographs of frog's tissue stained with silver nitrate and carmine demonstrated the intercellular stomata or openings necessary for diapedesis to occur. Figure 15 represents a photomicrograph of the external epithelium of frog's skin. Silver nitrate was used to stain the borders of the cells while the nuclei were brought into relief by staining with carmine in borax. The openings in the photomicrograph appear as little rings with black margins in the walls of the epithelial cells. Some of these rings are opacified by stain.

It is quite evident by now that ever since Vesalius, an extensive body of knowledge had

accumulated regarding the anatomical make-up of the heart and blood vessels. Further observations by anatomist-physiologists rendered the picture more complete. A different approach to anatomical study became more evident during the 19th century and this was to continue well nigh into the 20th century with the further imposition of a multi-disciplinary effort in basic research. It was no longer sufficient to render the elements of structure in a purely descriptive fashion. Anatomy, both gross and microscopic, had to be described and analyzed in terms of function. Harvey was the first to do this in a systematic manner, but it was during the 19th century that physiology began to assume a close working relationship with anatomy. Medical schools were now well established in both Europe and America so that they could easily incorporate and support the many physiologic laboratories that came into existence during the 19th century. Physiologists began to enrich anatomy through their application of more exacting methods of observation and experimentation. One of the first to do this was Johannes Mueller (1801–58). Carl Ludwig (1816–95) carried on this tradition. He discovered the ganglion cells in the interatrial septum as part of his physiologic experiments. This plus the discovery of the cardiac nerves helped define cardiac anatomy more completely.

Before turning to electron microscopy, let us remember with humility that not all anatomists meet the standards of the housewife. Figure 16 is a caricature by Thomas Rowlandson emphasizing how an anatomist need not necessarily be a good 'carver'.

REFERENCES

1. Herrick, J.B. (1942). *A Short History of Cardiology*, p. 16. (Springfield, Ill.: Charles C. Thomas)
2. McMurrich, J.P. (1930). *Leonardo da Vinci, the Anatomist*, pp. 149–67. (Baltimore, MD)
3. Favaro, G. (1914–15). *La struttura del cuore nel quarto Quaderno d Anatomia di Leonardo*. Atti del Regio Istituto Veneto, LXXIV, 895
4. Mettler, C.C. (1947). *History of Medicine*, p. 41–44 (Philadelphia: The Blackiston Co.)
5. Vesalius: (1974). *Encyclopaedia Britannica*, 15th edn., **19**, 94–5
6. Herrick, J.B. (1942). *Op. Cit.*, p. 18
7. Roth, M. (1892). *Andreas Vesalius Bruxellensis*, pp. 65, 125, 144. George Reimer
8. Baker, F. (1909). The two Sylviuses: an historical study. *Bull. Johns Hopkins Hosp.*, **20**, 331
9. *Ibid.* p. 333
10. Clendening, L. (1960). *Source Book of Medical History*, p. 142. (New York: Dover Publications, Inc.)
11. Vesalius, A. (1949). *The Epitome of Andreas Vesalius* (Lind, L.R., translator). (New York: The MacMillan Co.)
12. Singer, C. (1925). *The Evolution of Anatomy*, p. 135. (London: Kegan Paul)
13. Mettler, C.C. (1947). *Op. Cit.*, p.48
14. Fabricius, H. (1952). De Formatione Ovi et Pulli. In Adelman, H.B. (ed.) *The Embryological Treatises of Hieronymus Fabricius of Aquapendente*, p. 217. (Ithaca: Cornell University Press)
15. Arcieri, J.P. (1945). *The circulation of the blood and Andrea Cesalpino of Arezzo*, p. 27. (New York: S.F. Vanni)
16. Krumbhaar, E.B. (1929). Bibliographical matters pertaining to the discovery of the circulation. *Ann. M. Hist. N.S.*, **1**, 61
17. Willius, F.A. and Dry, T.J. (1948). *A History of the Heart and the Circulation*, p. 36. (Philadelphia: W.B. Saunders Co.)
18. Mettler, C.C. (1947). *Op. Cit.*, p. 36
19. Castiglioni, A. (1941). *A History of Medicine*, (Translated by E.B. Krumbhaar), p. 418. (New York: Alfred A. Knopf)
20. Garrison, F.H. (1929). *An Introduction to the History of Medicine; with Medical Chronology, Suggestions for Study and Bibliographic Data*, edn. 4, p. 224. (Philadelphia: W.B. Saunders Company)
21. Singer, C. (1925). *Op. Cit.*, p. 167
22. Mettler, C.C. (1947). *Op. Cit.*, p. 69
23. Aselli, G. (1627). *De lactibus, sive lacteis venis, quarto vasorum mesaraicorum genere, novo invento, dissertatio*, Milan
24. Paris, 1651. (1653). For an English translation see *New Anatomical Experiments by Which the Hitherto Unknown Receptacle of the Chyle and the Transmission from Thence to the Subclavial Veins by the Now Discovered Lacteal Channels of the Thorax Is Plainly Made Appear in Brutes*, London
25. Bartholin, T. (1653). *Vasa lymphatica, nuper Hafnial in animantibus inventa et hepatis exsequiae*, Copenhagen
26. Rudbeck, O. (1653). *Nova Exercitatio Anatomica, exhibens ductus hepaticos aquosos et vasa glandularum serosa*. Westeras
27. Nuck, A. (1691). *Adenografia Curiosa*. Lugdini, Batavorum, Luchtmans
28. Miller, W.S. (1914). Niels Stenson. *Bull. Johns Hopkins Hosp.*, **25**, 47
29. Steno, N (1664). *De musculis et Glandulis. Observatonum Specimen*
30. Lower, R. (1932). *Tractatus de Corde, item de Motu et Colore Sanguinis et Chyli in Transitu*, (1669). Translation by K.J. Franklin in *Early Science in Oxford*, R.T. Gunther, (ed.)
31. Donley, J.E. (1909). John James Wepfer, a Renaissance student of apoplexy. *Bull. Johns Hopkins Hosp.*, **20**, 5
32. Mettler, C.C. (1947). *Op. Cit.*, p. 67.
33. Vieussens, R. (1715). Nouvelles découvertes sur lé coeur, Toulouse, 1706, and Traité nouveau de la structure et des causes du mouvement naturel du coeur. In Oeuvres francoises de M. Vieussens, Toulouse
34. Major, R.H. (1932). Raymond Vieussens and his treatise on the heart. *Ann. M. Hist., N.S.*, **4**, 147

35. Malpighi, M. (1974). *Encyclopaedia Britannica*, 15th edn., **11**, 388–9

36. Malpighi, M. (1661). *De pulmonibus epistolae II ad Borellium*, Bologna

37. Foster, M. (1901). *Lectures on the History of Physiology*, pp. 96–7. (London and New York: Cambridge Univ. Press, the MacMillan Co.)

38. Middleton, Knowles W.E. (1985). An unpublished letter from Marcello Malpighi. *Bull. Hist. Med.*, **59**, 105–7

39. Stenn, F. (1941). Giorgio Baglivi, *Ann. M. Hist.*, **53**, 3, 183–94 (May)

40. Willius, F.A. and Dry, T.J. (1948). *Op. Cit.*, p. 72

41. Stenn, F. (1941). *Op. Cit.*, p. 185

42. Mann, R.J. (Nov. 1974). Historical vignette, Scarpa, Hodgson, and Hope, artists of the heart and great vessels. *Mayo Clin. Proc.*, **49**, 889–92

43. Herrick, J.B. (1942). *Op. Cit.*, p. 49

44. East, T. (1957). *The Story of Heart Disease*, p. 65. (London: Wm. Dawson and Sons, Ltd.)

45. D'Azyr, F.V. (1786). *Traite d'Anatomie et de physiologie avec des planches colories representant au naturel les organes de l'homme et des animaux*, Paris

46. D'Azyr, F.V. (1805). *Oeuvres de Vicq D'Azyr*, Paris, 6 Vols

47. Albinus, B.S. (1747–1753). *Tabulae sceleti et musculorum corporis humani, cum explanatio*, Leyden

48. von Haller, A. (1746–52). *Disputationes anatomicae selectae*, Goettingen, 7 Vols

49. Mettler, C.C. (1947). *Op. Cit.*, p. 81

50. Peachey, G.C. (1924). *A Memoir of William & John Hunter*, pp. 133–4. Plymouth

51. Owen, E. (1911). John Hunter and his museum. *Lancet*, **1**, 418

52. Paget, S. (1897). *John Hunter*, p. 179. London

53. Cruikshank, W. (1786). *The Anatomy of the Absorbing Vessels of the Human Body*, London

54. Mettler, C.C. (1947). *Op. Cit.*, p. 87

55. Stilling, B. (1857). *Neu Untersuchungen ueber den Bau des Rueckenmarks mit einem Atlas mikroskop*, Abbidlungen von 30 lith. Taf., Cassel

56. von Koelliker, R. (1850–54). *Mikroskopische Anatomie*, Leipzig, 3 Vols

57. von Koelliker, R. (1852). *Handbuch der Geivebelehre des Menschen*, Leipzig

58. Varcho, S. (1972). J.J. Woodward (1870) on the histology and photomicrography of minute blood vessels. *Am. J. Cardiol.*, **30**, 542–6

3   Role of electron microscopy

Long before Christ, the Assyrians were aware of the magnifying power of glass spheres. Apparently optics were known also to the Romans since Claudius Ptolemy did write a treatise on optics in the second century AD. Further development of knowledge concerning refraction and magnification remained somewhat stagnant until the invention of spectacles in the 14th century. History owes a great deal to the unknown inventor of those spectacles because this precipitated a renewed interest in magnification culminating in the development of the so-called Gallileo telescope of the 17th century. This instrument was a hollow tube into which were mounted lenses in a strategic fashion so that by looking through it at one end a telescopic effect was produced while looking through it at the other end produced a microscopic effect. Although Gallileo did use the instrument for biological observations he was more interested in its capabilities for the study of planets and stars. It was Johannes Faber, an entomologist, and a contemporary of Gallileo, who gave the microscope its name.

There are five men who are responsible for the profound effect of the microscope on the biological sciences. These are Malpighi, van Leeuwenhoek, Swammerdam, Grew, and Hooke. Jan Swammerdam, Nehemiah Grew, and Robert Hooke did not play any significant role in cardiology. Malpighi's description of the capillaries with its impact on solidifying the structural basis for Harvey's concepts on the physiology of circulation has already been mentioned. Antonie van Leeuwenhoek, although noted more for his discovery of animalcules with the consequent demolition of the theory of spontaneous generation, did contribute to further microscopic descriptions of the arteries and veins and also gave the first accurate description of the red blood cells.

Leeuwenhoek was a Dutchman born in Delft who was a haberdasher and draper but became so interested in lens making and conducting observations with his lenses that he seriously neglected his means of livelihood. He was no doubt an excellent lens maker, achieving with his single lenses, magnifications up to 270 diameters; no mean accomplishment with lenses ground by hand. Leeuwenhoek lived to the ripe old age of 90, famous throughout the world for his craftsmanship and observations in the biological arena.

The development of the achromatic lens around 1830, the design of a new achromatic compound microscope by Ernst Abbe of Germany, and the subsequent addition of a substage illumination system and condenser provided the impetus and the means for the important histologic studies of the 19th century. Figure 1 portrays a selection of the early microscopes. They are housed in the Museum of History of Science at Oxford. Figure 2 depicts Leeuwenhoek in his prime.

Despite the many sophisticated variants of optical microscopy, extreme magnification did not become possible until the invention of electron microscopy. This system involves the use of a stream of electrons passing through a series of magnetic fields. The enormous potentialities of this instrument have yet to be fully realized but it has allowed the anatomists of the 20th century to begin exploring the ultrastructure of the cardiovascular system correlating function with structure on a molecular level.

Although the fundamental physical concepts upon which electron microscopy is based can be traced back to the latter part of the 19th century, the true impetus for its development is to be found in the de Broglie theory and a demonstration by Busch. In 1924, de Broglie postulated that a moving electron could be considered as having the properties of a light-like wave. In 1926, Busch demonstrated that suitably shaped magnetic or electrostatic fields could be used as true lenses to focus an electron beam to produce an image. Dennis Gabor[1] stated that the electron microscope

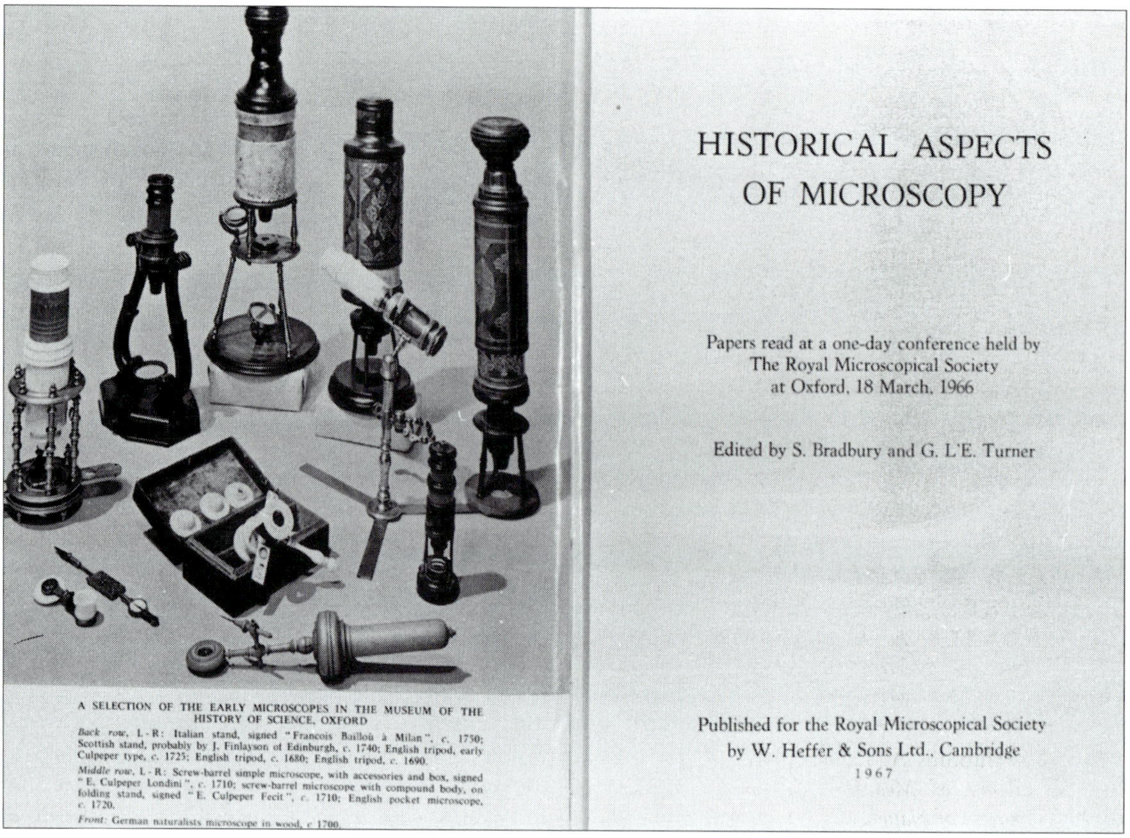
A SELECTION OF THE EARLY MICROSCOPES IN THE MUSEUM OF THE HISTORY OF SCIENCE, OXFORD
Back row, L-R: Italian stand, signed "Francois Baillou à Milan", c. 1750; Scottish stand, probably by J. Finlayson of Edinburgh, c. 1740; English tripod, early Culpeper type, c. 1725; English tripod, c. 1680; English tripod, c. 1690.
Middle row, L-R: Screw-barrel simple microscope, with accessories and box, signed "E. Culpeper Londini", c. 1710; screw-barrel microscope with compound body, on folding stand, signed "E. Culpeper Fecit", c. 1710; English pocket microscope, c. 1720.
Front: German naturalists microscope in wood, c 1700.
HISTORICAL ASPECTS
OF MICROSCOPY
Papers read at a one-day conference held by
The Royal Microscopical Society
at Oxford, 18 March, 1966
Edited by S. Bradbury and G. L'E. Turner
Published for the Royal Microscopical Society
by W. Heffer & Sons Ltd., Cambridge
1967

Figure 1 Selection of early microscopes in the Museum of the History of Science, Oxford. *Photo Source Royal College of Physicians. Literary Source Bradbury, S., Turner, G. L'E: Historical Aspects of Microscopy. W. Heffer & Sons, Ltd., Cambridge, 1967. With permission from The Royal Microscopical Society*

was an obvious invention. 'One has only to combine the fact that an axially symmetric electric or magnetic field is an electron lens with wave mechanics in order to see the possibility of an electron microscope'.

The results of the early work on cardiac muscle utilizing electron microscopy were plagued with distortions and inaccuracies due to tissue damage brought about not only by the electron beam itself but also by the fixation and embedding techniques then in use. This was evident in the publication of Bruno Kisch in 1951[2]. His book appears to be the first recorded observations regarding the histology of the heart with the electron microscope. In 1960, he published an amplification of the original text under the auspices of a different publishing house[3]. He was keenly aware of the necessity of utilizing sections of tissue no thicker than 0.1 and 0.2 μm in order to avoid blurring of detail. The development of the high-speed microtome by Gessler and his group helped a great deal in meeting this objective[4].

Kisch's work is outstanding not only because it represents a pioneering effort in expanding further anatomical knowledge of the heart on an ultrastructural basis but also because of the seminal influence it had on subsequent investigators. Kisch brought out how the electron microscope could lead to a clearer understanding of the inter-relationship between the contractile muscle fibril and enzyme bearing sarcosomes. He was able to show the excellent vascularization of the heart wherein individual muscle fibers were supplied by their own capillaries. He noted the presence of two types of fibril in heart muscle: Type A which he likened to a bamboo stick, and Type B which have a syncytial arrangement. He considered the bamboo stick fibril as the elementary unit of heart muscle. His observations also indicated the existence of a

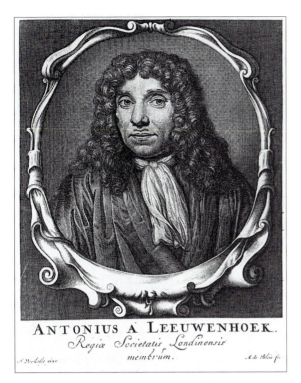

ANTONIUS A. LEEUWENHOEK.
Regiæ Societatis Londinensis membrum.

Figure 2 Antonius A. Leeuwenhoek. *Photo Source National Library of Medicine. Literary Source Photo Archives. Courtesy of National Library of Medicine*

kind of sarcolemma surrounding groups of bamboo stick fibrils and connected with Z bands. The Z band system was, in his opinion, an active part of the muscle fiber involved in the production of sarcosomes and playing a role in the electro-physiology of the muscle fiber.

Excellent preservation of tissue structure in most specimens was realized with the introduction of glutaraldehyde as the main primary fixative and the epoxy resins as the main embedding materials[5,6]. Technical problems of fixation and perfusion, however, still abound and the battle is far from won regarding the ideal methods, with each approach having its own limitations and distortions[7].

Cytochemical procedures as applied to electron microscopic studies of cardiac muscle were introduced in 1962 and 1964 to study phosphatase reactions at the cellular level[8,9]. These methods did reveal the presence of enzymes that split the various nucleoside phosphates but so far have failed to localize their precise anatomical location in the cell. Attempts at studying the three-dimensional geometry of cardiac muscle have also been hampered

by inadequate techniques. In 1975, L.D. Peachey was able to demonstrate the limited usefulness of high voltage electron microscopy in constructing three-dimensional views[10]. At about the same time, scanning electron microscopy was advanced as a means of investigating the structure of cardiac muscle[11]. Unfortunately, this technique also leaves a lot to be desired. Among the problems are distortion of images, difficulty in the proper interpretation of the images and the appearance of intracellular organelles as solid profiles.

The freeze-fracture technique introduced by Steere in 1972 has been very fruitful in providing more insight into the three-dimensional aspects of cardiac muscle cells[12]. Another successful advancement has been the theoretical and practical development of stereologic quantitation in the quantitative description of cardiac muscle[13]. Despite these approaches, significant errors in dimensions are still unavoidable, again because of present fixation and embedding procedures as well as the compression that ensues when cutting through the embedded tissues[14].

In all of this, the pericardium had not been neglected. Kluge and Hovig, in 1967, reported their observations on the ultrastructure of the pericardium in humans and rats utilizing transmission electronic techniques[15]. The pathology and surgical branches of the National Institute of Health reported their findings on patches of normal parietal pericardium removed from seven patients who had undergone cardiac surgery for cardiac lesions not involving the pericardium[16]. Their report was published in 1980. It described the histologic transmission and scanning electron microscopic anatomy and demonstrated some of the relationships between structure and function. The most important elements of the ultrastructure consist of microvilli on the serosal cells, actin filaments and cytoskeletal filaments. The microvilli presumably bear friction and facilitate fluid and ion exchange. Active change in the shape of the cells is mediated through the actin filaments while structural support is provided by the cytoskeletal filaments.

Prior to the Bethesda report, Miller and his co-workers described in 1971 the detailed ultrastructure of the cardiopericardial lymphatics[17]. They demonstrated that lymph from the myocardium first drains into the subepicardium and then ultimately to the mediastinum and right heart cavities. In congestive heart failure, fluid accumulates in the pericardial sac because the increase in central venous pressure interferes with the venous and lymphatic drainage from the myocardium[17]. At last, we have an anatomical basis for the pericardial effusion as seen in congestive heart failure.

The evolutionary steps in the development and application of electron microscopy have brought us to the stage where knowledge of the anatomical structure of the heart on a molecular basis is now possible. This is a far cry from the early beginnings of gross anatomy. We cannot, however, rest on our laurels. Further improvements are necessary to reduce to a bare minimum the deficiencies still present in the current procedures. We need to learn more about the ultrastructure of the sarcolemma, the intracellular components, the sarcoplasmic reticulum, the myofibrils themselves and the conduction fibers which are so important in maintaining the rhythm of the heart.

REFERENCES

1. Marton, L. (1968). *Early History of Electron Microscopy*. (San Francisco, California: San Francisco Press, Inc.)

2. Kisch, B. and Bardet, J.M. (1951). *Electron microscopic histology of the heart; an application of electron microscopic research to physiology*. (Brooklyn Medical Press)

3. Kisch, B. (1960). *Electronmicroscopy of the cardiovascular system*. (Springfield, Illinois: Charles C. Thomas)

4. Gessler, A.E. and Fullam, E.F. (1946). Sectioning for the electron microscope accomplished by the high speed microtome. *Am. J. Anat.*, **78**, 235

5. Sabatini, D.D., Bensch, K. and Barnett, R.J. (1963). Cytochemistry and electronmicroscopy. The preservation of cellular ultrastructure and enzymatic activity by aldehyde fixation. *J. Cell. Biol.*, **17**, 19–58

6. Luft, J.H. (1961). Improvements in epoxy resin embedding methods. *J. Biophysic. Biochem. Cytol.*, **9**, 409–14

7. Sommer, J.R. and Waugh, R.A. (1976). Cardiac cell muscle ultrastructure. *Am. J. Pathol.*, **1**, 192–221

8. Tice, L.W. and Barnett, R.J. (1962). Fine structural localization of adenosinetriphosphatase activity in heart muscle myofibrils. *J. Cell Biol.*, **15**, 401–16

9. Sommer, J.R. and Spach, M.S. (1964). Electron microscopic demonstration of adenosinetriphosphatase in myofibrils and sarcoplasmic membranes of cardiac muscle of normal and abnormal dogs. *Am. J. Pathol.*, **44**, 491–505

10. Peachey, L.D. (1975). Three-dimensional structure reconstruction by high voltage electron microscopy of biological specimens. In Bailey, G.W. (ed.) Proceedings of the 33rd Annual Meeting of the Electron Microscopy Society of America. (Baton Rouge: Claitors Publishing)

11. McCallister, L.P., Mumaw, V.R. and Munger, B.L. (1974). Stereo ultrastructure of cardiac membrane system in the rat heart. Scanning Electron Microscopy, (Part III) 1974. Proceedings of the Workshop on Advances in Biomedical Applications of the SEM. (Chicago: IIT Research Institute)

12. Steere, R.L. and Sommer, J.R. (1972). Stereo ultrastructure of nexus faces exposed by freeze-fracturing, *J. Microscopie*, **15**, 205–18

13. Page, E. and McCallister, L.P. (1973). Quantitative electron microscopic description of heart muscle cells: application to normal hypertrophied and thyroxin-stimulated hearts. *Am. J. Cardiol.*, **31**, 172–81

14. Sommer, J.R. and Waugh, R.A. (1976). *Op. Cit.*, p. 199

15. Kluge, T. and Hovig, T. (1967). The ultrastructure of human and rat pericardium, 1. Parietal and visceral mesothelium. *Acta. Pathol. Microbiol. Scand.*, **71**, 529–46

16. Ishihara, T., Ferrans, V.J., Jones, M., Boyce, S.W., Kawanami, O. and Roberts, W.C. (1980). Histologic and ultrastructural features of normal human parietal pericardium. *Am. J. Cardiol.*, **46**, 744–53

17. Miller, A.J., Pick, R. and Johnson, P.J. (1971). The production of acute pericardial effusion. The effects of various degres of interference with venous blood and lymph drainage from the heart muscle in the dog. *Am. J. Cardiol.*, **28**, 463–6

Section 2

Structural abnormalities

Part A   Acquired abnormalities

4   Panoramic view of cardiovascular pathology

Pathology is the study of structural changes in the body. These may be congenital or acquired. The altered structure forms the anatomical basis for the consequent disturbances in function. Structural changes are due to a wide range of causative factors, many of which have come to light only within the past half-century; a remarkably short span in the history of mankind. These include infectious, traumatic, genetic, metabolic or immunologic agents to mention but a few.

As with all else in medicine, the history of pathology dates back to primitive man. Unfortunately, our knowledge concerning the diseases afflicting the ancients is restricted to that gained from a study of their remains which in most cases is limited to a study of their bones. This is a rather meager and often unrewarding source since the finding of human archeologic remains is so utterly dependent upon climate, geographical location and the customs of the era during which the human remains were laid to rest.

As different civilizations arose throughout the eons, the written word became established so that eventually this medium took its place alongside the human remains as a concomitant source of information.

Although the Greeks and Romans were pre-eminent in the usage of the written word we are fortunate in being able to find many examples of written communication (whether it be in the form of hieroglyphics, drawings, carvings, tablets, etc.) left by civilizations as far back as the Babylo-Assyrians, Egyptians and Hebrews of biblical times. Custom and climate during the Egyptian era left us many artefacts of historical importance such as tombs, pottery, depictions, hieroglyphics and mummies. Mummification with its excellent preservation of viscera has proven a boon toward an appreciation of the diseases affecting the various organs during those times.

During the pre-Grecian era, especially among the Hebrews, but also among the Egyptians and Babylo-Assyrians, disease was thought to be primarily an affliction wrought by a vengeful deity. Rigid ritual laws were established and observed in an effort to propitiate whatever deity was in vogue at the time so as not to bring down his wrath. In addition, two other etiologic theories were entertained by these civilizations for the causation of non-traumatic illness. These were alimentary and meteorologically oriented. Seasonal changes in climate, variations of the prevailing winds, what one ate, and the disposal of excreta were all considered important factors. At first glance this seems to be quite a scientific approach, but, in reality, these were nothing else but notions with a magical or religious basis to them.

It was the Greeks who first began to inject some form of scientific basis into their approach towards disease. Their medical writings are replete with references to malformations and infection, while still retaining some aspects of the notions regarding some aspects of the meteorology. They emphasized the ill-effects of dietary indiscretion and the importance of water as a vehicle for spreading disease or as a means of maintaining a healthy body (as in baths) or ameliorating certain bodily dysfunctions as in hydrotherapy. The Romans developed this notion to a high art.

In time the gastro-etiologic factor in the causation of disease evolved into a fundamental body-fluid theory of pathology based upon digestion itself. It was felt that the ultimate product of digestion was a substance called 'coction', a nutrient that upon incorporation into the body became an important source of maintenance. So long as the various steps in the production of this 'coction' were undisturbed then the body was assured of a healthy state. Dysfunction was manifested via a humoral mechanism through the elaboration of the following four humors: blood, phlegm, yellow bile and black bile. The *Corpus Hippocraticum* embodies all of this while maintaining that meteorologic events exerted their effects through this digestive chain but explaining infection and contagion on a different basis.

The humoral theory was at variance with the views of Asclepiades. He adopted in its stead a modified Epicurean teaching based upon the atomism of Democritus. The atomic theory held to the belief that all matter was composed of particles of the same substance rather than four types of elements. In time, its followers became known as Methodists to distinguish them from the Pneumatists and Humoralists. Disease, according to the Methodists, was due to a disorderly arrangement of the atoms making up the human body. The disorderly arrangement occurred when the atoms became too tight or too loose. The whole body or variable portions of the body could be involved.

The Pneumatists created even more confusion during this era. Spearheaded by Athaneus, they added a fifth element to the previously described four humors. As the name of the school implies, this element was 'pneuma' or 'air-essence'. According to the Pneumatists, heat and moisture promoted health whereas heat and dryness resulted in an acutely diseased state. On the other hand, if it was cold rather than dry, a chronically diseased state ensued.

In the face of all these myths and fanciful theories swirling about, is it any wonder that no real contributions to pathology were made during this period of time? Unfortunately, the medical men of Rome perpetuated these falsehoods. Whatever medical advancements were made by them were due to governmental necessities for the political and geographical preservation of the military conquests rather than medical ingenuity and thought. 'Plagues' and other infectious disorders were being explained by the medical advisors on the basis of sidereal influences while the military officials were attempting to safeguard their troops and conquests with the application of sound public health principles that smack of modern times though in a somewhat abortive fashion.

Very good descriptions of pathologic alterations are to be found for the first time in the compilations of Celsus. His *De Medicina*, however, fails to disclose cardiac abnormalities, *per se*. Galen did not add much to cardiac pathology either. He did give, though, the first definition of aneurysm. An English translation of Galen's description as copied by Paulus Aegineta is to be found in F. Adams' *The Seven Books of Paulus Aegineta*[1]. It is as follows:

> Aneurism is a tumour soft to the touch and yielding to the fingers, having its origin from blood and spirits. Galen says 'an artery having become anastomosed (i.e. dilated) the affection is called an aneurism: it arises also from a wound of the same, when the skin that lies over it is cicatrized, but the wound in the artery remains, and neither unites nor is blocked up by flesh. Such affections are recognized by the pulsation of arteries; but, if compressed, the tumour disappears in so far, the substance which forms it returning back into the arteries'.

There was little or no advancement of knowledge in cardiac pathology in Europe during the Middle Ages. Mettler does mention that among the Arabic records an Ibn-Zuhr (1092–1162) wrote about serous pericarditis[2].

As dissection began to be practiced more frequently in Italy in the pursuit of anatomical knowledge, it was but a short step towards the usage of this method, initially for forensic reasons, and later for the study of structural changes themselves. This approach began to emerge by the end of the 13th century. However, the first definitive work on morbid anatomy based on actual postmortem dissections had to wait for the observations of Antonio Benivieni (1440–1502). He was the author of *De abiditis nonnullis ac mirandis morborum et sanationum causis*. East called it 'an odd little collection of curious cases'[3]. It was based on 20 necropsies. Although incomplete and rather inaccurate (probably because the author was ill-prepared) it served a purpose by stimulating others to continue on this logical road in the development of the pathological sciences. This was now at the time of the Renaissance with the intellectual activity of this era almost at its apogee and the rumblings against the humoral pathology of Galen becoming louder and louder.

Again, the genius of Leonardo da Vinci manifested itself; this time in the field of pathology but unnoticed as with his other contributions in medicine. He illustrated the arteries of a subject with arteriosclerotic changes remarkably accurately (Figure 1)[4].

Jean Fernel was also part of this era. He was professor of medicine at Paris. The second part of his book *Universa Medicina* published in 1554

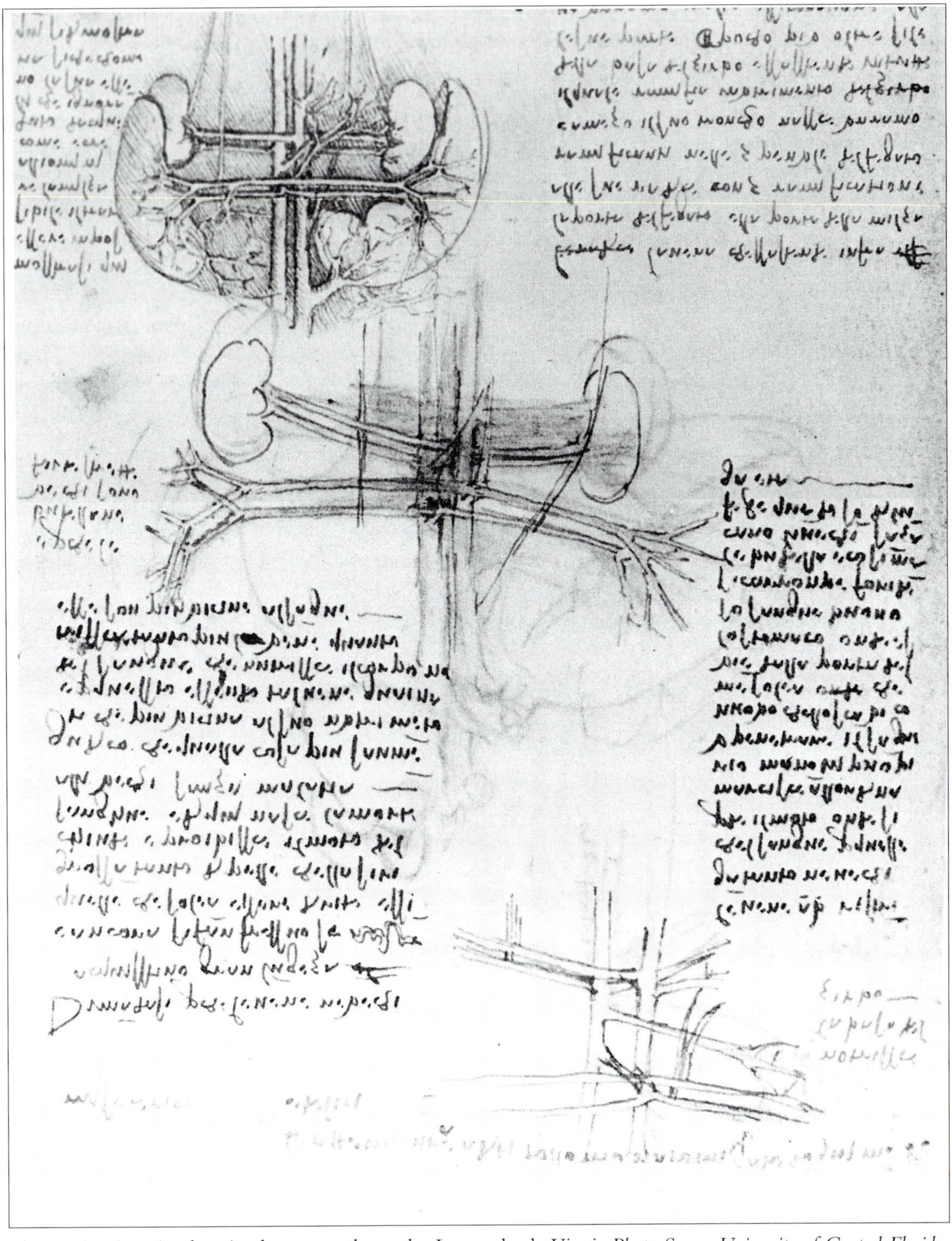

Figure 1 Arteriosclerotic changes as drawn by Leonardo da Vinci. *Photo Source University of Central Florida. Literary Source Quad. d'Anatomia, published by O.C.L. Vangensten, A. Fohnan, & H., Hopstock, Christiana, 1911–1916, folio 70 verso. Courtesy of University of Central Florida Library*

describes many of his observations in the field of pathology. He, along with others, such as Ambroise Paré (at a much later time), is credited with ascribing the cause of arterial aneurysms to syphilis which was pandemic during the Renaissance. Parés' description of a pulmonary aneurysm found at autopsy in a tailor and presumably due to syphilis is quoted by Zimmerman, as taken from Malgaigne's book on the complete works of Ambroise Paré[5,6]:

Aneurysms of the inner vessels are incurable and often appear in persons who have had the 'pox' (verolle) and who have been sweated many times. As a result of this treatment the blood is heated and the blood in the arteries attempts to escape causing a dilatation sometimes as large as a fist. I observed this condition in the body of one Belanger, a master-tailor on the Pont Saint Michel, near the Sign of the Cock, who had a large pulmonary aneurysm of which he died suddenly. Autopsy revealed a large amount of blood in the thorax and the artery was dilated to such an extent that one could place a fist within it. The inner tunic was bony. I demonstrated this before many people in the medical school where it caused much comment and later placed the specimen in my 'cabinet' among other monstrosities. Belanger had suffered from great throbbing of all of his arteries and complained that he experienced a sensation of extreme heat throughout his body and frequently felt faint. Sylvius, royal lecturer in medicine, had him stop drinking wine and substituted pure boiled water in its place. His food consisted of thoroughly churned cheese. In the evening he had pot barley to which barley flour and poppy seeds were added. A cataplasm was placed over the painful region and he occasionally took cooling clysters of pure cassia. Belanger told me that Sylvius had given him more relief than he had received from all the other physicians put together.

The large size of such aneurysms and the cause of their bony linings is due to the boiling blood since it causes the tunic of the artery to dilate and swell. Finally, it ruptures, absorbs material from neighboring parts to rebuild the lining and thus forms a large or small tumor depending upon the nature of the region involved.

Long and East mention several collators of information regarding pathology during the 16th century[7,8]. These were Marcello Donato, Rembert Dodoens, Felix Platter, and Johann Schenck von Grafenberg. But no new ground was broken in any of their works, and in particular, nothing of historical interest can be found in them. A large series was the one published by Felix Platter of Switzerland, 'who in 51 years dissected 300 bodies, was the teacher of Europe and left to posterity not one single truth'[9]. 'This', said Hermann Baar, 'is a fate shared with many others, for it is not everyone who can find truths'[9].

The 17th century continued in the same fashion insofar as the literature of pathology was concerned. The century produced works of compilation rather than discovery. In addition, although Malpighi had alerted the world to the benefits of microscopy, the application of this mode for studying morbid anatomy needed another century before it was to become an important and revealing tool.

Perhaps the most outstanding work in the field of pathology during the 17th century was the monumental tome of Theophile Bonet. Bonet's book was published in Geneva in 1679. It bore the grand title *Sepulchretum sine anatomia practica ex cadaveribus morbo denatis*. Long acknowledges that this work was outstanding but only in the sense that it is the greatest collection of data in the field of pathology up to that time being based on approximately 3,000 autopsies[10].

The pathologic descriptions are classified under the headings of clinical symptoms such as 'difficulty in breathing', 'abnormal pulses', and 'sudden death'. Of the two cases recorded concerning sudden death, one is that of an individual with a calcified stenotic aortic valve, and the other may very well be a description of sudden death due to coronary artery disease, though this is pure speculation.

Long's appraisal of the book is mostly derogatory. He decries the lack of judgement manifested by Bonet in his classification as well as in his indiscriminate acceptance of the opinions of the many authors that he cites such as Dodoens, von Grafenberg, and Ballonius.

An important contribution during this century was also made by Theodor Kerckring (1640–93). The so called 'polyps' found and described by earlier pathologists in the ventricles of the heart at autopsy and thought to be abnormal structures by them were correctly identified by Kerckring as being normal postmortem 'chicken-fat' clots.

The 18th century produced a multitude of important discoveries in the pathology of the heart.

The impetus was given by Giovanni Battista Morgagni, 'the father of systematic pathology'.

Giovanni Battista Morgagni was born in 1682 in Forli, a small town near Bologna, at that time a great center of learning. He was a precocious student, already manifesting, in his teens, an intense interest in such diverse subjects as poetry, philosophy and medicine. Throughout his life and apart from his scientific work, he was to maintain his interest in philosophy and literature along with history and archeology. This interest produced many papers on archeologic findings in the vicinity of Ravenna and Forli; letters to Lancisi on 'The Manner of Cleopatra's death'; and commentaries and notes on Celsus, Sammonicus, Varro, and a host of other ancient luminaries.

Morgagni graduated from Bologna at the early age of 19 and immediately began working for Valsalva as his prosector. This continued for several years during which time he published his first work on anatomy *Adversaria Anatomica Prima* which was presented before the Academia Inquietorum of which he had just been elected president.

He left Bologna for post-graduate study in anatomy at Padua and Venice. Upon completion of these studies he left academia to successfully engage in the private practice of medicine. Apparently this life did not suit him and as soon as the opportunity arose he accepted the chair of theoretical medicine at the University of Padua. This too did not last long because the death of Michaelangelo Monetti created a vacancy in the chair of anatomy at Padua to which Morgagni was appointed. He remained in this post until his death in 1771 at the age of 89, carrying on the splendid contributions of Vesalius and Fallopius, the previous occupants.

It was while at Padua that Morgagni published his second work on anatomy *Adversaria Anatomica Altera* as well as the classical and monumental work that immortalized him as the father of pathologic anatomy. Morgagni was already at the advanced age of 79 when he finished his *De sedibus et Causus Morborum per Anatomen Indagatis Libri Quinque*. This was the first attempt to correlate the clinical scenario with postmortem findings. The work was based on 640 necropsies most of which were performed by him but contained also some unpublished observations of Valsalva and Albertini[11].

A copy of the *De Sedibus* is in the American College of Physicians in Philadelphia. It was bequeathed by John Morgan, a prominent Philadelphian physician who received it as a gift from Morgagni upon the occasion of Morgan's visit to Morgagni at Padua in 1764. At this time Morgan was impressed with how young and vigorous Morgagni looked despite being 82 years old[12–14]. Castiglioni mentions the probability that because of the similarity of the names Morgagni and Morgan, a rumor was started about the two being related to each other[15].

Apparently, Morgagni's prolific output was not limited to his scientific endeavors. Despite a very active academic career he managed to sire 15 children, eight of whom were still living when he died.

Morgagni died suddenly, probably because of an acute myocardial infarction since the autopsy revealed a ruptured myocardium, an event about which Morgagni was well acquainted. The postmortem was conducted by Baglivi aided by Lancisi.

Morgagni's tome *De Sedibus* was the culmination of 20 years of labor and it correlated for the first time the clinical picture with the structural changes found at postmortem. The work was published in Venice in 1761. It consists of five books, the second of which deals with respiratory and cardiac dysfunctions. The idea for the book was spawned in 1740 while Morgagni was involved in a discussion of the deficiencies of Bonet's encyclopedic compilation. Morgagni at that time had agreed to write a series of letters to a young friend which were to resolve the various questions that were unsatisfactorily answered by Bonet and which would be written over the course of the years on the basis of Morgagni's own personal observations at the postmortem table. It took 20 years to accomplish and the resultant 70 letters represent Morgagni's answer to his friend over this period of time. In this work the relationship between symptomatology and structural changes removed pathology from the anatomical museum halls to the realm of the practicing physician and thus opened the door to a horde of future students eager to learn what bodily changes could be wrought by various diseases.

Benjamin Alexander of London translated Morgagni's work in 1769[16]. The preface of *De Sedibus* in his translation is as follows:

There are two sayings of C. Lucilius, as you have it in Cicero: I mean 'That he neither wished to have his writings fall into the hands of the most learned, nor of the most unlearned readers,' which I should equally make use of on the present occasion, if it were not my desire to be useful to the unlearned, as well as to be assisted by the learned reader, For I have had two views in publishing these writings; the first that I might assist the studies of such as are intended for the practice of medicine; the second, and this the principle view, that I might be universally useful though this cannot happen without the concurrence and assistance of the learned in every quarter. Theophilus Bonetus, was a man who deserved the esteem of the faculty of medicine in particular, and of mankind in general, in an equal degree with any other, on account of his publishing those books which are entitled the Sepulchretum. For by collecting in as great a number as possible and digesting into order, the dissections of bodies, which had been carried off by disease, he formed them into one compact body: and thereby caused those observations, which when scattered up and down through the writings of almost innumerable authors, were but of little advantage, to become extremely useful when collected together and methodically disposed.

Now then; in an affair wherein everyone is concerned, and not only in the present but in the future ages: in order to judge more easily what may be expected from me alone, and how far it is just to expect it, I must by no means conceal the circumstance which first gave occasion to my writing these books.

The anatomical writings of Valsalva being already published, and my epistles upon them, it accidently happened that being retired from Padua, as in those early years, I was wont frequently to do in the summer time, I fell into company with a young gentleman, of strict morals and an excellent disposition, who was much given to the study of the sciences and particularly to that of medicine. This young gentleman, having read those writings and those letters likewise, every now and then engaged me in a discourse, than in respect to my preceptors, and in particular Valsava and Albertini, whose methods in the art of healing, even the most trifling he was desirous to know; and he even sometimes enquired after my own observations and thoroughly as well as theirs. And having among other things, as frequently happens in conversations, opened my thoughts in regard to the Sepulchretum, he never ceased to entreat me by every kind of solicitation, that I would apply to this subject in particular: and as I had promised in my little memoir upon the Life of Valsalva, to endeavor that a great number of his observations, which were made with the same view, should be brought to public light, he begged that I would join mine together with them, and would show in both his and mine, by example as it were, what I should think wanting to complete a new edition of the Sepulchretum, which he perhaps, if he could engage his friends to assist him would at some time or another undertake.

With this view then I began upon returning to Padua to make a trial of that Nature, by sending some letters to my friend. And that he was pleased with them appears from two circumstances; the first that he was continually soliciting me to send him more and more after that till he drew me on so far as to the seventieth; the second, that when I begged them of him in order to revise their contents, he did not return them, till he had made me solemnly promise, that I would not abridge any part thereof.

Figure 2 is the frontispiece of *De Sedibus*.

Concerning the heart, early accounts are given of aneurysm, heart block, and valvular diseases. We are again indebted to Alexander's translation[16] for the following remarks on aneurysm:

A man who had been too much given to the exercise of tennis and the abuse of wine, was in consequence of both these irregularities, seized with a pain of the right arm, and soon after of the left, joined with a fever. After these there appeared a tumour on the upper part of the sternum, like a large boil: by which appearance some vulgar surgeons being deceived, and either not having at all observed, or used to bring these tumors to suppuration; and these applications were of the most violent kind. As the tumour still increased, others applied emollient medicines, from which it seemed to them to be diminished; that is, from the fibres being rubbed with ointments and relaxed; whereas they had been before greatly irritated by the applications. But as this circumstance related rather to the common integuments, than to the tumour itself, or to the coats that were proper thereto, it not only soon recovered its former magnitude, but

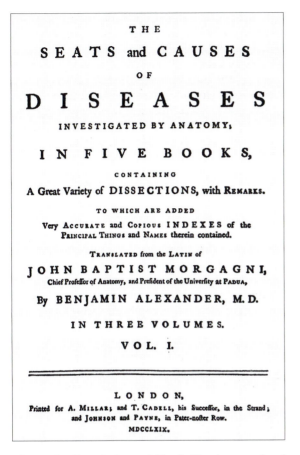

THE

SEATS and CAUSES

OF

DISEASES

INVESTIGATED BY ANATOMY;

IN FIVE BOOKS,

CONTAINING

A Great Variety of DISSECTIONS, with REMARKS.

TO WHICH ARE ADDED

Very ACCURATE and COPIOUS INDEXES of the
PRINCIPAL THINGS and NAMES therein contained.

TRANSLATED from the LATIN of

JOHN BAPTIST MORGAGNI,

Chief Profeſſor of Anatomy, and Preſident of the Univerſity at PADUA,

By **BENJAMIN ALEXANDER, M.D.**

IN THREE VOLUMES.

VOL. I.

LONDON,

Printed for A. MILLAR; and T. CADELL, his Succeſſor, in the Strand;
and JOHNSON and PAYNE, in Pater-noſter Row.
MDCCLXIX.

Figure 2 Frontispiece of 'De Sedibus' as translated by Benjamin Alexander. *Photo Source University of Central Florida. Literary Source Willius FA, Keys TE: Cardiac Classics. The C.V. Mosby Co., St. Louis, MO., 1941. Courtesy of the Mayo clinic*

even was, plainly, seen to increase every day. Wherefore, when the patient came into the Hospital of Incurables, at Bologna, which was, I suppose in the year 1704, it was equal in size to a quince; and what was much worse, it began to exude blood in one place; so that the man himself was very near having broken through the skin (this being reduced to the utmost thinness in that part, and he being quite ignorant of the danger which was at hand) when he began to pull off the bandages, for the sake of showing his disorder. But this circumstance being observed, he was prevented going on, and ordered to keep himself still, and to think seriously and piously of his departure from this mortal life, which was very near at hand, and inevitable. And this really

happened on the day following, from the vast profusion of blood that had been foretold, though not so soon expected by the patient. Nevertheless, he had the presence of mind, immediately as he felt the blood gushing forth, not only to commend himself to God, but to take up with his own hands a basin that lay at his bed-side; and, as if he had been receiving the blood of another person, put it beneath the gaping tumour, while the attendants immediately ran to him as fast as possible, in whose arms he soon expired.

In examining the body before I dissected it, I saw that there was no longer any tumour, inasmuch as it had subsided after the blood, by which it had been raised up externally, and had been discharged. The skin was there broken through, and the parts that lie beneath it with an aperture, which admitted two fingers at once. The membrana adiposa of the thorax discharged a water during the time of dissection, with which some vessels were also turgid, that were prominent, here and there, upon the surface of the skin in the feet and the legs. In both the cavities of the thorax, also, was a great quantity of water, of a yellowish color. And there was a large aneurism, into which the anterior part of the curvature of the aorta itself being expanded, had partly consumed the upper part of the sternum, the extremities of the clavicles which lie upon it, and the neighbouring ribs, and partly had made them diseased, by bringing on a caries. And where the bones had been consumed or affected with the caries, there not the least traces of the coats of the artery remained: to which, in other places, a thick substance every where adhered internally, resembling a dry and lurid kind of flesh, distinguished with some whitish points; and this substance you might easily divide into many membranes, as it were, one lying upon another, quite different in their nature from those coats to which they adhered, as they were evidently polypous. And these things being accurately attended to, nothing occurred besides that was worthy of remark.

The deplorable exit of this man teaches, in the first place, how much care ought to be taken in the beginning, that an internal aneurism may obtain to increase: and in the second place, if, either by the ignorance of the persons who attempt their cure, or the disobedience of the patient, or only by the force of the disorder itself, they do at length increase so that they are only covered by the common integuments of the whole body; that then we ought to take care lest the bandages, especially when they are already dried to the part, be hastily taken off: and finally, if the case proceed to such an extremity, that the rupture of the skin is every day impending, and bleeding, either on account of the constitution or infirmity of the patient, or on the score of other things which I have hinted at already, is dangerous; that every thing is to be previously studied, by which, for some days at least, life may be prolonged. That is to say, besides the greatest tranquility of body and mind, and the greatest abstinence that can be consistently observed, so that no more food be taken than is barely necessary for the preservation of life, and that in besides that situation of body, by which the weight of the blood being lessened, does not press upon the skin, and other things of the like kind; something ought to be thought of by the surgeon, by way doubled, were applied, or a bandage of soft leather; and the edges of this bandage were all daubed over with a medicine, by which they would be firmly glued down to the neighboring skin that lay around the tumour, and was as yet sound and entire.

In his 24th letter, he describes the findings at necropsy of a patient who had been admitted to the hospital at Padua because of an incarcerated hernia.

As I examined the internal surfaces of the heart, the left coronary artery appeared to have been changed into a bony canal from its very origin to the extent of many fingers breadth, where it embraces the greater part of the base. And part of that very long branch, also, which it sends down upon the anterior surface of the heart, was already become bony to so great a space as could be covered by three fingers placed transversely.

This is certainly a very good description of coronary artery disease due to arteriosclerosis. From the description it appears that both the left main coronary artery and its left anterior descending branch were involved, providing a perfect setting not only for angina but also for sudden death.

Morgagni also described lesions of all the cardiac valves and presented examples of mitral stenosis, calcific aortic stenosis and aortic regurgitation. The

myocardium received his attention with accurate descriptions of fibrous changes that he attributed to a degenerative process. This was an important deviation from the prevailing concept which persisted well into the first half of the 20th century that such changes were inflammatory. The probability is that Morgagni was describing the occlusive consequences of coronary artery disease because of the segmental location of these patches of fibrous tissue. He also recorded rupture of the heart (the event that killed him) in the presence of marked fatty changes in the myocardium.

The endocardium and pericardium also did not escape his attention with his description of vegetative endocardial lesions, pericardial effusion, adhesions and calcification. The congenital cardiac defects that he described included those that were characterized in life by cyanosis. Unfortunately he erred in believing that cyanosis was due to venous stasis rather than an improper admixture of venous and arterial blood.

De Sedibus spearheaded the development of a systematic approach to pathological anatomy and emphasized the importance of clinical correlation. Led originally by Morgagni and then in concert with him, a large group of his contemporary colleagues contributed towards the movement away from the humoral basis of disease that had been so firmly entrenched for more than a millennium. Morgagni was joined by such men as Jean Astruc (1684–1766), Raymond Vieussens (1641–1716), Jean-Baptiste Sénac (1693–1770), Giovanni Maria Lancisi (1654–1720), and Mathew Baillie (1761–1823).

Astruc's role in cardiac pathology was of no consequence; he being primarily interested in oncology and venereology. Vieussens, on the other hand, did describe rather clearly and with illustrations of high quality, mitral stenosis with calcification of the leaflets and dilation of the right heart. He also pointed out how pericardial adhesions restricted the pumping action of the heart, the occurrence of pleural effusion in heart disease, and that the structural changes of mitral stenosis were responsible for an increase in back pressure accounting for many of the clinical symptoms.

Vieussens must be regarded as one of the leading contributors to cardiology during the 18th century. His impact was felt not only in the description of the pathologic changes of the heart just outlined but also in the elucidation of many of the normal anatomical details of the heart as well as in his analysis of certain of the pathophysiologic processes affecting the cardiovascular system (as we shall see later)[17].

Jean-Baptiste Sénac was born in the district of Lombez in Gascony, France. Nothing is definitely known either about his early life or his family. There is also no documentation of where he received his medical degree although Montpellier and Reims are likely possibilities. Definite facts concerning his life begin with his first publication in 1724. It was a translation of Heister's anatomy and bore the title *L' Anatomie d' Heister avec des essais de physique sur l'usage des parties du corps humain*[18]. It was at this time too that he became an associate member of the Royal Academy of Sciences. Most of his interest over the next five years appeared to be centered on the respiratory organs. He published two memoirs on the subject both of which he presented before the Royal Academy of Sciences. The first Memoir was *On the Organs of Respiration* when he was elected to the Academy. A year later he presented a second memoir *On Drowning*.

His entry into political circles occurred in 1745 when he successfully cured the famous French general, Maurice, Count de Saxe, of a serious illness, and became part of the general's entourage. In several years, after the death of his patron, Sénac successively became chief physician, at first to the Duke of Orleans, and later to Louis XV. Sénac must have enjoyed royal favor because in due course he was appointed by the King as Counsellor of the State and Superintendent of the Mineral Waters and Medicinals of the Kingdom.

After 20 years of research, he published his now famous works that assured him an important niche in the history of cardiology. His *Traité de la Structure du Coeur de son Action et de ses Maladies* appeared in 1749 and consisted of two volumes. A posthumous edition appeared in 1777, seven years after the author's death[19,20]. Figure 3 is the frontispiece of Sénac's original text. His portrait is depicted in Figure 4.

The work is noteworthy primarily because of the many new and important observations it contains on the various diseased states that could affect the heart. Moreover, Sénac appreciated all too well the importance of pathology in clinical practice.

Corvisart quotes Sénac's position on the matter in his tome dealing with diseases of the heart[21]: 'If practitioners' [he said] 'do not understand diseases, they will pronounce with temerity of a multiplicity

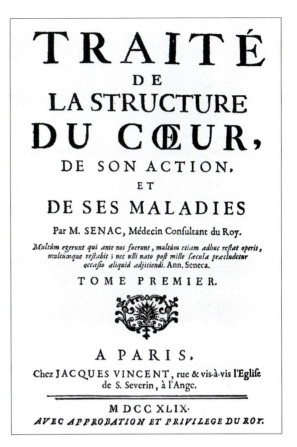

Figure 3 Frontispiece of Sénac's original text published in 1749. *Photo Source University of Central Florida. Literary Source Willius FA, Keys TE: Cardiac Classics. The C.V. Mosby Co., 1941. Courtesy of the Mayo clinic*

of cases; they will torment patients with remedies hurtful or useless; they will hasten death by treating alike ailments that are altogether different; they will be liable to be shamefully deceived on inspecting the dead; in fine, the danger will be near when they think it remote'.

It was Sénac's contention that dilatation was the most common expression of cardiac pathology. He also correlated the presence of hydrothorax with heart failure. There is a description in his book of how he evacuated six pints of fluid from the chest of a groom of the Royal Stables who had been complaining of marked difficulty in breathing. This could have been a case of massive pleural effusion due to heart failure. Sénac also described pericarditis and its frequent association with pleurisy

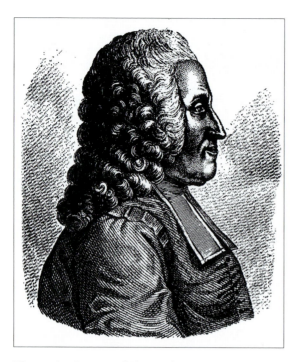

Figure 4 Portrait of Sénac. *Photo Source University of Central Florida. Literary Source Willius FA, Keys TE: Cardiac Classics. The C.V. Mosby Co., 1941. Courtesy of the Mayo Clinic*

and mediastinitis. His remark that 'the heart only fills itself with difficulty in diastole because it finds a barrier in its constricted envelope' shows a clear understanding of the mechanical effects of an adherent pericardium on the heart. He emphasized the fact that all the components of the heart were susceptible to inflammation contrary to the beliefs of earlier observers. He also described atrophy of the heart as well as the association of a ventricular aneurysm with coronary arteriosclerosis. Certain congenital defects were cited by him and they will be dealt with later. There was a good deal of skepticism on his part regarding the 'hairy' hearts described by earlier writers and the presence of stones and worms in the heart. Although not described as 'chicken-fat' clots he shared Kerckring's view that polyps of the heart formed at the time of death.

Probably the most authoritative writer on cardiac pathology during the 18th century was Giovanni Maria Lancisi. He is easily recognized as one of the leading figures of medicine during that century.

Lancisi was born in Rome, Italy in 1654, the scion of a wealthy bourgeois family[22]. While attending Collegio Romano he took courses in philosophy in preparation for the priesthood. He soon realized that his vocation lay in medicine and natural history. Abandoning theology, he pursued his medical studies at Sapienza receiving his medical degree from there at the age of 18; young even for those times. Lancisi continued his medical studies independently and began to advance quite rapidly in his profession. Just 3 years after graduation he was appointed to the staff of the Hospital Santo Spirito and in another 3 years he was nominated to membership in the Collegio del Salvatore. In 1684, at the age of 30, he was appointed professor of anatomy at his alma mater and remained there in this position for 13 years. In the meanwhile his relationship with the papal court became increasingly solidified with Lancisi finally being appointed by Pope Innocent IX in 1688 as pontifical doctor and as a representative of Cardinal Altieri to lead the pontifical committee for conferring degrees in the medical college of Sapienza. It was in 1706, while still serving as pontifical doctor that he was asked by the then reigning pontiff, Clement XI to investigate the causes for a mysterious increase in sudden deaths that had begun to assume epidemic proportions. After a year of conducting this work he published his first book. It contained his conclusions and comments derived from his observations on the large number of autopsies that he performed in carrying out the pope's mandate. The tract was entitled *De Subitaneis Mortibus, Libro duo*, and it became noted for the masterly manner in which it dealt with cardiac pathology. The author demonstrated that the sudden deaths in Rome were due to natural causes, and in particular, related to hypertrophy and dilatation of the heart as well as various types of valvular defects. He also mentioned that a cause of cardiac enlargement was calcified coronary arteries due to the obstructive nature of the disease. The mechanical barrier produced by narrowing of the valvular orifices was also recognized by him as a cause of cardiac enlargement. The ultimate emptying of the coronary arteries into the cardiac chambers was noted by him even before the findings of microscopic studies. Lancisi came to this conclusion when he noted the mercury appearing in the chambers of the heart after having been injected directly into the coronary arteries. He speculated that the mercury passed into the ventricular chambers via venous channels. Thus, he clearly anticipated the doctrine of myocardial perfusion through the coronary arterial system.

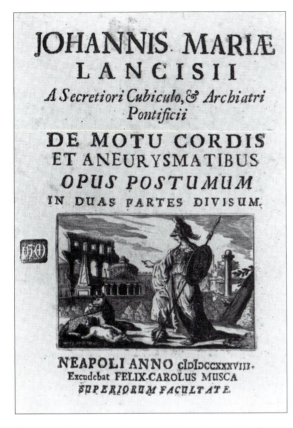

Figure 5 Frontispiece of De Motu Cordis et Aneurysmatibus by Lancisi. *Photo Source University of Central Florida. Literary Source East, T: The Story of Heart Disease. Wm. Dawson & Sons, Ltd. London, plate 9B, 1957. Public domain*

Lancisi's second tract *De Motu Cordis et Aneurysmatibus* was published in 1728, some eight years after his death. It is by far the better of the two. Figure 5 is an illustration of the frontispiece of this authoritative work. The highlights of the book are descriptions of warty vegetations and thickening of the valve cusps; the occurrence of so-called 'aneurysma gallicum' (a chronic dilatation of the heart as a sequel of lues); the relationship between valvular stenosis and cardiac alterations; and the differentiation between cardiac hypertrophy and dilatation. In discussing aneurysms of the heart, earlier observers meant global dilatation of a heart chamber or of the entire heart rather than segmental 'blistering' of the myocardial wall although this too was described.

Lancisi's main hobby apparently was the collection of books. During his lifetime he collected well over 20,000 volumes which he donated upon his death to the Hospital of Santo Spirito. The donation established in reality the library at this institution and for this reason it is named after Lancisi. The collection also contained Lancisi's personal papers and manuscript, and with further acquisitions over the years, the library has become an important source of historical data.

The English contribution to the literature of pathology could probably be said to have been initiated by John Hunter with his treatise published in 1794 and entitled *A Treatise on the Blood, Inflammation and Gunshot Wounds*. Although an eminent anatomist, as we have seen in the chapter dealing with anatomy, John Hunter, as a pathologist, left much to be desired. His treatise, in particular, lacked originality of thought or observation. His older brother also described certain cardiovascular pathologic abnormalities, but these were case reports selected for interest to a surgeon rather than as part of a grand design. An example of this is his description of arteriovenous fistula in his *Medical Observations and Inquiries* which appeared in London in 1762. This is probably the first description of an arteriovenous fistula, but again, from a purely surgical point of view. Still another example is the report of three cases of *Malformations of the Heart* that he published in 1784. One of these case reports seems to fit the structural abnormalities of the Tetralogy of Fallot, a condition about which we will say more later. The older Hunter must be credited, however, with advancing the notion that there was a tendency to multiplicity of congenital cardiac defects although he erred in the belief that pulmonary stenosis accounted for the multiple defects[23].

Matthew Baillie, the nephew of the Hunter brothers, also lacked originality in his writings, relying heavily on Morgagni and other European writers, but he surpassed his uncles by virtue of the fact that he, at least, served the useful function of introducing to England, Morgagni's systematic approach to pathology. The first of Baillie's works was published in London in 1793. He called it '*The Morbid Anatomy of Some of the most Important Parts of the Human Body*'. The title-page of this important work is illustrated in Figure 6. The second work, also on pathology, appeared six years later. It was entitled *A Series of Engravings to Illustrate the Morbid Anatomy of the Human Body*. In this tome he mentions rather casually the association of rheumatism and heart disease by quoting David

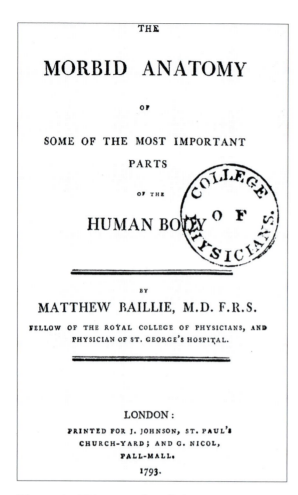

THE

MORBID ANATOMY

OF

SOME OF THE MOST IMPORTANT

PARTS

OF THE

HUMAN BODY

BY

MATTHEW BAILLIE, M.D. F.R.S.

FELLOW OF THE ROYAL COLLEGE OF PHYSICIANS, AND
PHYSICIAN OF ST. GEORGE'S HOSPITAL.

LONDON:
PRINTED FOR J. JOHNSON, ST. PAUL'S
CHURCH-YARD; AND G. NICOL,
PALL-MALL.
1793.

Figure 6 Title page of Baillie's treatise on morbid anatomy. *Photo Source Royal College of Physicians. Literary Source Bedford collection. Courtesy of the Royal College of Physicians*

Pitcairn's belief that 'enlargement was due to rheumatism attacking the organ'. Incidentally, the atlas was dedicated to Pitcairn, who, according to East, had passed the gold-headed Cane of the Royal College of Physicians to Baillie upon the latter's assumption of leadership of the Society[24]. The quotation attributed to Pitcairn indicates that he was one of the first to recognize a causal relationship between rheumatic fever and heart disease, although Pitcairn, himself, never put it in writing. More precise details regarding the pathologic alterations in the heart as a sequel to rheumatic fever had to await further observers, as we shall see in due course.

Baillie also published a paper in the Philosophic Transactions of the Royal Society of Medicine, which described a case of dextrocardia with complete situs inversus. It bore the title *A remarkable Transposition of the Viscera*. The paper was an amplification of a letter he had written to his uncle John on the subject in 1788. Baillie also described transposition of the great arterial trunks with the pulmonary artery arising from the left ventricle and the aorta from the right ventricle[25]. Finally, Baillie showed that death attributed to so-called cardiac polyps was, in reality, associated with intracardiac thrombi.

The above constitutes no mean contribution by an individual considered by some as an ordinary pathologist. True, he did not break new ground, but his mode of presentation and the clarity of his descriptions added in their own way to the fund of knowledge being accumulated in cardiac pathology.

Duffin expresses rather well the most important feature of the evolution of pathologic anatomy of the heart in the 18th century[26]. It changed from a description of 'graveyard specimens' to a vital discipline intimately linked with clinical medicine. This can best be appreciated by the change in titles of three of the century's significant publications in the field: Bonets' *Sepulchretum*, Morgagni's *De Sedibus et Causis Morborum per Anatomen Indagatis Libri Quinque*, and Antoine Portal's *Cours d'Anatomie Médicale*[27]. However, the pathway of transition was not easy nor even completely acceptable by all during the formative years of physical diagnosis.

Sénac expressed the problem of accurate correlation of the variable symptoms with organic changes, when he lamented the sorry prospects of detecting such changes before the patient died[28]. Duffin quotes him as saying 'But, how amongst so many false appearances, so many complications and varieties can one disentangle the heart diseases'. Portal went even further when he stated that clinicians did not make good pathologists and that pathologists were not good clinicians. Somehow or other, these two statements do not seem to reflect accurately what we know about the clinicians of the Parisian, and later the German and Viennese schools.

During the early part of the 19th century, Marie Francois Xavier Bichat was one of the most important supporters of morbid anatomy as part of the armamentarium of medical practice. He advocated a triangulated approach for the development of excellence in medicine wherein pathology was the base. Thayer quotes Bichat as follows: 'Dissect in anatomy, experiment in physiology, follow the disease and make the necropsy in medicine; this is the three-fold path, without which there can be no anatomist, no physiologist, no physician'[29]. These are certainly worthwhile criteria and still valid today despite our technological advancements. In the morbid anatomy of cardiology he did not leave any lasting contributions, but his plea above will always serve as a beacon for future generations of physicians regardless of their specialty. We shall meet him again.

The early years of the 19th century also saw throughout Europe the establishment of departments specifically devoted to pathology. The first chair was located at the University of Strasbourg, at that time a French school. Johann Lobstein was its first occupant. His most outstanding work was *Traite d'Anatomie Pathologique*. It was published in 1829 in incomplete form, and was never finished. For the first time, the term 'pathogenesis' was used. He employed it to describe the dynamic changes and alteration in function brought about by the structural changes in the organ. Lobstein is particularly remembered in cardiology for his very accurate description of arteriosclerosis[30,31].

Soon after, Paris established a chair in pathology with its first chairman being Jean Cruveilhier. Jean-Baptiste Bouillaud was indirectly instrumental in establishing the chair. Daremberg recounts how Bouillaud expressed in a footnote of his treatise on maladies of the heart the wish that a chair of pathologic anatomy be established as part of medical faculties, especially at Paris[32]. He is quoted as saying 'This would fill an enormous gap in our science'[33]. This wish was realized through a bequest by the illustrious French surgeon, Dupuytren. Prior to accepting the chair of pathology, Cruveilhier, a protege of Dupuytren, had been professor of surgery at Montpellier and later professor of descriptive anatomy at Paris.

It was only the force of his father's upper hand that propelled Cruveilhier in the direction of medicine. During his early training, Cruveilhier wanted to abandon medicine for the priesthood, presumably because of the shock he experienced upon witnessing his first autopsy[34].

During his tenure of thirty years as professor of pathology he contributed extensively to the field. His most important work was an atlas containing many colored illustrations and titled *Anatomie*

Pathologique du Corps Humain. Among those illustrations were those of myocardial infarcts. Unfortunately, he did not correlate these areas of necrosis with total occlusion of the coronary arteries[35,36]. He did contend, however, that they did not represent fatty metamorphosis. Cruveilhier also showed in his atlas examples of myocardial aneurysm and rupture of the myocardium, again, without recognizing their relationship to coronary artery disease.

Cruveilhier had a peculiar notion regarding the causation of morbid anatomical changes in general. Long states that Cruveilhier theorized that 'tissues were unalterable by themselves, that they were susceptible only to increase or diminution in their nutrition, and that all apparent organic alterations of texture were merely the expression of morbid as opposed to normal secretion within the interstices of the cellular tissue by an extraordinarily empowered capillary bed'[37]. In line with this theory, he felt that the capillary bed was the predisposing cause of all inflammatory reactions bringing about a phlebitis, which he asserted, erroneously, was then the precipitating cause of all pathologic processes. He further compounded the error by holding to the belief that phlebitis was not only the dominant force in pathology but also responsible for thrombosis in general. It remained for Virchow, as we shall see later, to unravel the confusion on thrombosis.

Jean Nicholas Corvisart was a contemporary of both Lobstein and Cruveilhier. He was primarily a clinician and one of the most sought after physicians of the era. As we shall see in the chapter dealing with physical diagnosis his main contributions centered on the popularization and refinement of the techniques of percussion and auscultation in bedside clinical diagnosis. His attention to and interest in morbid anatomy were motivated by his desire to explain the findings elicited through physical examination on the basis of the pathologic alterations of the organ being evaluated. His special fields of expertise were the heart and lungs. Much more will be said about this interesting person in connection with his role as a physical diagnostician.

Corvisart classified the pathologic entities of the heart into six categories[38]. They are as follows:

(1) Cardiac chamber enlargement with thickening of the wall. Under this group he

included four types of enlargement according to location: a) dilatation of the entire heart, b) dilatation of the left auricle, c) dilatation of the left ventricle, d) dilatation of the base of the aorta or of the right side of the heart.

(2) Cardiac chamber enlargement with thinning of the walls. This group also had four subdivisions in the same manner as in category 1.

(3) Decrease in cardiac chamber size. This was further subdivided into a) a decrease in the size of any one of the four cavities separately, b) simultaneous decrease of all four cavities, c) constriction at the origin of the great vessels.

(4) Lesions of the valves of the heart or great vessels with the following subclassification: a) hardening or calcification of the aortic valve, b) calcification of the mitral valve, c) stenosis of the auriculoventricular opening, d) calcification of the base of the aorta or of the right side of the heart.

(5) Cardiac disease due to foreign bodies. Under this he included: a) intracavitary polyps, b) calcification, c) vegetations on valvular surfaces.

(6) Abnormal perforations. This was his term for congenital malformations. He apparently recognized only two and he referred to them as: a) persistence or dilatation of the duct of Botallo (ductus arteriosus?) and b) perforation of the interventricular septum.

In later writings Corvisart added another category to the previous list under the general label of rupture of the heart. He recognized three varieties of rupture: a) rupture of a cavity of the heart, b) rupture of one or more of the 'columnae carnae', and c) rupture of an aneurysm of the great vessels.

Corvisart was particularly interested in aneurysms, the term being non-restrictive in that it was applied by him in describing dilatation of either the heart or blood vessels. He classified cardiac aneurysms into active and passive. The active aneurysms consisted of enlargement, dilatation and hypertrophy with the force of contraction increased while the passive types had no hypertrophy and a diminished force of contraction. In all of this, Corvisart emphasized the point that an enlarged heart was a diseased heart.

He described fibrinous pericarditis stating that 'the massive deposition of fibrin caused the pericardium to resemble the reticulum of the second stomach of the calf'[39]. Although his classification does not indicate it, Corvisart realized that pancarditis can and did occur. A close look at his cases of 'carditis', however, reflect that they consisted of a gamut of specific pathologic lesions. Some were endocarditis, probably bacterial in origin, others were pericarditis, and some of the myocardial lesions had the hallmarks of being areas of necrosis with fibrous tissue replacement due to coronary arterial occlusion.

Like all great men, he did have certain deficiencies. His most glaring one was his misconception that coronary sclerosis limited the development of cardiac hypertrophy and just as important was his failure to mention in his writings the clinical syndrome of angina pectoris in the presence of coronary artery sclerosis. Herrick's comments on this state of affairs are most interesting[40]. Herrick in a speculative mood offers several possibilities for Corvisart's failure to elaborate in any way on coronary artery disease: the lack of communication between France and England during the Napoleonic wars; the fact that Corvisart was a busy practitioner with little or no time for reading and therefore unaware of contemporary thought on the matter; the possibility of national pride on the part of Corvisart which induced him to 'conveniently' forget any contribution that was not French in origin; and his zest for living the good life at the expense of time that could have been devoted to reading. Any, or all of these could have been responsible. The very nature of Corvisart's interest in percussion and auscultation seems to me, however, reason enough for his failure to delve into coronary artery disease. These elements of physical diagnosis do not lend themselves to an objective evaluation of a subject with obstructive disease of the coronary arteries as readily as one with murmurs, enlargement of the heart or heart failure. What is even more surprising, taking into account Corvisart's commitment to physical diagnostic techniques, is his lack of significant contribution concerning the relationship between murmurs and valvular lesions. He certainly knew about the underlying pathologic alterations of diseased valves but he failed to utilize the same systematic approach with auscultation in the evaluation of these murmurs as he did with palpation and percussion when delineating abnormalities of other organs. He did, however, recognize that heart failure could ensue as a result of valvular lesions, describing this in detail in his major work *Essai sur les Maladies et les Lesions Organiques du Coeur et des Gros Vaisseaux*.

Despite the aforementioned deficiencies, Corvisart's importance in the development of cardiovascular pathology or his role as a clinical cardiologist remain unquestioned. He became an outstanding diagnostician because of his insistence upon postmortem confirmation. Herrick recounts how Corvisart, in his zealous adherence to this dictum, advanced a plan to write the 'inverse' of Morgagni's book with the suggested title of *De Sedibus et Causus Morborum per Signa Diagnostica Investigatis et per Anatomen Confirmatus* [41]. This would be entirely in keeping with Corvisart's 'quality control' of clinical diagnosis. However (I suppose with tongue in cheek) Corvisart added the remark 'for such a work, another Morgagni would be necessary'.

It is quite apparent by this time that up until now the evolution of our knowledge regarding the morbid anatomy of the heart, which had remained virtually stagnant for millennia, had suddenly entered an explosive phase. Indeed, the very possibility that the heart could be subject to pathologic changes was not even entertained by Hippocrates and those that followed because of the erroneous belief that the heart was immune to such changes. The advent of postmortem examinations made evident that pathologic changes could occur, but these lesions were either badly described or misinterpreted as to origin or significance. The world had to wait for Morgagni for a systematic and scientific approach to cardiac pathology as well as pathology in general. Clinical correlation took more time. The prestige and insistence of France's leading clinician of the late 18th and early 19th century were probably the pivotal factors in cementing this correlation. This was Corvisart's role.

Led by Corvisart, the Parisian school sponsored a number of leaders in a new movement that came to be characterized as 'anatomical diagnosis'. The newly introduced elements of percussion and auscultation formed the backbone of this movement. The whole cadre of the great Irish clinicians of the time soon joined forces with this movement, and in due time, the remainder of the 19th century saw the entry of the English, Danish and American clinicians in this new approach to pathology.

This seemingly scientific approach of the Parisian school had, however, one glaring defect. It regarded the structural change in the organ as being the disease itself and the clinical manifestation as being the outward expression of the lesion. It viewed the clinical significance of morbid anatomy in a static manner rather than realizing that the lesion could be only one manifestation of a broad underlying pathophysiologic process that accounts for the clinical picture. This is important to bear in mind, as we shall see later, because of the relationship that such a static approach had when attempting to understand the evolution of thought regarding the clinical significance of murmurs and cardiac enlargement, now being ascertained with increasing frequency, with the new art of physical diagnosis.

Despite this defect, the Parisian school played a very important and seminal role in the reinforcement of Corvisart's dictum of postmortem confirmation of clinical diagnosis. The adherents of this school cannot be faulted since at that time knowledge of the physiology of the heart and circulation was still in its infancy, and functional mechanisms had to be understood in more detail before one could appreciate the importance of disturbed function in producing disease processes.

It appears that the first American representative of the Parisian school was William Edmonds Horner (1793–1853) [42]. He was primarily an anatomist and surgeon. Horner wrote the first American textbook on pathology. Although the impact on cardiology was nil, his *Treatise on Pathological Anatomy*, published in 1829, was important in that it stimulated an interest in the study of pathology in general. Up until then, and as late as 1857, there was little or no teaching of pathology in the American schools of medicine.

Horner was the author of other textbooks besides the one on pathology. Middleton states that although they served their purpose well for the era in which they were published, they were criticized as being merely compilations and being stilted in style [43]. This is hardly justifiable criticism. By this time, the proliferation of scientific journals and transactions of the increasing number of learned societies made these the preferred means of communication regarding new ideas and observations. Textbooks were becoming compendia from these sources rather than the vehicles for the presentation of an individual's beliefs or experience. Moreover, the stilted style of Horner was the accepted mode of expression during his time and a reflection of his classical training.

Another representative of the Parisian school in America was William Wood Gerhard (1809–72). He published two important texts. These were *Clinical Guide and Syllabus of a Course of Lectures on Clinical Medicine and Pathology* in 1837 and *Lectures on the Diagnosis, Pathology and Treatment of Diseases of the Chest* in 1842. We shall meet him again in the chapter dealing with physical diagnosis.

The restrictions of 'anatomical diagnosis' were soon becoming apparent in Europe. In an attempt to circumvent them the Viennese, Rokitansky and Skoda adopted and fostered a physiologic approach to pathology[44]. In doing so, they influenced the many German pathologists that followed and who were so important in expanding the horizons of pathology during the 19th century. In reality, the Viennese were merely following the pathway established by Francois-Joseph-Victor Broussais (1772–1823) who was the first to voice objections against the identification of a disease process with a particular structural change.

Rokitansky was not free of error either. Although he contributed much to descriptive pathology, he entertained mistaken notions regarding the causation of disease and felt that the pathologic changes were due to abnormalities in the chemical constitution of the blood. He believed in spontaneous generation, a theory that espoused the ability of inert tissue fluids to generate, on their own, viable elements of the body; in other words, the transformation of a non-living substance into living matter.

Reduced to its simplest terms, the ultimate ill-effect of deranged structure is deranged function. In the heart this could mean a reduction in cardiac output (the basic expression of heart failure) or a cessation of cardiac output (a derangement incompatible with life). The disturbance in cardiac output may evolve over a period of time or may be sudden in onset. Sudden cessation of cardiac output is due to some catastrophic event. Examples of this would be rupture of the heart muscle, complete stoppage of blood flow through a major pulmonary arterial branch as in pulmonary embolism, or ineffectual twitching of the myocardium as a result of ventricular fibrillation.

Generally speaking, progressive reduction of cardiac output over a period of time is due to weakening contractility of the heart muscle. This is usually seen as an accompaniment of enlargement of the heart. The enlargement may involve one chamber or all chambers. It may be in the form of dilatation alone or it may be preceded by hypertrophy and then proceed to dilatation. An example of dilatation without hypertrophy is that brought about by myocarditis. Pressure overload is the usual *modus operandi* for the development of hypertrophy. An example of this would be hypertrophy of the left ventricle in the presence of stenosis of the aortic valve.

Not all of the pathologic alterations that can affect the heart will result in the scenario just outlined. Depending upon the nature of the lesions, other pathways of deranged function can be taken. In order to appreciate this more fully, a closer look is necessary at the historical background of our present knowledge concerning such specific anatomical components of the heart as the valves, endocardium, myocardium and pericardium. Some of it has already been touched upon in relationship to the contributions of those major personalities that have been presented so far. What follows is a more detailed version concerning the observations and thoughts of these and other contributors with respect to each component. It is hoped that these vignettes will form ultimately a scaffold upon which a kaleidoscopic appreciation of the whole historical picture can be achieved. Special attention will be paid to congenital disorders of the heart. Abnormalities concerning the electrophysiologic components will be discussed in the appropriate chapter in order to preserve the chronologic continuity of a complex subject.

REFERENCES

1. Adams, F. (1844–7). *The Seven Books of Paulus Aegineta*, **2**, 310. (London)

2. Mettler, C.C. (1947). *History of Medicine*, p. 247. (Philadelphia: The Blakiston Co.)

3. East, C.T. (1957). *The Story of Heart Disease*, p. 53. (London: Wm. Dawson and Sons Ltd.)

4. Bailey, P. (1911). A Florentine Anatomist. *Bull. Johns Hopkins Hosp.*, **22**, 141–2

5. Zimmerman, E.L. (1935). The Pathology of syphilis as revealed by autopsies performed between 1563 and 1761. *Bull. Inst. Hist. Med.*, **3**, 355–99

6. Malgaigne, J.F. (1840). *Oeuvres complètes d'Ambroise Paré*, 3 vols., **1**, 373–4. (Paris)

7. Long, E.R. (1928). *A History of Pathology.* (Baltimore: Williams & Wilkins)

8. East, C.T. (1957). *Op. cit.*, p. 55

9.   East, C.T. (1957). *Op. cit.*, p. 53
10. Long, E.R. (1928). *Op. cit.*
11. Adams, E.W. (1903). Founders of Modern Medicine: II. Giovanni Battista Morgagni (AD 1682–1771). *M. Libr. and Hist. J.*, **1**, 270–7
12. Long, E.R. (1928). *Op. cit.*
13. Nicholls, A.G. (1903). Morgagni, the father of modern pathology; an appreciation and a comparison. *Montreal M.J.*, **32**, 40–51 (Jan.)
14. Willius, F.A. and Keys, T.E. (1941). *Cardiac Classics; a Collection of Classic Works on the Heart and Circulation with Comprehensive Biographic Accounts of the Authors*, pp. 171–5. (St. Louis: C. V. Mosby Co.)
15. Castiglioni, Arturo. (1941). *A History of Medicine*. (Translated by E.B. Krumbhaar). (New York: Alfred A. Knopf)
16. Alexander, B. (1769). *The Seats and Causes of Diseases*. (London)
17. Vieussens, R. (1715). Traité Nouveau de la Structure et des Causes du Mouvements Natural du Coeur. In *Oeuvres Francoises de M. Vieussens dédi es à Nosseigneurs des états de la province de Languedoc*. (Toulouse)
18. Sénac, J.B. (1724). *L'Anatomie d'Heister avec des essais de physique sur l'usage des parties du corps humain*. (Paris)
19. Gillespie, C.C. (1970). *Dictionary of Scientific Biography*, Vol 12, pp. 302–3. (New York: Scribner)
20. Willius, F.A. and Keys, T.E. (1941). *Op. cit.*, pp. 159–160
21. Corvisart, J.N. (1812). *An Essay on the Organic Diseases and Lesions of the Heart and Great Vessels*. Trans. by J. Gates, p. 12. (Philadelphia)
22. Gillespie, C.C. (1970). *Op. cit.*, vol. VII, pp. 613–14
23. Pettigrew, T.J. (1940). William Hunter, MD. In *Medical Portrait Gallery; Biographical Memoirs of the Most Celebrated Physicians, Surgeons, etc. Who Have Contributed to the Advancement of Medical Science*, vol. 1. (London: Fisher, Son & Co.)
24. East, C.T. (1957). *Op. cit.*, p. 87
25. Willius, F.A. and Dry, T.J. (1948). *A History of the Heart and Circulation*, p. 92. (Philadelphia: W. B. Saunders Co.)
26. Duffin, J.M. (1989). Cardiology of RTH Laennec. *Medical History*, **33**, 42–71
27. Portal, A. (1804). *Cours d'Anatomie Médicale*, 5 vols. (Paris: Baudoin, AN XII)
28. Sénac, J.B. (1749). *Traité de la Structure du Coeur, de son action et de ses Maladies*, p. 34. (Paris: J. Vincent)
29. Thayer, S.W. (1903). *Bichat. Bull. Johns Hopkins Hosp.*, **14**, 197–201, p. 200
30. Castiglioni, A. (1941). *Op. cit.*, pp. 691–2
31. Garrison, F.H. (1913). *An Introduction to the History of Medicine*, pp. 843, 846. (Philadelphia: W. B. Saunders).
32. Daremberg, G. (1907). *Les Grands Médecins du XIX Siecle*, pp. 105–13. (Paris: Masson et Cie)
33. Herrick, J.B. (1942). *A Short History of Cardiology*, p. 160. (Illinois: Charles C. Thomas)
34. Willius, F.A. and Dry, T.J. (1948). *Op. cit.*. p. 123
35. Garrison, F.H. (1913). *Op. cit.*, pp. 445–6
36. Herrick, J.B. *Op. cit.*, pp. 222–4
37. Long, E.R. (1928). *Op. cit.*, p. 141
38. McDonald, A.L. The Aphorisms of Corvisart. *Am. M. Hist.*, 3rd. Ser., **1**, (1939), 374–387, 471–6, 546–63; **2**, (1940), 64–9
39. Willius, F.A. and Dry, T.J. (1948). *Op. cit.*, p. 108
40. Herrick, J.B. (1942). *Op. cit.*, pp. 78–9
41. Herrick, J.B. (1942). *Ibid.*, p. 75
42. Middleton, W.S. (1923). William Edmonds Horner (1793–1853). *Ann. M. Hist.*, **5**, 35
43. *Ibid.*, (1923). p. 36
44. Mettler, C. (1947). *Op. cit.*, p. 259

5   Endocardial lesions

As indicated before, the early observations regarding valvular deformities were confined to morbid changes with no reference to hemodynamic significance. The systematic study of valvular lesions needed not only clinical correlation but also a firmer understanding of the physiologic alterations that could ensue as a result of the structural changes.

The introduction of auscultation was probably the most important factor in sparking a clinical interest in valvulopathy. It provided a simple direct method for the detection of a valvular disturbance *in vivo*. For a while, the lesion itself, with its physical signs, became the all-consuming interest of the bedside clinician. It was only later that the hemodynamic consequences of such lesions began to assume their rightful role in the management of the patient. The advent of surgical techniques for the correction of these lesions further intensified the necessity for hemodynamic rather than structural evaluation *per se*. Handicapped by leakage, tightness of the orifice, or both, how did the patient under study cope with his valvular lesion? Could he tolerate physical activity, and to what extent? These became the logical questions that had to be answered. As we shall see, the current diagnostic procedures, both invasive and non-invasive, have removed a good part of the uncertainty from these questions so that surgical remedy can be staged, if indicated, and most importantly, at the proper time. One cannot wait for irreversible hemodynamic changes. At the same time one cannot intervene too early, taking into account the morbidity, complications and mortality associated with our current surgical techniques.

It is against this background that one must approach the evolution of our knowledge regarding valvular lesions. The pathologist, physiologist and clinician had to work, hand in hand, for the proper elucidation of morbid changes.

Valvular deformities are either acquired or congenital. This difference was not apparent to the early observers. In fact, true interest in congenital lesions of the heart did not develop until the publication of two textbooks, one by Farre in 1814, and the other by Peacock in 1858.

The earliest account of the pathologic anatomy of valvular lesions is to be found in the description of aortic stenosis by Riverius in 1674. The outstanding feature of the description was the calcareous deposits in the valve. Soon thereafter (1703) William Cooper (sometimes spelled Cowper) also described calcified aortic valves and recognized that leakage from such valves caused enlargement of the left ventricle. He described the left ventricle as 'being larger than in an ordinary ox'[1]. This antedates by many years the labeling of such ventricles as 'cor bovinum'. How such an important hemodynamic relationship could be lost over the years is difficult to understand.

Succeeding generations of observers added their descriptions. These included Haller (1749), Morgagni in two of his letters, one of which was No. 23, Baillie in his atlas (plate II), Corvisart, Hope, Abernethy, Chevers, and Peacock. Abernethy in 1808 described in detail the opaque appearance of the stenotic mitral valve and the associated thickening of the left atrium containing a clot[2]. This is a perfect presentation of a morbid anatomical setting for the development of embolic phenomena in mitral stenosis. In 1865, Peacock presented a comprehensive survey of the various types of valvular deformities in his Croonian lectures[3].

Ulcerations of the endocardial surface of the valves were noted by Fabrizio Bartoletti as far back as 1630. Since the science of bacteriology had not been established as yet, he failed to realize a possible relationship of these lesions to an infectious process. It was Bouillaud who first introduced the term 'endocarditis'[4]. Prior to this, Kreysig had been using the term 'carditis', advancing the thesis that the inflammatory process of 'carditis' was responsible for the narrowing of the valvular orifices[5]. Corvisart also noted endocardial valvular lesions though he had no idea that what he described were probably bacterial in origin. He called them vegetations, a term still used today. Joseph Hodgson preferred to call these wart-like excrescences 'fungus', a label that was also used by Heiberg in 1872[6-8].

During the latter half of the 19th century, the work of Pasteur and Koch had pretty well established that germs could cause an infectious process. Fortified by this concept, Winge of Oslo in 1867 demonstrated how microorganisms carried by the blood could attack the valves of the heart[9]. Thus, vegetations or 'fungus' (the 'pilzbildung' of Heiberg) seen at autopsy were now known to be caused by a bacterial invasion. East in his Fitzpatrick lectures before the Royal College of Physicians pointed out how Winge was anticipated in his conclusions by Kirkes of St. Bartholomew's Hospital in 1852. Kirkes at that time had indicated that there were different types of endocarditis, noting also that some of the vegetative lesions could fragment and embolize[10]. He described this in his paper, *On some of the Principal Effects resulting from the Detachment of Fibrinous Deposits from the Interior of the Heart and their Mixture in the Circulating Blood*. He probably had a very lenient editor since this is a rather long-winded title. In 1870, Wilks described the occurrence of multiple abscesses in the various organs as a result of such embolization. He used the expression 'arterial pyaemia as a result of endocarditis'[11].

The fact that bacterial infections carried by the blood targeted previously damaged or deformed valves was recognized as early as 1844 by Paget. But, it was Sir William Osler who pursued this further when in a series of publications he enlarged on the pathologic and clinical features of a syndrome that later came to be known as bacterial endocarditis. His first paper was entitled *Malignant Endocarditis*. It was published as part of his Gulstonian lectures in 1885[12]. In it he stated that the disease was capable of manifesting itself in an acute or chronic manner[12]. It was a good 24 years later (in 1909) that, on the basis of further experience, Osler identified, in a second paper on endocarditis, a subacute type[13].

The subacute type was also described by Schottmüller in 1910[14]. He called it 'endocarditis lenta'. He knew that *Streptococcus viridans* was, by far, the most frequent incriminating organism. By this time, bacteriologic culture techniques had become increasingly reliable. It was also in 1910 that Libman described a bacteria-free phase[15]. He also presented evidence of healing of the valvular lesions in some of the cases. It was he who renamed the 'endocarditis lenta' of Schottmüller as 'subacute bacterial endocarditis'[16].

Today, the bacterial endocarditides are classified under the umbrella term of infective endocarditis. The etiologic agents as well as the clinical spectrum have changed considerably. With the decline of rheumatic heart disease since the introduction of penicillin and the emergence of drug abuse, prosthetic valves, interventional strategies, and most recently AIDS, different etiologic factors have come into play and an entirely different clinical scenario has ensued. For some time, *S. viridans* was the usual incriminating organism. Today, an entirely different gamut of organisms can be responsible, including true fungi.

The past two decades have solidified more concretely our knowledge of the pathogenesis and various pathologic changes seen in valvular as well as in non-valvular endocarditis. It is now recognized that there are many portals of entry for the microorganisms as well as many predisposing factors for the initiation of the disease process. We have now come to recognize a variant known as non-bacterial thrombotic endocarditis. The term 'marantic endocarditis' is also used, but I find it confusing. We do know that it can be seen in patients who are chronically ill, especially those with a malignancy. We also know that the lesions on the valves consist of sterile thrombi that are capable of being dislodged and traveling to distant sites. It seems to me that this is another way of saying non-bacterial thrombotic endocarditis.

Be that as it may, we have come a long way since Osler gave his original paper on *Malignant Endocarditis* in 1885. Of all the contributors to our knowledge of infective endocarditis, it is my opinion, that the 'Golden Cane' belongs to him by virtue of this classical paper; a gem sparkling with clarity, accuracy and organization. It would seem fitting then at this point to present a more detailed picture of this 'compleat physician'. Canadian by birth, temporarily American by adoption, and finally British by choice, Osler was neither a pathologist nor a cardiologist. He was an internist with a vast range of interests but with a particular affinity for both pathology and cardiology.

William Bart Osler was born at Bond Head, Canada in 1849. He was the youngest son of an Anglican minister and enjoyed the privileges of an intellectual home environment and a good education. Following his graduation from Trinity University in Toronto he pursued his medical studies at McGill University, receiving his doctorate in Medicine in 1872. He then spent two years in postgraduate training in medicine at the acclaimed centers of the time in London, Berlin and Vienna. Upon his return to Canada in 1874, he was appointed to the medical faculty of McGill University. In 10 years' time he transferred to the University of Philadelphia as professor of clinical medicine where he remained until 1889. He was appointed professor of medicine at Johns Hopkins in 1889 and remained in this position until 1905, at which time he decided to accept the Chair as Regius Professor of Medicine at Oxford University. Osler served in this position until his death in 1919.

Osler was widely acclaimed throughout his lifetime. He received numerous honorary doctorates from the various universities of America, Canada and Great Britain. In 1911, he was created a baronet of the United Kingdom. He published numerous monographs and papers on medical and non-medical subjects. His major text was *The Principles and Practice of Medicine* which was first published in 1892 and enjoyed such wide acclaim that it went into many editions. Despite a rather congested schedule of activities, Osler also found time to edit a seven volume encyclopedia of medicine called *The System of Medicine*[17,18].

The greatness of Osler lies not in this prosaic summary. The stupendous magnitude of his life can be appreciated only in terms of his influence on generations of medical students, medicine in general, and the philosophical aspects of life. His literary output was the vehicle for his unremitting influence, and expressed the spiritual nature of this man.

There is no doubt that Osler's textbook of medicine was unquestionably an admirable one. But, there have been other equally excellent textbooks of medicine. In fact, during the same era, Strumpell's text was probably even more successful. There is no doubt that Osler deserves credit for a great deal of originality not only in clinical medicine, but also in allied fields. His contribution to cardiology has already been discussed at length. He was one of the first to describe blood platelets, and his name will remain associated with the clinical picture of a considerable number of diseases as long as eponyms remain in vogue.

All of these great accomplishments, individually and collectively, do not truly explain the man's greatness. His renown, as Sigerist suggests, lies in the sum total of his personality 'as a physician, as teacher, as man'[19]. Sigerist compares him to Boerhaave, the great European clinician of the early 18th century. Like Boerhaave, Osler 'was a magnet continually attracting pupils … He was a man who taught juniors how to watch and how to think at the bedside of the sick, and was one who inspired medical students with an enthusiasm for the healing art and filled them with the physician's ethos'[20].

Osler was the 'compleat physician' because he combined his interest in medicine with his love of the humanities. A collector of books, he read them all avidly, and with the knowledge gained from them he was able to write such penetrating essays as *Science and Immortality* (1904); *Counsels and Ideals* (1905); *An Alabama Student* (1908); *A Way of Life* (1914) and *The Student Life* (1913).

Figure 1 shows Osler giving a demonstration and lecture in the amphitheater at Johns Hopkins.

The relationship of deformed valves to rheumatic fever also had to await the latter part of the 18th century before being entertained. We have alluded already to Pitcairn's role in recognizing this relationship. Wells in 1812 indicated that Pitcairn in 1788 already knew about rheumatism and lesions of the heart but failed to leave a written record of this[21].

William Charles Wells (1757–1817) was an American who was born in Charleston, South Carolina, of Scottish immigrants. Wells studied initially at the University of Edinburgh, then returned to Charleston where he became apprenticed to a very respected practitioner in town, a Dr. Alexander Garden. Incidentally, the Gardenia is named after Wells' preceptor; this honor having been bestowed upon him by the great Swedish botanist, Linneaus, with whom Dr. Garden, also a botanist, had been keeping up a lively correspondence[22].

The family returned to England when the Revolutionary War broke out because Wells' father was sympathetic towards the Crown. Young Wells returned to Edinburgh to complete his medical training. He received his doctorate from that institution in 1780. Prior to this he had spent some time with John Hunter, the anatomist, and also some time at St. Bartholomew's Hospital as well as at Leyden University[23].

Apparently his personality left a great deal to be desired. He had very few friends, although he did seem to cherish his relationship with Pitcairn and

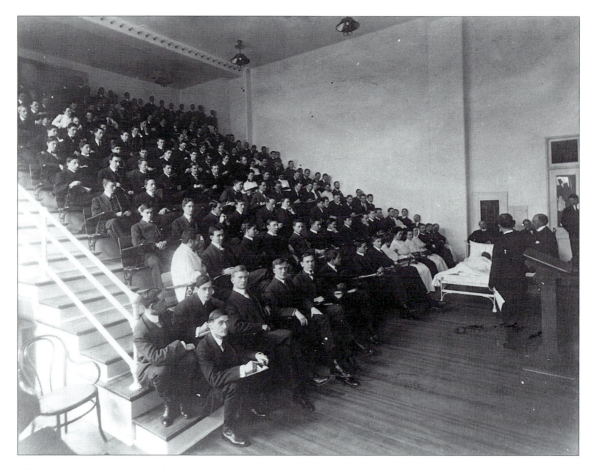

Figure 1 Sir William Osler giving a demonstration and lecture in the amphitheatre at Johns Hopkins University, School of Medicine; patient in bed, in front of Osler. *Photo Source National Library of Medicine. Literary Source Copied from photograph owned by C.L. Gemmill, M.D. Courtesy of National Library of Medicine*

Baillie. Herrick describes him as being irritable, pugnacious, impulsive, lonely and austere[24].

Wells' important contribution was his paper, *On Rheumatism of the Heart*. It was based on 14 cases, most of which were from his own practice. The paper describes in detail a clinical picture of what appears to be acute rheumatic fever. In one autopsy, excrescences on the mural and valvular endocardial surface are described. Contrary to what has been generally believed, this is not the first full account of rheumatic fever. Just four years earlier (1808) Dundas had published a paper based on nine cases in which the necropsies revealed enlarged hearts, adhesions in the pericardial sacs, and 'lymph on the mitral valves'. The relationship of these cases to rheumatism was underscored by Dundas by stressing 'the necessity of attending to the translation of

rheumatism to the chest'[25]. Wells' cases also showed thickening of the pericardium, so it appears that even during this early phase of recognition, rheumatic fever was known to affect other components of the heart besides the valvular structures.

Despite these observations by Dundas and Wells, two decades later, when J.B. Bouillaud published his *Traite Clinique des Maladies du Couer* in which he introduced the term endocarditis, he did not differentiate between an infective or rheumatic basis for the lesions that he observed at postmortem. He did say that there were two different types of endocarditis but this differentiation was based on the clinical picture rather than on morbid anatomy. The type characterized by protracted insidious manifestations was described by him as occurring in individuals with known disease of the valves, while the more fulminating or acute type was said by him to occur as part of a generalized septic process (as in pneumonia) with murmurs appearing during the clinical course and being indicative of the development of a valvular defect. This description was based on 13 cases that he culled from his own practice and appeared to be variations of a bacterial endocarditis. What is confusing is that included among the postmortem examples were valvular lesions with a warty (verrucous) appearance, and others that were indurated or calcified with or without narrowing of the orifices[26]. These, in the light of present knowledge, appear to be perfect examples of both infective and rheumatic endocarditis.

Presumably as he gained more experience, Bouillaud's interpretation of clinical events and postmortem correlation began to assume a more clarified position. It was just one year after his initial treatise on heart disease that Bouillaud published the first of his monographs on rheumatism[27]. It was entitled *Nouvelles Récherches sur le Rhumatisme*. This was truly the first comprehensive and accurate account of the relationship between heart disease and rheumatism. In it, he stated his 'law of coincidence' which is as follows: 'In the great majority of cases of acute generalized febrile articular rheumatism, there exists a variable degree of rheumatism of the fibrous tissue of the heart. This coincidence is the rule rather than the exception'[28]. In still another treatise published four years later and entitled *Traite Clinique du Rhumatisme Articulaire* he stated that if the articular manifestations were mild, then the concomitant occurrence of carditis did not prevail[29]. Later observations by others proved this statement to be quite erroneous since the clinical picture of rheumatic fever is notoriously variable, with the incidence of cardiac complications not at all dependent upon the presence or severity of the arthritis. Another error was his belief that myocarditis occurred independently of endocarditis and pericarditis.

Bouillaud described the endocarditis in his treatise on maladies of the heart as occurring in three stages. The first stage he characterized as being a period of 'sanguinary congestion, of softening, and of ulceration or suppuration'. The second phase is a 'period of organization of secreted products or of a portion of fibrinous concretions'. The final or third period is characterized by the formation of 'cartilaginous, osseous or calcareous

induration of the endocardium in general, and of the valves in particular, with or without narrowing of the orifices of the heart'.

He gives a very detailed description of the narrowing which he found, describing it as a common occurrence and a consequence of a prolonged chronic endocarditis.

> The degrees of narrowing of the orifices of the heart are very variable. In extreme degrees, one can hardly introduce the tip of the little finger, or even the tip of a writing pen, into the narrowed orifice. The opening which is left between the thick, indurated valves or those valves united by their neighboring borders, is permanent, or constantly open. It is sometimes rounded, oval or elliptic. It resembles in many cases a buttonhole or a glottis of which the lips are represented by the rounded borders of the thickened valve leaflets. This comparison applies particularly to certain narrowings of the left auriculo-ventricular orifice. In a few cases, the leaflets of the bicuspid valve have acquired an enormous thickening and protrude from the side of the auricle; then the retracted orifice may be compared to the orifice of the cervix uteri, and like this imitates a fish mouth. Seen from the auricular side, the circumference of the retracted auriculo-ventricular orifice presents a very pronounced folding, as if this circumference had been folded upon itself; this disposition gives it the appearance of the external circumference of the anus or the opening of a purse drawn together with cords[30].

How can anyone forget this description? It stands out as a classical example of pure descriptive pathology.

Jean Baptiste Bouillaud was born in 1796 at Bragette near Angoulême in France. He lived to the ripe old age of 85 during which time he achieved international fame in his chosen profession. Apparently he was quite patriotic. It is said that while studying medicine at Paris he joined the students of the École Polytechnique in an ineffectual resistance against the Allied forces marching against Napoleon's armies in Paris. Bouillaud actually manned the barricades at Clichy in 1814. Bouillaud continued to serve with Napoleon until the defeat at Waterloo, after which he resumed his medical studies at Paris.

During the post-Napoleonic period Paris once again enjoyed pre-eminence in medical training and research. Physicians and surgeons were held in great esteem and benefited in many ways from this acclaim. Honoré de Balzac also shared in this feeling and in the series of novels that constitute his 'La Comédie Humaine', a number of physicians, both obscure and famous, are portrayed by some of the leading characters. Among them was Bouillaud who according to Poynter is none other than Horace Bianchon, 'The wise and compassionate physician, always in demand'[31].

Poynter quotes the following description of Bianchon (Bouillaud) by Balzac when Bianchon first comes on the scene in 'La Pease de Chagrin' as a man of the future: '... the most distinguished perhaps of the new physicians, the good and modest representative of the young generation who are preparing to receive their heritage – the treasures amassed over fifty years by the school of Paris, and who will perhaps build the monument for which the preceding centuries had contributed so many diverse materials'.

Bouillaud was fortunate to have had many illustrious teachers including among them Corvisart and Bertin. He was only 35 years old when he was appointed professor of clinical medicine of the Faculté de Médicine of Paris. Soon after, while on the staff of Charity Hospital, he published his *Traité Clinique des Maladies du Coeur*. As already noted, it was in this work that Bouillaud introduced the term endocarditis. According to Rolleston, the expression 'Maladie de Bouillaud' was suggested by Trousseau as an eponym for endocarditis, since it 'was an almost unknown affliction until the illustrious professor of the Hôpital de la Charité drew the attention of the medical world to it in a description to which nothing can be added'[32,33]. 'Maladie de Bouillaud', however, remains as the term for acute articular rheumatism which Bouillaud described in such meticulous detail while establishing irrevocably its relationship to valvular lesions of the heart.

Bouillaud's brilliance as a clinician is beyond question, and his description of the morbid anatomy of the valvular lesions of endocarditis is a remarkable example of keen observation. It is sad but true that despite all this he was woefully inadequate in his approach to treatment. Bloodletting was his therapeutic tour-de-force.

Figure 2 is a portrait of Bouillaud. The frontispiece of his text 'Maladies du Coeur' is illustrated in Figure 3.

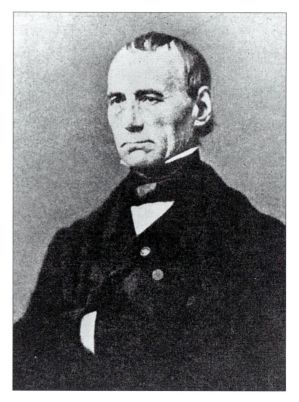

Figure 2 Portrait of Jean-Baptiste Bouillaud. *Photo Source University of Central Florida. Literary Source Herrick JB: A Short History of Cardiology. Charles C. Thomas, Springfield, Illinois. Taken originally from Brusquet & Gentz: Les Biographies Medicales. Paris, 1929–1931. With permission*

Many years after Bouillaud's description of endocarditis, Duroziez published a survey of pure mitral stenosis which is cited by East as being the best of its kind[34]. This paper describes both the clinical and pathologic aspects of mitral stenosis. He traces the fusion of the vegetations on the mitral valve which in due time creates the classical 'funnel' shaped appearance. The 'fish mouth' appearance of the valve initially described by Bouillaud also appears in Duroziez's paper[35,36].

Many years had to elapse after these important break-throughs (well into the 20th century) before it became definitely established that rheumatic fever was an inflammatory disease induced by an antecedent group A beta-hemolytic streptococcal pharyngitis.

The microbic origin of rheumatic fever was investigated as early as 1887 by A. Mantle[37].

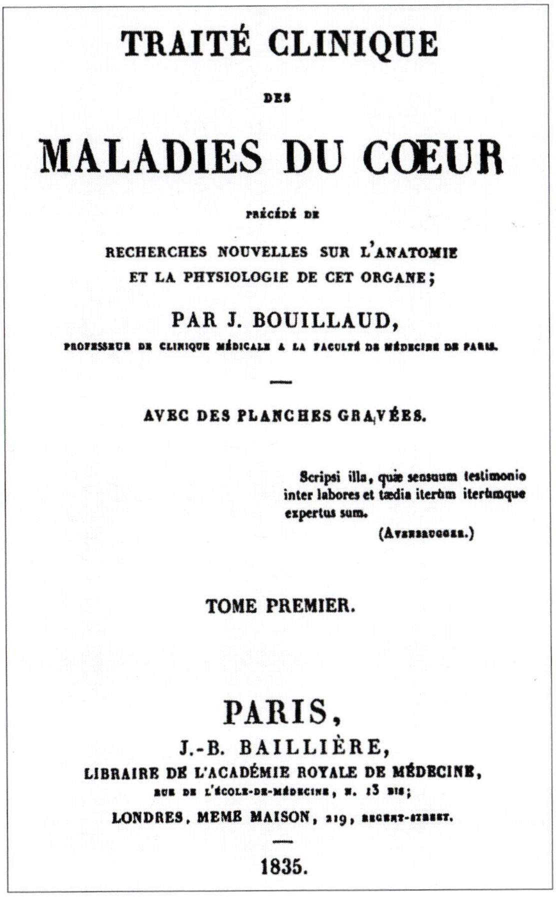

TRAITÉ CLINIQUE

DES

MALADIES DU COEUR

PRÉCÉDÉ DE

RECHERCHES NOUVELLES SUR L'ANATOMIE
ET LA PHYSIOLOGIE DE CET ORGANE;

PAR J. BOUILLAUD,

PROFESSEUR DE CLINIQUE MÉDICALE A LA FACULTÉ DE MÉDECINE DE PARIS.

—

AVEC DES PLANCHES GRAVÉES.

Scripsi illa, quæ sensuum testimonio
inter labores et tædia iterûm iterûmque
expertus sum.

(AVERRHOËS.)

TOME PREMIER.

PARIS,

J.-B. BAILLIÈRE,

LIBRAIRE DE L'ACADÉMIE ROYALE DE MÉDECINE,
RUE DE L'ÉCOLE-DE-MÉDECINE, N. 13 BIS;

LONDRES, MÊME MAISON, 219, REGENT-STREET.

1835.

Figure 3 Frontispiece of 'Maladies Du Coeur' by J. Bouillaud. *Photo Source University of Central Florida. Literary Source Willius FA, Keys TE: Cardiac Classics. The C.V. Mosby Co., 1941. Courtesy of the Mayo Clinic*

From then on, successive investigators provided repeated documentation of the relationship between the streptococcal organism and rheumatic fever[38–41]. In 1940, May G. Wilson published a monograph on rheumatic fever. It should be regarded as a classic work since for the first time it synthesized the accumulated knowledge of pathologic changes induced by rheumatic fever, emphasizing the etiology and epidemiology of the disease[42].

Although many questions still remain unanswered, recent observations have provided important insights into its pathogenesis. It appears that there may be only certain strains of streptococci that have a rheumatogenic capability. Rheumatogenicity is apparently related to the presence of a particular type of surface M protein.

An immune response is initiated against these strains of streptococci in a host that is genetically susceptible. We will examine the historical background of the genetic and immunologic aspects in the appropriate sections.

The foundation for the modern concept that Group A streptococcal pharyngitis is causally related to rheumatic fever rests upon two important developments in the field of bacteriology. These are the classification of streptococci introduced by Lancefield and the development of the antistreptolysin O titer by Todd.

E.W. Todd described the anti–hemolysin titers in hemolytic streptococcal infections and their significance in rheumatic fever in 1932[43]. R.C. Lancefield outlined the specific relationship of cell composition to biological activity of hemolytic streptococci during a series of Harvey lectures that he gave in 1940 and 1941[44].

Abreast of these developments, two keen clinicians, Coburn from the USA and Collis from England, appreciated the potentiality of their practical application and were the first to correlate them clinically with rheumatic fever[45,46].

World War II provided the opportunity to confirm these initial impressions. Utilizing bacteriologic and immunologic techniques, Rammelkamp and his associates documented the relationship of streptococcal epidemics and rheumatic fever[47]. The Streptococcal Laboratory of the Armed Forces Epidemiological Board at Warren Air Force Base in Wyoming and the Naval Research Unit No. 4 at Great Lakes Naval Training Center both played prominent roles in this classical investigation[48].

The most convincing evidence concerning the streptococcal basis for rheumatic fever was that afforded by the protective benefits of penicillin. The introduction of this therapeutic agent for the treatment and prevention of streptococcal infections began in the early 1950s and was initially reported by Stollerman and co-workers in the Journal of the American Medical Association in 1952, and again in the New England Journal of Medicine in 1955[49,50].

REFERENCES

1. Cooper, W. (1706). Valvular diseases. *Trans. R. Soc. London*, **5**, 218
2. Abernethy, J. (1808). Stenosis of the mitral valve. *J. Med. Chir. Trans.*, **1**, 27

3. East, C.T. (1957). *The Story of Heart Disease*, p. 78. (London: Wm. Dawson and Sons Ltd.)
4. Bouillaud, J.B. (1835). *Traité Clinique des Maladies du Coeur*, vol. 2, pp. 170–92. (Paris: J.B. Baillière)
5. Kreysig, F.L. *Die Krankheiten des Herzens*, vol. 2, p. 67
6. Hodgson, J. (1815). *Treatise on Diseases of Arteries and Veins*. (London)
7. East, C.T. (1957). *Op. cit.*, p. 79
8. Heiberg, H. (1872). Pilzbildung. *Virchow's Arch.*, **56**, 407
9. Winge, E. (1867). *Canstats Jahresbericht f.d. Jahr*, **2**, 240
10. Kirkes, W.S. (1852). On some of the principal effects resulting from the detachment of fibrinous deposits from the interior of the heart, and their mixture in the circulating blood. *Med. Chir. Trans.*, **35**, 281
11. Wilks, S. (1870). *Guy's Hosp. Rep.*, **15**, 3rd. ser. 29
12. Osler, W. (1885). Malignant endocarditis. Gulstonian Lectures. *Lancet*, **1**, 459
13. Osler, W. (1909). *Q. J. Med.*, **2**, 219
14. Schottmüller, E. (1910). *Münch Med. Wschr.*, **57**, 617
15. Libman, E. and Celler, H.L. (1910). *Am. J. Med. Sci.*, **140**, 516
16. Libman, E. (1913). *Am. J. Med. Sci.*, **146**, 625
17. Cushing, H. (1925). *The Life of Sir William Osler*, 2 vols. (Oxford)
18. Reed, G. (1931). *The Great Physician*. (Oxford)
19. Sigerist, H.E. (1933). *A Biographical History of Medicine*. (Translated by Eden and Cedar Paul). (Woking: Unwin Bros. Ltd.)
20. *Ibid.*
21. Wells, W.C. (1812). On rheumatism of the heart. *Tr. Soc. Improved Med. Chir. Knowledge*, **3**, 373–424
22. Beck, J.B. (1850). *An Historical Sketch of the State of American Medicine before the Revolution*, 2nd edn., 63 pp. (Albany, New York: Charles van Benthuysen)
23. Bartlett, E. (1849). *A Brief Sketch of the Life, Character, and Writings of William Charles Wells*. An address delivered before the Louisville Medical Society. December 7, 1849, 32 pp. (Louisville, Kentucky: Prentice and Weissinger)
24. Herrick, J.B. (1942). *A Short History of Cardiology*, p. 153. (Illinois: Charles C. Thomas)
25. East, C.T. (1957). *Op. cit.*, p. 87
26. Bouillaud, J.B. (1835). *Traité Clinique des Maladies du Coeur*, vol. 2, pp. 170–92. (Paris: J.B. Bailliére)
27. Bouillaud, J.B. (1836). *Nouvelles Récherches sur le Rhumatisme*. (Paris)
28. *Ibid.* (1836). p. 29
29. Bouillaud, J.B. (1840). *Traité Clinique du Rhumatisme Articulaire*. (Paris)
30. Bouillaud, J.B. (1835). *Traité Clinique des Maladies du Coeur*. Section Deuxieme, Histoire Générale de l'Endocardite, Article Premier, Paris, pp. 170–92. Translated by Erich Hausner, MD. (Amsterdam, New York)
31. Poynter, F.N.L. (1968). Doctors in the Human Comedy. *J.A.M.A.*, **204** (1), 105–8
32. Rolleston, J.D. (1931). Jean Baptiste Bouillaud (1796–1881). A Pioneer in Cardiology and Neurology. *Proc. R. Soc. Med.*, (Section of the History of Medicine) **24** (pt.2), 1253–62
33. Lereboullet, P. (1914). J. Bouillaud (1796–1881). *Paris Méd.*, **16**, 177–83
34. East, C.T. (1957). *Op. cit.*, p. 89
35. Duroziez, P.L. (1861). *Arch. Gén. de Méd.*, April, 417
36. Duroziez, P.L. (1877). *Arch. Gén. de Méd. Ciéme*, Ser. **30**, 32
37. Mantle, A. (1887). Etiology of rheumatism considered from a bacterial point of view. *Br. Med. J.*, **1**, 1381
38. Coburn, A.F. (1931). *The Factor of Infection in the Rheumatic State*. (Baltimore: Williams and Wilkins)
39. Paul, J. (1943). *The Epidemiology of Rheumatic Fever and Some of its Public Health Aspects*. (New York: Metropolitan Life Ins. Co.)
40. Rantz, L.A. (1952). *The Prevention of Rheumatic Fever*. (Springfield, Ill.: Charles C. Thomas)
41. Thomas, L. (1952). *Rheumatic Fever*. (Minneapolis: Univ. of Minnesota Press)
42. Wilson, M.G. (1940). *Rheumatic Fever*. (New York: The Commonwealth Fund)
43. Todd, E.W.L. (1932). Antihaemolysin titres in haemolytic streptococcal infections and their significance in rheumatic fever. *Br. J. Exp. Pathol.*, **13**, 248–59
44. Lancefield, R.C. (1941). Specific relationship of cell composition to biological activity of hemolytic streptococci. *Harvey Lectures 1940–41*, **36**, 251–90
45. Coburn, A.F. (1931). *The Factor of Infection in the Rheumatic State*. (Baltimore: Williams and Wilkins)
46. Collis, W.R.F. (1931). Acute rheumatism and hemolytic streptococci. *Lancet*, **1**, 1341–5
47. Rammelkamp, C.H., Denny, F.W. and Wannamaker, L.W. (1952). Studies on the

epidemiology of rheumatic fever in the Armed Services. In Thomas, L. (ed.) *Rheumatic Fever,* pp. 72–89. (Minneapolis: Univ. Minnesota Press)

48. Stollerman, G.H. (1975). *Rheumatic Fever and Streptococcal Infection*, p. 102. (New York: Grune and Stratton)

49. Stollerman, G.H. and Rusoff, J.H. (1952). Prophylaxis against Group A streptococcal infections in rheumatic fever patients. Use of new repository penicillin preparation. *J.A.M.A.*, **150**, 1571–5

50. Stollerman, G.H., Rusoff, J.H. and Hirschfeld, I. (1955). Prophylaxis against Group A streptococci in rheumatic fever. The use of single monthly injections of benzathine penicillin G. *N. Engl. J. Med.*, **252**, 787–92

6   Myocardial lesions

Tracing the evolution of knowledge regarding the spectrum of myocardial disease is a rather complex affair. First of all, the terminology is confusing and in the past it has been non-specific as well as notoriously inaccurate. This can be illustrated by the simple word myocarditis. The connotation today is vastly different from what was meant in the distant past. The other stumbling block is the sheer weight of newer pathological findings that are being uncovered with continued improvement of investigative techniques.

Historically, the most common characteristic of myocardial disease at postmortem has been enlargement of the heart. This being so, this would be as good a place as any to begin our story. Once this has been covered, the more prudent approach would be to use the most current classification of specific myocardial diseases and what is now generally termed the cardio-myopathies. No classification exists as yet that is completely acceptable on scientific grounds. But this need not deter us because what we need is merely some sort of scaffold upon which an historical outline can be built.

Corvisart was one of the first to recognize cardiac enlargement as a marker of myocardial disease. In his classification of cardiac lesions we have already seen that one of the groupings addresses itself to this phenomenon. He divided enlargement into two broad categories: hyper-trophy and dilatation.

On hypertrophy he remarked: 'The cavities acquire very often a thickness and force which makes the contractions extremely distinct'. Pressure overload as a cause of the hypertrophy was also recognized by him. But he did not realize that aside from a constricted valvular orifice, pressure overload could also exist in the presence of hypertension[1]. Recognition of high blood pressure as a common cause of hypertrophy of the left ventricle was to come at a much later date.

Aneurysm was Corvisart's term for enlargement of the cardiac chambers. He distinguished between two types: 'Active and passive dilatation'. In active dilatation, the walls were thickened and the vigor of contraction was increased. In passive dilatation there was diminished contractility with thinning of the wall.

Laénnec adopted all of Corvisart's classifications of enlargement except that he substituted the term 'hypertrophy' for Corvisart's 'active aneurysm'. As a matter of fact, it was Laénnec who coined the term hypertrophy of the myocardium and pointed out that it could exist without dilatation[2]. Duffin lists Laénnec's classification of diseases of the myocardium as indicated in Table 1[3]. It is not a logical arrangement but rather a collection of abnormalities that were encountered at the postmortem table.

In 1824, Bertin classified enlargement into three types:

(1) A simple hypertrophy with no alteration in the size of the chamber;

(2) An eccentric type of hypertrophy where both ventricular cavity and muscle were increased in size; and

(3) A type of hypertrophy characterized by increased muscle wall thickness with con-comitant decrease in the size of the chamber[4].

Hope knew of the different pathogenic mechanisms between dilatation and hypertrophy. He was well aware that in valvular leakage during diastole, the muscle wall softened due to volume overload and stretched with a resultant dilatation of the chamber. He agreed with Corvisart and others that a stenosed valve caused thickening of the muscle because of the increased force needed to drive the blood through the constricted orifice. He, too, was unaware of elevated blood pressure

Table 1 Laénnec's classification of diseases of the myocardium

---

Diseases of the myocardium
Hypertrophy: left, right, both
Dilatation: left, right, both
Dilatation with hypertrophy
Partial dilatation
Hardening
Softening: violet, yellow, white
Atrophy
Gangrene
Displacement
Prolapse
Congenital abnormalities
Carditis
Communication between right and left heart
Rupture
Fatty degeneration
Ossification of the myocardium
Tubercles
Cancers
Cysts: serous, acephalocysts
Inflammation of the internal membrane
Valves: induration and ossification
Detached eustachian valve
Mitral aneurysm
Polyps

---

as a common cause of hypertrophy[5]. Hope also said that myosclerosis caused enlargement. Here we come across our first semantic confusion. What did he mean by myosclerosis? Was the condition the result of an infarct? Was the hardening of the myocardium due to fibrosis, ossification or whatever? Careful study of his description fails to enlighten us.

Besides enlargement, Corvisart also described fatty infiltration as a myocardial lesion. Laénnec used the term fatty degeneration to describe the same process. Stokes felt that fatty degeneration of the myocardium provided the pathological basis for 'disturbances of vital phenomena'[6].

In 1968, the World Health Organization defined cardiomyopathy as conditions involving the muscle of the heart, frequently of unknown etiology but having as a dominant feature cardiomegaly and heart failure. This definition excluded any disorder of heart muscle due to valvular disease, coronary artery disease or systemic or pulmonary vascular disease. Table 2 represents the classification of cardiomyopathy and specific myocardial lesions as advocated by Shabetai[7] and in accordance with the recommendations of the World Health Organization. Another form of classification distinguishes between so-called primary and secondary cardiomyopathies. In the secondary type, the heart muscle abnormality is dependent upon a single cause or part of a systemic process while the primary is of unknown etiology and confined to the heart muscle alone. Still another schema is a functional classification which has three basic categories: dilated, hypertrophic and restrictive.

These remarks are intended to reinforce the nosologic complexity of myocardial diseases and the need to negotiate skilfully within the semantic maze that exists. Be that as it may, this text is not a suitable forum for debating the scientific merits of one classification over another. What we need for our purposes is a manageable vehicle for an orderly voyage through the historical background of myocardial lesions. It is for this reason that I now propose to dwell upon cardiomyopathy and myocarditis. The myocardial changes seen in coronary artery disease will be dealt with in Section 4.

For our purposes, the classification dividing cardiomyopathy into primary and secondary is probably the most useful because of its simplicity. We have already seen how the clinical significance of valvular deformities evolved with respect to their impact on the heart muscle. This would be, in this scheme, an example of secondary cardiomyopathy since the myocardial alteration can be ascribed to either volume or pressure overload on the basis of a valvular lesion. Let us turn now to primary cardiomyopathy and try not to get lost in the multiplicity of labels prior to the adoption of the term itself.

The concept that myocardial disease could exist independently of congenital or acquired lesions involving the valves, lungs, coronary arteries or hypertension is a relatively new one. It was Virchow who first labeled non-valvular heart disease as 'chronic myocarditis', with inflammation being the only cause of heart muscle disease[8]. Although since then it has become increasingly evident that almost any disease process, acute or chronic, may involve cardiac muscle, the label 'chronic myocarditis' became firmly entrenched in the clinical arena. This was especially so even as late

Table 2   Classification of cardiomyopathy and the specific myocardial diseases, according to Shabetai[7] and the World Health Organization

---

Idiopathic cardiomyopathy
    Acute
    Chronic, insidious onset
    Chronic, following acute
    Associated with
        Alcohol
        Peripartal state
        Familial predisposition
Chronic ischemic heart failure (due to coronary atherosclerosis)
    Associated with
        Overt myocardial infarction
        Covert myocardial infarction
        Diffuse scarring
Specific myocardial disease
    Myocarditis (inflammatory, infectious)
    Metabolic
    Infiltrative, granulomas, storage diseases
    Nutritional (deficiency)
    Amyloid
    Collagen vascular (connective tissue)
    Muscular dystrophies, neuromuscular disorders
    Toxic and sensitivity reactions

---

as the fourth and fifth decades of the 20th century. I remember many a death certificate assigning the cause of death to 'chronic myocarditis'. It was in reality a catch-all phrase for the ill-effects of hypertension and coronary artery disease since by this time the common occurrence of both hypertension and coronary artery disease was being recognized: the general feeling being that these two diseases were the causative factors for 'chronic myocarditis'. Old habits and attitudes among physicians are hard to change. The pervasive entrenchment of 'chronic myocarditis' persisted despite the fact that in 1933, Shields Warren, a pathologist, had documented the actual rarity of this lesion at autopsy[9]. Warren's paper did, however, stimulate a renewed interest in Krehl's work which had been reported as far back as 1891[10], and which concerned itself with non-valvular heart muscle disturbances that had no known etiology. The paper provided the spark for pathologists to search for all possible etiologic factors in any myocardial aberration that bore the label idiopathic or essential.

At a clinical level, it was Henry Christian in 1950 who widened the horizon by demonstrating that about one-third of non-inflammatory diseases of heart muscle could not be attributed to either hypertension or coronary artery disease[11]. The medical profession, initially skeptical, soon began to orient itself towards the valid existence of new categories of myocardial diseases with diverse etiologic factors and bearing no relationship to hypertension or coronary artery disease. In 1959, Thomas Mattingly reintroduced the term primary myocardial disease for this group of patients[12]. The term had been previously used by Josserand and Gallavardin of Lyon in 1901 but during the intervening years it had been consigned to obscurity[13].

Just two years before Mattingly, The Lancet published a paper written by Brigden describing uncommon myocardial diseases. Instead of calling them primary myocardial diseases, he introduced the label 'non-coronary cardiomyopathy'[14]. Soon after, Fowler and his group added their views to these pathologic entities but preferred to adopt Mattingly's label of primary myocardial disease[15]. There was further stirring of the pot with the appearance of other terms such as myocardiosis, myocardiopathy and cardiomyopathy. As more knowledge began to accumulate from such investigators as W.P. Harvey, Goodwin, Burch, Shabetai and many others, the term idiopathic myocardial disease was introduced to indicate a special category of myocardial alteration without known cause[16–19]. This, seemingly, resolved the semantic confusion by eliminating the word primary which had begun to have two connotations: primary as a synonym for idiopathic or as a label to denote the myocardium as being predominantly involved regardless of cause.

We are at the stage now where myocarditis is considered a specific myocardial lesion, and cardiomyopathy is the preferred term for any disease involving heart muscle. Cardiomyopathy can be subdivided further into primary or secondary. The primary type would be those lesions affecting the myocardium that have arisen *de novo* and independently of any systemic disturbance. Several of the known varieties are still called idiopathic, meaning without known cause. Secondary cardiomyopathy would represent disturbances of heart muscle in response to one or more diverse factors. These would include metabolic, endocrine, toxic, infiltrative or hypersensitivity determinants;

to present but a random selection within a constantly expanding etiologic base.

On pathological grounds, this distinction has helped to clear the way for greater precision in diagnosis by opening up multiple avenues of approach in the search for more and more etiologic factors. This, in turn, should hopefully eliminate eventually the idiopathic varieties and pave the way for a proper therapeutic modality.

For a long time myocarditis was, as Edens said, the 'stepchild of pathology'[20]. It is only within the past several decades, because of more intensive histologic studies and utilizing more rigid criteria, that this pathologic entity is now becoming better understood. Contrary to the connotations of old, amidst the confusion of the loosely used term 'chronic myocarditis', we now know that myocarditis is a specific myocardial lesion. It can be infectious or inflammatory in origin with a multitude of etiologic factors. The spectrum of the infectious agents ranges from the viral to the helminthic. The list is only as finite as the number of known organisms. The non-infectious inflammatory type of myocarditis is seen in collagen diseases and granulomatous processes.

Advancements in knowledge of the myocarditides have not been derived from the labors of one man or even a select group of men. Rather, these advancements have come about from the collective labors of numerous investigators from all over the world. It is impossible to single out one or even several outstanding individuals. The ease and rapidity of modern communications has helped in no small way to co-involve the efforts and expertise of many disciplines that transcend both academic and national boundaries.

A special word, however, must be said about the myocardial lesions of rheumatic fever. The cardiac lesions in this syndrome were always regarded as being localized to the endocardium or pericardium or both. It was not until the latter part of the 19th century that a few scattered reports began to appear concerning myocardial involvement as part of the disease. Among these were the reports of West[21] and Goodhart[22].

Although they did not describe the specific lesion of rheumatic fever, two German pathologists brought out and emphasized the important participation of the myocardium in the rheumatic fever syndrome as well as in other infections. Krehl published his report in 1890[23] and Romberg in 1894[24].

The specific myocardial lesion of rheumatic fever is the rheumatic nodule. Although it is known to us by the name Aschoff body, it was apparently described initially by F. J. Poynton in 1899[25]. Aschoff's description appeared in 1904[26]. Within the next decade, confirmations of Aschoff's description were quickly forthcoming. By 1914, a considerable body of literature had accumulated. At that time, Thalhimer and Rothschild wrote a review, including their own observations that served to establish the Aschoff body as a specific marker for rheumatic fever, past or present, regardless of the clinical history[27]. The Russian Talalaev, professor of pathology at Moscow University, also described in detail the pathogenesis and structural make-up of these rheumatic granulomas[28]. In Russia (naturally) they carry the eponym Aschoff-Talalaev granuloma.

The historical background of the more common cardiomyopathies may be found in those sections of this text dealing with separate disease entities or with the various factors known to affect the functional mechanisms of the circulatory system. I would like to devote the remainder of this chapter to an intriguing disturbance that is called, for lack of a better term, 'hypertrophic cardiomyopathy'.

Hypertrophic cardiomyopathy is an entity involving mainly the left ventricle and characterized by asymmetric or concentric hypertrophy. The cause is unknown. It is usually but not always associated with disarray of the myocardial fibers. Right ventricular involvement may occur either alone or in combination with the left ventricle. The pathophysiologic scenario and clinical manifestations are quite varied. Although ongoing studies continue to expand the clinical spectrum of hypertrophic cardiomyopathy, our knowledge concerning the basic cellular defect is still wanting.

The modern description of hypertrophic cardiomyopathy has evolved over the past 30 years or so. Prior to this, the gross anatomy of the syndrome was described by two 19th century French pathologists and an early 20th century German pathologist[29–31]. The French pathologists were Liouville and Hallopeau whose reports appeared in 1869. The German pathologist was A. Schmincke. His paper appeared in 1907. It was not until 1957 and 1958 that modern attention was drawn to this disease by the independent papers of Brock and Teare[32–34].

Brock wrote about the functional obstruction of the left ventricle caused by the asymmetrical hypertrophy of the ventricular septum in two papers; first in 1957 and then again in 1959. Both papers emanated from Guy's Hospital. In 1958, Teare reported on asymmetrical hypertrophy of the heart in young adults. His paper appeared in the *British Heart Journal* and was based on the postmortem findings of nine patients.

Subsequent to Teare's report, a number of papers appeared between the years 1959 and 1964 by many investigators among whom may be listed Brachfeld and Gorlin (1959)[35], Brent (1960)[36], Braunwald (1960)[37], Goodwin (1960)[38], Paré (1961)[39], Bjork (1961)[40], Menges (1961)[41], and Wigle (1962)[42].

These papers described variations of the cardiomyopathy under such descriptive terms as 'subaortic stenosis', 'idiopathic hypertrophic subaortic stenosis (IHSS)', 'obstructive cardiomyopathy', and 'hereditary cardiovascular dysplasia'[43]. As these papers indicate, Brock and Teare precipitated an intense interest in this peculiar disturbance of the myocardium.

Eight out of Teare's nine patients died suddenly. Postmortem findings revealed an asymmetrical hypertrophy of the interventricular septum. On histologic sectioning, short, plump hypertrophic myocardial fibers were seen arranged in a very haphazard manner. This started a stampede in support of the belief that the chaotic and bizarre architecture of the myocardial fibers in association with marked interstitial fibrosis was the specific pathological abnormality for hypertrophic cardiomyopathy.

The argument for specificity of the lesion now dubbed 'myocardial disarray' has been especially championed by the group at the National Institutes of Health in Bethesda, Maryland. A series of papers began to flow from this center written by Maron, Epstein, Ferrans, and W.C. Roberts, advancing the thesis that the myocardial disarray was a relatively sensitive and specific marker for hypertrophic cardiomyopathy[44].

Evidence against its specificity was marshalled by the following investigators: Paré (1961)[39], Stampbach (1962)[45], Snijder (1970)[46], Olsen (1971)[47], and Davies (1974)[48].

As more and more players entered the fray, it became evident that myocardial disarray could be seen in a variety of conditions, even congenital as well as in normal hearts. Van der Bel-Kahn documented its presence not only in normal hearts, but in such conditions as hypertension, cor pulmonale and coronary artery disease[49].

Further studies by the Bethesda group caused them to alter their initial statements with the revised claim that myocardial disarray can be considered as a highly sensitive and specific marker for obstructive cardiomyopathy *only* when considered in a quantitative rather than a qualitative fashion[50–52]. This is where we stand currently. Rest assured, more is yet to come.

Among the cardiomyopathies, there is a large group that has come to be called the dilated cardiomyopathies. These are distinct and separate from all the others. Dilated cardiomyopathy can occur during pregnancy or in the postpartum period; as a result of anthracycline; in chronic alcoholism and in selenium deficiency, among a host of etiologic agents. In many patients, however, the cause cannot be established and it is called idiopathic.

At necropsy, the most striking feature is the marked dilatation of both ventricular cavities. The heart is heavier than usual but there is no thickening of the muscle. On histologic study many of the muscle cells are larger than normal while others show atrophy. Electron microscopic studies have also demonstrated many changes at the ultrastructural level but, unfortunately, they are non-specific.

Knowledge of the morbid anatomy regarding this group of myocardial diseases shares the same historical background as the hypertrophic variety in its brevity and with essentially the same cast of investigators. There is one among them, however, who should be singled out for a more detailed presentation. He is George E. Burch of Tulane University.

George E. Burch was born in 1910 and died in 1986. He was a pioneer in the study of the cardiomyopathies, having made many contributions towards their pathologic anatomy including histochemical and electron microscopic studies[53]. His influence on the subject extended also to their classification by his descriptions of 'senile cardiomyopathy' and 'ischemic cardiomyopathy'[54,55].

George Burch received his medical degree from Tulane University in 1933 and strangely enough he was awarded the Bachelor of Science from the same university two years later. His entire professional life was spent at his alma mater. After postgraduate training at Charity Hospital in New Orleans and at the Rockefeller Institute in New York he returned to Tulane University in pursuit of his academic interests. At the age of 37 he was appointed Henderson Professor and Chairman of the Department of

Medicine, a position which he held until his retirement at the age of 65. He continued to work, however, until the day he died at the age of 76[56].

Burch was a prolific author and an accomplished investigator with wide interests. Although research always played a dominant role in his career, he was a teacher *par excellence*, and remained, forever, a clinician. Quality, accuracy, reliability, reproducibility and honesty were his basic tenets[56].

There are many aphorisms attributed to him. These are often referred to as 'Burchisms' or, as his medical students labeled them, 'quotations of Chairman George'[56]. These were concerned with food and eating, drugs and treatment, cardiac procedures, and a host of other topics. The following remarks on pathologists and pathology are in Roberts' biographical sketch[56]. 'Pathologists are like bankers. If Ludwig would come out of the grave, he could open his book and not be one day behind.' 'Nothing makes you more humble in medicine than the autopsy table.'

We shall come across this outstanding cardiologist of the 20th century several more times. He was responsible for a number of advancements in cardiovascular physiology. Although most of his interests concerned the veins, lymphatics and neurohumoral control of the circulation, he contributed a great deal towards an understanding of the climatic effects on the heart, electrocardiography and the cardiomyopathies. He was responsible also for the development of the technique of digital rheoplethysmography.

REFERENCES

1. Corvisart, J.N. (1818). *Essai sur les Maladies du Coeur*, 3rd. edn., p. 66

2. Laénnec, R. (1819). *De l'Auscultation médiate ou Traité de Diagnostic des Maladies des Poumons et du Coeur fondé Principalment sur ce Nouveau Moyen d'Exploration*, 2 vols., pp. 7–8. (Paris: Brosson and Chaudé)

3. Duffin, J.M. (1889). Cardiology of RTH Laénnec. *Medical History*, p. 49

4. Bertin, H.J. (1824). *Traité des Maladies du Coeur*, p. 283. (Paris)

5. Hope, J. (1834). *Principles and Illustrations of Morbid Anatomy*. (London)

6. Stokes, W. (1854). *Diseases of the Heart*, p. 302. (Dublin)

7. Shabetai, R. (1983). Cardiomyopathy: how far have we come in 25 years, how far to go? *J.A.C.C.*, **1**, 252–63

8. Virchow, R.L.K. (1858). *Die Cellularpathologie in ihrer Begründung auf physiologische und pathologische Geivebelehre*. (Berlin: A. Hirschwald)

9. Warren, S. (1933). The Pathology of Chronic Myocarditis. *N. Engl. J. Med.*, **208**, 573

10. Krehl, L. (1891). Beitrag zur Kentniss der idiopathischen Herzmushelk-rankungen. *Dtsch. Arch. Klin. Med.*, **48**, 414–31

11. Christian, H. (1950). Clinically the myocardium. *Arch. Intern. Med.*, **86**, 491–7

12. Mattingly, T.W. (1959). The clinical and hemodynamic features of primary myocardial disease. *Trans. Am. Clin. Climatol. Assoc.*, **70**, 132–41

13. Josserand, E. and Gallavardin, L. (1901). De L'Asystolie progressive des jeunes sujets per myocardite subaigue primitive. *Arch. Gen. Med.*, **6**, 684–704

14. Brigden, W. (1957). Uncommon myocardial diseases. The non-coronary cardio-myopathies. *Lancet*, **2**, 1179–243

15. Fowler, N.O., Gueron, M. and Rowlands, D.T. Jr. (1961). Primary myocardial disease. *Circulation*, **23**, 498–508

16. Harvey, W.P., Segal, J.P. and Gurel, T. (1964). The clinical spectrum of primary myocardial disease. *Prog. Cardiovasc. Dis.*, **7**, 17–42

17. Goodwin, J.F., Hollman, G.H., Gordon, H. and Bishop, A. (1961). Clinical aspects of cardiomyopathy. *Br. Med. J.*, **1**, 69–79

18. Burch, G.E., Walsh, J.J. and Block, W.C. (1963). Value of prolonged bed rest in management of cardiomegaly. *J.A.M.A.*, **183**, 81–7

19. Goodwin, J.F. (1982). The frontiers of cardiomyopathy. *Br. Heart J.*, **48**, 1–18

20. Edens, E. (1929). *Die Krankheiten des Herzens und der Gefässe*. (Berlin: Julus Springer)

21. West, S. (1878). Analysis of 40 cases of rheumatic fever. *St. Barth. Hosp. Rep.*, **14**, 221–3. (London)

22. Goodhart, J.F. (1879). Case of rapid enlargement of the heart. *Trans. Path. Soc.*, **30**, 279–81. (London)

23. Krehl, L. (1889–90). Beitrag zur Pathologie der Herzlappenfehler. *Dtsch. Arch. Klin. Med.*, **46**, 454–77. (Leipzig)

24. Romberg, E. (1894). Über die Bedeutung des Herzmuskels für die symptome und den Verlauf der acuten Endocarditis und der chronischen Klappenfehler. *Dtsch. Arch. Klin. Med.*, **53**, 144–88. (Leipzig)

25. Poynton, F.J. (1899). A case of rheumatic pericarditis and extreme dilatation of the heart. *Med. Chir. Trans.*, **32**, 355

26. Aschoff, L. (1904). Zur Myocarditisfrage. *Vehr. Dtsch. Ges. Pathol.*, **8**, 46–51

27. Thalhimer, W. and Rothschild, M.A. (1914). On the significance of the submiliary, myocardial nodules of Aschoff in rheumatic fever. *J. Exp. Med.*, **19**, 417–28

28. Talalaev, V.T. (1929). Acute rheumatism (pathogenesis, pathological anatomy and clinical anatomical classification) (Trans. from Russian). (Moscow-Leningrad)

29. Liouville, H. (1869). Retrecissement cardiaque sous aortique. *Gaz. Med.*, **24**, 161. (Paris)

30. Hallopeau, L. (1869). Retrecissement ventriculo-aortique. *Gaz. Med.*, **24**, 683. (Paris)

31. Schmincke, A. (1907). Ueber linksseitige muskulose conusstenosen. *Dtsch. Med. Woehenschr.*, **33**, 2082

32. Brock, R.C. (1957). Functional obstruction of the left ventricle. *Guys Hosp. Rep.*, **106**, 221–38

33. Brock, R.C. (1959). Functional obstruction of the left ventricle. *Guys Hosp. Rep.*, **108**, 126–33

34. Teare, R.D. (1958). Asymmetrical hypertrophy of the heart in young adults. *Br. Heart J.*, **20**, 1–8

35. Brachfeld, N. and Gorlin, R. (1959). Subaortic stenosis: a revised concept of the disease. *Medicine* (Baltimore) **38**, 415–33

36. Brent, L.B., Aburano, A. and Fischer, D.L. (1960). Familial muscular subaortic stenosis. An unrecognized form of 'idiopathic heart disease' with clinical and autopsy observations. *Circulation*, **21**, 167–80

37. Braunwald, E., Morrow, A.G., Cornell, W.P. *et al.* (1960). Idiopathic hypertrophic subaortic stenosis. *Am. J. Med.*, **29**, 924, 945

38. Goodwin, J.F., Hollman, A., Cleland, W.P. *et al.* (1960). Obstructive cardiomyopathy simulating aortic stenosis. *Br. Heart J.*, **22**, 403–14

39. Paré, J.A.P., Fraser, R.G. Pirozynski, W.J., Shanks, J.A and Stubington, D. (1961). Hereditary cardiovascular dysplasia: a form of familial cardiomyopathy. *Am. J. Med.*, **31**, 37–62

40. Bjork, V.O., Hultquist, G. and Lodin, H. (1961). Subaortic stenosis produced by an abnormally placed anterior mitral leaflet. *J. Thorac. Cardiovasc. Surg.*, **41**, 659–69

41. Menges, J.H. Bradenburg, R.D., Brown, A.L. Jr. (1961). The clinical, hemodynamic and pathological diagnosis of muscular subvalvular aortic stenosis. *Circulation*, **24**, 1126–36

42. Wigle, E.D., Heimbecker, R.O. and Gunton, R.W. (1962). Idiopathic ventricular septal hypertrophy causing muscular subaortic stenosis. *Circulation*, **26**, 325–40

43. Ciba Foundation Symposium (1964). *Cardiomyopathies*, pp. 49–69. (Churchill: London)

44. Maron, B.J. and Epstein, S.E. (1980). Hypertrophic cardiomyopathy. Recent observations regarding the specificity of three hallmarks of the disease: asymmetric septal hypertrophy, septal disorganization and systolic anterior motion of the anterior mitral leaflet. *Am. J. Cardiol.*, **45**, 141–54

45. Stampbach, O. and Senn, A. (1962). Die Idiopathische Hypertrophische Subaortenstenose. *Schweiz Med. Wochenschr.*, **92**, 125–30

46. Snijder, J., DeJong, J. and Meijer, A.E.F.H. (1970). Histopathological, enzyme-histochemical and electron-microscopical observations in hypertrophic obstructive cardiomyopathy. A preliminary report. *Pathol. Microbiol.*, **35**, 81–5. (Basel)

47. Olsen, E.G.J. (1971). *Morbid Anatomy and Histology of Hypertrophic Obstructive Cardiomyopathy.* In Wolstenholme, G.E.W. and O'Connor, M. (eds.) *Hypertrophic Obstructive Cardiomyopathy*, pp. 183–91. (Ciba Foundation Study Group 37). (London: Churchill Livingstone)

48. Davies, M.J., Pomerance, A. and Teare, R.D. (1974). Pathological features of hypertrophic obstructive cardiomyopathy. *J. Clin. Pathol.*, **27**, 529–35

49. Van der Bel-Kahn, J. (1977). Muscle fiber disarray in common heart diseases. *Am. J. Cardiol.*, **40**, 355–64

50. Maron, B.J., Sato, N., Roberts, W.C., Edwards, J.E. and Chandra, R.S. (1979). Quantitative analysis of cardiac muscle cell disorganization in the ventricular septum. Comparison of fetuses and infants with and without congenital heart disease and patients with hypertrophic cardiomyopathy. *Circulation*, **60**, 685–96

51. Maron, B.J., Anan, T.J. and Roberts, W.C. (1981). Quantitative analysis of the distribution of cardiac muscle cell disorganization in the left ventricular wall of patients with hypertrophic cardiomyopathy. *Circulation*, **63**, 882–94

52. Maron, B.J. and Roberts, W.C. (1981). Hypertrophic cardiomyopathy and cardiac muscle cell disorganization revisited; relation between the two and significance. *Am. Heart J.*, **102**, 95–110

53. Ferrans, V.J. (1989). Pathologic anatomy of the

dilated cardiomyopathies. *Am. J. Cardiol.*, **64**, 9C–10C

54. Burch, G.E. and Giles, T.D. (1972). Ischemic cardiomyopathy. *South. Med. J.*, **65**, 11–16

55. Burch, G.E. and Giles, T.D. (1971). Senile cardiomyopathy. *J. Chronic Dis.*, **24**, 1–3

56. Roberts, W.C. (1989). George Edward Burch, (1910–86). *Am. J. Cardiol.*, **64**, 3C–8C

7   Pericardial disease

Although we can trace the historical background of pericardial disease as far back as antiquity, the information throughout the centuries is, for the most part, a collection of isolated, usually vague, rather incomplete and often inaccurate observations. It was not until the 18th century with the publication of various compendia that any semblance of order began to emerge. But, as in so many other aspects of cardiology, it has been only within the past three decades or so that we have seen tremendous strides made in pericardial lore. The explosion in knowledge has been the result of the combined efforts of cardiologists, physiologists, pathologists and others from widely diverse disciplines. Among the modern cardiologists who have played a prominent role in this field we must include as major figures Fowler, Shabetai, Gunteroth, Reddy, Friedman and Spodick. Along with these men the members of the Bethesda group have been singularly important in their observations on the ultrastructure of the pericardium.

In an attempt to follow a chronological order and yet not get lost in the maze of descriptive terms with different meanings, it appears to me that a simplified but structured mode of presentation would be to follow, though not too rigidly, the classification of pericardial diseases currently in vogue. This classification consists of five major categories: acute pericarditis, pericardial effusion, constrictive pericarditis, specific forms of pericarditis and congenital absence or defects of the pericardium. In the specific form category this would include those types of pericardial disturbances that are due to infectious agents, neoplasms, radiation, renal failure, immunologic factors, and so on. This list gets longer and longer as time goes on.

Originally attention was drawn to the pericardium primarily by the finding at postmortem of fluid within the pericardial sac or of inflammatory lesions. Since inflammatory lesions so often induce effusion they can be presented together.

The first description of pericardial effusion is attributed to Galen who observed it in a monkey he was dissecting[1]. This was long after Hippocrates. It is not surprising that the works of Hippocrates fail to mention pathologic alterations of the pericardium. It must be recalled that Hippocrates held firmly to the belief that the heart was inviolate and could not be a target for disease. The Alexandrian, Erasistratus (c 310–250 BC) may have been the first to stray from this belief. His writings indicate that he was aware of both pleuritis and pericarditis. He searched for their causes but unfortunately his concepts regarding the causes of disease were based on the factor of plethora (hyperemia) and completely out of tune with reality.

Nothing more can be found on either pericarditis or effusion until the 12th century when Avenzoar described serofibrinous pericarditis[2–5]. He is also known as Ibn-Zuhr. Referred to often as the 'Famous Wise Man', he is probably one of the greatest of the Spanish Moslem physicians. Avenzoar was born in Cordova, Spain, in 1113. He spent most of his life in Arabia but finally returned to his native country, dying there in 1162. Six medical works are attributed to him but only three of them have survived. All of his references to the heart including his description of serofibrinous pericarditis are to be found in his *Theiser* which is the latinized form of *al Taysir fi al-Mudawak w-al-Tadbir*. This is the most popular of the three extant works although it is said to be a diffuse and rambling composition based upon Aristotelian premises. Avenzoar gained renown for not sharing the views of Galen and Avicenna. He apparently wrote the *Theiser* late in life at the request of his close friend, Averroes. The latter incorporated the *Theiser* into the great medical encyclopedia that he wrote and which was titled *Colliget*[6].

Another hiatus ensued until the 15th century when Antonio Benivieni, the noted surgeon of Florence and Padua, described examples of fibrinous pericarditis among the twenty postmortem examinations that constituted his posthumously published *De Abditis Nonnulus ac Mirandis Morborum ac Sanationum Causis*[7]. He described the fibrin as being thick and stringy and labeled the entire alteration as 'cor villosum'.

During the 16th century, Guillame de Baillou described pericardial effusion in his treatise *Consiliorum Medicinalum Libri II*. This was published in Venice 119 years after his death. De Baillou was born in 1538 and died in 1616. He was a student of Fernel at Paris, and after graduation remained there to become eventually dean of the faculty of medicine. When discussing palpitation, he mentioned that it was a manifestation of pericardial effusion. It seems strange but true – all his works were published after his death.

A case of hemorrhagic pericardial effusion was presented by William Harvey in his second essay, *De Circulatione Sanguinis*[8]. A ruptured myocardium was the cause of the blood escaping into the pericardial sac. Incidentally, this essay was dedicated to Jean Riolan of France.

Observations and interpretations on the pathology and impact of pericardial disease continued in the 18th century in a more systematic manner. Of course, the whole field was dominated by the great Morgagni with clinical correlation being increasingly emphasized[9]. Morgagni's observations, as outlined in Epistles 16, 22, 53(3), and 63 (4 and 5), led him to the conclusion that pericarditis was commonly associated with pleuritis. He described the clinical and pathological findings in 45 cases. Morgagni also observed and commented on hemopericardium. He was able to establish several causes for blood in the pericardial cavity. Ironically, he died from one of them, namely, rupture of the myocardium. In one of his cases, the hemopericardium was due to puncture of a coronary artery. He also pointed out that not all wounds of the heart were immediately fatal. The development and swiftness of a tamponade were, in his belief, the deciding lethal factors. This was a very shrewd conclusion since physiologists had yet to come to grips regarding pericardial effusion, *per se*, and cardiac tamponade.

During the same century, Sénac also described both pericarditis and pericardial effusion. He referred to the effusion as 'hydrops pericardii', and commented on the relationship between pericarditis, pneumonia, pleurisy, and mediastinitis[10].

No further reports of merit on the descriptive pathology of acute pericarditis appeared until the 19th century; a century of grandeur and remarkable advances in bedside clinical evaluation. Gabriel Andral (1797–1876), professor of pathology, presented in a clear manner the pathological picture of acute fibrinous pericarditis in his *Clinique Médicale* which was published from 1829–33. Although it added nothing new to the pathogenesis of acute pericarditis, even though it was written from the perspective of a pathologist, the work is, nonetheless, meritorious since it called attention to the fact that the chest pain in this disease can simulate that of angina pectoris[11].

William Stokes also reported his observations on acute fibrinous pericarditis but these were clinical rather than anatomical. He did bring out the occasional occurrence of pericarditis prior to the arthritis in rheumatic fever.

Corvisart was one of the first to conceptualize pancarditis. His observations on the pericardium are to be found in his *Essay*[12]. His analogy for the postmortem appearance of fibrinous pericarditis, as already noted, was the 'reticulum of the second stomach of the calf'. The *Essay* also contains an account of massive pericardial effusion in which the pericardial sac contained four liters of fluid. Corvisart also recognized the existence of what we would categorize today as specific forms of pericarditis, notably that form due to tuberculosis.

Laénnec, too, described the morbid anatomy of both pericarditis and pericardial effusion[13]. He recognized that pericarditis can be either acute or chronic. He recorded the occurrence of isolated and even localized pericarditis. Hydropericardium was his term for pericardial effusion. He coined the term 'pneumopericardium' as well as 'pneumohydropericardium', when fluid is present in association with air. We shall speak of both Laénnec and Corvisart again in connection with constrictive pericarditis.

In 1832, Hope's tome on cardiovascular physiology and clinico-pathologic correlations went into considerable detail on both inflammatory pericardial effusion and acute pericarditis[14]. It emphasized the association of both with rheumatic fever. The book was based on 1000 cases. It was so well accepted that it went into three editions, the third one being in 1839, in which the clinical aspects were amplified rather than the morbid anatomy.

The first description of a syndrome called idiopathic pericarditis was rendered by Hodges in 1854[15]. This was a clinical rather than a pathological description. A few years later another clinical description of the same syndrome was described by Bäumler[16]. He reported three cases, one of which was himself.

Knowledge concerning specific forms of pericarditis has evolved over the years in concert with the advances made in bacteriology, immunology and oncology. Among the earliest observers of specific forms of pericarditis was, as already mentioned, Corvisart. This he did with his description of tubercles in the pericardium and the resultant pericarditis in association with pulmonary and mediastinal tuberculosis. Laénnec too described tubercles in the pericardium. In his classification of diseases of the pericardium, one of his categories is 'accidental productions in the pericardium'[17], and it is therein that we find tubercles as an example of 'accidental productions'. The inclusion of tubercles under this category is somewhat confusing to me. His description of 'accidental productions' leads me to believe that Laénnec meant all new tissue that was non-inflammatory in origin. Yet, we know that a tubercle is a granuloma with an inflammatory component. He does admit that it is impossible to ascertain the nature of such 'morbid growths'. His description of this category is as follows:

Various species of accidental productions have been found between the pericardium properly so-called, and the pleura; also between it and the internal and serous membrane; and, lastly, between the serous membrane and the heart. In the Sepulchretum of Bonetus and other collections of cases, we find examples of what appear to be tubercles, cancerous tumours, or cysts, in the different situations just mentioned. But the imperfect knowledge of membranes before the time of Bichat, and the general confusion of all accidental productions under the names of Scirrhus, Carcinoma, Atheroma, etc., renders it impossible to ascertain precisely either the nature or site of such morbid growths: I have already noticed the fatty productions, in the form of a cock's comb, developed occasionally between the pleura and fibrous membrane of the pericardium. Twice or thrice I have found tubercles in the same situation, in subjects which exhibited a great number of these bodies in the lungs and elsewhere. I have also seen a tubercle

situated at the point of the origin of the pulmonary artery and beneath the serous membrane of the pericardium.

At least, the above description leaves no doubt that Laénnec was describing tuberculous pericarditis, a specific form of the malady.

An interesting type of specific pericarditis is that associated with uremia. It is a frequent and serious complication of chronic renal failure. Bright noted its presence in 8% of autopsied patients with chronic renal failure. He reported this from Guy's Hospital in 1836[18]. Uremic pericarditis is still seen quite often. Even the advent of dialysis has not diminished to any notable degree the frequency of its occurrence. It can occur even during the first few months of therapy with dialysis.

The list of investigators who have helped pinpoint the multitude of agents or factors responsible for the initiation of the various types of specific as opposed to idiopathic pericarditis is quite lengthy. It would serve no purpose to enumerate them, primarily because of the multidisciplinary approach of modern medical research, and secondarily because no new historical perspectives would be added in such an exercise.

Constrictive pericarditis is also known as pericardial adhesions or chronic pericardial adhesions. Stray references are to be found in earlier medical writings. The description varies according to the observer's background and powers of observation. As time went on, such terms as callous, calcified or ossified were used. A non-incriminating label used by some writers was 'concretio cordis cum pericarditis'. Another interesting label is the 'Hairy Hearts of Hoary Heroes' which Spodick uses in the title of his paper dealing with the medical history of the pericardium[19]. Finally, because of the widespread interest generated by Pick, the clinical syndrome was given the eponym, Pick's disease. The eponym is hardly used today with the preferred term being constrictive pericarditis.

One of the most striking features of adhesive pericarditis could be a shaggy appearance at postmortem. Since most of the observations of this abnormality in early times were made in men who died during battle, it required just a step to equate the shagginess with the hairy-chested appearance of these noble warriors, who, by dying in battle, displayed their valor and heroism. Spodick, in his classical paper on the medical history of the pericardium, recites in detail descriptions of this relationship in the writings of Valerius Maximus, Pliny and Homer[20]. The descriptions by Maximus and Pliny are actual but that of Homer appears to be purely literary rather than literal.

Quoting freely from Spodick's paper, the descriptions by Maximus and Pliny are as follows:

> More marvelous than his eyes was the heart of Aristomenes, the Messenian; this the Athenians cut out because of his extraordinary cunning and found it stuffed with hair, after he had been caught several times and had escaped by his slyness and they (finally) seized him (permanently).

The same story is given, with more detail, and in the context of an already established belief in the hairy hearts of heroes, by Pliny in his *Natural History* (published before AD 79):

> It is related certain men are born with hairy hearts, and that no others are of greater energy, for example, Aristomenes, The Messenian, who killed 300 Lacaedaemonians. Wounded and captured once, he escaped through a cave in a quarry, following the narrow passage used by foxes. Captured a second time, when his guards were overcome by sleep, he rolled to the fire and burned off his thongs together with (some of) his body. When he was captured a third time, the Lacaedaemonians cut out his heart while he still lived, and a hairy heart was found.

Boyd and Elias recount how several centuries later another description of a hairy heart is to be found in the writings of Hesychius of Alexandria. The cadaver this time was not a fallen soldier but a rhetorician known as Hermogenes[21]. Observations of the same sort were recorded by Muretti and Benivieni in the 16th century. Muretti attached the label 'cor hirsutism' while Benivieni described it as 'cors pilis refertum' (a heart stuffed with hair)[22]. Benivieni also correlated this finding with the subject's character during life. The corpse was that of a recidivistic thief. This led Benivieni to advance the opinion that the hairy heart represented a certain amount of indomitable will in a man guilty of turpitude[23].

Fabrizio Bartoletti (c 1630) presented many interesting clinical and pathological correlations in his *Methodus in Dyspnoeam Bononiae*, among which were his observations on pericardial adhesions and fatty accumulation in the pericardium[24]. A clearer presentation of correlation, however, was that of Richard Lower of Cornwall.

Richard Lower (1631–91), a physiologist and clinician rather than a pathologist, presented the limiting effect of pericardial adhesions on the muscular behavior of the heart. He wrote from the same physiologic perspective when he discussed the tamponade effect of pericardial effusion. In his description of the autopsy findings in a London woman of 30, he states that the pericardial sac, instead of being thin and translucent, had become 'thick, opaque and almost callous'. His treatment of both effusion and adhesions are to be found in his *Tractatus de Corde*, published in London in 1669[25].

His younger contemporary at Oxford, and a fellow Cornishman, John Mayow, also reported in 1674 a case of pericardial adhesions that he had personally observed. Mayow describes the heart as being nearly covered by cartilage, and 'adherent to its interior', impeding the flow of blood into the ventricle[26].

Another careful observer of the 17th century was the brilliant Parisian clinician, Theophile Bonet (Bonetus) (1620–89). Pericardial adhesions were thought by him to be the cause of palpitation. The term he used for palpitation was 'cordis tremor'. He also described the pulse in pericardial effusion as having an ant-like quality (formicans). By this he meant 'small and intermittent'. His famous opus *Sepulchretum sive Anatomia Practica ex Cadaveribus Morbo Denatis* was published, according to some sources, initially in 1679 and then again in 1706[27]. Is it too banal to discuss an apparent confusion of dates and spelling with regard to Bonet's tome? Some secondary sources place the publication date of the first edition in the year 1679. This would mean the work appeared three years before Morgagni was born. Other sources refer to the word 'Denatis' in the title as 'de natis' or 'Donatus'. Is all this important? Probably not, but in an attempt to be as accurate as possible, I refer the reader to Figure 1 which depicts the frontispiece of the tome. Please note that the word in the title is 'Denatis' and that the date of publication for Bonet's *Tomus Primus* is MDCC (1700).

Be that as it may, Bonet's tome was considered for many years as the standard reference work on pathologic anatomy. Despite this fact, and its excellence for the time, Morgagni was less than satisfied with it, and possibly for this reason attempted to improve the situation by recording his

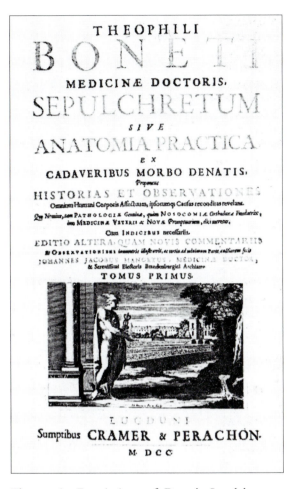

THEOPHILI
BONETI
MEDICINÆ DOCTORIS.
SEPULCHRETUM
SIVE
ANATOMIA PRACTICA
EX
CADAVERIBUS MORBO DENATIS.
HISTORIAS ET OBSERVATIONES

TOMUS PRIMUS

Sumptibus CRAMER & PERACHON.
M DCC

Figure 1 Frontispiece of Bonet's Sepulchretum. *Photo Source University of Central Florida. Literary Source East, T.: The Story of Heart Disease. Wm. Dawson & Sons, Ltd., London, Plate 8B, 1957. Taken from the Library of the Medical School, King's College Hospital, London. With Permission*

own observations, using the prevailing affectation of the time, namely, letters or epistles to a friend[28].

By the end of the 17th century, several other investigators added their observations on constrictive pericarditis. Among these was Giorgio Baglivi (1668–1706) who likened the calcification of the pericardium to a 'heart invested in a mortar sheath'[29]. Baglivi should be recalled as the celebrated student of Malpighi who, in turn, performed the autopsy on his mentor when Malpighi died as a result of a massive cerebral hemorrhage[30].

Both Vieussens (1641–1716) and Lancisi (1654–1720) straddle the latter part of the 17th and the early years of the 18th century. We will come across these two notables many times in this text. Both, as leading contributors to the field of cardiology, left legacies remarkable for their accuracy and prescience. Vieussens described the morbid anatomy of pericardial adhesions, commented on the impact that the condition had on cardiac function, and also elaborated on the diagnostic features of pericardial effusion. His description of how he removed a quart of fluid from the pericardial sac after the patient's face had become darker and the pulse thready and rapid should be read in the original to appreciate its vividness[31]. These observations were published in his *Traité Nouveau de la Structure et des Causes du Mouvement Natural du Coeur*.

Lancisi also described pericardial adhesions and stressed their importance as a cause of heart disease. There is no need to dwell further on his highly intellectual and fascinating personality since we have already dealt with him at some length elsewhere.

Another important figure of this period is Francesco Ippolito Albertini (1662–1738). Albertini had excellent credentials. Born near that great center of learning, Bologna, he became a pupil of Malpighi, had as his colleague and friend, Valsalva, and was a teacher of Morgagni. He too, stressed the importance of clinicopathologic correlation. Unfortunately, he added nothing new to constrictive pericarditis but he was, at least, frank enough to admit the difficulty of diagnosing the condition. His legacy was *De Affectionibus Cordis*, an outstanding work that appeared in 1726. It must be emphasized that during his career, the anchor sheet of diagnostic modalities consisted only of inspection and palpation. Therefore, this man's perspicacity and ability, as manifested in his work, become even more noticeable when one realizes how difficult it would be to have a high rate of accuracy in antemortem diagnosis with these primitive tools. Indeed, he proved to be quite humble when he admitted how difficult the diagnostic aspect of medical practice was when he wrote in 1726: 'I know from long attentive observation and experience in the dissection of bodies after death, that diagnosis is the branch of the healing art in which the greatest number of mistakes is made'. Fortunately, we have come a long way since then with our present array of technological aids.

During the 18th and 19th centuries, those who played a role in the morbid anatomy of constrictive pericarditis were Sénac, Haller, Morgagni, Corvisart,

Burns, Warren, Kreysig, Laénnec, Adams, Griesinger, Kussmaul and Wilks. Notice how the cast of players is increasing. In the general field of pathology, and in terms of pure description, Morgagni, as stated before, towers above them all, but he did not add much to this particular abnormality. Haller was more of a physiologist than a pathologist but his contribution here is still relevant. The others, as we shall see, added building blocks to the clinical edifice rather than new anatomical information.

Sénac we already know and will meet again because of his many contributions to other aspects of cardiology. On a clinical basis, he outlined the differential diagnosis between pericardial effusion and pleural effusion stressing the value of inspection and palpation. On pericardial adhesions he stressed the mechanical effects on the heart. Haller was not the first to describe calcification of the pericardium but he is credited as being the first to do so in a very detailed manner. The description is to be found in his *Opuscula Pathologica*. It is based on postmortem material that he personally observed[32]. The description as taken from Cardiac Classics is as follows[33]:

> … the pericardium of the heart and the pleura of the lungs were everywhere attached, and all over the surface of the pericardium were white hard masses, some firm and some filled with white material like pus. These hard swellings were totally and indissolubly united to the pericardium by bands. The semi-stone-like inferior part of the right ventricle was strongly adherent to the pericardium by a mass of tophaceous calculi like fine sand. The sinus between the two membranes of the aortic valve was hard and in part stony.

Figure 2 illustrates the title page of *Opuscula Pathologica*.

Morgagni also recognized and described pericardial adhesions and calcification of the pericardium. He did not subscribe to the view, held in some circles, that the adhesions could be congenital in origin.

During the discourse on acute pericarditis, I brought out Corvisart's comments on the massive deposition of fibrin and its similarity in appearance to the reticulum of the second stomach of the calf. Corvisart does not go into further detail, but is it possible that he was describing pericardial adhesions

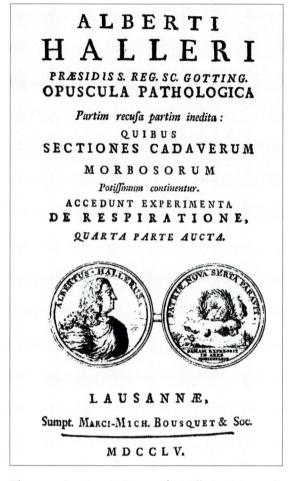

Figure 2 Frontispiece of Haller's 'Opuscula Pathologica'. *Photo Source University of Central Florida. Literary Source Willius FA, Keys TE: Cardiac Classics. The C.V. Mosby Co., St. Louis, MO., 1941. Courtesy of the Mayo Clinic*

rather than an acute fibrinous process? We do know that constrictive pericarditis is initiated by an acute process characterized by fibrin deposition and not all such cases need end up with dense scarring and calcification.

In 1809, Allan Burns described and discussed pericardial adhesions in his book, noting that, at times, the pericardium was completely matted to contiguous structures. This is the same Burns who, despite the lack of a medical degree, was able to command respect and admiration because of sheer ability. Apparently, the lack of a formal degree did not deter him from advising that on physical examination the possibility of adhesive pericarditis should be entertained 'where also no change takes place in the spot where the pulsation is felt in the chest when the patient turns from side to side, we are assisted in the diagnosis'[34].

Laénnec listed ossification as the last of the categories in his classification of diseases of the pericardium (see Table 1, Chapter 6). He came across ossification between the layers of the pericardium only once but the case intrigued him so much that he described the pathological findings in detail. The autopsy was done on a 65 year old man who died after a long illness characterized by breathlessness on exertion but without orthopnea, by dropsy and lips that were 'swollen and violet'. On postmortem,

> ... the heart was enlarged, and adhered throughout to the pericardium by means of very close cellular attachments. On first touching it, it seemed to be quite inclosed in a bony case, situated beneath the fibrous membrane of the pericardium; but on further examination this incrustation was found to be incomplete. Around the base of the ventricles there was a zone or band, partly bony and partly cartilaginous of from one to two finger's breadth of unequal thickness, flattened, yet somehow rough on its surface. This band projected into the angle between the ventricles and auricles, and extended along the interventricular septum on both sides, to near the apex of the heart. The whole of this production was contained between the fibrous membrane of the pericardium and the serous membrane which lines it internally[35].

Figure 3 is the frontispiece of Forbes' translation of Laénnec's text containing his comments on the pericardium.

This and Haller's description are quite vivid word-pictures of advanced and calcified chronic constrictive pericarditis. But, for those who are interested in 'tidbits' of medical lore, as found in the lay literature, what could be a more titillating morsel than Nathaniel Hawthorne's tale of the ultimate fate of Ethan Brand who truly had a 'heart of stone'[36].

> With his long pole in his hand, he (Bartram) ascended to the top of the kiln. After a moment's pause, he called his son. 'Come up here Joe!' he said. So little Joe ran up the hillock, and stood by his father's side. The marble was all burnt into perfect, snow-white lime. But on its surface, in

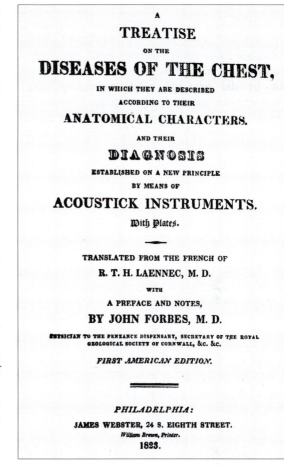

Figure 3 Frontispiece of Forbes' translation of Laénnec's text containing his comments on the pericardium. *Photo Source University of Central Florida. Literary Source Willius FA, Keys TE: Cardiac Classics. The C.V. Mosby Co., St. Louis, MO., 1941. Courtesy of the Mayo Clinic*

the midst of the circle, snow-white, too, and thoroughly converted into lime, lay a human skeleton, in the attitude of a person who, after long toil, lies down to long repose. Within the ribs strange to say was the shape of a human heart. 'Was the fellow's heart made of marble?' cried Bartram, in some perplexity at the phenomenon. 'At any rate, it is burnt into what looks like special good lime; and, taking all the bones together, my kiln is half a bushel richer for him', so saying, the rude lime-burner lifted his pole, and, letting it fall upon the skeleton, the relics of Ethan Brand were crumbled into fragments.

Robert Adams (of heart block fame) also observed and commented on pericardial lesions[37]. His view of why cardiac enlargement can be found in the presence of pericardial adhesions is most interesting. He believed that the increased vascularity brought about by the adhesions secondarily nourished the heart muscle causing it to enlarge. This was a fascinating bit of conjecture. Adams anticipated by about a century the anatomical rationale of Claude Beck's procedure for vascularizing the myocardium in coronary artery disease.

Stokes also observed that cardiac hypertrophy might accompany pericardial adhesions, but he did not feel that this enlargement was necessarily the case nor did it occur with absolute regularity as contended by Adams[38]. Hope shared the same opinion as Adams declaring, as Spodick recounts, that he had 'never examined after death a case of complete adhesion of the pericardium without finding enlargement of the heart'[15, 39]. Another view advanced by other observers was that the heart in constrictive pericarditis should be small because of the constricting effect of the adhesions. At around this time, Norman Chevers became involved in the controversy. He put forth the notion that pericardial adhesions could be either constricting or non-constricting. This, of course, is obvious to us today since the pathophysiologic effect on the heart is dependent upon the extent and severity of the adhesions. He, too, observed that, at times, the pericardial adhesions were accompanied by cardiac enlargement. In these cases, he maintained that the cause of the cardiac enlargement was independent of that for the pericardial adhesions. He went on to say that when the adhesions were extensive enough to exert a constricting effect on the heart, then atrophy of the heart would ensue. Chevers' observations and comments are to be found in a paper published in the Guy's Hospital Reports and is entitled *Observations on the Diseases of the Orifices and Valves of the Aorta*[40]. His remarks on the subject appear to be directed primarily to Hope who was held in such esteem by his contemporaries, that his words carried considerable clout. Chevers' comments read as follows:

> With deference of this high authority [referring to Hope], I must venture to suggest that the above remarks can be applied only to one class of case of this description – to those in which, super-added to adhesion of the pericardium

there is also disease of the valvular passages of the heart; these cases certainly are the most frequent, but I think a sufficient number of contrary instances have occurred under my own notice, to prove that where the valves are healthy, complete and close adhesion of the pericardial surface, far from producing hypertrophy of the heart and vessels, has a tendency to be followed by general diminution in the size of the heart and its vessels and contraction of its cavities …
> The principal cause of dangerous symptoms of the above description appears to arise from the occurrence of gradual contraction in the layer of adhesive matter which has been deposited around the heart, compressing its muscular tissue and embarrassing its systolic and diastolic movement, but more particularly the latter. The ventricles having become diminished in capacity, make up for this loss by the rapidity of their contractions …

Chever's conclusions are easier to accept by noting the logical presentation of his subject matter.

Further observations were made by Griesinger in 1854, Wilks in 1870–71, and Kussmaul in 1873. These papers, however, did not generate much interest. In fact, a long hiatus existed between the pathological descriptions of the early 19th century and those of Friedel Pick in 1896[41]. Pick's report originating from Pribam's clinic in Prague brought about such a resurgence of interest in constrictive pericarditis that a deluge of case reports emanated from many centers with controversial issues being raised as to its cause, relationship to tuberculosis and physiologic impact on the heart's function as a pump. Since, at times, the pericardial adhesions were noted in association with inflammatory changes in the peritoneum and with the frosted spleen and liver (Zuckergussleber) of Curschmann, the term polyserositis was suggested to denote the entire disease process[42].

Historically, tuberculosis was a leading cause of constrictive pericarditis. It is no longer the case. Unfortunately, most of the cases seen today are of unknown etiology. Some are seen with auto-immune diseases such as rheumatoid arthritis and systemic lupus erythematosus. Still others are found in association with malignancy or following mediastinal radiation. Charcot was the first to describe its occurrence in rheumatoid arthritis[43]. He reported the presence of pericardial fibrosis in 4 of 9 autopsied cases, presenting these findings at a meeting of the Sydenham Society in London in 1891.

During the early part of the 20th century further reports on the morbid anatomy and clinical correlates were made by Volhard (1923), Fischer (1926) and B. Schur (1934). Interest in the disease, however, had declined once more until the appearance of Paul D. White's series of papers beginning in 1935 and ending (in collaboration with co-workers) in 1948 with an analysis of a total of 53 cases[44-46]. White not only restimulated interest in constrictive pericarditis but he was also instrumental, along with Claude Beck, for laying the groundwork for surgical relief. In 1951, Burwell added his contribution to the pot by describing some of the effects on the pulmonary circulation[47].

Continuing research in the field is successfully reducing the number of so-called idiopathic cases. An example of this is the report by Lindsay and his co-workers which appeared in 1970, and which describes the occurrence of chronic constrictive pericarditis following uremic hemopericardium[48].

A few brief statements will suffice to cover congenital absence of the pericardium, the last category I loosely followed. It was first described by Realdus Columbus in 1559. The first antemortem diagnosis though was not made until 1959 (four hundred years later)[49]. Not to be outdone, Galen did mention congenital absence of the pericardium prior to Columbus[50]. However, Galen (like so many physicians, past, present, and future), 'often wrong, but never in doubt', mistook pericardial adhesions for congenital absence of the pericardium.

During the past 30 years or so, 5 major books have been published on the pericardium and its diseases. Brilliant advances have been made in the morbid anatomy of the ultrastructure, in the elucidation of the functional aberrations that occur, and in chipping away at the idiopathic mantle. I have mentioned already the major figures currently involved in this field. We are now in the last decade of the 20th century, and we can point with pride to all these achievements. Progress marches on! Or does it? Despite this attempt at closing on a high note, we must emphasize that physicians in their daily practice have yet to catch up in their diagnostic acumen with all the brilliant achievements described in these pages. Sir William Osler, as usual, stated a truism, which still prevails, when he wrote in 1892, 'no serious disease is so frequently overlooked by the practitioners as is pericardial heart disease'[51].

REFERENCES

1. Galen, C. *De Affectionibus Localis*, Book V and Book VII.

2. Castiglioni, A. (1941). *A History of Medicine*, pp. 276–7. (New York: Alfred A. Knopf)

3. Garrison, F.H. (1929). *An Introduction to the History of Medicine*, p. 132.

4. Herrick, J.B. (1942). *A Short History of Cardiology*, p. 11. (Illinois: Charles C. Thomas)

5. Vierordt, Hermann (1903). Geschichte der Herzkrankheiten. In Puschmann, Theodor (ed.) *Handbuch der Geschichte der Medizin*, vol. 2, pp. 632–3. (Jena: Gustav Fischer)

6. Mettler, C.C. (1947). *History of Medicine*, p. 359. (Philadelphia: The Blakiston Co.)

7. Benivieni, A. (1507). *De Abditis Nonnulus ac Mirandis Morborum ac Sanationum Causis*. (Florence: Giunta Press)

8. Harvey, W. (1649). *De Circulatione Sanguinis: Exercitatis Altera, Ad J Riolanum*. (Cambridge: Roger David)

9. Morgagni, J.B. (1756). *De Sedibus et Causis Morborum per Anatomen Indigatis*. (Louvain: Typographica Academica)

10. Sénac, J.B. (1778). *Traité de la Structure du Coeur, de son Action et de Ses Maladies*, 2nd edn. (Paris)

11. White, P.D. (1944). *Heart Disease*, p. 958. (New York: The MacMillan Co.)

12. Corvisart, J.N. (1812). *An Essay on the Organic Diseases and Lesions of the Heart and Great Vessels*, p. 50. (Philadelphia)

13. Laénnec, R.T.H. (1819). *De l'Auscultation médiate ou Traité de Diagnostic des Maladies des Poumous et du Coeur fondé Principalment sur ce Nouveau Moyen d'Exploration*. (Paris: Brosson and Chaudé)

14. Hope, J. (1839). *A Treatise on the Diseases of the Heart and Great Vessels, Comprising a New View of the Heart's Action*. 1st edn., 1832; 3rd edn. (London: W. Kidd)

15. Spodick, D.H. (1970). Medical history of the pericardium. *Am. J. Cardiol.*, **26**, 447–54

16. Bäumler, C. (1871). Drei Fälle von Perikarditis Acuta. *Clin. Soc. Trans.*, **5**, 8

17. Laénnec, R.T.H. (1819). *Op. cit.* Book Third, Chap. 2, Section Third. In Willius, F.A. and Keys, T.E. (1941). *Cardiac Classics*, p. 378. (St. Louis: C.V. Mosby Co.)

18. Bright, R. (1836). Tabular view of the morbid appearance in 100 cases connected with albuminous urine, with observations. *Guy's Hosp. Rep.*, **1**, 380

19. Spodick, D.H. (1970). *Op. cit.*, p. 447
20. *Ibid.*, p. 448
21. *Ibid.*, p. 448, Quoting Boyd, L.J. and Elias, H. (1955). Contributions to diseases of the heart and pericardium. 1. Historical introduction. *Bull. NY Med. Coll.*, **18**, 1–37
22. *Ibid.*, p. 448
23. Benivieni, A. (1507). *Op. cit.*
24. Vierordt, H. (1903). Geschichte der Herzkrankheiten. In Puschmann, Theodor (ed.) *Handbuch der Geschichte der Medezin*, vol. 2, pp. 634 and 642. (Jena: Gustav Fischer)
25. Lower, R. (1669). *Tractatus de Corde*. (London)
26. Mayow, J. (1674). Tractatus Quinque. *De Respiratione*. (Oxford)
27. Bonet, T. (1700). *Sepulchretum sive Anatomia Practica ex Cadaveribus Morbo Denatis*. (Geneva: Cramer and Perachon)
28. Willius, F.A. and Dry, T.J. (1948). *A History of the Heart and Circulation*, pp. 304–305. (Philadelphia: W.B. Saunders Co.)
29. *Ibid.*, p. 73
30. Stenn, F. (1941). Giorgio Baglivi. *Ann. M. Hist.*, **53**, **3**, 183–94
31. Vieussens, R. (1715). *Traité Nouveau de la Structure et des Causes du Mouvement Natural du Coeur*. (Toulouse: Guillamette)
32. Haller von, A. (1755). *Opuscula Pathologica*. Lausannae, Bousquet et soc., p. 135 (Translated by Maurice N. Walsh, MD, Mayo Clinic).
33. Willius, F.A. and Keys, T.E. (1941). *Op. cit.*, p. 170
34. Burns, A. (1809). *Diseases of the Heart*. (Edinburgh: Thomas Bryce & Co.)
35. Laénnec, R.T.H. (1823). *A treatise on the diseases of the chest, in which they are described according to their anatomical characters, and their diagnosis established on a new principle by means of acoustick instruments*. (Translated by John Forbes.) First American Edition, (3rd book, chap. 2, 3rd Section) p. 312, (Philadelphia: J. Webster)
36. Hawthorne, N. (1937). Ethan Brand. In *The Novels and Tales of Nathaniel Hawthorne*, p. 1196. (New York: Random House)
37. Adams, R. (1827). Cases of disease of the heart, accompanied with pathological observations. *Dublin Hosp. Rep.*, **4**, 353
38. Stokes, W. (1854). *Diseases of the Heart*, p. 302. (Dublin)
39. Hope, J. (1839). *Op. cit.*
40. Chevers, N. (1842). Observations on diseases of the orifice and valves of the aorta. *Guy's Hosp. Rep.*, **7**, 387
41. Pick, F. (1896). Über Pericarditische Pseudo-lebercirrhose (chronische, unter dem Bilde der Lebercirrhose verlaufende Pericarditis). *Zeitsch. f. Klin. Med.*, **29**, 385–410
42. Herrick, J.B. (1942). *Op. cit.* p. 189
43. Charcot, J.M. (1891). *Clinical Lecture on Senile and Chronic Diseases*, pp. 172–5. (London: Sydenham Society)
44. White, P.D. (1935). Chronic constrictive pericarditis (Pick's Disease) treated by pericardial resection. *Lancet*, **2**, 539, 597
45. Harrison, M.D. and White, P.D. (1942). Chronic constrictive pericarditis: a follow-up study of 37 cases. *Ann. Intern. Med.*, **17**, 790
46. Paul, O., Castleman, B. and White, P.D. (1948). Chronic constrictive pericarditis: a study of 53 cases. *Am. J. M. Sc.*, **216**, 361
47. Burwell, C.S. (1951). Some effects of pericardial disease on the pulmonary circulation. *Tr. A. Am. Physicians*, **64**, 74–9
48. Lindsay, J. Jr., Crawley, I.S. and Callaway, G.M. (1970). Chronic constrictive pericarditis following uremic hemopericardium. *Am. Heart J.*, **79**, 390
49. Ellis, K., Leeds, N.E. and Himmelstein, A. (1959). Congenital deficiencies in partial pericardium: review of two new cases including successful diagnosis by plain roentgenography. *Am. J. Roentgenology*, **82**, 125
50. Galen, C. *De Affectionibus Localis*, Book V and Book VII.
51. Osler, W. (1892). *The Principles and Practice of Medicine*. (New York: D. Appleton Co.)

8   Arterial lesions

Structural abnormalities of the arteries may arise from congenital defects, trauma, infectious agents or an atheromatous process. The most important of these in this century has been the atherogenic one. This was hardly the case in antiquity. Man did not live long enough to develop arteriosclerosis to any significant degree. Most of the arterial problems were traumatic in origin, and resulted either in death from hemorrhage, or in the formation of aneurysms. Aneurysms of the peripheral arteries were well known to Galen, and were described also by Aetius in the 6th century. These localized dilations were probably almost always due to injury. It was not until syphilis appeared in Europe during the latter part of the 15th century, and assumed epidemic proportions during the Renaissance that the arterial effects of this disease became evident and commonplace. Much dispute and time had to pass though before it became recognized that not only lues, but also other infectious agents were capable of causing arterial lesions. And it was not until the 18th century that atherosclerosis was found to be a common, and all-too pervasive affliction of the arterial tree.

Aside from the abnormalities that are mentioned in the section dealing with congenital malformations, perhaps the most important congenital lesion of the aorta is cystic medial necrosis. Erdheim is responsible for the name. The microscopic description was outlined in a paper called *Medionecrosis Aortae Idiopathica Cystica* published in 1930[1]. It is a histologic disorder that is seen frequently in Marfan's syndrome and other inherited connective tissue disorders. It has also been seen in those without a so-called phenotypic syndrome[2]! The importance of this histologic disorder lies in its propensity to cause aortic dissection or to form cylindrical dilatation of the ascending aorta.

Hypertension appears to be an important contributing factor for aortic dissection in an individual with cystic medial necrosis. About half of all aortic dissections that occur in women below the age of 40 are associated with pregnancy[3]. This relationship remains unexplained. The role of chemical toxins is also unknown.

This, in essence, is the clinical spectrum of cystic medial necrosis. What then is the historical background leading up to our current knowledge?

For centuries, aortic dissection was synonymous with aortic aneurysm. It has been only during the 20th century that a definite distinction between the two has emerged. One of the earliest descriptions of an aneurysm that is ascribed to pathological distention of all the layers of the arterial wall is to be found in Wishart's translation of Scarpa's treatise on aneurysms which appeared in 1808[4]. Scarpa attributes the description to Fernelius who wrote it in 1542. Not quite a century later, Sennertus in 1628 noted internal rupture and swelling of the adventitia in a case of aortic aneurysm believing that this was the pathogenic mechanism for the formation of aortic aneurysms in general rather than citing this as an example of aortic dissection *per se*[5].

Aortic dissection was described by Morgagni in 1761 in his *De Sedibus*[6]. But he, too, was not aware of its relationship to cystic medial necrosis, nor did he realize that it could occur independently of saccular aneurysms that were syphilitic in origin. Morgagni described the process as 'blood forcing its way by degrees through the wall and coming out under the external coat of the artery, first by drawing it from the internal coats and then by raising it as a large kind of ecchymosis'[7].

J.C. Leonard recounts the mode of death of George II of Great Britain with autopsy findings that graphically describes the gross anatomical changes. The following is a direct quotation from his paper[8, 9].

On 25 October 1760 George II, then 76, rose at his normal hour of 6 am, called as usual for his chocolate, and repaired to the closet-stool. The

German valet de chambre heard a noise, memorably described as 'louder than the royal wind', and then a groan; he ran in and found the King lying on the floor, having cut his face in falling. Mr. Andrews, surgeon to the household, was called and bled His Majesty but in vain, as no sign of life was observed from the time of his fall. At necropsy the next day Dr. Nicholls, physician to his late Majesty, found the pericardium distended with a pint of coagulated blood, probably from an orifice in the right ventricle, and a transverse fissure on the inner side of the ascending aorta 3.75 cm long, through which blood has recently passed in its external coat to form a raised ecchymosis, this appearance being interpreted as an incipient aneurysm of the aorta.

Forty-two years had to pass before Maunoir described the errant blood as 'dissecting through the circumference of the aorta'[10]. It was he who gave the first accurate and detailed description of aortic dissection. It appeared in his *Memoires Physiologiques, et Pratiques sur l'Aneuvrisme et la Ligature des artéres*[10]. 'The intima ruptures at one point and the adventitia forms a pocket and it alone resists the bloody effusion which progresses following dehiscence of the intima. The pocket enlarges, the blood dissects occasionally around the entire circumference of the artery which then lies in the center of the aneurysm, bathing in aneurysmal blood.' This is a perfect description of the 'double-barreled' aorta that forms as a result of the dissection.

Although Maunoir appeared to realize that aortic dissection was neither an initiating mechanism nor a usual component of all aneurysms, many clinicians in the early years of the 19th century were still adhering to the concept advanced by Sennertus in that dissection preceded all aneurysms and that both aneurysms and dissection were part of the same disease process. Laénnec too believed this when in 1826 he introduced the term 'dissecting aneurysm' in the second edition of his *Traite de L'Auscultation Médicale*. Laénnec's term is still in use today though it is obviously a misnomer since a hematoma is present rather than an aneurysm[11].

In 1822, Shekelton clearly described the distal re-entry phenomenon in the double-barreled aorta that allows the blood to flow back into the true lumen of the aorta. The re-entry phenomenon was recognized by several subsequent investigators among whom were Hope in 1833, Hodgson in 1834, Bouillaud in 1847, Schroder van der Kolk in 1849, Goupil in 1853 and von Recklinghausen in 1864[12]. Most of these investigators realized that the double-barreled aorta with the distal re-entry point represented a natural, albeit imperfect, method of restoring the circulation. Schroder van der Kolk, however, held the unique misconception that the entire anatomical abnormality was a congenital anomaly[13].

The nature of the internal tear was first described by Elliotson in 1830[14]. He noted that the rupture of the intima occurred in the transverse plane of the aorta with the dissection then progressing along a longitudinal path. Pennock, an American, demonstrated in 1839 that the dissection proceeded between the layers of the media[15]. Confirmation of this important anatomical detail was supplied independently several years later by Henderson of Edinburgh[16]. He, along with Pennock, were among the first to realize that the media was the site of the initial lesion. Henderson, at the same time, was the first to describe the lining found in the aneurysmal sac when the dissection entered the chronic phase. He noted that this lining was fibrous in nature.

We cannot end this historical survey of the morbid anatomy of aortic dissection without mentioning the observations of Burns and Hodgson. In their case reports, hemopericardium was the fatal complication. Burns' description is to be found in his book *Observations on some of the Most Frequent and Important Diseases of the Heart*. The hemopericardium was attributed by him to a rupture of the right atrium. He noted the presence of an irregular vent 1.25 cm long in the ascending aorta. It was his opinion that the blood passed through this vent into an aneurysmal sac that was bounded by 'the proper and cellular coverings' of the aorta and which extended from the root of the aorta to the origin of the innominate artery[17].

In Hodgson's case recorded several years later in his treatise on diseases of arteries and veins, the hemopericardium was said to be due to rupture of the right ventricle while at the same time describing findings in the ascending aorta similar to those in Burns' patient. The similarities between the two cases are striking. What is even more striking is what appears to be an erroneous conclusion by Burns that the blood escaped from the right atrium, and that of Hodgson who felt that in his case the blood came from rupture of the right ventricle.

Dr. Nicholls in his autopsy of George II was also in error when he suggested that His Majesty's hemopericardium arose 'from an orifice in the right ventricle'[18].

The morbid anatomy of dissecting aneurysm of the abdominal aorta was described by Shekelton in 1822[19]. In his two cases, the re-entry opening was found in the common iliac artery. Otto's case report two years later of a young girl who died within 24 hours after the onset of severe chest pain is interesting in that it represents the first description of coarctation of the aorta complicated by a dissecting aneurysm[20].

The first antemortem diagnosis of a dissecting aneurysm was reported by J. Swain of England. This case report was presented by Latham in a paper before the Pathological Society of London in 1855[21]. The patient died three months after the diagnosis was made. The postmortem examination showed an unruptured dissecting aneurysm of the distal end of the abdominal aorta extending to its bifurcation. The patient was said to have died because of congestive heart failure so that these findings at necropsy seem to indicate that the patient's lesion was an example of a so-called natural cure.

The pathogenesis of aortic dissection has been the subject of bitter debate ever since Scarpa wrote in 1804 that the predisposing elements were 'corrosion and rupture of the proper coats of the aorta'. He did realize that a hematoma resulted from the blood dissecting through the arterial wall and attributed the thickening of the adventitia to the hematoma. Burns, on the other hand, claimed that the thickened adventitia preceded the dissection and was the predisposing factor for the process. Rokitansky offered the opinion that the thickened adventitia was the result of chronic inflammation.

Thomas Peacock, the author of the splendid work on congenital malformations of the heart, entered the debate with two very commendable papers on dissecting aneurysm. The first paper appeared in 1843 and the second one 20 years later[22,23]. Leonard quotes Peacock as noting that the 'coats of the aorta are in a healthy state, capable of extreme distention, before giving way ... the rupture of the internal coats of the vessel ... must be ascribed to their being lacerable by disease'[24]. The last statement is an important clue regarding the initiation of the entire process.

Peacock's experiments in cadavers utilizing injections of fluid between the adventitia and media demonstrated that this was the anatomical pathway of the blood in its course during dissection and that this pathway tended to reopen into the original lumen at a variable distance from its point of origin rather than burst externally. He realized that the formation of this double-barreled lumen constituted a method of aborting the dissection resulting in 'an imperfect natural cure'. He also recognized clearly how death was more likely with the formation of a hemopericardium when the dissecting process involved the ascending aorta, since the blood was directed towards the heart rather than in the reverse direction as in those cases where the dissection begins past the aortic arch.

Thus, Peacock's concept of the pathogenesis of aortic dissection involved three stages. The first was rupturing of the intima (when this layer was 'lacerable'), with the second stage immediately following as the blood penetrated into the media, and with distal re-entry representing the third stage and occurring only occasionally as a natural means of allowing the patient to survive.

The etiology of aortic dissection has also been bandied about with numerous fallacies and acrimonious debate. When von Recklinghausen reported his case of long-standing dissection, he attributed the cause to molecular changes in the elastic tissue. Sanderson's account of the various etiological proposals is both concise and illuminating[25]. It begins with Boström's proposal in 1888 that trauma was the causative factor in all cases, and that if disease of the media were noted, it was to be considered an incidental finding. Flockemann in 1898 felt that trauma was rarely the cause and that a diseased aorta was never responsible. Rindfleisch advanced the theory that there were band-like thickenings between the ascending aorta and the pulmonary artery. He termed these thickenings 'vincula aortae', stating that they developed in later life. He claimed that most tears originated on the inner side of the aorta just proximal to the band-like thickening.

A return to Henderson's concept was voiced by Schede in 1908, but it was Babes and Mironescu in 1910 who first suggested that aortic dissection could occur without rupture of the intima[26]. They felt that a hemorrhage from the vasa vasorum into the media initiated the entire process which they labeled 'dissecting mesarteritis'. The possibility that this could be the initiating factor in some cases was supported by Kruchenberg in 1920 and Shennan in 1934[27].

Shennan's classical work *Dissecting Aneurysms* appeared in 1934. It attempted to elucidate the etiology and pathogenesis of aortic dissection based on a detailed study of more than 300 cases culled from the literature, existing museum specimens and from his own experience. He concluded that degeneration of the media was the most frequent finding and that neither atheroma nor lues were of importance in the etiology. Microscopic changes in the connective and elastic tissue of the media had already been demonstrated by Moriani in 1910 utilizing silver-staining techniques with light microscopy[28]. The word 'cystic' never appears in Shennan's text nor in any of the previous descriptions. Shennan's text does note a high incidence of associated coarctation of the aorta and he did comment on the role that hypertension and congenital diseases of the aorta played. During the 20th century the studies conducted by Edwards and later by Roberts from the National Institutes of Health led them to acknowledge and confirm a statistical association of aortic dissection with coarctation of the aorta. But both men expressed the view that the dissection is probably related to the coexistent hypertension or a congenitally bicuspid aortic valve rather than to the coarctation *per se*[29,30].

The association between a congenital bicuspid aortic valve and aortic dissection was first noted by Maude Abbott in 1927[31]. This association is not mentioned at all in a review by Wilson and Hutchins that appeared in 1982[32]. These two men collected necropsy reports of 204 subjects that spanned a period of 92 years. Their failure to mention this association is rather strange because just a year later Eric Larson and William Edwards, two pathologists from the Mayo Clinic, found that the risk of aortic dissection in persons with congenital bicuspid aortic valve was at least nine times greater than in subjects with normal valves[33]. This discrepancy can be explained perhaps by the fact that Larson and Edwards based their observations on actual specimens rather than relying on necropsy reports written by various observers which was the case with Wilson and Hutchins.

Wilson and Hutchins also proposed that atherosclerosis was an important risk factor predisposing to weakness of the medial layer of the wall and dissection. This view was not held by Hirst and his group when they published their review of the subject in 1958 based on an analysis of 505 cases[34]. The prominent American cardiac

pathologist, W. C. Roberts, also rejected atherosclerosis as a risk factor in his review which appeared in 1981[35].

It was not until 1943 that the association between Marfan's syndrome and aortic dissection was first recognized. This was brought out by Helen Taussig in the Bulletin of the Johns Hopkins Hospital with R.W. Baer as the leading author[36]. The original description by Marfan of the syndrome that bears his name does not mention associated cardiovascular disorders. In fact, all he described were the characteristic skeletal abnormalities of elongated extremities and skull deformities[37].

Marfan originally suggested the name 'dolichostenomelie' for the syndrome because of the long, thin extremities. Arachnodactyly is the term introduced by Achard six years after Marfan's report[38]. It aptly describes the 'spider fingers' that are so characteristic of the full-blown syndrome and it has replaced Marfan's 'dolichostenomelie' as a more popular designation for the skeletal manifestations. Achard also added to the clinical manifestations, the laxity of ligaments which is responsible for the excessive mobility of the joints. He was also the first to note a familial tendency.

Salle was the first to note the association of cardiovascular abnormalities[39]. These observations appeared in 1912. Fourteen years later Piper and Irvine-Jones described the association of congenital heart disease with arachnodactyly[40]. As already noted, it was not until 1943 that the initial reports of associated aortic lesions appeared. These include the congenital aneurysms already alluded to and described by Baer in collaboration with Helen Taussig[41], and the occurrence of dissecting aneurysm as described by Etter and Glover[42]. Pregnancy as another predisposing factor was first described by Schnitker and Bayer in 1944[43], followed by Pedowitz and Perrell in 1957[44].

The controversy regarding the pathogenesis of dissecting aneurysm in the majority of cases is by no means resolved. It was the observations of Gsell (1928) and those of Erdheim (1929) that initially focused attention on cystic medial necrosis as being the usual underlying cause of aortic dissection.

Butler in 1947 attempted to implicate atheroma as an important cause, but no other investigator has supported this view[45]. Schlicter and associates advanced the thesis in 1949 that the basic defect was in the vasa vasorum[46]; with continued narrowing of the lumen of these vessels resulting in ischemia of the arterial wall and leading eventually to dissection. Gore in 1952 considered medial necrosis as the sole mechanism in the older person while advocating that in younger people, especially those with Marfan's syndrome or congenital cardiac defects (such as coarctation of the aorta), fragmentation of the elastic laminae was the important initiating catalyst[47]. Giant-cell arteritis and syphilis have been implicated but these are rare causes. In 1973, Gore and Hirst suggested that rupture of the vasa vasorum initiated the entire dissecting process[48]. This was a different twist on Schlicter's thesis.

Schlatmann and Becker examined the aortas of 100 patients without evidence of dissection or aneurysmal dilation. They published their findings in 1977 concluding that medial necrosis, elastin fragmentation and cystic medial necrosis were not specifically concerned in the etiology of dissecting aneurysm[49]. They believed further that if any of these changes were found at autopsy, they were the result of the vessel's response to injury.

In a classical paper by Hasleton and Leonard in 1979, evidence was presented to indicate that no one factor can be implicated in the pathogenesis of dissecting aneurysm[50]. They published their findings in the American Journal of Cardiology concluding that medial necrosis, elastin fragmentation, and cystic medial necrosis in and of themselves are not more important than other predisposing factors.

Does this mean that 'cystic medial necrosis' is a misnomer? Hirst and Gore certainly thought so in 1976 when they continued the controversy in their paper that had as its title a question: *Is cystic medionecrosis the cause of dissecting aortic aneurysm?*[51]. Schlatmann and Becker certainly supported this view with their suggestion that 'medionecrosis represents an adaptation phenomenon rather than a cause'. My suggestion is that the reader be patient, with the hope that future studies will not compound further the present confusion.

Two other important anatomical abnormalities of the aorta are aneurysmal dilatation and idiopathic dilatation of the ascending aorta. According to Sigerist, arterial aneurysms must have been known to the Egyptians as far back as fourteen hundred years before Christ[52]. He based this assertion on the word content of the incantations in vogue at the time which presumably inferred that they were being invoked for the treatment of aneurysms, although neither the term aneurysm nor the site or nature of these lesions are to be found in any of the extant descriptions of these incantations. The probability that aneurysms of the peripheral arteries, but not those of the aorta, were encountered may be closer to the truth. The Ebers papyrus definitely lists aneurysms among the diseases mentioned[53]. It must be recalled that in mummification there was practically complete removal of the intrathoracic and intrabdominal organs. Only remnants of the aorta and its major branches remained for study by future pathologists. Arteriosclerosis was present during that era. Ruffer's description of arterial lesions, both in the aortic remnants and peripheral arteries, amply attests to this[54]. From the vantage point of current knowledge regarding arteriosclerosis as an important etiologic factor, aneurysms of the aorta must have occurred in those who managed to live long enough.

Galen is considered to be the first to have described and defined the arterial lesion itself. In *The Seven Books of Paulus Aegineta* translated by Adams[55], the following quotation is attributed to Galen: '... artery having become anastomosed (i.e., dilated) the affection is called an aneurism; it arises also from a wound of the same, when the skin that lies over it is cicatrized, but the wound in the artery remains, and neither unites nor is blocked up by flesh. Such affections are recognized by the pulsation of the arteries.'

Trauma, of course, was the major recognizable cause of aneurysm in that period of time, involving most commonly the peripheral and superficial arteries; they being readily accessible to injury during battle or gladiatorial jousts. Galen's position as physician to the gladiators afforded him a great deal of opportunity to observe, firsthand, aneurysms that were traumatic in origin. This gave him a rather biased outlook on the pathogenesis of aneurysms since he had no experience with the garden variety of aortic aneurysm that is so prevalent today.

No worthwhile descriptions of aortic aneurysm can be found until the 16th century. According to Garrison, Saporta gave the earliest description in 1554[56]. During the same year, however, Fernel's famous *Universa Medicina* appeared. We have already met Fernel in the early pages of this Section, but a few more words about him would not be amiss. He was born in 1506 and died in 1588. After graduating from the University of Paris, he occupied the chair of medicine at his alma mater for many years, while carrying on a successful practice. Fernel is regarded as one of the most outstanding physicians of the

French Renaissance. In line with the customs of the time Fernel's academic interests encompassed mathematics and philosophy as well as medicine. He was also known to dabble in astronomy. Fortunately for us, his interest in medicine outweighed all his other endeavors. Fernel was quite outspoken in deposing many of Galen's teachings, and very instrumental in marshalling about him a considerably sized group of vocal anti-Galenists.

Figure 1 is a portrait of Fernel while the frontispiece of his *Universa Medicina* is illustrated in Figure 2. The book consists of three sections dealing with physiology, pathology and therapeutics.

Fernel was well aware that aneurysms could be found in both the thoracic and abdominal cavities. Erichsen quotes him as claiming that 'aneurysms occurred in the chest, or about the spleen and mesentery where a violent throbbing is frequently observable'[57]. Aetius also claimed that they could occur in any part of the body and this was in the 6th century[58]. However, Vesalius must be given credit for specifically recognizing and describing in 1555 aneurysms of the thoracic and abdominal aorta rather than its branches.

Concerning the pathogenesis, since trauma was such a common cause of arterial aneurysms among the ancients, it was only natural for them to feel that the lesions were initiated by rupturing of the arterial wall. Arguments flew back and forth as to whether the rupture involved only the inner coat, outer coat, or all layers of the wall. Rupture as the initiating element remained a fixed concept even as observers of the 16th and 17th centuries realized that trauma was an infrequent cause of aortic aneurysms.

Some observers concluded that aneurysms were simply the result of dilation of the wall rather than rupture. This view was held by Antyllos in the second century AD, even though it appears that his experience involved mostly the traumatic type of aneurysm[59]. A word of caution is advisable regarding contributions of Aetius on this subject in the 6th century. In Erichsen's translation, it appears that Aetius may not have been describing aneurysms at all in some instances but rather lesions of a different nature and not vascular at all[60]. Moreover, the descriptions of Aetius were clinical rather than pathological.

In 1595, Guillemeau wrote that 'an aneurism is occasioned when the blood and spirits pass out of the vessels'. He felt that dilatation as a mechanism could apply only to small aneurysms, 'as it is

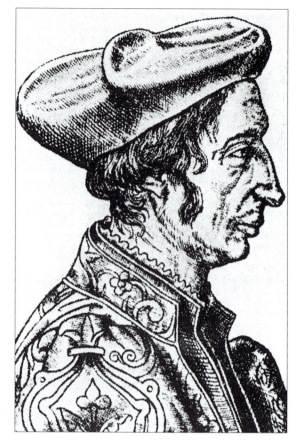

Figure 1 Portrait of Fernel. *Photo Source University of Central Florida. Literary Source Willius FA, Dry TJ: A History of the Heart and Circulation. W.B. Saunders Co. Philadelphia, p.92, 1948. Public domain*

impossible that the artery can really be dilated and enlarged to the size of the large aneurysms that are often met with'[61].

Fernel had also subscribed to the belief that aortic aneurysms arose from dilatation of the entire wall but he implicated lues as the major culprit in the process. Ambroise Paré also adhered to the concept of dilatation. We have already seen how he described aneurysms as being present in those with the 'pox' but attributed the cause to the treatment rather than the disease itself.

Throughout the Renaissance and well into the 20th century, until the discovery of penicillin initiated the antibiotic era, syphilis was an important cause of aortic aneurysms. Lancisi was also one of the first to recognize the relationship between aortic aneurysms and lues. East quotes several cases

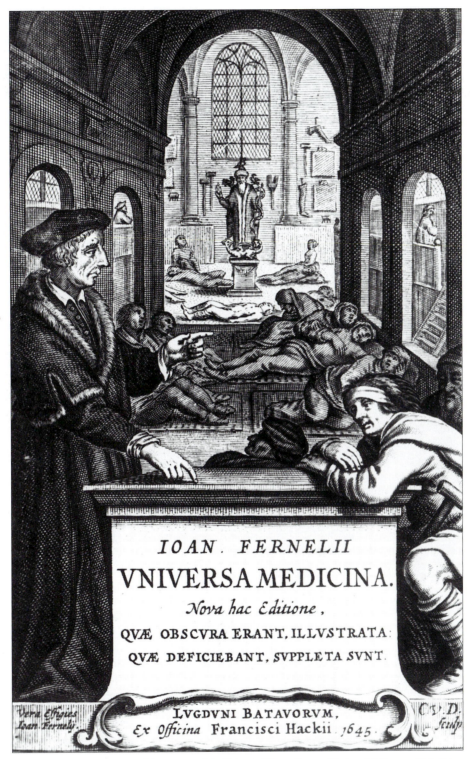

Figure 2 Frontispiece of 'Universa Medicina'. *Photo Source National Library of Medicine.*
Literary Source Photo Archives (copy of original). Courtesy of National Library of Medicine

mentioned by Lancisi in defense of this relationship[62]. These are worthy of reproduction here. There is the runner of thirty, 'nec minus in Studius, quam in Veneris palaestra exercitatus', who had an abdominal aneurysm that ruptured; and a running footman of thirty-three, 'similiterque athleta in Veneris palaestra', who had one in his left; and finally there is the fishmonger, 'Baccho nimirum, Dianaae, Neptuno ac Veneri frequenter indulgens'. These quotations are to be found in Lancisi's *De Motu Cordis et Aneurysmatibus*'. Lancisi believed that the luetic process was responsible for the dilatation. However, aside from syphilis, he cited that in some cases, the dilatation was due to an inherent defect in the wall which 'may be constructed by nature with fibers too slack and too small'[63]. Could he have been referring to the connective tissue disorder as seen in Marfan's syndrome?

In 1670, prior to Lancisi's posthumous publication, Giovanni Riva also had made notable contributions towards understanding the nature and character of aneurysms. Riva (1627–77), an eminent anatomist and pathologist in his own right, was Lancisi's teacher, and physician to both Louis XIV and Pope Clement X. It is a pity that most of the anatomic plates he made were destroyed. His legacy did remain, however, in the society of pathologists that he founded and in the anatomic museum that he began.

Not everyone subscribed to syphilis as the causative agent of aortic aneurysms. During the Renaissance, and for some time afterwards, there was a considerable body of physicians who felt that the aneurysms were due to the mercury used in the treatment rather than the luetic process itself. We have already seen how Paré's description appears to imply that the aneurysm was caused by 'the heated blood' rather than the 'pox'. East also recounts how Morgagni noted aneurysmal dilatation of the carotid artery in an old woman of Bologna with a full bounding pulse, and ascribed the cause of the aneurysm to gluttony and drunkenness rather than syphilis[64]. Despite this case report Morgagni did not reject lues as a causative factor in other cases.

Acquired immunodeficiency syndrome (AIDS) today has appeared to replace syphilis as the plague of sexual promiscuity. It, too, is accompanied by its own emotional accoutrement. The emotional elements of syphilis were politics and national bias as indicated by the name 'morbus gallicum', meaning that the French introduced the disease to Europe.

The high incidence of AIDS among homosexuals appears to underline the current political orientation towards the disease.

Before the end of the 17th century two other personalities figured prominently in the historical background concerning the pathogenesis of aneurysms. These were Wiseman and Bourdelot. Wiseman in 1676 believed that an aneurysm arose as a result of rupture of the entire wall and that the impetus was due either to the erosive quality of blood or to its impetuosity. Regarding the latter endogenous factor, Erichsen quotes Wiseman as saying 'The impetus may rise, first from the quantity of the blood, either when it is more than the vessel can contain or else when the blood is too forcibly driven forwards from the heart towards some peculiar artery, when the farther progress being (it may be) intercepted by some violent contraction of the muscles through which it must pass, it of necessity breaks the vessel'[65]. Bourdelot in 1681 suggested that the middle layer of the arterial wall gave way, the result of 'ebullition of the blood' with consequent dilatation[66]. It must be emphasized that these men were speaking of aneurysms in general rather than those arising from the aorta.

Aneurysms, in general, became the focus of interest of several investigators during the first half or so of the 18th century. These included Alexander and Donald Monro, Petit, the Hunter brothers and Home. They attempted to differentiate between true and false aneurysms, traumatic and non-traumatic. They also described arteriovenous aneurysms. Actually, none of them contributed anything original to the pathogenesis of any of these varieties. One of them, John Hunter, did conduct an experiment on a dog in an effort to elucidate the mechanisms. Home also conducted experiments on dogs. On the basis of their findings, both men were of the opinion that pre-existing disease of the arterial wall was necessary for the production of an aneurysm. Experiments such as these were a step in the right direction, but unfortunately not very enlightening at the time.

Baillie in his description of aneurysm of the aortic arch overlooked the arteriosclerotic changes in the vessel[67]. In 1770, Baillie did mention, however, the presence of laminated thrombus in some of the aneurysms. He considered this a natural cure.

The most important contributors towards an understanding of the morbid anatomy of aortic aneurysms were three men whose lives straddled the end of the 18th century and the beginning of the 19th. These three were Scarpa, Hope and Hodgson. They were remarkable in that all three were excellent illustrators as well as keenly observant morbid anatomists.

We have already met Antonio Scarpa as an anatomist of note. It was his close relationship with fellow anatomist, Vicq d'Azyr that afforded him the opportunity to observe and report on an unusual case of an aortic aneurysm which had eroded through the first rib and sternum of a 45 year old soldier. At autopsy, Scarpa was able to dissect this aneurysm, recording that the morbid anatomy revealed degeneration of the arterial wall. The findings and his comments were presented by him in a paper before the French Royal Society of Medicine[68]. Figure 3 is an illustration of this lesion and its eroding effect as drawn by Scarpa himself.

Scarpa had also observed four previous cases of aortic aneurysm. All of his observations on aneurysm were collated and presented in 1804 in his *Sull Aneurisma Riflessioni ed Osservazioni Anatomico-chirurgiche*. In his comments he stressed that pathologic degeneration of the arterial wall was the common denominator shared by all the cases. He apparently agreed with both Lancisi and Morgagni in alluding to the probable luetic origin of the degenerative changes in the wall of the artery[69]. He also, however, regarded arteriosclerosis as an important element besides syphilis in the etiology of aortic aneurysm. He was the first to regard arteriosclerosis as a lesion of the inner coats and contended that the intima and media were ruptured in the formation of the aneurysm.

James Hope's contributions are to be found in his doctoral thesis in medicine, *Aneurism of the Aorta*. Published in 1825, it contains many worthwhile observations fortified with his own artistic renditions of the morbid anatomy[70]. It is ironic that this great physician who described so well so many anatomical abnormalities in his 'Principles and Illustrations of Morbid Anatomy' had a marked repugnance towards anatomical dissection[71]. This along with his intense desire to perfect his artistic abilities are outlined by A.F. Hope[72]. The account reads as follows:

He compelled himself to make three or four drawings per week during the remainder of his stay in Paris; each drawing taking him from two to eight hours... This proved to be the most irksome task that he ever performed. His repugnance to anatomy [as a student, he always wore gloves when dissecting] though greatly subdued, was not totally eradicated, and this occupation was consequently so alien to his taste, that it was only by the strongest mental effort that he could compel himself to proceed. It was far, he used to say, from being a mere mechanical employment like copying; for in making original drawings, one paints with the head, not with the hand alone; every touch, every shade of colour is a thought, and thus the intellectual process is a severe one. Notwithstanding, he thus occupied himself five hours daily, and he satisfied himself so thoroughly with it, that he never afterwards could settle to drawing of any kind, except from pure necessity.

Hodgson's role is a very special one as we shall see. Before proceeding to him, I would like to elaborate still further on the thoughts regarding syphilis and arteriosclerosis. In 1864, Hasse authored a text called *An Anatomical Description of the Diseases of the Organs of Circulation and Respiration*[73]. The section on aneurysms presents the most detailed classification available up until that time. Among his comments was his assertion that atheroma predisposed to the development of aortic aneurysm. He did not agree with Scarpa's contention that rupture of the intima and media was necessary for aneurysmal dilatation. He postulated that the atheromatous process caused a degeneration of the intima and media with consequent loss of elasticity leading to dilatation of the entire wall.

Rokitansky also lent his talents to the subject. His observations and comments are to be found in his *Manual of Pathological Anatomy* which appeared in 1852[74]. He rejected laceration of the inner coats as an element in the process since he had never personally observed this phenomenon. He speaks of a 'special aneurismal diathesis' but does not elaborate on the role of syphilis or arteriosclerosis.

As the century wore on, there was still a great deal of confusion concerning the actual importance of syphilis in the entire process. Garrison claimed that final acceptance of syphilis as a causative agent was stimulated by Wilks' work in 1863[75]. It was Welch, however, who in 1875 finally differentiated the aortitis of syphilis from atheroma[76]. Welch was convinced that it was chiefly the inflammatory changes in the aorta produced by syphilis that was

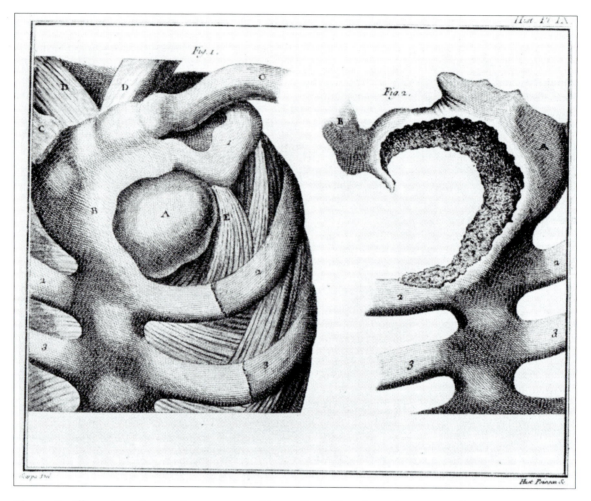

Figure 3 Illustration of an aortic aneurysm and its eroding effect, drawn by Scarpa. *Photo Source University of Central Florida. Literary Source Mann RJ: Historical Vignette. Scarpa, Hodgson, and Hope, Artists of the Heart and Great Vessels. Mayo Clinic Proceedings., 49:890–892, 1974. With Permission from Mayo Foundation*

responsible for the aneurysmal dilatation. He was probably right for that time period, but the microscopic studies of Coats and Auld that followed in 1983 were also of great importance in establishing arteriosclerosis as another major cause[77].

The discovery of penicillin has brought about the almost complete eradication of syphilis as an import cause of aortic aneurysm. Arteriosclerosis is currently the prime culprit in the pathogenesis of both thoracic and abdominal aortic aneurysms.

The other important anatomical abnormality of the aorta is idiopathic dilatation of the ascending aorta and aortic annulus, and this is where Hodgson figures more prominently. There is no saccular aneurysmal bulging of the aorta in this condition but rather a cylindrical type of dilatation. The current label for this abnormality is annuloaortic ectasia, a term introduced by Ellis and colleagues in 1961[78]. Since the initial report by Ellis, written with the collaboration of Cooley and DeBakey, the abnormality is being diagnosed with increasing frequency. Perhaps anywhere between 5 and 10% of patients today with pure aortic regurgitation fall in this category. Cystic medial necrosis is the common pathological feature.

Patients with annuloaortic ectasia appear to fall into three groups: those with classic Marfan's syndrome; those with the forme frusté of this connective tissue disorder; and those with no obvious underlying cause. As the media of the arterial wall continues to degenerate, the aorta widens in a cylindrical fashion. Extension of the degenerative process into the root of the aorta also affects the annulus so that it too widens. As the annulus widens the cusps of the aortic valve no longer coapt during diastole with consequent leakage of blood back into the ventricle.

It appears to me that, in terms of gross anatomy, this abnormality is exactly what Burns, and later, Hodgson described when they referred to cylindrical dilatation of the aorta with intact wall. The similarities are too great to think otherwise. It must be emphasized that neither of these men described the microscopic appearance of this abnormality.

We have already commented on the brilliance of Burns and gave a brief sketch of his life. In addition to cylindrical dilatation of the aorta, Burns also recorded his findings in 14 cases of aortic aneurysm that he personally dissected. I wonder what other contributions were in store for humanity if Burns had lived longer. Unfortunately, he died at the age of 31 from an abdominal abscess which ruptured into the cecum, and which, probably, arose from an acute bout of appendicitis that went undiagnosed[79].

Joseph Hodgson was born in 1788, the son of a Birmingham merchant. He first became interested in diseases of the arteries and veins while apprenticed to Dr. Freer, surgeon to the General Hospital. Hodgson drew some of the plates for his mentor's treatise on aneurysms. Hodgson's interest in vascular diseases continued unabated while studying in London for his MRCS, culminating in an essay on wounds and diseases of arteries and veins. He was awarded the Jacksonian Prize on the basis of this essay which, in a few short years, was expanded and finalized to form his *Treatise on Diseases of Arteries and Veins*. The treatise was published in 1815 when Hodgson was only 27 years old. Many of the drawings in his work were personally done by Hodgson. At a later date, these drawings, along with those by others, were collated in the form of an atlas. Both the atlas and the treatise enjoyed an international reputation. He was elected to the Royal College of Surgeons at the age of 49, served on its council, and became its first provincial president. He died at the age of 81, probably as a result of the complete heart block that he had developed one year prior to his demise[80].

Hodgson's classic description of cylindrical dilatation of the aorta without saccular aneurysmal bulging is to be found in his treatise[81]. It is as follows:

Scarpa acknowledges the existence of that state of praeternatural dilatation of an artery which I have described, and mentions the frequency of its occurrence in the ascending aorta … The disease to which I allude consists in a praeternatural dilatation of the whole circle of an artery and not in a partial or lateral distension of its coats. The root of an aneurismal sac however never or very rarely commences on one side by a neck which is in most instances narrower than the body of the tumour. An artery is sometimes praeternaturally dilated without any morbid alteration having taken place in the texture of its coats. On the other hand, the structure of most aneurismal sacs differs essentially from that of a dilated artery. The former in general possesses a smooth membranous surface lined with coagulum, and in an advanced state of the disease it exhibits no traces of the coats of the vessel; whilst the latter possesses an uniformity of structure, and is evidently composed of the coats of the artery, which are generally in a morbid condition. The passage of the blood is not so materially interrupted in a dilated artery as when it passes into the recess of an aneurismal sac, and consequently grumous clots and lamellated coagulum, which are almost constantly deposited in aneurisms, are never met with in dilated arteries. These observations show that there is an essential difference between the praeternatural dilatation of the whole circle of an artery and an aneurismal sac, whether it originated in the destruction or partial dilatation of the coats of the vessel.

The preceding account was so impressive that the French conferred upon this abnormality the eponym *Maladie de Hodgson*. The frontispiece of Hodgson's treatise is illustrated in Figure 4.

The inflammatory lesions of the aorta can be grouped for ease of presentation under the generic term of aortic arteritis syndromes. These would include as specific types: Takayasu's arteritis, giant-cell arteritis and the aortic root inflammatory lesions with concomitant aortic regurgitation that can be seen in association with a category of diseases currently classified as manifestations of an autoimmune mechanism. All of the last group has some form of arthritis as part of the clinical syndrome.

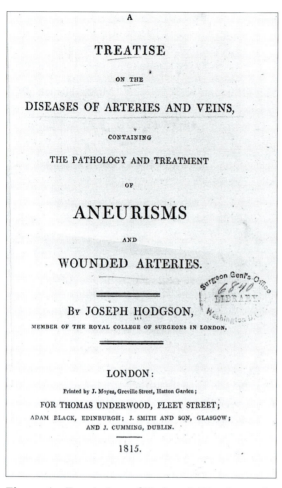

A

TREATISE

ON THE

DISEASES OF ARTERIES AND VEINS,

CONTAINING

THE PATHOLOGY AND TREATMENT

OF

ANEURISMS

AND

WOUNDED ARTERIES.

By JOSEPH HODGSON,
MEMBER OF THE ROYAL COLLEGE OF SURGEONS IN LONDON.

LONDON:

Printed by J. Moyes, Greville Street, Hatton Garden;

FOR THOMAS UNDERWOOD, FLEET STREET;

ADAM BLACK, EDINBURGH; J. SMITH AND SON, GLASGOW;
AND J. CUMMING, DUBLIN.

1815.

Figure 4 Frontispiece of Hodgson's 'Treatise on the Diseases of Arteries and Veins'. *Photo Source National Library of Medicine. Literary Source Photo Archives (copy of original). Courtesy of National Library of Medicine*

It was a Japanese ophthalmologist, Takayasu, who, in 1908, first described the arteritis that carries his name. The various clinical features of this entity that were subsequently described have caused it to be endowed with a number of diverse designations such as 'aortic arch syndrome', 'pulseless disease', 'young female arteritis', and 'occlusive thromboaortopathy'. Takayasu's report concerned a young woman with cataracts who also manifested 'wreathlike arteriovenous anastomoses surrounding the optic papillae'[82]. It was his colleagues, however, who called attention to two other patients that came under their care with similar ocular findings but absent radial pulses[83]. It was not until 1956 that Shimizu and Sano applied

the term 'pulseless disease' to this syndrome because of involvement of the brachiocephalic arteries[84]. Further reports by Inada[85]. in 1962 and a year later by Nasu[86] greatly expanded the pathologic and clinical spectrum with evidence that the disease was not confined to the arch alone but could involve the entire aorta in an indiscriminate manner. This accounts for the various names subsequent to Takayasu's original description. Nasu gave a rather detailed description of the pathologic changes and the degree to which the aorta could be involved in his paper in 1963[86].

An arteriographic-pathologic correlation was presented by Laude and LaPorta in 1976[87]. It was based on one case with the histopathologic findings at necropsy described by them in the greatest detail. The possibility that Takayasu's arteritis may have an autoimmune basis was discussed by Nako and his colleagues in 1967[88].

It is quite apparent that most of the substantial contributions of this disease have come from the Japanese community. Scattered reports from the rest of the world including those of the Japanese bring the total number of detailed autopsy observations to well over 100[89]. Among these reports are at least five that should be mentioned. The first is that by Tanaka, who in 1979, presented echocardiographic evidence of widening of the aortic root[90]: Then there is the clinical study of 107 cases by Lupi-Herrera and his group citing involvement of the pulmonary artery in 50% of their series[91] and in 1983 that of Acar and associates which reported a 5–19% incidence of aortic insufficiency as a complication[92]. A well-documented study of 32 North American patients was published by Hall and co-workers from the Mayo Clinic in 1985[93]. They stressed that the histopathologic spectrum included overlapping features of a granulomatous and sclerosing aortitis, and that these changes were indistinguishable from giant-cell arteritis. Moreover, all their patients manifested multiple sites of arterial involvement with various combinations of stenosis, luminal irregularity and aneurysm formation. Three of their patients had aortic insufficiency but only one needed the valve to be replaced.

It was Paulley and Hughes who first suggested that giant-cell arteritis be called arteritis of the aged. They commented that 'when elderly patients begin to fail mentally or physically, giant-cell arteritis is one of the first diseases to consider, not one of the last'. This was in 1960[94]. The advanced age of almost all of the patients described to date is certainly the most consistent feature of this unusual form of arteritis.

Knowledge concerning the association of aortic root inflammation complicated by aortic insufficiency in the autoimmune diseases has an historical background that is quite recent in onset. It begins with Jacquet's report from Paris in 1897[95]. In his case report, he described the complication in an individual with what is now known as Reiter's syndrome. Paronen published a paper in 1948 recording his observations in 344 cases of Reiter's syndrome[96]. There is no mention of aortic insufficiency in this rather large series. Scattered case reports originating primarily from Finland, Great Britain and the USA have appeared since then noting the presence of cardiac and aortic root lesions in Reiter's syndrome. Most of them were clinical descriptions with auscultatory evidence of aortic insufficiency. These were under the authorship of Dixon in 1960[97], Neu and associates[98], also in 1960, Csonka and associates[99] in 1961, Weinberger[100] in 1962, Rodnan and his group[101] in 1964, Ford[102] in 1970, Cliff[103] in 1971 and Paulus[104] in 1972. Among all these only Rodnan, Cliff and Paulus were able to correlate their clinical findings with postmortem examination. Up until the publication of the paper by Paulus, well-documented evidence of aortic insufficiency was present in only 10 cases. Paulus added five more to the list, and in addition, his paper was the first to describe the early aortic lesion in this syndrome[104].

The association of aortitis and aortic insufficiency was brought out by Graham and Smythe in 1958[105]. They described as well the carditis that can occur in this disease. During the same year, Ansell and his group added their description of the aortic lesion in ankylosing spondylitis. Further reports appeared in 1959 by Toone[106], in 1963 by the Mayo group headed by Davidson[107], in 1966 by Weed and co-workers[108] and in 1969 by Malette and associates[109]. All of these reports revealed a much higher incidence of cardiac lesions in ankylosing spondylitis than in Reiter's syndrome.

The association with ulcerative colitis was brought out by Zvaifler and Weintraub in 1963[110] as part of a reappraisal of aortitis and aortic insufficiency in chronic rheumatic disorders. Pearson and his group[111] described the occurrence of aortic aneurysms as well in a case of relapsing polychondritis in 1967.

REFERENCES

1. Erdheim, J. (1930). Medionecrosis aortae idiopathica cystica. *Virchow's Arch. Path. Anat.*, **276**, 187

2. Leoppky, C.B., Alpert, M.A., Hamel, P.C., Martin, R.H. and Saab, S.B. (1981). Extensive aortic dissection from combined-type cystic medial necrosis in a young man without predisposing factors. *Chest*, **79**, 116

3. Pumphrey, C.W., Fay, T. and Weir, I. (1986). Aortic dissection during pregnancy. *Br. Heart J.*, **55**, 106

4. Scarpa, A. (1808). *A Treatise on the Anatomy, Pathology and Surgical Treatment of Aneurysm.* Trans. by J.H. Wishart, p. 1503. (Edinburgh: Dorg and Stevenson)

5. Sennertus (1650). Cited by Shennan, T. (1934). Dissecting Aneurysms. *Medical Research Council Special Report Series*, **193**, 138

6. Morgagni, G.B. (1761). *DeSedibus.* Ep. 26, Art 17 (Ep48), F50. (Venice)

7. Morgagni, G.B. (1769). *The Seats and Causes of Diseases investigated by Anatomy*, Vol. I. Trans. B. Alexander, A. Miller, T. Cadele, p. 808. (London)

8. Leonard, J.C. (1979). Thomas Bevill Peacock and the early history of dissecting aneurysm. *Br. Med. J.*, **2**, 260–2

9. Trench, C.C. (1973). *George II*, p. 298, (London: Allen Lane)

10. Maunoir, J.P. (1802). *Mémoires Physiologiques et Pratiques sur l'Aneuvrisme et la Ligature des Artéres.* (Geneva: Paschond)

11. Sanderson, C.J., Cote, R.J., Levett, J.M., Beere, P. and Anagnostopoulos, C.E. (1982). Acute aortic dissection. An historical review, *J. R. Coll. Surg. of Edinburgh*, **27**, 195–9

12. *Ibid.*, p. 196.

13. Shennan, T. (1934). Dissecting aneurysms. *Medical Research Council Special Report Series*, **193**

14. Elliotson, J. (1830). *On Recent Improvements in the Art of Distinguishing Diseases of the Heart, being the Lumleian Lectures delivered before the Royal College of Physicians in the Year 1829.* (London: Longman, Rees, Orme, Brown and Green)

15. Pennock, C.W. (1839). Aortic dissection. *Am. J. Med. Sci.*, **23**, 13

16. Shennan, T. (1934). *Op. cit.*

17. Burns, A. (1809). *Observations on Some of the Most Frequent and Important Diseases of the Heart*, p. 231. (Edinburgh: Boyce)

18. Nicholls, F. (1761). *Philosophical Transactions B*, **52**, 265

19. Shekelton, J. (1822). Dissecting aneurysms of abdominal aorta. *Dublin Hosp. Rep.*, **3**, 221

20. Otto, G. (1824). *Neve Seltene*, p. 66. (Berlin: Beobachtungen)

21. Latham, P.M. (1855–6). *Transactions of the Pathological Society of London*, **7**, 106

22. Peacock, T.B. (1843). *Edinburgh Medical and Surgical Journal*, **60**, 276

23. Peacock, T.B. (1863). *Monthly Transactions of the Pathological Society of London*, **14**, 87

24. Leonard, J.C. (1979). *Op. cit.*, p. 260

25. Sanderson, C.J., Cote, R.J. et al. (1982). *Op. cit.*, p. 196

26. Shennan, T. (1934). *Op. cit.*

27. *Ibid.*

28. *Ibid.*

29. Edwards, J.E. (1973). Aneurysms of the Thoracic Aorta complicating coarctation. *Circulation*, **48**, 195–201

30. Roberts, W.C. (1981). Aortic dissection: anatomy, consequences, and causes. *Am. Heart J.*, **101**, 195–214

31. Abbott, M.E. (1927). Congenital cardiac disease. In McCrea, T. (ed.) *Osler's Modern Medicine*, vol. 4, 3rd. edn., p. 747. (Philadelphia: Lea and Febiger)

32. Wilson, S.K. and Hutchins, G.M. (1982). Aortic dissecting aneurysms: causative factors in 204 subjects. *Arch. Path. Lab. Med.*, **106**, 175–80

33. Larson, E.W. and Edwards, W.D. (1984). Risk factors for aortic dissection: a necropsy study of 161 cases. *Am. J. Cardiol.*, **53**, 849–55

34. Hirst, A.E. Jr., Johns, V.J. Jr. and Kline, S.W. Jr. (1958). Dissecting aneurysm of the aorta: a review of 505 cases. *Medicine*, **37**, 217–79

35. Roberts, W.C. (1981). *Op. cit.*, p. 196

36. Baer, R.W., Taussig, H.B. and Oppenheimer, E.H. (1943). *Bulletin of the Johns Hopkin's Hospital*, **72**, 309

37. Marfan, A.B. (1896). Un cas de déformation congénitale des quatres membres plus prononcée aux extrémites characterisée par l'allongement des os avec un certain degré d'amincissement. *Bull. et Mém. Soc. Méd. Hôp.*, *Paris*, **13**, 220

38. Achard, C. (1902). Arachnodactylie. *Bull. Mém. Soc. Méd. Hôp.*, *Paris*, **19**, 834–40

39. Salle, V. (1912). Über einen Fall von angelborner abnormer Grösse der Extremitäten miteinen an Akromegalie erinnernden Symptomenkomplex. *Jahrb. Kinderheilkd.*, **75**, 540–50

40. Piper, R.K. and Irvine-Jones, E. (1926). Arachnodactylia and its association with congenital heart disease. *Am. J. Dis. Child.*, **31**, 832–9

41. Baer, R.W., Taussig, H.B. and Oppenheimer, E.H. (1943). Congenital aneurysmal dilatation of aorta associated with arachnodactyly. *Bull. Johns Hopkins Hosp.*, **72**, 309–31

42. Etter, L.E. and Glover, L.P. (1943). Arachnodactyly complicated by dislocated lens and death from rupture of dissecting aneurysm of aorta. *J.A.M.A.*, **123**, 88–9

43. Schnitker, M.A. and Bayer, C.A. (1944). *Annals of Internal Medicine*, **20**, 486

44. Pedowitz, P. and Perell, A. (1957). *Am. J. Obstet Gynecol.*, **73**, 720

45. Hasleton, P.S. and Leonard, J.J.C. (1979). Dissecting aortic aneurysms: a clinicopathological study. II Histopathology of the aorta. *Q. J. Med.*, New Series XLVIII, **189**, 63–76

46. Schlicter, J.G., Amromin, G.D. and Solway, A.S.L. (1949). The pathogenesis of aortic dissection. *Arch. Int. Med.*, **84**, 558

47. Gore, I. and Seiwert, V.J. (1952). Dissecting aneurysms of the aorta. *Arch. Pathol.*, **53**, 121

48. Gore, I. and Hirst, A.E. Jr. (1973). Dissecting aneurysms of the aorta. Clinico-pathologic correlations. In Brest, A. (ed.) *Cardiovasc. Clin.*, p. 239. (Philadelphia)

49. Schlatmann, T.J.M. and Becker, A.E. (1977). Pathogenesis of dissecting aneurysm of aorta. *Am. J. Cardiol.*, **39**, 21

50. Hasleton, P.S. and Leonard, J.C. (1979). *Op. cit.*, pp. 63–76

51. Hirst, A.E. and Gore, I. (1976). Is cystic medionecrosis the cause of dissecting aortic aneurysm? *Circulation*, **53**, 915–16

52. Sigerist, H.E. (1951). *A History of Medicine*, p. 1, 273. (New York: Oxford University Press)

53. Major, R.H. (1954). *A History of Medicine*, p. 51. (Illinois: Charles C. Thomas)

54. Ruffer, M.A. (1911). On arterial lesions found in Egyptian mummies. *J. Pathol. Bacteriol.*, **15**, 453

55. Adams, F. (1846). *The Seven Books of Paulus Aegineta*, translated from the Greek with a commentary, II, p. 311. (London: Sydenham Society)

56. Garrison, F.H. (1943). Revised by L.T. Morton: *A Medical Bibliography*, p. 173. (London: Grafton & Co.)

57. Erichsen, J.E. (1844). *Observations on Aneurism*, pp. 4–5. (London: Sydenham Society)

58. *Ibid.*, p. 4

59. Castiglioni, A. (1941). *A History of Medicine*. Translated from the Italian and edited by

E.B. Krumbhaar, p. 247. (New York: Alfred A. Knopf)

60. Erichsen, J.E. (1844). *Op. cit.*, p. 4
61. *Ibid.*, p. 6
62. East, C.T. (1957). *The Story of Heart Disease*, p. 81. (London: Wm. Dawson and Sons, Ltd.)
63. Lancisi, G.M. (1952). *De Aneurysmatibus Opus Posthumum*, revised with translation and notes by W.C. Wright. (New York: The Macmillan Co.)
64. *Ibid.*, p. 81
65. Erichsen, J.E. (1844). *Op. cit.*, pp. 11–14
66. *Ibid.*, pp. 207–13
67. *Ibid.*, pp. 175–9
68. Scarpa, A. (1780–81). Sur un Anéurisme de l'Arcade de l'Aorte, avec érosion de la Premiére Côte & du Sternum. *Hist. Soc. Roy. Med.*, **4**, 290–4
69. Osler, W. (1907). Aneurism. In *Modern Medicine, Its Theory and Practice*, vol. 4, pp. 448–502. (Philadelphia: Lea and Febiger)
70. Mann, R.J. (1974). Historical Vignette. Scarpa, Hodgson, and Hope, Artists of the Heart and Great Vessels. *Mayo Clin. Proc.*, **49**, 890–2
71. *Ibid.*, p. 890
72. Hope, A.F. (1848). *Memoir of the Late James Hope, MD Physician to St. George's Hospital*, 4th edn., pp. 30, 40–1, 44. (London: J. Hatchard and Son)
73. Hasse, C.E. (1846). *An Anatomical Description of the Diseases of the Organs of Circulation and Respiration*, translated and edited by W.E. Swaine, pp. 83–97. (London: Sydenham Society)
74. Rokitansky, C. (1852). *A Manual of Pathological Anatomy*, translated by G.E. Day, IV, pp. 275–2. (London: Sydenham Society)
75. Garrison, F.H. (1943). *Op. cit.*, p. 142
76. Long, E.R. (1933). In Cowdry, E.V. (ed.) *Arteriosclerosis*, p. 23. (New York: The Macmillan Co.)
77. Coats, J. and Auld, A.G. (1893). Preliminary communication of the pathology of aneurysms with special reference to atheroma as a cause. *Br. Med. J.*, **II**, 456–60
78. Ellis, P.R., Cooley, D.A. and DeBakey, M.E. (1961). Clinical considerations and surgical treatment of anulo-aortic ectasia. *J. Thorac. Cardiovasc. Surg.*, **42**, 363
79. Bedford, D.E. (1967). The Surgeon Cardiologists of the 19th Century. *Br. Heart J.*, **29**, 461–8
80. *Ibid.*, pp. 463–4
81. Hodgson, J. (1815). *A Treatise on the Diseases of Arteries and Veins, Containing the Pathology and Treatment of Aneurysms and Wounded Arteries*, p. 58–9, 89. (London: T. Underwood)
82. Takayasu, M. (1908). Case with unusual changes of the central vessels in the retina. *Act. Soc. Opthalmol. Japan*, **12**, 554
83. Braunwald, E. (1988). *Heart Disease. A Textbook of Cardiovascular Medicine*, 3rd. edn., p. 1563. (Philadelphia: W.B. Saunders Co.)
84. Shimizu, L. and Sano, K. (1956). Pulseless disease. *J. Neuropathol. Clin. Neurol.*, **1**, 37–47
85. Inada, K., Shimizu, H. and Kokoyama, T. (1962). Pulseless disease and atypical coarctation of the aorta with special reference to their genesis. *Surgery*, **52**, 433–43
86. Nasu, T.O. (1963). Pathology of pulseless disease. *Angiology*, **11**, 225–42
87. Laude, A. and La Porta, A. (1976). Takayasu arteritis. An arteriographic-pathological correlation. *Arch. Pathol. Lab. Med.*, **100**, 437–40
88. Nako, K., Iheda, M., Kimata, S. *et al.* (1967). Takayasu's arteritis. *Circulation*, **35**, 1141–55
89. Lande, A. and La Porta, A. (1976). *Op. cit.*, p. 337
90. Tanaka, H., Mihara, K., Ookura, H. *et al.* (1979). Echocardiographic findings in patients with aortitis syndrome. *Angiology*, **30**, 620
91. Lupi-Herrera, E., Sanchez-Torres, G., Marchshamer, J., Mispireta, J., Horwitz, S. and Vela, J.E. (1977). Takuyasu arteritis. Clinical study of 107 cases. *Am. Heart J.*, **93**, 94
92. Acar, J., Laurent, B., Slama, M. *et al.* (1983). Insuffisance aortique et maladie de Takayasu. *Annu. Med. Interne.*, Paris, **134**, 606
93. Hall, S., Barr, W., Lie, J.T. *et al.* (1985). Takayasu arteritis. A study of 32 North American patients. *Medicine*, **64**, 89–99
94. Paulley, J.W. and Hughes, J.P. (1960). Giant-cell arteritis, or arteritis of the aged. *Br. Med. J.*, **2**, 1562
95. Jacquet, L. (1897). Ghika: Sur un cas d'arthro blennorhagisme avec troubles trophiques. *Bull. Soc. Méd. Hôp.*, Paris, **14**, 93
96. Paronen, I. (1948). Reiter's disease. A study of 344 cases observed in Finland. *Acta Med. Scand.*, Suppl. **212**, 1
97. Dixon, A.S.G. (1960). 'Rheumatoid arthritis' with negative serological reaction. *Ann. Rheum. Dis.*, **19**, 209
98. Neu, L.T. Jr., Reider, R.A. and Mack, R.E. (1960). Cardiac involvement in Reiter's disease: report of a case with review of the literature. *Ann. Intern. Med.*, **53**, 215
99. Csonka, G.W., Litchfield, J.W., Oates, J.K. and Wilcox, R.R. (1961). Cardiac lesions in Reiter's disease. *Br. Med. J.*, **1**, 243

100. Weinberger, H.J. (1962). Reiter's syndrome re-evaluated. *Arthritis Rheum.*, **5**, 202

101. Rodnan, G.P., Benedek, T.G., Shaver, J.A. and Fennell, R.H. Jr. (1964). Reiter's syndrome and aortic insufficiency. *J.A.M.A.*, **189**, 889

102. Ford, D.K. (1970). Reiter's syndrome. *Bull. Rheum. Dis.*, **20**, 588

103. Cliff, J.M. (1971). Spinal bony ridging and carditis in Reiter's disease. *Ann. Rheum. Dis.*, **30**, 171

104. Paulus, H.E., Pearson, C.M. and Pitts, W. Jr. (1972). Aortic insufficiency in five patients with Reiter's syndrome. *Am. J. Med.*, **53**, 464–72

105. Graham, D.C. and Smythe, H.A. (1958). The carditis and aortitis of ankylosing spondylitis. *Bull. Rheum. Dis.*, **9**, 171

106. Toone, E.C. Jr., Pierce. E.L. and Hennigar, G.R. (1959). Aortitis and aortic regurgitation associated with ankylosing spondylitis. *Am. J. Med.*, **26**, 255

107. Davidson, P., Bagenstoss, A.H., Slocumb, C.H. and Daugherty, G.W. (1963). Cardiac and aortic lesions in rheumatoid spondylitis. *Proc. Mayo Clin.*, **36**, 427

108. Weed, C.L., Kulander, B.G., Mozzarella, J.A. and Decker, J.L. (1966). Heart block in ankylosing spondylitis. *Arch. Int. Med.*, **117**, 800

109. Malette, W.G., Eiseman, B., Danielson, G.K., Mazzoleni, A. and Rams, J.J. (1969). Rheumatoid spondylitis and aortic insufficiency. An operable combination. *J. Thorac. Cardiovasc. Surg.*, **57**, 471

110. Zvaifler, N.J. and Weintraub, A.M. (1963). Aortitis and aortic insufficiency in chronic rheumatic disorders – a reappraisal. *Arthritis Rheum.*, **6**, 241

111. Pearson, C.M., Kroening, R., Verity, M.A. and Getzen, J.H. (1967). Aortic insufficiency and aortic aneurysm in relapsing polychondritis. *Trans. Ass. Am. Physicians*, **80**, 71

9   Atherosclerosis (arteriosclerosis)

Before delving into the historical background of this very complex scourge of humanity, a few words about terminology would be most appropriate. The need for this will become more apparent as the historical details change from an early descriptive phase with unsubstantiated attempts at pathogenesis to the subsequent introduction of various theories concerning the how and why of atherosclerosis in the light of more precise observations and experimentation. The initial descriptions emphasized the bone-like changes and accounted for the usage of such terms as ossification and petrification. Later observers noted that there were other lesions in the spectrum of the morbid anatomy which were characterized as being soft and containing 'gruel-like' material.

The term arteriosclerosis was introduced by Lobstein in 1833, and it eventually evolved into the generic label for hardening of the arteries[1]. It was not until 1904 that its pre-eminence as a generic designation was challenged. In that year, in an attempt to incorporate both ends of the pathologic spectrum, Marchand presented a paper at the 21st Congress for Internal Medicine in Leipzig wherein he recommended the adoption of the term 'atherosclerosis'[2]. This seemed like a reasonable semantic approach since in Greek, 'athero' means gruel and 'sclero' stands for hardening. Many pathologists, however, were not inclined to embrace atherosclerosis as a generic term for a number of reasons, but especially because it did not address the specific layer of the blood vessel that was involved. Moreover, it did not take into account the observations that Virchow had published in 1856. Two years after Marchand's original proposal, Klotz, in an effort to resolve the issue, urged a return to Lobstein's 'arteriosclerosis' as the generic designation for the entire process[3]. The various stages or entities could then be subdivided into atheromatosis, hyperplastic arteriosclerosis and Mönckeberg sclerosis which was a unique variety characterized by calcification of the media.

The terminology remained at this level until 1971 when Haust and More, in discussing the development of modern theories on the pathogenesis of this common vascular abnormality, went to considerable length in support of what they felt would be a more precise terminology[4]. They recommended a re-adoption of Marchand's 'atherosclerosis' as the generic term embracing all or any given stage of the disease. Since the medial calcinosis of Mönckeberg appears to have an entirely different pathogenesis, it was excluded from their classification. Under their schema, subsidiary terms would be atheromatous lesion, atheroma, advanced lesions and complicated lesions. The early atheromatous lesion would be 'fatty dots and streaks,' and atheroma would refer to the atherosclerotic plaque whose inner core would contain necrotic proteinaceous and fatty substances. In the advanced lesion, there would be fibrous plaques as well. The complicated lesion would manifest any or all of the following: ulceration, calcification, hemorrhage and thrombosis.

I do not wish the reader to be smug about the return of the pendulum to Marchand's original proposal. The semantic debate is still far from over. The use of the term atherosclerosis has been a bone of contention itself because it, as well as arteriosclerosis, has become synonymous with arteriopathy. On a clinical basis this is not necessarily true. Although all people in time will develop atherosclerosis only a certain proportion of them will manifest ill-effects from the process.

I am personally in favor of the nomenclature recommended by Haust and More simply because it incorporates, as the complete historical background will reveal, the various stages of the process, and the types of lesions that are produced during each stage. Current knowledge has definitely established atherosclerosis as involving metabolic, hemodynamic, hematologic, and genetic factors. The one parameter that can be visually appreciated and classified is the resultant arterial tissue change, and this nomenclature serves the purpose well.

Atherosclerosis must have been present long before the lifetimes of Aristotle, Galen and Celsus. There is no doubt that it was present among the early Egyptians. Proof of this was supplied by Ruffer and Shattuck, independently of each other. Marc Armand Ruffer was a member of the medical faculty at Cairo when, in 1911, he published his observations involving an extensive macroscopic and microscopic study of the arterial lesions of Egyptian mummies. Although most of the intrathoracic and intra-abdominal arteries were destroyed during the almost complete evisceration of the body while undergoing mummification, enough remnants remained both there and in the limbs for Ruffer to describe in detail the lesions of atherosclerosis in various stages of development and appearance[5]. These included the soft atheromatous lesions, the calcified plaques, the ulcers and even the type of sclerosis that Mönckeberg described so well in 1903. Ruffer was also able to demonstrate that the sclerotic changes were not the exclusive prerogative of the elderly. Utilizing Aristotle's method of estimating age on the degree of hardening of the cartilaginous tissues, he was able to roughly assess the age of the mummy under study, and thus noted atherosclerotic lesions even in younger people.

Ruffer's work followed by only three years Shattuck's description of atherosclerotic lesions in the mummy of Menephtah.

This Egyptian Pharaoh was probably an old man when he died; death being attributed to natural causes and not from drowning in the Red Sea during the Hebrew exodus[6]. Long recounts how the body was found in the tomb of Amenhotep II, and unwrapped by G. Eliot Smith who sent a piece of the aorta to S. G. Shattuck in London[6].

Utterly on their own, and with no knowledge of what the Egyptian mummies would reveal in the 20th century, Aristotle and his contemporaries left descriptions of 'bone-in-the-heart' as well as elsewhere that were highly suggestive of atherosclerosis[7]. It was looked upon as a natural consequence of advancing age with no perception of its significance in terms of disrupting normal physiological functions or as a causative factor in the demise of individuals.

Subsequently, a total silence persisted on the subject for more than a millennium. Despite the dissections that went on in Alexandria by men trained in the Aristotelian tradition, neither their writings nor those of Galen and Celsus contain any mention of human atherosclerosis. Significant descriptions of atherosclerotic lesions did not begin to appear until the 1500s. The earliest report begins with Benivieni, dated 1507[8], followed by Fallopio in 1575[9]. Benivieni's description bears all the characteristics of the lesion that we now label as atherosclerosis although he did not designate it as such. It is found in his treatise on the hidden causes of disease. Fallopio's description is that of a woman whose arteries at one side had become bony. Ossification was the term both men used for the hardening process.

A strange omission is that of Jean Fernel. The reader will recall how he described aneurysms at some length in his celebrated *Medicina*, but there is little or no reference to atherosclerosis. At the end of the 16th century, Schenck von Grafenberg in his *Observationum Medicarum Rararum* referred to atherosclerotic lesions many times but these are compilations of descriptions from various sources rather that the result of his own observations[10].

During the 17th century, Bellini and Bonet were among the first to add their descriptions. Bellini in 1662 called the arterial lesions petrifications (again, referring to the stone-like hardness) and was one of the first to speculate on the cause[11]. He held the opinion that it was due to an inflammatory process, and referred to the calcified plaque as a 'crust'. Bonet's contribution was merely a compilation of previous descriptions with no original observations[12]. By the end of the century, an observation of prescient significance was made by William Cowper. He noted the restriction of blood flow in thickened arteries[13].

In the first half of the 18th century, Johann Brunner described an aorta that had unmistakable signs of softening as well as petrification[14]. He is therefore credited as being probably the first to record softening as part of the morbid anatomy of atherosclerosis up to that time, although it was the bony hardness rather than the softening that attracted the most attention. The human interest aspect of Brunner's publication is, to me, far more intriguing. The aorta that Brunner described was that of his father-in-law, Johann Jacob Wepfer, who was the first to incriminate cerebral hemorrhage as a cause of apoplexy. Figure 1 depicts Wepfer's aorta, opened in a longitudinal manner. It can be found in Wepfer's *Observationes Medico-Practicae de Affectibus*

Capitis Internis et Externis which was published in 1727, 32 years after his death[15]. Morgagni's *De Sedibus* which appeared 15 years after Brunner's original report refers to Brunner's description of the aorta in the following words: '... the internal coat in several places was ruptured, lacerated and rotten like fruit, and hurt the fingers when thrust in it, from the roughness of the bones'[16].

As the 18th century progressed, there was a considerable increase in the number and extent of descriptions that appeared regarding the vascular changes of atherosclerosis. In addition, this century saw the promulgation of the first theories on pathogenesis. However, instead of really advancing knowledge the majority of these writings merely added to the confusion; being heavily weighted with fallacies and misconceptions. Illustrative of this is Crell's treatise which appeared in 1740 and dealt particularly with atherosclerosis of the coronary arteries[17].

Johann F. Crell was from Helmstadt. Although his description of the coronary lesions was good, it was his concept of the pathogenesis that was erroneous. Following Bellini's footsteps he referred to the atheromatous lesions as 'incrustations' rather than ossifications. He was of the belief that they were derived from pus. In the course of time, as the fluid portion of the pus evaporated, the remaining material thickened and hardened. There is no mention of calcification so that, in reality, Crell considered the atheromatous plaque as being tophaceous rather than bony in nature. He was right in one respect: namely, that the lesion could be found in any age group.

Another concept in pathogenesis was that offered by Boerhaave of Leyden[18]. He was of the opinion that the entire process was due to failure of the vasa vasorum to nourish its segment of the arterial wall. The loss of blood supply (he reasoned) was due to obliteration of the lumen of the vasa vasorum brought about by constriction as a result of the hardening of fibers surrounding the vessel. That segment of the arterial wall dependent upon the affected vasa vasorum would then harden over time into a solid firm nodule. This concept was rejected by his famous pupil, Albrecht von Haller. Haller envisaged the evolution of the atheromatous lesion as a continuous process beginning with the formation of a soft plaque and ending as a hard bone-like lesion. Haller stressed the softening process rather than the ossification and did not agree at all

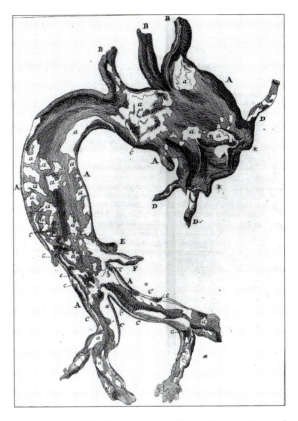

Figure 1 Wepfer's aorta. *Photo Source National Library of Medicine. Literary Source Wepfer, John-Jacobi: Observationes Medico-Practicae de Affectibus Capitis. Courtesy of National Library of Medicine*

with his teacher's view concerning the mechanism of closure of the lumen of the vasa vasorum nor the role this played in the atherosclerotic process. We shall come across both Boerhaave and Haller again, in the chapter dealing with functional mechanisms. At that time we will speak of them at greater length since their main contributions to cardiology were in the realm of physiology.

Morgagni's comments on atherosclerosis appeared in his *De Sedibus*[19]. It was, by far, a more extensive treatment of the subject than any that had been published before. He called attention to several important relationships: senility was not an invariable setting since he cited the case of a 90 year old woman who had minimal evidence of sclerotic changes; atheromatous plaques were often seen in association with dissecting aneurysms; and there was an association between antemortem complaints of 'chest pain' and the postmortem presence of 'ossification of the arteries of the heart'. Morgagni did comment on the obstructive potentiality of the lesions but failed to recognize the relationship between this and necrosis as a result of the occlusive process.

Scarpa's contribution to the field, as we have seen, was his recognition of the role played by atherosclerosis besides syphilis in the formations of aneurysms. Although he did suggest a relationship between syphilis and atherosclerosis, he softened this error somewhat by emphasizing the etiologic potentiality of atheromatous ulcers in the formation of aneurysms.

The early 19th century marked the end of the era of pure description and the beginning of a concerted attempt to be more precise in elucidating the nature and significance of atherosclerosis. As the century unfolded, attention was being drawn to the newer histopathologic observations, the pathophysiologic effects and to various concepts of pathogenesis. The chief participants were the English, French, German and Viennese schools. The scenario was cacophonous rather than orderly. Debate, often acrimonious, was the rule rather than the exception.

Beginning at the very start of the century, Bichat considered the lesions a degenerative process, and a natural consequence of aging. This placed him in direct opposition to Morgagni's view, as well as the view of others who found the lesions in various age groups[20]. Bichat, who was part of the French school, never used a microscope, but on the basis of meticulous dissection, advanced the opinion that the site of the initial lesion was in the intima and that ossification progressed from this initial lesion. The reputation of Bichat was such that a good part of the Parisian school of the time adhered to his view. His pupil, Laénnec, however, placed the lesions between the intima and the media. During this time, Cruveilhier focused his attention on intravascular clotting[21]. He reasoned that thrombosis was a repair mechanism in response to the inflammatory reaction of the arterial wall at the site where the circulatory blood deposited putaceous material from an atheromatous lesion located elsewhere. Although his reasoning and conclusions were erroneous, he must be given credit for at least being astute enough to regard thrombosis as an important element in the atherosclerotic process.

The early concepts of the pathophysiologic effects on the heart already had emerged in the latter part of the preceding century with Heberden's classical account of angina pectoris. But we are going to reserve this and other aspects of the historical background of ischemic heart disease for that section dealing with this disease entity. At this point, I should like to continue with that part of the English influence during the 19th century that was in the hands of Hodgson, Carswell and Hope.

We have already met Hodgson in his role with the pathologic entity of dissecting aneurysm. His impact on the broader aspects of atherosclerosis was also of an important magnitude. Concerning the pathophysiologic effects, Hodgson was well aware that the atherosclerotic lesions not only could induce angina pectoris but also could result in gangrene of the extremities or apoplexy from rupture of the cerebral vessels. The chemical make-up of the calcareous deposits was also delineated by his research and that of his staff. These studies led him to the conclusion that such deposits were not true bone. The beginnings of experimentation in atherosclerosis are inherent in this approach. Hodgson also described the ulcerative complication that is part of the spectrum of the sclerotic lesion. Hodgson, as was pointed out, was an excellent illustrator. His atlas contains many excellent depictions of atherosclerotic changes. He also gave a clear description of that unique type of arterial hardening which bears the eponym of Mönckeberg – having observed them in the peripheral arteries of the legs. Hodgson, too, did not agree with Bichat's contention that atherosclerosis was a natural consequence of aging. He helped pioneer the concept that atherosclerosis was a disease and not a natural phenomenon.

Hope's involvement with atherosclerosis centered primarily on its association with aortic aneurysms and there is no need to elaborate again on this.

Robert Carswell expounded his views through his book *Illustrations of the Elementary Forms of Disease* which appeared in 1837[22], just six years after Hope's opus on diseases of the heart and vessels. Carswell's text demonstrates a thorough knowledge of the morphologic characteristics known at the time, but he too was in error as to the how and why of the process. Thomas Smith recounts how Carswell illustrated a case of gangrene of the toes, attributing it to ossification of the arterial wall but mistakenly believing that the blood supply to the toes was cut off by deposition of fibrin alone within the lumen of the feeding artery[23].

Further developments during the 19th century were marked by the appearance of histopathologic studies that were not merely isolated presentations but rather an integral part of the various approaches attempting to delineate the pathogenesis of atherosclerosis. The historical background of this aspect began with the Viennese school but gradually expanded to include other European centers. American investigators did not begin to play an important role until the early years of the 20th century. Throughout all this, we shall see the shift from independent personalities to a team approach. We shall also see how the descriptive approach underwent reinforcement through the use of experimentation. And, finally, it will become quite evident that the evolving knowledge has become increasingly dependent on a multi-disciplinary approach utilizing the expertise from such seemingly unrelated fields as pathology, biochemistry, genetics and epidemiology.

The number of theories that have been proposed on pathogenesis since the earliest descriptions are almost legion. Out of this prolific output, several have prevailed. The most important of them are the thrombogenic theory, the inflammatory theory of Virchow, the insudation theories of Rössle and Doerr, and the lipid theory. Numerous other concepts have also been introduced but they have been proven completely invalid or absorbed into the key theories just outlined. No matter what, all have played a role in the solidification of current concepts and therefore deserve to be included in any historical survey.

The thrombogenic theory is the oldest among the key theories proposed prior to the era of experimentation. It is also known as the encrus-tation theory taking its name from the descriptions of Bellini and Crell. The outline of the theory was developed by Rokitansky in 1841. In his discussion of the extensive deposits seen on the inner layer of the arterial wall, he proposed that they were derived primarily from fibrin and other blood elements rather than being the result of a purulent process[24]. Rokitansky attempted to place atherosclerosis within his schema of 'stases and crases'. He postulated that the atheroma resulted from degeneration of the fibrin and other blood proteins that had been deposited on the intima of the artery as a result of a pre-existing 'crasis' of the blood. The metamorphosis of these initial deposits saw them converted either into a pulpy mass containing cholesterol crystals and fatty globules or into an ossified mass[25].

Cruveilhier, on the other hand, attempted to include the atherosclerotic process within his own schema, namely, that most pathologic lesions were the result of an inflammatory process[26]. He therefore considered the arterial clots, when present, as the result of an arteritis. He also felt that the calcareous incrustations were part of a protective mechanism to prevent dilatation and aneurysm formation.

Rokitansky's view became the dominant one until it came under attack by Virchow not many years later. Although badly battered by Virchow's assault, Rokitansky's thrombogenic concept was never completely discarded. It remained 'on the back burner', as it were, until the American pathologist, F. B. Mallory, reactivated it in his Harveian lectures in 1923[27]. He too was impressed with the fibrin-like material in the plaques and expressed the view that it was derived from blood proteins.

Twenty years later, Clark and his group published a paper on thrombosis of the aorta and coronary arteries wherein they made special reference to 'fibrinoid' lesions[28]. On the basis of their histologic observations, they expounded the view that the thrombotic process began with deposits on the surface of the intima which then gradually became covered with endothelium and finally underwent a transition to collagenous tissue containing fibroblast. Since some plaques consisted of stratified layers of fibrin-staining material alternating with fibrous tissue they proposed that the deposition of blood elements at any particular site was a repetitive process.

The next decade saw no further interest in the thrombogenic theory until the publication of a series of papers by Duguid beginning in 1946. His initial paper concerned itself with thrombosis as a factor in the pathogenesis of coronary atherosclerosis. Three years later he published his classic paper on *Pathogenesis of arteriosclerosis*[29]. In it, he attempted to buttress the validity of the thrombogenic theory with the principles of vascular physiology. Thus, the fibrous thickening was not a reaction to a degen-erative process but actually represented a stage in the morphologic transition from the initial surface deposits due to hemodynamic factors. In other words, the reactive fibrosis that Virchow advocated could not be accepted as valid. Since the arterial wall expands and recoils during the ebb and flow of the cardiac cycle, and since this depends on the inherent elasticity of the arterial wall, then any loss of elasticity through a reactive fibrotic replacement would result in dilatation of the artery rather than the narrowing that is so commonly seen.

The baton in favor of the thrombogenic theory was taken up during the next few years by a number of investigators among whom may be listed Harrison[30] (1948), Heard[31] (1952), McLetchie[32] (1952), Barnard[33] (1953), Hand and Chandler[34] (1962) and Mustard and his group in 1963[35].

There are still many supporters of the theory but, unfortunately, it cannot account for all the features of atherosclerosis, nor can it account for the initial deposition of thrombi. Duguid's revival of interest in the concept, however, did have an important spin-off. It helped stimulate such an intensive interest in the field of thrombosis that considerable progress has been made in our knowledge of the subject. As we shall see, the new knowledge gained has provided the foundation for many of the modern therapeutic approaches in the management and prevention of thrombotic episodes.

Incidentally, a little known but interesting fact is that while Rokitansky's thrombogenic theory was at the height of its popularity, there was one lone voice in America who ignored fibrin and identified cholesterol as the major constituent of atherosclerotic plaques. The voice was that of J. Vogel. His remarks appeared in his text *The Pathological Anatomy of the Human Body*, which was published in 1847[36].

The inflammatory theory owes its origin to Virchow[37]. His approach to the problem stemmed from his detailed study of the complex histologic features of the atherosclerotic lesion in all its stages. Prior to his involvement, nobody had studied the subject to such an extent and depth. He was truly obsessed with the most minute detail. The major fruit of his labors was the recognition that the lesion was actually situated within or underneath the intimal lining and that the primary deposit occurred by imbibition of certain blood elements through this lining as the blood coursed through the channel. He described the next stage in the process as a softening of the connective tissue matrix at the site of deposition followed by an active proliferation of this same tissue within the intima. Concomitant with progressive softening of the ground substance in the affected area, a fatty metamorphosis of the connective tissue cells ensued which led to localized thickenings.

In attempting to explain the nature of the process, Virchow applied the term 'endarteritis deformans'. By this he meant that the atheroma was the product of an inflammatory process within the intima, and that the fibrous thickening evolved as a consequence of a 'reactive fibrosis' induced by proliferating connective tissue cells within the intima. Virchow maintained that the irritative stimulus was initiated by mechanical forces and that the 'endarteritis' was part of a repair mechanism. Once the process began the continued softening of the ground substance eventually led to erosion of the localized thickening while the constantly proliferating connective tissue cells assumed an almost neoplastic intensity of growth.

Virchow's inflammatory theory has elements that are acceptable to current investigators in the field, but it also has features that have been invalidated. The master did recognize two morphologic forms: the early fatty dots and streaks which he called 'atherosis' and the later sclerotic plaques. The theory does not provide an explanation of how the 'atherosis' progresses to the sclerotic plaques nor does it take into account the importance of mural thrombosis as an element in the entire process. We also know today that the fibrous cap of the atherosclerotic lesion is not a purely reactive fibrosis. Currently, it is commonly accepted that it represents an organization of various blood proteins that either enter or are deposited on the intima with a portion derived, as a secondary source, from microscopic hemorrhages, as some of the newly-formed, thin-walled intimal capillaries rupture. Most importantly, his 'fibroblasts' are really smooth muscle cells, a histologic feature about which he was in error, and an important ingredient of the current views on pathogenesis. However, Virchow's concept of local intimal injury as the initiating 'irritative' stimulus is still widely held though considerably extended to include other factors besides those of a mechanical nature.

Rudolph Virchow was a giant among the German pathologists. Small in stature he has been described as 'an elastic, professional figure, with snappy black eyes, quick in mind and body, with a touch of the Slav, something of a martinet in the morgue or lecture room, often transfixing inattention or incompetence with a flash of sarcasm'[38]. He was born in 1821 in Schivelbein, Pomerania. His medical degree was granted by the University of Berlin, immediately following which he began his lifelong career as a pathologist.

Only four years after graduation, he began with his friend, Benno Reinhardt, a new journal, *Archiv für pathologische Anatomie und Physiologie, und für klinische Medezin*. Virchow continued as the sole editor long after Reinhardt's death. The journal is now known as Virchow's Archives. Virchow also published a weekly paper *Die Medezinische Reform*. The paper, which lasted for only five years, had a markedly political orientation, and apparently its editorial comments as well as its articles displeased the authorities to the extent that Virchow was relieved of his position as prosector at the Charité. Although reinstalled just a fortnight later, Virchow left Charité to occupy the newly-formed chair of pathologic anatomy at Würzburg. He spent seven years there establishing a reputation as a brilliant teacher and researcher. During his tenure at Würzburg, Virchow had already begun to formulate his theory of cellular pathology. He not only was the author of many papers on pathological anatomy but also had begun the publication of his monumental *Handbuch der speziellen Pathologie und Therapie*. In 1856, he returned to Berlin where he occupied the chair of pathological anatomy and the post of director of the newly established pathological institute. Both positions and the institute were created especially for him[39].

Virchow's interests were wide and varied; a characteristic that we have seen quite often in men of exceptional ability. Aside from his medical pursuits, he became actively involved as a political reformer, serving at first in the Prussian lower house and then for many years in the Reichstag. Honor upon honor was bestowed upon him for his numerous accomplishments in pathology, legislation, sanitation, teaching and cultural activities. Even in old age he continued to work on various sociopolitical and scientific projects at an undiminished pace. Just three years before his death, he dedicated the celebrated pathological museum to which he had donated his own personally assembled collection of more than 23 000 specimens.

Virchow's opus magnum *Cellular Pathology as based upon Physiological and Pathological Histology* was published in 1858. He was only 37 years of age at the time. The text is really a series of 20 lectures that he gave during the year of its publication. It reflects throughout its pages, his unified concept of the 'sick cell' as being the essence of all disease. Garrison quotes Virchow as saying the body is 'a cell-state in which every cell is a citizen, disease being merely a conflict of citizens in this state, brought about by the action of external forces'[40].

Virchow's disputatious sorties were not confined to politics. They were the very fiber of his being whether the confrontations were in politics or in scientific debate. The highlights of his scientific confrontations were those he had with Rokitansky's 'crasis' theory, the views of Hugh Bennet regarding leukemia, and his opposition to Cruveilhier's doctrine of phlebitis as the source of all pathologic lesions.

Of course, Virchow made many errors during his lifetime. All men who are on the cutting edge of knowledge share this human defect. Among his erroneous positions were his opposition to Darwin's theory of evolution and his stance against the toxin–antitoxin concepts of Koch and Behring.

After a long and fruitful life, Virchow died in 1902 at the age of 81, probably because of an accident he suffered nine months earlier. He was the 19th century version of a true Renaissance man in every sense of the word. Figure 2 is a photograph of Virchow and Figure 3 is a depiction of the frontispiece of his *Cellular Pathology*.

The inflammatory theory of Virchow continued to be promulgated by his pupil, Edward Rindfleisch, with certain modifications[41]. He distinguished between Virchow's proliferative degeneration and ordinary fatty degeneration of the intima without a preliminary overgrowth of connective tissue[42]. Rindfleisch considered the degenerative process as consisting of two stages: a fatty degeneration of the connective tissue cells with marked softening of the intercellular ground substance and a stage characterized by the impregnation of the ground substance with calcium salts[43].

Histologic techniques underwent considerable improvement during the last few decades of the 19th century. Armed with these technological innovations, Jores in 1898 investigated more thoroughly the role of elastic tissue. His investigations led him to ascribe to it a prominent role in the vascular regenerative process[44,45]. He demonstrated its influence on the organization of thrombi in the intact artery and classified the types of elastic tissue into regenerative and hyperplastic.

By the end of the 19th century, the inflammatory theory of Virchow was gradually being abandoned. This was especially true among the German pathologists, who substituted in its stead, several conflicting theories of their own. Prominent among them was Richard Thoma of Heidelberg. He was active in the field for a long time;

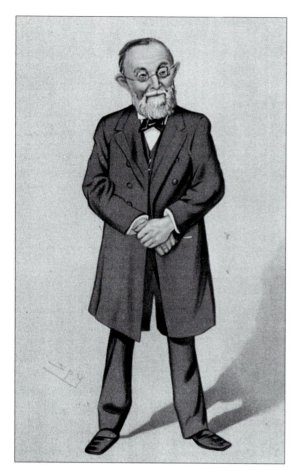

Figure 2 Rudolph Virchow (1821–1902). *Photo Source National Library of Medicine. Literary Source Photo Archives. Courtesy of National Library of Medicine*

his impact secured by a series of papers appearing over a span of 40 years. In 1883, he summarized his entire view on the subject in a paper published in Virchow's own periodical[46]. Thoma looked upon the intimal proliferation not as an initiating factor at all. He considered it to be a compensatory mechanism in response to loss of elasticity of the middle coat of the artery. He attributed the loss of elasticity to a natural consequence of age which in turn weakened the wall's ability to withstand the constant pounding by the intra-arterial pressure so that it would tend to dilate. In an effort to prevent the artery from dilating unduly, nature responded by thickening of the intima. Since the process was a continuing one, the thickening of the intima would reach a point where it outgrew its nutritional supply and then enter a stage of deterioration

culminating in the characteristic fibrotic, atheromatous and calcific lesions.

Although Thoma had many supporters, his concept was doomed to failure. It had an insurmountable major flaw in that it did not explain the lipid deposits in the lesion.

We have already met Oscar Klotz because of his attempt in 1906 to introduce his own classification of atherosclerosis in opposition to that of Marchand. Several years later in a monograph on diseases of the media and their relation to aneurysm, he stressed the concept of 'medial arteriosclerosis'[47]. The work describes two types of medial disease: the productive and degenerative. On the basis of this classification, he attributed their cause to such diverse factors as advancing age, hard work, infections and poisons. Arguing from a histological base, he ventured the opinion that Marchand's term 'atherosclerosis' could not be utilized as a generic designation since true atheroma did not occur in the media except as an extension of the process from the intima and therefore the term was inapplicable to all types of medial disease.

The last few years of the 19th century and the first decade or so of the 20th were conspicuous by the recurrent debates and speculation concerning the relationship between arteriosclerosis and hypertension and the role of the kidneys in the matter. By this time, the continuing evolution of the sphygmomanometer made blood pressure measurements easier and quite accurate and therefore clinical studies could be done on a firmer basis regarding this diagnostic modality.

The confusing element during these years continued to be the vexing role of the kidney. A significant breakthrough was provided by Frederick Akbar Mahomed of Guy's Hospital, London. In a series of papers published between 1874 and 1881, he demonstrated that high blood pressure could exist for some time without any overt renal damage[48–50]. This was the first indication that hypertension and renal disease need not co-exist. Having established that hypertension could exist independently of kidney disease, the debate continued regarding its role in atherosclerosis. Von Basch as late as 1893 had assumed that high blood pressure was the result of atherosclerosis[51–53]. On the other hand, Allbutt in 1895 and again in 1915 claimed that it was the high blood pressure that brought about arteriosclerosis[54,55]. Once it was recognized that more than one disease entity constituted atherosclerosis/arteriosclerosis, then it became apparent that a definite relationship with hypertension did exist but in a complex manner. This will be dealt with in the section on hypertension.

The turn of the century marked the beginning of intensive experimentation in the field to seek the initiating cause and utilizing widely divergent methods. Mechanical injury as the precipitating stimulus was investigated by Malkoff (1899)[56], Andriewitsch[57] (1901), Fabris[58] also in 1901, Jones[59] again in 1902 and Sumikawa[60] in 1903. They utilized ligation, pinching, wounding and cauterization of the arteries in animal models. Czyhlarz and Helbing[61] (1897), Jores[59], and Marchand[62] (1904) reported arterial changes after irritating or severing certain nerves but these findings were never confirmed. The lipid era began with the implications that certain constituents in the diet exercised an influence on the development of atherosclerosis. This gradually led to the knowledge that it was probably cholesterol. Further advances led to the knowledge that it was the cholesterol in transit that was being deposited along the arterial highway. It soon became apparent that cholesterol was transported with different types of 'cargo vehicles' called lipoproteins and these different lipoproteins could be separated by ultra-centrifuge and categorized as very low density, (VLDL), low density (LDL) and high density (HDL). Later developments targeted the LDL component as the culprit factor with HDL cholesterol playing a benevolent role. Biochemical studies indicated that the LDL cholesterol had to undergo oxidation before it could incite the development of atherosclerosis. Concomitant with these developments was the recognition of the important role genetics played in the entire process by supplying adequate receptors on the lipoproteins.

Thus, knowledge developed along three main lines: dietary, metabolic and genetic with epidemiologic confirmation of all three. The dietary aspect was initiated by Ignatovski, the metabolic by a host of investigators and the genetic by Brown and Goldstein.

The year 1908 marks the beginning of the dietary era in the story of atherosclerosis. The key to a whole new approach in delineating the pathogenesis of atherosclerosis was supplied by A. I. Ignatovski of the Russian Imperial Military Medical Academy. His findings and hypothesis

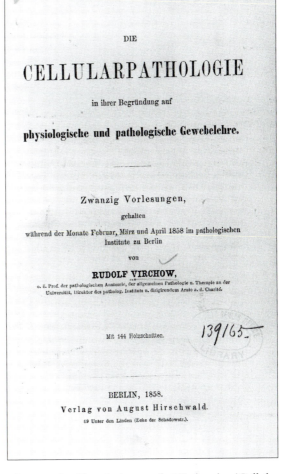

Figure 3 Frontispiece of Virchow's 'Cellular Pathology'. *Photo Source National Library of Medicine. Literary Source Photo Archives (copy of original). Courtesy of National Library of Medicine*

stimulated an unprecedented output of laboratory, clinical and epidemiologic investigations.

Ignatovski conducted the first experiments that lay the foundation for subsequent investigations. He reported that when rabbits were fed milk and egg yolk, they developed severe arteriosclerosis[63]. Like a bolt of lightning, this was an extraordinary approach to the atherosclerotic problem. Ignatovski was already aware from his own observations and those of others that there was a statistical difference in the incidence and severity of atherosclerosis among peoples of different socio-economic strata and occupations. This led him to formulate the hypothesis that the occurrence of atherosclerosis in humans was influenced to a significant degree by diet, and that the culprit ingredients of that diet were milk and eggs. It took more than 40 years before this revolutionary hypothesis of Ignatovski was confirmed by epidemiological studies, but in no time at all his experimental technique was exploited by his Russian colleagues, and for a while, the Russians occupied a dominant position in experimental atherosclerosis. Over the next several years following Ignatovski's paper, Stuckey, Wesselkin, Chalatov and Anischkov reported their results on the dietary influence in the evolution of the atherosclerotic lesion. The importance of diet is stressed in Figure 4. It is sarcastically labelled 'The Physician's Friend'.

Stuckey experimented with different types of fat and found that egg yolk and brain were more effective than milk in producing arterial lesions in rabbits whereas none could be seen following the ingestion of fish-oil, meat or sunflower-seed oil[64]. In 1908, Saltykow claimed that atherosclerosis could be produced by the administration of a staphylococcal–alcohol combination[65]. He did not realize at the time that his animals were being fed large quantities of milk, a food substance very rich in cholesterol and saturated fat. In 1913, he acknowledged his error in two papers and emphasized that it was not protein or any other lipid but rather the cholesterol in the diet that was important[66,67]. The high cholesterol content of the experimentally produced atheromatous lesions, as demonstrated by the studies of Windaus in 1910 provided additional evidence of a dietary correlation[68]. Wesselkin and Chalatov also showed that cholesterol-rich foods caused cholesterol-rich deposits in tissues[69]. In 1913, Anischkov and Chalatov went a step further by adding pure cholesterol to the diet of their rabbits[70]. These experiments were repeated and confirmed by Bailey of Stanford University just three years later[71].

Despite these experiments there was still considerable skepticism concerning the role of cholesterol. It was not until Timothy Leary and Anischkov published their individual views in the 1930s that any degree of certainty began to prevail. The identity of the actual culprit dietary ingredient and the type of animal model used continued to be the subject of debate.

Some investigators still held to the belief that the lesions were induced by feeding animal proteins to herbivores. In 1916, Kon and Yamada presented their view based on an analysis of the methodology utilizing the dietary approach[72]. They noted that liver had become the most commonly used food in many dietary experiments presumably as a source of protein. They also realized that liver has a very high cholesterol content. Though not referring to Saltykow by name, they implied that the objectors to the cholesterol hypothesis were guilty of the same error that he originally committed in 1908. In other words, it was the high cholesterol in the liver and not the protein that produced the atherosclerotic lesions.

Concomitant with the above, the species of animal model used also loomed large as a topic of debate during these early formative years of the lipid theory. Guinea pigs, dogs and chickens were found to be excellent animal models. The resultant histologic changes in the various species did reveal similarities and dissimilarities among them and between them and man. Some points were clear. The experimental lesions were infiltrative from the deposition of cholesterol, and the amount of cholesterol being deposited was far beyond any amount that might be derived from pre-existing tissue. It was soon realized that these early infiltrative deposits led to the full-blown atherosclerotic lesion. Finally it became apparent that the cholesterol had to be fed rather than injected. However, the marked dissimilarity between the lesions produced in rabbits and those seen in man led to increasing objections to use of this animal in further experiments. Anischkov, himself, conceded this.

In 1944, Dauber reported on the occurrence of spontaneous arteriosclerosis in chickens[73]. The use of chickens as an experimental model had already been suggested by the Japanese team Yamagiwa and Adachi as far back as 1914[74]. Dauber wrote that 'of all animals, birds have arteriosclerosis most closely resembling human arteriosclerosis.' Moreover, the chick was omnivorous removing a significant objection to the use of herbivores. In 1956, Fillios and associates reported on the use of rats[75]. Over the course of time, primates also were added to the list of animal models.

Anischkov emerges as one of the most influential figures in the field of experimental atherosclerosis. His original investigations contributed a good deal of light on the subject, and he remained active in the field well into the 20th century with many of his pupils continuing with their own significant contributions.

In 1933, Anischkov surveyed the history of experimental arteriosclerosis and wrote a classical paper which summarized the state of knowledge up to that time[76]. His comments in that paper included conclusions derived from his own experiments and many of his observations served as a guide for future experimentation.

He considered atherosclerosis as an infiltrative rather than a degenerative process. 'The process always begins with the accumulation of lipoid substances in the intercellular substance of the innermost layers of the arterial walls.' Using trypan blue as a colloidal stain, he noticed that, normally, a constant stream of liquid passes from the lumen of the artery through all the coats of its wall. This was a significant point of positive evidence that the infiltrative concept had a physiologically valid basis. He also acknowledged that the parenteral introduction of cholesterol did not produce any atherosclerotic change even when injected intravenously as a colloidal suspension.

Anischkov cautioned at the time against the blind acceptance of hypercholesterolemia as 'the cause' of arteriosclerosis. He proposed that atherosclerosis did not result from a single cause such as cholesterol but rather from modifications of physiological mechanisms involving 'internal secretions (hormones) and other local factors at the site of the lesion. He preferred to look upon the lesion as a disease of 'metabolic disturbance'.

Timothy Leary's paper followed that of Anischkov by two years[77]. Both papers went a long way towards convincing clinicians of the pervasive influence of diet in the arteriosclerotic process regardless of the uncertainty of the actual mechanisms involved and the realization that not all animals and humans responded in the same way to dietary manipulations. An apparent reason for this variable response was supplied by the investigations of Li and Freeman in 1946[78]. They noticed a striking and exceedingly important difference between the rabbit or chick and the higher mammals. They found that in dogs, a diet rich in both fat and cholesterol produced high levels of cholesterol in plasma whereas neither cholesterol feedings alone nor high fat diet alone had any appreciable effect. Herein was the clue as to why, on the same diet, some individuals or strains of animals show blood cholesterol levels much lower or higher than average. Subsequent investigators delineated this difference even further and accumulated enough evidence to prove that rabbits and chicks absorb cholesterol efficiently on diets low in fat, but that dogs, monkeys and humans could not absorb

dietary cholesterol unless the diet contained sufficient fat. Epidemiologic studies, in time, were to confirm this in man and serve as an important springboard for therapeutic intervention.

Anischkov alluded to this when he commented in the same paper of 1933:

> It should be mentioned that the various investigators prepared their cholesterin solutions with different vegetable oils. It is not impossible that the particular kind of oil used for this purpose might have some influence on the absorption of cholesterin from the intestine, and also on the rapidity and intensity of the atherosclerotic changes in the arteries[79].

Ignatovski's choice of food in his initial experiments was fortuitous in that the amount of saturated fat in the foods he selected was not important for the absorption of cholesterol in rabbits. If the reverse were true, it would be interesting to speculate on what the subsequent course of events would have been. Be that as it may, Anischkov was trying to simulate the diet (high in fat) of rich Russians in contrast to the low unsaturated fat content of the diet of the poor.

It was Isidore Snapper who first suggested that unsaturated fat protected against arteriosclerosis. This is to be found in his book 'Chinese Lessons to Western Medicine' which appeared in 1941[80]. Snapper was originally from Holland but spent many years in north China so he was quite conversant with the dietary make-up of both regions. Proof that diets high in unsaturated fat lowered blood cholesterol was then provided by two groups in 1952 working independently of each other. Groen headed one group[81], and Kinsell headed the other[82]. But it was Ahrens who provided the most convincing experimental proof in humans[83]. He and Hellman later showed through isotope studies that saturated fat increases absorption of cholesterol by reducing the loss through the bile derived fecal sterol[84].

Epidemiologic studies since the middle of the 20th century have shown repeatedly that in industrialized countries a positive relationship exists between increasing levels of plasma cholesterol and an increased risk of developing coronary artery disease. The earliest convincing proof that diet could cause human coronary artery disease was provided by Lober in 1953[85]. In the same year an equally convincing report was that of the Armed Forces Institute of Pathology demonstrating the existence of coronary artery disease among the youthful war dead in Korea[86].

More recently, metabolic studies have definitely shown that plasma cholesterol levels almost always increase with a more saturated fat diet. There is a striking correlation between intake of saturated fats and coronary artery disease. Numerous animal studies including those with non-human primates during the past decade have consistently demonstrated that lowering cholesterol through dietary and other means stops or actually reverses the disease process.

Probably the most important statistical study linking lower cholesterol levels and lower incidence of coronary artery disease was that conducted by the Lipid Research Clinics Coronary Primary Prevention Trial (LRC-CPPT). Held under the auspices of the National Institutes of Health, it had Basil Rifkind as the program officer in charge. He called the study results 'conclusive'. For the die-hard statistician this seems to be a reasonable statement since the data were analyzed by several statistical methods, all of which gave essentially the same results.

Prior to this there were a number of seminal epidemiologic studies convincingly proving an association between dietary fats and serum lipid concentrations. These studies had been based on geographic, retrospective, prospective and cross-cultural factors. Most of them had been conducted during the past 40 years or so. As late as 1958 there was still a great deal of resistance in accepting the role of lipids in the pathogenesis but it is no longer the case. Of course it is not the only factor, but it is undoubtedly a major one as these studies have proven.

As currently stated, the lipid theory holds that persistently elevated levels of plasma LDL contribute to the accumulation of cholesterol in the spaces between the endothelial cells of the arteries. How the LDL gets into these spaces, and what transpires after its infiltration have been the major focus of research interest during the past two decades or so. It is an interesting story emphasizing the multidisciplinary approach of modern medical research. No single individual is entirely responsible nor can any one center or country claim complete credit. Although many problems and questions still remain, and not all of the co-factors have been delineated, medical science has come a long way since Ignatovski supplied the original clue with his rabbit experiments.

A good deal of the current knowledge concerning the pathway of atherogenesis has been derived from studies in non-human primates (macaque monkeys), swine, and Watanabe heritable hyperlipidemic rabbits[87]. The use of such models has helped address the major failing of the lipid theory which was its inability to explain the focal distribution of atheromas. Two corollaries to the lipid theory have emerged during the past decade to explain not only this but also several other key questions. The corollaries are the concepts of lipid infiltration and endothelial injury. These have been formulated to address the following key questions:

(1) What is the connection between fatty streaks and fibrous plaques;

(2) What are the earliest structural or functional changes that initiate the atherosclerotic process;

(3) What are the various factors besides hypercholesterolemia that contribute towards the development of the lesion; and

(4) What precipitates occlusion of the arteries?

Normally, the endothelial lining is an effective barrier against the infiltration of unwanted substances. The endothelial damage hypothesis states that atherosclerotic lesions develop only after chronic injury to the endothelial lining. This was brought out by Ross and Glomsett in the *New England Journal of Medicine* in 1976[88,89]. The means of injuring the endothelium can be derived from at least three sources. These are hemodynamic, immunologic and biochemical. Historically, certain vascular sites have been known to be prone to atherosclerotic lesions. These are sites of arterial branching, flow dividers and curvature. This suggests that the fluid dynamics of the circulation at these sites create an area of turbulence which in turn injures the endothelial lining so that it becomes more permeable to the circulating lipoprotein. It is not too difficult to appreciate how an elevated blood pressure could intensify the pounding against the arterial wall and provide a hemodynamic accelerator to the injurious process. The list of possible biochemical sources is not entirely known. It includes serotonin, angiotensin, and catecholamine, all known for increasing blood pressure. Hypoxia, blood-borne toxins and antigens such as viruses have also been identified as possible sources of injury. The last two bring us back to

Virchow's inflammatory theory. However, the most important of the biochemical factors is the LDL level itself. It must be persistently high to take advantage of the injurious process. The immunologic factors operate in the transport and deposition of the cholesterol attached to the low density lipoprotein.

Although fatty streaks have been known to exist throughout the ages, not all of them are transformed into plaques. The response to injury hypothesis attempts to unveil the mechanisms for the transformation. It too was formulated by Ross and Glomsett in the same two papers that advanced their endothelial damage hypothesis[88,89]. They recently refined their concepts in an article published in 1986[90]. Accordingly, the first step in plaque formation occurs when the endothelial cells covering these fatty streaks begin to separate, exposing the streaks and surrounding connective tissue to the circulation. Two things can happen now. The circulating platelets clump together at the denuded site to form a clot and/or smooth muscle cells may proliferate. The proliferation of smooth muscle cells occurs under the stimulus of a 'platelet-derived growth factor'. Chemotactic proteins also come into play to help attract circulating monocytes to the site of injury. The most important of these proteins are derived from the smooth muscle cells. Once inside the subendothelial space, the monocytes become transformed into macrophages which act as scavengers.

An historical landmark was supplied by Goldstein, Brown and co-workers in 1979 when they offered evidence to indicate that these scavenger cells take up and degrade LDL through an oxidative mechanism, and then continue to play a key role in foam cell formation and cellular toxity[91]. As the process of atherogenesis proceeds, macrophages are eventually converted into foam cells by holding onto the oxidized low-density lipoprotein particles via a genetically inherited receptor. As the 20th century nears its end, how sophisticated the lipid theory has become. Notice too, how it now embodies elements from both the thrombogenic and inflammatory theories.

The third key theory that we have to touch upon is the insudation theory. It was originally proposed and formulated by Rössle between the fourth and fifth decade of this century, describing the process as one of 'serous inflammation'[92]. Rössle's theory was based on observations made by Ribbert as early as 1904[93]. Doerr expanded Rössle's original formulation and substituted the term perfusion for serous inflammation[94,95].

The theory is important because it antedates the endothelial damage hypothesis of the lipid theory. It proposed that the endothelium is damaged by injurious elements which Rössle called 'noxious agents of blood'. This precipitates a serous inflammatory response at the site of injury manifesting itself initially as the presence of an insudate derived from blood. The inflammatory fluid is called an insudate rather than an exudate because it does not accumulate outside the wall. If the injury is severe enough, the fluid becomes organized into avascular connective tissue.

In 1970, Haust extended the theory even further[96,97]. It became so all-embracing that it could be easily utilized as a vehicle for the incorporation of the valid points of the thrombogenic, inflammatory and lipid theories. Haust and More in 1972 gave this description of the mechanisms involved on the basis of the insudation theory[98]:

Thus, if an 'agent' injures the endothelium in a given area, this may result either in increased permeability, microthrombus deposition, or both. The composition and amount of the insudate will be determined by the severity of the injury and by the composition of blood, e.g., the more severe the insult, the more fibrin will enter the intima in the insudate; the more lipids in the plasma, the richer in fat content will be the entering fluid. The insudate, even relatively fat-free, when not absorbed quickly may impair the metabolism of the native smooth muscle cells with ensuing fatty metamorphosis. Should the insudate be ultimately absorbed, the fatty changes may regress, provided the cells have not reached the stage of 'no-return.' The lipid content of the insudate is one of the two important determinants (the other being fibrin) of its fate; the large, metabolically inert lipoprotein can be neither efficiently drained from the avascular intima nor catabolized. The organization of the proteins contained in the insudate contributes to the fibrous component of the emerging advanced lesion, and the lipid content contributes to the lipid component. Other elements, both local and derived from blood, contribute to either one or both main components of atherosclerotic plaque.

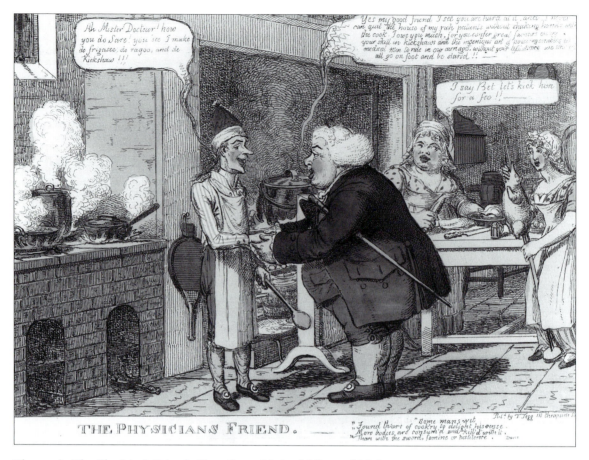

Figure 4 The Physician's Friend. *Photo Source National Library of Medicine. Literary Source T. Tegg, Cheapside. Courtesy of National Library of Medicine*

The main value of this extended form of Rössle's original theory according to the authors themselves is that it would serve as a starting point for the identification of the factors responsible for the initial injury to the endothelium.

In addition to the major theories just outlined, numerous other concepts have been introduced to describe the pathogenesis of atherosclerosis. Some have been proven invalid and others absorbed into the previous theories. Among them are anoxemia, senescence and the theory of intimal hemorrhages. The oldest is the senescence theory which advocated that fats and calcium were deposited as advancing age rendered connective tissue into a hyalinized state. This theory was promulgated by Aschoff in 1909, followed by Hueck in 1920 and then by Bürger in 1928[99–101]. Although it is now obsolete, it did teach us that the connective tissue of

the arterial intima does age rapidly and can become hyalinized at an early stage in life.

Hypoxia as an initiating factor has certainly been established as an important cofactor within the lipid theory. In this sense Hueper's theory on anoxemia certainly represents a contribution to the overall picture[102]. Although microhemorrhages do occur in atherosclerotic lesions, especially in hypertensive patients, the theory of intimal hemorrhages has not been generally accepted[103,104]. As the initiating factor, it was proposed originally by Winternitz and co-workers in 1938[105]. They proposed that the process begins with rupture of those capillaries of the arterial wall which connect with the lumen. The escaping blood would then deposit both lipid and fibrous components to form the resultant plaque. It is now known that microhemorrhages do occur in atherosclerotic lesions and that though they do not represent the initiating factor, they nevertheless contribute in some way to the formation of the plaque.

This, in essence, is the historical background of atherosclerosis as it evolved from the purely descriptive to the most recent work concerning pathogenesis. A few words at this point on arteriolosclerosis should round out the historical data pertaining to the arteries.

It was during the latter part of the 19th century that interest was also focused on the smaller blood vessels in the arteriosclerotic process. The most influential workers in the field were George Johnson of London and the team of Gull and Sutton. Johnson, as early as 1852, called attention to the abnormal thickening of the arterial walls of the kidney in chronic Bright's disease[106]. He claimed that the thickening in these vessels was due to muscular hypertrophy as a compensatory response to renal damage, and that this response was also widespread throughout the body. This concept was elaborated by him in a series of lectures delivered during 1873 on the diagnosis, pathology and treatment of Bright's disease[107]. It was also during the same period of time that Gull and Sutton were conducting their own microscopic studies on blood vessels both on healthy and diseased subjects. In their paper on the morbid anatomy of Bright's disease, they rejected Johnson's view of muscular hypertrophy suggesting instead that the thickened walls were due to 'a hyalin–fibroid rearrangement'[108].

Obviously, the changes described are totally different from the constellation of lesions seen in atherosclerosis of the larger arteries. Arteriolosclerosis represents a separate and distinct entity, apart from atherosclerosis despite their frequent association. It deserves a special category in the classification of arterial lesions just as the medial calcinosis of Mönckeberg deserves its own.

REFERENCES

1. Lobstein, J.G. (1933). *Tratie d'anatomie pathologique*, Paris
2. Marchand, F. (1904). *Über Arteriosklerose (atherosklerose)*. Verhandlungen des Kongress für innere medizin 21st Kongress, Leipzig
3. Klotz, O. (1906). Experimental Production of arteriosclerosis. *Br. Med. J.*, **2**, 1767
4. Haust, M.D. and More, R.H. (1972). Development of modern theories on the pathogenesis of atherosclerosis. In Wissler, R.W., Geer, J.C. and Kaufman, N. (eds.) *The Pathogenesis of Atherosclerosis*, (Baltimore: Williams and Wilkins Co.)
5. Ruffer, M.A. (1911). On arterial lesions found in Egyptian mummies. *J. Pathol. Bacteriol.*, **15**, 453
6. Long, E.R. (1967). Development of our knowledge of arteriosclerosis. In *Cowdry's Arteriosclerosis*, edited by Blumenthal, H.T., p. 6, 2nd edn. (Springfield, Ill.: Charles C. Thomas)
7. Aristotle, Historia animalium. *De generatione animalium*. (Greece) (ca. 364 BC)
8. Benivieni, A. (1507). *De abditis nonnullis ac mirandis norborum et sanationum causes*. (Florence)
9. Fallopio, G. (1575). *Lectiones de partibus similaribus humani corporis, Noribergae, Gerlach*
10. Schenck von Grafenberg, J. (1584–97). *Observationum Medicarum Raraum Libri VII*
11. Bellini, L. (1662). *Exercitatio Anatomica*. (Florence)
12. Bonet, T. (1679). *Sepulchretum sive Anatomia Practica*
13. Long, E.R. (1967). *Op. cit.*, p. 8
14. Brunner, J.S. (1746). *Dissertatio Inauguralis Medica Sistens Gravissimam Anginae Speciem*. (Magdenburg)
15. Wepfer, J.J. (1727). *Observationes Medico-Practicae de Affectibus Capitis Internis et Externis*
16. Morgagni, G.B. (1761). *De Sedibus et Causes Morborium per Anatomen Indignatis*. (Venice)
17. Crell, J.F. (1740). *Observatio De Arteria Coronaria instar essis Indurata*, Vimbergae, Reinhold
18. Boerhaave, H. *Praelectiones ad Institutione*, cited by Morgagni, ref. 16.
19. Morgagni, G.B. (1761). *Op. cit.*
20. Bichat, M.F.X. (1800). *Anatomie Generale*. (Paris)
21. Cruveilhier (1833). *Anatomie Pathologique du Corps Humain*. (Paris)
22. Carswell, R. (1837). *Illustrations of the Elementary Forms of Disease*. (London)
23. Smith, T.H.F. (1960). A chronology of atherosclerosis. *Am. J. Pharm.*, Nov., 390–403
24. Rokitansky, C. (1841). *Lehrbuch der Pathologischen Anatomie*. (Wien)
25. Rokitansky, C. (1852). *Über einige der wichtigsten krankheiten der arterien*
26. Cruveilhier, J. (1833). *Op. cit.*
27. Mallory, F.B. (1913). The infectious lesions of blood vessels. In *Harvey Lectures*, p. 150. (Philadelphia: J.P. Lippincott Co.)
28. Clark, E., Graef, I. and Chasis, H. (1936). Thrombosis of the aorta and coronary arteries.

With special reference to the 'fibrinoid' lesions. *Arch. Pathol. (Chicago)*, **22**, 183

29. Duguid, J.B. (1949). Pathogenesis of arteriosclerosis. *Lancet*, **2**, 925

30. Harrison, C.V. (1948). Experimental pulmonary arteriosclerosis. *J. Pathol. Bacteriol.*, **60**, 289

31. Heard, B.E. (1952). An experimental study of thickening of the pulmonary arteries of rabbits produced by the organization of fibrin. *J. Pathol. Bacteriol.*, **64**

32. McLetchie, N.G.B. (1952). The pathogenesis of atheroma. *Am. J. Pathol.*, **28**, 413

33. Barnard, P.J. (1953). Experimental fibrin thromboembolism of the lungs. *J. Pathol. Bacteriol.*, **65**, 129

34. Hand, R.A. and Chandler, A.B. (1962). Atherosclerotic metamorphosis of autologous pulmonary thromboemboli in the rabbit. *Am. J. Pathol.*, **40**, 469

35. Mustard, J.F., Rowsell, H.C., Murphy, E. and Downe, H.G. (1963). Intimal thrombosis in atherosclerosis. In Jones, R.J, (ed.), *Evolution of the Atherosclerotic Plaque*, p. 183. (Chicago: Univ. of Chicago Press)

36. Vogel, J. (1847). *The Pathological Anatomy of the Human Body*. (Philadelphia: Lea and Blanchard)

37. Virchow, R. (1856). Plogose und thrombose im Gefäss-system. Gesamelte Abhandlungen zur wissenschaftlichen Medicin. (Frankfurt: Medinger, Son and Co.)

38. Garrison, F.H. (1929). *An Introduction to the History of Medicine*, pp. 569–72. (New York: W.B. Saunders Co.)

39. Virchow, R. (1974) *Encyclopaedia Britannica*, vol. 19, pp. 150–1

40. Garrison, F.H. (1929). *Op. cit.*, p. 570

41. Rindfleisch, E. (1867). *Lehrbuch der pathologischen Gewerbelehre zur Einführung in das Studium der pathologischen Anatomie.* (Frankfurt: Medinger, Son and Co.)

42. Smith, T.H.F. (1960). *Op. cit.*, p. 394

43. Long, E.R. (1967). *Op. cit.*, p. 12

44. Jores, L. (1898). Über die Neubildung elastischer Fasern in der Intima bei Endarteritis. *Beiträge zur pathologischen Anatomie und zur allgemeinen Pathologie*, **24**, 458

45. Jores, L. (1903). *Wesen und Entwicklung der Arteriosklerose.* (Weisbaden: Bergmann)

46. Haust, M.D. and More, R.H. (1972). *Op. cit.*

47. Klotz, O. (1911). *Arteriosclerosis: Diseases of the Media and their Relation to Aneurysm.* Univ. of Pittsburgh, School of Medicine. (Lancaster, Pa.: New Era Print Co.)

48. Mahomed, F.A. (1874). The etiology of Bright's disease and the prealbuminuric stage. *Med. Chir. Trans.*, **57**, 197

49. Mahomed, F.A. (1879). Some of the clinical aspects of Bright's disease. *Guy's Hosp. Rep.*, **39**, 363

50. Mahomed, F.A. (1881). Chronic Bright's disease without albuminuria. *Guy's Hosp. Rep.*, **40**, 295

51. Basch, S.S. (1880). Ueber die Messung des Blutdrucks am Menschen. *Ztschr. klin. Med.*, **2**, 79

52. Basch, S.S. (1881). Einige Ergebnisse der Blutdruckmessung und Gesunden und Kranken. *Ztschr. klin. Med.*, **3**, 502

53. Basch, S.S. (1893). Ueber latente Arteriosclerose. *Wiener med. Presse*, **34**, 761, 808, 818, 891, 1102, 1142, 1184

54. Allbutt, T.C. (1915). *Diseases of the Arteries, Including Angina Pectoris.* (London: Macmillan)

55. Allbutt, T.C. (1895). Senile plethora or high arterial pressure in elderly persons. *Trans. Hunterian Soc.*, p. 38

56. Malkoff, G. (1899). Bedentung der traumatischen Vertletzung von Arterien für die Entwicklung der wakren Aneurysmen und der Arteriosklerose. *Beiträge zur path. Anatomie und zur allgemeinen Pathologie*, **25**, 431

57. Andriewitsch, A.N. (1901). *Zür Frage der Arterienveränderungen bei Wandreizung.* (Petersburg)

58. Fabris, A. (1901). Experimentelle Untersuchungen Über Pathologenese von Aneurysmen. *Virchow's Arch. für pathologische Anatomie und Physiologie*, **165**, 439

59. Jores, L. (1903). *Verhalten der Blutgefässe im Gebiete durchschnittener Nerven.* In ref. no. 45

60. Sumikawa, T. (1903). Ein beitrag zur Genese der Arteriosklerose. *Beiträge zur path. Anatomie und zur allgemeinen Pathologie*, **34**, 242

61. von Czyhlarz, E.B. and Helbing, C. (1897). Experimentielle Unterschungen über die Beziehung von Nervenläsionen zu Gefässveränderungen. *Centralblatt für allgemeine Pathologie und pathologische Anatomie*, **8**, 849

62. Marchand, F. (1904). *Op. cit.*

63. Ignatovski, A.I. (1908). On the influence of animal food on the tissues of the rabbit. *Reports of the Imperial Military Medical Academy, St. Petersburg*, **16**, 154

64. Dock, W. (1958). *Research in Arteriosclerosis – The First Fifty years*, **49**, 699–705

65. Saltykow, S. (1908). Atherosklerose bei Kaninchen nach weiderholten staphylokokken-injectionen. *Beiträge zur path. Anatomie und zur allgemeinen Pathologie*, **43**, 147

66. Saltykow, S. (1913). Experimentelle Athero-sklerose. Beiträge zur path. *Anatomie und Physiologie*, **57**, 415

67. Saltykow, S. (1913). Zur Kenntniss der alimentären Krankheiten der Versuchstiere. *Virchow's Archiv für path. Anatomie und Physiologie*, **213**, 8

68. Windaus, A. (1910). Über den Gehalt normaler und atheromatöser Aorten an Cholesterin und Cholesterinester. *Ztschr. f. Physiol. Chem.*, **67**, 174

69. Dock, W. (1958). *Op. cit.*, p. 699

70. Anischkov, N. and Chalatov, S. (1913). On experimental cholesterol steatosis and its significance in the development of various pathologic processes. *Centralbl. f. allg. Path. u. Path. Anat.*, **24**, 1

71. Bailey, C.H. (1916). Atheroma and other lesions produced in rabbits by cholesterol feeding. *J. Exp. Med.*, **23**, 69

72. Kon, Y. and Yamada, H. (1916). Weitere Untersuchungen über Fütterung mit Leberpulver und Eiglieb. *Trans. Japan. Pathol. Soc.*, **6**, 98

73. Dauber, D.V. (1944). Spontaneous arteriosclerosis in chickens. *Am. Med. Assoc. Arch. Pathol.*, **38**, 46

74. Yamagiwa, K. and Adachi, O. (1914). Über die Arteriosklerose bei Hünnern. *Virhandlungen der Japanische pathologischen Gesellschaft*, **4**, 55

75. Fillios, L.C., Andrus, S.B., Mann, G.V. and Stare, F.J. (1956). Experimental production of arteriosclerosis in the rat. *J. Exp. Med.*, **104**, 539

76. Anischkov, N. (1933). Experimental athero-sclerosis in animals. In *Cowdry's Arteriosclerosis*. (New York: Macmillan)

77. Leary, T. (1935). Atherosclerosis, the important form of arteriosclerosis, a metabolic disease. *J. Am. Med. Assoc.*, **105**, 475

78. Li, T.W. and Freeman, S. (1946). Experimental lipemia and hypercholesterolemia produced by protein depletion and by cholesterol-feeding in dogs. *Am. J. Physiol.*, **145**, 660

79. Anischkov, N. (1933). *Op. cit.*

80. Snapper, I. (1941). *Chinese Lessons to Western Medicine*, pp. 30 and 160. (New York: Interscience Publishers, Inc.)

81. Groen, J., Tjong, B.K., Kamminga, C.E. and Willebrands, A.F. (1952). The influence of nutrition, individuality and some other factors, including various forms of stress on the serum cholesterol, and experiment of nine months duration in 60 normal human volunteers. *Voeding*, **13**, 56

82. Kinsell, L.W., Partridge, J., Boling, L., Margen, S. and Michaels, G. (1952). Dietary modification of serum cholesterol and physpholipid levels. *J. Clin. Endocrinol.*, **12**, 909

83. Ahrens, E.H. Jr, Blankenhorn, D.H. and Tsaltas, T.T. (1954). Effect on human serum lipids of substituting plant for animal fat in diet. *Proc. Soc. Exp. Biol. Med.*, **86**, 872

84. Hellman, L., Rosenfeld, R.S., Insull, W. Jr and Ahrens, E.H. Jr (1957). Regulation of plasma cholesterol levels by fecal sterol excretion. *Circulation*, **16**, 497

85. Lober, P.H. (1953). Pathogenesis of coronary sclerosis. *Am. Med. Assoc. Arch. Pathol.*, **55**, 357

86. Enos, W.F., Holmes, R.H. and Beyer, J. (1953). Coronary disease among United States soldiers killed in action in Korea. *J. Am. Med. Assoc.*, **152**, 1090

87. Small, D.M. *et al.* (1984). Physicochemical and histological changes in the arterial wall of nonhuman primates during progression and regression of atherosclerosis. *J. Clin. Invest.*, **73**, 1590–605

88. Ross, R. and Glomsett, J.A. (1976). The pathogenesis of atherosclerosis (first of two parts). *N. Engl. J. Med.*, **295**(7), 369–77

89. Ross, R. and Glomsett, J.A. (1976). The pathogenesis of atherosclerosis (second of two parts). *N. Engl. J. Med.*, **295**(8), 420–5

90. Ross, R. (1986). The pathogenesis of atherosclerosis – an update. *N. Engl. J. Med.*, **314**(8), 488–500

91. Goldstein, J.L. *et al.* (1979). Binding site on macrophages that mediates uptake and degradation of acetylate low density lipoprotein, producing massive cholesterol deposition. *Proc. Natl. Acad. Sci. USA*, **76**(1), 333–7

92. Rössle, R. (1944). Über die serösen Entzün-dungen der Organe. *Virchow Arch. [Path. Anat.]*, **311**, 252

93. Ribbert, H. (1904). Ueber die Genese der arteriosklerosen Veränderungen der Intima. *Verh. Deutsch. Ges. Path.*, **8**, 168

94. Doerr, W. (1963). Perfusionstheorie der Arteriosklerose. In Bargmann, W. and Doerr, W. (eds.) *Zwanglose Abhandlungen aus dem Geiet der Normalem und Pathologischen Anatomie*, Heft 13. (Stuttgart: Georg Thieme Verlag)

95. Doerr, W. (1970). Arteriosclerose. In *Allgemeine Pathologie der Organe des Kreislaufes*, p. 568. (New York: Springer-Verlag)

96. Haust, M.D. (1970). Injury and repair in the pathogenesis of atherosclerosis. In Jones, R. J. (ed.) *Atherosclerosis*, p. 12. (New York: Springer-Verlag)

97. Haust, M.D. (1971). Arteriosclerosis. In Brunson, J.G. and Gall, E.A. (eds.) *Concepts of Disease: A Textbook of Human Pathology.* (New York: The Macmillan Company)

98. Haust, M.D. and More, R.H. (1972). *Op. cit.*, pp. 11–12

99. Aschoff, A. (1909). Über Entwicklung-, Wachstumsund Altersvorgänge an den Gefässen von Muskuläarem und Elastischem Typ. (Jena: Gustav Fischer)

100. Hueck, W. (1920). Anatomisches zur Frage nach Wesen und Ursache der Arteriosklerose. *München. Med. Wschr.*, **67**, 535, 606

101. Bürger, K. (1928). Bedeutung chemischer Geweb-suntersuchungen für die Altersforschung. *Klin. Wschr.*, **7**, 1944

102. Hueper, W.C. (1945). Arteriosclerosis. A general review. *Arch. Path. (Chicago)*, **38**, 162, 245, 350, 1944; **39**, 51, 117, 187

103. Paterson, J.C. (1936). Vascularization and hemorrhage of the intima of arteriosclerotic coronary arteries. *Arch. Path. (Chicago)*, **22**, 313

104. Paterson, J.C., Mills, J. and Lockwood, C.H. (1960). The role of hypertension in progression of atherosclerosis. *Canada Med. Ass. J.*, **82**, 65

105. Winternitz, M.C., Thomas, R.M. and Le Compte, P.M. (1938). *The Biology of Arterio-sclerosis.* (Springfield, Ill.: Charles C. Thomas)

106. Johnson, G.J. (1852). *Diseases of the Kidney*

107. Johnson, G.J. (1873). Lectures on the pathology, diagnosis and treatment of Bright's disease. *Br. Med. J.*, **1**, 161

108. Gull, W. and Sutton, H. (1872). On the pathology of the morbid state commonly called Bright's disease with contracted kidney. *Med. Chir. Trans.*, **55**, 273

10   Primary tumors of the heart

Primary tumors of the heart are rare. Two thirds of them are benign, and more than half are myxomas. The remainder of the primary tumors are malignant with a sarcomatous base. The word benign here is used purely in its pathologic sense. That is, tumors of this kind, unlike cancer, do not send out seeds to other parts of the body. In a physiologic sense, there is certainly nothing benign about a tumor in the heart. Its very location will not only create a marked functional disturbance but will almost certainly be lethal.

Metastatic tumors of the heart are much more common. The majority arise for the most part from carcinoma (especially from the lung), melanomas, and the leukemias or lymphomas. Metastatic tumors of the heart are found in at least 10% of all patients dying of a malignancy. Scott and Garvin reported in 1939 that their observations indicated the heart was commonly involved in this metastatic process by malignant cells acting as emboli, entering the heart via the coronary arteries[1]. The next most common mode of involvement is by direct extension from a tumor in the lungs or mediastinal lymph nodes, and the least common is by retrograde invasion through the lymphatics of the heart[2,3].

Recorded observations of primary tumors of the heart date as far back as the 16th century[4]. The first correct antemortem diagnosis has been attributed to Barnes and his group. Their report appeared in the American Heart Journal in 1934[5]. Göttel on the other hand cites Pawlowski as having made the diagnosis during life of a primary tumor of the auricle in 1895[6]. Göttel was probably right in assigning to Pawlowski priority for an antemortem diagnosis. However, if one reads Pawlowski's original paper, the tumor that he describes is actually in the left auricle[7], while Yater states in his monumental review that 'Göttel gave Pavlovsky credit for the diagnosis during life of a primary tumor of the left auricle, which in reality was in the right auricle'[8]. This follows by several pages Yater's discussion of how mitral stenosis and mitral regurgitation may be simulated by tumors in the left auricle. I quote from Yater's paper: 'Göttel quoted Pavlovsky's case of a primary sarcoma of the right auricle, in which during life the diagnosis of a primary tumor of the left auricle had been made, because the signs were those of stenosis when the patients' body was vertical and those of regurgitation when horizontal'[9]. I am still confused.

In 1924, Rösler's report[10] appeared on the antemortem diagnosis of metastatic invasion of the heart. Six years later, Willius and Amberg[11] then reported two cases of secondary tumor of the heart in children, in one of which the diagnosis was made during life.

It is difficult to establish priority of postmortem recognition of primary cardiac tumors in the earlier writings simply because there is no convincing evidence that the author was actually capable of distinguishing between a thrombus and a tumor. It was not until the early 19th century that Thomas Hodgkin made the first clear distinction between an intramural tumor and a thrombus.

The subject of his description was a 55 year old woman. The following quotation is from Raeburn who in turn quoted it from King's paper on Hodgkin's contribution which appeared in The Lancet in 1845[12–14].

In the left auricle, close to the margin of the foramen ovale, was attached a large polypiform body of about the size of a pullet's egg. The surface by which it was attached was nearly the size of a shilling. Though rather dark and discoloured in some parts, it was generally of a light yellow, and semi-transparent, with some opaque white specks dispersed through it, having some resemblance to the opaque points in soft soap, but rarer and smaller. It was firmer than the ordinary fibrinous concretions which are found in the heart, and was especially so about its root.

On fine injection being thrown into the coronary arteries, minute vessels were seen beautifully ramifying through the transparent substance. This polypoid concretion was covered by a thin membrane continuous with that of the lining membrane of the auricle. Though its substance was not disposed in layers, some appearance in it (as, for instance, darkish points of a brownish colour) had a trace of arrangement equidistant from the surface.

This is quite a vivid detailed word picture of the tumor. I am particularly impressed with the analogy to soft soap and how Hodgkin showed the blood supply to the tumor being derived from the coronary arteries. He leaves no doubt that the lesion in the left auricle is a tumor and not a 'polyp' or clot. This should be compared to the case report by Bricheteau which appeared in 1837, and apparently without the author having any knowledge of Hodgkin's work[15].

The left atrial lesion described by Bricheteau was thought by him to be a tumor formed originally by a blood clot. Semantics now enters the picture. Tumor being derived from the latin, 'tumere' means a swelling and this may be actually the sense in which Bricheteau used the word. On careful study of his description, I am quite convinced that the lesion was actually a thrombus rather than a true neoplasm, and that the patient had long-standing rheumatic mitral disease with left atrial enlargement; a well-known predisposing combination for the formation of a left atrial thrombus. Carl Bartecchi wrote a paper published in 1982 which dealt with the historically elusive nature of primary cardiac tumors[16]. In this brief communication he attempted to put forth the likelihood that the 'atrial tumor' as described by Bricheteau was 'compatible with an actual tumor'. The following words are taken from Bartecchi's paper and are Bricheteau's original description. There is nothing in the morbid anatomy to support Bartecchi's view.

The pericardium contained a little citron-coloured serum. The heart was pale, flaccid, somewhat large, and sunk down into the shape of a birding-pouch (en forme de gibeciere). The right cavities were in a sound state. The left ventricle was as large as the right, and the thickness of their parietes was the same. The mitral valves were hard and cartilaginous; and, when applied back to back, two small apertures resulted, of the size of a quill, separated from each other by the tendon of the internal valve. The left auricle was greatly dilated, and could have contained a large hen's egg; it inclosed some black blood, and a kind of champignon or fungous growth of a red colour: the form of this body cannot be better compared than to that of the Lycoperdon, commonly called vesse-de-loup (puff-ball). This fungus had no pedicle, but was feebly adherent to the inner surface of the auricle, from which it could be separated without any force. It was situated at the left upper part of the auricle, which presented, at the point of adhesion, inequalities that appeared to have served for a kind of incrustation. This species of tumor, quasi free in the auricle, was more than an inch in diameter; it had a central cavity communicating with others of smaller size, filled with a reddish, manifestly purulent, fluid; it was of fibrinous appearance, and hard and coriaceous, except at the point of adhesion, which was a little softened. The pulmonary veins were dilated and filled with black blood.

This case is not simply remarkable in respect to the lesion of the mitral valves, which reduced the auriculo-ventricular orifice to two apertures of less than a line each in diameter, and by their insufficiency offered an obstacle to the circulation; it also presented a tumour floating, as it were, in the left auricle, a tumour which was probably formed originally by a clot of blood, which had afterwards become the centre of an inflammatory process, and a suppuration in which the auricle had taken no part. This fungus presents, then, a rare example of disease of the blood, which is susceptible, it seems, of becoming the seat of different changes as yet but little determined. From the appearance of the parts, it was impossible to establish any relation by continuity between the inner surface of the auricle and the tumour; the latter was simply agglutinated to it, but was not attached to it by any 'pedicle.'

My purpose in presenting the preceding at some length is to illustrate and emphasize how careful one must be in assessing the validity and accuracy of the historical descriptions of the past that purport to be those of primary cardiac tumors.

Several recent investigators have also maintained that many tumors reported as fibromas or fibromyxomas are really organized clots. This position compounds the dilemma further. The lack of authenticity that surrounds the true anatomical nature of the lesions described as primary neoplasms has also created confusion with respect to the validity of the total number of cases reported to date. The bias of the compiler in accepting or rejecting the accuracy of the reported cases has played a most disconcerting role in this regard. Thus Tedeschi[17] in 1893 compiled 86 cases while, during the same year, Berthenson[18] acknowledged only 30 as valid. In a similar fashion, Hagedorn[19] in 1908 counted 46 and a few months later Link[20] compiled 91.

Against this background, it appears that Realdus Columbus may have been the first to recognize the existence of tumors of the heart. The description is to be found in his *De Re Anatomica* published in 1562[21]. Zollicofferus wrote a dissertation in 1685 that bore the title *De Polypo Cordis*[22]. Postmortem descriptions are also to be found in the writings of Bonet (1700) and in those of Morgagni (1762)[23]. In fact, Morgagni in his *De Sedibus* refers to the contributions of Zollicofferus.

Yater's classic paper in 1931 was the first general review of the subject in the English literature. There are some errors in it and some of his remarks are rather confusing because of a lack of preciseness in his phraseology. Despite this minor flaw, it is a monumental piece of scholarship and deserving of wide acclaim. An even more comprehensive treatment of cardiac tumors was the monograph by Mahaim which appeared in 1945[24]. The extensive bibliography alone places this review among the best ever presented. Another distinctive asset of the review was the author's vast personal experience in the subject matter.

The first authenticated case of a primary tumor of the heart is ascribed by many pathologists to Albers. His report appeared in 1835 and the tumor he described was a fibroma[25, 26]. It is the second most common cardiac tumor in infants and children. Waaler and co-workers reported on the common occurrence of calcification in these tumors in 1972[27]. Multiple fibromas in the same heart were first described by Luschka in 1855[28]. Since then it has been reported only twice (in 1979 and 1980)[29,30].

Cardiac lipoma is another example of a so-called benign tumor of the heart. It is extremely rare, and according to Heath only 30 cases are to be found in the literature[31]. The tumor arises from the epicardial or pericardial fat. The first description of a cardiac lipoma is attributed to Paget who reported finding it in a sheep. This was published in 1870 in his book entitled *Lectures on Surgical Pathology*[32].

Rhabdomyoma refers to a non-malignant tumor arising from muscle. Cardiac rhabdomyoma was first described by von Recklinghausen in 1862[33]. Since then more than 110 cases have been reported in the literature, and in at least 50% of the time, tuberous sclerosis was also present[34]. It is the most common cardiac tumor in both infants and children. There is still controversy regarding the neoplastic nature of cardiac rhabdomyoma. The strong association with tuberous sclerosis is consistent with Heath's concept, advanced by him in 1968, that the growth is a hamartoma[35]. A hamartoma is a malformation in which the tissue components are normally found in the affected organ. In 1984, Reece and his group also found evidence of an association between rhabdomyoma and tuberous sclerosis[36]. The importance of these tumors, or any ventricular tumor for that matter, in the causation of ventricular arrhythmias, was stressed as recently as 1974 by Engle and co-workers[37]. Fenoglio and his group described in the same year the electron microscopic appearance of cardiac rhabdomyoma, and in their clinico-pathologic correlation they commented on the fact that the site of the ectopic rhythm did not always correlate with the site of the lesion[38]. When strategically located, cardiac rhabdomyoma is capable of producing a subaortic stenosis. This was described by Kidder in 1950[39], Kuehl in 1970[40], Shaker in 1972[41], and again by Reece in 1984[42].

The most interesting of the benign primary tumors of the heart is the myxoma. The first clinical description of the tumor was written by King in 1845[43]. It is a rare tumor and for years it was merely a medical curiosity. Isolated case reports of its occurrence were left to gather dust on library shelves. The controversy over whether or not it is a true neoplasm, the ease with which it can be diagnosed today, and the high success rate for its complete removal, thanks to modern surgical techniques, are all contributing factors towards the resurgence of interest in this lesion. The diagnostic accuracy of angiocardiography and echocardiography is a triumph of modern technology. Prior to the introduction of these techniques, the varied and bizarre clinical pictures that this tumor can create, confounded even the most astute of diagnosticians. Goldberg and associates were the first to utilize angiocardiography as a diagnostic modality[44].

Prior to this no one had diagnosed the presence of an intracardiac myxoma during life. Their report was published in 1952, and, perhaps, was the prime catalyst for removing the myxoma from a 'dead-house curiosity' to the clinical arena amenable to diagnosis *in vivo*.

Yater, in his review, stated that myxoma was the most debated type of tumor of the heart[45]. More than half a century has passed since this comment appeared in print with the debate still in force today. It revolves around whether they are true neoplasms or thrombi that have imbibed plasma to become swollen clots in various stages of organization. The view that the myxoma was thrombotic in nature was advanced by Karrenstein in 1908[46], followed by Stahr[47] in 1910, Thorel[48] in 1915 and Husten[49] in 1922. The opposition was led by Ribbert[50] who, in 1924, claimed that it was not all that difficult to differentiate the growth from a thrombus. Yater in his review favored the neoplastic origin. Most of the recent reports on the subject have adhered to the view held by Ribbert and Yater.

There are four reports in the literature which strongly suggest a tendency for myxoma to affect certain families. The first is that of Krause and associates[51]. They described its occurrence in two brothers. One had a myxoma of the pulmonic valve and the other in the left atrium. I will leave to the pathologists the possibility that the lesion on the pulmonic valve may have actually been an example of the so-called papillary tumor rather than a true myxoma. In 1973, two years after the report by Krause, two papers appeared independent of each other. The leading author in one was Kleid[52]. Heydorn headed the second report though Kleid was among the authors[53]. Both reports dealt with two teenage brothers. Farah's description appeared in 1975[54]. It involved a brother and sister. A year later, Siltanen and his group from Finland described a family in which the mother and three of seven children underwent surgery for atrial myxoma[55].

The possibility that cardiac myxomas can recur even after apparently adequate surgical removal was first brought out by Gerbode and his group in 1967 in an article that concerned itself with the surgical management of cardiac tumors[56]. Moreover, despite its supposedly benign nature, evidence of its metastatic potentiality was provided by Read and associates in 1974[57], and later by Rankin and his group in 1978[58]. Embolism of tumor particles from the mother lesion had already been described by

Ringerts in 1942[59], and reiterated by Heath and MacKinnon in 1964[60] with the development of pulmonary hypertension as a result of recurrent emboli from a right atrial tumor.

During the 20th century, several opinions were advanced to account for the rarity of primary tumors of the heart. Adami[61] in 1908, wrote in his *Principles of Pathology*, that the relative immunity of the heart to neoplastic disease 'is probably attributed to the fact that the heart, above all organs, is constantly in a state of great efficiency, well-nourished, well-innervated, and functionally always active'. This sounds like Galenism, although couched in physiological terms. Yater, however, in 1931, suggested the lack of mitotic activity in the cardiac muscle as being responsible for the rarity of primary tumors of the heart[62]. Unfortunately, this opinion too offers no better explanation.

A few final words are necessary regarding a lesion of heart valves known as papillary tumor. Heath described it as a gelatinous papillary mass resembling a 'sea anemone' growing on one or more of the heart valves[63]. There has been considerable controversy and confusion regarding the neoplastic nature of these masses. Curtis, as early as 1871, thought they were probably an inflammatory lesion[64]. Koechlin[65] in 1908 was positive in the assertion that they were nothing else but unusually large excrescences of Lamble. Lamble's excrescences are formed by the organization of small deposits of fibrin where the endothelial lining has been damaged. Pomerance added fuel to the debate in 1961 when she expressed the belief that the so-called tumors 'originated in and grew from the close approximation of excrescences'[66]. Heath expressed agreement with her views in 1967[67]. Pomerance's view that these lesions were small, harmless bodies was similar to that of Bohrod who had already referred to them as such in 1929[68]. An interesting feature of Bohrod's paper was his statement that the lesion was described in the past under a bewildering array of names depending on the predominant tissue seen in the specimen. Thus, they could have been designated as myxoma, fibroma and so on. He added to the litany by introducing the term hemangio-fibroma. Currently, there is a general consensus that papillary tumors of the heart valves bear a close histologic similarity to cardiac myxomas. This was brought out by Heath in 1968[69]. However, the issue as to their true nature is far from settled.

REFERENCES

1. Scott, R.W. and Garvin, C.F. (1939). Tumors of the heart and pericardium. *Am. Heart J.*, **17**, 431–6

2. Aubertin, C. (1905). Sur un cas de thrombose neoplasique du coeur droit. *Arch. de Med. Exp.*, **17**, 197

3. Wolf and Giet (1922). Lymphosarcome mediastinal: envahissement du myocarde. *Bull. Soc. Anat.*, **92**, 340

4. Mahaim, L. (1945). *Les Tumeurs et les Polypes de Coeur: Étude Anatamo – Clinique*. (Paris: Masson)

5. Barnes, A.R., Beaver, D.C. and Snell, A.M. (1934). Primary sarcoma of the heart: report of a case with ECG and pathological studies. *Am. Heart J.*, **9**, 480

6. Göttel, L. (1919). Ein Fall von Primären Herztumor. *Deutsche Med. Wchnschr.*, **45**, 937

7. Pawlowski, R.A. (1895). Beitrag zum studien den symtomatologie der neubildungen des Herzens. Polypose neubildungen des linken Vorhofs. *Berl. Klin. Wchnschr.*, **32**, 393

8. Yater, W.M. (1931). Tumors of the heart and pericardium. Pathology, symptomatology and report of nine cases. *Arch. Int. Med.*, **48**, 627–66

9. *Ibid.*, p. 647

10. Rösler, O.A. (1924). Vier seltenere Herzbefunde, un Beitrag zur Herz Diagnostik. *Zentralbl. f. Herz. u. Gefässkr.*, **16**, 261

11. Willius, F.A. and Amberg, S. (1930). Two cases of secondary tumor of the heart in children, in one of which the diagnosis was made during life. *Med. Clin. N. Am.*, **13**, 1307

12. Read, C.R. (1980). Cardiac myxoma and surgical history. *Ann. Thorac. Surg.*, **29**, 395–6

13. Raeburn, C. (1952). The histogenesis of four cases of angiomyxoma of the auricle. *Clin. Pathol.*, **5**, 339

14. King, T.W. (1845). On simple vascular growths in the left auricle of the heart. *Lancet*, **2**, 428–30

15. Bricheteau, I. (1837). Pericarditis and aneurism of the heart. Case VI. *Medical Clinics of the Hospital Necker*, pp. 118–20

16. Bartecchi, C.E. (1982). Primary cardiac tumors: historically elusive lesions. *Southern Med. J.*, **75**, 1250–1

17. Tedeschi, A. (1893). Beitrag zum studium der herz-geschwülste. *Prag. Med. Wchnschr.*, **18**, 121

18. Berthenson, L. (1893). Zur frage von der diagnose primärer neoplasmen des herzens, myxom des linken Vorhofes. *Arch. f. Path. Anat. u. Physiol. u. f. klin. Med.*, **132**, 390

19. Hagedorn, O. (1908). Über primäre herztumor. *Centraebl. f. allg. Path. u. Path. Anat.*, **19**, 825

20. Link, R. (1909). Die Klinik der primären neubildungen des herzens. *Ztschr. f. klin. Med.*, **67**, 272

21. Columbus, M.R. (1562). *De Re Anatomica*, Libri XV, p. 402. (Paris)

22. Beck, C.S. and Thatcher, H.S. (1925). Spindle cell sarcoma of the heart. *Arch. Intern. Med.*, **36**, 830

23. Perlstein, J. (1918). Sarcoma of the heart. *Am. J. M. Sci.*, **156**, 214

24. Mahaim, L. (1945). *Les Tumeurs et les Polypes du Coeur: Étude Anatomoclinique*. (Paris: Masson et Cie)

25. Straus, R. and Merliss, R. (1945). Primary tumor of the heart. *Arch. Path.*, **39**, 74

26. McAllister, H.A. and Fenoglio, J.J. (1978). *Tumors of the Cardiovascular System, Atlas of Tumor Pathology*, Vol. 15 (Washington, DC: Armed Forces Institute of Pathology)

27. Waaler, P.E., Svendsen, S. and Halvorsen, J.F. (1972). Intramural calcified fibroma of the heart. *Acta Paediatr. Scand.*, **61**, 217–22

28. Luschka, H. (1855). Fibroma in the heart muscle. *Virchows Arch.*, (*Pathol. Anat.*), **8**, 343–7

29. Zander, R. (1980). Fibroma of the heart. *Virchows Arch.*, (*Pathol. Anat.*), **80**, 507–10

30. Fernando, S.S.E. (1979). Cardiac fibroma (fibrous hamartoma) of infancy. Two case reports. *Pathology*, **11**, 111–17

31. Heath, D. (1968). Pathology of cardiac tumors. *Am. J. Cardiol.*, **21**, 315–27

32. Paget, S.J. (1870). In Turner, W. (ed.) *Lectures on Surgical Pathology*, 3rd. edition, p. 447. (London: Songman)

33. Von Recklinghausen, F. (1862). Verhandlungen der Gesellschaft für Gerburtshulfe, Herr V. Recklinghausen tegt der Gesellschaft ein Herz von einem Neugeborenen. *Monatsear Geburtsk.*, **20**, 1–2

34. Reece, I.J., Cooley, D.A., Frazier, O.H., Hallman, G.L., Powers, P.L. and Montero, C.G. (1984). Cardiac tumors. Clinical spectrum and prognosis of lesions other than classical benign myxoma in 20 patients. *J. Thorac. Cardiovasc. Surg.*, **88**, 439–46

35. Heath, D. (1968). *Op. cit.*, p. 321

36. Reece, I.J. (1984). *Op. cit.*, p. 441

37. Engle, M.A., Ebert, P.A. and Redo, S.F. (1974). Recurrent ventricular tachycardia due to resectable cardiac tumor. Report of two cases in two-year-olds with heart failure. *Circulation*, **50**, 1051–7

38. Fenoglio, J.J., McAllister, H.A. and Ferrans, V.J. (1974). Cardiac rhabdomyoma. A clinico-pathological and electron microscopic study. *Am. J. Cardiol.*, **38**, 241–51

39. Kidder, L.A. (1950). Congenital glycogenic tumors of the heart. *Arch. Pathol.*, **49**, 55–9

40. Kuehl, K.S., Perry, L.W., Chandra, R. and Scott, L.P. (1970). Left ventricular rhabdomyoma. A rare cause of subaortic stenosis in the newborn. *Pediatrics*, **46**, 464–8

41. Shaker, R.M., Farina, A., Alley, R., Mansen, P. and Bishop, M. (1972). Congenital subaortic stenosis in infancy caused by rhabdomyoma of the left ventricle. *J. Thorac. Cardiovasc. Surg.*, **63**, 157–63

42. Reece, I.J. (1984). *Op. cit.*, p. 441

43. King, T.W. (1845). *Op. cit.*

44. Goldberg, H.P., Glenn, F., Dotter, C.T. and Steinberg, I. (1952). Myxoma of the left atrium. Diagnosis made during life with operative and postmortem findings. *Circulation*, **6**, 762–7

45. Yater, W.M. (1931). *Op. cit.*, p. 632

46. Karrenstein (1908). Ein Fall von Fibroclasto-myxom des Herzens und Kasuistisches zur Frage der Herzgeschwülste besonders der Myxome. *Virchows Arch. f. Path. Anat.*, **194**, 127

47. Stahr, H. (1910). Ueber sogenannte Endokarddtumoren und ihre Entstehung. *Virchows Arch. f. Path. Anat.*, **199**, 162

48. Thorel, C. (1915). Pathologie der Kreislauforgane des Menschen. *Ergebn. d. allg. Path. u. Path. Anat.*, **11**, 90

49. Husten, K. (1922). Ueber Tumoren und Pseudotumoren des Endocards, *Beitr. z. path. Anat. u. z. allg. Path.*, **71**, 132

50. Ribbert, H. (1924). *Die Endokardtumoren, in Henke and Lubarsch: Handbuch der speziellen Pathologie, Anatomie und Histologie*, vol. 2, p. 276. (Berlin: Julius Springer)

51. Krause, S., Adler, L.N., Reddy, P.S. *et al.* (1971). Intracardiac myxoma in siblings. *Dis. Chest.*, **60**, 404–6

52. Kleid, J.J., Klugman, J., Haas, J. *et al.* (1973). Familial atrial myxoma. *Am. J. Cardiol.*, **32**, 361–4

53. Heydorn, W.H., Gomez, A.C., Kleid, J.J. *et al.* (1973). Atrial myxoma in siblings. *J. Thorac. Cardiovasc. Surg.*, **65**, 484–6

54. Farah, M.G. (1975). Familial atrial myxoma. *Ann. Intern. Med.*, **83**, 358–360

55. Siltanen, P., Tureteri, L., Noris, R. *et al.* (1976). Atrial myxoma in a family. *Am. J. Cardiol.*, **38**, 252–6

56. Gerbode, F., Kerth, J.W. and Hill, D.J. (1967). Surgical management of tumors of the heart. *Surgery*, **661**, 94

57. Read, R.C., White, H.J., Murphy, M.L. *et al.* (1974). The malignant potentiality of left atrial myxoma. *J. Thorac. Cardiovasc. Surg.*, **68**, 857

58. Rankin, L.I. and DeSousa, A.L. (1978). Metastatic atrial myxoma presenting as intracranial mass. *Chest*, **74**, 451

59. Ringerts, N. (1942). Uber sog endokard-myxome. *Pathol. Microbiol. Scand.*, **199**, 262

60. Heath, D. and MacKinnon, J. (1964). Pulmonary hypertension due to myxoma of the right atrium. *Am. Heart J.*, **68**, 227

61. Adami, J.G. and Nichols, A.G. (1908–9). *The Principles of Pathology*, p. 158. (Philadelphia: Lea and Febiger)

62. Yater, A.M.(1931). *Op. cit.*

63. Heath, D. (1968). Pathology of cardiac tumors. *Am. J. Cardiol.*, **21**, 315–27

64. Hertzog, A.J. (1936). Papillary fibroma of cardiac valve. *Arch. Pathol.*, **22**, 222

65. Koechlin, E. (1908). *Über primaren tumoren und papillomatose exkreszenzen der herzklappen.*

66. Pomerance, A. (1961). Papillary 'tumors' of the heart valves. *J. Pathol. Bacteriol.*, **81**, 135

67. Heath, D. (1968). *Op. cit.*

68. Bohrod, M.G. (1929). Multiple hemangiofibroma of the pulmonary valve. *Arch. Pathol.*, **8**, 68

69. Heath, D. (1968). *Op. cit.*, p. 321

11 Anatomical changes due to neurologic disorders

The interplay between cardiac disturbances and neurologic disorders is highly complex and varied. The clinical variations may be described as follows[1]: major hereditary disorders of a neuromyopathic nature having cardiac disease as an integral and constant feature[2]; less common neuromyopathic diseases in which cardiac dysfunction can occasionally be seen[3]; cardiomyopathy as the presenting feature of a neuromuscular disturbance[4]; cardiac denervation *per se*; and acute cerebral disorders in association with cardiovascular abnormalities[5].

There are three major categories of heredofamilial neuromyopathic disorders: the X-linked progressive muscular dystrophies; the limb-girdle dystrophy of Erb; and the facioscapulohumoral dystrophy of Landouzy-Déjérine. Duchenne dystrophy and Becker muscular dystrophy are sub-types within the progressive muscular dystrophy category. The Duchenne dystrophy has an early onset and is rapidly progressive while the Becker subtype is late in onset and slowly progressive.

Despite the eponym, Duchenne's progressive muscular dystrophy was first described clinically by Meryon in 1852[1]. The histological changes in the skeletal muscle were first described by Erb in 1891[2]. The first one to recognize involvement of the myocardium in this disease was Ross in 1883[3,4]. This was published as a case report of pseudohypertrophic paralysis in the *British Medical Journal*. Further reports of cardiac involvement in Duchenne's dystrophy were few and far between and consisted of isolated descriptions. The occurrence of chronic fibrous myocarditis was noted by Bunting in 1908[3]. Up until 1923 only ten cases had been reported in the literature. At this time Globus added one of his own while reviewing the previous ten[4]. His findings were similar to those of Bunting. In addition, his patient manifested left ventricular hypertrophy and fatty infiltration of the myocardium. Bevans, 22 years later, added her case report[5]. She was particularly impressed with the extensive deposition of fibrotic changes in the subepicardial area. Bunting had also noted this, and these findings were to be confirmed in later years by James, Batsakis, and Frankel and Rosser. Frankel and Rosser, in their paper which appeared in *Human Pathology* in 1976, were 'struck by the distinctive, peculiar nature of the myocardial fibrosis. Fibrosis begins at the junction between the epicardial fat and the outer myocardium'. They suggested that the 'vectorcardiogram and electrocardiogram in patients with Duchenne's progressive muscular dystrophy can best be explained by considering the myocardial involvement as a form of the generalized myopathy with degeneration and fibrosis occurring in a peculiar and characteristic fashion'[6].

It is now known that heart disease in Duchenne dystrophy is unique and characterized by a genetically determined predilection for the postero-basal and lateral left ventricular wall[7,8]. Historically, this has been well documented by the necropsy studies just described, and as recently as 1978 by Sanyal and associates[9]. These investigators also described the ultrastructural basis for the distinctive electrocardiographic pattern seen in this disease. It was Rubin and Buchberg who, in 1952, first described the abnormalities of the QRS complex that are so characteristic of this disease[10]. According to Sanyal, the ultrastructural hallmark of the cardiomyopathy is a myofibrillar lysis involving both the thick and thin myofilaments.

The importance of myocardial scarring in the etiology of cardiac arrhythmias in this disease was initially stressed by Northacker in 1950[11]. Systematic studies of specialized cardiac tissues in Duchenne's dystrophy are, however, rather sparse. T.N. James in 1962 recorded his observations in a paper published in *The American Heart Journal*[12]. These were light microscopic studies of the cardiac conduction system. The patient died suddenly, apparently of a cardiac arrhythmia. Arteriopathy of the cardiac nodes with degeneration of the nodal fibers were the outstanding pathologic changes, which could easily account for the disturbances in rhythm.

Another histological study appeared in 1982. The paper, written by Nomura and Hizawa, was based on 23 hearts obtained at autopsy[13]. Only the distal conduction system, i.e. the Purkinje fibers, was involved in their patients. The fibers showed necrobiotic changes resembling those of the skeletal and cardiac contractile muscles. The SA node was intact. No vascular changes were noted. Apparently, these two observers were not acquainted with the work of T.N. James since they lay claim to being the first to describe histologic changes in the cardiac conduction system. Ultrastructural observations on the specialized cardiac tissues were presented in 1961 by Skyring and McKusick but these were minimal and inconclusive[14].

Electron microscopic evidence pointing to a basic or early abnormality in the plasma membrane of the muscle fiber was first provided by Mokri and Engel in 1975[15]. In 1980, Sanyal and his group published another paper which delineated the ultrastructural abnormalities that were responsible for the mitral valve prolapse that is so often seen in Duchenne's dystrophy[16]. They described dystrophic changes similar to the ones they reported in their initial paper of 1978. However, in those subjects with mitral valve prolapse, these changes did not involve the mitral valve leaflets, its chordae or annulus, but rather, were confined to the papillary muscle and ventricular myocardium.

In Becker's dystrophy, cardiac involvement differs from that seen in the Duchenne subtype. All four chambers are incriminated with dilatation and failure of the ventricles. The dystrophy was described by Becker in 1962 as a 'benign sex-linked recessive muscular dystrophy'[17]. The associated dilated cardiomyopathy was described in detail by Perloff and associates in 1966[18]. They also described anatomical changes in the His bundle and infranodal conduction tissue which account for the bundle branch block or complete heart block that can complicate the cardiac status. Further reports concerning the cardiomyopathic process and disturbances in conduction appeared from various centers in following years. The most prominent among them are the papers having as their leading authors Katijar (1977)[19], Hassan (1979)[20], and Vrints (1983)[21].

In the limb-girdle dystrophy of Erb, cardiac involvement is relatively infrequent and seldom severe with arrhythmias or disturbances in con-

duction being the main manifestations. These electrophysiologic disturbances were brought out by Lambert and Fairfax in two separate papers in 1976[22,23]. The occurrence of congestive cardiomyopathy was also noted by an Italian group led by Svetoni in 1984[24].

Permanent paralysis of the atria (atrial standstill) is the chief cardiac abnormality in the facioscapulohumeral dystrophy of Landouzy-Déjérine. Permanent atrial standstill was initially well described by Chavez in 1946[25]. Cushny had experimentally produced standstill of the atria in 1897[26]. It can occur in at least three clinical settings, one of which is in association with a variety of neuromuscular disorders. In the neuromuscular setting, it was originally described in patients with the facioscapulohumeral muscular dystrophy by Bloomfield in 1965[27], Caponnetto in 1968[28] and then by Baldwin in 1973[29].

In addition to these, other isolated case reports appeared from Japan, France and Italy. Bloomfield's report is well documented, that of Baldwin is rather hazy. Although the patient described by Baldwin did indeed have facioscapulohumeral muscular dystrophy, neither a necropsy nor a biopsy was performed. This appears to me to be a critical point since the patient had received sulfonamide for a 'flu-like' syndrome and a sulfonamide myocarditis was not ruled out[29].

Later, atrial standstill was found to occur in other neurologic disorders such as Charcot-Marie muscular dystrophy by Bensald in 1971[30], and X-linked humeroperoneal neuromuscular disease by Waters in 1975[31], Emery-Dreifuss muscular dystrophy by Rowland in 1979[32], and limb-girdle muscular dystrophy by Rapelli in 1969[33] and J. Antonio in 1978[34].

Myotonic muscular dystrophy was first recognized as a distinctive hereditary disease by Steinert in 1909[35]. Posterity remembers him with the eponym 'Steinert's disease', despite the fact that during the same year, the entity was also described by Batten and Gibb[36]. Although Steinert's paper called attention to the slow pulse which was later confirmed by Griffith in 1911[37], the frequency of cardiac involvement was not widely appreciated until 1944, then again in 1950, and later, in the subsequent decades, when the usage of electrocardiography in this disease became routine[38,39].

It is now recognized that cardiac involvement in Steinert's disease is an integral part of the disorder with the genetic marker targeting the infranodal (His bundle-Purkinje) conduction system, the sinus node, and lastly, the myocardium. All of this was brought out by Perloff and his associates in a paper published in 1984 in the *American Journal of Cardiology*[40]. They noted also that the myocardial involvement results in dystrophy rather than myotonia, and that the process involves all four chambers when present. Many necropsy and biopsy studies have been published beginning with that by Keschner and Davidson in 1933 who described in their patient fatty infiltration into both ventricular walls[41]. Black and Ravin's paper was published in the *Archives of Pathology* in (1947)[42]. Their findings were based on five cases that came to autopsy. Observations utilizing light microscopy including theirs and subsequent ones have varied from few or no changes to focal or diffuse fatty infiltration and fibrosis in all four chambers[43]. Electron microscopic studies were first reported by Bulloch in 1967[44], followed by Uemura in 1973[45], Tanaka in 1973[46], Ludatscher in 1978[47] and Motta in 1979[48]. These studies have revealed, for the most part, abnormalities of the sarcoplasmic reticulum and the mitochondria.

Familial mitral valve prolapse also occurs in this disease and it appears that the first to describe this association was Winters and his group in 1976[49].

The list of contributors could go on and on but, besides being a boring recital of names, it would serve no purpose from the perspective of history. What we should appreciate from this brief discussion, and in other sections of this text, is that the research efforts of the 20th century, except on rare occasions, are no longer in the hands of a single individual but rather dependent upon contributions from groups situated in centers all over the world. From this vast amount of material, I have attempted to select those who I thought were the most important contributors.

In this regard, certain Japanese groups have been outstanding in their zeal to uncover the structural changes of the heart in Steinert's disease. I was particularly impressed with a paper by Hiromasa and his co-workers which appeared in 1986 in the *American Heart Journal*[50]. This paper summarized very nicely the histopathologic changes described to date utilizing both light and electron microscopy. In doing so, it attempted to furnish a structural basis for the clinical manifestations. I quote the pertinent remarks from this paper:

... the AV and intraventricular conduction disturbances observed in the present cases are most likely due to a direct involvement of the specialized conducting system by the dystrophic process. On light microscopic examination, the cardiac tissue from cases of myotonic dystrophy usually show nonspecific histologic changes including irregularities in cell size, hypertrophy, fiber disarray, uneven nuclei, increased interstitial fibrosis, and interstitial fatty infiltration. Electron microscopic studies have often revealed various abnormalities, even in those hearts showing no significant changes on light microscopy. For instance, irregularity, indistinctness, and partial loss of the sarcolemma, degeneration of the myofibril, swelling and degeneration of the mitochondria, and marked vacuolation of the sarcoplasmic reticulum have been observed. Although not directly demonstrated by endomyocardial biopsy in the present cases, these histopathologic changes would damage the ionic channels of the sarcolemma, increase the intracellular resistivity, and impair cell-to-cell electrical coupling, thereby causing those electrophysiologic abnormalities described above.

Friedreich's ataxia is essentially a neurological rather than a myopathic disorder[51]. Yet, the incidence of cardiac involvement exceeds 90% with death often the result of cardiac dysfunction[52]. Although hypertrophic cardiomyopathy is seen, concentric or asymmetrical, septal cellular disarray is either absent or focal at necropsy. This may explain the lack of lethal ventricular arrhythmias in these people in contradistinction to the genetic type of hypertrophic cardiomyopathy. At times, global hypokinesia of the left ventricle is seen with a flabby myocardium and normal wall thickness at autopsy. Thus, the postmortem findings point to two basically different types of anatomical derangement in the heart.

In his original publication, Friedreich described the cardiac findings in the three patients that he subjected to necropsy as consisting of 'severe fatty degeneration of the musculature of the left ventricle'[53]. It was not until 1887, however, that Pitt of London described the clinico-pathologic correlation of the heart and the disease[54]. Subsequent postmortem studies by Hewer in 1969[55], and Boyer several years before[56], have shown that all patients in their series revealed diffuse interstitial fibrosis of the heart and considerable focal degeneration of muscle fibers. The first detailed histologic characteristics of the heart in Friedreich's ataxia were reported by Unverferth and his group in 1987 in a paper published in the *American Journal of Medicine*[57]. On histologic grounds, they ascribed the thickness of the ventricular walls to hypertrophy of the myocytes as well as increased fibrosis. The occurrence of intimal proliferation in the small intramural coronary arteries was stressed in 1963 by T.N. James[58].

He suggested that the focal fibrosis and degeneration, which constitute the basic structural changes in the so-called 'myocarditis' of Friedreich's ataxia, could possibly be due to progressive occlusion of these small arteries. James also noted intimal proliferation in the smaller branches of the pulmonary arterial tree. His report appears to be the first to describe the pulmonary arterial changes. Apparently, the arteriopathy can involve peripheral vessels as well, since Pitt described an extensive 'obliterative endarteritis' of the upper extremities in Friedreich's ataxia back in 1887.

Observations similar to those of James were reported by Nadas in 1951[59] and by Ivemark and Thorén in 1964[60]. Nadas described considerable narrowing of the lumen of the coronary arteries due to intimal proliferation. In addition, he noted medial hypertrophy. The patient in the case report was only 16 at the time of death.

Four patients were described by Ivemark and Thorén[60]. They ranged in age between 21 and 50. Narrowing of the lumen of the coronary arteries was also seen by them but they involved the large and medium sized arteries and appeared to be due to patchy, subintimal fibrosis.

Amplification of these pathologic data of the arteries as well as in the myocardium were supplied by Hewer in his well-documented paper *The Heart in Friedreich's Ataxia* in 1969; the details of which were based on necropsy in 27 patients gathered from different centers in the United Kingdom[61].

It was Loiseau in 1938 who first suggested the catecholamine hypothesis in the pathogenesis of cardiomyopathy[62]. A lively debate ensued since then regarding the role of catecholamines not only in Friedreich's ataxia but also in genetic hypertrophic cardiomyopathy. Norepinephrine is known to stimulate hypertrophy of the myocytes. Pasternac and Merkel both reported in 1982, the presence of increased plasma catecholamines in Friedreich's ataxia[62,63].

Despite the enormous amount of effort already expended as this historical survey suggests, two basic questions still remain unanswered. Why are the morphologic changes expressed by two different pathways (dystrophy or hypertrophy), and why are there such morphologic changes to begin with? If Goodwin's 'catecholamine hypothesis', proposed by him in 1974, is valid in the pathogenesis of hypertrophic cardiomyopathies in general, then the documentation of a hyperadrenergic state in Friedreich's ataxia could certainly explain, at least, the hypertrophic pathway[62,63].

Several less common neuromyopathic diseases have been found to be associated with heart disease. Among these are myasthenia gravis, peroneal muscular atrophy and the Kearns-Sayre Syndrome.

Gibson in 1975 attempted to implicate the myocardium in myasthenia gravis on the basis of clinical, electrocardiographic and vectorcardiographic data[64]. Specific cardiac involvement, however, still remains unproven in the absence of confirmatory pathologic changes.

In 1901, Weigert described groups of abnormal cells in the epicardium and myocardium of a patient who had died of myasthenia gravis[65]. At autopsy a thymoma was also found. Weigert was of the opinion that the abnormal cells in the heart were metastatic from the thymoma. Buzzard in 1905 identified and categorized as a cardiac lesion in myasthenia gravis the presence of so-called lymphorrhages[66]. Lymphorrhages are clusters of lymphocytes. Other isolated case reports describing histopathologic changes in the heart appeared subsequent to Buzzard's paper. These were authored by Marie and associates[67], Mella[68], and Barton[69], spanning the years between 1921 and 1937. In 1942, Rottino and his co-workers reviewed the entire literature up to that date and described the myocardial lesions in their case[70]. They described such microscopic changes as myofibrillar necrosis, inflammatory changes with edema, hemorrhage, lymphocytic infiltration and large irregular histiocytes. They also contested on histopathologic grounds the malignant nature of the thymoma in Weigert's case. Assuming the validity of their contention (and their paper appears to present adequate evidence in support of this view) then metastases were not possible and the cells that Weigert described were lymphorrhages rather than metastatic thymoma cells. Be that as it may, Weigert's paper should still be given priority as being the first to have presented evidence of structural changes in the heart regardless of the true nature of these changes.

The changes noted by Rottino and his group were also reported by subsequent investigators, among whom were Mendelow[71], Russell[72], Rowland[73] and Huvos[74]. The common denominator of all the lesions described by all of these investigators was their lack of specificity. This was emphasized by Russell in her paper in 1953[72]. These studies did, however, establish the association of myocardial pathology with thymoma. In addition, they also brought out the existence of changes highly suggestive of myocarditis. I do hope the next historical survey will delineate, in a specific fashion, the significance and role of these changes in myasthenia gravis.

Beginning with Leak's report in 1961[75], followed in the ensuing two decades by those of Littler (1970)[76], Kay (1972)[77], Isner (1979)[78] and Lowry (1983)[79], the sporadic occurrence of cardiac conduction tissue disease in peroneal muscular atrophy has been amply demonstrated. Kay described the ultrastructure of the myocardium in familial heart block and peroneal muscular atrophy in the *British Heart Journal* and eleven years later Lowry and Littler published their paper on peroneal muscular atrophy associated with cardiac conduction tissue disease in the *Postgraduate Medical Journal*.

The first case report of a dilated cardiomyopathy in association with this neuromyopathic syndrome was reported by Martin Du-Pan and colleagues in 1984[80].

Chronic progressive external ophthalmoplegia was first described by von Gräfe in 1868[81]. The first confirmed report of cardiac involvement was that by Sandifer in 1946[82]. The combination of chronic progressive external ophthalmoplegia with atypical retinitis pigmentosa and AV block was described by Kearns and Sayre in 1958[83]. This combination now carries the eponym 'Kearns-Sayre Syndrome'. Seven years later, Kearns reviewed the syndrome and described nine cases, only one of which came to autopsy[84]. His and subsequent postmortem examinations both grossly and histologically with light microscopy failed to reveal any specific anatomical abnormality. However in 1975, Clark and his associates did describe at necropsy, morphological changes in the distal portion of the His bundle as far as the origins of the bundle branches[85]. This was a convincing structural basis for the impaired infranodal conduction in this syndrome.

Confirmation of a morphologic basis for abnormal infranodal conduction was also demonstrated by Roberts and Perloff in 1979. Their paper written in conjunction with Kark revealed 'extensive histologic changes in the distal portion of the His bundle extending to the origins of the bundle branches'[86].

In 1981, Charles and his group described ultrastructural abnormalities of the myocardium not previously observed in this condition[87], and which could account for the development of an irreversible and potentially lethal heart block in these patients. The newly observed abnormalities were in the mitochondria and were associated with accumulations of glycogen.

These changes underscore the need for prophylactic pacemakers in this syndrome.

Poliomyelitis would be an example of a neuromuscular disorder that at times could present itself with cardiomyopathy as the prominent feature. There are, of course, many other examples, some of which we have already reviewed. In poliomyelitis, the earliest reports of associated cardiac conduction defects are those by Singsen in 1976[88] and Gottdiener in 1978[89]. They described degeneration and fibrous replacement of the SA node, His bundle and both bundle branches.

There have been a host of reports documenting the relationship between cardiomyopathy and a number of well-recognized neurologic disorders in which skeletal muscle weakness is a prominent feature. Comments on skeletal muscle involvement in idiopathic cardiomyopathy date back to Evans in 1949[90]. We have already noted the contributions of Perloff and his group in 1966 with regard to progressive muscular dystrophy. Another important contribution was the paper by Prystowsky and co-workers which appeared in *Circulation* in 1979[91]. They outlined the natural history of conduction system disease in myotonic muscular dystrophy. It was Norris, however, who in 1966, first reported four cases of cardiomyopathy in whom the skeletal muscle on histologic examination demonstrated a dystrophic process with an increase in endomysial fibrosis along with fatty infiltration and replacement of muscle tissue in the sections under scrutiny[92].

In 1972, Shafiq and associates presented the first detailed pathologic study of skeletal muscle in idiopathic cardiomyopathy[93]. Isaacs and Munche in 1975[94] conducted electron microscopic studies in three patients which showed ultrastructural abnormalities of mitochondria, myofibrillar loss and vacuolization.

In 1984, Dunnigan and her co-workers presented histologic and biochemical analysis of skeletal muscle biopsies in 10 patients with cardiac and skeletal myopathy associated with cardiac dysrhythmias[95]. At the ultrastructural level the biopsies also showed an increased amount of endomysial fibrosis as well as abnormalities of mitochondrial morphology.

The association between cardiovascular abnormalities and overt acute cerebral events such as intracranial hemorrhage, cerebral thrombosis or embolism and subdural hematoma has been known for almost a century[96].

Cardiovascular abnormalities in severe head injury have also long been recognized. In 1934, Bramwell proposed a relationship between cardiac arrhythmia and head trauma[97]. Myocardial damage in response to cerebral injury was stressed by McLeod in 1982, and Sciarra in 1984. The study by McLeod and his group appeared in the British Heart Journal[98]. The paper presented evidence that even young and healthy subjects who have had a severe head injury, are at risk from secondary myocardial damage. Only one case was autopsied, however, and this revealed a focal area of myocardial necrosis. The remainder of the paper is based on clinical evidence of hyperadrenergic stimulation which appears to be an accepted mechanism for myocardial necrosis. Sciarra's observations and comments parallel those of McLeod and were recorded in *Merritt's Textbook of Neurology*[99]. Cardiovascular changes after severe cranial injury were also described by Brown in 1967[100]. Clifton in 1981 reported the occurrence of subendocardial hemorrhage as found on autopsy studies[98]. The relationship between sympathetic nervous system hyperactivity and myocardial changes was described by a number of investigators between 1974 and 1980. They include Neil-Dwyer[101] and Wilmore[102] in 1974, Benedict[103] in 1978 and Hörtnagl in 1980[104].

Since so many donor hearts for cardiac transplantation are taken from victims of trauma, it is interesting to speculate on what consequences, if any, we can expect on cardiac function if these transplanted hearts have microscopic necrotic lesions of the myocardium. In addition, what effect would these have on the immune response in the recipient?

Ever since coronary thrombosis emerged as a clinical entity, stroke has been recognized as an important complication. This was initially brought out by Levine and Brown in 1929 in a monograph published in *Medicine*[105]. The coexistence of acute cardiac and brain infarction as established by postmortem studies is a relatively recent observation beginning with Grant's report in 1980[106], followed by von Arbin[107], Badui[108], and Moles[109], all in 1982.

The most common cause of cardiac denervation is cardiac transplantation. The historical survey will be found in the chapter dealing with the procedure. The other important cause of cardiac denervation is Chagas' disease, and a few words regarding the cardiac manifestations of Chagas' disease would be appropriate at this point.

Chagas' disease is caused by a parasite, *Trypanosoma cruzi*. It is endemic in Brazil and gains entry into the human body via the gastro-intestinal tract or through broken skin. The earliest pathologic descriptions of the myocardium in this disease were those by Vianna and Torres. These studies were reported by Vianna in 1911[110] and Torres between 1917 and 1941[111–113]. They served as a model for all subsequent studies of the morbid anatomy of the heart in this disease. Although the clinical manifestations appear to be those of myocarditis, the actual derangement is to be found in the destruction of the parasympathetic ganglia within the myocardium. The same changes are found in the gastrointestinal tract. When located in the esophagus, it results in megaesophagus, and when in the colon, the condition is called megacolon. The destruction of the ganglia in the heart results in an unchallenged overdrive by the sympathetic system. It was Köberle who, in a series of papers beginning in 1956, demonstrated the alterations involving the ganglion cells. His output on the problem was prodigious and continued for several years. I have selected two of his papers for reference since I feel they are most representative of his work on the pathologic changes involving the heart[114,115]. Mott and Hagstrom summarized the pathologic lesions of the cardiac autonomic nervous system in chronic Chagas' myocarditis in their paper published in *Circulation* in 1965[116]. Their own observations clearly confirmed the presence of numerous inflammatory and degenerative lesions of the ganglia in chronic Chagas' myocarditis.

REFERENCES

1. Meryon, E. (1852). On granular and fatty degeneration of the voluntary muscles. *Med. Clin. Tr. London*, **35**, 73

2. Erb, W.H. (1891). Dystrophia muscularis progressive. Klinische und pathologis-chanatomische studien. *Deutsch Z. Nevenheilk.*, **1**, 13–94, 173–261

3. Bunting, C.H. (1908). Chronic fibrous myocarditis in progressive muscular dystrophy. *Am. J. Med. Sci.*, **135**, 244

4. Globus, J.H. (1923). The pathologic findings in the heart muscle in progressive muscular dystrophy. *Arch. News. Psych.*, **9**, 59

5. Bevans, M. (1945). Changes in the musculature of the gastrointestinal tract and in the myocardium in progressive muscular dystrophy. *Arch. Pathol.*, **40**, 225

6. Frankel, R.A. and Rosser, R.J. (1976). The pathology of the heart in progressive muscular dystrophy: epimyocardial fibrosis. *Human Pathol.*, **7**, 375–86

7. Perloff, J.K., de Leon, A.C. and O'Doherty, D. (1966). The cardiomyopathy of progressive muscular dystrophy. *Circulation*, **36**, 625

8. Perloff, J.K., Roberts, W.C., de Leon, A.C. and O'Doherty, D. (1967). The distinctive electrocardiogram of Duchenne's progressive muscular dystrophy. *Am. J. Med.*, **42**, 179

9. Sanyal, S.K., Johnson, W.W., Thapar, M.K. and Pitner, S.E. (1978). An ultrastructural basis for the electrocardiographic alterations associated with Duchenne's progressive muscular dystrophy. *Circulation*, **57**, 1122–9

10. Rubin, I.L. and Buchberg, A.S. (1952). The heart in progressive muscular dystrophy. *Am. Heart J.*, **43**, 161

11. Northacker, W.G. and Netsky, M.G. (1950). Myocardial lesions in progressive muscular dystrophy. *Arch. Pathol.*, **50**, 578

12. James, T.N. (1962). Observations on the cardiovascular involvement, including the cardiac conduction system, in progressive muscular dystrophy. *Am. Heart J.*, **63**, 48–56

13. Nomura, H. and Hizawa, K. (1982). Histopathological study of the conduction system of the heart in Duchenne's progressive muscular dystrophy. *Acta Pathol.*, **32**, 1027–33

14. Skyring, A. and McKusick, V.A. (1961). Clinical, genetic and electrocardio-graphic studies in childhood muscular dystrophy. *Am. J. Med. Sci.*, **242**, 54–67

15. Mokri, B. and Engel, A.G. (1975). Duchenne dystrophy. Electron microscopic findings pointing to a basic or early abnormality in the plasma membrane of the muscle fiber. *Neurology*, **25**, 1111

16. Sanyal, S.K., Johnson, W.W., Dische, M.R., Pitner, S.E. and Beard, C. (1980). Dystrophic degeneration of papillary muscle and ventricular myocardium. A basis for mitral valve prolapse in Duchenne's muscular dystrophy. *Circulation*, **62**, 430–8

17. Becker, P.E. (1962). Two new families of benign sex-linked recessive muscular dystrophy. *Rev. Can. Bio.*, **21**, 551

18. Perloff, J.K., de Leon, A.C. and O'Doherty, D. (1966). *Op. cit.*, p. 625

19. Katijar, B.C., Soman, P.N., Mischra, S. and Chaterji, A.M. (1977). Congestive cardio-myopathy in a family of Becker's X-linked muscular dystrophy. *Postgrad. Med. J.*, **53**, 12

20. Hassan, Z., Fastabend, C.P., Mohanty, P.K. and Isaacs, E.R. (1979). Atrioventricular block and supraventricular arrhythmias with X-linked muscular dystrophy. *Circulation*, **60**, 1365

21. Vrints, C., Mercelis, R., Vanagt, E., Snoeck, J. and Martin, J.J. (1983). Cardiac manifestations of Becker-type muscular dystrophy. *Acta Cardiol.*, **38**, 479

22. Lambert, C.D. and Fairfax, A.J. (1976). Neurological associations of chronic heart block. *J. Neurol. Neurosurg. Psychiatry*, **39**, 571

23. Fairfax, A.J. and Lambert, C.D. (1976). Neurological aspects of sinoatrial heart block. *J. Neurol. Neurosurg. Psychiatry*, **39**, 576

24. Svetoni, N., Spargi, T., Ballantonio, M. and Lanzetta, T. (1984). Erbs muscular dystrophy and congestive myocardiopathy. *G. Ital. Cardiol.*, **14**, 59

25. Chavez, I., Brumlik, J. and Pollares, D.S. (1946). Sobre un Caso Extraordinaris de Paralisis Auricular Permanente con Degeneracion del Nudulo de Keith y Flack. *Arch. Inst. Cardiol., Mex.*, **16**, 159–81

26. Cushny, A.R. (1897). On the action of substances of the digitalis series on the circulation in mammals. *J. Exp. Med.*, **2**, 333

27. Bloomfield, D.A. and Sinclair-Smith, B.C. (1965). Persistent atrial standstill. *Am. J. Med.*, **39**, 335–9

28. Caponnetto, S., Pastorini, C. and Tirelli, G. (1968). Persistent atrial standstill in a patient affected with facioscapulohumeral dystrophy. *Cardiologia*, **53**, 341–50

29. Baldwin, B.J., Talley, R.C., Johnson, C. and Nutter, D.O. (1973). Permanent paralysis of the atrium in a patient with facioscapulo-humeral muscular dystrophy. *Am. J. Cardiol.*, **31**, 649–53

30. Bensald, J., Gilgenkrantz, J. and Fernandez, F. (1971). Paralysie Auriculaire Permanents Familial en Fapport Probable avec une Maladie Génetique du Type Charcot-Marie. *Arch. Mal. Coeur*, **65**, 935–53

31. Waters, D.D., Nutter, D.O., Hopkins, L.C. and Dorney, E.R. (1975). Cardiac features of an unusual X-linked humeroperoneal neuro-muscular disease. *N. Engl. J. Med.*, **293**, 1017–22

32. Rowland, L., Fetell, M., Olarte, M., Hays, A., Singh, N. and Wanat, F. (1979). Emery-Dreifuss muscular dystrophy. *Ann. Neurol.*, **5**, 111–17

33. Rapelli, A., Gagna, C. and Fabris, F. (1969). Standstill Atrial Permanente in un Paziente affetto da Distrofia Muscolare Progressive e da Diabete Mellits. *Minerva Cardioangiol.*, **17**, 63–8

34. Antonio, J., Diniz, M.C. and Mirand, D. (1978). Persistent atrial standstill with limb-girdle muscular dystrophy. *Cardiology*, **63**, 39–46

35. Steinert, H. (1909). Über das Klinische und Anatomische Bild des Muskelschwundes der Myotoniker. *Deutsche Ztschr Nervenh.*, **37**, 38–104

36. Batten, F.E. and Gibb, H.P. (1909). Myotonia atrophica. *Brain*, **32**, 187–205

37. Griffith, T.W. (1911). On myotonia. *Q. J. Med.*, **5**, 229

38. Evans, W. (1944). The heart in myotonia atrophica. *Br. Heart J.*, **6**, 41–7

39. De Wind, L.T. and Jones, R.J. (1950). Cardiovascular observations in dystonia myotonica. *J.A.M.A.*, **144**, 299–303

40. Perloff, J.K., Stevenson, W.G., Roberts, N.K., Cabeen, W. and Weiss, J. (1984). Cardiac involvement in myotonic muscular dystrophy (Steinert's disease). A prospective study of 25 patients. *Am. J. Cardiol.*, **54**, 1074

41. Holt, J.M. and Lambert, E.H.N. (1964). Heart disease as the presenting feature in myotonia atrophica. *Br. Heart J.*, **26**, 435

42. Black, W.C. and Ravin, A. (1947). Studies in dystrophia myotonica. VII. Autopsy observations in five cases. *Arch. Pathol.*, **44**, 176–91

43. Perloff, J.K., Stevenson, W.G., Roberts, N.K., Cabeen, W. and Weiss, J. (1984). *Op. cit.*, p. 1080

44. Bulloch, R.T., Davis, J.L. and Hara, M. (1967). Dystrophia myotonica with heart block. A light and electron microscopic study. *Arch. Pathol.*, **84**, 130–40

45. Uemura, N., Tanaka, H., Niimura, T., Hashiguchi, N., Yoshimura, M., Terashi, S. and Kanehisa, T. (1973). Electrophysiological and histological abnormalities of the heart in myotonic dystrophy. *Am. Heart J.*, **86**, 616–24

46. Tanaka, N., Tanaka, H., Takeda, M., Nimura, T., Kanehisa, T. and Terashi, S. (1973). Cardiomyopathy in myotonic dystrophy. A light and electron microscopic study of the myocardium. *Jpn. Heart J.*, **14**, 202–12

47. Ludatscher, R.M., Kerner, H., Amikam, S. and Gellel, B. (1978). Myotonia dystrophica with heart involvement. An electron microscopic study of skeletal, cardiac and smooth muscle. *J. Clin. Pathol.*, **31**, 1057–64

48. Motta, J., Guilleminault, C., Billingham, M., Barry, W. and Mason, J. (1979). Cardiac abnormalities in myotonic dystrophy. Electrophysiologic and histopathologic studies. *Am. J. Med.*, **67**, 467–73

49. Winters, S.J., Schreiner, B., Griggs, R.C., Rowley, P. and Nanda, N.C. (1976). Familial mitral valve prolapse and myotonic dystrophy. *Ann. Intern. Med.*, **85**, 19

50. Hiromasa, S., Takayuki, I., Kubota, K., Takata, S., Hattori, N., Nishimura, M. and Watanabe, Y. (1986). A family with myotonic dystrophy associated with diffuse cardiac conduction disturbances as demonstrated by His bundle electrocardiography. *Am. Heart J.*, **111**, 85–91

51. Butterworth, R.F., Shapcott, D., Melancon, S., Breton, G., Geoffroy, G., Lemieux, B. and Barbeau, A. (1976). Clinical laboratory findings in Friedreich's ataxia. *J. Can. Sci. Neurol.*, **3**, 335

52. Child, J.S., Perloff, J.K., Bach, P.M., Wolfe, A.D., Perlman, S. and Kark, R.A.P. (1986). Cardiac involvement in Friedreich's ataxia. *J. Am. Coll. Cardiol.*, **7**, 1370

53. Perloff, J.K., de Leon, A.C. and O'Doherty, D. (1966). *Op. cit.*, p. 625

54. Pitt, G.N. (1887). On a case of Friedreich's disease; its clinical history and post-mortem appearances. *Guy's Hosp. Rep.*, **44**, 369

55. Child, J.S., Perloff, J.K. *et al.* (1986). *Op. cit.*, p. 1370

56. Brooke, M.H. (1979). *A Clinician's View of Neuromuscular Diseases*. (Baltimore: Williams and Wilkins)

57. Unverferth, D.V., Schmidt, W.R., Baker, P.B. and Wooley, C.F. (1987). Morphologic and functional characteristics of the heart in Friedreich's ataxia. *Am. J. Med.*, **82**, 5–10

58. James, T.N. and Fisch, C. (1963). Observations on the cardiovascular involvement in

Friedreich's ataxia. *Am. Heart J.*, **66**, 164–75

59. Nadas, A.S., Alimurung, M.M. and Sieracki, L.A. (1951). Cardiac manifestations of Friedreich's ataxia. *N. Engl. J. Med.*, **244**, 239

60. Ivemark, B. and Thorén, C. (1964). The pathology of the heart in Friedreich's ataxia. *Acta Med. Scand.*, **175**, 227

61. Hewer, R.L. (1969). The heart in Friedreich's ataxia. *Br. Heart J.*, **31**, 5–14

62. Pasternac, A., Wagniart, P., Olivenstein, R. *et al.* (1982). Increased plasma catecholamines in patients with Friedreich's ataxia. *J. Can. Sci. Neurol.*, **9**, 195–203

63. Merkel, A.D. and Barbeau, A. (1982). Plasma catecholamines in Friedreich's ataxia assayed using high performance liquid chromatography with electrochemical detection. *J. Can. Sci. Neurol.*, **9**, 205–8

64. Gibson, T.C. (1975). The heart in myasthenia gravis. *Am. Heart J.*, **90**: 389

65. Weigert, C. (1901). Pathologisch-anatomischer Beitrag zur Erb'schen Krankheit (myasthenia gravis). *Neurol. Zentralbl.*, **20**, 597

66. Buzzard, E.F. (1905). The clinical history and post-mortem examination of five cases of myasthenia gravis. *Brain*, **28**, 438

67. Marie, P., Bouttier, H. and Bertrand, L. (1921). Étude anatomo-clinique d'un cas grave de myasthénie de ErbGoldflam. *Ann. Med. Paris*, **10**, 173

68. Mella, H. (1923). Irradiation of the thymus in myasthenia gravis. *Med. Clin. North Am.*, **7**, 939–49

69. Barton, F.E. and Branch, C.F. (1937). Myasthenia gravis. Report of a case with necropsy. *J.A.M.A.*, **109**, 2044

70. Rottino, A., Poppiti, R. and Rao, J. (1942). Myocardial lesions in myasthenia gravis. Review and report of a case. *Arch. Pathol.*, **34**, 557

71. Mendelow, H. (1958). Pathology. In Osserman, K.E. (ed.) *Myasthenia Gravis*, pp. 10–43. (New York: Grune & Stratton, Inc.)

72. Russell, D.S. (1953). Histological changes in the striped muscles in myasthenia gravis, *J. Pathol. Bacteriol.*, **65**, 279

73. Rowland, L.P., Hoefer, P.F.A., Aranow, H. Jr. and Merritt, H.H. (1956). Fatalities in myasthenia gravis. A review of 39 cases with 26 autopsies. *Neurology Minneap.*, **6**, 307

74. Huvos, A.G. and Pruzanski, W. (1967). Smooth muscle involvement in primary muscle diseases. III. Myasthenia gravis. *Arch. Pathol.*, **84**, 280

75. Leak, D. (1961). Paroxysmal atrial flutter in peroneal muscular atrophy. *Br. Heart J.*, **23**, 326

76. Littler, W.A. (1970). Heart block and peroneal muscular atrophy. *Q. J. Med.*, **39**, 431

77. Kay, J.M., Littler, W.A. and Meade, J.B. (1972). Ultrastructure of the myocardium in familial heart block and peroneal muscular atrophy. *Br. Heart J.*, **34**, 1081

78. Isner, J.M., Hawley, R.J., Weintraub, A.B. and Engel, W.K. (1979). Cardiac findings in Charcot-Marie-Tooth disease. *Arch. Intern. Med.*, **139**, 1161

79. Lowry, P.I. and Littler, W.A. (1983). Peroneal muscular atrophy associated with cardiac conduction tissue disease. *Postgrad. Med. J.*, **59**, 530

80. Martin Du-Pan, R.C., Juse, C. and Perrenoud, J.J. (1984). Congestive cardiomyopathy and pyruvate elevation in a case of Charcot-Marie-Tooth disease. *Schweiz Med. Wochenschr.*, **5**, 114

81. Von Gräfe, A. (1868). Verhandlungen Arztlicher Gesellschaften. *Berl. Klin. Wochenschr.*, **5**, 125

82. Sandifer, P.H. (1946). Chronic progressive ophthalmoplegia of myopathic origin. *J. Neurol. Neurosurg. Psychiatry*, **9**, 81

83. Kearns, T.P. and Sayre, G.P. (1958). Retinitis pigmentosa, external ophthalmoplegia and complete heart block. *Arch. Ophthalmol.*, **60**, 280

84. Kearns, T.P. (1965). External ophthalmoplegia, pigmentary degeneration of the retina and cardiomyopathy. A newly recognized syndrome. *Trans. Am. Ophthalmol. Soc.*, **63**, 559

85. Clark, D.S., Myerburg, R.J., Morales, R.R., Befeler, B., Hernandez, F. and Gelband, H. (1975). Heart block and Kearns-Sayre: electrophysiologic-pathologic correlation. *Chest*, **68**, 727

86. Roberts, N.K., Perloff, J.K. and Kark, R.A.P. (1979). Cardiac conduction in the Kearns-Sayre syndrome (a neuromuscular disorder associated with progressive external ophthalmoplegia and pigmentary retinopathy.) *Am. J. Cardiol.*, **44**, 1396–400

87. Charles, R., Holt, M.B. Kay, J.M., Epstein, E.J. and Rees, J.R. (1981). Myocardial ultrastructure and the development of atrioventricular block in Kearns-Sayre syndrome. *Circulation*, **63**, 214–19

88. Singsen, B., Goldreyer, B., Stanton, R., Hanson, V. (1976). Childhood poliomyelitis with cardiac conduction defects. *Am. J. Dis. Child.*, **131**, 71

89. Gottdiener, J.S., Sherber, H.S., Hawley, R.J. and Engel, W.K. (1978). Cardiac manifestations in poliomyelitis. *Am. J. Cardiol.*, **41**, 1141

90. Evans, W. (1949). Familial cardiomegaly. *Br. Heart J.*, **11**, 68

91. Prystowsky, E.N., Pritchett, E.L., Roses, A.D. and Gallaghher, J. (1979). The natural history of conduction system disease in myotonic muscular dystrophy as determined by serial electrophysiologic studies. *Circulation*, **60**, 1360–4

92. Norris, F.H. Jr., Moss, A.J. and Yu, P.N. (1966). On the possibility that a type of human muscular dystrophy commences in myocardium. *Ann. NY Acad. Sci.*, **138**, 342–53

93. Shafiq, S.A., Saude, M.A., Carruthers, R.R., Killip, T. and Milborat, A.T. (1972). Skeletal muscle in idiopathic cardiomyopathy. *J. Neurol. Sci.*, **15**, 303

94. Isaacs, H. and Munche, G. (1975). Idiopathic cardiomyopathy and skeletal muscle abnormality. *Am. Heart J.*, **90**, 767–73

95. Dunnigan, A., Pierpont, M.E., Smith, S.A., Breningstall, G., Benditt, D.G. and Benson, D.W. (1984). Cardiac and skeletal myopathy associated with cardiac dysrhythmias. *Am. J. Cardiol.*, **53**, 731–7

96. Vanderark, G.D. (1975). Cardiovascular changes with acute subdural hematoma. *Surg. Neurol.*, **3**, 305

97. Bramwell, C. (1934). Can head injury cause auricular fibrillation? *Lancet*, **1**, 8

98. McLeod, A.A., Niel-Dwyer, G., Meyer, C.H.A., Richardson, P.L., Cruickshank, J. and Bartlett, J. (1982). Cardiac sequelae of acute head injury. *Br. Heart J.*, **47**, 221–6

99. Sciarra, D. (1984). Head injury. In Rowland, L.P. (ed.) *Merritt's Textbook of Neurology*, 7th edn., p. 277. (Philadelphia: Lea and Febiger)

100. Brown, R.S., Mohr, P.A., Carey, J.S. *et al.* (1967). Cardiovascular changes after cranial cerebral injury and increased intracranial pressure. *Surg. Gynecol. Obstet.*, **125**, 1205–11

101. Neil-Dwyer, G., Cruickshank, J., Stott, A. *et al.* (1974). The urinary catecholamine and plasma cortisol levels in patients with subarachnoid hemorrhage. *J. Neurol. Sci.*, **22**, 375–82

102. Wilmore, D.W., Long, J.M., Mason, A.D. Jr. *et al.* (1974). Catecholamines. Mediator of the hypermetabolic response to thermal injury. *Ann. Surg.*, **180**, 653–69

103. Benedict, C.R. and Loach, A.B. (1978). Clinical significance of plasma adrenaline and noradrenaline concentrations in patients with subarachnoid hemorrhage. *J. Neurol. Neurosurg. Psychiatry*, **4**, 113–17

104. Hörtnagl, H., Hammerle, A.F., Hackl, J.M. *et al.* (1980). The activity of the sympathetic nervous system following severe head injury. *Intensive Care Med.*, **6**, 169–77

105. Levine, S.A. and Brown, C.L. (1929). Coronary thrombosis: its various clinical features. *Medicine*, **8**, 245–418

106. Grant, A.P. and Dowey, K.E. (1980). The association of acute stroke and myocardial infarction in elderly medical emergencies. *Ir. J. Med. Sci.*, **149**, 15–18

107. Von Arbin, M., Britton, M., de Faire, U., Helmers, C., Miah, K. and Murray, V. (1982). Myocardial infarction in patients with acute cerebrovascular disease. *Eur. Heart J.* **3**, 136–41

108. Badui, E., Estenol, B. and Garcia, R.D. (1982). Coincidence of cerebrovascular accident and silent myocardial infarction. *Angiology*, **33**, 702–9

109. Moles, K.W., Grant, P. and Biggart, J.D. (1982). The coincidence of infarcts of the heart and brain: an analysis. *Ir. J. Med. Sci.*, **151**, 145–50

110. Vianna, G. (1911). Contribuicão para o estudo da anatomia pathológica da 'moléstia de Carlos Chagas'. *Mem. Inst. Cruz.*, **3**, 276

111. Torres, C.M. (1917). Estudos ds miocardio na moléstia de Chagas (forma aguda). I. Alteracões da fibra muscular cardiaca. *Mem. Inst. Cruz.*, **9**, 114

112. Torres, C.M. (1923). A Trypanosomose Americana e sua anatomia pathológica. *Folha Med.*, **4**, 25

113. Torres, C.M. (1941). Sôbre a anatomia pathológica da doenca de Chagas. *Mem. Inst. Cruz.*, **36**, 391

114. Köberle, F. (1956). Pathologische Befunde an den muskulären Hohlorganen bei der experimentellen Chagaskrankheit. *Zentralbl. Allg. Path.*, **95**, 321

115. Köberle, F. (1958). *Cardiopatia chagásica Hospital Rio*, **53**, 311

116. Mott, K.E. and Hagstrom, J.W.C. (1965). The pathologic lesions of the cardiac autonomic nervous system in Chagas' myocarditis. *Circulation*, **31**, 273–86

12 Anatomical changes due to endocrine and nutritional factors

ACROMEGALY AND THE HEART

As a disease entity, acromegaly was first described by Marie in 1886[1]. Enlargement is the major cardiac anatomical change in acromegaly. Historically, several mechanisms have been postulated to account for this. It was Huchard in 1895 who first suggested that the cardiomegaly occurred either as a part of the generalized enlargement of the organs that is seen in this disease or as a result of the accompanying arteriosclerosis[2]. The associated hypertension was brought out by G. Alessandri in 1908[3]. This was confirmed time and again in the succeeding decades. In 1967, J.V. Souadijian and A. Schirger summarized the existing knowledge of this association and reported that systemic hypertension occurred in about 30% of acromegalic patients[4]. Still another mechanism was advanced by Davis in 1934. He felt that since the thyroid was enlarged in at least half of the 166 cases he studied, hyperthyroidism was the most probable mechanism for producing what he termed 'myocardial insufficiency' leading to cardiac enlargement[5].

In those cases of acromegaly where hypertension is not present several investigators have postulated that the cardiomegaly was due to a direct myocardial effect of the increased hormone secretion. This was advocated by Hejtmancik and associates in 1951[6], and again by Carl Pepine in 1970[7]. Experimental confirmation of this thesis was supplied by De Grandpre and Raab in 1953[8]. They were able to produce cardiac hypertrophy in non-hypertensive hypophysectomized rats by the administration of growth hormone.

Histologic studies of the heart were reported by Rossi and his group in an individual who died suddenly after exhibiting cardiac arrhythmias for some time[9]. They found degeneration of the AV node and inflammatory as well as degenerative changes in the sinoatrial perinodal nerve plexus. These findings were published in *Chest* in 1977.

In 1980, Lie and Grossman reported their observations from 27 autopsied patients[10]. Another paper by Lie a year later stressed the histopathologic features of acromegalic heart disease[11]. Both papers described the presence of non-specific myocardial hypertrophy and interstitial fibrosis, a lymphocytic infiltrative type of myocarditis and small vessel disease as well as intramural coronary arterial wall thickening.

Despite this background of historical data and observations, the pathogenesis of cardiac enlargement in acromegaly still eludes us. Out of the numerous reports of markedly enlarged acromegalic hearts, there is one case that stands out above all others. This is the report by Levene and Miller in 1942, where the patient had a perfectly normal sized heart[12]. How come?

PHEOCHROMOCYTOMA

This neoplasm of adrenal chromaffin tissue, although rare, is an important lesion because it is a remediable cause of hypertension. It was first described by Frankel in 1886 and later given its name by Pick in 1912[13]. The cardiovascular complications arise from the excessive amount of catecholamines produced by the tumor.

In 1906, R.M. Pearce presented the first experimental evidence in animals that histologic changes in the myocardium could be induced with intravenous injections of adrenalin[14]. The ability of norepinephrine to produce similar changes was than brought out by Szakács and Mehlman in 1960[15], almost a half-century later. Further confirmation that catecholamines can induce a cardiomyopathy in animals was supplied by Franz (1937)[16], Raab (1943)[17] and Reichenbach and Benditt in 1970[18].

The initial reports describing the presence of myocardial lesions in association with pheochromocytoma were those of Szakács and Cannon in 1958[19], and Kline in 1961[20]. Several years later (1966), Van Vliet and his colleagues from the Mayo Clinic reported their findings on necropsy in 26 patients[21]. In addition, these workers produced experimental lesions in the myocardium of rats and compared these lesions with those of the 26 patients. The number of patients studied is quite large for so rare a disease. A good number of them had evidence of active myocarditis, while the majority showed an increased amount of fibrous tissue replacing the myocardial fibers. The fibrotic process was noted particularly around the small vessels, and in the inner two-thirds of the myocardium. The authors applied the term 'catecholamine myocarditis' to those histopathologic alterations that were compatible with an active process. Histologically similar evidence of active myocarditis was striking in the rats that were injected with norepinephrine. As a matter of fact, their most important observation was that the myocarditis seen in their patients was similar to those in other patients with pheochromocytoma, as well as in those who had received norepinephrine therapeutically before death, and in several species of laboratory animals after injection of various catecholamines.

Myocardial infarction is another myocardial change that has been reported in association with pheochromocytoma. It was described as one of the cardiac complications by Radtke and his group in 1975[22]. In 1981, Levister and Taylor described a patient with pheochromocytoma who clinically had evidence of physiological hypertrophic subaortic stenosis and who, at necropsy, was found to have subendocardial infarction[23].

Oakley and Goodwin in 1974, independently called attention to the development of hypertrophic cardiomyopathy in the presence of pheochromocytoma[24,25]. The possibility that a pheochromocytoma could induce a hypertrophic cardiomyopathy by virtue of chronic norepinephrine stimulation was advanced by Blaufuss in 1975 utilizing the dog as the animal model[26].

Pheochromocytoma need not be confined to the adrenal gland itself. Although extremely rare, it has been found arising within the intrathoracic cage itself. It is difficult to prioritize the observers or even to present them in a chronological manner. The reports are sparse, isolated, difficult to find, and written by teams of authors rather than individuals.

The earliest report that I could find of an intrathoracic pheochromocytoma was that by Peiper and Golestan in 1963[27]. A malignant primary cardiac pheochromocytoma was described by Voci and his associates in 1982[28]. Pericardial sites of origin were also reported by Besterman[29] in 1974, and Saad[30] with his group in 1983. The first report of a pheochromocytoma involving the posterior wall of the left ventricle and coronary sinus was that of David and co-authors in 1986[31].

My obsession with trying to make this text as historically complete as possible is my only excuse for having presented this boring concatenation.

THYROID

The first one to call attention to cardiac involvement in thyrotoxicosis was Parry. It is to be found as part of a collection of unpublished writings which appeared in 1825[32]. The collection spans a period of 39 years. Eight patients in all are described with the first of the patients having been seen by him in 1786. All of them demonstrated exophthalmic goiter, edema, cardiac enlargement and irregularity of the pulse. Parry's observations were confirmed by several other clinicians during the remaining part of the 19th century. They were Graves[33] in 1835, von Basedow[34] in 1840, Lockridge[35] in 1879, and Moebius[36] in 1896. Although Graves' name is eponymously attached to thyrotoxicosis with exophthalmic goiter, Parry's description of the disease predates that of Graves by 49 years.

Parry's case no. 1 is worthy of quotation since it embodies the most pertinent clinical elements of the syndrome[32].

There is one malady which I have in five cases seen coincident with what appeared to be enlargement of the heart, and which, so far as I know, has not been noticed, in that connection by medical writers. This malady to which I allude is enlargement of the thyroid gland.

The first case of this coincidence which I witnessed was that of Grace B., a married woman, aged thirty-seven, in the month of August, 1786. Six years before this period she caught cold in lying-in, and for a month suffered under a very acute rheumatic fever; subsequently to which, she became subject to more or less palpitation of the heart; very much augmented by bodily exercise, and gradually increasing in force and frequency till my attendance, when it was so vehement, that each systole of the heart shook the whole thorax. Her pulse was 156 in a minute, very full and hard, alike in both wrists, irregular as to strength and intermitting at least once in six beats. She had no cough, tendency to fainting, or blueness of the skin, but had twice or thrice been seized in the night with a sense of constriction and difficulty of breathing, which was attended with a spitting of a small quantity of blood. She described herself also as having frequent and violent stitches of pain about the lower part of the sternum.

About three months after lying-in, while she was suckling her child, a lump of about the size of a walnut was perceived on the right side of her neck. This continued to enlarge till the period of my attendance, when it occupied both sides of her neck, so as to have reached an enormous size, projecting forwards before the margin of the lower jaw. The part swelled was the thyroid gland. The carotic arteries on each side were greatly distended; the eyes were protruded from their sockets, and the countenance exhibited an appearance of agitation and distress, especially on any muscular exertion, which I have rarely seen equalled. She suffered no pain in her head, but was frequently affected with giddiness.

For three weeks she had experienced a considerable degree of loss of appetite, and thirst, and for a week had edematous swelling of her legs and thighs, attended with very deficient urine, which was high coloured, and deposited a sediment. Until the commencement of the anasarcous swellings, she had long suffered night sweats, which totally disappeared as the swellings occurred. She was frequently sick in the morning, and often threw up fluid tinged with bile[37].

Caleb Hillier Parry was born on October 21, 1755, the son of a minister. He was the first of ten children. Parry pursued his medical studies at the University of Edinburgh in two stages. Upon completion of the second year of study, he left the university and moved to London where he spent the next two years as a preceptee of a Dr. Thomas Dunham, an obstetrician of much local renown. He then re-entered the University of Edinburgh, and at the end of one year, he was admitted to the M.D. degree. His doctoral dissertation was entitled *De rabie contagiosa vulgo canina*. Parry married during the same year he received his doctorate, and settled in Bath, England, where he remained until his death.

Ten years after establishing his practice, Parry became a licentiate of the Royal College of Physicians of London. He had four sons. Charles, the first son, followed in the father's footsteps as a physician. Another son, called William, became renowned as the arctic explorer.

Parry's avocation during the early years of his career centered about fossils. In pursuing this interest he acquired an admirable collection as well as enough data to form the basis of a publication called *Proposals for a History of Fossils of Gloucestershire*. Parry's first paper on a medical subject appeared in 1792. The subject matter had already been presented by him three years earlier before the Medical Society of London. He then published an important study on angina pectoris in 1799. The paper was a clinicopathologic analysis with illustrations of the morbid anatomy as derived from dissections. Parry's opus magnum was his *Elements of Pathology and Therapeutics*. He was able to finish only the first of the projected two volumes. It appeared in 1815. He suffered a stroke a year after its publication, and was never able to continue with the work. The unfinished second volume was published by his son Charles in 1825 in conjunction with the republication of the first volume. Charles had also assembled the entire collection of his father's unpublished writings, all of which were published during 1825, three years after his father's death[38].

There has been considerable controversy over the years concerning the precise role of hyperthyroidism in the genesis of the cardiovascular abnormalities. Quite a number of authorities have stoutly maintained that the thyrotoxic state, itself, is capable of causing heart disease. These include Magee and Smith[39], who presented their views in 1935, followed by Likoff and Levine in 1943 with similar views[40] and Griswold and Keating[41] in 1949.

On the other side of the controversy are such luminaries as Willius, Boothby and Wilson[42], who presented the first cogent evidence for the adversarial position in 1923, followed a year later by Lahey and Hamilton[43] from Boston, and in turn, by Hurxthal[44] in 1928, and Friedberg and Sohval[45] in 1937. This entire group has maintained the position over the succeeding years that when heart disease is present in thyrotoxicosis, it is due to an independent process such as rheumatic fever, hypertension or coronary artery disease.

In 1958, a well documented paper appeared in the *Quarterly Journal of Medicine* authored by G. Sandler and G.M.Wilson[46]. It analyzed a very large group of thyrotoxic patients that had been treated with radioactive iodine. As part of their study, they considered the role of thyrotoxicosis in producing heart disease. Autopsies were done in several cases. On the basis of this rather detailed study, they concluded that 'although thyrotoxicosis may not be the sole cause of the cardiac disability, in many patients with thyrotoxicosis and heart disease, it is nevertheless, the predominant factor'.

Concerning structural changes in the heart and hyperthyroidism, a marked difference of opinion has also emerged on the histopathologic pattern. The first studies directed towards the problem were reported by Fahr in 1916[47]. He found focal necrosis and interstitial myocarditis in five fatal cases of thyrotoxicosis. Two more cases with similar findings were described by Hashimoto in 1921[48]. Wilson reported on 18 cases in 1923[49]. He concluded that 'in patients with long-sustained pronounced hyperthyroidism, the myocardium shows more advanced fat changes than in individuals of the same age without hyperthyroidism.' But two important studies, both reported in 1932, failed to establish any relationship between the clinical manifestations of hyperthyroidism and structural changes in the heart. These were the work of Rake and McEachern based on 27 autopsies[50], and that of Weller and his associates from an analysis of 35 fatal cases[51]. Reversible changes in the mitochondria as demonstrated by electron microscopic studies were reported in animals by Callas and Hayes in 1974[52].

Apart from these histologic studies, a lively debate has been going on for many years regarding the ability of excess thyroid hormone to cause myocardial hypertrophy in formerly normal hearts. This question has never been truly resolved in the human. However, in a number of different species of animals at least, the debate appeared to be laid to rest through the efforts of Skelton and Sonnenblick. They demonstrated in 1974 that hypertrophy of the myocardium can indeed come about under the influence of excess thyroid hormone[53]. Furthermore, they demonstrated the reversibility of the hypertrophy once the excess thyroid hormone was eliminated.

Cardiac involvement in myxedema was first recorded by Zondek in 1918[54]. The histological characteristics and their clinical correlates have also merited attention beginning with Fahr's report in 1925[55]. Over the succeeding years, a number of investigators added their findings to those of Fahr. The major figures have been Campbell and Suzman (1934)[56], Means (1937)[57], Fournier (1942)[58], Bustamente and his group (1955)[59], and Hamilton and Greenwood in 1957[60]. The structural changes of myocardial damage were described initially by Hallock in 1933[61], and the term cardiomyopathy gradually surfaced as the generic label for the structural changes. Means also was instrumental in focusing attention on the gross anatomical changes. His comments are to be found in his textbook *The Thyroid and its Diseases*; a classic that served as a major source of reference on the thyroid for many years[62]. In 1952, Ellis and his associates published a rather descriptive paper on the morbid anatomy of the heart in myxedema and which appeared in the *American Heart Journal* (at that time, probably the leading American journal in cardiology)[63]. Along with their histologic descriptions, Hamilton and Greenwood also elaborated on the gross morbid anatomy in their paper on myxedema heart disease in 1957[64].

Pericardial effusion is another characteristic and frequent complication of myxedema. The association was originally brought out by Freeman in 1934[65]. It was a case report describing the existence of chronic pericardial effusion in an individual with myxedema. Further case reports then appeared from both sides of the Atlantic. Marzullo and Franco reported theirs in 1939[66]; Boivin from France in 1945[67]; a year later Schnitzer and Gutmann[68] presented their findings in *The British Heart Journal*. Pericardial effusion as a constant, early and major factor in the cardiac syndrome of hypothyroidism was stressed by Kern and his group in 1949[69].

Radiologic evidence of cardiomegaly, whether due to hypertrophy or pericardial effusion was described in a series of reports beginning with Hallock when he wrote about myocardial damage in 1933[61]. Practically all of the previous investigators were involved in this diagnostic feature. Scherf and Boyd elaborated on the X-ray findings in their text on cardiovascular diseases, published in 1939[70].

Throughout all this evolving knowledge, the burning question has been: are the cardiac changes a direct effect of the hypothyroidism or mediated through the accelerated development of arteriosclerosis because of the hypercholesterolemia that is so constantly associated with myxedema? A long series of isolated case reports have linked hypothyroidism with coronary artery disease. These begin with the case report by A.M.Fishberg that appeared in the *Journal of the American Medical Association* in 1924[71]. In 1963, Aber and Thompson analyzed the clinical records of 53 myxedematous patients from the medical units of two Liverpool Hospitals in England. It was their contention on clinical grounds that the cardiac enlargement is not necessarily a component of the myxedematous process[72]. They concluded that when seen it may be due in part to advancing age and the concomitant presence of hypertension and/or coronary artery disease, and that the elevated blood cholesterol level is an important factor in the development of atherosclerosis. The first systematic study based on necropsy evidence was conducted by A.D. Steinberg in 1968[73]. The findings were culled from the autopsy records of 38 women with myxedema and a pathologic diagnosis of chronic thyroiditis or thyroid atrophy and fibrosis. He showed that statistically, myxedema did not appear to predispose to coronary artery disease unless hypertension was present.

This is where we currently are in the relationship between myxedema and the heart. In Steinberg's words, 'Although clinical studies have suggested a correlation between myxedema and coronary artery disease … a final answer will come only from a controlled prospective study with careful pathologic examination of injected hearts'[74].

PARATHYROID

Knowledge concerning the effects of hyperparathyroidism on the heart has evolved only within the past several decades or so. It is now known that primary hyperparathyroidism is almost invariably associated with myocardial hypertrophy. In the 1950s, Hellstrom advanced the belief that the hypertrophy was due to the hypertension that occurs in the hyperparathyroid state, and that, in fact, hypertension and hypertensive cardiovascular disease were the major causes of disability and death in this disorder[75]. The validity of this statement has been refuted time and again by subsequent investigators. First of all, cardiac hypertrophy in

hyperparathyroidism is seen even in the absence of hypertension.

The cardiac hypertrophy associated with the hyperparathyroid state can be symmetric, asymmetric or in the form of hypertrophic cardiomyopathy. It was in 1978, that McFarland and co-workers first suggested that it was the prolonged hypercalcemia which provided the stimulus for the development of hypertrophic cardiomyopathy[76]. That this too was not true was shown by Symons and his group in 1985. Their study was a purely clinical one with no postmortem observations. It was the first time that a pattern of cardiac muscle hypertrophy could be clearly related to a hormonal abnormality. Their paper presented rather convincing evidence that the various forms of myocardial hypertrophy seen in hyperparathyroidism, including hypertrophic cardiomyopathy, were the effect of the increased concentration of parathyroid hormone itself. Four years before this clinical study, Katoh and his colleagues had already demonstrated the positive inotropic effect of parathyroid hormone on the rat heart which could be blocked by verapamil (the first of the calcium-channel blocking agents)[78]. During the same year, Bogin and his associates, utilizing rat heart cells in culture, had reported not only the positive chronotropic effect that parathyroid hormone had on these cells but also that this action could be duplicated with calcium ionophore and blocked by verapamil[79]. These experimental data indicated that the direct effect of parathyroid hormone on the myocardium is mediated through an influx of calcium at the cellular level and is independent of the extracellular concentration of calcium.

How then does hypercalcemia fit into all of this? Apparently, elevated levels of calcium in the blood do have an effect but a different morphologic alteration is produced rather than the myocardial hypertrophy of parathyroid hormone. This was brought out by W. Roberts and B. Waller from the National Institutes of Health in 1981. It is somewhat amazing that 1981 saw the publication of several landmark papers in this relatively narrow field of study by investigators focusing on different aspects of the problem and working independently of each other.

The study by Roberts and Waller was prompted by the lack of necropsy data in the clinical setting of chronic hypercalcemia. They evaluated the postmortem cardiac findings on 18 patients in whom there was unequivocal evidence of elevated blood calcium levels for a year or more. Their study demonstrated that 'chronic hypercalcemia is associated with accelerated deposition of calcium in the cardiac annuli and valvular cusps, in the media and intima of the coronary arteries and in individual myocardial fibers (dystrophic calcification), and that coronary intimal calcification may be associated with or produce luminal narrowing, especially in patients with total serum cholesterol over 200 mg/dl' [80].

The possibility of some relationship between chronic parathyroid insufficiency and myocardial damage was first suggested by Rose in 1943 [81]. His conclusion was based on a patient that he followed for 16 years who had developed an otherwise unexplained congestive heart failure after a surgically induced hypoparathyroidism. Prior to this, Hegglin (1939) had reported on the effects of hypocalcemia on the heart [82].

Since these initial studies, very few scattered case reports have appeared linking hypoparathyroidism with cardiomyopathy. The leading authors of these papers are Evans (1945) [83], Jernigan (1953) [84], Schulman (1955) [85], Grieve (1955) [86], Weill (1967) [87] and Giles [88] in 1981. Giles' comments are interesting in that he includes the hypomagnesemia along with the hypocalcemia as mechanisms for the development of the dilated cardiomyopathy.

OBESITY AND THE HEART

The ill effects of obesity on survival have been well recognized since the days of Hippocrates. In aphorism 44, he clearly brought out the shortened life expectancy of the obese when compared to those who were slender. To think that he came to this conclusion without benefit of the computerized actuarial statistics so beloved by the life insurance companies of today... Celsus also was an astute observer. His statement that fat people are very subject to acute diseases may be found in his eleventh aphorism [89].

The cardiovascular consequences of severe obesity are well known today. The historical background concerning the morbid anatomical changes of the heart in the obese individual should start with William Harvey. He was probably the first to publish observations on the 'fatty heart' [90]. This was in the 17th century and the heart that he described was that of a very obese man. It was so

completely covered with fat that Harvey called it 'cor adipe plane tectum'. In addition, in his essay concerning the anatomical examination of the body of Thomas Parr, Harvey describes Parr's heart as being large, thick and fibrous, and encased, as it were in a considerable amount of adherent fat [90].

Quite a number of prominent clinicians beginning with Sprengall in 1708, and followed by Senac (1783), Corvisart (1806), Ormerod (1849), and Quain in 1850, recognized and commented on the relationship between obesity and cardiac dysfunction.

Sprengall pointed out that it was Celsus who described rather vividly the labored respirations of obese people [91]. In Senac's famous treatise on the heart, he describes a case of sudden death 'in which the fat spreading over the heart extinguished its movement' [92]. Corvisart believed that the heart was smothered in obese people by the immense amount of fat that enveloped it [93]. He, too, described fatty changes in the muscle of the heart saying that it was analogous to the fatty changes seen in the voluntary muscles of the elderly.

In 1818, when Cheyne described that type of respiration known eponymously as Cheyne-Stokes respiration, the cardiac findings at necropsy in that patient were dubbed by Cheyne as being those of 'fatty degeneration'. His case report was entitled 'A case of apoplexy in which the fleshy part of the heart was converted into fat', and his conclusion was that the patient's peculiar type of breathing was a sine qua non of a fatty heart [94].

Laénnec devoted an entire chapter to fatty heart in his treatise on mediate auscultation [95]. He also discussed it in his treatise on diseases of the chest [96]. Laénnec also distinguished between accumulation of fat on the epicardial surface and fatty degeneration of the myocardium. He described the degeneration grossly as being characterized by a yellowish pallor, like dead leaves [95]. Paget later emphasized that fatty degeneration implied fat not on but in the muscular fibers which became converted into fatty tubes [97]. Ormerod's observations were published in the London Medical Gazette and concerned themselves primarily with the clinical history and pathology of one form of fatty degeneration of the heart [98].

Quain's reputation as the leading authority of the time on the 'fatty heart' was established with the appearance of his monograph on the subject in 1850 [99]. Careful anatomical studies were lacking until those of Quain and Rokitansky. Those of

Rokitansky were recorded in his manual of pathological anatomy which appeared in 1852[100]. Quain's paper made such an impression that for many years thereafter, it was 'de rigeur' to blame sudden death on the 'fatty heart'. Quain also distinguished between fatty degeneration of the muscle fibers and fatty infiltration between them. He characterized the infiltration as a 'surcharge of fat spreading over the surface of the heart'. He even described in his monograph the clinical features of a fatty heart. These included labored breathing, chest discomfort, 'languid, feeble circulation', syncopal episodes, coma, and sudden death with rupture of the heart[99]. Probably, Quain's most important contribution, according to Bedford, was his recognition that localized fatty change was associated with obstruction of that branch of the coronary arterial tree feeding that segment of myocardium[101]. Morgan brought out in 1968 that most of Quain's cases were actually examples of coronary artery disease or ruptured hearts as a result of an acute infarction[102].

The belief that the 'fatty heart' was the most important form of myocardial disease held sway well into the latter part of the 19th century, and even in the first decade or so of the 20th century. Most of the standard texts on cardiology during this span of time stressed the frequency and importance of the fatty heart in terms of morbidity and mortality. Throughout the early part of the 20th century, as I indicated in the section dealing with myocardial lesions, 'chronic myocarditis' supplanted the 'fatty heart' as the most common diagnosis of heart disease. Obviously in both cases, the true nature of the pathologic changes was not recognized. As Bedford points out in his historical survey of the fatty heart, the medical world needed Herrick's second paper, published in 1919, to finally realize the role of coronary artery disease in what was misinterpreted as initially the 'fatty heart' and later 'chronic myocarditis'[101,103].

Alcohol was often mentioned as a cause of fatty heart, especially in those who favored London gin. I wonder if this bit of trivia would have any deterrent effect on our current 'antecebum martini afficionados'. Many clinical signs were advanced as manifestations of the underlying pathologic abnormality. Some were to the point of absurdity. An example of this would be Fothergill's contention that those with a fatty heart had a guarded, quiet and distrustful gait[104]. Persistent confusion with the cardiac effects of atherosclerosis was the inclusion of arcus senilis as one of the clinical signs.

Gallavardin's review of the subject in 1900 remains a classic[105]. He did not confuse the fatty degeneration at postmortem with coronary occlusion and myocardial infarction. This was an important step since in doing so he was able to put the morbid anatomy of the 'fatty heart' into its proper niche; a step that Quain had failed to follow to its logical conclusion. Gallarvardin found fatty degeneration to be common in those dying with cachectic, anoxemic and anemic states; an anatomical change distinctly different from the fatty heart of the obese or those with myocardial changes secondary to the ischemia of coronary artery disease. Gallavardin recognized two forms of fatty degeneration based on their detection with the naked eye or with a microscope. The microscopic type was a diffuse process while the macroscopic variety presented itself as endocardial speckling with islets of fatty changes[105].

It was not until a year after Gallavardin's review that attention was drawn to the microscopic changes in the heart with relationship to obesity *per se*. The view advanced by Rosenfeld[106] and Herxheimer[107], each working independently of each other, was that the fat content within the myocardial cell was an infiltrative rather a degenerative phenomenon. In a paper on 'Adiposity of the Heart' which appeared in 1933[108], Smith and Willius expressed their agreement with this view. Their findings were derived from a clinical and pathological study of 136 patients. The only criterion utilized by these authors for inclusion in the study was obesity. They also pointed out that they too were in agreement with the position held by Beattie and Dickson who, in 1909, stated 'that an increase in the amount of fat in the subepicardial connective tissue and in the connective tissue lying between the muscle bundles and muscle fibers is best designated as adiposity of the heart[109].

A very recent study (1984) on the morphologic characteristics of the heart in obesity was that conducted by C. Warnes and W. Roberts from the National Institutes of Health[110]. They studied 12 patients, all of whom had massive obesity, weighing between 312 and 500 lbs; equivalent to 88–268% increase over so-called ideal body weight. The degree of excess body weight in the study by Smith and Willius varied between 13 and 170% with an average of 45%. All the hearts in the series cited by

Warnes and Roberts were heavier than normal. Nine of them had increased amounts of subepicardial adipose tissue. These findings, along with those of the much earlier investigators from Harvey to Smith and Willius are in marked contrast to those of Amad and his associates. They too studied 12 patients, reporting their findings in 1965[111]. Strangely, none of their patients showed any evidence of fatty infiltration in the myocardium, nor grossly visible foci of myocardial necrosis or fibrosis, or right ventricular hypertrophy, either isolated or predominant. It should be pointed out that all but one of the patients described by Warnes and Roberts showed dilated right and left ventricular cavities. This is an important descriptive element since long-standing obesity is known to have a dampening effect on the bellows action of the lungs.

The restrictive effect of obesity on the bellows action of the lungs leads to decreased alveolar-capillary gas exchange – with consequent hypoxia and retention of CO_2. Hypoxia is now known to induce constriction of the pulmonary arterioles. Persistent hypoxia with unremitting arteriolar constriction creates the stage for a chronic pressure overload on the right ventricle so that eventually one can expect to find evidence of right ventricular hypertrophy and dilatation. In addition, the hypoxia serves as the biochemical basis for the hypersomnia and sleep apnea that is so commonly seen in morbidly obese individuals. Interestingly enough, of the 12 patients studied by Warnes and Roberts, one had hypersomnia and three had sleep apnea.

All of this brings to mind how clinically observant Charles Dickens was with his astute and detailed portrayal of Joe, the fat boy in the Pickwick papers. In the vignette relevant to Joe, I have selected a few of the remarks and word-pictures that should stamp Dickens as an observer beyond reproach.

Fastened up behind the barouche was a hamper of spacious dimensions … and on the box sat a fat and red-faced boy, in a state of somnolency, whom no speculative observer could have regarded for an instant without setting down as the official dispenser of the contents of the before mentioned hamper, when the proper time for their consumption should arrive.

'Come along, sir. Pray, come up' said the stout gentleman. 'Joe-damn that boy, he's gone to sleep again. Joe, let down the steps.' The fat boy rolled slowly off the box, let down the steps, and held the carriage door invitingly open.

As Dickens proceeds to describe the noise and excitement surrounding everyone in the barouche while watching the staged military action being unfolded before them, he notes that

Everybody was excited except the fat boy, and he slept as soundly as if the roaring of cannon were his ordinary lullaby … 'Joe, Joe!' said the stout gentleman, when the citadel was taken, and the besiegers and besieged sat down to dinner. 'Damn that boy, he's gone to sleep again. Be good to pinch him, sir in the leg, if you please; nothing else wakes him thank you. Undo the hamper, Joe' … 'Now, Joe knives and forks' … 'Plates, Joe plates' … Now, Joe, the fowls. Damn that boy; he's gone to sleep again. Joe! Joe!' (Sundry taps on the head with a stick, and the fat boy, with some difficulty, roused from his lethargy.) 'Come, hand in the eatables' … There was something in the sound of the last word which roused the unconcious boy. He jumped up: and the leaden eyes, which twinkled behind his mountainous cheeks, leered horribly upon the food as he unpacked it from the basket…

'Damn that boy,' said the old gentleman, 'he's gone to sleep again.'

'Very extraordinary boy, that' said Mr. Pickwick, 'does he always sleep in this way!'

'Sleep!' said the old gentleman, 'he's always asleep. Goes on errands fast asleep, and snores as he waits at the table'.

'How very odd!' said Mr. Pickwick. 'Ah! odd indeed,' returned the old gentleman; 'I'm proud of that boy, wouldn't part with him on any account, he's a natural curiosity! Here, Joe, Joe, take these things away, and open another bottle d'ye hear?'

The fat boy rose, opened his eyes, swallowed the huge piece of pie he had been in the act of masticating when he last fell asleep, and slowly obeyed his master's orders gloating languidly over the remains of the feast, as he removed the plates, and deposited them in the hamper…

As the Pickwickians turned round to take a last glimpse of it, the setting sun cast a rich glow on the faces of their entertainers, and fell upon the form of the fat boy. His head was sunk upon his bosom; and he slumbered again'[112].

The hypersomnia of marked obesity is so like that of our fat boy, Joe, that it begged for the sobriquet 'Pickwick Syndrome'.

MALNUTRITION AND THE HEART

There has been a prevalent but poorly documented belief that structural changes in the heart do not occur during long periods of starvation. One has only to witness the impaired cardiac performance in beri-beri heart disease to realize that structural changes must be present to account for the heart failure.

Beri-beri heart disease was originally described by Wenkebach in 1928. His paper was entitled 'St. Cyre's lecture on heart and circulation in a tropical avitaminosis[113]. The presence of structural changes in this disease was first described by Benchimol and Schlesinger in 1953. Their autopsy observations revealed interstitial and perivascular edema, some of which had progressed to myocardial fibrosis and necrosis[114].

Nutritional forms of heart disease other than the thiamine deficiency of beri-beri were reported in malnourished Bantus and Ceylonese in a number of papers beginning with that of Gillanders in 1951[115], followed a year later with another paper written in collaboration with his associate, Higginson[116], and then with the contribution by Obeyesekere in 1968[117]. The hearts of those that came to autopsy were dilated and hypertrophied with only minute foci of myocardial fibrosis[116]. But the cases described by Gillanders and Obeyesekere were associated with severe end-stage liver disease, and the effect of this entity on cardiac structure, separate and distinct from malnutrition alone, could not be assessed accurately.

An overall decrease in heart weight in fasting humans was reported by Bloom and co-workers in 1966[118]. Three years later, Alleyne and his group demonstrated a decrease in heart weight in children who died of malnutrition[119]. The term 'cardiac cachexia' was introduced in 1976 by Abel and associates to describe those states of chronic congestive heart failure of varied etiology that are accompanied by protein-calorie malnutrition[120]. In 1979, Abel and his group then presented experimental evidence of marked myocardial atrophy in dogs subjected to a prolonged state of protein-calorie malnutrition[121].

Endocardial fibroelastosis is a cardiomyopathy of unknown origin. There is hypertrophy and dilatation of the heart, especially of the left ventricle. Myocardial contractility is impaired, and at autopsy the endocardium is milky white and thickened. In 1981, Tripp and co-workers studied a family in which cardiomyopathy developed in four of five children, three of whom died suddenly and were found at autopsy to have endocardial fibroelastosis[122]. Their paper presented sound evidence to substantiate their contention that the cause of this unique type of cardiomyopathy in this family was systemic carnitine deficiency. Carnitine is an essential co-factor for transportation of long- chain fatty acids into mitochondria for oxidation. Depletion of carnitine results in depressed mitochondrial oxidation of fatty acids and in cytoplasmic accumulation of lipids. Carnitine deficiency in humans was first described by Engel and Angelini in 1973[123].

REFERENCES

1. Marie, P. (1886). Sur deux cas d'acromegalie; hypertrophie singuliere non congenitale des extremities superieures, inferieures et cephalique. *Rev. Med. Paris*, **6**, 297

2. Huchard, H. (1895). Anatomie pathologique, lesions et troubles cardiovasculaire de l'acromegalie. *J. Praticiens*, **9**, 249

3. Alessandri, G. (1908). Acromegalia con polso raro ed enorme ipertensione arteriosa. *Policlinico*, **15**, 913

4. Souadijian, J.V. and Schirger, A. (1967). Hypertension in acromegaly. *Am. J. Med. Sci.*, **254**, 398

5. Davis, A.C. (1934). The thyroid gland in acromegaly. *Proc. Staff Meet., Mayo Clin.*, **9**, 709

6. Hejtmancik, M.R., Bradfield, J.Y. and Hermann, G.R. (1951). Acromegaly and heart: a clinical and pathologic study. *Ann. Intern. Med.*, **34**, 1445

7. Pepine, C.J. and Aloia, J. (1970). Heart muscle disease in acromegaly. *Am. J. Med.*, **48**, 530

8. De Grandpre, R. and Raab, W. (1953). Interrelated hormonal factors in cardiac hypertrophy. Experiments in nonhypertensive hypophysectomized rats. *Circ. Res.*, **1**, 345

9. Rossi, L., Thiene, G., Caregaro, L. *et al.* (1977). Arrhythmias and sudden death in acromegalic heart disease. *Chest*, **72**, 495–8

10. Lie, J.T. and Grossman, S.J. (1980). Pathology of the heart in acromegaly: anatomic findings in 27 autopsied patients. *Am. Heart J.*, **100**, 41

11. Lie, J.T. (1981). Acromegaly and heart disease. *Primary Cardiology*, **7**, 53

12. Levene, G. and Miller, L.C. (1942). Acromegalic gigantism without cardiac enlargement: report of a case. *J. Clin. Endocrinol.*, **2**, 403

13. Manger, W.M. and Gifford, R.W. (1977). In *Phaeochromocytoma*, p. 5. (New York: Springer)

14. Pearce, R.M. (1906). Experimental myocarditis: study of histologic changes following intravenous injections of adrenalin. *J. Exp. Med.*, **8**, 400–9

15. Szakács, J.E. and Mehlman, B. (1960). Pathologic changes induced by L-norepinephrine: quantitative aspects. *Am. J. Cardiol.*, **5**, 619–27

16. Franz, G. (1937). Eine seltene Form von toxischer Myokardschädigung. *Virchow's Arch. f. Path. Anat.*, **298**, 743–52

17. Raab, W. (1943). Pathogenic significance of adrenalin and related substances in heart muscle. *Exp. Med. Surg.*, **1**, 188–225

18. Reichenbach, D.D. and Benditt, E.P. (1970). Catecholamines and cardiomyopathy: the pathogenesis and potential importance of myofibrillar degeneration. *Hum. Pathol.*, **1**, 125–50

19. Szakács, J.E. and Cannon, A. (1958). L-norephinephrine myocarditis. *Am. J. Clin. Pathol.*, **30**, 425–34

20. Kline, I.K. (1961). Myocardial alterations associated with phaeochromocytomas. *Am. J. Pathol.*, **38**, 539–51

21. Van Vliet, P.D., Burchell, H.B. and Titus, J.L. (1966). Focal myocarditis associated with phaeochromocytoma. *N. Engl. J. Med.*, **274**, 1102–8

22. Radtke, W.E., Kazmier, F.J., Rutherford, B.D. and Sheps, S.G. (1975). Cardiovascular complications of phaeochromocytoma crisis. *Am. J. Cardiol.*, **35**, 701–5

23. Levister, E.C. and Taylor, J.B. (1981). Physiological hypertrophic subaortic stenosis and subendocardial infarction in a patient with phaeochromocytoma. *J. Natl. Med. Assoc.*, **73**, 357–61

24. Oakley, C.M. (1974). Clinical recognition of the cardiomyopathies. *Circ. Res.*, **34**–II, 152–67

25. Goodwin, J.F. (1974). Prospects and predictions for the cardiomyopathies. *Circ. Res.*, **50**, 210–19

26. Blaufuss, A.H., Laks, M.M., Garner, D. *et al.* (1975). Production of ventricular hypertrophy simulating idiopathic hypertrophic subaortic stenosis (IHSS) by subhypertensive infusion of norepinephrine in the conscious dog. *Clin. Res.*, **23**, 77A

27. Peiper, H.J. and Golestan, C. (1963). Intrathorakeles phaeochromocytoma. *Thorax*, **10**, 517

28. Voci, V., Olson, H. and Beilin, L. (1982). A malignant primary cardiac phaeochromocytoma. *Surg. Rounds*, **9**, 88

29. Besterman, E., Bromley, L.L. and Peart, W.S. (1974). An intrapericardial phaeochromocytoma. *Br. Heart J.*, **36**, 318

30. Saad, M.F., Frazier, O.H., Hukey, R.C. and Samaan, N.A. (1983). Intrapericardial phaeochromocytoma. *Am. J. Med.*, **73**, 371

31. David, T.E., Lenkei, S.C., Marquez-Julio, A. *et al.* (1986). Phaeochromocytoma of the heart. *Ann. Thoracic. Surg.*, **41**, 98–100

32. Parry, C.H. (1825). *Collections from the Unpublished Writings of the late Caleb H. Parry, MD London*, **2**, p. 111

33. Graves, R.J. (1835). *London Med. Surg.*, **7**, 516

34. Basedow von, K. (1840). *Wschr ges Heilk.*, **6**, 197, 220

35. Lockridge, J.E. (1879). *Am. Practit.*, **19**, 287

36. Moebius, P.J. (1896). *Die Basedow'sche Krankheit.* Wien

37. Major, R.H. (1932). *Classic Descriptions of Disease.* (Springfield, Ill.: Charles C. Thomas)

38. Willius, F.A. and Keys, T.E. (1941). *Cardiac Classics*, pp. 385–6. (St. Louis: C.V. Mosby Co.)

39. Magee, H.R. and Smith, H.L. (1935). *Am. J. Med. Sci.*, **189**, 683

40. Likoff, W.B. and Levine, S.A. (1943). *Am. J. Med. Sci.*, **206**, 425

41. Griswold, D. and Keating, J.H. Jr. (1949). *Am. Heart J.*, **38**, 813

42. Willius, F.A., Boothby, W.M. and Wilson, L.P. (1923). *Trans. Assoc. Am. Phys.*, **38**, 137

43. Lahey, F.H. and Hamilton, B.E. (1924). *Surg. Gynec. Obstet.*, **39**, 10

44. Hurxthal, L.M. (1928). *Am. Heart J.*, **4**, 103

45. Friedberg, C.K. and Sohval, A.R. (1937). *Am. Heart J.*, **13**, 599

46. Sandler, G. and Wilson, G.M. (1959). The nature and prognosis of heart disease in thyrotoxicosis. A review of 150 patients treated with [131]I. *Q. J. Med.*, **28**, 347

47. Fahr, T. (1916). *Zbl. Allg. Path. Anat.*, **27**, 1

48. Hashimoto, H. (1921). *Endocrinology*, **5**, 579
49. Willius, F.A., Boothby, W.M. and Wilson, L.B. (1923). *Op. cit.*, p. 144
50. Rake, G. and McEachern, D. (1932). *Am. Heart J.*, **8**, 19
51. Weller, C.V., Wanstrom, R.C., Gordon, H. and Bugher, J.C. (1932). *Am. Heart J.*, **8**, 8
52. Callas, G. and Hayes, J.R. (1974). Alterations in the fine structure of cardiac muscle mitochondria induced by hyperthyroidism. *Anat. Rec.*, **178**, 539–50
53. Skelton, C.L. and Sonnenblick, E.H. (1974). Heterogeneity of contractile function in cardiac hypertrophy. *Circ. Res.*, **34** & **35**, *Suppl.* **2**, 11, 83, 96
54. Zondek, H. (1918). Das Myxödemherz. *Münch Med. Wschr.*, **65**, 1180
55. Fahr, G. (1925). Myxedema heart. *J. Am. Med. Assoc.*, **82**, 345
56. Campbell, M. and Suzman, S.S. (1934). The heart in myxedema. *Guy's Hosp. Rep.*, **84**, 281
57. Means, J.H. (1937). *The Thyroid and Its Diseases.* (Philadelphia: Lippencott)
58. Fournier, J.C.M. (1942). The circulating apparatus in myxedema. *Proc. Mayo Clin.*, **17**, 212
59. Bustamente, R., Perez Stable, E., Casas Rodriquez, R. and Mateo De Acosta (1955). Corazón mixedematosa: estudio clinico de 34 casos. *Rev. Cuba Cardiol.*, **16**, 405
60. Hamilton, J.D. and Greenwood, W.F. (1957). Myxedema heart disease. *Circulation*, **15**, 442
61. Hallock, P, (1933). The heart in myxedema with a report of two cases. *Am. Heart J.*, **9**, 196
62. Means, J.H. (1937). *Op. cit.*
63. Ellis, L.B., Mebane, J.G., Maresh, G. *et al.* (1952). The effect of myxedema on the cardiovascular system. *Am. Heart J.*, **43**, 341
64. Hamilton, J.D. and Greenwood, W.F. (1957). *Op. cit.*
65. Freeman, E.B. (1934). Chronic pericardial effusion in myxedema: report of case. *Ann. Intern. Med.*, **7**, 1070
66. Marzullo, E.R. and Franco, S. (1939). Myxedema with multiple serous effusions and cardiac involvement (myxedema heart); case report. *Am. Heart J.*, **17**, 368
67. Boivin, J.M. (1945). Histoire d'un épanchement péricardique récidivant asséché par e'extrait thyröiden. *Arch. Mal. Coeur*, **38**, 289
68. Schnitzer, R. and Gutmann, D. (1946). Myxoedema with pericardial effusion. *Br. Heart J.*, **8**, 25
69. Kern, R.A., Soloff, L.A., Snape, W.J. and Bello, C.T. (1949). Pericardial effusion: a constant, early and major factor in the cardiac syndrome of hypothyroidism (myxedema heart). *Am. J. Med. Sci.*, **217**, 609
70. Scherf, D. and Boyd, L.J. (1939). *Cardiovascular Diseases.* (St. Louis: Mosby)
71. Fishberg, A.M. (1924). Arteriosclerosis in thyroid deficiency. *J.A.M.A.*, **82**, 463
72. Aber, C.P. and Thompson, G.S. (1963). Factors associated with cardiac enlargement in myxoedema. *Br. Heart J.*, **25**, 421–3
73. Steinberg, A.D. (1968). Myxedema and coronary artery disease – a comparative study. *Ann. Intern. Med.*, **68**, 338–44
74. *Ibid.* p. 343
75. Hellstrom, J. (1950). Clinical experiences of twenty-one cases of hyperparathyroidism with special reference to prognosis following parathyroidectomy. *Acta Chr. Scand.*, **100**, 391
76. McFarland, K.F., Stefadouros, M.A., Abdulla, A.M. and McFarland, D.E. (1978). Hypercalcemia and idiopathic hypertrophic subaortic stenosis. *Ann. Intern. Med.*, **88**, 57–8
77. Symons, C., Fortune, F., Greenbaum, R.H. and Dandona, P. (1985). Cardiac hypertrophy, hypertrophic cardiomyopathy and hyperparathyroidism – an association. *Br. Heart J.*, **54**, 539–42
78. Katoh, Y., Klein, K.L., Kaplan, R.A., Sanborn, W. and Kurokawa, K. (1981). Parathyroid hormone has a positive inotropic action in the rat. *Endocrinology*, **109**, 2252–4
79. Bogin, E., Massry, S.G. and Harary, I. (1981). Effect of parathyroid hormone on rat heart cells. *J. Clin. Invest.*, **67**, 1215–27
80. Roberts, W.C. and Waller, B.F. (1981). Effect of chronic hypercalcemia on the heart: an analysis of 18 necropsy patients. *Am. J. Med.*, **71**, 371–84
81. Rose, E. (1943). Hypoparathyroidism. *Clinics*, **1**, 1179–96
82. Hegglin, R. (1939). Herz und hypokalzamie. *Helv. Med. Acta*, **5**, 584–90
83. Evans, J.A. and Elliott, F.D. (1945). Multiple vitamin deficiencies including beri-beri heart with congestive failure. *Lahey Clin. Bull.*, **4**, 173–81
84. Jernigan, J.A. and Sadusk, J.F. Jr. (1953). Idiopathic hypoparathyroidism: discussion and presentation of a case. *Stanford Med. Bull.*, **11**, 266–71
85. Schulman, J.L. and Ratner, H. (1955). Idiopathic

hypoparathyroidism with bony demineralization and cardiac decompensation. *Pediatrics*, **16**, 848–56

86. Grieve, S. and Sehamroth, L. (1955). Idiopathic hypoparathyroidism. *S. Afr. Med. J.*, **29**, 232–34

87. Weill, J., Bouchard, R., Antebi, L. *et al.* (1967). La cardiomégalie liée àune hypocalcémie chronique. *Soéiete Medicale des Hopitaux de Paris*, **118**, 659–67

88. Giles, T.D., Iteld, B.J. and Rives, K.L. (1981). The cardiomyopathy of hypoparathyroidism. *Chest*, **79**, 225–8

89. Pratt, J.H. (1904). On the causes of cardiac insufficiency. *Bull. Johns Hopkins Hosp.*, **15**, 301 (Oct.)

90. Harvey, W. (1847). Anatomical examination of the body of Thomas Parr. In Harvey, William, *Works of William Harvey*, translated from the Latin by Robert Willis, p. 589. (London: Sydenham Society)

91. Sprengall, C.J. (1708). *The Aphorisms of Hippocrates and the Sentences of Celsus.* (London: R. Bonwick (and others))

92. Senac, J.B. (1783). *Traite de la Structure du Coeur, de son Action, et de ses Maladies*, 2nd edn., Vol. 2, p. 384. (Paris: Mequignon)

93. Corvisart, J.N. (1812). *An Essay on the organic diseases and lesions of the heart and great vessels*, p. 153. (Philadelphia: A. Finley)

94. Cheyne, J. (1818). A case of apoplexy in which the fleshy part of the heart was converted into fat. *Dublin Hosp. Rep.*, **2**, 216

95. Laénnec, R.T.H. (1819). *De l'Auscultation Médiate on Triate du Diagnostic des Maladies des Pomnons et du Coeur*, vol. 2, p. 295. (Paris: Brosson and Chaudé)

96. Laénnec, R.T.H. (1838). *A Treatise on Disease of the Chest*, p. 682. (New York: S.S. and W. Wood)

97. Paget, J. (1847). Lectures on nutrition, hypertrophy, and atrophy. *J. London Med. Gazette*, **5**, 227

98. Ormerod, H.L. (1849). Observations on the clinical history and pathology of one form of fatty degeneration of the heart. *London Med. Gazette*, **9**, 739

99. Quain, R. (1850). Fatty diseases of the heart. *Med. Chir.*, **33**, 120

100. Rokitansky, C. (1852). *A Manual of Pathological Anatomy*, vol. 4. p. 204. (London: Sydenham Society)

101. Bedford, E. (1972). The story of fatty heart. A disease of Victorian times. *Br. Heart J.*, **34**, 23–8

102. Morgan, A.D. (1968). Some forms of undiagnosed coronary disease in nineteenth-century England. *Med. History*, **12**, 344

103. Herrick, J.B. (1919). Thrombosis of the coronary arteries. *J. Am. Med. Assoc.*, **72**, 387

104. Fothergill, J.M. (1879). *The Heart and its Diseases*, 2nd edn. (London: Lewis)

105. Gallavardin, L. (1900). *La dégénerescence Graisseuse du Myocarde.* (Paris: J. B. Baillière)

106. Rosenfeld, G. (1901). Über die Herzverfettung des Menschen. *Zentralbl. f. inn. Med.*, **22**, 145, (Feb. 9)

107. Herxheimer, G. (1901). Über Fettfarbstoffe. *Deutsche med. Wchnschr.*, **27**, 607

108. Smith, H.L. and Willius, F.A. (1932). Adiposity of the heart. *Arch. Intern. Med.*, **59**, 911–31

109. Beattie, J.M. and Dickson, W.E.C. (1909). *A Text-Book of Special Pathology*, p. 522. (London: Rebman)

110. Warnes, C. and Roberts, W. (1984). The heart in massive (more than 300 pounds or 136 kilograms) obesity: analysis of 12 patients studied at necropsy. *Am. J. Cardiol.*, **54**, 1087–91

111. Amad, K.H., Brennan, J.C. and Alexander, J.K. (1965). The cardiac pathology of chronic exogenous obesity. *Circulation*, **32**, 740–5

112. Dickens, C. (1944). *The Pickwick Papers*, pp. 43–9. (Dodd, Mead and Co. Inc.)

113. Wenkebach, K.F. (1928). St. Cyre's lecture on heart and circulation in a tropical avitaminosis (beri-beri). *Lancet*, **2**, 265

114. Benchimol, A.B. and Schlesinger, P. (1953). Beriberi heart disease. *Am. Heart J.*, **46**, 245

115. Gillanders, A.D. (1951). Nutritional heart disease. *Br. Heart J.*, **13**, 177

116. Higginson, J., Gillanders, A.D. and Murray, J.F. (1952). The heart in chronic malnutrition. *Br. Heart J.*, **14**, 213

117. Obeyesekere, I. Idiopathic cardiomegaly in Ceylon. Congestive cardiac failure, cardio-megaly, hepatomegaly and portal fibrosis. *Br. Heart J.*, **30**, 226–35

118. Bloom, W.L., Azar, G. and Smith, E.G. Jr. (1966). Changes in heart size and plasma volume during fasting. *Metabolism*, **15**, 409

119. Alleyne, G.A.O., Halliday, D. and Waterlow, M.C. (1969). Chemical composition of organs of children who died from malnutrition. *Br. J. Nutr.*, **23**, 783

120. Abel, R.M., Fischer, J.E., Buckley, M.J. *et al.* (1976). Malnutrition in cardiac surgical patients. *Arch. Surg.*, **111**, 45

121. Abel, R.M., Grimes, J.B., Alonso, D. *et al.* (1979). Adverse hemodynamic and ultra-structural changes in dog hearts subjected to protein – calorie malnutrition. *Am. Heart J.*, **97**, 733–44

122. Tripp, M.E., Katcher, M.L., Peters, H.A. *et al.* (1981). Systemic carnitine deficiency presenting as familial endocardial fibroelastosis. *N. Engl. J. Med.*, **305**, 385–90

123. Engel, A.G. and Angelini, C. (1973). Carnitine deficiency of human skeletal muscle with associated lipid storage myopathy: a new syndrome. *Science*, **179**, 899–902

Section 2

Structural abnormalities

Part B   Congenital abnormalities

13   Congenital abnormalities

Knowledge concerning congenital defects of the heart can be traced as far back as Aristotle in the 4th century BC[1]. Subsequent to this, significant observations were made over the succeeding centuries by a number of people. Among them were Fabricius, von Haller, Morgagni, Senac, Hunter, Spallanzani, Baillie, Rokitansky, Roger, Sandifort, Fallot, Eisenmenger and Mall[1]. The list is by no means complete, and it would serve no purpose to make it so. The important point is that these were isolated descriptions presented by independent observers as part of their other observations, and in an incidental or casual manner. None of them constituted a link, as it were, for forging a panoramic view of the entire spectrum of congenital defects. Moreover, many of these observations remained buried and forgotten in dust-covered manuscripts only to be resurrected or rediscovered when an interest in congenital cardiac defects finally began to prevail. This did not occur until the 19th century with the publication of two textbooks, one by Farré, and the other by Peacock. Of the two, it appears that Peacock's text had the greater impact. However, a truly definitive appreciation of the pathologic alterations in the various forms of congenital cardiac defects did not come about until the appearance of Maude Abbott's *Atlas of Congenital Cardiac Disease* in 1936[2]. Prior to this, whatever interest prevailed was confined to those congenital defects manifested by cyanosis. Now, non-cyanotic as well as the cyanotic varieties were being studied with equal fervor. Abbott's monumental work was based on an analysis of 1,000 personally observed cases. It bridged the gap between the purely descriptive presentation of the previous observers and the modern 20th century stance that paved the way for an understanding of the resultant pathophysiologic changes. It was another woman, Helen Brooke Taussig, who was to supply the complete pathophysiologic scenario[3–6]. Again, explaining function and dysfunction in terms of anatomical structure and alterations provided the means for the appropriate therapeutic measures. In this case, surgery would provide the modern corrective approach.

Let us look first at some of the more important isolated descriptions and their observers. It is generally accepted that Aristotle was probably the first embryologist. The punctum saliens, vitelline and allantoic veins were described by him. Aristotle was a contemporary of Hippocrates, and like that noble physician also of Asclepiad stock.

The first recorded instance of dextrocardia is attributed to Alessandro Benedetti of Padua (1460–1525). Hieronymus Fabricius (1537–1619) amplified Aristotle's work with his own studies on the formation of the chick in the egg. Giulio Aranzio (1530–1619) discovered the ductus arteriosus of the fetus. Others give priority to Botallo. Castiglioni, however, is of the opinion that Botallo had confused the foramen ovale with the ductus[7]. The general conformation of the fetal heart and the presence of the foramen ovale were described by Arcangelo Piccolimini (1525–86) of Ferrara. Giambattista Carcano(1536–1606), also of Ferrara, added his own description of both the foramen ovale and ductus arteriosus. The first description of the foramen ovale in an adult heart is ascribed to Pierre Gassendi (1592–1655), but Leonardo da Vinci may have superseded Gassendi in this. In fact, da Vinci may have also superseded all others by being the first to describe a congenital lesion in a human heart. Figure 1 is taken from the *Quaderni d' Anatomia* which dates from 1513, and in which Leonardo wrote in his mirror script 'I have found from a, left auricle, to b, right auricle, a perforating channel from a to b which I note here to see whether this occurs in other auricles of other hearts'. This description certainly fits in with the presence of a patent foramen ovale and thus appears to antedate Pierre Gassendi's description in 1640 of the same type of lesion that he observed in an adult cadaver[8].

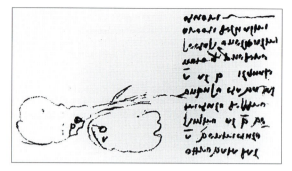

Figure 1 Leonardo da Vinci's drawing of a patent foramen ovale. *Photo Source National Library of Medicine. Literary source Rashkind WJ: Historic Aspects of Congenital Heart Disease. Birth Defects: Original Article Series. Vol. VIII, no. 1, Feb. 1972 (Fig. 13) and taken from Quaderni d'Anatomia. Courtesy of National Library of Medicine*

The recorded observations of Sénac are to be found in a short chapter on cardiac malformations in his treatise on diseases of the heart. They include a case of a three-chambered heart (cor triloculare) due to complete absence of the interventricular septum. The patient was obviously cyanotic during life although Sénac does not say so. Incidentally, Sénac, in discussing the state of cyanosis, rightfully attributed it to an admixture of venous and arterial blood. He also realized that at times the 'true oval' and 'canal arterial' failed to close[9].

Haller's contribution was, strictly speaking, not in pathology but rather in his demonstration that the heart of the chick embryo pulsated before any other structure manifested evidence of dynamic function.

Among the congenital defects described by Morgagni was his account of a girl with cyanosis who at postmortem revealed a patent foramen ovale, large enough to admit a finger; stenosis of the pulmonary valve with an orifice smaller in size than a 'lentil'; and a markedly enlarged right auricle and right ventricle. Morgagni was of the opinion that the cyanosis in this case was due to stagnation of the venous blood rather than due to an admixture of venous and arterial blood. He reasoned that the venous stasis in both the right auricle and ventricle was due to blockage of blood flow through the tight pulmonary valve and with the increased stasis on the right side of the heart, the valve of the foramen ovale was pushed open allowing the blood to pass into the left side of the heart[10]. For a while the congenital abnormality just

described was called by the French the 'trilogy of Fallot'.

Much more common as a cause of cyanosis is the multiple defect that carries the eponym 'Tetralogy of Fallot'. It consists of pulmonic stenosis, interventricular septal defect, hypertrophy of the right ventricle and dextroposition of the aorta. It is now uniformly acknowledged that Niels Stensen was the first to describe this common cause of blue babies as far back as 1672, and that Sandifort and Fallot added their contributions at a much later date. Under the latinized name of Steno his account of the malformation is to be found in a paper published in *Acta Medicine et Philosophia* under the title 'Anatomicus Regij Hafniensis Embryo Monstro affinis Parisiis dissectus'[11]. East in a Fitzpatrick lecture[12] quotes him as follows:

... before other things there attracted my attention and wonder the unusual form of the arteries projecting from the heart, and I specially observed that the pulmonary artery to be far narrower than the aorta, and to seem to be of no use; therefore I opened from the right heart chamber direct into the hilus of the lungs and there I saw that the canal that leads into the aorta from the pulmonary artery was completely wanting. Then I opened the right ventricle afterwards, and found the sound, which went far up and onwards along the side of the partition of the ventricles, went directly into the aorta, with the same ease with which it passed up the aorta from the left ventricle. There were therefore three openings from the right ventricle; one into the right auricle, and the other two were into the arteries. The same aortic canal that was common to both heart chambers formed, together with the chamber's partition a double opening.

The description then ends with the following words:

There was a cleft palate and hare-lip on the right side, and the mother attributed this anomaly to the fact that she was fond of rabbit stew ... the unusual form of the arteries arising from the heart attracted the chief attention and called for admiration. In particular, the pulmonary artery was much narrower than the aorta ... when I opened the right ventricle, the probe that was passed forward and upward along the interventricular septum entered directly into the aorta just as readily as the probe passed from the left ventricle.

Niels Stensen was not only a great anatomist; he was also a student of geology, physiology and theology. He was appointed to the Bishopric of Titiopolis after having defected from Lutheranism to the Roman Catholic Church. Incidentally, this defection cost him his chair in anatomy at Copenhagen. Apparently this created no state of depression since he devoted a good deal of his time later to proselytizing his newly adopted religious persuasion. It was during one of these missions that he died. Aside from the contribution just described, Stensen also proved that the heart was a muscular organ. This important observation was the first European recording to consider the heart as a purely muscular organ. It is to be found in his treatise *De musculis et Glandulous Observationem Specimen, cum Epistolis duabus Anatomicus*[13]. Prior to this, reference to the muscular nature of the heart is to be found in the works of Hippocrates and believed to be written by an unknown Alexandrian[14].

Edward Sandifort, who was professor of physiology at Leyden University, described the Fallot malformation in his book *Observationes Anatomicae et Pathologicae* which was published in 1777, more than a century later[15]. The description is found in the chapter entitled *De Rarissimo Cordis Vitio*, and concerns a boy who died at the age of 12½, and who, during his short life, manifested cyanosis, extreme fatigue, fainting spells, palpitations, and pedal edema[16].

Sandifort's vivid description of the autopsy findings is as follows:

> This artery (pulmonary), having been cut above the valves, showed these to be very small almost rigid … so that only a very small space was left, which, permitting the entrance of the point of a rather thin stylus, proved (to be) the passageway for this to the right ventricle, and transmitted the same with some difficulty from the ventricle to the artery … the right (ventricle), if not thicker, had the same thickness as the left … But how great was the surprise of the onlookers, how great equally was my own surprise, when we saw the point of the finger (inserted in the right ventricle) to stretch into the aorta, which is not at all accustomed to maintain communication with the right ventricle, in conformity with otherwise constant laws of nature! … the arterial aorta … showed the same edge, by which the orifice was divided into a larger part, connecting with the right ventricle, and into a smaller part, ascribed to the left ventricle. And thus the arterial aorta was springing from both ventricles, and had to receive all the blood from both.

This description is equally as good as that of Stensen and can stand on its own; not only because of this but also because the chapter presents the first good account of the clinical picture with post-mortem confirmation.

In 1784, William Hunter described three examples of pulmonary stenosis or atresia with multiple defects. Willius and Dry quote an adaptation from Pettigrew's biography of Hunter which illustrates that Hunter's cases fit the features of Tetralogy of Fallot[17].

> Three cases of Mal-conformation of the Heart … The second case … the pulmonary artery was so small at its beginning, that it would barely give passage to a small probe; and the septum cordia was deficient, or perforated at the basis of the heart, so as to allow Dr. H's thumb (a small one), to pass across from one ventricle to the other, the orifice of the aorta being close to the perforation, so as to receive the blood from the right ventricle as well as from the left. This child lived thirteen years. The third case was of a still-born child at six months, the preparation of which was in Dr. H.'s museum. There was an opening of communication between the two ventricles, by which the blood of one cavity could pass into the other, without going through the usual circuit of the vessels.

Hunter erroneously believed that all the multiple defects were a consequence of the pulmonary stenosis. Other notables who recognized this common congenital defect were Farre in 1814, Gintrac in 1824, Peacock in 1866 and Roger in 1879.

The eponym 'Tetralogy of Fallot' was applied after Fallot presented the most comprehensive account of what the French originally called 'maladie bleue'. Fallot was well aware of the prior literature on the subject. His main contribution lies in the fact that he demonstrated the feasibility of a diagnosis before death, an important step in the proper management of this entity[18]. Fallot's paper was titled *Contribution à l'Anatomie Pathologique de la Maladie Bleue (Cyanose Cardiaque)*[19]. It is remarkable for its precise and terse presentation. A few lines from his paper will illustrate this:

... we see from our observations that cyanosis, especially in the adult, is the result of a small number of cardiac malformations well determined. One of these cardiac malformations is much more frequent than the others. This malformation consists of a true anatomopathologic type represented by the following tetralogy: (1) Stenosis of the pulmonary artery; (2) Interventricular communication; (3) Deviation of the origin of the aorta to the right, (4) Hypertrophy, almost always concentric, of the right ventricle. Failure of obliteration of the foramen ovale may occasionally be added in a wholly accessory manner.

One cannot, at present, attribute cyanosis to the persistence of the foramen ovale ... It seems to be much more logical and more in conformity with the laws of physiology to regard the whole series of cardiac changes enumerated as wholly the result of pulmonary stenosis.

Very little is known about the life of Etienne-Louis Fallot. We do know that he was born in Cette, France in 1850, that he was a very good student and that he received his medical degree from the École de Medicine at Marseille. Throughout his professional life he remained at the University of Marseille where he served first as interim professor of medicine and then as professor of hygiene and legal medicine until his death in 1911. His interest in congenital lesions of the heart was apparently aroused during his temporary tenure in charge of the course in pathologic anatomy[20,21].

Fallot (like Hunter) erred greatly in his delineation of the pathogenesis of the multiple defects. He felt that all the defects were consequences of the pulmonary stenosis rather than of an aberration in development during the embryonic stage.

Cyanosis, one of the more important clinical signs of congenital heart disease, has long been of interest and an object of speculative thought among medical observers. Through the ages it has been referred to as 'morbus coeruleus', 'maladie bleue' or 'Blausucht'; all meaning the blue disease. It had been described by the Egyptians as far back as 3000 years ago. Artistic representations have also been found in the works of several ancient cultures such as the Indian and Persian. The Indian God, Krishna, is generally portrayed with a blue skin[22].

Figure 2 is thought to be the earliest illustration of a blue skinned person[22]. Its approximate date is 2000 BC and it is taken from the tomb of Osiris. The Smith papyrus which has already been described in Chapter 1 presents convincing evidence that cyanosis was observed even earlier than this illustration indicates. The Smith papyrus is 5000 years old, dating back to 3000 BC. Figure 3 shows a hieroglyph from this papyrus; B in the figure describes a color that is reddish while C indicates a color that is bluish. Rashkind quotes Prof. Luckhardt, a physician and Egyptologist, as being inclined to the view 'that the color meant is the one medical men had in mind when they say the person is cyanotic. It is a mixture of a red and a blue'[23].

Coarctation of the aorta was described by Morgagni in his 18th letter of *De Sedibus*. He noted the presence of a constricted aorta in association with a huge left ventricle. The letter also refers to a similar case reported by the elder Meckel in 1750. Coarctation of the aorta was again described by Paris in 1791[24]. He was the first to point out the existence of a collateral circulation in this condition. Paris had already taken note of the presence of markedly dilated intercostal arteries in the female cadaver he was dissecting. He confirmed that these dilated arteries were collateral channels by utilizing an injection technique[25]. Two decades or so after the original description by Paris, the circumvention of reduced flow to those parts of the body distal to the narrowed aorta were elaborated upon by another Meckel (1827)[26], Raynaud (1828)[27], and Jordan (1830)[28]. They all recognized the importance of the intercostal arteries in providing the bypass to the coarctation.

Several observers throughout the latter half of the 19th century also added to the general knowledge of coarctation of the aorta. These were Bertin in 1824, Craigie in 1841, Peacock in 1860, Barie in 1886, and Vierordt in 1898. They emphasized, however, the clinical manifestations rather than the pathologic aberration, *per se*.

Bertin described the case of a young boy where the heart was markedly enlarged ('double in volume') and the ascending aorta was 'almost 4 inches across'. He further described the subclavian as having the appearance of a dilated aorta, the presence of dilated intercostal arteries and that the descending aorta was 'entirely obliterated for several lines'[29]. Even Laénnec observed a postmortem example of coarctation likening the constriction to the size of a 'swan's or even a goose's quill'[30]. In 1827, Albrecht Meckel, the third

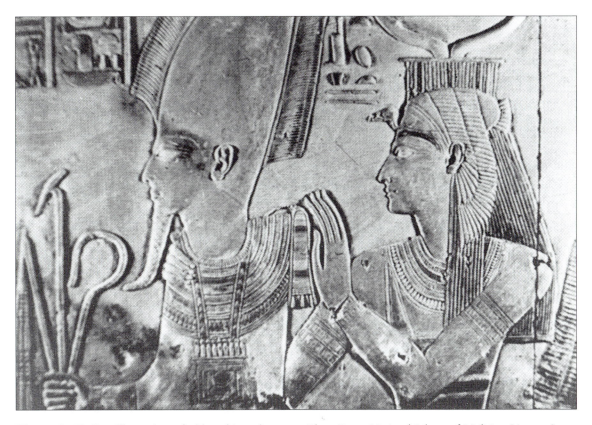

Figure 2 Earliest illustration of a blue-skinned person. *Photo Source National Library of Medicine. Literary Source Rashkind WJ: Historic Aspects of Congenital Heart Disease. Birth Defects. Original Article Series. vol. VIII, no. 1, Feb., 1972 (Fig. 5). Courtesy of National Library of Medicine*

generation of the Meckel dynasty (in anatomy), presented a case report of a miller from Bern who died suddenly from a ruptured heart and who at autopsy showed the notches on the upper surface of the 3rd and 4th ribs bilaterally caused presumably by the constant pounding of the collateral intercostal arteries[30].

Craigie was the first to suggest that coarctation of the aorta was caused by obliteration of the ductus arteriosus[31]. Barié utilized the autopsied cases of Rokitansky in his review of congenital lesions[32]. In 1903, L.M. Bonnet published a definitive work that dwelt upon the previously reported cases while adding a considerable number of his own[33]. He classified coarctation of the aorta into infantile and adult types. Thirty years later Sir Thomas Lewis added his observations and views including the utility of the more modern diagnostic techniques in vogue during his time.

'Maladie de Roger' is characterized by a ventricular septal defect. The eponym was imposed upon posterity by Dupré in 1891. Campbell laments the imposition since in his opinion 'the blind acceptance of the view by Roger that all lone ventricular septal defects produced striking physical signs but no symptoms is one of the most curious medical errors'[34]. Campbell goes on to say that the view was 'based on a few patients Roger had seen and his memory of a necropsy about 18 years before on a boy', and finally that, 'it was 12 years before there was necropsy proof of such a case that had been diagnosed in life by Dupré; all rather shaky ground for suggesting the unfortunate name 'maladie de Roger'[35]. The view generally held today is that the natural history of a ventricular septal defect is predicated upon the size of the opening and the degree of pulmonary vascular resistance. If the defect is small then Roger's view is correct.

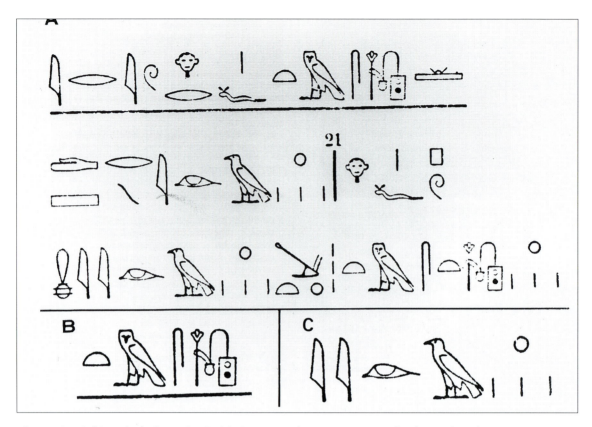

Figure 3   A hieroglyph from the Smith Papyrus. *Photo Source National Library of Medicine. Literary Source Rashkind WJ: Historic Aspects of Congenital Heart Disease. Birth Defects. Original Article Series. vol. VIII, no. 1, Feb., 1972 (Fig. 8). Courtesy of National Library of Medicine*

A little known contributor to the pathologic anatomy of congenital cardiac defects was Allan Burns, a man who, we saw, never received a degree in medicine, and yet should be regarded with esteem because of his advanced ideas, clarity of thought and the logical conclusions of his observations. Burns lived for only 32 years (1781–1813), but during this short span of time he was able to accomplish a great deal. Unable to practice medicine because of the lack of a medical degree, young Burns was permitted to assist his formally accredited older brother John, as a lecturer in John's anatomy classes. This afforded Allan the opportunity to make a number of astute observations which he collected and recorded in his book *Observations on some of the most frequent and important Diseases of the Heart; on Aneurism of the Thoracic Aorta; on Preternatural Pulsation in the Epigastric Region; and on the Unusual Origin and Distribution of some of the Large Arteries of the Human Body, illustrated by Cases*[36]. A rather long-winded title to say the least.

In this book, Burns classified the diseases of the heart into three basic groups, the second of which was composed of congenital defects and malformations which result in the admixture of arterial and venous blood. He further divided the congenital groups into six basic types: those in which the aorta arises from both the right and left ventricles; those in which the foramen ovale and the ductus arteriosus are open; a third type in which the ductus arteriosus is closed but the foramen ovale is patent or instead there is a defect in the interventricular septum; a fourth type characterized by closure of the pulmonary artery at its origin but with the artery able to accept blood from the aorta through a patent ductus arteriosus; a type consisting of a two-chambered heart; and finally, a type with congenital stenosis of the mitral valve[37]. This is a remarkable piece of work from an individual without a formal academic background but exemplary of the heights one can achieve when adhering to high standards of investigation. As a further illustration of the clarity of his thinking, Burns was opposed to the view held by some authorities of the time that people with patent foramen ovale or atrial septal defect made good divers. This was based on the notion that because the fetus survived in amniotic fluid with a patent foramen ovale, those with an atrial septal defect were able to resist the watery elements much longer than others.

The two most common malformations of the tricuspid valve are Ebstein's anomaly and atresia. Ebstein described the anomaly that bears his name in 1866, and it consists of a downward displacement of the tricuspid valve into the right ventricle due to an anomalous attachment of the tricuspid leaflets. More than half the cases are associated with an atrial septal defect of the ostium secundum variety or with a patent foramen ovale. Tricuspid atresia is characterized by an absence of a tricuspid orifice in association with underdevelopment of the right ventricle and a communication between the atria and the ventricles.

In comparison to other congenital defects, the incidence of Ebstein's anomaly is not at all common. But, as often happens in medicine, a rare disease may generate contributions to knowledge far beyond that offered by the patient afflicted with it. This is the case with Ebstein's anomaly. Studies of this defect have been responsible for many advances in electrocardiology, circulatory hemodynamics and pulmonary function.

Ebstein was a renowned clinician and investigator with a catholicity of interests in medicine. Even against this background, with many and diverse contributions in the general field of medicine to his credit, the major source of Ebstein's fame rests on his classic paper that bears his name[38,39]. It was published early in his career and remained in obscurity until after his death. Ebstein's clinical expertise rested on an excellent foundation of pathology as he trained under Virchow. The paper he published was based on an autopsy he performed on a 19 year old laborer in whom a diagnosis of a congenital but unidentified cardiac defect had been made antemortem by the attending physician, a Dr. Kornfeld[40].

On examining the right ventricle, Ebstein saw

an extremely abnormal appearance of the tricuspid valve. A membrane ... originated from a quite normally developed right annulus fibrosus ... It ... was related to both the anterior ... and posterior ... walls of the right ventricle and blended with the posterior half of the endocardium of the ventricular septum ... This membrane, together with markedly opacified and thickened posterior half of the endocardium of the ventricular septum, formed a sac ...

Fifteen mm. below the right annulus fibrosus, and directly under the membranous portion of the ventricular septum, a (malformed) leaflet about the size of a 40 cent piece [?] took its origin from the endocardium[41].

Ebstein wrote that of the three cardiac anomalies in the case:

(1)   a severe malformation of the tricuspid valve,

(2)   absence of a thebesian valve, and

(3)   a patent foramen ovale,

the first was the most important. He concluded that a tricuspid valve as such did not exist and that development of a malformation of the tricuspid valve probably occurred at the time the atrioventricular valves developed in the third month of gestation.

After a careful search of the literature, Ebstein could not find a similar case. In discussing the case, Ebstein went into detail concerning the circulatory disturbances that resulted from the anomaly[42]. The description is an excellent example of the post-mortem method of confirmation of the clinical diagnosis espoused by the Parisian school.

In 1900, William G. MacCallum, professor of pathology at Johns Hopkins, described a museum specimen that had all of the characteristics of Ebstein's defect. This was the first pathologic description of Ebstein's anomaly to appear in the American literature[43]. The eponym was used by Yater and Shapiro in 1937 in their landmark paper on the subject[44]. The crucial paper, however, on Ebstein's disease was the one written by Mary Allen Engle and her colleagues. It was comprehensive in scope and appeared in the first volume of *Circulation* in 1950[45]. The paper originated from Johns Hopkins Hospital during Helen Taussig's tenure as chief of the pediatric cardiac clinic.

Laubry and Pezzi in 1921 credited the earliest description of tricuspid atresia to Henriette, Ferber, and Hiffe (1860)[46]. This is at variance with the well documented statements made by W.J. Rashkind in his historical review of tricuspid atresia published in 1982[47]. Rashkind's research of the literature puts the earliest report of a 'probable' case of tricuspid atresia as having been published in 1812. The pitfalls of any historical survey and the obstacles to be surmounted in searching for early case reports are well summarized by him and are worthy of emphasis. These include ignorance of the original language, incomplete descriptions in early writings and the burden of approaching early works with a mind 'cluttered by modern concepts'.

Bearing these valid remarks in mind, Rashkind is convinced (while offering documentary evidence) that Kreysig in 1817 was the first to describe a 'true' case rather than a 'probable' one[48]. He further documents that the first usage of the word 'atresia' for an absent tricuspid orifice is to be found in Schuberg's paper published in 1861[49]. As part of the title indicates, this paper describes the effect of atresia on the right venous ostium. The term 'atresia' did not begin to appear again until 1872 when Döbner reintroduced it in his paper[50]. Expressions such as 'no tricuspid valve', 'complete obliteration of the tricuspid valve', and 'absent tricuspid valve' were used instead. It was not until the early part of the 20th century that atresia became the generally accepted term.

Holmes in 1824 had described a case of malformation of the heart which has since become known as the Holmes Heart[51]. This heart showed no communication between the right auricle and the right ventricle, and for this reason, it was thought to represent an early case report of tricuspid atresia. On careful analysis of Holmes' description as well as the accompanying illustrations, it has since become quite obvious that the Holmes Heart is not an example of tricuspid atresia but rather one of a single left ventricle with an infundibular outflow chamber and with atresia of the mitral valve rather than tricuspid. The drawing definitely shows the right atrium communicating with the left ventricle via a tricuspid valve[52]. The malformation is actually a case of cor biatriatum triloculare. Maude Abbott's atlas of 1936 has an illustration of a heart with this morphologic configuration under the heading of biatriatum triloculare (p. vii).

The same error was committed by Henriette, Ferber and Hiffe in 1860. Their case was also an example of biatriatum triloculare rather than tricuspid atresia as claimed by Laubry and Pezzi.

Lost in all this maze of errors is the paper published at the same time as that of Holmes. It is Brown's clinicopathologic report which appeared in the London Medical Repository. The description of the heart fulfills the classical anatomical criteria of true tricuspid atresia but not as an isolated phenomenon as can be seen by the following quotation from Brown's paper[53].

> ... The auricles were much larger than usual (particularly the left) and communicated with each other by an open foramen ovale. The auriculo-ventricular opening on the right side was wanting (and consequently no communication could be traced from the right auricle to the right ventricle). The pulmonary artery arose from a very small cavity on the right side of the heart, and appeared, with its semilunar valves healthy. This cavity communicated by a small opening in the muscular fibres with the left ventricle; it had none of the characters of ventricle, having neither carneae columnae nor chordae tendineae.

The first American report of the anomaly was provided by Worthington in 1833 followed by Fearn in 1834[54,55]. Additional case reports appeared in the literature throughout the subsequent years, emanating especially from England, Germany and France. Peacock in his 2nd edition of *Malformations of the Human Heart* erroneously attributed one of these case reports to Claude Bernard, the outstanding French physiologist, but it was really published by Charles Bernard in *L'Union Medicale* in 1860[56].

It is difficult to trace the historical background of congenital aortic stenosis. Prior to Thomas Peacock, the isolated descriptions of calcified aortic valves made no distinction between acquired or congenital types. Words such as ossification are repeatedly found in these descriptions but again no detail is given regarding the number of cusps present on these deformed valves or even whether or not the deformities were rheumatic or infective in origin.

Aortic valvular stenosis in the presence of a bicuspid make-up was first clearly described by Peacock. He ventured the opinion that the bicuspid aortic valve (which is the basic congenital lesion) was very prone to inflammation and calcification. He also noted the frequent association of bicuspid aortic valves with coarctation of the aorta.

One of the earliest descriptions of stenosis of the aortic valve is the one by Lazare Riviere (Riverius) of Montpellier[57]. This is to be found in his work *Opera Medica Universa* published in Frankfurt in 1674. But again, there is no mention as to whether or not the lesion was thought to be congenital. Even earlier than this, the term 'ossification of the aortic valves' can be found in Fabrizio Bartoletti's work on clinicopathologic correlations *Methodus in Dyspnoeam* (circa 1630).

Theophile Bonet (Bonetus) was a brilliant Parisian clinician who has won critical acclaim for his exacting observations and analysis of post-mortem correlates and which are to be found in his book *Sepulchretum sive Anatomia Practica ex Cadaveribus Morbo de Natio* initially published in Geneva in 1679, and then again in 1706. In his text *Heart Disease*, published in 1951, Paul D. White attributes the following description of sudden death in a man with calcific aortic stenosis to Bonet as recorded in the *Sepulchretum*[58]. 'A Parisian tailor, not yet old, having dined and left his house had walked hardly 40 paces when he suddenly fell to the ground and expired. His body was opened and no disease was found except that the three semilunar cusps leading to the aorta were bony'.

The only evidence advanced by White that the aortic lesion was congenital in origin was that the subject was young. This is hard to accept since congenital calcific aortic stenosis is usually found in aortic valves that are bicuspid, unicuspid or quadricuspid and Bonet's description clearly states that there were three semilunar cusps. Note that the word bony is used, the same adjective that Morgagni used when he described the occasional finding of calcified aortic valves in his *De Sedibus*, published in 1761.

Wing recounts an interesting story regarding the first American description of calcific aortic stenosis[59]. It is a clinical and pathological description, presented by a Doctor Joshua Brackett in 1785, and based on the autopsy he performed on his brother-in-law, General William Whipple. The General was one of the signers of the Declaration of Independence. During the last five years of a previously healthy and active life, he experienced recurrent episodes of 'strictures of the breast', distressing palpitations of the heart after little exertion and fainting spells. He also complained of orthopnea. Against this background, the General gave permission that upon his death, his body should be subjected to an autopsy to determine the anatomical basis for his distress. He died suddenly on November 10, 1785. Brackett's description of the autopsy is rather terse:

> His body [Whipple] was opened, and it was found that ossification had taken place in his heart; the valve was united to his aorta, only a small aperture, the size of a knitting needle was open, through which all of the blood flowed in its circulation, and when any sudden motion gave it new impulse, it produced the palpitation and faintness to which he was liable.

There is no doubt that the patient had calcific aortic stenosis. The classical course of his history against a previously healthy life and the age at which he died do point to the probability that the stenosing calcification developed on a bicuspid valve. The weak link, of course, is that no mention is made of the cuspal configuration of the valve.

The first book to treat in depth the various malformations of the heart was Farre's small text entitled *Pathological Researches. Essay 1. On Malformations of the Human Heart*[60]. It was published in 1814. As stated before, Farre's book played an important role in stimulating interest in congenital lesions of the heart, but not to the extent as Peacock's text which appeared some 44 years later.

Farre's book describes aortic stenosis (ostium aortae) in a case of sudden death in a young pregnant female who at necropsy revealed a markedly calcified bicuspid aortic valve. Note the descriptive bicuspid but no comments are made as to its congenital basis. The book also describes patent foramen ovale as an isolated lesion or in association with patent ductus arteriosus, with pulmonary atresia or with stenosis of the 'ostium arteriae pulmonalis'. The essay describes still other abnormalities such as solitary pulmonary stenosis, transposition of the great vessels, ventricular septal defect and the finding of the pulmonary artery or aorta being common to both ventricles. All in all, it proved to be quite an illuminating compendium.

During the greater part of the 19th century there were two outstanding workers in congenital cardiac abnormalities. They were Thomas Peacock, whom we have already met, though briefly, and Carl von Rokitansky (1804–78).

Rokitansky was the renowned professor of pathological anatomy at Vienna, who, along with Skóda, was mainly responsible for that school's prestigious position during that era. Rokitansky shall always be accorded an important niche in cardiology because of his great book wherein there are detailed descriptions of the morbid anatomy of atrial and ventricular septal defects so elegantly illustrated with highly accurate and artistically executed drawings[61]. The book was called *Die Defecte der Scheidewände des Herzens*. It was published in 1875. The distinctive differences between the ostium primum and ostium secundum types of atrial septal defect are clearly delineated for the first time. We shall come across Rokitansky again in other sections of this book.

Thomas Bevill Peacock was born in 1812 and died in 1882. After serving as apprentice to John Fothergill, he received further training at the University College Hospital in London and then his MD degree at Edinburgh[62]. At the age of 37 he was elected assistant physician to St. Thomas' Hospital. Although primarily a clinician he had a marked and sustained interest in pathology. Most of his important writings were concerned with this interest and utilized a personal collection of pathologic specimens consisting mostly of the heart and great vessels. This interest in pathology dated back to when he was house physician and pathologist at the Edinburgh Royal Infirmary while preparing for his doctorate in medicine. At that time he already manifested his investigative bent with the publication of a paper illustrating the mode of formation of dissecting aneurysms by injecting fluids between the external and middle coats of the aorta removed from young cadavers[63].

Peacock wrote his monograph on congenital and acquired malformations of the heart in 1858[64]. The treatise became a standard of reference and,as stated repeatedly, it provided the spark plug for a renewed interest in congenital abnormalities of the heart. It was divided into five sections with the malformations classified into those that resulted from arrested development during the early stages of fetal life; those that had malformations which prevented postnatal development; and those which, although they did not interfere with the function of the heart, nevertheless provided the nidus for clinical disturbance in later life.

Almost a decade prior to this treatise, Peacock had written a paper published in the *Transactions of the Pathological Society of London* describing the Tetralogy of Fallot[65].

In this case there existed extreme contraction of the orifice of the pulmonary artery, with a deficiency in the interventricular septum, and the aorta arose in chief part from the right ventricle. The right auricle and ventricle were of large size, and the walls of the latter thick and very firm. The left ventricle was, on the contrary, small, and its walls thin and flaccid. The left auricle was also small. The foramen ovale and ductus arteriosus were both closed. The heart was taken from a child two years and five months old, who had exhibited well-marked symptoms of cyanosis, which commenced three months after birth … The intensity of the cyanosis, and the duration of life in these cases, bears a general relation to the amount of contraction of the pulmonary orifice and the freedom of communication between the right and left cavities of the heart, through the medium of the open foramen ovale and the aperture in the interventricular septum.

The above description antedates that of Fallot by 40 years. Elsewhere, Peacock acknowledged that he was not the first to describe this anomaly.

Although we owe a marked debt of gratitude to Peacock for his collation and clarification of the existing knowledge regarding the congenital abnormalities of the heart, the world was even more fortunate when Maude Abbott was born. Endowed with extraordinary energy, Canada's gift to the medical profession demonstrated throughout her professional career the ability to present in a logical manner conclusions drawn from detailed analysis of relevant data. Her total contribution in the form of a comprehensive, organized and systematized knowledge of congenital heart disease made her a world authority. In all she wrote 41 papers, case reports and book chapters on the subject. Her interests also included history, medical museums, and (of course) women in medicine; again with an extraordinary output of publications in these areas[66].

Maude Elizabeth Seymour Abbott was born in 1869 in St. Andrews, East Quebec. Maude was only 7 when her mother died of tuberculosis. More misfortune occurred when Maude's father, the Reverend Jeremiah Abbott, abandoned his family. Maude and her older sister were then adopted and reared by their grandmother.

Even as a youngster, Abbott manifested a keen interest in knowledge. Her diary documents this quite frequently. Taking advantage of McGill

University's new policy of admitting women to their Arts program, she pursued her undergraduate studies there graduating with high honors in 1890. Unfortunately, the faculty of medicine at McGill was not as open-minded towards women studying medicine, and despite persistence on her part she was repeatedly refused admission to the medical school. Bishop's College of Medicine saw fit to accept her and in 1894 she received her doctorate while walking away with the highest marks and the senior anatomy prize. It was during her clerkship at Montreal General Hospital that Abbott first came under the stewardship of McGill professors who shared a teaching affiliation with the Bishop's College faculty. Her enthusiasm and competence soon cemented a professional relationship with McGill that was to continue for the rest of her career. It is ironic that the school that rejected her in 1890 would recognize her in 1910 with an honorary doctorate of medicine.

At the time of Maude Abbott's graduation from medical school, the mecca for post-graduate study was Europe, especially Vienna. Initially her interests lay in gynecology and obstetrics but she soon became enamored of internal medicine and pathology. In her autobiographical notes[67] she stated:

> In the consensus of opinion then (and I believe still) the greatest things to be had there [Vienna], by far, were the pathology with Kolisko and Albrecht and the Internal Medicine courses with Ortner in Neusser's clinic … it was the grounding in internal medicine and pathology … that determined my bent and made possible my later work at McGill.

Upon returning from Europe, the bright well-trained physician engaged in private practice but did so in a rather desultory fashion, pursuing with greater vigor and attention her role in the department of pathology as assistant curator of the McGill University medical museum. In just a matter of months she was named curator of the museum. Under Abbott's leadership, the museum was transformed from a dust-laden collection of jarred specimens into an amphitheater of teaching. Despite a temporary setback caused by a fire that destroyed the medical building and severely damaged the museum collection, Maude continued to collect, identify and catalogue the various specimens. She was aided in this by donations of museum specimens from many parts of the academic world. By 1915, the first installments of a massive descriptive catalogue were published.

Although Maude Abbott had already known of Osler, in part through his generous support of the museum, and esteemed him in almost a reverential fashion, her first meeting with him occurred in December of 1898 during a trip to the United States, while visiting museums of pathology at various institutions. After accompanying Osler and his retinue, as a guest, on staff rounds at Johns Hopkins, Abbott accidentally crushed her finger in a door. She not only received prompt and sympathetic attention from Osler himself but also an invitation to join him at dinner that evening with his students and interns. Segall, a former student and later a close friend of Abbott, describes Maude's recollection of the conversation immediately subsequent to Osler's medical ministrations as follows: At that time she asked the great teacher for a reprint of his *Internal Medicine as a Vocation*. 'Oh, you like reprints', he said, 'come in here'. In a small room off his study, lined with reprints arranged in piles on the shelves, he handed a blue pamphlet to her saying 'this is the one I like better than anything else I have written'. It was *The Alabama Student*[68]. At the dinner that evening, in the company of his interns and students, he remarked to her 'What a wonderful opportunity it was to be at McGill museum'. He told her to go home and look up the *British Medical Journal* for 1893 and read the article by Mr. Jonathan Hutchinson on *A Clinical Museum*. This is what he calls his museum in London, and it is the greatest place I know for teaching students in pictures of life and death together, wonderful!' 'This was the gentle seed that was dropped and that dominated all my future work'[68,69].

Seven years after this meeting, Osler invited Abbott to write a section on congenital heart disease for the text *System of Modern Medicine* co-edited by him and McCrae. This chapter was written on a statistical basis in accordance with Osler's advice. Initially it was a small chapter of only 22 pages involving an analysis of the 412 cases then extant in her collection. Subsequent editions saw this chapter grow to 200 pages utilizing a data base that now comprised 1000 cases. Osler described the original chapter as being 'far and away the very best thing ever written on the subject in English, possibly in any language'[70].

The statistical data and classification of the various congenital abnormalities, though presented on the basis of anatomical characteristics, invoked physiological concepts to some degree in explaining the clinical signs and symptoms. This was a marked change from the purely morphological descriptions of the past. This approach was to be amplified in 1947 by Helen Taussig.

Despite her intense loyalty to McGill, Abbott spent some time away from her beloved McGill to occupy the chair of pathology at the Women's Medical College in Philadelphia. During her tenure there, she wrote, in collaboration with William Dawson, acting professor of physiology at the same institution, a paper entitled *The Clinical Classification of Congenital Heart Disease, with remarks upon its Pathological Anatomy, Diagnosis and Treatment*. In this article, the physiological approach was emphasized to an even greater degree. It advanced the argument that physicians should approach the management of congenital lesions of the heart in terms of three major types: acyanotic, delayed cyanotic, and cyanotic[71].

The culmination of Maude Abbott's life-long interest and dedication to unlocking the secrets of congenital cardiac abnormalities was to be the grand tome that she labored over for many years. It was published in 1936, bearing the title *Atlas of Congenital Cardiac Disease*[72]. The atlas analyzed the 1000 cases personally studied by her and included a review of the development and comparative anatomy of reptilian, amphibian and mammalian hearts. Kathleen Smith quotes Abbott as saying that the atlas 'came out as preliminary to a larger volume on congenital heart disease which the author has under preparation'[73]. Unfortunately, death in 1940 prevented Abbott from realizing this.

In the forward to the *Atlas*, Paul Dudley White wrote that 'Maude Abbott fired by a spark from Osler made the subject of congenital heart disease, one of such general and widespread interest that we no longer regard it with either disdain or awe, as a mystery for the autopsy table alone to discover or to solve'.

Abbott's classification of the various abnormalities as mentioned provided insight into the pathophysiologic pathways. This enabled the surgeons to devise a rational surgical method for correction or amelioration of the altered physiology. Herein lies Abbott's greatness and that of Helen Taussig. They provided the key for correction of nature's mistakes. We shall elaborate on this later in the chapter dealing with surgical intervention.

The surgical approach, however, required a long and tortuous path for its realization. The very nature of the procedures involved required a complex supportive technology. I am sure this was not far from Abbott's mind when she began to concern herself with the causes and mechanism of abnormal cardiac morphogenesis. Obviously answers to these would provide a rational basis for their prevention; a far better method of approach than the complex one of surgical intervention once the malformation has been established.

In the past, myths and misconceptions abounded as to the causation of these abnormalities. Note how both Hunter and Fallot believed it was the pulmonic stenosis that produced the multiple defects of the Tetralogy syndrome. What caused the pulmonic stenosis, itself? Remember the mother who thought that her child's hare lip was due to her fondness for rabbit stew! In essence, no one really addressed the problem in a scientific manner.

In search for the causes, Abbott asked six basic questions[74]:

(1) Is it a fault in the germ plasm? It is well known that chromosomal disorders are frequently associated with cardiac disease. An example of this is Down's syndrome (trisomy 21) where a 10% incidence has been reported.

(2) Can the abnormalities be truly inherited? Dominant, X-linked and multifactorial forms of inheritance have been demonstrated.

(3) Is it due to an altered environment of the embryo? The fetotoxicity of alcohol, thalidomide and other drugs has been well documented.

(4) Is it a disease state of maternal tissues or secretions? Diabetes, enzyme disorders and heritable blood diseases such as hemophilia have been incriminated.

(5) Diseases of the early embryo? Rubella as a cause of patent ductus arteriosus as well as other malformations is a classic example. Other viruses have been found to be teratogenic.

(6) Fetal trauma or exhaustion of a parturient uterus? Evidence to-date indicates there is no increased risk with a birth disorder when corrected by maternal age.

All of these questions were answered in whole or in part by the Baltimore Washington Infant study conducted between 1981 and 1986[75]. Thus a multifactorial etiology appears to be responsible for the congenital aberrations. In posing all these questions, Abbott stressed the importance of congenital infections *in utero* as of singular importance. It is of interest that Thomas Peacock stressed this also in 1858[76]. Most recently Wagner (1981) has reactivated awareness of intra-uterine infections as an important cause[77].

Canada gave us Maude Abbott and we are grateful. Not to be outdone, New England obliged us with Helen Taussig. Abbott was the pathologist and Taussig was the clinician. Abbott unfortunately died before she was able to realize the surgical fruits of her labor while Taussig lived to see and appreciate the technological explosion and surgical advancements of the 20th century. Abbott contributed a systematic anatomical approach while Taussig was the clinician's delight in her pathophysiologic analysis. Each patient was viewed by Taussig as a 'crossword puzzle' that had to be solved with the information at hand and with practically no technological assistance other than the fluoroscope and electrocardiogram. Abbott and Taussig were both strong beacons of light complementing each other in so many ways. Above all, as Abbott transformed the gloomy museum of specimens into an orchestrated presentation of knowledge so did Taussig convert the 'dead-end' outlook of congenital abnormalities into an optimistic attitude for relief or correction.

Helen Brooke Taussig was born in Cambridge, Massachusetts, in 1898. Although a very bright student, she suffered the same ignominious rejection from the medical school of her first choice as Abbott experienced. Harvard Medical School refused to accept her as a matriculating student simply because the doors were closed to females at that time. The Boston University School of Medicine was much more liberal and this is where Helen began her medical studies. She, however, transferred to Johns Hopkins, obtaining her medical degree in 1927. The young Dr. Taussig was to spend her entire professional career at her alma mater.

Soon after completing an internship in pediatrics she was appointed as the director of a newly established cardiac clinic at Johns Hopkins. At the suggestion of Dr. Edwards A. Park she concentrated on those cardiac diseases that were congenital. Her approach to each case was from a functional point of view. This was the Viennese and German physiological approach to pathology in contra-distinction to the Parisian school. Each case was studied with the most meticulous attention to detail. Her studies culminated in the publication of her first edition of a monumental text that took 10 years to write. Aptly titled *Congenital Malformations of the Heart*, it analyzed each pathological abnormality on the basis of the hemodynamic changes that ensued and that were responsible for the clinical picture. The text was fortified with clearly detailed anatomical drawings and schematic diagrams shaded from red to blue to indicate varying degrees of oxygenation. It also contained many pertinent radiographs[78].

This text removed the whole spectrum of congenital heart disease from a museum of pathologic curiosities to a vibrant clinical entity that could be approached and evaluated on the basis of physiologic alterations. It complemented and augmented Maude Abbott's *Atlas*. The magnitude of Taussig's contribution can be appreciated even more keenly when one realizes that all of this work was accomplished with just three tools: the elements of physical diagnosis, fluoroscopy and electrocardiography.

Taussig's functional approach was the springboard for the surgical amelioration of that common cyanotic defect known as the Tetralogy of Fallot. This too was a monumental step since cardiac surgery at that time was virtually non-existent, or, at any rate, quite crude and primitive compared to the sophisticated level of today's surgical techniques.

After being summarily rejected by Gross of Boston, she was fortunate in being able to share her enthusiasm and interest with Alfred Blalock who had already been working on the surgical correction of coarctation of the aorta. As the newly appointed chief of surgery, he was able to give Taussig his unhindered and full collaboration. In due time their conjoint effort resulted in the publication of a paper entitled *The Surgical Treatment of Malformations of the Heart*. History was made! It described in detail the Blalock-Taussig procedure for the alleviation of cyanosis in Tetralogy of Fallot.

Dietrich outlines an interesting anecdote regarding the surgical technician who worked with Blalock and Taussig on the animals prior to the first human application of the above procedure[79]. His name was Vivian Thomas. He was a very big black man with very little formal education but apparently, because of his intelligence and dexterity, he commanded a great deal of respect from both Blalock and Taussig. Dietrich tells that at one of the early blue baby operations, an anatomic variant was found that had not been seen before during the animal surgical experiments. 'Drs. Blalock and Taussig turned to Thomas and asked 'What do we do now, Vivian?' Mr. Thomas later became Dr. Thomas.

Taussig's clinic continued to grow at a phenomenal rate following the success of the Blalock-Taussig procedure. Patients were being referred from all over the world. In 1952, she was able to report on the results of 1000 patients who had undergone the Blalock-Taussig procedure. Pediatric cardiology was virtually non-existent when Taussig started. By the time she was ready to retire she had trained more than 60 physicians from all over the world. Many of them established their own training programs at various medical centers. Honorary degrees, major awards, prizes and lectureships came from far and wide. But strangely, Johns Hopkins did not promote her to a full professorship until 4 years prior to retirement. This is a sad commentary on the politics of academia.

Helen Taussig was one of the brightest stars in a medical firmament that was dominated by men. Vincent Gott, a cardiac surgical colleague once said of her, 'although she was the most honored and respected woman of medicine she remained a warm, completely approachable, unpretentious lady'. Some of her reminiscences were published in a very short article in 1981 and excerpts from this are worthy of quote since they give us an unadulterated insight into her personality and dedication[80].

After a 1-year fellowship in cardiology and 1½ years in pediatrics, Dr. Park put me in charge of the cardiac clinic. My friends said, 'Why go into such a narrow field as pediatric cardiology?' To me it was a great opportunity to combine pediatrics and cardiology. I vowed then and there not to get into a rut in this 'narrow' field. Dr. Park gave me the tools to work with: an electrocardiograph, a technician secretary and a social worker. All for $4,000, including my salary! He arranged to have x-rays taken without cost to the patient and installed a fluoroscope in Harriet Lane Home for the use of the pediatric staff.

Dr. Park firmly believed that new tools brought new knowledge. In 1930 a fluoroscope was a new tool. It proved to be my most useful one.

When I began to write a book on the subject, friends gasped, 'Why waste your time on such a trivial subject!' I replied as I would today, 'If you stay in academic medicine and learn anything, you are morally obligated to make that knowledge available to others'. I cared for those cyanotic infants in the clinic and followed them to the autopsy table. There I learned that infants with pulmonary atresia died as the ductus closed and those with severe pulmonary stenosis became markedly worse. The obvious problem was how to keep the ductus open. 'When Drs. Robert Gross and John Hubbard showed it was possible to ligate a patent ductus, I immediately thought that it must be possible to build a ductus. I consulted Dr. Gross in Boston. He said he had built many ductuses but as he was in the full glory of the successful ligation of a patent ductus arteriosus, to build a ductus seemed foolish. He was not in the least interested in my idea. I returned to Baltimore and waited for Dr. Alfred Blalock.

I knew Dr. Blalock was interested in thoracic surgery. He had operated successfully on three patients with a patent ductus arteriosus. When Dr. Blalock performed his first operation at Hopkins on a child with a patent ductus, I said to him, 'I stand in awe and admiration of your surgical skill but truly a great day will come when you build a ductus for a cyanotic child'. Dr. Blalock took the problem to the laboratory. His work there is a separate story. Two years later he told me that he was convinced that he knew how to build a ductus. Our first two patients were severely incapacitated. Both survived and were improved, but not until the third child did we see a dramatic change. That little boy was 6 years old, deeply cyanotic, miserably unhappy; he could no longer walk. When Dr. Blalock finally completed the anastomosis and released the clamps, he said he felt a beautiful thrill and almost simultaneously the anesthesiologist said, 'He's a lovely color now'. I walked to the head of the table and saw his face with lovely pink cheeks and cheery red lips. The child woke up in the operating room and asked to get up. We knew we had won.

Taussig, like Abbott, was also interested in pinpointing the origin of cardiac defects. Even during retirement she continued working and developing the hypothesis that the origin of isolated cardiac malformations was more likely genetic than teratogenic[81,82]. This problem took her to the cardiac embryology laboratory at Johns Hopkins where she meticulously studied bird hearts in an attempt to find possibly a common genetic background. She also worked hard at combating the many social problems of the era. The vocal outbursts of the antivivisectionists had to be addressed and nullified. New funding was needed for the continued care of the patients. When the thalidomide disaster broke out she became heavily involved with the problem both from the scientific and legislative points of view. She realized full well the need for more extensive testing of drugs and for stricter control by the Federal Drug Administration.

All of this, reflective of a long and fruitful life, was cut short when she 'apparently did not see an approaching car as she turned from a parking area into a main road'[83]. How ironic! After giving new light to so many children without the aid of modern technology, it was technology itself that snuffed out her flame.

REFERENCES

1. Adams, F.H. Some notes on the history of congenital heart disease. Cited in Adams, F.H. (1968). Development of pediatric cardiology. *Am. J. Cardiol.*, **22**, 452–5

2. Abbott, M. (1936). *Atlas of Congenital Cardiac Disease.* (New York: American Heart Association)

3. Adams, F.H. (1968). Development of pediatric cardiology. *Am. J. Cardiol.*, **22**, 452–5

4. Willius, F.A. and Dry, T.J. (1948). *A History of the Heart and Circulation*, pp. 237–8. (Philadelphia: W.B. Saunders Co.)

5. Herrick, J.B, (1942). *A Short History of Cardiology*, p. 160. (Illinois: Charles C. Thomas)

6. East, C.T. (1957). *The Story of Heart Disease*, p. 54. (London: Wm. Dawson and Sons Ltd.)

7. Castiglioni, A. (1941). *A History of Medicine.* (New York: Alfred A. Knopf)

8. Rashkind, W.J. (1972). Historic aspects of congenital heart disease. *Birth Defects*, Original Article Series, vol. VIII, no.1

9. Campbell, M. (1971). Early anatomical knowledge of cardiac malformation. *Br. Heart J.*, **33**, 169–72

10. Morgagni, J.B. (1761). *De Sedibus et Causis Morborum.* (Venice)

11. Steno, N. (1671). Anatomicus Regij Hafniensis Embryo Monstro affinis Parisiis dissectus. *Acta Med. et Philosophia, Hafminsia*, **I**, 200

12. East, C.T. (1957). *Op. cit.*, p. 57

13. Willius, F.A. and Dry, T.J. (1948). *Op. cit.*, p. 61

14. Lutz, J.G. (1904). Nicholas Steno. *M. Library and Hist. J.*, **2**, 166–82

15. Sandifort, E. (1777). Observationes Anatomical et Pathologicae. *Lib. I*, **I** (Translated by Bennet, L.R. Sandifort's 'Observations', Chapter 1, concerning a very rare disease of the heart). *Bull. Hist. Med.*, **20**, 539–70

16. Duke, M. (1984). Whose tetralogy is it? A short history of the tetralogy of Fallot. *Connecticut Med.*, **48**(2), 103–4

17. Willius, F.A. and Dry, T.J. (1948). *Op. cit.*, p. 83

18. Duke, M. (1984). *Op. cit.*, p. 103

19. Fallot, A. (1888). Contribution – l'anatomie pathologique de la maladie bleue (cyanose cardiaque). *Marseille Med.*, **25**, 77, 138, 207, 341, 403

20. Olmer, D. (1929). 'Etienne-Louis Arthur Fallot' in lecon d'ouverture de la chaire de clinique médicale. *Marseille Méd.*, **66**, 741–59

21. Willius, F.A. and Keys, T.E. (1941). *Cardiac Classics; a Collection of Classic Works on the Heart and Circulation with Comprehensive Biographic Accounts of the Authors*, pp. 687–90. (St. Louis: C.V. Mosby Co.)

22. Rashkind, W.J. (1972). Historic aspects of congenital heart. *Birth Defects*, Original Article Series, vol.VIII, no.1

23. *Ibid.* (1972). p. 3

24. Paris, M. (1791). Rétrécissement considérable de l'aorte pectoral observeé à l'Hôtel Dieu de Paris. *Journal de Chirurgie* (Desault), **2**, 107

25. East, C.T. (1957). *Op. cit.*, p. 71

26. Meckel, A. (1827). Verschliessung der Aorta am vierten Brustwirkel. *Archiv für Anatomie and Physiologie*, p. 345

27. Raynaud, A. (1828). Observation d'une oblité-ration presque complète de l'aorte, etc. *Journal Hebdomadaire de Médecine*, **1**, 161

28. Jordan, J. (1830). A case of obliteration of the aorta. *N. Engl. Med. Surg. J.*, **1**, 101

29. East, C.T. (1957). *Op. cit.*, p. 68

30. *Ibid.* (1957). p. 68

31. Craigie, D. (1841). Instance of obliteration of the aorta beyond the arch, illustrated by similar

cases and observations. *Edinburgh Med. Surg. J.*, **56**, 427

32. Barié, E. (1886). Du rétrécissement congénital de l'aorte descendante. *Rev. Méd.*, **6**, 343, 409, 501

33. Bonnet, L.M. (1903). Sur la lesion dite stenose congénitale de l'aorte dans la Région de l'Isthme. *Rev. Méd.*, **23**, 108, 255, 335, 418, 481

34. Campbell, M. (1971). *Op. cit.*, p. 170

35. Dupré, E. (1891). Communication congénitale des deux coeurs par inocclusion du septum interventriculaire. Premiére observation de la lésion, reconnue pendant la vie et vérifiée aprés la mort. *Bulletins de la Société Anatomique de Paris*, **66**, 404 (5 méser 5)

36. Herrick, J.B. (1935). Allan Burns 1781–1813; anatomist, surgeon and cardiologist. *Bull. Soc. M. Hist. Chicago*, **4**, 457–83 (Jan.)

37. Burns, A. (1809). *Observations on some of the most frequent and important diseases of the heart; on aneurism of the thoracic aorta; on preternatural pulsation in the epigastric region; and on the usual origin and distribution of some of the large arteries of the human body*, p. 332. (Edinburgh: Bryce & Co)

38. Burchell, B.H. (1979). Ebstein's disease. *Mayo Clin. Proc.*, **54**, 205–7 (Editorial)

39. Ebstein, W. (1866). Über eine sehr seltenen Fall von Insufficienz der Valvula Tricuspidalis, bedingt durch eine angeborene hochgradige missbildung derselben. *Arch von Reichert Bois-Reymond*, **2**, 238–54

40. Seward, J.B., Tajik, A.J., Feist, D.J. and Smith, H.C. (1979). Ebstein's anomaly in an 85-year old man. *Mayo Clin. Proc.*, **54**, 193–6

41. Schiebler, G.L., Gravenstein, J.S. and Van Mierop, L.H.S. (1968). Ebstein's anomaly of the tricuspid valve: translation of original description with comments. *Am. J. Cardiol.*, **22**, 867–73

42. Sekelj, P. and Benfey, B.G. (1974). Historical landmarks: Ebstein's anomaly of the tricuspid valve. *Am. Heart J.*, **88**, 108–14

43. MacCallum, W.G. (1900). Congenital malformations of the heart as illustrated by the specimens in the pathological museum of the Johns Hopkins Hospital. *Johns Hopkins Hosp. Bull.*, **11**, 69–71

44. Yater, W.M. and Shapiro, M.J. (1937). Congenital displacement of the tricuspid valve (Ebstein's disease): review and report of a case with electrocardiographic abnormalities and detailed histologic study of the conduction system. *Ann. Intern. Med.*, **11**, 1043–62

45. Engle, M.A., Payne, T.P.B., Bruins, G. and Taussig, H.B. (1950). Ebstein's anomaly of the tricuspid valve; report of three cases and analysis of clinical syndrome. *Circulation*, **1**, 1246–60

46. Laubry, C. and Pezzi, C. (1921). *Traité des Maladies Congénitales du Coeur.* (Paris: Bailliere)

47. Rashkind, W.J. (1982). Tricuspid atresia: a historical review. *Pediatr. Cardiol.*, **2**, 85–8

48. Kreysig, F.L. (1817). Die Krankheiten des Herzens. *Dritte Thiel*, p. 104. (Berlin: A.W. Hayn)

49. Schuberg, W. (1861). Beobachtung von Verkümmerung des rehten Herzventrickels in Folge von Atresie dest Ost. venos. dextr.; Perforation des Herzscheidewand und dadurch Bildung eines Canales, der durch den rudimentären rechtaen Ventrickel in die Art. pulmon. führt. *Virchows Arch. Pathol. Anat.*, **20**, 294–6

50. Döbner. (1872). Zur Kausistik der Missbildungen des Herzens. *Wiener Medizinoche Presse*, **13**, 603–5, 629–31

51. Holmes, W.F. (1824). Case of malformation of the heart. *Trans. Med. Chir. Soc. Edinburgh*, **1**, 252

52. *Ibid.*

53. Brown, B. (1824). Case of singular malformation of the heart. *London Med. Repository*, **1**, 127

54. Worthington, W. (1833). Case of malformation of the heart. *Am. J. Med. Sci.*, **22**, 131

55. Fearn, S.W. (1834–5). Singular malformation of the heart. *Lancet*, **1**, 312

56. Bernard, C. (1860). Note sure en cas de vice de conformation du coeur, qui etaite divise en-deux cavites seulement, et observe chez un Engant ayant vecu un mois. *L'Union Medicale N.S.*, **5**, 612

57. Castiglioni, A. (1941). *Op. cit.*, p. 560

58. White, P.D. (1951). *Heart Disease*, p. 692. (New York: MacMillan)

59. Wing, E.S. (1983). First American description of calcific aortic stenosis. *Rhode Island Medical J.*, **66**, 243–5

60. Farre, J.R. (1814). *Pathological researches. Essay I. On malformations of the human heart.* Longman

61. von Rokitansky, C. (1875). *Die Defecte der Scheidewände des Herzens.* (Vienna: Braumüller)

62. Porter, I.H. (1962). The nineteenth-century physician and cardiologist, Thomas Bevill Peacock, 1812–82. *Med. Host.*, **6**, 240

63. Peacock, T.B. (1843). An account of some experiments illustrative of the mode of formation of the dissecting aneurisms. *Lond. Edinburgh J. Med. Sci.*, **3**, 871

64. Peacock, T.B. (1858). *On Malformations of the Human Heart.* (London: J. Churchill)

65. Peacock, T.B. (1846–7). Malformation of the

heart, consisting in contraction of the orifice of the pulmonary artery with deficiency at the base of the interventricular septum. *Trans. Path. Soc. Lond.*, **1**, 25

66. Dobell, A.R.C. (1988). Maude Abbott. *Clin. Cardiol.*, **11**, 658–9

67. Abbott, M.E.S. (1959). Autobiographical sketch. *McGill Med. J.*, **28**, 127

68. Segall, H.N. The genesis of Canadian cardiology. In *Pioneers of Cardiology in Canada, 1820–1970*

69. McDermott, H.E. (1941). *Maude Abbott: A Memoir.* (Toronto: The MacMillan Co. of Canada, Ltd.)

70. Dobell, A.R.C. (1988). *Op. cit.*, p. 659

71. Abbott, M.E. and Dawson, W.T. (1924). The clinical classification of congenital cardiac disease. *Int. Clin.*, **4**, 156–88

72. Abbott, M.E. (1936). Atlas of congenital cardiac disease. (American Heart Association)

73. Smith, K. (1982). Maude Abbott: pathologist and historian. *C.M.A. Jour.*, **27**, 774–6

74. Abbott, M.E. (1932). Congenital heart disease. *Nelson Looseleaf Medicine IV*, 220

75. Ferencz, C. (1989). Origin of congenital heart disease: reflections on Maude Abbott's work. *Can. J. Cardiol.*, **5**(1), 4–9

76. Peacock, T.B. (1858). *Op. cit.*, p. 114

77. Wagner, H.R. (1981). Cardiac disease in congenital infections. In Plotkin, S.A. and Stuart, E.S. (eds.) *Clinics in Perinatology: Symposium on Perinatal Infections*, **8**, 481–497. (Philadelphia: W.B. Saunders)

78. Dietrich, H.J. (1986). Helen Brooke Taussig. *Trans. and Studies of the College of Physicians of Philadelphia*, Ser. 5, vol. 8, no. 4, 261–5

79. *Ibid.* p. 267

80. Taussig, H.B. (1981). Little choice and a stimulating environment. *J.A.M.W.A.*, **36** (2), 43–44

81. McNamara, G. (1986). Helen Brooke Taussig: 1898–1986. *Pediatric Cardiol.*, **7**, 1–2

82. Clark, E.B. (1988). The origin of common cardiac defects. *J.A.C.C.*, **12**, 1807

83. Dietrich, H.J. (1986). *Op. cit.*, p. 265

Section 3

Functional mechanisms

14 Earliest physiological observations to present concepts

INTRODUCTION

Cardiovascular physiology is a rather complex component of cardiologic lore. Knowledge concerning it evolved very slowly, needing initially, for its proper development, a sound foundation in anatomy, both gross and microscopic. For years notions concerning the circulation were based, as everything else in cardiology, on myth, theological distortions, misconceptions and authoritarianism. Harvey's role was pivotal but by no means the only important one. As we shall see, many personalities were involved, especially in the maturation of this discipline from his epochal observations and insight to the stupendous advances made during the 19th century and continuing to the current one. The 19th century saw the initiation of a truly experimental approach and with the technological superiority of the 20th century, a veritable explosion of knowledge occurred that served to remove the physiological basis of cardiologic practice from uncertainty to one based on well-established and documented principles.

The functional mechanisms of the heart and vessels embrace the laws of contraction and relaxation that account for the pumping action of the heart, the electrophysiologic principles that initiate and regulate the rhythm of the heart, the nuances of blood pressure regulation, and the relationship between the cardiovascular system and the other systems of the body. The last include the lungs, kidneys, endocrine, hematologic and nervous systems. The very extent of these related factors accounts for the complexity of the problem and the slowness with which our knowledge concerning the circulatory system evolved over the centuries. Though we have come a long way this knowledge is still incomplete. No doubt further advances will continue to be made, and, as in all else in science, they will be realized only by perching ourselves on the shoulders of the giants that preceded us.

Blood is the main constituent of the cardiovascular system. It is responsible for carrying the necessary nutrients and oxygen to the innermost recesses of the body and carrying away the waste products of metabolism to the lungs, liver and kidneys for proper disposal. The essential purpose of the circulation is to see that the blood does indeed accomplish this mission.

The nutrients are derived from ingested food. The gastrointestinal tract is simply a highway with the ability to transform the ingested food in transit into a substance that can be metabolized. The oxygen necessary for metabolizing these substances is derived from the lungs. This is rather a simple concept but one that took millennia before its details could be delineated.

EARLY CONTRIBUTORS

Animal figures found painted on the walls of caves and dating back to primitive man often show representations of the heart. No evidence of its physiological role, however, can be deduced from these simplistic animal drawings. The first inklings of the functional purpose of the heart may be found in the Egyptian Papyri though the evidence for this is rather tenuous. The Ebers and Brugsch Papyri describe the heart as a well from which vascular conduits extend to the limbs[1,2]. A later manuscript, the Edwin Smith, describes the heart as the center in a system of distributing vessels. Key and colleagues use the words 'pumping force'[3]. Although the pulse was recognized and counted at this time, no specific statements are to be found in this or any other papyrus that the heart acted as a pump.

The ancient Chinese also appear to have had some knowledge of the circulation. Evidence for this can be found in the *Neiching* which dates back to 1000 BC. It described the liver as a storehouse for blood and the heart as a repository for the pulse.

The blood contained the soul while the pulse was the spirit. The lungs were the seat of energy (breath), and the kidneys for the principle[4]. This work is also known as *Nei Ching, Internal Classic* or *Canon of Medicine*. The Yellow Emperor, Huang Ti, is thought to be the author but this is based on tradition rather than historical documentation. At any rate, several statements in the Canon reveal an astonishing recognition of the principles of circulation while another passage is totally absurd in its description. This latter passage describes the circulation of blood as originating in the foot and traveling from there to the kidneys, heart, lungs, liver and spleen. From the spleen it went back to the kidneys with no explanation as to why and no description of its further transit[5]. Against the background of this absurdity, the following statements appear to be a marvel of perspicacity.

> The blood current flows continuously in a circle and never stops ... The blood cannot but flow continuously like the current of a river, or the sun and moon in their orbits. It may be compared to a circle without beginning or end ... The blood travels a distance of three inches during inhalation and another three inches during exhalation, making six inches with one respiration[6].

These statements were obviously unknown to the early Greeks or if known, were completely disregarded. Like the early Chinese, however, the great Grecian philosophers of the pre-Christian era also believed that blood contained a basic substance of great importance. The Chinese called it soul while the Greeks referred to it as the vital essence. Unlike the Chinese, the Greeks spent a great deal of time in the identification of this vital essence. The idea that inspired air had something to do with vital essence was born in that cradle of Greek science called Ionia. It was here that the view arose that the vital essence was the result of a mixture of air and blood, and that this coupling occurred in the lungs. These early philosophers were not scientists, and at best, they were crude experimentalists, depending mostly on visual observations for their conclusions. As philosophers they were quite adept, however, at debating, and this they did without end when it came to determining the nature of a First Principle.

One of them was Anaximenes, who lived in the 6th century BC. It was he who called the First Principle pneuma[7,8]. Diogenes of Apollonia then gave to pneuma the property of being essential to life[9].

Empedocles of Agrigento, Sicily, elaborated further on the relationship between blood and pneuma by stating that pneuma was the source of health, and carried to the various parts of the body by blood which at the same time was the carrier of innate heat. Empedocles' concept of circulation was one of tides and pulsations. He espoused the notion that the blood issued from the heart with both air and its innate heat and that it returned to the heart by moving backwards rather than by a closed loop of vessels[7,8]. At least he recognized that blood vessels originated from the heart; an anatomical detail that had been previously advanced by Alcmeon of Croton[9], who is thought to be the first Greek to have gained his knowledge of anatomy through dissection.

'Motion of blood in a circle' had to wait for Harvey for its full elucidation. However, the first suggestion that blood does circulate in this manner can be found in the Hippocratic Corpus. The following paragraph from this work appears to substantiate this premise:

> The vessels communicate with one another and the blood flows from one to another. I do not know where the commencement is to be found, for in a circle you can find neither commencement nor end, but from the heart the arteries take their origin and through the vessel, the blood is distributed to all the body, to which it gives warmth and life; they are the sources of human nature and are like rivers that purl through the body and supply the human body with life; the heart and the vessels are perpetually moving, and we may compare the movement of the blood with courses of rivers returning to their sources after a passage through numerous channels[9].

This paragraph not only demonstrates a loop concept but in the analogy of 'courses of rivers returning to their sources after a passage through numerous channels', it also provides a clear picture of the microscopic anatomy of the capillaries. Later on, Erasistratus also anticipated the need for a capillary circulation when he postulated the existence of intercommunications between the finest ramifications of the arteries and veins.

Another Hippocratic document, *On the Heart*, also describes several physiological notions pertaining to the cardiovascular system:

The auricles regulate respiration ... the vessel originating from the right ventricle supplies the lung with blood which serves as its nourishment ... the blood leaks back through a weak pulmonary valve allowing some air to pass through in small quantity [10].

These statements are remarkable in that they antedate Galen's conceptions by five centuries. However, the authenticity of the authorship of the document is very much in doubt. Leboucq, a French Hellenist of repute, claimed it was a compendium of student notes derived from lectures given by Philiston of Locroi, a disciple of Empedocles [10]. Michel on the other hand felt that it was a later addition to the Hippocratic Corpus [11].

Plato had his own ideas about the heart and circulation. Some of these were, no doubt, transmitted to his most famous student, Aristotle. Willius and Dry quote Plato's views as follows:

For when respiration is going in and out, the fire, which is first bound within, follows it ever and anon moving to and from, enters the belly and reaches the meat and drink, it dissolves them, and dividing them into small portions, and guiding them through the passages where it goes, pumps them as from a fountain into the channels of the veins, and makes the stream of the veins flow through the body as through a conduit [12].

This quote serves to underscore Plato's recognition that the blood is in constant motion, although he is rather fuzzy as to the source of the pumping action responsible for blood flow.

Aristotle also maintained that the blood was responsible for distributing 'transformed food' throughout the body. According to Sarton, Aristotle believed the propelling force for moving the blood was the heart [8]. Despite this, he was no different from his predecessors in that he, too, had no clear conception of the circulation. Aristotle believed the brain prevented the heart from overheating. He also thought the heart was the first organ to come to life and the last to die. From the viewpoint of organ systems, isn't this the way it truly is?

Aristotle's disciple, Praxagoras, conceived the notion that the left ventricle and arteries carried only air while the right ventricle and veins transported only blood. His student, Herophylus did not accept this teaching in its entirety, especially after he demonstrated that the arteries contained blood only during life, and that it was after death that they became flat and devoid of blood. He taught that the heart transmitted its blood to the lungs via the pulmonary artery, which he called arterial vein. This was part of his concept of a dual system for transport of blood and air. According to him the lungs absorbed fresh air and then distributed it through the body. The lungs also collected the air returning from the body for evacuation to the exterior. Though stated crudely, this teaching contains the rudiments of our current views regarding the relationship between respiration and respiratory gas transport.

Erasistratus advanced this thesis further by formalizing the dual concept of blood and air transport. His two basic elements of the vital processes were blood and pneuma. Blood nourished the body with the natural spirit that it carried. Pneuma was derived from ambient air. In the body pneuma existed in two forms – vital and animal. After being inspired by the lungs, it was brought to the left ventricle via the vein-like artery which had been described by Herophylus, his former mentor, as the venal artery. The transformation of the pneuma into vital spirit occurred in the left ventricle, from whence it was distributed throughout the body via the aorta and arteries. The portion of the vital spirit that reached the brain underwent a further transformation into animal spirit which now traveled through 'hollow' nerves emanating from the brain to nourish also all parts of the body. The blood with its natural spirit was manufactured by the liver. Most of it was distributed throughout the body including the right ventricular chamber via the veins. Since he felt that the tricuspid valve functioned only in a unidirectional manner this portion of the blood after being propelled through the pulmonary artery (the arterial vein of Herophylus) to the lungs could not reflux back through the vena cava. Erasistratus also attributed a unidirectional function to the pulmonary and mitral valves. Thus, blood was prevented from going back into the right ventricle via the pulmonary valves. This mechanism assured the lungs of nourishment from the natural spirit of the blood held up in this manner. Meanwhile the pneuma that arrived in the left ventricle from the lungs was prevented from returning by a closed mitral valve. One of the major errors in this schema was his assumption that blood moved from the right ventricle into the lungs during diastole. He was, however, correct when he taught that the blood with pneuma entered the left ventricular cavity also during this phase of the cardiac cycle. In hindsight, although Erasistratus assumed that an intercommunication existed between the finest ramifications of the arteries and veins, he could not visualize the circulatory system as a closed loop because of his adherence to the concept that blood was the source of matter, that pneuma was the source of energy and that since they originated from different sources, they required two separate systems of transportation. It should be noted that both Herophylus and Erasistratus were fortunate in having lived during the reign of Ptolemy I Soter, one of Alexander's generals, who proclaimed himself King right after Alexander's death. He was a patron of the intellectual activities of the time, freeing scholars from the constraints of religious bondage. To him belongs the credit for allowing these two great physicians to take advantage of this intellectual freedom.

Galen came on the scene four centuries later, at which time he added his own thoughts to the teachings of the two Alexandrian physicians. Galen also did not subscribe to the belief that the arteries contained only air, and yet his notions of the circulation were also wrong. Galen was not only an anatomist and experimental physiologist, but a highly successful practitioner as well. These three attributes helped cement his unshakable authority for at least 12 centuries. Just as Galen's pervasive influence retarded the growth of anatomical knowledge (see Chapter 1), so did it affect in the same manner the elucidation of the physiologic basis of heart action and circulation.

Galen also believed in three types of spirit: natural, vital and animal. He was of the opinion that food was transported via the portal vein from the intestine to the liver, where it became blood endowed with natural spirit, thus providing the body with nutrition and ability to grow. Part of the blood in the liver was then transported to the right ventricle, from which it was carried to the lungs via the *vena arterialis*. This blood lost its impurities through exhalation, and the purified blood now ebbed to and fro for purposes of nutrition while remaining on the venous side. A small part of the blood within the right ventricular chamber passed to the left ventricle through pores within the left ventricular chamber. In the left ventricle this blood

became charged with vital spirit by mixing with air that had been brought from the lungs via the *arteria venalis*. The blood loaded with vital spirit provided the organs with function by ebbing to and fro within the arteries. The blood was charged with animal spirit while in the brain. The animal spirit was also known as the breath of the soul. It was brought to the brain via the nerves which he also thought were hollow. From the brain, the blood now properly charged with animal spirit was carried to the various organs to cause sensation, motion and other functions. This entire scenario was simply a variation of the theme espoused by Erasistratus.

In essence, Galen conceived the circulatory system as consisting of two components (arterial and venous) joined together through invisible pores in the interventricular septum. Even Leonardo da Vinci as late as 1500 accepted this anatomical concept with his drawings depicting these invisible pores[13]. Although Galen recognized the unidirectional characteristics of the cardiac valves, he did not grasp the true schema of the circulation by his adherence to the ebb and flow motion of the blood. Galen placed a great deal of reliance on these interventricular pores but he also visualized the same sort of pore communication between the pulmonary artery and the pulmonary vein if the following quotation is interpreted correctly. Although attributed to Galen, the quotation is taken from Fulton[14]:

There is generally a mutual anastomosis or joining of the arteries and veins, and transfer blood and spirit equally from each other by invisible and very small passages. If the mouth of the pulmonary artery always stayed open and nature had no way of closing it when necessary or of opening it again, the blood could not transfuse these invisible and delicate pores in the arteries during contraction of the thorax. All things are not equally attracted or expelled. Something light is more easily drawn in by the distention of the part, and pushed out in contraction than something heavy. Likewise anything is more quickly passed through a wide tube than through a narrow one. When the thorax contracts, the pulmonary veins, strongly compressed on all sides, quickly expel some of the spirits in them, and take some blood from these tiny mouths. This could never happen if blood could flow back through the large opening of the pulmonary artery. Thus, its return through this great hole being blocked, and being compressed on every side, some of it filters into the arteries through these small pores.

At this point a few words have to be said about sources of confusion in the translations of the Galenical writings. In regard to this historical background of the circulation, they have to do with interpretations of such key words as pneuma and arteries.

Pneuma was a part of the Stoic doctrine. The word 'pneuma' as a technical term was originally used by Chrysippus (281–201 BC). It was meant to signify the 'active principle' as opposed to the 'passive principle'. The active principle was made up of the contents and qualitative elements of all matter. In a philosophical tone, active principle imparted life and purpose to the universe. It made sure that preordained development was fulfilled. On the other hand, the passive principle had no character of its own. It was unqualified and dormant matter, being merely the recipient of the characteristics of the active principle.

Most often, pneuma was represented as being composed of air and fire. This was part of Empedocles' doctrine of the four elements: air, fire, water and earth. These were the root of things in Stoic doctrine. Occasionally, however, pneuma was used as a synonym for air which in turn was used as a synonym for 'breath'. Departure from its original stoical definition created an ambiguity that led to confusion among translators of the early Grecian works. Galen's writings were not immune so that when Galen referred to 'life-giving spirit' translators assumed that he meant air rather than the Stoic term itself. Galen never meant that pneuma carried by the arteries was air. He was referring to the vital spirit mixed with the blood in the arteries.

Another source of confusion was the term 'artery'. Initially the term was used to designate the trachea and bronchi which were thought to be the conduits for the transport of ambient air to the heart (pneuma). When, later, dissections revealed that some of the vessels originating from the heart were found to be empty of blood, they too were called arteries, the implication being that they were primarily carriers of pneuma.

Be that as it may, Galen still passed on to posterity several errors that were difficult to correct because of the lack of courage on the part of innumerable generations of physicians to challenge the entrenched authority of Galen. Although Galen agreed with Erasistratus regarding the anatomical basis for the distribution throughout the body of each of the three spirits (natural, vital and animal), he departed from Erasistratus when he affirmed that blood was carried in the arterial system as well as in the venous. This major point of disagreement was not in error but his anatomical explanation for the presence of blood in the arteries most certainly was: Galen contended that the blood within the right ventricular chamber was transmitted to the left ventricular chamber via invisible pores in the interventricular septum. These along with the other pulmonary arterial-venous pores assured the mixing of the pneuma arriving from the lungs. Since Galen did not view the heart as a true muscle, he introduced another error by claiming that the mixed blood in the left ventricular chamber was sucked into the aorta and arteries through the 'pulsific' properties of these vessels. The third error so clearly stated by Cournand was that

> inspired air in some form or other, or some quality derived from air, was transferred from the lung through the venous artery into the left cavity of the heart by means of the diastolic active dilatation of the left ventricle, and that there was a movement of waste products in the opposite direction, from left ventricle to the lung through which they were expired[15].

Cournand ends this passage with a quotation from Galen as expressed in the translation by C.G. Kühn[16]:

> The venous artery [pulmonary vein] has no advantage of being closed since it has rather the mission of letting pass from the heart into the lungs the sooty residues which the natural heat necessarily produces in that organ [the heart] and which have no shorter means of exit. This discharge is made possible by the comparative weakness of the mitral valve.

Still, in another segment of his *Opera Omnia* (De usu partium 6, X), his views on the movement of blood within the lungs are as follows:

> If the great orifice of the arterial vein were always open, and if Nature had not invented a

means for alternately closing it and opening it at appropriate times, the blood would not penetrate into the pulmonary arteries on contraction of the thorax. When the thorax contracts, the pulmonary arteries with their veinlike structure, crowded and pushed from all sides with great force, instantly expel the Pneuma which they contain and in return are filled through these narrow channels with particles of blood … as it is, the blood, finding its passage cut off through the great orifice of the arterial vein on the side of the heart penetrates in the form of minute drops into the arteries … otherwise the blood would always be coming and going, to no purpose and without end like tides in a strait[16].

This all seems rather confusing. At one point Galen describes the movement of blood as an ebbing and flowing; and yet, in another paragraph he talks of blood penetrating the 'pulmonary arteries' (our pulmonary veins) in the form of 'minute drops' because otherwise the blood would be coming and going without purpose. Cournand cites Fleming as showing that Galen's usage of the metaphor of ebb and flow was his means of illustrating 'the kind of absurdity that nature would not fall into'[15,17]. My own conception of what Galen is trying to say is that the movement of blood simulates somewhat the segmental mixing of intestinal contents known to occur in the intestinal tract prior to their transmission from one segment to another. This is not ebb and flow but rather a temporary halt of movement while the pertinent physiological activities go on.

If this be so, then Galen, although definitely obscure on this point, may have also antedated the discovery in 1661 of the pulmonary capillaries when he wrote of invisible pores between the pulmonary arteries and the pulmonary veins. The previously quoted passages do suggest these pores as a coexisting pathway rather than having the blood move from right to left only through the interventricular septum.

Ironically, Key mentions a little-known fact, namely, that Galen subsequently abandoned the idea that a significant amount of blood passed through the pores in the interventricular septum[3]. Even more ironic is that it was this particular point in Galen's schema that came under attack later on, especially by Harvey.

As Galen's system percolated throughout the civilized portion of the European and African

continents it was made known eventually to the Moslem physicians through Avicenna's famous *Canon*. We have already met Avicenna in Chapter 1 regarding his contributions to anatomical knowledge. The general impression is that Avicenna swallowed all of Galen's teachings without reservation. This is not so, according to Muhammad Ilyas[18]. Although Avicenna (Ibn Cena) was for the most part a strict adherent of Galenical doctrine he did not support Galen's concept of blood passing through the pores of the interventricular septum. Ilyas states that Avicenna did believe that a communication existed between the atria but only in infancy and via the foramen ovale rather than septal pores[18]. Ilyas also states that Avicenna postulated the circulation of blood in the extremities through arterial-venous anastomoses. The validity of these claims must rest on the accuracy with which Ilyas translated Avicenna's words. Since Arabic is the native language of Ilyas, I can reasonably assume that Ilyas had no difficulty either in interpreting or translating this section of the *Canon*.

Unquestionably, however, the first true challenge to Galen among the early Moslem physicians was the one proposed by Ibn al-Nafis regarding the pulmonary circulation. Ibn al-Nafis was the precursor of the Renaissance man. This Damascene physician born in 1210 was also a philosopher, linguist, Moslem theologian and rhetorician. Though it is probable that, like his contemporaries, his medical 'bible' was Galen's writings, he rejected the great master's invisible pores in the interventricular septum while accepting the existence of such pores in the pulmonary vascular tree. Nafis contended that the blood passed through these pores during its passage in the lungs and entered the left ventricle via the pulmonary vein. This was a major departure in emphasis from the views of Galen who was rather obscure on the significance of the pulmonary arterial pores. There can be no equivocation on what Nafis was saying as this passage from his manuscript so clearly states: 'The blood passes through the vena arteriosa to the lung, spreads through its substance, mixes with the air and becomes completely purified; then it passes through the arteria venosa to reach the left chamber of the heart'[19]. The pores turned out to be the capillary communications between the arterial and venous sides of the pulmonary circulation.

The mere fact that Ibn al-Nafis thought of this was not only a manifestation of a learned man's brilliant insight but also a daring assault on

Galenical doctrine. The manuscript wherein his views were expressed was entitled *Commentary on the Anatomy of Avicenna's Canon*. The following words illustrate his departure from Galen's authority: 'We had to rely on statements made by our predecessors in this field, particularly Galen whose books were by far the best in this respect, except in a few points which we suspect were errors committed by scribes, or information obtained by him that was not the result of actual experimentation'[12]. The wording is rather polite and even deferential but without equivocation.

Figure 1 is a page from the manuscript of Ibn al-Nafis describing the lesser circulation.

Was it insight alone that led Ibn al-Nafis to describe the pulmonary circulation so accurately or did he do so on the basis of his own dissections? That he did practice dissection can be inferred from his description of a method for suffocating animals by immersing them in a 'liquid to avoid exterior lesions while obtaining the engorgement of the veins'[20].

In a letter to the editor of *The Lancet*, S.A. Khulusi of the Bodleian Library of Oxford asserted that Ibn al-Nafis was not alone in his description of the lesser circulation. He claimed that Ibn al-Quff (1233–86), a contemporary of Ibn al-Nafis, also explained the function of the 'capillaries' between the pulmonary arteries and veins. He attributed the conclusions reached by al-Quff to pure logic based on anatomical observations. He also marveled at the ability of al-Quff to conceptualize this relationship 400 years before Malpighi demonstrated the very existence of such capillaries with the microscope. He concluded his letter by stating that al-Quff was also aware of the unidirectional function of the cardiac valves and those in the veins[21–23].

Be that as it may, it is the *Commentary* by Ibn al-Nafis[24] that has enjoyed the historical limelight rather than the comments of al-Quff. Since this is so, the burning question is when did the *Commentary* become available to the Western World?

This is important in determining the priorities of description and the sources for such description by the luminaries of the 16th century. These men were Servetus, Valverde, Colombo and Cesalpino. Did they arrive at their conclusions independently of Ibn al-Nafis, of each other, or did they rely on the *Commentary* for their views? Moreover, Moslem translators claim that it was this document that initiated the antigalenical trend at the University of Padua in the 16th century. If this be true it was

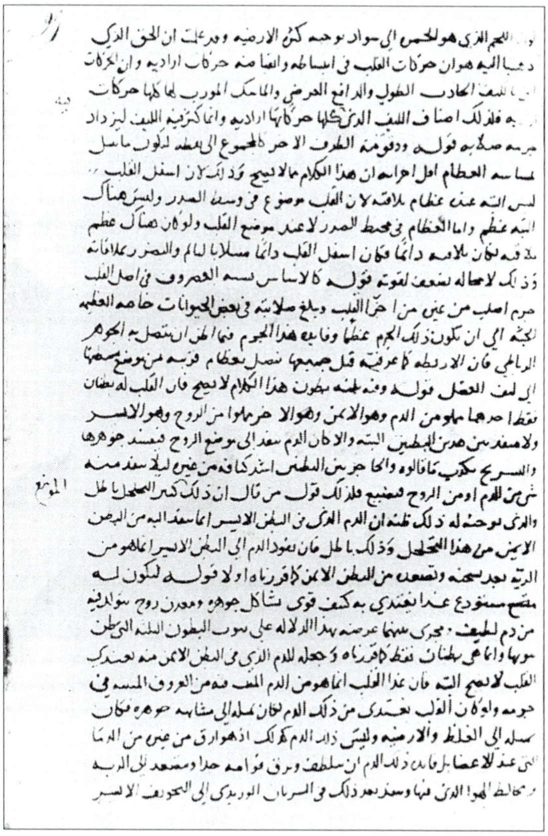

Figure 1 A page from the manuscript of Ibn al-Nafis, describing the lesser circulation. *Photo Source University of Central Florida. Literary Source Fonds arabe. no. 2939.f.95r. This was found in Ghaliourrgui P: Four landmarks of Egyptian cardiology. Journal of the Royal College of Physicians, vol. 18, no.3, p.185, July,1984. Taken from Fonds arabe, no. 2939.f. 95r. Bibliotheque Nationale. With Permission from Bibliotheque Nationale*

known to the Western world long before 1922 when it was 'discovered' by Muhyi el din At Tatawi, an Egyptian medical student. He came across the manuscript among the archives of the Prussian State Library while researching the literature in preparation for his baccalaureate thesis in medicine for the University of Freiburg[25].

There is no doubt that the Damascene physician described the pulmonary vascular circuit in the 13th century. The date of his manuscript speaks for itself. The question is why did Western medicine have to wait until the 16th century before the pulmonary circulation was described *de novo* or was it really *de novo*? The answer probably lies in the fate that usually befalls documents rarely understood or read by Westerners. This could have been the case with the *Commentary*. Nafis' manuscript, written in the Arabic tongue, could have come into the hands of some unknown scholars, consigned to the various 'home libraries' of these scholars, copied and transferred probably to other libraries, remaining buried in the stacks of these repositories of silent knowledge, and rediscovered serendipitously as in the case of the Egyptian medical student.

The pivotal point here could be the translation of the *Commentary* by Andrea Alpago. On the other hand, Arabic may have been more widely understood and known than we are inclined to believe. Even Vesalius apparently knew the language if his translation of Rhazes is true as reported by Jalili[26]. A.Z. Iskandar catalogued in 1967 Arabic manuscripts on medicine and science. They are in the Wellcome Historical Medical Library. Among them is a manuscript of Ibn al-Nafis describing the lesser circulation. It is now housed in the Paris Bibliothèque Nationale[27]. This is similar to the other manuscript found by Tatawi at the Prussian State Library. The presence of these two manuscripts in the libraries of the Western world offers circumstantial evidence that these or others, yet to be discovered, may have been known by Servetus and those who immediately followed him.

Of course, this is pure speculation on my part, but as Coppola states:

> Future research along these lines eventually may show that the theory of the pulmonary circulation propounded by Ibn an-Nafis in the thirteenth century was not forgotten, and that centuries after his death it may have influenced the direction of the anatomical investigations of Colombo and Valverde, who finally announced it to the Western world as a physiological fact susceptible to experimental proof[28].

To return to more concrete facts, the translation of the *Commentary* by Albago appeared in Venice in 1547. Unfortunately, it does not contain the section concerned with the anatomy, and this, according to Cournand, is rather crucial to the hypothesis that Albago was the link between the 16th century anatomists and Ibn al-Nafis[29]. Coppola, however, in my opinion, advances enough evidence in his essay to substantiate a linkage of sorts, though tenuous at best[30].

Andrea Albago is sometimes called Andrea Bongajo or Mongajo[31]. He was born in Belluno around 1450 from a family that was part of the minor nobility. He received his doctorate in medicine from the University of Padua.

Albago spent many years in Damascus and over this period of time he became quite familiar with the Arabic language. His duties were confined to the medical needs of the Venetian consulate in Damascus. In accordance with the times, Albago exercised his brand of nepotism by having as his assistant his own nephew Paolo, who, in the eyes of a Venetian consul, was a physician of 'very little experience'[32]. At any rate, Wüstenfeld depicts Albago as having acquired an excellent knowledge of Arabic, and that with the help of his nephew, he collected, translated and edited the works of various Arabic medical writers[33]. After 33 years of absence he and his nephew returned to their homeland carrying with them all the Arabic manuscripts they had collected during this time.

Although Albago's translation does not contain any reference to the anatomy, a crucial point, nevertheless, there is enough evidence to indicate that he had read other works of Ibn al-Nafis. Coppola is inclined towards this view. 'It is evident that Albago knew of Ibn al-Nafis, that he had read his exposition on the fifth canon of Avicenna, his exposition on the book of Samarcandi, and that he was familiar with certain of Ibn an-Nafis' ideas concerning the cardiovascular system. Beyond this we cannot go. If he had read Ibn an-Nafis' account of the pulmonary circulation, he makes no mention of it'[34]. Despite these remarks, he goes on to say, however, and with this I do agree, that Albago's long sojourn in the East makes it reasonable to assume that he may have come across this account. Although it has not been found as yet, there is a possibility that among the unpublished manuscripts of Albago, many of which over successive generations became widely scattered, there may yet be found one that translates Ibn al-Nafis' description of the lesser circulation.

Another key to a possible linkage may also lie in Paolo, the elder Albago's nephew who, after his uncle's death, enjoyed an esteemed position of his own at Padua. Paolo's activities at Padua may have been sufficient in themselves to transmit the teachings of al-Nafis to Vesalius and Colombo. Intrigued by these revelations, these men could have delved into the matter further with observations of their own.

Did Michael Servetus know about the *Commentary*? Why not? He was at Padua for a time and had access to the translation by Albago and to the academic discussions on campus. If this be so, then why did Servetus not acknowledge his sources. According to Binet and Herpin, acknowledgement of this kind was not generally followed at this time[35]. Meyerhof offers the following comment in this regard: 'It is as though the Arabic work had been translated a bit freely into Latin'[36]. This comment was provoked by Meyerhof's discernment that certain essential phrases in the writings of Servetus and Ibn al-Nafis resembled each other quite closely. This is what Chehade had to say: 'Attention has recently been called in the writings of Ibn al-Nafis to a description of the lesser circulation which is strangely reminiscent (even word for word) of the description given by Michael Servetus in the 16th century in his 'Christianismi Restitutio'[37].

Haddad, 19 years before, had already attempted a linkage when he noted a similarity between the writings of Servetus and Ibn Nafis' *Epistle on the Perfect Man*. 'He who reads the work of Servetus cannot help noticing that it is almost a literal translation of a passage in Ibn Nafis' *Epistle on the Perfect Man*[38]. Although the Epistle does not describe the pulmonary circulation at all, the implication is that if Servetus knew of this work, he was no doubt familiar with the *Commentary*. This appears to me to be a reasonable assumption. Temkin was quite certain, however, that Servetus was completely ignorant of the existence of the *Commentary* either in the original or in the later translation by Albago[39].

All debate aside, the first description of the pulmonary circulation to appear in print in the West was that of Michael Servetus. This was in 1553. The next to appear was that of Valverde in 1556. Colombo's description appeared in 1559. Juan Valverde's description appeared in a book on anatomy written in Spanish. He was a prosector for Colombo, and in this book he acknowledges Colombo as being the source of his description of the pulmonary circulation. An Italian translation of this book was published the same year that Colombo's *De re Anatomica* appeared. Twelve years later, Andrea Cesalpino, a pupil of Colombo, reiterated in his monograph *Quaestionum Peripateticarum* what his mentor had said[40,41]. The word circulation is found for the first time in this publication. Cesalpino was referring to the circular motion of the blood as observed with his experiments with vein ligatures similar to those of Harvey. In his second book, *Quaestionum Medicarum*, published 22 years after his first, Cesalpino emphasized again the important role of the cardiac valves and the pumping characteristics of the ventricles[41].

It is generally believed that Colombo and Servetus attained their knowledge of the pulmonary circulation independently of each other. Coppola states that at best the evidence for plagiarism on the part of either one is purely speculative. In fact, at no time did Colombo ever attribute any obligation to Servetus. Was this because of the cloud of heresy surrounding Servetus? It is because of this that the finger of plagiarism was pointed at Colombo. After all, they were contemporaries and did have Vesalius as a common link. On the other hand, some authors contend that Colombo could not have read any part of the *Restitutio*. This is hard to believe since not all the copies of the monograph were destroyed. Moreover, preprinted copies were also available[42].

Servetus is a sad figure – an outstanding intellectual who dared to oppose the powerful theological bigots of the time and who became a martyr in the process. His outspoken views were in support of religious reformation and the newly emerging movement against the doctrine of the Holy Trinity. Even while being consumed by flames he had the courage of his conviction by exclaiming 'Jesus, son of the Eternal God' rather than 'Jesus, the Eternal son of God'[43].

Miguel Servede was born into a family of lawyers in the province of Navarre, Spain in 1511. He was first and foremost a philosopher-theologian and only secondarily a physician. While in the service of Carlos V of Spain, Servetus had already expressed in seven books his views against the trinitarian doctrine. This cost him the support of his family and regal patron. He left Spain and worked for a while in a printer's shop in France under the pseudonym 'Villanovanus'. On the basis of his recompilation of Ptolemy's geography, Servetus established a reputation in this field, and because of this he was invited to lecture on the subject in Paris. It was during this time that he was befriended by an elderly physician, a Dr. Champier, who guided him through his medical studies. He counted among his teachers Sylvius, Fernel, and Guenther of Andernach. It was at this time that he met Vesalius who was also a student of Guenther.

There is some confusion as to whether or not Servetus accompanied Vesalius when the latter left Paris for Padua. Michel and Donath think so but Cournand says there is no binding evidence[11,42]. To me this is an important detail since if Servetus did go to Padua he would have had the opportunity (as we have seen) of becoming acquainted with Nafis' work on the pulmonary circulation.

Regardless of how Servetus came to describe the pulmonary circulation, his views were outlined in the suicidal theological work that he called *Christianismi Restitutio*. Although it was published anonymously, it was well known that he and he alone was the author. He was soon charged by both the Calvinists and the Roman Inquisition with heresy and in a very short time he was burned at the stake for his opposition to established Christian doctrine. There is a stone tablet in Geneva, marking the spot where Servetus died for his beliefs. He therefore shares with Girolamo Savonarola of Florence a martyrdom at the altar of religious expression. Figure 2 is the title page of Christianismi Restitutio. The photograph is taken from a copy preserved at the Bibliothèque Nationale in Paris. Of the thousand books printed, only three authentic copies are extant, all others either destroyed or lost. Servetus, himself, died with a copy in his hand. The copy housed in the National Library in Paris is said to have belonged to Colladin, a friend of Calvin, and the chief witness against Servetus. How it wound up in the archives of the National Library is unknown. Its existence was revealed by an Englishman, Wolton, more than a century after the death of Servetus … He saw the copy with his own eyes only after having obtained a transcription of it from an English surgeon[44].

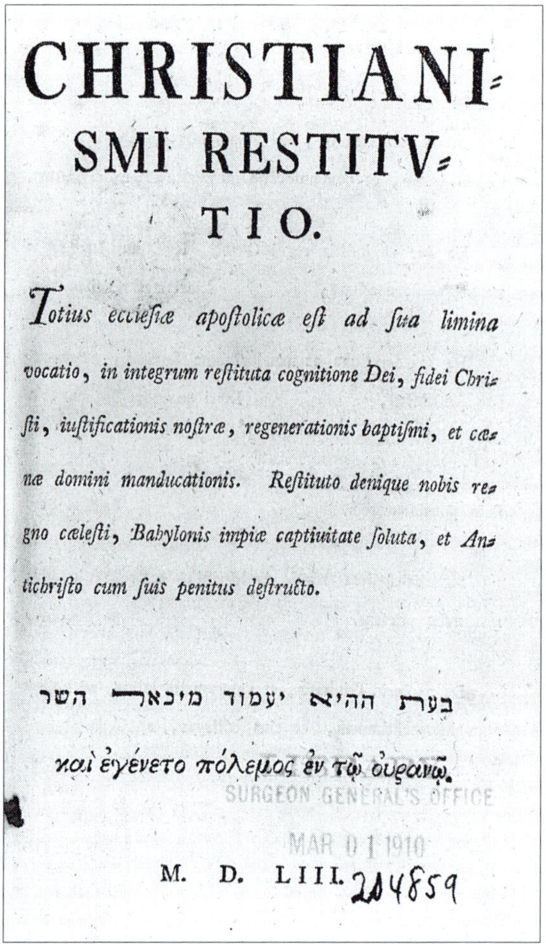
CHRISTIANI-
SMI RESTITV-
TIO.

Totius ecclesiæ apoſtolicæ eſt ad ſua limina vocatio, in integrum reſtituta cognitione Dei, fidei Chri- ſti, iuſtificationis noſtræ, regenerationis baptiſmi, et cœ- næ domini manducationis. Reſtituto denique nobis re- gno cœleſti, Babylonis impiæ captiuitate ſoluta, et An- tichriſto cum ſuis penitus deſtructo.

בעת ההיא יעמוד מיכאל השר

καὶ ἐγένετο πόλεμος ἐν τῷ οὐρανῷ.

M. D. LIII.

Figure 2 Title page of 'Christianismi Restitutio' by Michael Servetus. *Photo Source National Library of Medicine. Literary Source Photo Archives (copy of original). Courtesy of National Library of Medicine*

The passage that is important to us is in chapter V. It was translated by C.D. O'Malley and it reads as follows[45].

> It is not said that the divine spirit is principally in the walls of the heart, or in the body of the brain or of the liver, but in the blood, as is taught by God Himself in Gen. 9, Levit. 8, Deut. 12.
>
> In this matter there must first be understood the substantial generation of the vital spirit which is composed of a very subtle blood nourished by the inspired air. The vital spirit had its origin in the left ventricle of the heart, and the lungs assist greatly in its generation. It is a rarefied spirit, elaborated by the force of heat, reddish-yellow (flavo) and of fiery potency, so that it is a kind of clear vapor from very pure blood, containing in itself the substance of water, air, and fire. It is generated in the lungs from a mixture of inspired air with elaborated, subtle blood which the right ventricle of the heart communicates to the left. However this communication is made not through the middle wall of the heart, as is commonly believed, but by a very ingenious arrangement the subtle blood is urged forward by a long course through the lungs; it is elaborated by the lungs, becomes reddish-yellow and is poured from the pulmonary artery into the pulmonary vein.

Then in the pulmonary vein it is mixed with inspired air and through expiration it is cleaned of its sooty vapors. Thus finally the whole mixture, suitably prepared for the production of the vital spirit, is drawn onward to the left ventricle of the heart by diastole.

That the communication and elaboration are accomplished in this way through the lungs we are taught by the different conjunctions and the communication of the pulmonary artery with the pulmonary vein in the lungs. The notable size of the pulmonary artery confirms this; that is, it was not made of such sort or of such size, nor does it emit so great a force of pure blood from the heart itself into the lungs merely for their nourishment; nor would the heart be of such service to the lungs, since at an earlier stage, in the embryo, the lungs, as Galen teaches, are nourished from elsewhere because those little membranes or valvules of the heart are not opened until the time of birth. Therefore that the blood is poured from the heart into the lungs at the very time of birth, and so copiously, is for another purpose. Likewise, not merely air, but air mixed with blood, is sent from the lungs to the heart through the pulmonary vein; therefore the mixture occurs in the lungs. That reddish-yellow color is given to the spiritous blood by the lungs; it is not from the heart.

In the left ventricle of the heart there is no place large enough for so great and copious a mixture, nor for that elaboration imbuing the reddish-yellow color. Finally, that middle wall, since it is lacking in vessels and mechanisms, is not suitable for that communication and elaboration, although something may possibly sweat through. By the same arrangement by which a transfusion of blood from the pulmonary artery to the pulmonary vein occurs in the lung. If anyone compares these things with those which Galen wrote in Books VI and VII, *De usu partium*, he will thoroughly understand a truth which was unknown to Galen.

The last paragraph reveals only too clearly that the break from Galen was not complete 'although something may possibly sweat through' when Servetus refers to the interventricular septum: Servetus had no idea that he would go down in posterity as one of the discoverers of the pulmonary circulation. The passage just quoted was merely incidental to his main theme, the Trinity. He was strongly influenced by the ancient ideas of pneuma (or spiritus in Latin), and he used them as a theological point of departure for his main theme. Unwittingly, his theological views caused his death but it was his physiological concept of the lesser circulation that remained as his legacy.

Apart from the anatomical basis of his description, Servetus recognized the importance of ambient air in the production of the vital spirit and that the act of respiration was an important element in the process. This relationship was clarified even more by Realdo Colombo in his book *De re Anatomica*, and also by his protege, Valverde.

Colombo's contributions were anticipated by his pupil, Juan Valverde. As already noted, Valverde's original description, in Spanish, appeared three years before that of Colombo. Did Valverde try to upstage his mentor? There is some controversy about Valverde's role, revolving especially about his self-perception and his relationship to Colombo.

Bainton affirms that Valverde presented his teacher's concepts as his own[46]. He cites as an example Valverde's brazen declaration that he was the first to point out the lack of pores in the interventricular septum: '... but no blood passes from one ventricle to the other, as they say who have written of it until now'[47]. Of course, we all know otherwise. In fact, in Chapter 1 we have already seen how Vesalius was the first among the Renaissance anatomists to depart from Galen on this matter. Coppola, however, feels that the following passage reveals Valverde's acknowledgement that Colombo was the source of his inspiration: 'All that is useful that will result from this book of mine, is not less to be attributed to Andreas Vesalius, than to Realdo Colombo, my preceptor in this faculty'[48,49].

Valverde's close collaboration with Colombo is revealed by another passage wherein he refutes the Galenical notion that the pulmonary vein contains pneuma:

> According to all those who have written before me, the function of the pulmonary artery is that of nourishing the lungs, and the function of the pulmonary vein is to bring air from the lungs to the left ventricle of the heart, it appearing to them that there could not be blood in this vein under any circumstance. But, if they had experimented on this, as I have done many times with Realdo, both in live animals and in dead ones, they would have found that this

vein is no less full of blood than is any other vein[50].

The relationship to respiration is delineated clearly in the following sentence:

> I believe with certainty that the blood oozes from the pulmonary artery into the substance of the lung where it is thinned and prepared in order to be more easily converted into spirit. It is then mixed with air which, entering through the branches of the trachea, accompanies it to the pulmonary vein and thence to the left ventricle of the heart. Here it is mixed with the somewhat thicker blood which passes from the right ventricle of the heart to the left, if any at all does pass.

In this passage, Valverde does not mention Colombo as the source or collaborator, but it must have originated with Colombo as his *De re Anatomica* reveals.

De re Anatomica was published posthumously. Where Valverde equivocated or appeared to be still somewhat hesitant to free himself completely from the shackles of Galen, his mentor, Colombo was much more certain of his position. Colombo's description attests to this quite clearly:

> Between these ventricles there is a septum through which almost everyone believes there opens a pathway for the blood from the right ventricle to the left, and that the blood is rendered thin so that this may be done more easily for the generation of vital spirits. But they are in great error, for the blood is carried through the pulmonary artery to the lung and is there attenuated; then it is carried, along with air, through the pulmonary vein to the left ventricle of the heart. Hitherto no one has noticed this or left it in writing, and it especially should be observed by all[51].

De re Anatomica not only recognizes the impermeability of the interventricular septum but also denies unequivocally Galen's doctrine of the excretion of sooty vapors by the trachea via the pulmonary vein while emphasizing that the lungs contained arterial blood. Figure 3 depicts the frontispiece of *De re Anatomica* libri XV, 1559.

De re Anatomica consists of fifteen books. Actually only the first book can be correctly called a book. The others are really chapters, some of them only a few pages in length. Book seven deals with the pulmonary circulation and book fourteen contains observations obtained at vivisection. The publication was based on more than one thousand autopsies spanning a period of fourteen years, and on numerous vivisections performed on dogs. It was published during the Renaissance, a time in Italy blessed with an increasingly amiable relationship between church and science; so much so that Colombo dedicated book 14 to Pope Paul IV.

Matteo Realdo Colombo was born in Cremona, the son of an apothecary. Initially, he was to follow in his father's footsteps, but while pursuing the study of philosophy and liberal arts at Milan, his interests turned to surgery. At that time no formal academic degree was necessary to enter the surgical ranks. An apprenticeship with a surgeon, however, was required. Colombo's father was friendly with the eminent Venetian surgeon, Giovanni Plato, and because of this young Colombo was placed with him to fulfill this requirement. After spending seven years with Plato, Colombo went to Padua to pursue his medical studies. It was there that Colombo met Vesalius, and soon became his prosector.

There was evidently at first a relationship of mutual respect and affection between Colombo and his mentor, Vesalius. In the first edition of the *Fabrica*, Vesalius refers to Colombo as *mihi admodum familiaris Realdus Columbus, nunc sophistces apud Patavinos professor, Anatomes studiosissimus*[52]. This relationship cooled considerably over the succeeding years, so much so, that in the second edition of the *Fabrica*, Vesalius no longer refers to Colombo in such friendly terms. This, no doubt, had something to do with the fact that Vesalius held two chairs of surgery at Padua and with the progress of Colombo up the academic ladder.

Under the patronage of an important university authority, Joannes Schilinus, Colombo was selected to replace Vesalius for the second chair. Colombo was denied the position by the Venetian Senate possibly because of opposition from Vesalius who did not want to vacate it. Colombo did succeed to the chair later, but only by a stroke of luck. This occurred when Vesalius was in Basel away from his teaching duties, and Colombo was appointed on an interim basis to teach anatomy during this absence. The appointment gave Colombo the opportunity to display his proficiency so that soon after, when Vesalius left Padua permanently, the Venetian Senate elected Colombo as lecturer in anatomy and surgery.

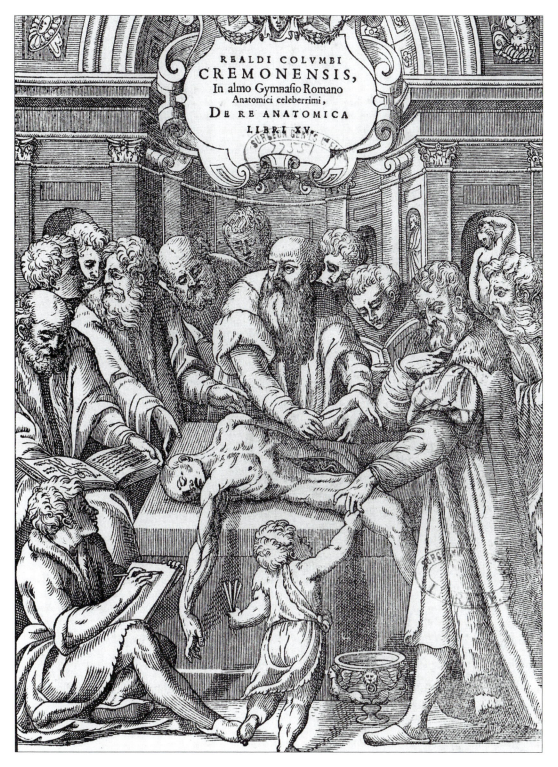

Figure 3 Frontispiece of De re Anatomica, libri XV by Realdi Columbi Cremonensis. *Photo Source National Library of Medicine. Literary Source Photo Archives (copy of original). Courtesy of National Library of Medicine*

191

Colombo held this position for less than the two years stipulated by his contract. He left to assume the chair of anatomy at the University of Pisa, newly reorganized under the patronage of the duke of Tuscany, Cosimo Medici. Colombo thus became the first full-time teacher of anatomy at Pisa[53]. In just two years, however, Colombo left Pisa for Rome, at first temporarily and then permanently. Cosimo I allowed him to do so initially because Colombo's intent for traveling to Rome was to enlist the services of Michelangelo. Colombo was preparing at the time his *De re Anatomica*, a book that was intended to correct many of the errors of the *Fabrica*, and that was to surpass Calcar's illustrations with anatomical drawings by the great Michelangelo himself[54]. This dream was never realized. Colombo returned to Pisa and remained for only a short time. He left again for Rome where he taught at Sapienza until his death in 1559.

As Tollin so aptly put it, Colombo was not the simpleton that Vesalius stated him to be, neither was he a genius as had been suggested by Harvey's admirers. 'He was highly critical not only of earlier authorities in his field, but he also criticized Vesalius – his master – for his description of the muscles. 'Unlike Aristotle who considered the heart to be the most important organ of the human body, Colombo advocated the primacy of the brain'[57].

The last of the Paduan anatomists to be involved with the pulmonary circulation prior to Harvey was Andrea Cesalpino. As a pupil of Colombo he was thoroughly grounded in anatomy and dissection. After his master's death he continued to expand anatomical knowledge with his own studies at the dissecting table. As stated previously, he was the first to use the term 'circulation'. The passage in his *Quaestionum Peripateticarum* containing the word circulation reads as follows:

Therefore the lung draws the warm blood from the right ventricle of the heart through a vein resembling an artery [the pulmonary artery] and returns it through the venous artery [the pulmonary vein] to the left ventricle of the heart ... To this *circulation* of the blood from the right ventricle of the heart through the lungs into the left ventricle of the same, [the findings] from dissection fully correspond ... Thus the whole system is beautifully ordered. Since it is necessary to have heat in the blood of the heart in order to bring about the perfection of the

nutriment ... blood is transmitted from the right side of the body to the left, partly through the septum and partly through the inner tissue of the lungs, for the sake of being cooled[56].

This book was published in 1571. He wrote another book that was published in 1593 and entitled *Quaestionum Medicarum*. It too mentions the pulmonary circulation. Notice, though, that he still felt that part of the blood passed through the septum.

Cesalpino's writing style was ponderous and vague. Some historians claim that he came close to Harvey in importance. This is disputed by others who regard him as merely another figure in the long line of Paduan anatomists, and one too slavishly devoted to Aristotle, thus precluding any originality of thought on his part[57,58].

There is still another figure that immediately preceded Harvey's revelations. He is Carlo Ruini, a relatively unknown figure in medical circles but apparently appreciated by veterinarians. He is remembered by them for his book on *The Anatomy and Diseases of the Horse*. Originally published in 1598, shortly after Ruini's death, the book apparently was widely acclaimed by the veterinarians for whom it was intended and republished well into the 18th century. He stated in this book that the function of the right ventricle was to propel the blood and nourish the lungs while the function of the left ventricle was to receive the blood from the lungs and send it to the rest of the body[59-61].

Almost three decades of the 17th century had to pass before one of the most significant contributions to medicine made its appearance. It did so in a very quiet fashion with no indication at all that it would change significantly and forever the face of cardiovascular physiology. The contribution came in the form of a slender book, badly printed and on poor paper. It came from the presses of William Fitzer of Frankfort, Germany. The year was 1628, the author was William Harvey and its title was *De Motu Cordis*. The book represented a distillation of thought based on observations from controlled and repeated experiments that once and for all demolished the entrenchment of galenical error in cardiovascular physiology. Harvey was able to incorporate the teachings of others into a comprehensive system that logically defined and delineated the physiological mechanisms of the circulation based on scientifically derived data. This in essence was Harvey's unique contribution.

William Harvey first saw the light of day in 1578 in the coastal fishing town of Folkstone. His father was a yeoman farmer and landowner who later in life joined the ranks of the gentry as a result of his gainful pursuits in commerce. The effects of the Renaissance were all about him at the time of his birth and the age he was to live in was to be one of even greater tumult and achievement. Shakespeare's maturity coincided with Harvey's youth. Tintoretto and Rembrandt were to pour out their souls in their magnificent paintings. Galileo was a contemporary from whom Harvey learned about the circulatory motion of planets and the importance of quantification and measurement [62].

As a youngster, Harvey acquired the usual public school background in classics while attending the King's school at Canterbury in Kent. He then enrolled at Gonville and Caius College, Cambridge, as a commoner. Almost immediately he became the recipient of a Mathew Parker scholarship. After being awarded a Bachelor of Arts in 1597 Harvey remained at Cambridge for another two years before enrolling at Padua. At that time, Padua was one of the leading universities of the continent. It had developed as an offshoot of the University of Bologna, but for more than two centuries it basked in the limelight of its own prestigious faculty in medicine, especially anatomy. Among them were the men we have already met in the dismantling of Galen's hold on the pulmonary circulation. It was here that Harvey enjoyed also an intellectual association with Gabriel Fallopius and Girolamo Fabricius of Aquapendente.

Padua was a student-controlled university. The students elected the instructors as well as the Rector, and had the last word on the curriculum. Cambridge, on the other hand, was under the control of the faculty and for this reason it was referred to as a 'Magistral University' [63]. Padua's fame was such that it attracted students from many nations. This ethnic diversity caused fellow countrymen to group together in order to protect and foster their own interests. Harvey was elected to be the English students' 'Consilarius'. Although Harvey was described as being short tempered and inclined to be choleric, his personality must have still been engaging enough to have caused him to be selected by his fellow Englishmen as their representative.

Harvey spent several years at Padua, receiving his doctorate in physic from there in 1602. That same year he returned to England where he received his doctoral degree in medicine from Cambridge. The diploma from Padua is interesting. In typical Italian hyperbole, it states how Harvey had shown such skill, memory and learning that he had 'far surpassed even the great hopes that his examiners had for him' [64].

While at Padua young Harvey was one of the most diligent students of Fabricius of Aquapendente. Later on Harvey was to acknowledge the enormous influence this brilliant man had on his thinking. During his tenure Fabricius continued to perpetuate Padua's reputation as a great school of anatomy. It was difficult to fill the shoes of such notable predecessors as Vesalius, Colombo and Cesalpino, but Fabricius did so quite admirably. In relationship to Harvey, perhaps, the most notable of Fabricius' contributions was his description of the valves in the veins. He was not the first to know of their existence since Vesalius already knew about them, ascribing their discovery to Canano. What was important, as Harvey, himself, told Robert Boyle, the noted chemist, years later, was that Fabricius' work on the venous valves was the source of Harvey's interest in the nuances of the circulation [65].

William Harvey began to practice medicine in London. Although I do not intend to detract in any way from Harvey's ability, his social and professional standing were no doubt aided by his marriage to the daughter of Lancelot Browne, physician to Queen Elizabeth and James I. In a few short years he was elected to the Royal College of Physicians and appointed physician to St. Bartholomew's Hospital where he remained for thirty-six years. The succeeding years saw him appointed Lumleian lecturer, an honor that he held for 41 years. In due time, he also became physician-in-ordinary to Charles I. This last position was to prove to be both a benefit and a detriment when for a time the vicissitudes of political turmoil and his loyalty to the king found him in the ranks of the undesirables [66].

Throughout his rise to these positions of prominence Harvey was actively engaged in research and in the process of formulating his views on the circulation. Although he first presented his concepts at the Lumleian lecture delivered in 1616, it was not until 1628 when he finally felt secure enough in his views to allow his book to be published. His tenets were succinctly worded in his introduction when he affirmed that incorrect beliefs should be made right by anatomical study, repeated experimentation, and careful observation [67].

Despite the fact that the book appeared without fanfare, it soon stirred up a great deal of controversy, especially among the Galenists of the day. One of the most vitriolic of the critics was the Parisian anatomist, Jean Riolan, who, to his dying day, refused to give up the erroneous teachings of Galen[68]. Many years later William Hunter also tried to demolish Harvey's image when he said:

> Harvey's rank must be low indeed. So much had been discovered by others that little more was left for him to do than to dress it up into a system; and that required no extraordinary talent. Yet, easy as it was, it made him immortal. But none of these writings show him to have been a man of uncommon abilities[69].

Harvey referred to his critics as 'crack-brained' and believed that most of the criticism was due to envy rather than scientifically based opposition. Harvey was fortunate in that he lived long enough after the publication of his book to realize as Hobbes (a friend) says in his book *De Corpore*: 'He is the only man perhaps that ever lived to see his own doctrine established in his own lifetime'[69,70].

William Harvey was noted for his contemplative nature. It seems he was always curious about anatomical facts, and especially appreciative of the relationship between structure and function. His book *De Insectis* illustrates this very clearly. It took many years to prepare, being based on numerous dissections. Indeed, prior to becoming the Lumleian lecturer, Harvey had already dissected and observed more than eighty species of animals[71]. Many of Harvey's early papers were destroyed depriving us of much needed information as to his other contributions. Harvey was an intense loyalist and throughout the rebellion against Charles I, he remained with his king suffering as a consequence the loss of many of his belongings and papers. When his important papers on comparative anatomy were destroyed by the Puritan forces, he commented in a tone of resignation, so alien to his temperament: 'Let gentle minds forgive me, if recalling the irreparable injuries I have suffered, I here give vent to a sigh'. However, much later in life, he did manage to compile his views on embryology and comparative anatomy in a book entitled *Exercitationes de Generatione Animalium*. This was just six years before his death at the age of 79[72–76]. Figure 4 is the title page of this work which some consider as the forerunner of modern embryology.

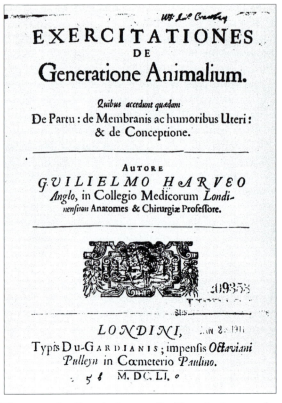

Figure 4 Frontispiece of 'Exercitationes de Generatione Animalium' by William Harvey. *Photo Source National Library of Medicine. Literary Source Photo Archives (copy of original). Courtesy of National Library of Medicine*

Aubrey, who knew Harvey well, wrote a very interesting and personalized life that is both entertaining and incisive in its revelations[77–79]. He describes how Harvey's penmanship and Latin were both bad. '*The Circuitis Sanguinis* (Circulation of the Blood) was, as I take it, done into Latin by Sir George Ent'[77]. Aubrey also brings out how Harvey loved to spend time contemplating in the dark. He went so far as to have caves made in the earth surrounding a house he owned in Surrey so that he could enter them in the summertime and meditate away from the distractions of the outside world. Although not a bigot or consciously arrogant, he was still 'wont to say that man was but a great, mischievous baboon'. His views on womanhood would not set well with the feminists of today. 'He would say that Europeans knew not how to order or governe our woemen, and that the Turks were the only people used them wisely … I remember he kept a pretty young wench to wayte on him, which I guesse he made use of for warmth-sake as King Daniel did, and tooke care of her in his will, as also of his manservant'[77].

Aubrey also describes him as 'not tall, but of the lowest stature, round faced, olivaster complexion; little Eie, round, very black, full of spirit; his haire was black as a Raven, but quite white 20 years before he dyed'.

Anatomy was no doubt his forte, since accounts of his therapeutic ability leave much to be desired. Again, we are indebted to Aubrey for this description:

All his Profession would allow him to be an excellent anatomist, but I never heard of any that admired his therapeutic way. I knew several practisers in London that would not have given 3d for one of his Bills; and that a man could hardly tell by one of his Bills what he did aime at. (He did not care about Chymistrey, and was wont to speake against them with an undervalue.

For a good part of his adult life, Harvey suffered greatly from the gout. His method for obtaining relief during an acute episode was quite unique to say the least. He would place his legs in a pail of cold water until 'he was almost dead with cold and then betake himself to his stove, and so t'was gone'[77]. There is an erroneous perception that Harvey might have died from an overdose of opium, taken because of a particularly painful episode. The truth of the matter is that he had a stroke and ended his days in this manner. Aubrey was at his funeral and helped to carry him into the vault[76,80–82]. The Royal College of Physicians removed his remains from the family vault in 1883. They now lie in a grand sarcophagus in Hempstead Church, Essex. The epitaph reads:

The Remains of William Harvey
Discoverer of the Circulation of the Blood
Were Reverentially Placed in this Sarcophagus by
The Royal College of Physicians of London
in the Year 1883.

Figure 5 is a portrait of William Harvey. The artist did manage to convey the piercing eyes in a scowling face. The close relationship between Harvey and his king is revealed in Figure 6 depicting Harvey explaining the circulation of blood to Charles I. Figure 7 is a photograph of the frontispiece of Harvey's *Anatomica de Motu Cordis et Sanguinis*. There are seventeen chapters in all.

Harvey's motives for writing the book are outlined in Chapter 1 entitled *The Authors Motives for Writing:*

When I first gave my mind to vivisections, as a means of discovering the motions and uses of the heart, and sought to discover these from actual inspection, and not from the writings of others, I found the task so truly arduous, so full of difficulties, that I was almost tempted to think, with Fracastorius, that the motion of the heart was only to be comprehended by God. For I could neither rightly perceive at first when the systole and when the diastole took place, nor when and where dilatation and contraction occurred, by reason of the rapidity of the motion, which in many animals is accomplished in the twinkling of an eye, coming and going like a flash of lightning; so that the systole presented itself to me now from this point, now from that; the diastole the same; and then everything was reversed, the motions occurring, as it seemed, variously and confusedly together. My mind was therefore greatly unsettled, nor did I know what I should myself conclude, nor what believe from others; I was not surprised that Andreas Laurentius should have said that the motion of the heart was as perplexing as the flux and reflux of Euripus had appeared to Aristotle.

At length, and by using greater and daily diligence, having frequent recourse to vivisections, employing a variety of animals for the purpose, and collating numerous observations, I thought that I had attained to the truth, that I should extricate myself and escape from this labyrinth, and that I had discovered what I so much desired, both the motion and the use of the heart and arteries; since which time I have not hesitated to expose my views upon these subjects, not only in private to my friends, but also in public, in my anatomical lectures, after the manner of the Academy of old.

These views, as usual, pleased some more, others less; some chid and calumniated me, and laid it to me as a crime that I had dared to depart from the precepts and opinion of all anatomists; others desired further explanations of the novelties, which they said were both worthy of consideration, and might perchance be found of signal use. At length, yielding to the requests of my friends, that all might be made participators in my labours, and partly moved by the envy of others, who, receiving my

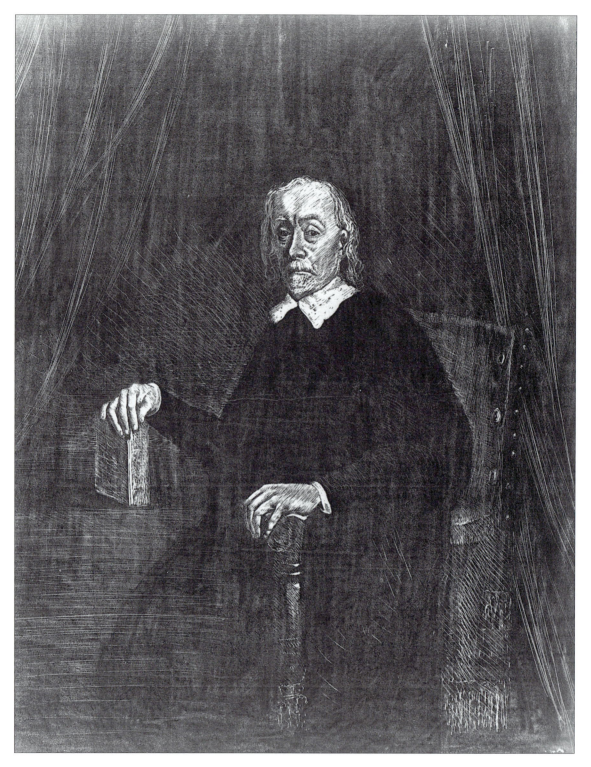

Figure 5   Portrait of William Harvey. *Photo Source National Library of Medicine. Literary Source Photo Archives. Courtesy of National Library of Medicine*

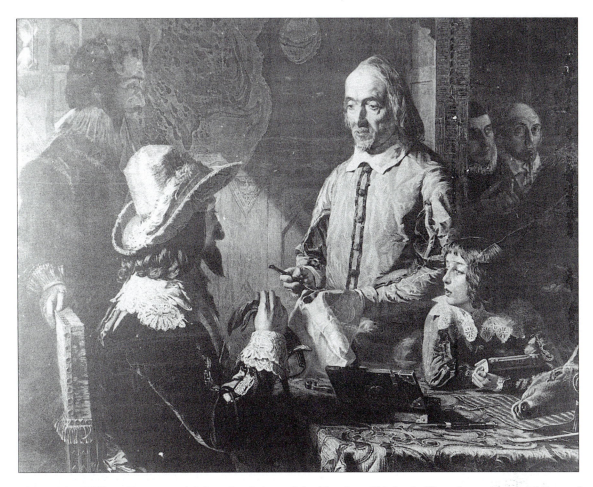

Figure 6 William Harvey explaining circulation of the blood to Charles I. *Photo Source National Library of Medicine. Literary Source Photo Archives. Courtesy of National Library of Medicine*

views with uncandid minds and understanding them indifferently, have essayed to traduce me publicly, I have been moved to commit these things to the press, in order that all may be enabled to form an opinion both of me and my labours. This step I take all the more willingly, seeing that Hieronymus Fabricius of Aquapendente, although he has accurately and learnedly delineated almost every one of the several parts of animals in a special work, has left the heart alone untouched. Finally, if any use or benefit to this department of the republic of letters should accrue from my labours, it will, perhaps, be allowed that I have not lived idly, and, as the old man in the comedy says:

For never yet hath any one attained
To such perfection, but that time, and place,

And use, have brought addition to
his knowledge;
Or made correction, or admonished him,
That he was ignorant of much which he
Had thought he knew; or led him to reject
What he had once esteemed of highest price.

So will it, perchance, be found with reference to the heart at this time; or others, at least, starting from hence, the way pointed out to them, advancing under the guidance of a happier genius, may make occasion to proceed more fortunately, and to inquire more accurately[83].

He arrived at a formulation of the general principles of the circulation in a truly scientific manner. His experiments were all simple but critical and models of design. Harvey's time at

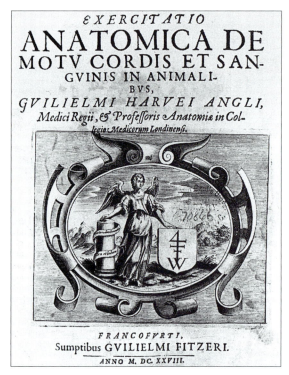

Figure 7 Frontispiece of 'Anatomica de Motu Cordis et Sanguinis' by William Harvey. *Photo Source National Library of Medicine. Literary Source Photo Archives. Courtesy of National Library of Medicine*

Padua exposed him to much of Galileo's teachings so that in pursuing his studies he applied the geometrical method of Galileo[84]. It was in the form of a triad consisting of:

(1) analysis of a phenomenon to determine the principle involved,

(2) deduction of its consequences, and

(3) test by further experiment.

After careful analysis of his innumerable observations, he proposed the following schema for the circulation:

It has been shown by reason and experiment that blood by the heat of the ventricles flows through the lungs and heart and is pumped to the whole body. There it passes through pores in the flesh into the veins through which it returns from the periphery everywhere to the center, from the smaller veins into the larger ones, finally coming to the vena cava and right auricle. This occurs in

such an amount, with such an outflow through the arteries and such a reflux through the veins, that it cannot be supplied by the food consumed. It is also much more than is needed for nutrition. It must therefore be concluded that the blood in the animal body moves around in a circle continuously, and that the action or function of the heart is to accomplish this by pumping. This is the only reason for the motion and beat of the heart[67,85].

In writing about the pulmonary circulation, his dissections led him to conclude that the only possible way for blood to enter the pulmonary vein was through the lungs. Since Harvey had no knowledge of the existence of capillaries he reasoned that the blood was pushed through the porous substance of the lung by the forceful action of the lung. He knew there was a communication between the pulmonary arteries and veins similar to the peripheral circulation but he did not know that the anatomical linkage was through capillaries. This had to wait for Malpighi and the microscope. Harvey relied on perfusion experiments to demonstrate the communication. To him, the lungs functioned as a filtering system for the venous blood reaching them from the right ventricle. As to the possibility of pores in the interventricular septum, he was rather vehement when he wrote: 'But, damn it, no such pores exist nor can they be demonstrated'[86].

The physiological basis for the passage of blood through the lungs also escaped him. He relied entirely on Galen when he wrote that the 'hot blood is carried to and through the lungs, to be tempered by the inspired air, and to be freed from bubbling to excess'. He later modified these views somewhat in his *Exercitationes de Generatione Animalium* when he wrote: 'Those who consider more closely the nature of air will, I think readily grant that air is given to animals neither for cooling nor as a nutriment'[87]. Just four years before the publication of this book, he had already broken away from the doctrine of pneuma. In his second disquisition to Riolan he had written:

Persons of limited information, when they are at a loss to assign a cause for anything, very commonly reply that it is done by the spirits … Some speak of corporeal, others of incorporeal spirits; and they who advocate the corporeal spirits will have the blood, or the thinner portion of the blood, to be the bond of union with the soul, the spirit being contained in the blood as the flame is in the smoke of a lamp or candle, and held admixed by the incessant motion of the fluid ... There is nothing more uncertain and questionable, then, than the doctrine of the spirits ...[88]

Harvey proved that mathematically it was impossible for the blood in the body to do anything but circulate. This is what he had to say about it:

Let us assume, either arbitrarily or from experiment, the quantity of blood which the left ventricle of the heart will contain when distended, to be, say, two ounces, three ounces, or one ounce and a half ... Let us assume further how much less the heart will hold in the contracted than in the dilated state; and how much blood it will project into the aorta upon each contraction ... and let us suppose as approaching the truth that the fourth, or fifth, or sixth, or even but the eighth part of its charge is thrown into the artery at each contraction; this would give either half an ounce, or three drachms, or one drachm of blood as propelled by the heart at each pulse into the aorta ... Now in the course of half an hour, the heart will have made more than one thousand beats ... Multiplying the number of drachms propelled by the number of pulses, we shall have either one thousand half ounces, or one thousand times three drachms, or a like proportional quantity of blood, according to the amount which we assume is propelled with each stroke of the heart .... a larger quantity in every case than is contained in the whole body![89]

Harvey revised and reformulated the old splanchnic circulatory scheme. Though, in doing so, he still adhered to the galenic concepts of innate heat produced by the heart and all the three forms of pneuma (animal, vital and natural), he substituted the heart for the liver as the center of the vascular system. 'Just as the king is the first and highest authority in the state, so the heart governs the whole body!'

As far as the cerebral circulation was concerned, he used its largeness to refute the notion that the function of the right ventricle was to nourish the lungs. 'It is altogether incongruous to suppose that the lungs need for their nourishment so large a supply of food, so pulsatorily delivered, and also so much purer and spiritous (as being supplied directly from the ventricles of the heart). For they cannot need such more than the extremely pure substance of the brain'[90].

Harvey was also cognizant of the role of the coronary circulation. When Riolan objected to the existence physiologically of a two-fold system (pulmonary and systemic) Harvey wrote in *De Circulatione Sanguinis*:

It was possible for the learned gentleman here to add a third, very short circulation; namely, from the left ventricle to the right one driving a portion of the blood round through the coronary arteries and veins, which are distributed with their small branches through the body, walls and septum of the heart,

and later,

for what should the coronary arteries pulsate in the heart save to drive blood on by that impulse? And why should there be coronary veins except to acquire blood from the heart? Add further that a valve is very commonly found in the opening of the coronary vein preventing entry into it, but favouring egress from it. So a third circulation must certainly be admitted by one who admits a general circulation passing through both lungs and brain[91].

Finally, his entire schema of the circulation was solidified by a series of observations utilizing the simple technique of ligation and the demonstration that the valves in the veins functioned in a unidirectional manner preventing the return of blood from whence it came (Figure 8). He noted that the heart became purple and dilated when the aorta was compressed with a tight ligature, and remained so until the ligature was released. A tight ligature on the arm could also effectively obliterate the pulse below it and, at the same time, render the hand cool. These two maneuvers are a testimonial to his exquisitely designed and simple experiments. No enormous governmental grants were needed nor was there a lack of confidence in the observations because of the absence of modern technological gadgetry. The full impact of Harvey's simple and yet brilliant approach can be appreciated even more by carefully reading the few paragraphs devoted to how the blood finds its way back to the heart. It is in Chapter XIII:

Thus far we have spoken of the quantity of blood passing through the heart and the lungs in

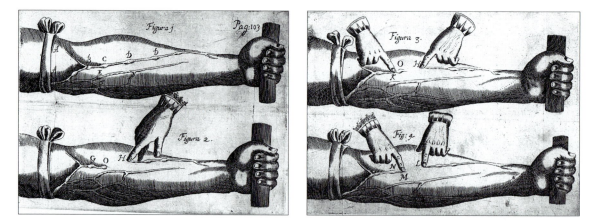

Figure 8   Illustrations (Figures 1–4) from folding leaf in Harvey's 'De Motu Cordis'. *Photo Source Mayo Medical Library. Literary Source The 1643 edition owned by the Mayo Medical Library. Courtesy of the Mayo Medical Library*

the center of the body, and in like manner from the arteries into the veins in the peripheral parts and the body at large. We have yet to explain, however, in what manner the blood finds its way back to the heart from the extremities by the veins, and how and in what way these are the only vessels that convey the blood from the external to the central parts; which done, I conceive that the three fundamental propositions laid down for the circulation of the blood will be so plain, so well established, so obviously true, that they may claim general credence. Now the remaining position will be made sufficiently clear from the valves which are found in the cavities of the veins themselves, from the uses of these, and from experiments cognizable by the senses.

The celebrated Hieronymus Fabricius of Aquapendente, a most skilful anatomist, and venerable old man, or, as the learned Riolan will have it, Jacobus Sylvius, first gave representations of the valves in the veins, which consist of raised or loose portions of the inner membranes of these vessels, of extreme delicacy, and a sigmoid or semilunar shape. They are situated at different distances from one another, and diversely in different individuals; they are connate at the sides of the veins; they are directed upwards or towards the trunks of the veins; the two for there are for the most part two together regard each other, mutually touch, and are so ready to come into contact by their edges, that if anything attempt to pass from the trunks into the branches

of the veins, or from the greater vessels into the less, they completely prevent it; they are farther so arranged, that the horns of those that succeed are opposite the middle of the convexity of those that precede, and so on alternately.

The discoverer of these valves did not rightly understand their use, nor have succeeding anatomists added anything to our knowledge: for their office is by no means explained when we are told that it is to hinder the blood, by its weight, from all flowing into inferior parts; for the edges of the valves in the jugular veins hang downwards, and are so contrived that they prevent the blood from rising upwards; the valves, in a word, do not invariably look upwards, but always towards the trunks of the veins, invariably towards the seat of the heart. I, and indeed others, have sometimes found valves in the emulgent veins, and in those of the mesentery, the edges of which were directed towards the vena cava and vena portae. Let it be added that there are no valves in the arteries [save at their roots], and that dogs, oxen, etc., have invariably valves at the division of their crural veins, in the veins that meet towards the top of the os sacrum, and in those branches which come from the haunches, in which no such effect of gravity from the erect position was to be apprehended. Neither are there valves in the jugular veins for the purpose of guarding against apoplexy, as some have said; because in sleep the head is more apt to be influenced by the contents of the carotid arteries. Neither are the valves present, in order that the blood may be retained in the divarications of smaller trunks and minuter branches, and not to be suffered to flow entirely into the more open and spacious channels; for they occur where there are no divarications; although it must be owned that they are most frequent at the points where branches join. Neither do they exist for the purpose of rendering the current of blood more slow from the center of the body, for it seems likely that the blood would be disposed to flow with sufficient slowness of its own accord, as it would have to pass from larger into continually smaller vessels, being separated from the mass and fountain head, and attaining from warmer into colder places.

But the valves are solely made and instituted lest the blood should pass from the greater into the lesser veins, and either rupture them or cause them to become varicose; lest, instead of advancing from the extreme to the central parts of the body, the blood should rather proceed along the veins from the center to the extremities; but the delicate valves, while they readily open in the right direction, entirely prevent all such contrary motion, being so situated and arranged, that if anything escapes, or is less perfectly obstructed by the cornua of the one above, the fluid passing, as it were, by the chinks between the cornua, it is immediately received on the convexity of the one beneath, which is placed transversely with reference to the former, and so is effectually hindered from getting any farther.

And this I have frequently experienced in my dissections of the veins: if I attempted to pass a probe from the trunk of the veins into one of the smaller branches, whatever care I took I found it impossible to introduce it far any way, by reason of the valves; whilst, on the contrary, it was most easy to push it along in the opposite direction, from without inwards, or from the branches towards the trunks and roots. In many places two valves are so placed and fitted, that when raised they come exactly together in the middle of the vein, and are there united by the contact of their margins; and so accurate is the adaptation, that neither by the eye nor by any other means of examination can the slightest chink along the line of contact be perceived. But if the probe be now introduced from the extreme towards the

more central parts the valves like the floodgates of a river, give way, and are most readily pushed aside. The effect of this arrangement plainly is to prevent all motion of the blood from the heart and vena cava, whether it be upwards towards the head, or downwards towards the feet, or to either side towards the arms, not a drop can pass; all motion of the blood, beginning in the larger and tending towards the smaller veins, is opposed and resisted by them; whilst the motion that proceeds from the lesser to end in the larger branches is favoured, or, at all events, a free and open passage is left for it.

But that this truth may be made the more apparent, let an arm be tied up above the elbow as if for phlebotomy (A,A, Figure1) [See Figure 8 for Figures 1 through 4 in quoted chapter]. At intervals in the course of the veins, especially in labouring people and those whose veins are large, certain knots or elevations (B,C,D,E,F) will be perceived, and this not only at the places where a branch is received (E,F), but also where none enters (C,D): These knots or risings are all formed by valves, which thus show themselves externally. And now if you press blood from the space above one of the valves, from H to O (Figure 2), and keep the point of a finger upon the vein inferiorly, you will see no influx of blood from above; the portion of the vein between the point of the finger and the valve O will be obliterated; yet will the vessel continue sufficiently distended above that valve (O,G). The blood being thus pressed out, and the vein emptied, if you now apply a finger of the other hand upon the distended part of the vein above the valve O (Figure 3), and press downwards, you will find that you cannot force the blood through or beyond the valve; but the greater effort you use, you will only see the portion of vein that is between the finger and the valve become more distended, that portion of the vein which is below the valve remaining all the while empty (H,O, Figure 3).

It would therefore appear that the function of the valves in the veins is the same as that of the three sigmoid valves which we find at the commencement of the aorta and pulmonary artery, viz., to prevent all reflux of the blood that is passing over them.

Farther, the arm being bound as before, and the veins looking full and distended, if you press at one part in the course of a vein with the point of a finger (L, Figure 4), and then with another finger streak the blood upwards beyond the next valve (N), you will perceive that this portion of the vein continues empty (L N), and that the blood cannot retrograde, precisely as we have already seen the case to be in Figure 2; but the finger first applied (H, Figure 2, L, Figure 4), being removed, immediately the vein is filled from below, and the arm becomes as it appears at D C, Figure 1. That the blood in the veins therefore proceeds from inferior or more remote to superior parts, and towards the heart moving in these vessels in this and not in the contrary direction, appears most obviously. And although in some places the valves, by not acting with such perfect accuracy, or where there is but a single valve, do not seem totally to prevent the passage of the blood from the center, still the greater number of them plainly do so; and then, where things appear contrived more negligently, this is compensated either by the more frequent occurrence or more perfect action of the succeeding valves or in some other way: the veins, in short, as they are the free and open conduits of the blood returning to the heart, so are they effectually prevented from serving as its channels of distribution from the heart.

But this other circumstance has to be noted: The arm being bound, and veins made turgid, and the valves prominent, as before, apply the thumb or finger over a vein in the situation of one of the valves in such a way as to compress it, and prevent any blood from passing upwards from the hand; then, with a finger of the other hand, streak the blood in the vein upwards till it has passed the next valve above, the vessel now remains empty; but the finger being removed for an instant, the vein is immediately filled from below; apply the finger again, and moving in the same manner streaked the blood upwards, again remove the finger below, and again the vessel becomes distended as before; and this repeat, say a thousand times, in a short space of time. And now impute the quantity of blood which you have thus pressed up beyond the valve, and then multiplying the assumed quantity by one thousand, you will find that so much blood has passed through a certain portion of the vessel; and I do now believe that you will find yourself convinced of the circulation of the blood, and of

its rapid motion. But if with this experiment you say that a violence is done to nature, I do not doubt but that, if you proceed in the same way, only taking as great strength of vein as possible, and merely remark with what rapidity the blood flows upwards, and fills the vessel from below, you will come to the same conclusion[86].

Let us turn our attention now to the evolution of further knowledge regarding the passage of blood through the lung. The pulmonary circulation was now clearly outlined in the broadest of terms. The anatomical confirmation of the existence of the capillaries was supplied by Marcello Malpighi (see Chapter 1). What was needed now was someone to correlate the existing information with the minutiae of respiration. That is, what was the *raison d'être* for the passage of blood through the lungs? Almost three hundred years were to elapse before the complete physiological role of the pulmonary circulation would be finally delineated. During this time, knowledge evolved as a result of the contributions of physicists and chemists as collated and interpreted by physiologists. In due time, physiology was to develop as a separate disclipine and establish itself as the motherlode of cardiovascular knowledge.

Although Malpighi demonstrated that the alveoli communicated with both the bronchi and the pulmonary capillaries, he did not suspect the true function of this anatomical arrangement.

Concerning the use of the lungs, I know that many views are held from the ancients onwards, and about them there is very much dispute especially about the cooling which is taken to be the principle purpose when it strives with the imagined excessive heat of the heart, which may require eventation; wherefore these things have made me diligently inquisitive in the investigation of another purpose, and from these things which I subjoin I can believe that the lungs are made by nature for mixing the mass of blood[92].

Richard Lower picked up the clue eight years after Malpighi's description. This is how he reported his findings:

For if the trachea (of a dog) is exposed in the neck and divided, a cork inserted and the trachea ligatured tightly over ... then the blood flowing from a simultaneous cut in the cervical artery will be seen as completely venous and dark in colour as if it had flown from a wound in the jugular vein

… This being so we must next see to what the blood is indebted for this deep red colouration … If the anterior part of the chest is cut away and the lungs are continuously insufflated by a pair of bellows inserted into the trachea and they are also pricked with a needle in several places to allow free passage of air through them, then, on the pulmonary vein being cut near the left auricle the blood will flow completely bright red in colour[93].

He concluded from these observations that 'this red color is entirely due to the penetration of particles of air in to the blood'.

Richard Lower was at first a pupil and then a research associate of Thomas Willis. Throughout his earlier years at Oxford he was associated with that brilliant group of Oxonian natural scientists that included not only Willis but also Boyle, Black and Wren. Upon leaving Oxford, he settled in London where he developed a quite successful practice. His political affiliations, however, ultimately caused the loss of his position as the court physician and a large portion of his practice, forcing his retirement to Cornwall. As a confirmed Whig, he suffered when James II succeeded to the throne.

His treatise *Tractatus de Corde* appeared in 1669. It contained the first experimental study of the heart after Harvey[94]. In it he described the arrangement of the muscle fibers in the ventricles, and how exercise increased the heart rate, attributing the increase in blood flow, however, to the pumping action of the skeletal muscles. He also described the movement of chyle and how edema could be produced by ligating the veins. Lower was one of the first to transfuse blood from a dog into a man[95].

The color of the blood is the subject of the second portion of the subtitle of the treatise. It was based on both *in vivo* and *in vitro* experiments. The affinity of venous blood for air (later identified as oxygen) was demonstrated by a simple *in vitro* experiment[96,97].

Indeed, if the cake of blood is turned over after remaining stationary for a long while, its outer and uppermost layers takes on the red colour in a short space of time (provided the blood is still fresh). It is a matter of common knowledge that venous blood becomes completely red when received into a dish and shaken up for a long time to cause a thorough penetration of air into it.

On this account it is extremely probable that the blood takes in air in its course through the lungs, and owes its bright colour entirely to the admixture of air. Moreover, after the air has in large measure left the blood again within the body and the parenchyma of the viscera, and has transpired through the pores of the body, it is equally consistent with reason that the venous blood, which has lost its air, should forthwith appear darker and blacker.

Lower first made known his interest in the effect of air on blood in a letter to Robert Boyle in 1664[98]. Five years later, and after much investigation he published *De Corde* (see Figure 9) in the hope that there was now sufficient evidence to substantiate the thesis that the function of the pulmonary circulation was to add a substance to venous blood. He thought the substance found in air was a nitrogenous gas calling it 'spiritus aeris nitrosus'. In his introductory paragraph, he acknowledges his previous erroneous beliefs and his intention not to 'attack the opinions and beliefs of others, or to bring scorn on myself by challenging my own, but what is suggested by reason and confirmed by experience carries more weight with me and always have my allegiance'.

He is also quite candid and honest in acknowledging his indebtedness to Robert Hooke for help in conducting a crucial experiment by 'keeping the lungs continually dilated for a long time without meanwhile endangering the animal's life'. It was this experiment that led him to realize that he was wrong when he had written earlier 'about blood withdrawn from the pulmonary vein being like venous blood'. At that time 'all the air had been forced out of the lung before I was able to seize and to lance the pulmonary vein'.

If you ask me for the paths in the lungs, through which the nitrous spirit of the air [spiritus aeris nitrosus] reaches the blood, and colours it more deeply, do you in turn show me the little pores by which that other nitrous spirit, which exists in snow, passes into the drinks of gourmets and cools their summer wines. For, if glass or metal cannot prevent the passage of this spirit, how much more easily will it penetrate the looser vessels of the lungs? Finally, if we do not deny the outward passage of fumes and of serous fluid, why may we not concede an inward passage of this nitrous foodstuff into the blood through the same or similar little pores?

On this account it is extremely probable that the blood takes in air in its course through the

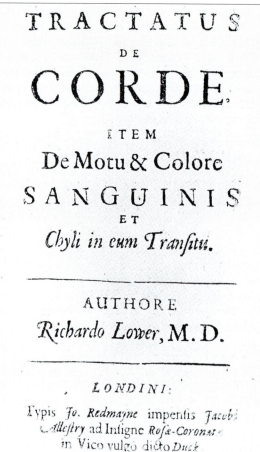

TRACTATUS

DE

CORDE,

ITEM

De Motu & Colore

SANGUINIS

ET

Chyli in eum Transitu.

AUTHORE

Richardo Lower, M.D.

LONDINI:

Typis Jo. Redmayne impensis Jacob: Allestry ad Insigne Rosæ-Coronæ in Vico vulgo dicto Duck lane. MDCLXIX

Figure 9 Title page of 'Tractatus de Corde' by Richard Lower. *Photo Source National Library of Medicine. Literary Source Lower R.: Tractatus de Corde. Allestry, London, 1669. Courtesy of National Library of Medicine*

lungs, and owes its bright colour entirely to the admixture of air. Moreover, after the air has in large measure left the blood again within the body and the parenchyma of the viscera, and has transpired through the pores of the body, it is equally consistent with reason that the venous blood, which has lost its air, would forthwith appear darker and blacker.

From this it is easy to imagine the great advantage accruing to the blood from the admixture of air, and the great importance attaching to the air taken in being always healthy and pure; one can see, too, how greatly in error are those, who altogether deny this intercourse of air and blood.

Without such intercourse, any one would be able to live in as good health in the stench of a prison as among the most pleasant vegetation. Wherever, in a word, a fire can burn sufficiently well, there we can equally well breathe[93,99].

The disciplines of physics and chemistry were needed to give substance to Lower's views. The chemists were already looking for a unifying agent to replace the traditional concept of the four elements. They were replaced by a mythical universal chemical agent called phlogiston which was released into the ambient air during the course of combustion. No one saw it, no one measured it. It was as ethereal as its theoretical roots. Van Helmont of Belgium (1566–1644) had already labeled it 'gas sylvestre'. Cornelius Drebbel (1527–1633) prepared a gas capable of maintaining life by decomposing potassium nitrate (nitre), a well-known fertilizer and explosive.

This was the uncertain complex of ideas that the awesome collection of brilliant men had to unravel during the golden period of the natural sciences at Oxford. Lower thought the substance was a nitrogenous gas (his spiritus aeris nitrosus) but his contemporaries at home and abroad were to zero in on the true nature of this vital substance.

Robert Boyle played an ancillary role at this time both as Lower's teacher and through his own experiments which delineated in a more precise fashion the physical properties of air and its role in combustion and respiration.

Singer called the second half of the 17th century the era of physical experiment. Many things happened as a result of this that had ultimately a favorable impact on the elucidation of cardiovascular physiology. Natural phenomena were being scrutinized and explained by experiments exquisitely designed and simple in approach. The vagueness of alchemy was being supplanted with accurate observations. Mathematics and physics were emerging as rigorous disciplines. Boyle was one of the leading natural philosophers of this era which included among so many such great figures as Descartes, Sanctorius, Borelli, Galileo and Kepler. The iatrochemical group also played a prominent role equal in every respect to that of the physicists and mathematicians. It was led by van Helmont of Belgium, Sylvius of Leiden and Willis of Oxford.

Robert Boyle was born in Lismore, County Waterford, Ireland in 1627. He was the 14th child to be born into a family that had wealth and the social advantages of nobility. After having studied in England, France, Switzerland and Italy, he lived for a while in Dorset where he wrote moral essays. One of them is said to have been the source of inspiration for *Gulliver's Travels* by Jonathan Swift.

Boyle was an intensely devout Protestant. His religious beliefs fueled his enthusiasm for experimental science for he was determined to show that the results obtained through experimentation furnished irrefutable proof of the greatness of God. Most of his experimental work was conducted while he was at Oxford between 1656 and 1668. He had the good fortune while there to have as his assistant, an equally brilliant man, Robert Hooke. Using an air pump designed with the aid of Hooke, Boyle carried out a series of experiments that helped delineate the physical properties of air, and the essential role it played in combustion, respiration and the transmission of sound. This work was described in his book *New Experiments Physio-Mechanicall, Touching the Spring of the Air and its Effects*. The first edition appeared in 1660. The second edition which appeared two years later contained his report of 1661 to the Royal Society of London. That is now known to us as Boyle's law. It states that at a constant temperature the volume of a gas is inversely proportional to the pressure.

After leaving Oxford he spent the remainder of his life in London pouring out many scientific and religious writings. Just one year before his death, Boyle presented his theological views in *The Christian Virtuoso*. The work revolved around the theme that the study of nature was a religious duty and oriented towards the adoration of God, the creator of all things. He held to the view that at the beginning of time God set into motion all the natural phenomena and left them to function according to secondary laws which science was able to identify[100].

Among the contemporaries of Boyle, Hooke and Lower, there was a younger man whose role is somewhat controversial. Was he really a brilliant and original thinker who deserves a prominent niche in the evolution of cardiology? Or, was he an extremely capable individual who was quite proficient in assimilating the ideas of others, and unethical enough to present them later on as his own? Most of the balanced information about him was provided by T.S. Patterson[98,101] and J.F. Fulton[102]. This controversial figure is none other than John Mayow.

According to these two historians, many of the comments found in Mayow's *Tractatus duo* and *Tractatus quinque* were presented as his own but were really adopted by Mayow from the works published by Boyle, Hooke and Lower while a contemporary of theirs at Oxford[103,104]. These comments run the gamut from the multiple components of air with the presence of a vital substance similar to that found in nitre and nitric acid to the deduction that this substance (nitro-aerial spirit) was necessary to life. Many of the experiments that he describes in both treatises were really not his own but those of Boyle, Hooke and Lower.

Mayow did legitimately demonstrate, however, two important facts:

(1)   He proved that during respiration there was a reduction in the known amount of air from the donor vessel, and

(2)   He extended the application of Boyle's law to hydrogen and nitric oxide.

Further studies on the properties of air and its relationship to the pulmonary circulation were carried out in the succeeding years by several men. The most prominent among them were Stephen Hales, Joseph Black, Henry Cavendish, Joseph Priestley and Antoine Lavoisier.

Stephen Hales is considered by most scholars as the founder of quantitative gasometry though he is remembered mostly for his blood pressure experiments. The latter are treated in depth in Section 5. Insofar as the pulmonary circulation is concerned he developed several devices that were able to measure the quantity of air 'absorbed or fixed or generated by the breath of living animals'[105]. He was also able to define the site of absorption of the inspired air[106]. In his initial experiment he concluded that:

> … some of the elasticity of air which is inspired is destroyed and that chiefly among the vesicles…whence probably … acid spirits … are conveyed in the blood which we see by an admirable contrivance spread into a vast expanse commensurate to a large surface of air from which it is parted by very thin partitions; so very thin as thereby probably to admit the blood and air particles…within the reach of each other's attraction, whereby a continued succession of fresh air must be absorbed by the blood.

These comments are recorded in the first volume of his *Statical*[107]. When he published the second volume he was able to report the measurements made by direct observation of the rate of flow in the lung capillaries of frogs.

Chemists now moved into the scene with their studies on the characteristics of gas. Experiments by Joseph Black, the Scottish chemist, pointed to the presence of a fixed gas in expired air which later was identified as carbon dioxide. Joseph Priestley, a self-taught chemist, conducted a series of experiments that enabled him to conclude the presence of two types of gas in atmospheric air. These were described in his *Experiments and Observations in Different Kinds of Air*[108]. One gas which he labeled 'dephlogisticated air' allowed a candle to be 'burned with remarkably vigorous flame' and prolonged the life of mice when they were placed in a receptacle containing it. This turned out to be oxygen. The other gas which he named 'phlogisticated air' was later found to be nitrogen. He demonstrated that it was the 'dephlogisticated air' that was essential for the maintenance of life. Unfortunately, he did not extrapolate these findings to what went on at the alveolar-capillary level of the lung. He still adhered to the erroneous concept that 'the function of the blood is not to receive the phlogiston of the air, or to meet with the phlogisticated air while it circulates, but to communicate phlogiston to air'[109].

Moreover, he insisted that respiration and putrefaction were identical. He regarded the act of respiration as being a dephlogistication of phlogisticated air. Venous blood contained the phlogiston and during its passage through the lung the phlogiston was removed. Priestly was too pre-occupied with the phlogiston theory, otherwise he might have learned more about the objective characteristics of oxygen.

A talented Swedish pharmacist by the name of Scheele also isolated a gas in atmospheric air analogous to the 'dephlogisticated air' of Priestley. He called it 'fire air', obviously because it had the same flame supporting property[110]. The properties of this 'fire gas' were described in a lost letter to Lavoisier[111]. It has been suggested that this letter plus a thorough knowledge of Priestley's work put Lavoisier on the path that ultimately led him to resolve the problems of combustion, calcination and respiration[109,111].

Lavoisier's first report was in the form of a sealed note to the Académie des Sciences in 1772[112]. It contained his observations on the weight gained

by sulfur and phosphorous by burning. He ascribed the gain in weight to 'prodigious quantities of air which are fixed'[112]. At a subsequent meeting of the Academy three years later he described his experiments and conclusions regarding the process of calcination[113]. Based on a series of experiments using mercuric red oxide, as suggested by Priestley during a conversation with him, Lavoisier concluded that 'the principle, called up to now 'fixed air', is the combination of the portion of eminently respirable air liberated by heating the calx with the carbon'. This conclusion served as the basis for his idea that respiration was a form of combustion.

In 1777, just two years later, and again, at a meeting of the Academy, he presented his essay on *Experiments on the respiration of animals and on the changes affecting air in its passage through the lungs*[114]. This contained his perception of respiration that was just short of solidification. 'Eminently respirable air that enters the lungs, leaves it in the form of chalky aeriform acid'. He was still not sure as to the source of the 'chalky aeriform acid'. He was of the opinion that the inspired air underwent a reaction in the lung similar to that observed in the combustion of carbon, and that in the process the chalky aeriform acid was formed[115].

His final views on the mechanism of respiratory combustion were expressed in a paper he wrote in collaboration with A. Séguin. It was entitled *Premier Mémoires sur la respiration des animaux*[116]. 'Respiration is a slow combustion of carbon analogous to that operating in a lamp or in a lighted candle, and that from this point of view animals which breathe are really combustible substances burning and consuming themselves ... The atmospheric air supplies the oxygen and the caloric; but since, in respiration it is the substance itself of the animal, the blood which supplies the combustible, if the animals were not replacing usually by food what they lose by respiration, the lamp would be short of oil, and the animal perish, just as the lamp goes out when it lacks nourishment' ... He also held to the view that 'carbonic acid is formed by digestion, introduced in the circulation by lymphatics, finally that reaching the lung, it is released from the blood while oxygen combines with it (the blood) by means of superior affinity'[116].

It took almost another fifty years before Gustav Magnus was able to measure the concentration of oxygen, nitrogen and carbon dioxide in the blood. He found that arterial blood had a higher concentration of oxygen than venous blood whereas venous blood had a higher concentration of carbon dioxide than arterial blood. These observations led him to conclude that combustion occurred in the body tissues and not in the lungs[117].

It should be noted that the comments of Lavoisier include for the first time the word oxygen. He used it as a substitute for the vague phlogiston. He actually called it the 'principle oxygine', meaning that which forms acid. Finally, the vital air of Galen was now known to be oxygen.

In 1760 Albrecht von Haller reported some experiments on the perfusion of frog lungs with dye, that demonstrated greater pulmonary blood flow when the lungs were moderately inflated in contrast to the diminished flow when the lungs were in a collapsed state[118]. These observations gave the first inkling of a definite relationship between pulmonary blood flow and phase of respiration. Haller's conclusions were ardently supported by Francois Magendie more than eight decades later[119].

In 1875 Cohnheim and Litten anticipated our current thinking with respect to alveolar ventilation and capillary perfusion. They noted that there was a marked variability in perfusion and blood volume among the many ramifications of the pulmonary vasculature. This led them to conclude that local blood flow was dependent upon the degree of resistance offered by the lungs in that area[120].

J. Poiseuille (1799–1869), who was both a physicist and physician, was not in accord with the views held by Haller and supported by Magendie. His experiments demonstrated that blood flow was, in fact, slower when the thoracic cage was distended[121]. These disparate views were finally reconciled twenty-one years later by Lichtheim[122]. He proved that natural inspiration and forced insufflation under positive pressure had opposite effects on pulmonary arterial pressure. This was crucial since Poiseuille's conclusions were based on the false premise that an artificially induced positive pressure inflation of the lungs was equal in every respect to inflation produced by natural inspiration of air.

In 1877 Jacques Arséne d'Arsonval, an assistant of Claude Bernard, contributed another bit of evidence in favor of Haller's original thesis. This was just one year after Lichtheim's report. D'Arsonval varied the capacity of the thoracic cage in the intact animal by exerting variable degrees of traction on the diaphragm. Blood was perfused through the inferior vena cava throughout the maneuvers. These experiments constituted the basis of his inaugural thesis and they demonstrated that 'the largest amount of air in the lungs coincides with the largest amount of blood present'[123].

Almost three years later, two Belgian physiologists, Héger and Spehl, also confirmed Haller's observations regarding the degree of pulmonary blood flow and the inflationary status of the lungs[124,125]. Employing a technique devised by Claude Bernard they were able to conduct their experiments in rabbits after closure of their chests, thus simulating natural conditions. They also estimated pulmonary blood volume during inspiration and expiration. It is to their credit that their results were found to be quite accurate when reassessed by more precise methods of quantitation based on anatomical measurements[126].

It is obvious by now that, again, national boundaries were non-existent in the continuing expansion of knowledge regarding the pulmonary circulation. In addition to the preceding personalities other figures emerged during the 19th century that were to contribute one or several significant facts governing the various physiological mechanisms involved with the circulation as a whole. At this juncture we shall continue to explore only those contributions relevant to the pulmonary circulation. The basic ingredients had already been supplied by the previously mentioned investigators of both the 18th and 19th centuries. The remaining contributors of the 19th century were those involved with the further introduction of graphic methods that not only recorded circulatory events but also registered the various phenomena in a quantitative manner. In a sense then, the 19th century could be regarded as the precursor of the technological era of the 20th century. Although relatively crude in retrospect, the graphic methods of the time were harbingers of more precise observations and measurements. The other investigators begin with Carl Ludwig's group in the first half of the 19th century and end with Henderson and his coterie, with part of their work being done in the closing years of the century and the remainder spilling over into the 20th century.

Ludwig's manometer (see Section 5) had already been in use for a few years when one of Ludwig's students, A. Beutner, used it to record the pressures in the pulmonary artery of rabbits, cats and dogs[127]. He found the mean blood pressure in the pulmonary artery to vary between 12 and 23 mmHg. The variability in these presumably normal animals was ascribed to the size of the animal being studied. More importantly, the mean pulmonary arterial pressure was seen to be much lower than the aortic pressure.

We will meet again, in Section 4, two great French physiologists who through their experiments were instrumental in exploring the techniques of cardiac catheterization long before Werner Forssmann. One was a veterinarian by the name of Auguste Chauveau (1827–1917), and the other Etienne Jules Marey (1830–1904), a brilliant Parisian physician, who was to do so much in furthering graphic methods in physiological experimentation (see Section 5)[128]. By virtue of their cardiac catheterization technique they were able to measure the pressures in both the left and right ventricles. The fully-awake horse was their experimental animal. Entry into the right ventricle was gained through the jugular vein while the carotid artery allowed them to gain access to the left ventricle by passing a specially designed catheter in a retrograde fashion. The systolic pressure in the right ventricle was found to measure 27 mmHg; that in the left ventricle averaged 129 mmHg. They also confirmed in later experiments the much lower pulmonary artery pressure in comparison to the aorta.

As a result of these studies, it was now becoming apparent that the pulmonary circulation was harboring many secrets that begged for unveiling. The details of the physiological mechanisms, however, had to await the development of precise methods for the delineation of gas exchange at the alveolar-capillary level.

Germany and Austria now led the way with their cadre of brilliant physiologists well-versed in physics and chemistry. Ludwig's laboratory in Vienna played a singularly important role in fostering these studies and in spawning physiologists of superb stature who would independently and collectively remain on the cutting edge of knowledge in cardiovascular physiology.

As we have seen, Gustav Magnus was the first to show that arterial blood had a higher concentration of oxygen than venous blood and that venous blood, in turn, had a higher concentration of carbon dioxide. The crucial question to be answered was the source of both the oxygen and carbon dioxide. Although Priestley had shown that oxygen was an essential ingredient of atmospheric air, the prevailing opinion at the time was that the oxygen in the blood came from the lung tissue itself.

The initial studies centered about hemoglobin. This proteinaceous element of red blood cells was discovered by Otto Funke in 1851[129,130]. Its affinity for oxygen was established by Lothar Meyer in 1857[131] as part of the intense physiological research being carried out by Carl Ludwig's group in Vienna. Hoppe-Seyler amplified Meyer's findings by demonstrating that the hemoglobin-oxygen combination was a rather loose one, capable of being easily separated[132,133].

But, where did the carbon dioxide come from? Answers to this were provided through the efforts of Mayer, Liebig and Pflüger. In 1845 Mayer had shown that oxidative processes at the systemic tissue level were responsible for providing energy[134]. The chemical components of these processes and part of the spectrum of cellular metabolism were unraveled by Liebig[135]. Pflüger added the final touch to all this in 1872[136].

Another product of Ludwig's laboratory was Christian Bohr of Copenhagen. He, in turn, trained August Krogh and K.A. Hasselbalch, both of whom played an important role along with their mentor in elucidating the physico-chemical basis for gas exchange at the alveolar-capillary level. Bohr worked on the problem of respiratory gas exchange for twenty years, first in Ludwig's laboratory and then in his own laboratory at Copenhagen. The results of these efforts were made known in a paper published in 1904 and written in collaboration with Krogh and Hasselbalch[137]. He erred, however, in still thinking that the blood received its oxygen through active secretion from the pulmonary epithelium[138]. Krogh later realized the error of this conclusion by showing that oxygen passed into blood at the alveolar-capillary level through the simple process of diffusion[139]. This was a major piece in the jig-saw puzzle. Krogh worked on this problem for six years. He was fortunate to have as his collaborator, his wife, Marie. Their paper, jointly co-authored, was published in 1910 under the title *On the rate of diffusion of carbonic oxide in the lungs of man*[139]. This was a pivotal report with far-reaching implications. It proved forever that the pulmonary circulation and the lungs were merely vehicles for the interchange of oxygen and carbon dioxide, and that this occurred at the capillary-alveolar level under certain well-defined physical laws.

As the 20th century evolved, Krogh's student, G. Liljestrand started his own series of experiments on the effects of hypoxia and hypercapnia on pulmonary vascular resistance and pulmonary blood flow. In 1946, he published a paper in conjunction with von Euler that demonstrated an increase in pulmonary vascular resistance in the presence of hypoxia and hypercapnia[140]. He felt that this was the most important mechanism responsible for regulating local vascular resistance. In a paper published two years later he presented the thesis that a homeostatic relationship was maintained between local alveolar ventilation and blood perfusion by virtue of varying the local vascular resistance as mediated by the partial pressure of respiratory gases in both the alveoli and capillary blood[141].

The role of the sympathetic nervous system in the control of pulmonary vascular resistance had also come under investigation during the latter part of the 19th century. The impetus for these studies was provided by the discovery of the sympathetic nerve supply to the lungs by Brown-Séquard in 1972. Badoud was the first to demonstrate a relationship[142]. While working in Fick's laboratory he showed that stimulation of the sympathetic supply produced a rise in pulmonary arterial pressure. Although the importance of this observation was questioned since it was thought to be part of a generalized vasoconstriction and therefore of no local significance, later investigation indicated this reaction might be a key point in the homeostatic mechanisms governing pulmonary blood flow. In retrospect, one can readily see how important blood flow is in transferring the oxygen of inspired air to the blood stream.

Charles Emile Francois-Franck (1849–1921) reinforced Badoud's observations by his method of eliminating the effects, if any, of simultaneous constriction of the systemic arterioles under sympathetic stimulation. He did this by selective stimulation of the sympathetic ganglia and their branches so that only the pulmonary vessels were constricted. His observations were presented at a meeting of the Sociéte de Biologié in 1880[143]. This mode of stimulation produced a rise in the systolic pressure within the right ventricle accompanied by a drop in the left atrial pressure. In order to magnify the pressure recordings form the left atrium, Francois-Franck modified his manometer by merely substituting sodium sulphate for the mercury[144,145].

Francois-Franck also used another graphic method in his experiments, that of oncography, a means of recording variations in the size of an organ[144,145]. This brought out a paradoxical finding that he did not explain in a satisfactory manner. The oncography revealed that there was an increase in pulmonary blood volume during sympathetic stimulation.

During this time two English physiologists were also engaged in experiments on the sympathetic nervous system and pulmonary blood flow. They too reached conclusions identical to those of Francois-Franck. They were the first to notice, in addition, a relationship between pulmonary vascular resistance and deprivation of oxygen. They noted that during asphyxia there was a rise in pulmonary arterial pressure[146]. This could have provided them with the opportunity to place in proper perspective the negligible role of the sympathetic nervous system in controlling pulmonary vascular resistance and hence pulmonary blood flow. Fifty-four years had to elapse before Liljestrand and von Euler formulated with convincing proof the currently accepted hypothesis that the partial pressure of the respiratory gases in the alveoli and capillary blood regulated the vascular resistance and not the sympathetic nervous system.

There are enormous implications in this since it embraces the potential for local vasomotor control capable of adjusting alveolar blood flow to alveolar ventilation. Thus, 'disturbances that can cause local alveolar hypoventilation would automatically divert blood from poorly ventilated areas, thereby protecting the oxygenation of blood'[147]. It is now well known that hypoxia is the most powerful pulmonary vasoconstrictor known with acidosis as an important contributory factor. The exact role of the sympathetic nervous system has yet to be defined. Most recent research points to the possibility that the vasoconstrictive capability of the sympathetic nervous system may come into play as an over-reactive phenomenon in the face of catastrophic pulmonary disturbances such as pulmonary embolism[148].

As the 20th century progressed the limelight of progress now shifted to the British Isles and the USA. Taking advantage of the groundwork established by the giants of continental Europe, four men stand out during this period. They are Haldane, Barcroft, Henderson and Cournand. The first three were basic scientists furthering the nuances of the physical chemistry of blood while

209

Cournand left his mark in the clinical arena through his brilliant advances in cardiac catheterization.

Haldane's work, unfortunately, was marred by his persistent belief that the secretion of oxygen by the lungs was the mechanism by which blood was oxygenated[149]. Apart from this, his brilliant investigations involving carbon dioxide and oxygen, their interrelationship and their role in respiration led to an important discovery regarding the absorption and dissociation of carbon dioxide in blood[150]. The discovery by Haldane and his associates on the effect of oxygenation of blood upon its carbon dioxide dissociation curves was the final factor that led Henderson to conclude that 'every one of the variables involved in the respiratory exchanges of blood must be a mathematical function of all the others'[151].

Joseph Barcroft (1872–1947), a Dubliner by birth, spent most of his career at Cambridge. He measured oxygen dissociation curves and demonstrated the effects of salts and acids on these curves. He is remembered mostly for his splendid contributions in high altitude physiology. Cournand was quite impressed with Barcroft, knowing him personally as part of the spirited circle that met religiously whenever the Physiological Society convened. This is what Cournand had to say of him:

> His enterprise, his free and prolific imagination, and his experimental skill were joined with an unfailing kindness and a whimsical and gay good humor. Barcroft's charming and lovable character set the tone for this entire group of kindred spirits. Their relations were spirited, friendly, stimulating, and argumentative, and they all enjoyed themselves immensely. Who could forget those meetings of the Physiological Society, when Barcroft's little terriers were scampering around the laboratory, their externalized spleens alternately swelling in contentment, or shrinking with excitement; especially when Barcroft would bring forth a cat at an appropriate moment, just to add zest to their canine emotions?[152]

Lawrence J. Henderson (1878–1942) was the American arm of this outstanding triumvirate of basic scientists. For years he worked with his assistants at Harvard, developing the initial concepts of the acid–base balance in biological systems[153–155]. When he had finally outlined the generalities of the system, he entered into a fruitful collaborative relationship with Donald van Slyke of The Rockefeller Institute. After three years of intensive investigation van Slyke and his associates published a monograph which described the system in terms of simple equations[156]. The joint efforts of both Henderson and van Slyke were responsible for putting together all the pieces of the mosaic that constitutes the physico-chemical basis of respiration and its effects on the constituents of the blood.

Henderson described the panorama of respiration as begining at the alveolar-capillary interchange when hemoglobin picks up the oxygen while giving up its carbon dioxide. The entire panoply for the normal state was then summarized by Henderson in the form of a nomogram that took into account the chloride concentration in plasma and cells, cell volume, percent water in cells, base bound to protein, cell and plasma bicarbonate, total CO_2, CO_2 tension, plasma pH, cell pH, respiratory quotient, oxygen tension, oxygen saturation, and hemoglobin concentration. Henderson then developed nomograms that took into account changes that take place during exercise, and many diseased states[157].

Andre F. Cournand has been aptly called the father of clinical cardiopulmonary physiology[158]. He opened the door with his development of right heart catheterization techniques for the systematic study of the pulmonary circulation under natural conditions and without the distortions of anesthesia.

It began while he was chief resident on Dr. Miller's chest service at Bellevue Hospital, Columbia University division. At that time, Cournand was asked by Dr. Miller to develop a laboratory for the study of cardiopulmonary function in normal humans and in patients with pulmonary disease. The details of this mandate and its subsequent course are outlined in Section 5. His contributions to cardiopulmonary physiology were ancillary results of this endeavor, one that was to occupy him for his entire professional career.

Initially, he and Dickinson W. Richards attempted to follow Henderson's proposal for the investigation of gas exchange. This was in 1932. Four years later, and after many frustrations, Cournand learned of Werner Forssmann's self-experiment. When he became convinced of its potential value and safety, he and his colleagues, Richards and Darling, began a systematic investigation of cardiac catheterization as a research tool. He spent four years ironing out the pitfalls using as subjects human cadavers, dogs and also a chimpanzee. It was 1940 when he finally subjected the first human to the procedure.

The physiology of the pulmonary circulation and cor pulmonale were to become his special field as a result of his intensive studies on the subject between the years 1944 and 1960. A landmark paper on the matter was presented by him in 1950 at a meeting of the American Heart Association. The title was *Some Aspects of the Pulmonary Circulation in Normal Man and in Chronic Cardiopulmonary Diseases*. It was the theme of the Fourth Walter Wile Hamburger Memorial Lecture[159].

When he shared the Nobel Prize with Richards and Forssmann in 1956, he gave the concluding lecture. It was concerned with the relationship between pressure and flow in the pulmonary bed. It is strange that he made no mention of the work of Liljestrand and von Euler on hypoxia. Although he acknowledged the acquisition of some understanding between pressure and flow, he lamented the poorly understood mechanism of action of hypoxia on the pulmonary vasculature[160].

Cournand was the ideal clinical scientist. He had compassion, was markedly ethical in his research efforts and refreshingly candid when he declared that it was absolutely necessary for the scientist to declare his errors without reservation. He expressed this nicely in a paper he co-authored with Zuckerman in 1970 when he wrote: 'The point of such confessions is not the parading of one's humility but the reaffirmation of the values of reason and experience'[161].

This section on the pulmonary circulation should end with a few words on the non-respiratory functions of the pulmonary circulation. The first discoveries on this aspect began to appear with the 1960s[162]. Surfactant was identified as a metabolic product of the type 2 alveolar cell. Certain substances circulating in the blood were also found to be modified by the alveolar endothelium during their passage through the lungs. Among these are angiotensin I, serotonin and norepinephrine. Most of angiotensin I appears to be converted to angiotensin II during passage.

These discoveries relevant to the nonrespiratory functions of the pulmonary circulation are but a tip of the iceberg. At the least, they have created a whole new approach to unraveling still further the myriad physiological phenomena that occur while blood is coursing through the lungs.

The crude methods of Harvey opened the gates in the 17th century, the more refined methods of the 20th century opened them a bit further, but it will probably be the technological advancements of the 21st century that will burst open these gates to flood capacity.

REFERENCES

1. Breasted, J.H. (1930). *The Edwin Smith Surgical Papyrus*, vol. 1, **13**, 64–5, 106–9. (Chicago: Univ. Chicago Press)
2. Willius, F.A. and Dry, T.J. (1948). A *History of the Heart and Circulation*, pp. 6–9. (Philadelphia: W.B. Saunders)
3. Key, J.D., Keys, T.E. and Callahan, J.A. (1979). Historical development of concept of blood circulation. *Am. J. Cardiol.*, **43**, 1026–32
4. Willius, F.A. and Dry, T.J. (1948). *Op. cit.*, p. 10
5. Wong, K.C. and Wu, Lien-teh. (1936). History of Chinese medicine: being a chronicle of medical happenings in China from ancient times to the present period, second edition. *Nat. Quarantine Serv.*, p. 35. (China: Shanghai)
6. *Ibid.*, p. 35
7. Sarton, G. (1927). *Introduction to the History of Science, VI. From Homer to Omar Khayyam.* (Baltimore: Williams and Wilkins)
8. Sarton, G. (1952). *A History of Science, I. Ancient Science through the Golden Age of Greece.* (Cambridge, Mass.: Harvard University Press)
9. Wiberg, J. (1937). The medical science of ancient Greece: the doctrine of the heart. *Janus*, **41**, 225
10. Leboucq, G. (1944). Une anatomie antique du coeur humain. Philiston de Locroi et le Timée de Platon. *Rev. Et. Grecques*, **57**, 7
11. Michel, P.H. (1957). La Science Hellène. In *Histoire Générale des Sciences. I. La Science Antique et Médiévale (des origines à 1450)*, p. 288. (Paris: Presses Universitaires de France)
12. Willius, F.A. and Dry, T.J. (1948). *Op. cit.*, p. 11.
13. Cole, J.S. (1977). A historical review of the concept of the left ventricle as a pump. *Catheterization Cardiovascular Diagn.*, **3**, 155–70
14. Fulton, J.F. (1932). *Readings in the History of Physiology*, pp. 41–2. (Springfield)
15. Cournand, A. (1982). In Fishman, A.P. and Richards, D.W. (eds.) *Circulation of the Blood, Men and Ideas*. p. 14. (Baltimore Md.: American Physiological Society, Waverly Press Inc.)
16. Galen, Claudius (1822). *Opera Omnia*. Tr. by C.G. Kühn. Lipsiae, Cnoblochii, v. 3, p. 460

17. Fleming, D. (1955). Galen on the motion of the blood in the heart and lungs. *Isis*, **46**, 14

18. Ilyas, M. (1985). Cardiovascular medicine, Islamic heritage: concepts and contributions. *J.P.M.A.*, September

19. Meyerhof, M. (1933). Ibn-an-Nafis und seine Theorie des Lungenkreislaufs. *Quell, u. Stud. Gesch. der Naturwiss. u. der. Med.*, **4**, 37

20. Al-Dabbagh, S.A. (1978). Ibn-al-Nafis and the pulmonary circulation. *Lancet*, May 27, p. 1148

21. Khulusi, S.A. (1978). Arab medicine and circulation of the blood. *Lancet*, p. 131, June 17

22. Ulmann, M. (1978). *Islamic Medicine*, p. 690. (Edinburgh)

23. Hayes, J.R. (ed.) (1978). The genius of Arab civilization. *Source of Renaissance*, p. 154. (Oxford)

24. Ibn-al-Nafis. *Commentary on Avicenna's Anatomy*, Manuscript no. 2939, fol. IV. (Paris: Bibliothèque National)

25. Tatawi, M.E.D. (1925). Der Lungenkreislauf nach el Koraschi, Dissertation, Freiburg im Breisgau

26. Jalili, M. (1982). *Histoire des Sciences Médicales*, vol. XVII

27. Iskandar, A.Z. *A Catalogue of Arabic Manuscripts on Medicine and Science.* (London: Wellcome Historical Medical Library)

28. Coppola, E.D. (1935). The discovery of the pulmonary circulation: a new approach. *The William Osler Medal Essay.* Based on an MD thesis submitted to the Yale University Department of the History of Medicine, May

29. Cournand, A. (1982). *Op. cit.*, p. 17

30. Coppola, E.D. (1935). *Op. cit.*, p. 74

31. Saccardo, P.A. (1895). La botanica in Italia. (Venezia: tipografia Carlo Ferrari)

32. Wüstenfeld, F. (1877). *Die Übersetzungen Arabischer Werke in das Lateinische seit dem XI. Jahrhundert.* (Göttingen: Dieterich'sche Verlags-Buckhandlung)

33. *Ibid.* p. 123

34. Coppola, E.D. (1935). *Op. cit.*, p. 70

35. Binet, L. and Herpin, A. (1948). *Bull. Acad. Nat. Méd.*, **132**, 541

36. Meyerhof, M. (1935). Ibn al-Nafis (XIIIth cent.) and his theory of the lesser circulation. *Isis*, **23**, 100

37. Chehade, A.K. (1955). Ibn al-Nafis et la découverte de la circulation pulmonaire. *Institut Francaise de Dames*, p. 49

38. Haddad, S. (1936). Who is the discoverer of the lesser circulation? *Muktataf J.*, **89**, 264

39. Temkin, O. (1940). Was Servetus influenced by Ibn al-Nafis? *Bull. Hist. Med.*, **8**, 731

40. Caesalpinus, A. (1571). Quaestionum peripateticarum libri quinque. Venetiis, Iuntas

41. Caullery, M. (1957). Les grandes étapes des sciences biologiques. In Dumas, M. (ed.) *Histoire de la science des origines au XXe siécle. (Encylopédie de la Pléiade)*, pp. 1224–45, 1232. (Paris: Gallimard)

42. Donath, T. (1984). Who was the first to describe the pulmonary circulation? *Gegenbaurs morph. Jakrb. Leyzig*, **130**, 827–34

43. Bainton, R.H. (1953). *Hunted Heretic, the Life and Death of Michael Servetus, 1511–1533.* (Boston: Beacon Press)

44. Wolton, W. (1694). *Reflections upon Ancient and Modern Learning.* (London: J. Leake for P. Buck)

45. Servetus, M. (1953). A translation of his geographical, medical and astrological writings. Tr. by C.D. O'Malley, *Am. Philos. Soc. Mem.*, v. 34. (Philadelphia)

46. Bainton, R.H. (1931). The smaller circulation: Servetus and Colombo. *Sudhoffs Arch. Gesch. Med.*, **24**, 371

47. Valverde, J. (1559). Anatomia der corpo humano. *Ant. Salamanca et Antonio Lafrerj*, p. 105b. (Rome)

48. Coppola, E.D. (1935). *Op. cit.*, p. 60

49. Valverde, J. (1559). *Op. cit.*, **1**, A3

50. *Ibid.*, **1**, 131

51. Colombo, R. (1559). *Realdi Columbi Cremonenses, in almo gymnasio Romano anatomici celeberrimi, de re anatomica libri XV*, p. 177. (Venice: Nicolò Bevilacqua)

52. Vesalius, A. (1543). *De humani corporis fabrica*, p. 56. (Basel: J. Oporinus)

53. Fabroni, A. (1791). *Historiae Academiae Pisanae*, p. 74. (Pisa: Caietanus Mugnainius)

54. Condivi, A. (1928). *Michelangelo: la vita raccolta dal suo discepolo Ascanio Condivi.* (Milan: Gustavo Modiano)

55. Tollin, H. (1880). Matteo Realdo Colombo. Ein Breitag zu seinem Leben aus seinem L. XV de re anatomica. *Pflüger's Arch.*, **22**, 262–90

56. Graubard, M. (1964). *Circulation and Respiration. The Evolution of an Idea.* pp. 112–13. (New York: Harcourt Brace and World)

57. Nordenskiöld, E. (1928). *The History of Biology: A Survey*, pp. 112–14. (New York: Alfred A. Knopf)

58. Graubard, M. (1964). *Op. cit.*, pp 103–17

59. Morton, L.T. (1970). *A Medical Bibliography (Garrison and Morton): An Annotated Check-List of Texts Illustrating the History of Medicine*, third edition, p. 50. (London: Andre Deutsch)

60. Bayon, H.P. (1935). The authorship of Carlo Ruini's 'anatomia del cavallo'. *J. Comp. Pathol. Ther.*, **48**, 138–48

61. Dyce, K.M. and Merlen, R.H.A. (1953). Carlo Ruini and 'l'anatomia del cavallo', *Br. Vet. J.*, **109**, 385–90

62. Bloch, H. (1979). Discovery of blood circulation: some dependence factors in evolution of a discovery. *N.Y. State J. Med.*, **79**, 1940–3

63. Bonnabeau, R.C. Jr and Bonnabeau, M.M. (1981). William Harvey revisited. *Minnesota Med.*, Jan., pp. 28–33

64. Key, J.D., Keys, T.E. and Callahan, J.A. (1979). *Op. cit.*, p. 1027

65. Poynter, F.N.L. and Keeler, K.D. (1961). *A Short History of Medicine*, p. 34. (London: Mills & Boon)

66. Silverman, M.E. (1985). William Harvey and the discovery of the circulation. *Clin. Cardiol.*, **8**, 244–6

67. Harvey, W. (1928). *Exercitatio Anatomica de Motu Cordis et Sanguinis in Animalibus.* (English translation with annotations by C.D. Leake), p. 7. (Springfield, Illinois: Charles C. Thomas)

68. Keynes, G. (1953). *A Bibliography of the Writings of Dr. William Harvey,* 2nd edn., pp. 38–43. (Cambridge: Cambridge Univ. Press)

69. Dormandy, T.L. (1978). Harvey at 40. *Lancet,* pp. 708–9, April 1

70. James Geraint, D. (ed.) (1978). *Circulation of the Blood.* (London: Pitman Medical)

71. Silverman, M.E. (1985). *Op. cit.*

72. Prieur, G.O. (1952). William Harvey. *Hist. Bull. Calgary Clin.*, **17**, 21

73. Sigerist, H.E. (1958). *The Great Doctors.* (Garden City: Doubleday)

74. Wells, L.A. (1978). William Harvey and the convergence of medicine and science. *Mayo Clin. Proc.*, **53**, 234

75. Willius, F.A. and Dry, T.J. (1948). *A History of the Heart and the Circulation,* pp. 294–8. (Philadelphia: W.B.Saunders Company)

76. Zeman, F.D. (1963). The old age of William Harvey. *Arch. Intern. Med.*, **111**, 829

77. *Aubrey's Brief Lives* (1975). Edited from the original manuscripts and with an introduction by Dick, Oliver Lawson, 3rd edn., pp. 128–33. (London and Edinburgh: Morrison and Gibb Ltd.)

78. Jarcho, S. (1958). William Harvey described by an eyewitness (John Aubrey). *Am. J. Cardiol.*, **2**, 381

79. Keynes, G. (1949). *The Personality of William Harvey – the Linacre Lecture delivered at St. John's College.* (Cambridge: Cambridge Univ. Press)

80. Sigerist, H.E. (1958). Great doctors: a biographical history of medicine. (Garden City: Doubleday)

81. Gillespie, C.C. Editor-in-chief. *Dictionary of Scientific Biography*, vol. XI. (New York: Charles Scribner's Sons)

82. Keynes, G. (1966). *The Life of William Harvey.* (London: Cheswick Press)

83. Willius, F.A. and Keys, T.E. (1941). *Cardiac Classics.* Translation of De Motu Cordis by Robert Wills, Barnes, Surrey, England, pp. 27–8. (St. Louis, Mo.: C.V. Mosby Co.)

84. Galilei, Galileo (1914). *Dialogues concerning two new sciences.* Tr. by H. Crew and A. de Salvio. (New York: Macmillan)

85. Randall, J.H. Jr. (1940). The development of scientific method in the school of Padua. *J. Hist. Ideas,* **1**, 177

86. Harvey, W. (1847). *The Works,* Tr. by R. Willis, v. 10, p. 597. (London: Sydenham Society Publication)

87. Marcus, R.B. (1962). *A New Book by an Old Master, William Harvey.* (New York: Franklin Watts)

88. Dawes, G.S., Mott, J.C. and Widdicombe, J.G. (1955). Closure of the foramen ovale in newborn lambs. *J. Physiol. (Lond.),* **128**, 384

89. Harvey, W. (1938). *On the Motion of the Heart and Blood in Animals.* Tr. by Robert Willis, Harvard Classics, Collier, vol. 38, pp. 75–149.

90. Barcroft, J., Barrow, D.H., Cowie, A.T. and Forsham, P.H. (1940). The oxygen supply of the foetal brain of the sheep and the effect of asphyxia on foetal respiratory movement. *J. Physiol. (Lond.),* **97**, 338

91. Bedford, D.E. (1968). Harvey's third circulation. De Circulo Sanguinis in Corde. *Br. Med. J.,* **4**, 273–7

92. Malpighi, M. (1661). *De Pulmonibus, Observationes Anatomical.* (Bologna)

93. Gunther, R.T. (1968). *Early Science in Oxford,* Vol. IX. (London: Dawson)

94. Fishman, A.P. and Richards, D.W. (1964). *Circulation of the Blood.* (New York: Oxford Univ. Press)

95. Editorial (1967). Richard Lower (1631–1691). Physiologic cardiologist. *J. Am. Med. Assoc.,* **199**, 146–7

96. Bailey, H. and Bishop, W.J. (1959). *Notable Names in Medicine and Surgery.* (London: Lewis)

97. Young, R.A. (1939). *Harveian Oration – The*

Pulmonary Circulation (London)

98. Patterson, T.S. (1931). John Mayow in contemporary setting: a contribution to the history of respiration and combustion. *Isis*, **13**, 47

99. Lower, R. (1669). *Tractatus de Corde*. (London: Allestry)

100. Fulton, J.F. (1932). *A Bibliography of the Honourable Robert Boyle*. (Oxford: Oxford Univ. Press)

101. Patterson, T.S. (1931). John Mayow in contemporary setting. II. Mayow's views on combustion. *Isis*, **13**, 504

102. Fulton, J.F. (1935). *A Bibliography of Two Oxford Physiologists, Richard Lower, 1631–1691, John Mayow, 1643–1679.* (Oxford: Oxford Univ. Press)

103. Mayow, J. (1668). *Tractatus Duo: De Respiratione, De Rachitide.* (Oxford: Hall)

104. Mayow, J. (1674). *Tractatus Quinque: De Sal Nitro et Spiritu – Aero, De Respiratione, Foetus in Utero et Qvo, de Motu Muscularis et Spiritibus Animalibus, De Rachitide.* (Oxford)

105. Hales, S. (1731). A specimen of an attempt to analyze the air by a great variety of chymostatical experiments which were read at several meetings before the Royal Society. In his *Statical Essays*, vol. I, *Vegetable Staticks*, 2nd edn. (London: Woodward and Peale)

106. *Ibid.*

107. Hales, S. (1733). *Statical Essays*, vol. II. *Haemastaticks.* (London)

108. Conant, J.B. (1957). The overthrow of the phlogiston theory. In his *Harvard Case Histories in Experimental Science*. (Cambridge, Mass.: Harvard Univ. Press)

109. Priestley, J. (1777–80). *Expérience et observations sur differentes espéces d'air*, Tr. by H. Gibelin, vol. 2, p. 290. (Paris)

110. Beklund, U. (1957–58). A lost letter from Scheele to Lavoisier. *Lychnos*, p. 39

111. Viallard, R. and Daumas, M. (1957). L'Edification de la science classique. In Daumas, M. (ed.) *Histoire de la science des origines au XXe siécle. (Encyclopédie de la Pléaide)*, p. 883. (Paris: Gallimard)

112. Lavoisier, A.L. (1862). Analyse du mémoire sur l'augmentation du poids des métaux par la calcination. In his *Ouvres, Tome II. Mémoires de chimie et de physique*, p. 97. (Paris: Imprimerie Impériale)

113. Lavoisier, A.L. (1862). Mémoire sur la nature du principe qui se combine avec les métaux pendant leur calcination et qui en augmente le poids. In his *Ouvres, Tome II. Mémoires de chimie et de physique*, p. 122. (Paris: Imprimerie Impériale)

114. Lavoisier, A.L. (1862). Expériences sur la respiration des animaux et sur les changements qui arrivent – l'air en passant par leur poumon. In his *Ouvres. Tome II. Mémoires de chimie et de physique,* p. 174. (Paris: Imprimerie Impériale)

115. Lavoisier, A.L. (1862). Mémoire sur la combustion en général. In his *Ouvres, Tome II. Mémoires de chimie et de physique,* p. 225. (Paris: Imprimerie Impériale)

116. Lavoisier, A.L. and Séguin, A. (1862). Premier mémoires sur la respiration des animaux. In his *Ouvres, Tome II. Mémoires de chime et de physique*, p. 688. (Paris: Imprimerie Impériale)

117. Magnus, G. (1837). Über die im Blute enthaltenen Gase. Sauerstoff, Stickstoff und Kohlensäure. *Ann. Phys. Chem.*, **12**, 583

118. von Haller, A. (1760). *Elementa physiologiae corporis humani*, vol. 3. (Lausanne: Bousquet)

119. Magendie, F. (1842). *Phénoménes physiques de la vie, Leçons professées au Collège de France.* (Paris: Baillière)

120. Cohnheim, J. and Litten. (1875). Über die Folgen der Embolie der Lungenarterien. *Virchow's Arch. path. Anat.*, **65**, 99

121. Poiseuille, J.J. (1855). Recherches sur la respiration. *C.R. Acad. Sci. (Paris),* **41**, 1072

122. Lichtheim, L. (1876). *Die Störungen des Lungenkreislaufs und ihr Einfluss auf den Blutdruck.* (Breslau: Jungfer)

123. D'Arsonval, J.A. (1877). *Recherches théoriques et expérimentales sur la rôle de l'élasticité du poumon dans les phénoménes de la circulation.* (Paris: Thèse)

124. Héger, P. (1880). Recherches sur la circulation du sang dans les poumons. *Ann. Université Libre Bruxelles, Fac. Med.*, **1**, 117

125. Héger, P. and Spehl, E. (1881). Recherches sur la fistule péricardiques chez le lapin. Ligature des vaisseaux de la base du couer pendant la respiration naturelle: évaluation de la quantité de sang contenue dans les poumons. *Arch. Biol.*, **2**, 153

126. Cournand, A. (1982). *Op. cit.*, p. 52

127. Beutner, A. (1852). Über die Strom – und Dückkräfte des Blutes in der Arteria und Vena pulmonalia. *Z. rat. Med., N.F.*, **2**, 97

128. Chauveau, A. and Marey, J. (1861). Détermination graphique des rapports du choc du couer avec les mouvements des oreillettes et des ventricules: expérience faite – l'aide d'un appareil enregistreur (sphygmographe). *C.R.*

Acad. Sci. Paris, **53**, 622

129. Funke, O. (1851). Über das Milzvenenblut. *Z. rat. Med., N.F.*, **1**, 172

130. Funke, O. (1852). Neue Beobachtungen über die Krystalle des Milzvenen und Fisch – Blutes. *Z. rat. Med., N.F.*, **2**, 198

131. Meyer, L. (1857). Die Gase des Blutes. *Z. rat. Med.*, **8**, 256

132. Hoppe-Seyler, F. (1864). Über di chemischen und optischen Eigenschaften des Blutfarbstoffes. Zweite Mitthheilung. *Virchow's Arch. Path. Anat.*, **29**, 233

133. Hoppe-Seyler, F. (1864). Über die chemischen und optischen Eigenschaften des Blutfarbstoffes. Dritte Mittheilung. *Virchow's Arch. Path. Anat.*, **29**, 597

134. Mayer, R. (1845). *Die organische Bewegung in ihrem zusammenhange mit dem Stoffwechsel.* (Heilbronn)

135. von Liebig, J. (1845). *Familiar Letters on Chemistry.* (London: Taylor and Walton)

136. Pflüger, E. (1872). Über die Diffusion des Sauerstoffs, den Ort und die Gesetze der Oxydationsprocesse im thierischen Organismus. *Pflügers Arch. ges. Physiol.*, **6**, 43

137. Bohr, C., Hasselbalch, K. and Krogh, A. (1904). Über einen in biologischer Beziehung wichtigen Einfluss den die Kohlensäure – spannung des Blutes auf dessen Sauerstoffbindung übt. *Skand. Arch. Physiol.*, **16**, 402

138. Bohr, C. (1909). Über die spezifische Tätigkeit der Lungen bei der respiratorischen Gasaufnahme und ihr Verhalten der durch die Alveolar-Wand statfindenen Gasdiffusion. *Skand. Arch. Physiol.*, **22**, 221

139. Krogh, A. and Krogh, M. (1910). On the rate of diffusion of carbonic oxide in the lungs of man. *Skand. Arch. Physiol.*, **23**, 236

140. von Euler, U.S. and Liljestrand, G. (1946). Observations on the pulmonary arterial blood pressure in the cat. *Acta Physiol. Scand.*, **12**, 301

141. Liljestrand, G. (1948). Regulation of pulmonary arterial blood pressure. *Arch. Intern. Med.*, **81**, 162

142. Badoud, E. (1876).Über den Einfluss des Hirns auf den Druck in der Lungenarterie. *Arb. Physiol. Lab. Würzburg*, **3**, 237

143. Francois-Franck, C.É. (1880). Sur l'innervation des vaisseaux des poumons et sur les effets produits dans la circulation intracardiaque et aortique par le resserement de ces vaisseaux. *Séances et Mémoires, Soc. Biol.*, 7e serie, **2**, 231

144. Francois-Frank, C.É. (1895). Nouvelles recherches sur l'action vasoconstrictive pulmonaire du grand sympathique. *Arch. physiol. norm. path.*, ser. 5, **7**, 744

145. Francois-Frank, C.É. (1895). Nouvelles recherches sur l'action vasoconstrictive pulmonaire du grand sympathique. (2e mémoire). *Arch. physiol. norm. path.*, ser. 5, **7**, 816

146. Bradford, J.R. and Dean, H.P. (1894). The pulmonary circulation. *J. Physiol. (Lond.)*, **16**, 34

147. Fishman, A.P. (1978). The pulmonary circulation. *J. Am Med. Assoc.*, **239**, 1299–301

148. Szidon, J.P. and Fishman, A.P. (1969). Autonomic control of the pulmonary circulation. In Fishman, A.P. and Hecht, H.H. (eds.) *The Pulmonary Circulation and Interstitial Space*, pp. 239–65. (Chicago: Univ. Chicago Press)

149. Haldane, J.S. (1922). *Respiration*. (New Haven: Yale Univ. Press)

150. Christiansen, J., Douglas, C.G. and Haldane, J.S. (1914). The absorption and dissociation of carbon dioxide by human blood. *J. Physiol. (Lond.)*, **48**, 244

151. Henderson, L.J. (1928). *Blood: a Study in General Physiology.* (New Haven: Yale Univ. Press)

152. Cournand, A. (1982). *Op. cit.*, p. 60

153. Henderson, L.J. (1906). Equilibrium in solutions of phosphates. *Am. J. Physiol.*, **15**, 257

154. Henderson, L.J. (1908). The theory of neutrality regulation in the animal organism. *Am. J. Physiol.*, **21**, 427

155. Henderson, L.J. (1909). Gleichgewicht zwischen Basen und Säuren im tierischen Organismus. *Ergebn. Physiol.*, **8**, 254

156. Van Slyke, D.D., Wu, H. and McLean, F.C. (1923). Studies of gas and electrolyte equilibria in the blood V. Factors controlling the electrolyte and water distribution in the blood. *J. Biol. Chem.*, **56**, 767

157. Henderson, L.J. (1928). *Blood: a Study in General Physiology.* (New Haven: Yale Univ. Press)

158. Franch, R.H. (1986). André F. Cournand: father of clinical cardiopulmonary physiology. *Clin. Cardiol.*, **9**, 82–6

159. Cournand, A. (1950). Some aspects of the pulmonary circulation in normal man and in chronic cardiopulmonary diseases. *Circulation*, **2**, 641

160. Sourkes, T.L. (1966). *Nobel Prize Winners in Medicine and Physiology 1901–1965.* (New York: Abelard-Schuman)

161. Cournand, A.F. and Zuckerman, H. (1970). The code of science. Analysis and some reflections on its future. *Stud. Gen.*, **23**, 941

162. Fishman, A.P. (1977). Nonrespiratory functions of the lungs. *Chest*, **78**, 84–9

15   The heart as a pump

Who was the first to compare the action of the heart to a pump? It was certainly not Galen because he believed that the forward flow of blood from the right ventricle through the lungs was due to the rhythmic respiratory movements of the thorax. There is some controversy as to whether or not Harvey was the first to compare the hearts action to a pump. Hamilton and Richards seem to favor this view[1]. It is based on their interpretation of Harvey's remarks in *De Motu Cordis*. Similar interpretations are presented by Webster[2] and Basalla[3]. In 1967, Siegel initiated a debate with contrary views[4].

Siegel claimed that Harvey used the simile of the water bellows not to describe the movements of the heart but to indicate the action of the lungs and diaphragm. He further asserted that Harvey believed that these organs (lungs and diaphragm), much like the 'two sides of a bellows', exerted a pumping effect on both the thoracic blood vessels and the heart[5,6]. Siegel marshaled several bits of evidence in favor of the thesis that Harvey did not regard the heart as a pump. Among them are the following:

(1) When referring to Galen, Harvey placed a great deal of emphasis on the effect of the thoracic excursions on the forward flow of blood through the lungs[7];

(2) Harvey's comparison of blood flow through the arteries as being similar to the effect of a siphon[8]; and

(3) Harvey's comparison of the action of the heart to the motion of a snake ('contracting along its length like a worm in its constrictive phase')[9].

On the other hand the earliest inkling that Harvey did indeed regard the heart as a pump can be found in the following quotation from his notes for the Lumleian lecture of April 17, 1616, long before his *De Motu Cordis*:

It is plain from the structure of the heart that the blood is passed continuously through the lungs to the aorta as by two clacks of a water bellows to raise water. It is shown by application of a ligature that the passage of blood is from the arteries into the veins. Whence it follows that the movement of the blood is constantly in a circle, and is brought about by the beat of the heart. It is a question, therefore, whether this is for the sake of nourishment or of heat, the blood cooled by warming the limbs, being in turn warmed by the heart[10].

These notes had been lost for almost 300 years. They were found in the British Museum in 1886[11]. Figure 1 illustrates a page from these notes.

In Chapter 2 of *De Motu Cordis* Harvey describes how the heart contracts in systole and that the blood is expelled during contraction. The pulmonary artery and aorta are seen to dilate during systole. This is described in Chapter 3. Chapter 5 describes how both auricles contract sending blood into the ventricles, followed by ventricular contraction sending blood to the arteries. Moreover, the actual words, 'pump' and 'pumping', are seen several times. Do we need any more proof of what he meant? Careful review of Siegel's paper leads me to believe that his entire argument rests on his own personal interpretation of what Harvey actually wrote. Being purely subjective, it must of necessity be biased so that I cannot accept his purported evidence as proof for his views.

We have already seen how Richard Lower ascribed the increase in blood flow during exercise to the pumping action of the skeletal muscles rather than the heart. Concerning cardiac output, Lower's contribution was not a direct one. Without being aware of it, he did establish a structural basis for a pump when he described the arrangement of the muscle fibers in the ventricles. His dissections of the heart revealed that the inner and outer muscle

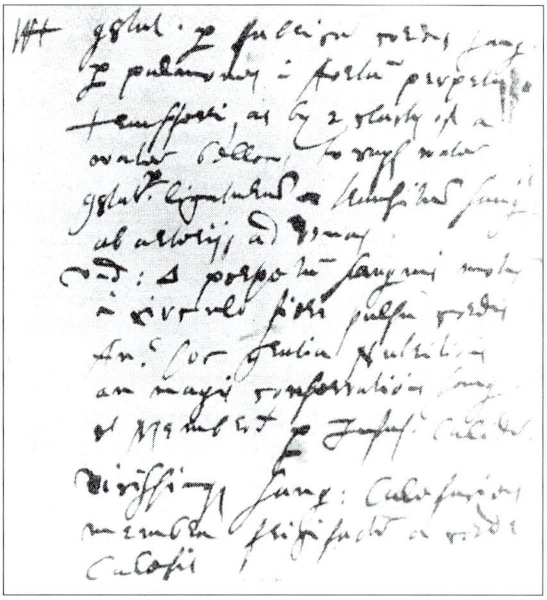

Figure 1 A page from Harvey's Lumleian lecture notes on April 16, 1616. *Photo Source University of Central Florida. Literary Source Fishman, A.P. and Richards, D.W. Circulation of the Blood, Men and Ideas. American Physiological Society. Printed in USA by Waverly Press, Inc., Baltimore, Maryland 21202. Originally published by Oxford University Press in 1964. Illustration is Figure 2 on p.73. Taken from the British Museum, London. With permission*

layers of the ventricles were arranged in an oblique manner and that around the apex they assumed a whorl-like configuration. His *in vivo* experiments demonstrated that as ventricular contraction proceeded, the apex of the heart moved closer to the base. These statements are to be found in his *Tractatus de Corde*[12].

As we shall see in Section 5, Stephen Hales' main contributions were in the presentation of a broad concept of blood pressure, blood flow and blood velocity based on quantitative measurements and calculations. However, he did provide an estimate of cardiac output in the horse. He did this by first exsanguinating the animal and then filling the left ventricle with melted beeswax. He then assumed that the left ventricular chamber had been completely emptied just prior to death. Since he knew the normal pulse rate of a healthy horse at rest, he calculated the cardiac output per minute by multiplying the measured volume of the left

ventricular chamber by the pulse rate. He also noted that systole occupied only one-third of the cardiac cycle and concluded that the run-off was accomplished by the elasticity of the large vessels[13].

Further advances in the mechanisms underlying the pumping action of the heart did not take place until the time of Carl Ludwig with his invention of the kymograph and his leadership role in experimental physiology. Fielding Garrison called him 'perhaps the greatest teacher of physiology who ever lived'. Again, he and his school undoubtedly played the most prominent role during the 19th century in expanding the frontiers of cardiovascular physiology. We have seen how one of his students, A. Beutner, utilized the kymograph for the recording of pulmonary arterial pressure. But he was only one among the many investigators who trained under Ludwig and later contributed their own pieces to the mosaic of physiology in general. Ludwig helped usher in the era of graphic methodology in physiological research and the time was now ripe to use his kymograph and other graphic methods for studying the hemodynamics of the circulation.

Ludwig was a firm believer in the interdependence of function and structure. Moreover, he was well aware of the potentialities of physics, chemistry and its subdivision of biochemistry in all aspects of physiology. Firmly grounded in these disciplines he led the academic world in merging them towards the unearthing of physiological phenomena.

Most of Ludwig's work was done at Leipzig where he was the head of the Institute of Physiology, established in 1865 for his use and under his direction. Prior to this he had spent 10 years at Vienna and 6 years at Zurich. His relationship with Adolph Fick began while he was professor of anatomy and physiology in Zurich. Rosen described him in such superlative terms that it is hard to imagine that Ludwig was indeed a human being[14]. His qualities included a fertile imagination, an awesome knowledge of anatomy, his almost boyish enthusiasm for his work, especially with each new discovery, and his loyalty, humor and generosity. What attributes for a man whose photograph (depicted in Figure 2) reveals a rather plain face with a disproportionately large nose and yet with a hint of kindliness in those eyes framed by spectacles.

The gamut of physiological studies conducted by him and his students (while working with him or

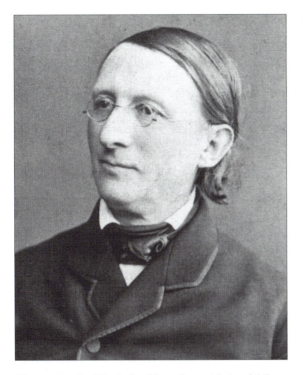

Figure 2 Carl Ludwig. *Photo Source National Library of Medicine. Literary Source Photo Archives. Courtesy of National Library of Medicine*

later on their own) was truly phenomenal. Their scope encompassed the role of the nervous system, circulatory hemodynamics, capillary blood pressure, blood gases and a host of other investigations that looked into every nook and cranny of physiology. No aspect was considered insignificant. Ludwig's greatness was duly recorded and brought into sharp focus with the publication of a Festschrift by his former students in honor of his 70th birthday. Therein, lies his greatest contribution – the master teacher who spawned a huge family of physiologists, renowned in their own right[15].

In 1867, Ludwig and Dogiel invented the stromuhr, a double vessel on a swivel for the measurement of volume flow. In 1874, Ludwig and Bowditch discovered the 'all-or-none' and 'staircase' phenomena of cardiac muscle; two crucial elements in the understanding of cardiac output[16].

Let us now turn our attention to Adolph Fick, perhaps the brightest of the stars in Ludwig's firmament; a man who has been labeled by E. Shapiro as the forgotten genius of cardiology[17]. His interest in cardiology started when he accepted a prosectorship with Carl Ludwig in Zurich. Fick was a mathematician and physicist as well as a physiologist. As a youth, he demonstrated an exceptional talent for mathematics and physics and it is said that it was his brother Heinrich's prescience that persuaded young Adolph to become learned in these disciplines before embarking on a medical career[18]. Fick's contributions to physiology were no doubt attributable to his skills in mathematics and physics. They were to prove quite useful, especially in his experiments regarding the physiology of muscular contraction. This particular subject was to occupy his efforts for 30 years, all of them spent at Würzburg where he was chairman of the department of physiology and finally rector of the university. He retired on his 70th birthday and died of apoplexy just one year later.

Fick was the first to realize that a relationship existed between blood flow and gas exchange in the lungs. This was to become the basis for his formula in the calculation of cardiac output. The following is his much-quoted paragraph which gives us the insight as to how he arrived at what is now known as Fick's principle; all the more remarkable because it was the product of pure reasoning in the hands of a keen mathematician and physicist.

It is astonishing that no one has arrived at the following obvious method by which [the amount of blood ejected by the ventricle of the heart with each systole], may be determined directly, at least in animals. One measures how much oxygen an animal absorbs from the air in a given time, and how much carbon dioxide it gives off. During the experiment one obtains a sample of arterial and venous blood; in both the oxygen and carbon dioxide content are measured. The difference in oxygen content tells how much oxygen each cubic centimeter of blood takes up in its passage through the lungs. As one knows the total quantity of oxygen absorbed in a given time one can calculate how many cubic centimeters of blood passed through the lungs in this time. Or if one divides by the number of heart beats during this time one can calculate how many cubic centimeters of blood are ejected with each beat of the heart. The corresponding calculation with the quantities of carbon dioxide gives a determination of the same value, which controls the first[19].

The physical law that underlies Fick's principle is the one that says matter can neither be created nor destroyed. Thus, the volume of oxygen taken up by the lungs must be equal to the amount of oxygen used by the tissues.

Fick's principle is expressed by the following equation:

$$\text{Cardiac output} = \frac{\text{oxygen consumption}}{\text{arteriovenous oxygen difference}}$$

This principle, though great in itself, and used daily by cardiologists throughout the world, is but one example of his application of physics to medical investigation. His pioneering efforts in this regard led to many innovative instruments and physiological laws. Many of these were presented by him in his monograph *Medizinische Physick*, published in 1856 when he was only 27 years old. It was the first book of its kind. Medicine had to wait almost a century before it was superseded by Otto Glasser's monumental *Medical Physics*[20]. Fick's book deals with the hydrodynamics of circulation, the diffusion of gases and water, sound recordings of circulatory events, optics, color vision, and bioelectric phenomena. The extent of his knowledge is astounding; truly a match for Leonardo da Vinci.

The major portion of Fick's efforts was focused on the mechanics of skeletal muscle. It was during the course of these studies that he conceptualized and defined the terms isometric and isotonic in relation to muscular contraction. An extension of these studies led him to investigate myocardial mechanisms. This in turn led Starling and Frank to formulate their law of the heart.

Among the many instruments that Fick devised, some of those that had an impact on cardiovascular physiology were the plethysmograph, the pneumograph, and his version of the aneroid manometer. These were in the tradition of Ludwig, that of adding precision to physiological experimentation.

As I stated before, when Fick presented his principle on cardiac output he had no experimental proof of its validity in man. Cardiac catheterization was not available yet. Despite this he was still able to arrive at a reasonably accurate estimation of resting cardiac output in man by utilizing the arteriovenous difference obtainable for the dog and the total carbon dioxide output for man, both of which were easily obtainable. The arteriovenous difference in the dog was obtained by Scheffer in Ludwig's laboratory. Fick's excuse for not obtaining experimental proof was that the method required two gas pumps, and he

simply did not have them. This reason seems rather specious and smacks of some arrogance on his part for placing complete reliance on mathematical and physical laws. At any rate, experimental proof was supplied by other investigators and it came many years after Fick first published his famous paragraph in the proceedings of the *Würzburg Physickalische-Medizinische-Gesellschaft*[21].

Grehant and Quinquad were the first to demonstrate the validity of Fick's formula. This was in 1886. They utilized dogs for their measurements of blood flow[22]. Twelve years later and just three years before Fick died, Zuntz and Hagemann added their experimental proof[23]. Their animal model was the horse. Samples of blood were taken from the right atrium utilizing the right heart catheterization techniques introduced by Chauveau and Bernard (see Section 5). The results were published in a paper noteworthy for its detailed documentation. Measurements of cardiac output were obtained at rest, during exercise and after eating.

In 1903, Loewy and von Schrötter attempted to overcome the problem in humans in obtaining an estimate of the gases in the blood entering the right heart without resorting to cardiac catheterization, which at that time was still a laboratory procedure restricted to horses. Their method, an indirect one, did not bear fruit[24]. A much simpler and more practical method was introduced by J. Plesch six years later[25]. It was described in his monograph *Hämodynamische Studien*. He obtained mixed venous values by rebreathing gas mixtures out of a bag until the blood coming into the lung was in equilibrium with the lung–bag system. This came to be known as the indirect Fick method for determining cardiac output. In a short time the procedure was modified so that the arterial carbon dioxide value was obtained by arterial puncture rather than by measuring alveolar carbon dioxide tension. Still another modification was the one introduced by Henderson and Prince in 1917[26]. This consisted in having a high concentration of oxygen in the rebreathing mixture. The idea behind this was to allow the CO_2 equilibrium to take place with oxygenated blood and plotting the oxygenated mixed venous tension samples on the oxygenated CO_2 dissociation curve of blood.

There were too many sources for error in the other modifications of the indirect Fick procedure. The results from different centers varied markedly because of the variability of the human factor in conducting the procedure as well as in the baseline conditions. Even the method introduced by Zuntz and his co-workers in 1911 did not eliminate the sources for error[27]. Their method was based on the absorption of nitrous oxide into the pulmonary bloodstream by inhaling it and re-breathing it from a bag.

Verification of the Fick principle in man utilizing a direct approach was initially accomplished in 1930. This was made possible through the daring exploits of Baumann and Grollman[28]. They were able to obtain samples of mixed venous blood by inserting a spinal-tap needle just to the right of the sternum entering the right ventricular chamber by puncturing its wall. Their comments on this maneuver long before the cloud of malpractice suits descended upon the medical profession are of some interest.

> If one carries out the entire procedure involved in removing blood from the right heart during the period of a single circulation of the blood and the subject is unaware of the nature of the contemplated procedure the effect of psychic disturbance is avoided … Hence, the arterial puncture necessary in applying the direct Fick's principle always followed the heart puncture[29].

During the same year Klein obtained his samples of mixed venous blood by entering the right heart with a rubber tube inserted through the median basilic vein. This was one year after Forssmann's self-catheterization and eleven years before Cournand and his associates began their observations with catheterization of the right heart.

Hamilton, Moore and Kinsman applied to man in 1929 an indicator dilution method that had a good deal of success in experimental animals[30]. This technique stemmed from the use of an intravenous salt solution for determining circulation time developed by George Neil Stewart in 1897[31]. Henrique modified Stewart's method by using a thiocyanate solution instead of salt and injecting this in the form of a bolus instead of a constant flow infusion. Hamilton and his associates further modified the technique by substituting vital red or blue dye, T-1824, as the indicator[32]. This dye dilution method was slow in gaining acceptance among physiologists as being a valid indirect method of measuring cardiac output. The acetylene method of Grollman was more popular. It was introduced by him in 1932[28]. The

values for cardiac output were erroneous because his assumed circulation times in man were not valid. Despite this, and its relative insensitivity, Grollman's method became the standard indirect method for estimating cardiac output until the advent of cardiac catheterization and the trail blazing contributions of Andre Cournand. The direct Fick principle for measuring cardiac output was now feasible in the human. Cournand and his associates provided a rather complete hemodynamic study utilizing measurements of volume flow combined with recordings of pressures and blood volume[33]. In 1948, Warren demonstrated that samples of mixed venous blood were drawn with more certainty from the pulmonary artery.

Notwithstanding the popularity of Grollman's approach, Hamilton and his colleagues continued experimenting with their dye dilution technique. In 1948, they collaborated with Cournand in a series of experiments that compared their method with the direct approach of cardiac catheterization. The resultant paper, authored by members of both teams, reported good agreement between both methods[34].

Further modifications in the injection method were made as a means of overcoming the tedious necessity of analyzing too many samples of blood. One important innovation was the use of a photoelectric cell and a light source to sense dye T-1824 as the blood containing it passed between them[35]. Again, in an attempt to overcome the invasive nature of cardiac catheterization, and in an attempt to find a satisfactory clinical tool to measure cardiac output and its fractional components, echocardiography and nuclear imaging techniques were utilized as they became available. Of the two, nuclear imaging appeared to have the upper hand in accuracy since measurements are based on volume rather than wall motion changes *per se*. This issue became a critical one among the experts in these two modalities when it soon became evident that segmental wall motion abnormalities impose a serious flaw with the echocardiographic approach.

Heart beat and stroke volume are important factors regulating cardiac output. These, in turn, are dependent upon the molecular physiology of muscular contraction. The secrets of myocardial contraction at the cellular level were uncovered only within the latter half of the 20th century. The gross parameters of heart beat and stroke volume were the first to be delineated, and this came about through the efforts of Otto Frank, Wiggers, Hill and Ernest Starling.

Otto Frank, another of Carl Ludwig's proteges, was the one who presented a synthesis of the factors involved in atrial and ventricular contraction. He had the same background in mathematics and physics as his mentor and therefore was well prepared to carry on this work. Most of the work was done during his tenure as chair of the department of physiology at Munich, a position he held for 26 years.

Frank's observations were published in 1895 in his classical paper *Zur Dynamik des Herzmuskels* [36]. He describes in this paper how he measured and recorded the pressures, chamber volume and output of the frog's heart perfused with diluted ox blood. Stopcocks were used to regulate inflow and outflow. His experiments were simple but detailed, delineating the features of isometric contraction against varying initial aortic pressures; the rapid buildup of chamber pressure during the early systolic phase of ventricular contraction, and the presence of residual blood in the ventricular chamber at the end of systole.

He evaluated the isometric curves of the ventricle by plotting the atrial and ventricular pressures against varying levels of ventricular filling. These curves led him to conclude that 'the maximal tension of isometric contraction at first increases with augmentation of the initial length or initial tension but beyond a certain level of filling, the peaks decline' [37]. Similar findings were obtained during the isotonic phase of contraction.

Cole rightfully pointed out that Frank was well-aware of the significance of end-diastolic volume and the probable relationship between this and pressure or compliance though his experimental model could not delineate the relationship in a quantitative manner [38].

... Tension rises as filling increases ... it (tension) would furnish a measure of filling if one knew the distensibility curve of resting heart muscle. The determination of this relationship would be helpful in connection with many problems of cardiac filling, which itself cannot be measured directly. Initial tension could be used to deduce the volume of the heart in relaxation. As already mentioned, the relationship cannot be determined from my observations [37].

The simplicity of his experimental model is a testament to his brilliance and straightforward approach to a physiological problem. It is illustrated in Figure 3A. The pressure curves are shown in Figure 3B.

Just 11 years before Frank's paper appeared, Howell and Donaldson had reported their observations derived from a series of experiments upon the heart of a dog with reference 'to the maximum volume of blood sent out by the left ventricle in a single beat, and the influence of variations in venous pressure, arterial pressure and pulse-rate upon the work done by the heart' [39]. Howell was working at the time in Newell Martin's laboratory at Johns Hopkins University, and had already begun to establish himself as someone who was to contribute significantly to the rapidly expanding discipline of physiology. This was, of course, borne out by his brilliant investigations in coagulation as we shall see in Section 6.

Howell and Donaldson used a heart-lung preparation as their experimental model. The cardiac output was measured via a cannula inserted directly into the ascending aorta. They noted that the stroke work changed in concert with the changes in arterial pressure. This is how they expressed it: 'The work done by the left ventricle of the dog's heart varies directly as the arterial pressure against which it works within the limits named above' [39]. They also brought out that a decrease in pulse-rate 'causes an increase in the quantity of blood thrown out from the ventricle at each systole and consequently an increase in the work done at each systole, and vice versa' [39]. The relationship between central venous pressure and stroke volume and work was also demonstrated by them.

One particular sentence in their paper stands out purely because of its prescience, and long before the discovery of the electron microscope and advances in the molecular physiology of cardiac muscle.

... an explanation more in accordance with what is known of the physiology of ordinary muscle is found in the supposition that as the load increases a greater amount of energy is liberated, in consequence of some change in the molecular state of the ventricular muscle associated with increased tension at the commencement and during the early stages of its contraction [39].

It is rather strange that this paper has never enjoyed a more important role in the evolution of cardiovascular physiology. When it is read carefully, it can easily be seen that its relegation historically to

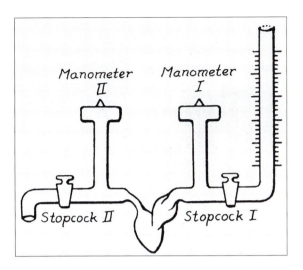

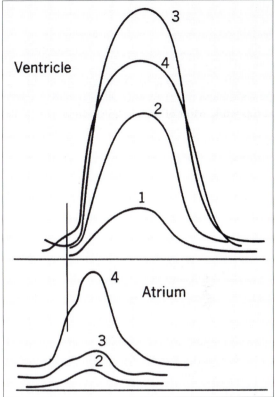

Figure 3 (left) Isolated frog heart preparation used by Otto Frank; (right) Atrial pressure recorded from manometer I and ventricular pressure from manometer II. *Photo Source National Library of Medicine. Literary Source Cole, J.S. (1977). A historical review of the concept of the left ventricle as a pump. Catheterization and Cardiovascular Diagnosis, vol.3, pp.155–70. Wiley–Liss, Inc., 41 East 11th Street, New York, NY 10003. With permission*

a secondary role is the result of neglect and lack of appreciation rather than fact. These two men along with Otto Frank clearly identified many of the observations that Starling later described.

In 1906, Yandell Henderson published a paper, also overlooked in the general enthusiasm generated by Starling's presentation[40]. According to Cole, it represents the first publication measuring simultaneously pressure and ventricular volume curves under varying physiologic conditions. Henderson used the dog as his experimental animal.

In 1914 Ernest H. Starling and his associates published three papers concerning the regulation of the heart beat and the mechanical factors determining the output of the ventricles[41–43]. These represented the culmination of 25 years of research.

Starling's work on the heart deserves credit as one of the great achievements in cardiovascular physiology. It is true that there were others before him who were familiar with the relationship between muscle fiber length and strength of contraction but as O'Rourke pointed out in 1984 Starling's 'work is classic because it described a simple basic mechanism that applied also to skeletal muscle, while explaining

comprehensively the heart's behavior under different circumstances, because Starling qualified its application to the intact heart, anticipating subsequent developments, and because he foresaw an ultrastructural basis for the law, a basis which has subsequently been described'[44]. This is not to say that the principle as enunciated by him was in its final form. It was further crystallized through the work of Wiggers, Straub, Katz and Krayer[45–47]. Starling was born in 1866 in London and spent most of his life in that remarkable city. He graduated from Guy's Hospital Medical School where he had come under the influence of a young physiologist, Charles Wooldridge, another product of Ludwig's laboratory[48,49]. Wooldridge managed to transmit to Starling, only 9 years his junior, the enthusiasm that characterized Ludwig, and that was to be indelibly stamped on all of his students. This interest on the part of Starling was reinforced when he spent a summer in that quintessential university town of Heidelberg soaking in the knowledge and Germanic preciseness offered by Willy Kühne and his staff. Only two years after he had returned to Guy's Hospital as a demonstrator in physiology, Starling was suddenly given a lectureship due to the premature death of his friend and mentor, Charles Wooldridge. Starling later married his mentor's widow.

One year later Starling left Guy's Hospital to work with W. M. Bayliss in the physiology department of University College. This move was prompted by the greater opportunities available at University College in terms of equipment and funding. A close relationship also developed between Bayliss and Starling. This relationship was cemented even further when Bayliss married Starling's sister.

In less than 10 years Starling was appointed Jodrell Professor of Physiology. During this short period of time, the fruits of his labors at University College were such that he had already established a reputation for his work in capillary filtration and lymph flow and for his introduction of the concept of chemical mediators. It was he who discovered secretin in 1902, and in fact, he was the first to use the word 'hormone'. He used this term for chemical mediator in his Croonian lecture in 1905 on *The Chemical Correlation of the Functions of the Body*[44,50].

Starling was a physiologist with a clinical outlook. His interest in experimental physiology was awakened and nourished primarily because of his perception that the results of such investigations would prove to be of value with respect to clinical situations. His work was conducted on animals but his orientation was always towards the patient. In a sense, he preceded Cournand in this respect, who, however, was primarily a clinician, and whose contributions were derived mainly from humans.

Cole relates an interesting anecdote about Starling and his chief, Bayliss. Though friendly to each other, they were far apart temperamentally. Bayliss was quiet and completely absorbed in his experiments whereas Starling is described as being 'brisk, ambitious, and too forthright and impatient to be diplomatic'. The anecdote concerns the famous 'brown dog' case. Cole recounts how Starling goaded Bayliss (who preferred to ignore the situation) into suing the antivivisectionist, Stephen Coleridge for challenging their experimental work. Bayliss won the case and donated the £2000 he was awarded to University College[38].

Starling's entire life seems to have been compressed into a relatively very short span. He acquired fame at a very early age, and he died at what is considered today an early age. He was only 61 when he died in 1927 of heart failure vaguely attributed to a dilated heart that he was said to have contracted while climbing in the Dolomites.

The paper that outlines the whole issue of what is now called Starling's law of the heart occupied the entire issue of the *London Journal of Physiology*[43]. It was authored by Patterson, Piper and Starling in that order. This slight detail is an indication of Starling's character. He was willing to take a back seat and give the privilege of leading authorship to his younger colleagues. Most of the paper is devoted to an explanation of previous experimental work and 'a reconciliation with previous theories and research from skeletal muscle'[38]. The paper does refer to Otto Frank's work but there are only indirect comments with regard to the contributions of Howell and Donaldson. The paper illustrates the law of the heart with a modification of Frank's figure as it appeared in Frank's *Zur Dynamik des Herzmuskels*. The modified figure substitutes volume for filling pressure on the abscissa. Starling later presented the law as the major theme in his Linacre lecture on the law of the heart[51]. Many historians cite this lecture when writing about Starling's contribution when in reality the original work is in the paper he wrote in 1914 in conjunction with his colleagues.

Starling's experiments were conducted with a canine heart preparation. It is illustrated in Figure 4. It is far more complicated than Frank's frog heart preparation. It should be noted that Newell Martin was the first to develop an effective mammalian heart-lung preparation, and that this was done while he held the chair in physiology at Johns Hopkins.

Newell Martin attended University College and while there he attended the physiology lectures being given by Michael Foster, a well-known investigator and teacher of the late 19th century. These lectures were voluntary and only the better students were willing to attend them since they were not part of the formal curriculum. Sewall recounts how Foster first met Martin and how Martin in time went to Johns Hopkins to establish a department of physiology in that new university.

These lectures on physiology were absolutely voluntary, and only the better students were willing to give up the time needed to get a more thorough grasp of physiology. Well, I appointed a time to see the few who wished to spend some time in this new study, this study of luxury, and there came to me a boy nothing more than a boy, who said: 'I am very sorry, sir; I should like to take your course if I could, but you see my parents are not very well off, and I get my board and lodging by living with a doctor close by … I have, in return for my board, to dispense all the doctor's medicines, and that dispensing takes me from two to five; now your lectures begin at four. I cannot come for the first hour; I will work hard and will try to make up the lost time.' I said, 'certainly, certainly'. So he came in, came in regularly late. He came in regularly at five o'clock, and he worked with such purpose that in the examination which I had at the end of the course I awarded him the prize. Well, his name was Henry Newell Martin, and I was so much struck with him that I asked him to assist me in my course, and he became my demonstrator. After we had been at University College together I think two or three years, Martin carrying on his duties and at the same time helping me, he came one day to me in great trouble because he could not make up his mind. He obtained what they call a scholarship at Christ College at Cambridge and he could not make up his mind to accept it and go there. He said he didn't want to leave me. But I was able to tell him what nobody else knew at that time, that in October in which his scholarship would take him to Cambridge I was going to Cambridge too, having been invited to lecture there … And after a career of considerable brilliancy of some years at Cambridge there came to him an invitation to the Johns Hopkins University at Baltimore. So if I have done nothing more, at all events I sent Henry Newell Martin to America[52].

Most of Martin's research dealt with cardiovascular research and the work of Howell and Donaldson was but one example of the many cardiovascular experiments going on his laboratory. Sewall who was also an assistant in Martin's laboratory describes in the same article recounting Foster's impressions of Martin, how the effective mammalian heart-lung preparation came about. This is what he said:

I very well remember one morning, I think it was in the Fall of 1880, Martin said to me, in effect, 'I could not sleep last night and the thought came to me that the problem of isolating the mammalian heart might be solved by getting a return circulation through the

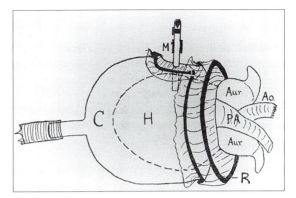

Figure 4 Starling's canine heart preparation. *Photo Source University of Central Florida. Literary Source Patterson, S.W., Piper, H. and Starling, E.H. (1914). The regulation of the heart beat. J. Physiol.(London)* **48**, *465. With permission*

coronary vessels'. The idea seemed reasonable and at the close of the day's work we anesthetized a dog, prepared him for artificial respiration and then Professor Martin opened the chest and ligatured one by one the venae cavae and the aorta in such a way as to leave a sufficient amount of blood in the heart itself. The heart continued to beat in a normal manner, the circuit made by the blood being from the right side, through the lungs to the left side and back through the coronary vessels in the heart wall to the right auricle again. Thus heart and lungs were completely isolated from the rest of the body and could be studied unaffected by the interference of factors foreign to itself … It was thought necessary to furnish the heart with an artificial supply of blood and accordingly defibrinated calf's blood was used and fed to the heart from a Mariotte's flask. The body of the dog and all the materials used in the experiment were inclosed within a glass walled hood of ample dimensions movable by ropes and pulleys over a shallow pan of zinc in which water was kept heated at a body temperature. In such an apparatus the isolated heart could be kept beating in a fairly normal fashion for upwards of five hours[53].

Martin is remembered chiefly for his method of isolating the heart in mammals[54]. But he should be remembered also for the many fine American physiologists who trained under him and for his efforts in founding the American Physiological Society in 1887.

As the illustration in Figure 5 indicates, blood entered the right atrium from the reservoir, the amount controlled by means of a pinch-clamp. Strategically placed manometers measured the various pressures. Cardiac output was measured at X utilizing a graduated cylinder. Resistance to outflow was controlled by varying the diameter of R1. Starling constructed the well-known curve by varying the venous flow and measuring the cardiac output[42].

The law of the heart is described as follows:

The behavior of the heart must be the sum of the behavior of the muscle fibers of which it is composed …the longer the muscle therefore (within physiological limits) the greater the amount of chemical energy, heat production and tension set up when the muscle passes from the resting to the active condition … these results can be transferred unreservedly to heart muscle making only certain modifications that are necessitated by the anatomical arrangements of the organ … In the heart we have no means of measuring directly either the length or the tension of the muscle fibers, but on the length of the muscle fibers depends the capacity or volume of the heart while tension of the muscle fibers determines the intracardiac pressure... the law of the heart is therefore the same as that for skeletal muscle, namely that the mechanical energy set free on passage from the resting to the contracted state depends on the area of chemically active surface, i.e. on the length of the muscle fibres. This simple formula serves to explain the whole behavior of the mammalian heart[43].

Although current concepts as to the mechanisms of congestive heart failure are indeed much more elaborate, Starling, nevertheless, did bring out the common denominator that is present in all cases, namely, an increase in venous pressure. Actually, he traced the failure to a loss of pumping ability on the part of the heart which causes more blood to remain in the chambers at the end of systole, and which, in turn, prevents adequate venous return. Volume overload in the cardiac chambers is reflected in a backward manner by an increase in venous pressure. The rise in venous pressure is therefore a passive phenomenon and incapable of increasing preload and hence cardiac output.

These are his words on venous pressure in congestive heart failure:

If for any reason the heart fails in its pumping action, the blood will remain in the auricles and ventricles and will prevent the further entry of blood from the reservoir. The heart will dilate more and more after each inefficient systole, while the pressure in the great veins will rise steadily: but this rise of pressure will be associated not with increased output from the ventricles but with diminished output. We have therefore to distinguish between a rise in venous pressure which is effective in dilating the heart during diastole and increasing its output and a rise of venous pressure which is passively induced by failure of the pumping action of the heart[43].

These words contain the fundamental reason why reduction in blood volume in congestive heart failure through diuretics or blood-letting can be so efficacious in holding in abeyance the dire consequences of heart failure … 'the only way to save such a heart is to diminish the inflow and allow the heart time to empty itself and time to recuperate after its exertions'[43].

Tinsley Harrison was the first clinician to explain the clinical features of congestive heart failure on the basis of Starling's physiological concepts[50]. Fye was certainly stating a truism when he wrote in 1983 that 'The physiologic principles relating to control of cardiac output described by Starling more than a half century ago took on new clinical relevance as the hemodynamic approach to the management of congestive failure and acute myocardial infarction' was introduced[50]. Today, the flow directed balloon-tipped Swan-Gans catheter is a regular feature in the bedside management of these and other clinical situations.

The transition period between the 19th and 20th centuries also saw contributions by another great physiologist, the notable Carl Wiggers. Not the least of his contributions was his modification of the manometer that recorded more accurately pressure variations. It was an optical device capable of a much greater frequency response than those previously available. The vessels and cardiac chambers were cannulated directly and high fidelity pressure tracings were obtained with a series of light-reflecting mirrors. The clarity of his pressure recordings was indeed phenomenal, so much so that they are equally as good as any of the tracings

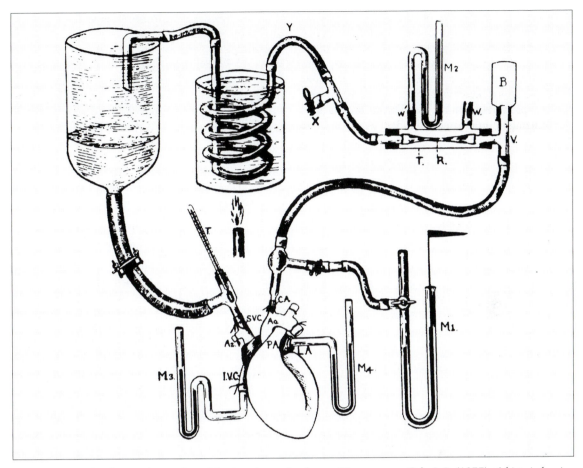

Figure 5 Starling's experimental model using the canine heart. *Literary source Cole, J. S. (1977). A historical review of the concept of the left ventricle as a pump. Catheterization and Cardiovascular Diagnosis, 3, 155–70. With permission*

obtained with our current level of technological development.

Wiggers' experiments with adrenaline brought out the observation that as the heart rate increased, there was initially a reduction of intraventricular pressure followed by a steep short rise during the isometric period. This is our well-known dp/dt parameter which refers to the maximum rise of pressure per unit time and which is ultimately dependent on the force of myocardial contractility. Cole quotes Wiggers regarding the variable quality and accuracy of records that shows a refreshing candor on the part of Wiggers, an attribute sorely lacking in many investigators.

While synchronous events and different curves can be established without difficulty in such records as are used to illustrate this paper, it must

be frankly acknowledged that I have many tracings in my possession in which adherence to strict corrective processes, such as outlined above, would force one to admit that a condition of dynamic chaos exists in the cardiovascular mechanisms, and one could point out many dynamic absurdities in published records of other investigators were one inclined to be critical[55].

Starling's successor to the chair of physiology at University College was Archibald Vivian Hill. Prior to this he too enjoyed an enviable reputation. Hill was widely acclaimed not only for his work in physiology but also for his significant contributions in the field of physical chemistry. His work in physical chemistry culminated in his formulation of the oxyhemoglobin dissociation curve. This was but an interlude from his main interest which involved studying the mechanisms of muscular contraction. These studies started in 1909 and restarted after a five year hiatus in 1919. All of this work was carried out at Cambridge, his alma mater. He was awarded the Nobel Prize for his studies on muscle contraction in 1922. His paper, *The heat of shortening and the dynamic constants of muscle* provided the background for the modern era of muscle mechanics and metabolism. It was published in 1938[56].

> The hope was recently expressed that with the development of a more accurate and rapid technique for muscle heat measurement, a much more consistent picture might emerge of the energy relations of muscles shortening and doing positive work. This hope has been realized, and some astonishingly simple and accurate relations have been found; relations, moreover, which (among other things) determine the effect of load on speed of shortening, allowing the form of the isometric contraction to be predicted and are the basis of the so-called 'visco-elasticity' of skeletal muscle[56].

It was Starling and Visscher in 1927 who had discovered that cardiac metabolism increased as its work increased[57]. It was this that set the stage for studies that would help define the interplay between work, metabolism and mobilization of energy in accomplishing this. Starling, unfortunately, died before he could continue with this breakthrough. Fenn had discovered in 1923 that during isometric contraction, a certain amount of energy is liberated as heat[58]. Furthermore, if work is performed by that muscle, although the same amount of heat is produced, total energy generated is increased[59]. These observations led to the view that work was accomplished through a mobilization of energy. The paper published by Hill in 1938 represented then an extension of Fenn's studies. Hill summarized his studies by stating that there were three types of mobilized energy: activation or maintenance heat, shortening heat with the amount dependent on degree of muscle shortening, and work heat. These physiological parameters offered a satisfactory mechanism for the observations by Starling and Visscher that cardiac metabolism increased as work increased.

Fenn and Marsh and Hill also formulated a force–velocity relationship in muscle which Mommaerts later suggested is based on chemical reactions occurring during contraction[56,60,61]. All

these studies were obviously leading the physiologists to an elucidation of the molecular mechanisms responsible for the contraction of the myocardial fibers. However, before we delve into the historical background of our current ideas of what goes on at the molecular level, let us trace first the evolution of the observations regarding the mechanical features of the problem at the macroscopic level.

The studies again begin with Hill in 1924[62-64]. Through his efforts and those of Ritchie and Wilkie, it was ascertained that tension develops almost instantaneously and remains at full force for a certain period of time and then declines[65-67]. Also, they showed that the force of the contractile elements is transmitted through the elastic components that have initially undergone stretching, and that all this occurs in a repetitive fashion so that to the eye the whole process appears as a twitch. The longer the duration of the state of tension, the stronger the twitch until anaerobic fatigue sets in, at which time the intensity of contraction decreases.

Another mechanical phenomenon visible to the eye is the staircase recording described by Bowditch as far back as 1871[68]. He was an American physiologist who also received his early training in Ludwig's laboratory. The term 'staircase' was applied because the tracings of the muscular contractions had the appearance of ascending stairs. It can be elicited by rhythmic stimulation of the myocardial preparation at regular intervals. As the myocardium responds to each stimulus of equal strength, it does so with increasing vigor until it reaches the highest level of response characteristic for that preparation.

Bowditch also described in the same paper the 'all-or-none' principle of the heart. Ranvier called it the 'hearts motto' when he elaborated on this phenomenon in 1880[69]. The principle states that once an impulse is received, the heart will respond either maximally or not at all. It is not the strength of the stimulus itself that elicits the all-or-none response, but rather the circumstances under which the heart perceives the stimulus. The general outline of this phenomenon remained unchanged ever since its formulation, until 1958 when Whalen pointed out an apparent exception[70]. He demonstrated that if the intensity of the stimulus is increased greatly, the heart muscle will respond with more forceful contractions, and that as regular threshold stimulation is resumed the force of contraction declines also.

The preceding paragraphs have given us a brief survey of the gross mechanical features of cardiac muscle contraction. As previously implied, the mechanics of contraction are ultimately due to the mobilization of energy produced by the metabolic activity of the cell. Nägeli was one of the earliest workers in the field of biological analysis on the molecular level. He was a botanist who was active during the mid-19th century[71]. Mommaerts states that Nägeli was the one who introduced the term molecular physiology, but that over the years its use became restricted to mechanisms of biosynthesis and heredity until Mommaerts revived it with its broader meaning, in 1950, by using it as the title of a book on the contraction mechanisms in muscle[71,72].

The belief that oxidation took place in the lungs, and only there, prevailed for a long time ever since Lavoisier and LaPlace published the results of their studies in 1780[73]. It was not until the first half of the 19th century that our current concepts of intracellular oxidation began to emerge. These concepts were not solidified, however, until the early 20th century and came about mostly through the efforts of Warburg and Wieland[74,75].

Warburg focused on the mechanism through which oxygen, the final hydrogen or electron acceptor, entered cellular metabolism. He assumed that a respiratory enzyme was necessary for this reaction. He called it 'Atmungsferment'. This turned out to be cytochrome oxidase, one of many pigments found in cells[76]. A. Szent-Györgyi and H. A. Krebs went on to delineate the steps involved in the complete oxidation of metabolites into CO_2 and H_2O[77,78]. Since then the Krebs cycle has become the bane of generations of students, and, unfortunately, because of its complexity and additions by other workers, just as easily forgotten. During the 1930s, a host of investigators added their contributions to the general scheme so that we have currently a fairly comprehensive knowledge regarding the metabolism of carbohydrates, lipids and proteins[79–85].

The importance of phosphorylation was brought out in the 1930s when adenosine triphosphate (ATP) was recognized as an essential coenzyme in the process[86]. Lippman introduced his concept of high-energy phosphate compounds in 1941 with ATP as the prototype. When ATP is hydrolyzed a large amount of energy is released. It was later determined that ATP was formed from adenosine diphosphate (ADP) under the influence of certain tissue enzymes which donate their phosphate group to ADP.

These fundamental biochemical reactions began to be perceived as part of the mechanism of myocardial contraction along with the unveiling of other physiological events at the molecular level. This began with the application of the polarization microscope by W. J. Schmidt in 1937[87]. His studies suggested that at the submicroscopic level the muscle had a filamentous structure arranged longitudinally with respect to the direction of the myofibrils. The publications by von Muralt and Edsall in 1930 indicated that myosin consists of long particles that lend themselves to making up the filamentous structure of the sarcomere[88,89]. Myosin filaments were then actually prepared by Weber and Noll in 1934[90,91].

Engelhardt and Ljubimova discovered in 1939 that myosin contained the catalytic enzyme involved in the hydrolysis of ATP[92]. This opened a whole new field of experimentation. Needhams' group was the first to focus on this pathway but our present concepts are derived from the detailed contributions of Szent-Györgyi[93]. He recognized first of all that myosin preparations available at the time had variable properties because they were actually a complex containing two types of protein: myosin and actin. Actin was discovered by Straub in 1942[94]. Further experimentation by Szent-Györgyi and others led to the development of a stable actomyosin fiber that could serve as a model for studying contractile mechanisms[95,96]. A relaxation factor was discovered by Marsh in 1952 and confirmed by Bendall a year later[97,98]. This can cause reversal of contraction in the fiber preparation. The possibility that this reversal is partially dependent on an enzyme capable of restoring the hydrolyzed ATP was then raised.

Electron microscopic studies were being conducted concurrently with the studies just mentioned. They began with Szent-Györgyi's group, Hall and his associates and the team of Draper and Hodge[99–101]. They were later amplified with technical refinements by Hanson and Huxley, and Sjöstrand[102–104]. These studies led to the view that contraction occurs when the actin rods move inwards into the A region (myosin) of the sarcomere. Mommaerts and his associates developed a freezing method to confirm this concept in 1955. Their muscle preparations were frozen at any given moment of activity and the preparation then subjected to molecular– morphological study[105].

Efforts were then directed towards elucidating the biochemical mechanisms at the cellular level that regulate muscle contraction. It became apparent that it was a complex affair involving an interplay between hormone receptors, ions and metabolic pathways. In due time the concept of excitation-coupling emerged. Bing called this concept 'the most important development in the history of cardiac metabolism'[106].

As far back as 1882, Ringer was the first to focus attention on the role of calcium in muscle contraction[107]. He showed that cardiac contraction depended on the external calcium ion concentration. In 1955 the 'relaxing factor' was identified by Kumugai, Ebashi and Takedo as a granular factor that contained the calcium binding cardiac microsomes[108]. Many years later Schwartz demonstrated that these microsomes have a sufficient capacity for calcium binding to accept a role for the sarcoplasmic reticulum in cardiac relaxation[109]. In 1965, Ebashi, following up on his previous investigations, isolated, in collaboration with Kodama, troponin as the calcium-binding protein responsible for the calcium sensitivity of the native myofibrils[110]. In 1974 Heilbrun and Wiercinski injected calcium into the muscles to initiate contraction.

Meanwhile, the discovery of the existence of receptors for catecholamines and acetylcholine set the stage for understanding the role of the autonomic nervous system in cardiac contraction. Raymond Ahlquist, a young pharmacologist at the Medical College of Georgia, became intrigued with the paradoxical effects of catecholamine administration[111]. This started him on a series of experiments that ultimately led to the identification of two distinct types of catecholamine receptors, alpha and beta. His paper on the subject which appeared in 1948 carried the following salient remarks: 'There are two distinct types of adrenotropic receptors ... the alpha is associated with most of the excitatory functions; the beta is associated with most of the inhibitory functions and one excitatory function (myocardial stimulation)'[112]. In Section 6, we shall see that Ahlquist's neurophysiologic concept was not only important in clarifying the apparent paradoxical responses to catecholamine stimulation but also served as the basis for the later development of a new class of cardiac pharmaceutical agents collectively known as beta-blockers.

Other investigators then showed that cholinergic receptors were involved in muscarinic stimulation.

In due time it became evident that the adrenergic receptors are modulated by a variety of molecular processes, and that both types of receptors are under the influence of regulatory proteins[113]. These proteins were called G-proteins because they contain guanine nucleotide. They act by coupling the hormone receptors to ion channels or enzymes. Dohlman and his associates identified the stimulatory proteins in cardiac muscle as G_S, noting further that they are responsible for coupling both $beta_1$ and $beta_2$ adrenergic receptors to adenylate cyclase[114]. Fain and his group presented evidence indicating that alpha adrenergic receptors are coupled to the enzyme phospholipase C[115]. The muscarinic receptors, on the other hand, were found to couple with atrial potassium ions by still another regulatory G-protein which was labeled G_K[116]. Elucidation of these receptor–effector pathways has created the hope that in due time specific pharmaceutical agents could be developed either to dampen or to enhance them. As yet no such agent has been found.

Two things occurred in the 1960s and 1970s that furthered our knowledge of the intracellular biochemical regulatory mechanisms. In the 1960s we began to recognize the role of the cyclic nucleotides as second messengers. Cyclic adenosine monophosphate (AMP) and cyclic guanosine monophosphate (GMP) were identified as part of this system. Albert Wollenberger presented evidence at the 1973 meeting of the International Society for Heart Research that cyclic AMP induced increased calcium uptake by the heart cell[117]. The frog myocardium was used as the model for their experiments. He and his group also showed that cyclic GMP had an opposite effect. These findings were confirmed by Brooker the very same year[118]. Current thinking holds the view that cyclic AMP mediates its effect through the sympathetic system while cyclic GMP acts through the cholinergic receptors.

In the 1970s, the role of calmodulin was unveiled by Means and his team[119]. The discovery of both calmodulin and the cyclic nucleotides led to a delineation of the various steps leading ultimately to muscle contraction. It is called the phosphoinositide pathway using calmodulin as the calcium ion receptor, and a phosphorylation process for the formation of two intermediary metabolites (diacylglycerol and inositol phosphate)[120].

Another major line of development was the pioneering efforts of Richard Bing beginning in

1947[121]. He took advantage of the relatively new technique of cardiac catheterization that was beginning to take hold in clinical practice. He was able to determine the substrate and metabolic uptake of the human heart *in situ* by analyzing samples of blood from the coronary sinus taken in this manner. By 1954 he was able to present in his Harvey lecture on *The Metabolism of the Heart*, the major substrates of the human heart stressing the major contribution of non-carbohydrate substrates in the metabolic process[122]. Fatty acids constituted the major portion of the non-carbohydrate substrates.

Although still incomplete, a rather complex scenario has developed since the original observations of the pioneers in cardiovascular physiology. This has been especially so at the molecular level, and it is primarily for this reason that I would like to provide at this time an overall integrated conceptual view of what we now believe to be the salient mechanisms as they relate to myocardial contraction at the ultrastructural and molecular level.

The fundamental individual contractile unit is the sarcomere. It is responsible for the pumping activity of the heart. The ventricle consists of bundles of muscles arranged essentially in a spiral fashion. Each bundle is composed of muscle cells all lined up in the same direction within a given bundle. In turn, each muscle cell (or fiber) has multiple parallel rows of longitudinal myofibrils which traverse the entire length of the cell. Each myofibril consists of several of the basic contractile units, the sarcomeres. The sarcomeres are joined serially end-to-end in a single line.

The sarcomere itself is composed of specific arrangements of two sets of overlapping myofilaments. The myofilaments are contractile proteins. They are divided into thick and thin filaments. The thick filaments are made up of myosin molecules, and the thin filaments of actin molecules. It is the biochemical and biophysical interactions between these strands of actin and myosin that ultimately produce contraction for the pumping effect of the ventricles. During the cardiac cycle the length of the sarcomere varies depending on the degree of end-diastolic fiber stretch and the extent of shortening during contraction. The principal morphologic changes in chronic excessive dilatation of the ventricle are slippage and malalignment of the myofibrils.

The actin and myosin filaments have distinct structural and functional properties. Each myosin filament has a globular cross bridge which interacts with actin to produce contraction. The energy for this contractile process is supplied by the enzyme activity of myosin adenosine triphosphatase (ATPase). That enzyme splits the phosphate bond of ATP and thereby liberates the energy for the contractile process. Actin enhances the enzymatic action of ATPase. It also combines with the myosin cross bridges in a 1 : 1 ratio. It is this coupling that forms the mechanical basis for contraction.

There is also a superficial membrane system. It consists of the sarcolemma membrane which covers the whole myocardial cell (or fiber); intercalated discs which lock each myocardial cell end-to-end; and the transverse tubular system (T system). The T system is formed by a deep vertical invagination of the sarcolemma into the interior of the cell at frequent intervals. The T system acts as a conduit for the transport of sodium, potassium and calcium ions during the electrical events of contraction and relaxation, and for the ingress and egress of metabolites and drugs so that these substances can come near to the contractile elements even if they do not actually cross the membrane.

The sarcoplasmic reticulum is an extensive intracellular tubular membrane system. It complements the transtubular T system in support of the process of excitation–contraction coupling and mechanical relaxation. The T system is in contact with the extracellular environment while the sarcoplasmic reticulum is entirely within the cell and at right angles to the T system. The reticulum has lateral sacs which store calcium for use as needed by the contractile process. In addition, the lateral sacs abut with the intercalated discs thereby providing the structural coupling for the dissemination of the excitation–contraction process.

The mitochondria contain the aerobic biochemical systems of the fiber. They are the metabolic power plants in which oxygen and appropriate substrates are utilized to form ATP, the final direct energy source for myocardial contraction. Anaerobic glycolysis goes on in the surrounding sarcoplasm from the glycogen that has been stored there.

All the processes in myocardial metabolism have as their goal two end points: excitation and contraction. The normal heart muscle has an obligatory need of large amounts of oxygen because it is dependent on aerobic metabolism for its energy supply. Myocardial oxygen extraction is near maximal at body rest; when more oxygen is needed coronary flow increases. Myocardial oxygen consumption requirements on the other hand are governed by three major and three minor determinants. The major determinants are intra-myocardial tension, myocardial contractility and heart rate. The minor determinants are fiber shortening (Fenn effect), energy required for activation and relaxation, and basal diastolic energy requirements. These determinants are all interrelated so that a change in one produces a domino effect.

Myocardial energy metabolism is directed towards aerobic production of ATP in the mitochondria since it is ATP that provides the immediate energy source for the contractile apparatus and biochemical reactions elsewhere in the cell. It does this by substrate oxidation and oxidative phosphorylation. Substrate oxidation involves the dehydrogenation of citric acid intermediates within the Krebs cycle. In oxidative phosphorylation the inorganic phosphate acquires a high-energy bond and combines with ADP to form ATP. The substrate fuels for this synthesis of ATP are fatty acids, glucose and lactate. Fatty acids are the most important. They must all be broken down to acetyl-CoA which then enters the Krebs cycle for aerobic ATP production. The lactate that is used as a fuel comes from the blood and its concentration is higher after prolonged skeletal muscle exercise. The heart muscle produces lactate only in the presence of hypoxia.

The importance of anaerobic glycolysis as a source of energy varies with the state of oxygenation of the myocardium. Glycolysis increases as hypoxia increases but it provides very few molecules of ATP compared to the breakdown of glucose *per se*. This makes it a very poor source for maintaining energy supply. Moreover, during hypoxia the pyruvate is reduced to lactate and this is not consumed as rapidly as it is produced so that during this state the coronary sinus blood will contain more lactate than systemic arterial blood. This is the basis for an important test for myocardial ischemia. Creatine phosphate functions as a limited reservoir of high-energy phosphate to maintain ATP levels.

Cyclic AMP is synthesized in the sarcoplasm from ATP through the influence of the enzyme adenylate cyclase. The activity of this enzyme can be enhanced by beta-adrenergic stimulation. Cyclic AMP increases skeletal muscle and myocardial glycogenolysis.

The entire pathway of contraction is activated when the adrenergic or muscarinic cholinergic receptors are bound to their respective hormones. The G proteins regulate the process by initially activating the enzyme phospholipase C. Once activated, phospholipase C in turn catalyzes the formation of two intermediary metabolites involving phosphorylation under the influence of protein kinase C. The two intermediary metabolites have been identified as inositol phosphates and diacylglycerol. The ultimate effect is to release calcium ions from the sarcoplasmic reticulum. The calcium ions diffuse within the sarcomere where they bind with the specific troponin calcium-receptor protein on the thin actin filament. This binding of the calcium to troponin is the direct activator of mechanical contraction. It does this by overcoming the inhibition of actin and myosin interaction that prevails during the resting phase. With the inhibition removed actin-myosin electrostatic cross bridges are formed and contraction occurs.

The process of contraction takes place by the sequential making and breaking of actin-myosin interconnections with consequent sliding of actin centrally along the fixed myosin filaments producing force development and shortening of the sarcomere. The electrostatic links between actin and myosin are broken in this sequence of events by the action of an enzyme called myosin ATPase. This enzyme breaks down ATP to ADP and inorganic phosphate. The making and breaking of these cross-linkages is a repetitive sequence during the entire course of ventricular contraction.

During relaxation, calcium is removed from the sarcoplasm and returned extracellularly to the depots in the sarcoplasmic reticulum lateral sacs. The calcium is pumped back into these sacs by the action of a relaxing factor. This factor has been identified as an enzyme called sarcotubular pump ATPase. The enzymatic reaction uses very little energy.

Contraction cannot occur without calcium. The greater the rate and quantity of calcium delivered to troponin, the faster the rate and the greater the number of activated interactions between actin and myosin. This results in a more rapid rate of tension development, greater maximum tension and increased contractility.

There are two basic mechanisms that control the force of myocardial contraction. These are the extent of diastolic stretch of the myofilaments, also known as preload, and the force of contractility itself which is related to the intensity of the interactions between the myofilaments.

The length of the sarcomere at end diastole governs the degree of overlap of the movable actin and fixed myosin contractile filaments and thereby determines the number of interaction sites. The strongest contraction occurs when there is maximum overlap since there are here many more sites available for interaction between actin and myosin. The weakest force of contraction occurs in the presence of minimum overlap. This relationship between sarcomere length and developed force is the ultrastructural basis for the Frank-Starling principle.

As the heart muscle contracts it develops tension. This is known as active tension and is a factor in the amount of force being developed during contraction. The degree of active tension is also dependent on the length of the sarcomere during the resting state. Again, it has been documented that optimal active tension occurs when there is optimal individual resting sarcomere length. This has been estimated as being 2.2 μm. When the sarcomere becomes too long or too short, overlap between the thick and thin filaments is no longer ideal and consequently adversely affects the force of contraction.

Heart muscle also generates a passive tension during diastole. This is caused by stretching of the myocardium as blood flows into the ventricular chamber. The stretching is known as distensibility or compliance since by so doing the ventricular cavity can accommodate the increasing volume of blood entering it without undue rise in intracavitary pressure.

REFERENCES

1. Hamilton, W.F. and Richards, D.W. (1982). The output of the heart. In Fishman, A.P. and Richards, D.W. (eds.) *Circulation of the Blood, Men and Ideas*. (Baltimore, Md.: Waverly Press, Inc.)

2. Webster, C. (1965). William Harvey's conception of the heart as a pump. *Bull. Hist. Med.*, **39**, 508

3. Basalla, A. (1962). William Harvey and the heart as a pump. *Bull. Hist. Med.*, **36**, 467

4. Siegel, R.E. (1967). Why Galen and Harvey did not compare the heart to a pump. *Am. J. Cardiol.*, **20**, 117–20

5. Ibid., p. 118

6. O'Malley, C.D., Poynter, F.N.L. and Russell, K.F. (1961). *William Harvey: Lectures on the Whole Anatomy, an Annotated Translation*, p. 152. (Berkeley and Los Angeles: Univ. California Press)

7. Harvey, W. (1957). *De Motu Cordis et Sanguinis*, Chap. 1. Translated by Franklin, K.J. (Oxford: Blackwell Scientific Publ.)

8. Ibid., p. 170

9. Ibid., p. 68

10. Franklin, K.J. (1933). *A Short History of Physiology*. (London: Bale)

11. Ibid.

12. Lower, R. (1669). *Tractatus de Corde*. (London: Allestry)

13. Hales, S. (1733). *Statical Essays, vol. II. Haemastaticks*. (London: Innys and Manby)

14. Rosen, G. (1936). Carl Ludwig and his American students. *Bull. Inst. Hist. Med.*, **4**, 609

15. Franklin, F.J. (1933). *Op. cit.*

16. Ibid.

17. Shapiro, E. (1972). Adolph Fick – forgotten genius of cardiology. *Am. J. Cardiol.*, **30**, 662–5

18. Ibid.

19. Fick, A. (1870). Uber die Messung des Blutquantums in der Herzventrikeln. *SB Phys-Med. Ges. Würzburg*, July 9. (Note: Fick's publications have been collected in Schenk, F. (1903–05). *Adolf Fick Gesammete Abhandlungen, Wurzburg*, 4 volumes)

20. Shapiro, E. (1972). *Op. cit.*, p. 665

21. Fick, A. (1870). Ueber die Messung des Blutquantums in den Herzventrikeln. *S.B. Phys-Med. Ges. Würzburg*, July 9

22. Grehant, N. and Quinquad, C.E. (1886). Recherches expérimentales sur la mesure du volume de sang qui traverse les poumons en un temps donné. *C.R. Soc. Biol. Paris*, **36**, 285

23. Zuntz, N. and Hagemann, O. (1898). Untersuchungen über den Stoffwechsel des Pferdes bei Ruhe und Arbeit. *Landw. Jb.*, **27** (Ergänz. Bd. 3)

24. Loewy, A. and von Schrötter, H. (1903). Ein Verfahren zur Bestimmung der Blutgasspannungen, der Kreislauf – geschivindigkeit und des Herzschlagvolumens am Menschen. *Arch. Anat. Physiol. Abth.*, p. 304

25. Plesch, J. (1909). Hämodynamische Studien. *Z. Exp. Path. Ther.*, **6**, 380

26. Henderson, Y. and Prince, A.L. (1917). Application of gas analysis. II. The CO_2 tension of the venous blood and the circulation rate. *J. Biol. Chem.*, **32**, 325

27. Markoff, I., Müller, F. and Zuntz, N. (1911). Neue Methode zur Bestimmung der im menschliken Körper umlaufenden Blutmenge. *Z. Balneol.*, **4**, 373, 409, 411

28. Grollman, A. (1932). *The Cardiac Output in Man in Health and Disease*, p. 11. (Springfield, Ill.: Charles C. Thomas)

29. *Ibid.*

30. Kinsman, J.M., Moore, J.W. and Hamilton, W.F. (1929). Studies on the circulation. I. Injection method: physical and mathematical considerations. *Am. J. Physiol.*, **89**, 322

31. Stewart, G.N. (1897). Researches on the circulation time and on the influences which affect it. IV. The output of the heart. *J. Physiol. (London)*, **22**, 159

32. Moore, J.W., Kinsman, J.M., Hamilton, W.F. and Spurling, R.G. (1929). Studies on the circulation. II. Cardiac output determinations. Comparison of the injection method with the direct Fick procedure. *Am. J. Physiol.*, **89**, 331

33. Cournand, A. (1945). Measurement of the cardiac output in man using the right heart catheterization. Description of technique, discussion of validity and of place in the study of the circulation. *Fed. Proc.*, **4**, 207

34. Hamilton, W.F., Riley, R.L., Attyah, A.M., Cournand, A., Fowell, D.M., Himmelstein, A., Noble, R.P., Remington, J.W., Richards, D.W. Jr., Wheeler, N.C. and Witham, A.C. (1948). Comparison of the Fick and dye injection methods of measuring the cardiac output in man. *Am. J. Physiol.*, **153**, 309

35. Wood, E.H. (1950). Special instrumentation problems encountered in physiological research concerning the heart and circulation in man. *Science*, **112**, 707

36. Frank, O. (1895). Zur Dynamik des Herzmuskels. *Z. Biol.*, **32**, 370

37. Frank, O. (1969). 'On the dynamics of cardiac muscle (1895)'. Chapman, C.B. and Wasserman, E. *Am. Heart J.*, **58**, 282–317, 467–78

38. Cole, J.S. (1977). A historical review of the concept of the left ventricle as a pump. *Catheterization Cardiovascular Diagn.*, **3**, 155–70

39. Howell, W.H. and Donaldson, F. Jr. (1884). Experiments upon the heart of the dog with reference to the maximum volume of blood sent out by the left ventricle in a single beat, and the influence of variations in venous pressure, arterial pressure, and pulse-rate upon the work done by the heart. *Philos. Trans. Pt. I.*, 139

40. Henderson, Y. (1906). The volume curve of the ventricles of the mammalian heart, and the significance of this curve in respect to the mechanics of the heart-beat and the filling of the ventricles. *Am. J. Physiol.*, **14**, 325–67

41. Markwalder, J. and Starling, E.H. (1914). On the constancy of the systolic output under varying conditions. *J. Physiol. (London)*, **48**, 348

42. Patterson, S.W. and Starling, E.H. (1914). On the mechanical factors which determine the output of the ventricles. *J. Physiol. (London)*, **48**, 357

43. Patterson, S.W., Piper, H. and Starling, E.H. (1914). The regulation of the heart beat. *J. Physiol. (London)*, **48**, 465

44. O'Rourke, M.F. (1984). Starling's law of the heart: an appraisal 70 years on. *Aust. NZ. J. Med.*, **14**, 879–87

45. Wiggers, C.J. (1952). Determinants of cardiac performance. In his *Circulatory Dynamics, Physiologic Studies.* (New York: Grune and Stratton)

46. Straub, F.B. (1942). *Actin Stud. Inst. Med. Chem. Szeged*, **2**, 3

47. Straub, F.B. (1943). *Actin II Stud. Inst. Med. Chem., Szeged*

48. Chapman, C.B. (1962). Ernest Henry Starling, the clinician's physiologist. *Ann. Intern. Med.*, **57** (suppl. 2), 1

49. Colp, R. Jr. (1952). Ernest H. Starling: his contribution to medicine. *J. Hist. Med.*, **7**, 280

50. Fye, W.B. (1983). Ernest Henry Starling, his law and its growing significance in the practice of medicine. *Circulation*, **68**, 1145–7

51. Starling, E.H. (1918). *The Linacre Lecture on the Law of the Heart.* (London: Longmans, Green and Co.)

52. Sewall, H. (1911). Henry Newell Martin. *Bull. Johns Hopkins Hosp.*, **22**, 329–30

53. *Ibid.*, p. 332–3

54. Martin, H.N. (1881). A new method of studying the mammalian heart. *Stud. Biol. Lab. Johns Hopkins University*, **2**, 119–30

55. Wiggers, C.J. (1914). Some factors controlling the shape of the pressure curve in the right ventricle. *Am. J. Physiol.*, **33**, 382–96

56. Hill, A.V. (1938). The heat of shortening and the dynamic constants of muscle. *Proc. R. Soc. London*, **126**, 136–95

57. Starling, E.H. and Visscher, M.B. (1927). The regulation of the energy output of the heart. *J. Physiol. (London)*, **62**, 243

58. Fenn, W.O. (1923). A quantitative comparison between the energy liberated and the work performed by the isolated sartorius muscle of the frog. *J. Physiol. (London)*, **58**, 175

59. Fenn, W.O. (1924). The relation between work performed and the energy liberated in muscular contraction. *J. Physiol. (London)*, **58**, 373

60. Fenn, W.O. and Marsh, B.S. (1935). Muscular force at different speeds of shortening. *J. Physiol. (London)*, **85**, 277

61. Mommaerts, W.F.H.M. (1982). Heart muscle. In Fishman, A.P. and Richards, D.W. (eds.). *Circulation of the Blood, Men and Ideas*, p. 159. (Balitimore: Waverly Press, Inc.)

62. Gasser, H.S. and Hill, A.V. (1924). The dynamics of muscular contraction. *Proc. R. Soc. B.*, **96**, 398

63. Hill, A.V. (1949). The abrupt transition from rest to activity in muscle. *Proc. R. Soc. B.*, **136**, 399

64. Hill, A.V. and MacPherson, L. (1954). The effect of nitrate, iodide and bromide on the duration of the active state in skeletal muscle. *Proc. R. Soc., B.*, **143**, 81

65. Ritchie, J.M. (1954). The effect of nitrate on the active state of muscle. *J. Physiol. (London)*, **126**, 155

66. Wilkie, D.R. (1954). Facts and theories about muscle. *Progr. Biophys.*, **4**, 288

67. Wilkie, D.R. (1956). The mechanical properties of muscle. *Br. Med. Bull.*, **12**, 177

68. Bowditch, H.P. (1871). Ueber die Eigenhümlichkeiten der Reizbarkeit welche die Musskelfasern des Herzens zeignen. *Ber. Math.-Phys. Sächs. Ges. Wiss. Leipzig*, **13**, 652

69. Ranvier, L.A. (1880). Leçons d'anatomie générale faites au Collége de France. *Année 1877–78*. (Paris: Bailliére)

70. Whalen, W.J. (1958). Apparent exception to the 'all or none' law in cardiac muscle. *Science*, **127**, 468

71. Mommaerts, W.F.H.M. (1982). *Op. cit.*, p. 168

72. Mommaerts, W.F.H.M. (1950). *Muscular Contraction. A Topic in Molecular Physiology.* (New York: Interscience)

73. Lavoisier, A.L. (1780). LaPlace: Mémoire sur la chaleur. *Mém. Acad. Sci. (Paris)*, p. 355

74. Warburg, O. (ed.). (1948). *Wasserstoffübertragende Fermente.* (Berlin: W. Saenger)

75. Wieland, H. (1932). *On the Mechanism of Oxidation.* (New Haven: Yale Univ. Press)

76. Keilin, D. (1925). On cytochrome, a respiratory pigment, common to animals, yeast and higher plants. *Proc. R. Soc. B.*, **98**, 312

77. Szent-Györgyi, A. (1937). *Studies on Biological Oxidation and Some of its Catalysts.* (Leipzig: Barth)

78. Krebs, H.A. (1954). The tricarboxylic acid cycle. In Greenberg, D.M. (ed.) *Chemical Pathways of Metabolism*, **1**, 109. (New York: Academic Press)

79. Harden, A. (1932). *Alcoholic Fermentation*, 4th. edn. (New York: Longmans, Green)

80. Embden, G., Deuticke, H.J. and Kraft, G. (1932). Über die intermediären Vorgänge bei der Glyckolyse in der Muskulatur. *Klin. Wschr.*, **12**, 213

81. Kluyver, A.J. (1931). *The Chemical Activities of Micro-organisms.* (London: Univ. London Press)

82. Meyerhof, O. (1930). *Die chemischen Vorgänge im Muskel und ihr Zusammenhang mit Arbeitsleistung und Wärmebildung.* (Berlin: Springer)

83. Meyerhof, O. (1937). Über die Intermediarvorgänge der enzymatischen Kohle hydratsplatung. *Ergebn. Physiol.*, **39**, 10

84. Parnas, J.K. (1937). Der Mechanismus der Glykogenlyse im Muskel. *Ergebn. Enzymforsch.*, **6**, 57

85. Cori, C.F. (1946). Enzymatic reactions in carbohydrate metabolism. *Harvey Lect.*, **61**, 253

86. Mommaerts, W.F.H.M. (1950). *Op. cit.*

87. Schmidt, W.J. (1937). *Die Doppelbrechung von Karyoplasma, Zytoplasma, und Metaplasma.* (Berlin: Borntraeger)

88. von Muralt, A.L. and Edsall, J.T. (1930). Studies in the physical chemistry of muscle globulin. III. The anisotropy of myosin and the angle of isocline. *J. Biol. Chem.*, **89**, 315

89. von Muralt, A.L. and Edsall, J.T. (1930). Studies in the physical chemistry of muscle globulin. IV. The anisotropy of myosin and double refraction of flow. *J. Biol. Chem.*, **89**, 351

90. Noll, D. and Weber, H.H. (1934). Polarisationsoptik und molekularer Feinbau der

Q-Abschnitte des Froschmuskels. *Pflügers Arch. Gen. Physiol.*, **255**, 234

91. Weber, H.H. (1934). Der Feinbau und die mechanische Eigenschaften des Myosinfadens. *Pflügers Arch. Gen. Physiol.*, **235**, 205

92. Engelhardt, W.A. and Ljubimova, M.N. (1939). Myosin and adenosinetriphosphatase. *Nature (London)*, **144**, 668

93. Banga, I., Erdös, M., Gerendas, W.F., Mommaerts, W.F.H.M. and Straub, F.B. (1942). Szent-Györgyi: myosin and muscular contraction. *Stud. Inst. Med. Chem. Szeged*, **I**

94. Straub, F.B. (1942). Actin. *Stud. Inst. Med. Chem. Szeged*, **2**, 3

95. Szent-Györgyi, A. (1951). *Chemistry of Muscular Contraction*, 2nd edn. (New York: Academic Press)

96. Weber, H.H. and Portzehl, H. (1952). Kontraktion, ATP-Cyclus und fibrilläre Proteine des Muskels. *Ergebn. Physiol.*, **47**, 369

97. Marsh, B.B. (1952). The effects of adenosinetriphosphate on the fibre volume of a muscle homogenate. *Biochem. Biophys. Acta*, **9**, 247

98. Bendall, J.R. (1953). Further observations on a factor (The 'Marsh' factor) effecting relaxation of ATP – shortened muscle – fibre models, and the effect of Ca and Mg ions upon it. *J. Physiol. (London)*, 121–232

99. Rosza, G., Szent-Györgyi, A. and Wychoff, R.W.G. (1949). The electron microscopy of F-actin. *Biochim. Biophys. Acta*, **3**, 561

100. Hall, C.E., Jakus, M.A. and Schmitt, F.O. (1946). An investigation of cross striations and myosin filaments in muscle. *Biol. Bull.*, **90**, 32

101. Draper, M.H. and Hodge, A.J. (1949). Studies on muscle with the electron microscope. I. The ultrastructure of toad striated muscle. *Aust. J. Exp. Biol. Med. Sci.*, **27**, 465

102. Hanson, J. and Huxley, H.E. (1955). The structural basis of contraction in striated muscle. *Symp. Soc. Exp. Biol.*, **9**, 228

103. Huxley, H.E. (1957). The double array of filaments in cross-striated muscle. *J. Biophys. Biochem. Cyto.*, **3**, 631

104. Sjöstrand, F.D. and Andersson, E. (1939). The ultrastructure of skeletal muscle myofilaments. In *Proc. First European Regional Conference on Electron Microscopy, Stockholm*, 1957, p. 204. (New York: Academic Press)

105. Mommaerts, W.H.F.M. and Schilling, M.O. (1955). Interruption of muscular contraction by rapid cooling. *Am. J. Physiol.*, **182**, 579

106. Bing, R.J. (1973). From organisms to the cell: the history of metabolism: In Dhalla, N.S. (ed.) *Recent Advances in Studies on Cardiac Structure and Metabolism*, vol. 3, *Myocardial Metabolism*, pp. 3–9. (Baltimore: University Park Press)

107. Ringer, S. (1882). A further contribution regarding the influence of the different constituents of the blood on the contraction of the heart. *J. Physiol. (London)*, **4**, 30

108. Katz, A. and Rephe, D.I. (1967). Quantitative aspects of dog cardiac microsomal binding and calcium uptake. *Circ. Res.*, **21**, 153–62

109. Schwartz, A. (1971). Calcium and the sarcoplasmic reticulum. In Harris, P. and Opie, L.H. (eds.) *Calcium and the Heart*, pp. 66–92. (London: Academic Press)

110. Opie, L.H. (1980). Cardiac metabolism: catecholamines, calcium, cyclic AMP, and substrates. In Tajuddin, M., Das, P.K., Tariz, M. and Dhalla, N.S. (eds.) *Advances in Myocardiology*, vol. I, pp. 3–19. (Baltimore: University Park Press)

111. Wenger, N.K. and Greenbaum, L.M. (1984). From adrenoceptor mechanisms to clinical therapeutics: Raymond Ahlquist, PhD, 1914–1983. *J.A.C.C.*, **2**, 419–21

112. Ahlquist, R.P. (1948). A study of the adrenotropic receptors. *Am. J. Physiol.*, **153**, 586–600

113. Gilman, A.G. (1987). G-proteins: transducers of receptor-generated signals. *Annu. Rev. Biochem.*, **56**, 615–49

114. Dohlman, H.G., Carow, M.C. and Lefkowitz, R.J. (1987). A family of receptors coupled to guanine nucleotide regulatory proteins. *Biochem.*, **26**, 2658–64

115. Fain, J.N., Wallace, M.A. and Wajikiewicz, R.J.H. (1988). Evidence for involvement of guanine nucleotide-binding regulatory proteins in the activation of phospholipases by hormones. *FASEB J.*, **2**, 2569–74

116. Neer, E.J. and Clapman, D.E. (1988). Roles of G-proteins in transmembrane signaling. *Nature (London)*, **333**, 129–34

117. Opie, L.H. (1980). *Op. cit.*, p. 8

118. Brooker, G. (1973). Change in myocardial adenosine 3'5' cyclic monophosphate during the contraction cycle. In Dhalla, N.S. (ed.) *Recent Advances in Studies on Cardiac Structure and*

Metabolism, Vol. 3. *Myocardial Metabolism*, pp. 207–12. (Baltimore: University Park Press)

119. Means, A.R. and Dedman, J.R. (1980). Calmodulin – an intracellular calcium receptor. *Nature (London)*, **285**, 73–7

120. Berridge, M.J. (1987). Inositol triphosphate and diacylglycerol: two interacting second messengers. *Annu. Rev. Biochem.*, **53**, 159–93

121. Bing, R.J., Vandam, L.D., Gregoire, F., Handelsman, J.C., Goodale, W.T. and Eckenhoff, J.E. (1947). Catheterization of coronary sinus and middle cardiac vein in man. *Proc. Soc. Exp. Biol. Med.*, **66**, 239–40

122. Bing, R.J. (1954–55). The metabolism of the heart. *Harvey Lecture Series*, pp. 27–70. (New York: Academic Press, Inc.)

16   The electrophysiologic control of the heart

Electricity is the phenomenon brought about by a relationship between positively and negatively charged particles. The theories and laws governing the entire spectrum have been formulated only during the last two centuries. Knowledge concerning the electrical field, which is the space surrounding the charged particle, did not evolve until the latter part of the 19th century.

Electricity forms an integral part of the physical properties of matter, and is most intimately involved with the uniquely interesting phenomenon of magnetism. However, despite this known relationship, magnetism was discovered independently of electricity. Later, the development of modern technology occurred with the discovery that electric currents produce magnetic fields and that changing magnetic fields produce electric effects[1]. The electromagnet is an example of this physical law while gamma rays and X-rays are possible only because of this relationship.

Biological processes such as the heart beat, nerve transmission, and muscle action are all dependent on electrical phenomena, and these in turn can be measured and observed through electromagnetic means. The electrocardiograph which is essentially a galvanometric device is an example of how such observations can be made.

The early history of electrical phenomena should be explored simply because it serves as the fountainhead from which current knowledge of the electrophysiologic control of the heart emerged. Every schoolchild in America is introduced to these phenomena with Benjamin Franklin's kite and terrestrial lightning experiments; but observations of electrical phenomena were made long before Franklin. In fact, electrical and magnetic phenomena were known to the ancients, but, again, that is all they were. Observations were based on chance occurrences with explanations derived from conjecture and mythical beliefs. Systematic investigations did not really begin until the late Middle Ages.

The initial observations were made from such banal sources as the electric ray or torpedo fish, rubbed amber, and the lodestone. It took millennia before it became apparent that observations made in connection with these sources had a common link that would eventually lead to the development of electrophysiology as a major discipline of cardiology. As with all else in cardiology, it required first the integration of basic principles with a firm foundation in anatomy, especially at the microscopic level, and now at the ultrastructural level.

The ancients were acquainted with two types of fish that manifested electrical properties. These were the electric catfish (*Malapterurus electricus*) and the torpedo fish (*Torpedo mamorata*) also known as the electric ray. Both are aptly named since the sting from either one is capable of inducing at the minimum an electrical shock or, even worse, a state of torpor[2]. The Greeks were well acquainted with these creatures and tried to turn their electrical potentialities to their advantage in the treatment of headaches, and in the management of epilepsy or even labor pains[2].

Amber was also known to the Greeks. It is a fossil tree resin occurring in various shades of yellow, orange or brown and even white. The white variety should not be confused with the morbid intestinal secretions of the sperm whale, and which also carries the name, ambergris. The resin itself is found all over the world with the largest deposits currently along the shores of the Baltic Sea. These deposits are used for making a variety of articles such as cigarette holders, pipe stems, beads and rosaries.

Amber has a unique property. When rubbed it becomes electrified so that it attracts and holds on to light objects. This property caused the Greeks to name it electron. The Arabs later gave it the name anbar. The Greeks were not the first to discover this property. Some historians assert that it was familiar during the reign of Emperor Hoang-Ti in 2635 BC[3].

The first systematic investigations of electrical phenomena were in magnetism and began with Petrus Peregrinus de Maricourt in Picardie. This French crusader of the 13th century was the first to describe the phenomena associated with natural magnetism. He used lodestone, a natural magnet, as the model for his studies. De Maricourt was responsible for developing the notions of North and South poles and polarization; notions that still survive and that are known to play an important role in electromagnetism[4].

Lodestone is a magnetic oxide of iron. It literally means 'waystone' from its later usage as a compass for guiding mariners. The initial name for it was the magneta stone or stone from Magnesia in Thessaly. There are two opinions as to the derivation of the name magneta. The most obvious source is the name of the province where it was mined. Lucretius, the Roman author of the long, contemplative poem, *De rerum natura*, put forth this view[5]. On the other hand, Pliny the elder ascribes the name to its alleged discoverer, the shepherd Magnes in these words: 'The nails of whose shoes and the tip of whose staff stuck fast in a magnetic field while he pastured his flocks'[6].

The Lodestone was certainly known at least since the Periclean Age. Plato used it as the major theme in his discourse on the reading of Homer[7]:

> For as I was saying just now, this is not an art in you, whereby you speak well on Homer, but a divine power, which moves you like that in the stone which Euripedis named Magnetis, but most people call Heraclea. For this stone not only attracts iron rings but also imparts to them a power whereby they in turn are able to do the very same thing as the stone, and attract other rings; so that sometimes there is formed quite a long chain of bits of iron and rings suspended one from another; and they all depend for this power on that one stone[7].

When Lucretius described its properties he noted that at times iron particles were repelled rather than attracted. This led him to formulate what appears to be the first theoretical basis for magnetism. He attributed the attraction to the presence of a sort of vacuum around the Lodestone causing iron particles to swoop in and fill it.

The historical relationship of the lodestone to the compass is shrouded in obscurity. Some authors suggest that this relationship was known to the Chinese as early as 2600 BC. Others maintain that the compass is of Italian or Arabian origin and that it was introduced to China as late as the 13th century. We do know that de Maricourt described through experimental investigation the relationship between the lodestone and the magnetic excursions of the compass. This information could have been passed on then to the Chinese. However, Alexander Neckam (1157–1217) clearly described the use of the magnetic needle in navigation many years before de Maricourt's report. He was a school teacher who revealed his observations and views in both of his books, *De utensilibus* and *De naturis rerum*. Beasley quotes him as saying: 'Mariners at sea when, through cloudy weather in the day which hides the sun, or through the darkness of the night, they lose the knowledge of the quarter of the world to which they are sailing, touch a needle with the magnet, which will turn around till, on its motion ceasing, its point will be directed toward the north'[8]. Neckam's needle was suspended on a pivot. The earliest Italian compasses were needles lying on reeds and floating freely in water.

Further experimentation on magnetism was not conducted to any significant degree until the arrival of William Gilbert in the late 16th century. He was a product of Cambridge, one of the earliest in their long line of distinguished scientists. Gilbert was one of the great English physicians of the 16th century. Throughout his career he maintained a keen interest in electricity and magnetism. His observations, extending over many years and based on rigid experimentation, were collated and explained in his treatise published in 1600, just three years before his death. It bore the rather long title *De Magnete, magneticisque corporibus, et de magno magnete tellure; physiologia nove, phirimis et argumentis et experimentis demonstrata*[9].

Gilbert recognized that the earth itself is a magnet because of its similarity in magnetic behavior to the spherical lodestone. It was he who coined the terms 'electric' and 'charged body'. He can be considered as the father of electromagnetism. He not only gave a systematic discussion of magnetism but also considered the force between two objects charged by friction. Electric was the term he used for the force. Gilbert attributed the electrification of a body by friction to the removal of 'humour' which then left an 'effluvium' around the body. 'Humour' is equivalent to what is currently called 'charge', and 'effluvium' has been renamed 'electric field'.

Figure 1 illustrates his method of magnetizing a bar of metal by holding it in the direction of the earth's magnetic field while subjecting it to repeated blows of the hammer.

The succeeding two centuries saw an increasing interest in electrostatic effects, magnetism and electricity in general. The result was a marked advancement of knowledge that would soon serve as the springboard for the delineation of electrophysiologic principles. National boundaries were again transcended by contributions from the European continent, England and the New World.

The first electric machine came into being through the genius of the German Otto von Guericke. It was a simple machine consisting of a rotating globe, initially of sulphur and then of glass, that became electrified when rubbed against the hand[10]. Electrical conductors were discovered by Stephen Gray of England in 1729, showing that they were distinctly different from insulators. Many years later Benjamin Franklin, the peripatetic genius from Philadelphia, suggested to Priestley the probability that when a hollow conducting vessel is electrified no electric force acts on objects in its interior. When Priestley did actually show this to be true, he put forth the view that 'the attraction of electricity is subject to the same laws with that of gravitation, and is therefore according to the (inverse) squares of the distance'[11]. This discovery completed the laws of electrostatics.

The gardener to the king of France, Charles Francois de Cisternay Du Fay, showed that in order to electrify conductors they had to be insulated or supported by non-conductors. More importantly he developed the thesis that there was a repellant electric force in addition to the well-known attractive one. These observations were further organized and systematized by the largely self-taught American, Benjamin Franklin. He enunciated the law known as the conservation of charge. This states that the net sum of a charge (plus and minus) within a region is always constant.

The Bishop of Pomerania, Ewald von Kleist, demonstrated in 1745 that the charge from an electric machine could be transferred to a glass bottle and stored there[12]. The Bishop may also have been one of the earliest victims of shock from static electricity. Although primitive, these early electric machines, once charged, stored a powerful amount of static electricity. One day, after pushing an iron rod through the cork of a bottle filled with mercury, he held the rod to the conductor of an electric machine. The bishop accidentally touched the conductor and immediately experienced a violent shock to his arm. Von Kleist's rude jolt was soon experienced by physicists at the University of Leyden who were also conducting experiments with charged bottles under the direction of Pieter van Musschenbroek (1692–1761). His account of the experiences of his staff piqued the interest of the Abbé Nollet who, at the same time, immediately grasped the potential ramifications of these accidents. Jean-Antoine Nollet is responsible for naming the glass bottle, the Leyden jar, and to this day the name and jar survive albeit with numerous improvements[10]. The Leyden jar became an important investigative tool over the succeeding years. The improvements made the jar so powerful that it could produce sparks large enough to be transmitted through long circuits of wire and water. Its lethal capabilities were soon realized in the death of small animals. The jar was also utilized as a source of entertainment. Cohen recounts how all 700 monks from the Convent du Paris were shocked by a spark from the jar as they were joined together by clasping each other's hands[13]. Who, among us, can ever forget our own experiences when we were initiated into the secrets of physics during our formative student days?

Coding, clarification and mathematical expression of the various laws of electricity and magnetism were accomplished by Henry Cavendish, Charles-Augustin Coloumb and Poisson during the 18th and early part of the 19th centuries. Poisson's mathematical equation published in 1813 and Franklin's law of the conservation of charge constitute the sum and substance of the laws of electrostatics. Henry Cavendish investigated the power of a material to conduct static electricity and made measurements of electrical capacity[10]. Although Cavendish anticipated the fundamental law of electric flow, its final and surviving clarification was accomplished by George Simon Ohm, a German physicist.

Ohm published his famous and very simple law in 1827. Coloumb's contributions were expressed in the law he formulated. This was arrived at through experiments conducted with a magnetic torsion balance. It is the inverse square law of force between both magnetic poles and electric charges. In each case, like poles repel each other while unlike poles attract each other[14]. These and other

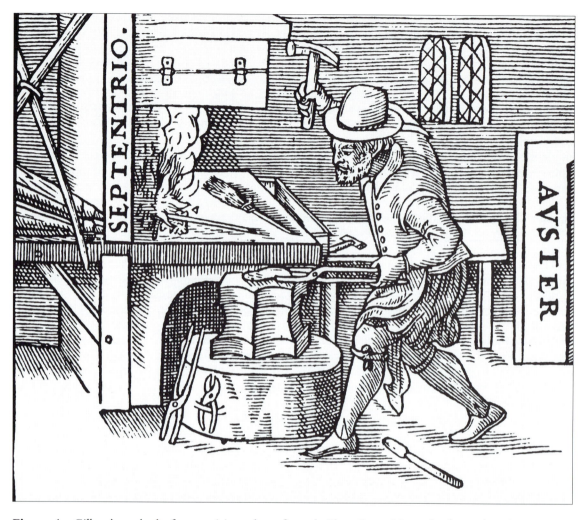

Figure 1   Gilbert's method of magnetizing a bar of metal. *Photo Source National Library of Medicine. Literary Source Gilbert, W. (1900). On the Magnet, Magnetic Bodies also on the Great Magnet, the Earth. Tr. by S.P. Thompson, Chiswick, London. With permission*

formulations of electricity and magnetism, both theoretical and mathematical, occupied the rest of the 19th century. Concomitant with all these contributions by the physicists, other investigators were exploring the mysteries of animal electricity with the Leyden jar playing a significant role.

More than sixteen centuries had elapsed before the strange powers of the torpedo fish were to interest anyone again. The first tentative attempts at investigating this phenomenon were those of E. Bancroft in 1676[3]. He advanced the view that the sting of the torpedo fish was electrical in origin. Almost another 100 years were to pass before others took up this work. This was in 1773

when two papers appeared in the same issue of the Royal Society. One was an anatomical and physiological study by John Walsh attributing the shock to release of 'compressed electrical fluid'[15]. The title is of interest in that it referred to torpedoes found on the coast of England, a rather convenient source of fish for his studies. In essence, he said that the shock was similar to that from the Leyden jar. The other paper written by John Hunter, the noted anatomist, described observations identical to those of Walsh[16]. Observations with an artificial model were reported by Henry Cavendish in 1777. His artificial torpedo was made of wood and leather. When it was submerged in salt water and then electrified with a charge from the Leyden jar, Cavendish noted that electric shocks were produced similar to those with the live fish.

Leopoldo Caldani (1725–1813), professor of anatomy at Bologna, turned to the frog for his experiments. He was able to excite the isolated nerve and muscle preparation from a frog with a spark from the Leyden jar[17]. His student, Luigi Galvani, participated in these studies. It was almost 24 years later when Galvani started his own series of experiments with most of the work carried out in his dissection room during his tenure as professor of anatomy at Bologna. Galvani's studies were actually an extension of Caldani's preliminary work with the electric machine and animal tissues. His own efforts were prompted by his desire to unveil the true nature of the phenomenon as determined by rigorous experimentation. There were too many conjectures and theoretical assertions stirring about in academic circles at the time. His goal was to fathom the mechanisms, once and for all, and, as in so many discoveries in medicine, he was placed on the right path by an accidental observation. Details of the first experiment were described by Galvani in the following words:

The course of the work has progressed in the following way. I dissected a frog and prepared it. Having in mind other things, I placed the frog on the same table as an electrical machine so that the animal was completely separated from and removed at a considerable distance from the machine's conductor. When one of my assistants by chance lightly applied the point of a scalpel to the inner crural nerves suddenly all the muscles of the limbs were seen so to contract that they appeared to have fallen into violent tonic convulsions. Another assistant who was present when we were performing electrical experiments thought he observed that this phenomenon occurred when a spark was discharged from the conductor of the electrical machine. Marvelling at this, he immediately brought the unusual phenomenon to my attention when I was completely engrossed and contemplating other things. Hereupon I became extremely enthusiastic and eager to repeat the experiment so as to clarify the obscure phenomenon and make it known. I myself, therefore, applied the point of the scalpel first to

one then to the other crural nerve, while at the same time one of the assistants produced a spark; the phenomenon repeated itself in precisely the same manner as before. Violent contractions were induced in the individual muscles of the limbs and the prepared animal reacted just as though it were seized with tetanus at the very moment when the sparks were discharged[18].

Galvani's experiment was crucial in that he confirmed the observation that electrical stimulation could induce muscle contraction. His other crucial experiments had to do with the action of a combination of dissimilar metals when placed in contact with the muscles of a frog. These studies were carried out initially as an attempt to demonstrate the influence of atmospheric electricity on the muscles of a frog. It was again purely fortuitous that this observation was made.

Both series of experiments were described in his monograph, *Die vivibus electricitatis in motu commentarius*[19]. It was published in 1791, eleven years after he had started the investigations. Figure 2 is an illustration of Galvani's experimental models to demonstrate the presence of animal electricity.

Galvani's explanation for the mechanism underlying the dissimilar metal effect was challenged by Alessandro Volta and became a drawn out controversial issue between Galvani and his contemporary at the University of Pavia. Galvani was of the opinion that the muscles were able to store electricity and that this stored electricity caused the electrical stimulation after being released by contact with the dissimilar metals. Volta rejected this mechanism and substituted the view that the electrical stimulation was caused by the direct coupling of the dissimilar metals, and not to any discharge of stored electricity. Volta happened to be correct in the light of subsequent events.

Alessandro Volta is now remembered and honored as the founder of electrochemistry. He was not an anatomist but rather professor of natural philosophy at the equally prestigious University of Pavia. Volta was never able to demonstrate to his satisfaction the presence of animal electricity. This was actually the bone of contention between him and Galvani. His letter to Sir Joseph Banks of the Royal Society in 1800 leaves no doubt as to his position on the matter[20]. Volta considered Galvani's frog-leg preparation as an electrometer conducting the electricity reaching it as it was being produced

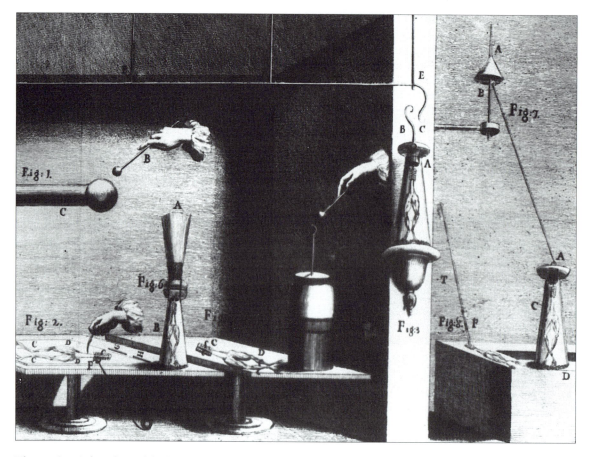

Figure 2 Galvani's models demonstrating animal electricity. *Photo Source National Library of Medicine. Literary Source Galvani L: De viribus electricitatis in motu musculari commentarius. De bononiensi scientarium et artium instituto at que academia commentarii, 7:363–418, 1791. Courtesy of National Library of Medicine*

by the dissimilarity between the two metals, one metal with a positive charge and the other with a negative charge.

Galvani attempted to resolve the controversy with a different approach. Three years after his initial monograph he published the results of his experiments without metal demonstrating that if the nerve of a nerve-muscle preparation is placed along an injured point on another muscle, the first muscle would contract[21]. This paper was called *Dell'uso e dell'attività dell'Arco conduttóre nelle contrazioni dei muscoli.* Although an important contribution for other reasons, these experiments without metal did not cause Galvani to reject his theory. He still held to the view that animals possessed electricity and that this electricity was to be found especially in the nerves and particularly in the brain. The passage of time indicated that both

men were correct but not realizing they were talking about two different phenomena. Volta was correct in stating that Galvani's electrical stimulation with two dissimilar metals was due to bimetallic coupling and Galvani was also correct in stating that animals indeed have their own storehouse of electricity but incorrect in viewing this as the source of electrical stimulation with bimetallic coupling. Alexander von Humboldt pointed this out in his *Versuche über die gereizte Muskel und Nervenfaser*[22].

It was Volta's interest in the electrophysical properties of metal that caused him to pursue a line of investigation that would eventually lead to the creation of his famous pile. In the process he initiated the new science of electrochemistry. Basing his conclusions on a series of experiments with dissimilar metallic conductors he formulated a law in 1795 that still survives today. Simply put, it states that when two dissimilar metallic conductors are placed in contact with each other and a moist conductor, a flow of electricity takes place. Four years later in another letter to the Royal Society addressed to Sir Joseph Banks, he described how he came to the construction of the now famous 'voltaic pile'[20].

After a long silence, for which I shall offer no apology, I have the pleasure of communicating to you, and through you to the Royal Society, (of which I am a Fellow), some striking results I have obtained in pursuing my experiments on electricity excited by the mere mutual contact of different kinds of metal, and even by that of other conductors, also different from each other, either liquid or containing some liquid, to which they are properly indebted for their conducting power. The principle of these results, which comprehends nearly all the rest, is the construction of an apparatus having a resemblance in its effects (that is to say, in the shock it is capable of making the arms, Etc. experience) to the Leyden flask … The apparatus to which I allude, and which will, no doubt, astonish you, is only the assemblage of a number of good conductors of different kinds arranged in a certain manner. Thirty, forty, sixty, or more pieces of copper, or… silver, applied each to a piece of tin, or zinc, which is much better, and as many strata of water, or any other liquid, which may be a better conductor, such as salt water, lye, Etc. or pieces of pasteboard, skin, Etc. well soaked in these liquids; such strata interposed between every pair of combination of two different metals in an alternate series, and always in the same order of these three kinds of conductors, are all that is necessary for constituting my new instrument …

To this apparatus, much more similar fundamentally, as I shall show, and even such as I have constructed it, in its form, to the natural electric organ of the torpedo or electric eel, Etc., than to the Leyden flask and electric batteries, I would wish to give the name of the artificial electric organ.

Figure 3 depicts a voltaic pile. He discovered that with an extended pile he could obtain an electric shock by touching the first copper plate and the last zinc plate. He confirmed that the effects of his pile were in every way equivalent to those of static electricity. He was wrong, however, in thinking

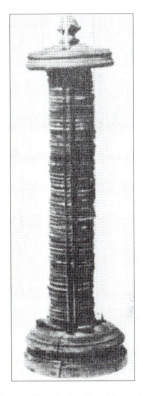

Figure 3 Galvani's voltaic pile. *Photo Source Wellcome Institute Library. Literary Source Photo Archives. By courtesy of the Wellcome Trustees*

that the electrical difference between the end plates of the pile was due to the contact itself between the different metals. The electrochemical basis for the electromotive force produced by this arrangement in his 'artificial electric organ' was correctly described by a number of later investigators that included among them Faraday, Davy and Oersted. Like the Leyden jar, it became a versatile tool in the hands of numerous researchers[23]. Volt (from Volta) is the word we now use when referring to electromotive force.

In 1820 Hans Oersted, a Danish physicist, discovered that the needle of a magnetic compass could be influenced by currents in neighboring conductors[24,25]. He used the voltaic pile for his source of electricity. Oersted correctly perceived that the change in the direction of the needle was due to the presence of a magnetic field around the conductors. The same discovery had been made and reported by an Italian jurist, Gian Domenico Romagnosi in 1802. It was reported in the Gazetta di Trentino but apparently the scientific community was not privy to this journal since interest in the subject was aroused only with Oersted's report. At any rate, several months after Oersted had made his announcement, the French physicist, André Ampère, became interested in Oersted's observations and showed that two parallel wires would be attracted to each other if the current in both of them flowed in the same direction, and that these two wires would repel each other, if their respective currents flowed in opposite directions. In the meanwhile, Ampère's co-national Francois Arago demonstrated that a current acts like an ordinary magnet. It could not only attract iron filings, it could also induce permanent magnetism in iron needles. Both men, in a collaborative effort, demonstrated that steel needles became more strongly magnetic inside a coil carrying an electric current. Ampère then went on to establish quantitative laws of magnetic force between electric currents.

These studies now took two different pathways. One was based on classical physics attracting in succession the interests of Faraday, Henry, Maxwell and Curie. The other pathway led to the development and refinement of the galvanometer and to the exploration of the phenomena associated with cardiac electrophysiology including electro-cardiography. The evolution of electrocardiography is described in Section 5.

As in electrocardiography, the evolution of electrophysiology also begins with Schweigger[26]. He was not alone because Poggendorff also conceived on his own a method of multiplying the action of electricity on the magnetized needle[27,28]. Schweigger's device was a simple one, consisting of insulated copper wire wound around a wooden frame. The greater the number of turns, the greater the action of the electricity on the magnetic needle. This is why it was called the multiplicator. Actually, it was a galvanometer that would eventually serve as a model for future ones (see Section 5).

The first one to move in the direction of muscle electrophysiology with the multiplicator was the Florentine, Leopoldo Nobili (1784–1834)[26]. He modified it with an astatic system so that by neutralizing the force of the earth's magnetism, he was able to increase many-fold the power of Schweigger's original model. It was now possible to measure the amount of current passing through a Galvani frog-leg preparation[24]; and this is what Nobili proceeded to do. His observations with this improved device were instrumental in starting Carlo Mateucci on his own investigations with the frog.

Mateucci was professor of physics, first at Bologna, then at nearby Ravenna, and finally at Pisa.

Mateucci's experiments were of singular significance because of their simplicity of design, their attention to detail, their use of improved instrumentation, and their trail-blazing impact. He found an electrical current of contraction in both the skeletal and cardiac muscle of the frog. This was later confirmed by Du Bois-Reymond. His 'rheoscopic' frog was unique. In this experiment he was able to show that when the nerve of a nerve-muscle frog preparation was placed in direct contact with the contracting muscle of another preparation, the muscle of the donor nerve would also contract. This demonstrated rather forcefully that an electrical force was being transmitted from the contracting muscle to the resting one via the resting muscle's nerve. In still another interesting series of experiments, he duplicated Volta's pile with frogs instead of dissimilar metals and pasteboard[29]. The leg of one frog was placed on top of the exposed nerve of the frog below. This was repeated until several layers were formed. He was able to get the muscles to contract by applying a potassium solution to the point of contact between a muscle and a nerve in the next layer. He also demonstrated that during the process an electrical current was generated and that the strength of this current could be measured by means of his modified galvanometer connected to both ends of the pile; the bigger the pile, the stronger the current.

We think of today as being the era of lightning-fast communications. Indeed, it is true, but there must have been among the academicians of the early 19th century, a system of communication, at least as efficient, if not as fast. All of Mateucci's efforts were known to Johannes Müller of Berlin while they were still in progress or soon after. Be that as it may, Mateucci's work aroused such an interest in Müller that he immediately placed a bright young assistant by the name of Du Bois-Reymond in charge of exploring further Mateucci's observations.

Emil Du Bois-Reymond (1818–96) was to spend a lifetime studying the electrophysiology of muscle, adding, during this time, many significant contributions. As soon as he confirmed Mateucci's observations on the flow of current in injured muscle, Du Bois-Reymond went on to contribute a number of firsts. Just two years after beginning his studies he found that there is a current of rest in muscle, and that with the onset of contraction, the intensity of this current diminishes. He proposed that this current was produced by 'electromotive molecules' arranged in series to form an unbroken circuit. Despite the error of his view concerning the mechanism his selection of the term 'action potential' for this negative fluctuation still survives in our current theory of depolarization[30].

His second contribution came 12 years later with his invention of the rheotome or current interrupter. It was a two-position switching device operated by a rocker arm that was able instantly and sharply to cut off the stimulus to the tissue under study. A galvanometer, previously connected to the tissue, would now be able to detect any electric current after the stimulus was cut off. Obviously, the detection of any current then could only mean that it was arising from the tissue itself. The instrument can be regarded as the first device capable of quantitating and graphically analyzing the time, course and amplitude of the action current in nerve and muscle[26]. R. Marchand in 1877 and T. W. Englemann, a year later, used it to chart the electrocardiogram. The rheotome was also used by Burdon-Sanderson and Page to study the nature of the T wave[31,32]. Most importantly, they were able to study the order of excitation, the nature of the excitatory process, and the duration of the excitatory state in the frog's ventricles[32]. The rheotome also became an important tool in the hands of Bernstein, whom we shall meet later, in his development of the 'membrane' theory in bioelectrical phenomena.

As these creative achievements in magnetism, electrical currents and instrumentation were going on we must not forget that before, during and after these advances, other investigators were also busily working so that eventually a synthesis of the whole picture began to emerge that ultimately attempted to explain all electrophysiologic phenomena on a cellular basis. Foremost among them were the anatomists. Other widely diverse disciplines were tapped through the introduction of the electron microscope, newer chemical methods of protein characterization, genetic coding and the delineation of metabolic events with isotope tracers. In fact, I can say without fear of contradiction, that anatomy led the way, simple visual observations opened the door a bit further, proper instrumentation expanded the view to panoramic dimensions, and that our current level of knowledge was cemented through the cooperative efforts of scientists from a multitude of disciplines. This brings us now to the origin and perpetuation of the heart beat, which, after all, is what electrophysiology is all about. Ever since Galen first demonstrated that an animal's heart would continue to beat even after removal from its host, the origin of this rhythmicity became an object of attention throughout the succeeding centuries. Recognition of this phenomenon became common knowledge but an understanding of its mechanism eluded the medical profession until Michael Foster's pupils set to work on the problem. Their objective was to resolve the debate centered around a myogenic versus a neurogenic origin for the heart beat.

Galen himself perceived the ability of the heart to beat without being tethered to its nerves when he wrote: 'The power of pulsation has its origin in the heart itself', and when he went on to say: 'The fact that the heart, removed from the thorax, can be seen to move for a considerable time is a definite indication that it does not need the nerves to perform its own function'[33,34]. Aristotle modified the myogenic basis for the beat by advancing the view that cardiac contraction was initiated by the blood within the heart[35].

Volcher Coiter (1534–76) described the beat in the living heart of a new-born kitten[36]. He noted that the ventricles contracted after the auricles. He also noted that during systole the heart was lengthened while during diastole it was shortened. His electrophysiologic contribution was his observation that when the heart was excised, different parts continued to beat with that part from the base of the heart beating the longest. This is a description of automaticity, one of the fundamental properties of heart muscle. Coiter, a Hollander, was a comparative anatomist and embryologist. He was like Harvey in the multiplicity of animal species that he subjected to study. It is strange how so little is written about him.

Harvey reported his observations on the heart beat in his *De generatione animalium*. His views appear to coincide with those of Aristotle when he wrote 'the cardiac auricle from which the pulsation starts, is excited by the blood'[37].

On the opposite side of the debate were those who advocated a neurogenic basis. Thomas Willis, in particular, was at the forefront of this view. The investigations of Galvani, Volta, and the others that followed, had already established an apparently logical framework for this mechanism with their observations of the nerve–muscle link. The reputation of Willis was such that many physicians joined his fold when he claimed that cardiac contraction occurred as a response to a 'nervous liquor' produced in the cerebellum and brought to the heart via the appropriate nerves[38,39].

The pendulum swung to the myogenic view again as a result of Albrecht von Haller's studies. In reality, all he did was repeat Galen's experiments, albeit with refined techniques. He made sure that all connections, nerves and otherwise, were severed. Aristotle's influence was still pervasive when Haller espoused the belief that blood flow through the heart triggered its intrinsic rhythmicity[40,41]. Despite the brilliance of von Haller and the world-wide respect he enjoyed, there were still a hard core of physiologists ready to battle his myogenic stance with their neurogenic one. One of them was the French physiologist, Cesar Legallois. While studying the functions of the spinal cord in animals, he noted that the heart stopped beating as soon as he crushed the spinal cord. Back and forth went conflicting reports. Experiments were devised with increasing complexity, relying more and more on the new instruments that were being introduced such as the multiplicator. Although these investigations revealed that heart muscle would contract in response to other stimuli besides electricity such as heat, cold or trauma, it soon became evident that a unique property of heart muscle was its ability to initiate its own beat. Anatomical observations joined with physiological ones in unraveling its mechanism. The principal workers in the field were now the French and German physiologists. In France, Francois Magendie carefully dissected away the entire sympathetic nerve supply to the heart including the first dorsal ganglion. While the animal was still alive, and the heart remaining in situ, he noted that the heart still kept beating. This was part of Magendie's attempts to eliminate ethereal 'vital forces' from all physiological phenomena and substitute in their stead concrete facts through carefully designed experimentation.

Johannes Müller also took up the challenge a few years later. Müller stands out as one of the great physiologists of all time, meriting the same respect and admiration that is accorded to Haller, Ludwig and so many of the other leading figures. His *Handbuch der Physiologie des Menschen* summarized practically all the physiologic knowledge up until 1840. The book is considered by many historians as a classic and a worthy successor to the encyclopedic tome of Haller. Müller's book presented a rather formidable analysis of the movements of the heart, the origin of the apex beat and the dynamic mechanisms involved with ventricular filling. Concerning the heart beat, Müller reviewed the experiments of Legallois in 1812 and restated Legallois' concept of a controlling spinal motor center. He acknowledged the intrinsic nature of cardiac rhythm so amply documented by the continued beating of the frog heart even after removal from the body. He also noted that once this excised heart stopped beating, it could be restarted by passing a weak constant current through it. This reinforced his belief that, *in vivo*, the nerve supply to the heart acted in the same manner as the electric current. He went on to say that 'The cardiac nerves concerned are partly the vagi with their admixture of Accessorius fibers and partly the first thoracic ganglia of the sympathetic system'[42].

Müller's pupil, Robert Remak discovered in 1839 the presence of ganglion cells in the sinus venosus of the frog. In a very short time, Friedrich W. Bidder, another pupil of Müller, found that ganglion cells were also in the atrioventricular junction while Ludwig identified them in the interatrial septum as well. In Müller's mind, the presence of these ganglia in the heart and other organs gave credence to his position that the sympathetic nervous system supplied the stimuli for the initiation and perpetuation of the heart beat in the living body. He proposed that a certain amount of nervous energy accumulated in the ganglia until it exceeded a critical level at which time it would trigger the heart beat. This was an attempt to explain the periodic beating of the heart in the presence of a constant flow of nervous energy as supplied by the sympathetic nerves via the ganglia.

The concept that the cardiac beat originates in the cells of Remak's ganglion was strengthened in 1852 by an experiment designed by Hermann Stannius. He applied a ligature around the sinoatrial junction of the frog's heart. Although the atria and the ventricles stopped beating, the sinus portion was still contracting rhythmically. He then put a second ligature around the atrioventricular junction. The ventricles now resumed beating. Stannius was at a loss to explain the latter observation. The site of origin for the heart beat was no doubt in the sinus portion. Conrad Eckhard

(1822–1902) suggested that the second ligature increased the excitability of Bidder's ganglion cells, and that this was responsible for the resumption of the ventricular beats. This was pure conjecture on the part of Eckhard since he did not advance any proof in support of his hypothesis[43].

The inhibitory influence of the vagus nerve was brought out in 1845 by Edward and Ernst Weber[44]. A mechanism for the neurogenic control of the heart beat in vivo was now beginning to emerge. In 1831, Faraday had paved the way for their discovery by his invention of an apparatus capable of delivering repetitive electric shocks. The Weber brothers capitalized on Faraday's invention by using it as a model in designing a rotatory electromagnetic induction machine. Based on a series of beautifully designed experiments, they advanced the thesis that the sympathetic system, acting through the intracardiac ganglia, caused the heart to beat and that the vagus nerve could slow or even stop the heartbeat. Fye quotes Geison, an historian as claiming that these discoveries meant 'the entire cardiovascular system could now be seen as a sort of muscular puppet whose strings were controlled by agents in the sympathetic nervous system'[45,46].

The Webers' observation of faradic excitation was also reported (and almost at the same time) by Julius L. L. Budge (1811–80). Wiggers rightfully points out that 'priority of discovery belongs not to the investigator who merely 'sees' a phenomenon but to the one who 'sees through it''[42]. The Weber brothers rather than Budge had the 'perspicacity in deducing that nerves can exert a suppressing as well as an excitatory effect on visceral activities'[42].

The concept of the refractory period helped explain the true basis for the periodic nature of the heartbeat and did away with any necessity to rely on Müller's explanation. Moritz Schiff (1823–96), a pupil of Magendie, was the first to demonstrate the existence of the refractory period[47,48]. He held to the view, however, that the vagi are motor nerves and that prolonged or strong stimulation from the vagi induced fatigue and thus blocked further impulses. Hugo Kronecker (1839–1914), while at Ludwig's famous laboratory at Leipzig, showed that the frog's heart is refractory to stimulation during systole. Jules Marey also confirmed the existence of the refractory period.

In 1862 Albert von Bezold (1826–68), while at Jena, reported an increase in heart rate concomitant with a rise in mean blood pressure when the cephalic end of the sectioned thoracic cord was subjected to faradic stimulation. In response to Ludwig's criticism that the rise in blood pressure may have been actually responsible for the increase in heart rate, Bezold designed further experiments that demonstrated that the cardiac acceleration was primarily due to stimulation by the sympathetic system and mediated via the stellate ganglion[42].

Another fraternal duo became involved in electrophysiologic studies. This was the Russian brothers, Elie Cyon and M. Cyon. Both had joined Ludwig's group at Leipzig. They showed that excision of the stellate ganglion eliminated the sympathetic cardiac accelerator effect. Meanwhile, Ludwig had discovered the depressor nerve in rabbits. There was now a beehive of activity in Ludwig's laboratory with men from various countries spending variable periods of time there under the masterful leadership and encouragement of Ludwig. Experiments on the sympathetic system were being conducted with pharmacologic agents as well as with electrical stimulation. In 1868 Bezold and Hirt showed that veratrine caused bradycardia and a drop in blood pressure. Young Oswald Schmiederberg, later director of his own pharmacologic laboratory, mapped out the pathway of sympathetic accelerator fibers in the dog. Pavlov during his tenure there started his investigations that led him to demonstrate augmentation of ventricular contractions by stimulating some cardiac sympathetic strands. This was later to be confirmed by other physiologists both in Europe and America. Among them were Francois-Franck (1890), Roy and Adami (1892), Howell and Dukes (1896) and Reid Hunt (1897)[42].

The era of graphic recordings and improved electrical instrumentation was obviously paying dividends. The intellectual ferment of the times readily lent itself to frenzied and sustained activity. The time was ripe for the jackpot. It was about to be realized with the entry into the field of the Englishman, Michael Foster and his coterie of brilliant proteges in a laboratory similar in orientation to that of Ludwig.

Michael Foster studied under another of the outstanding physiologists of the 19th century, William Sharpey of University College, London. His first publication on the heartbeat appeared in 1859[49]. Using a snail as his model, Foster described how small pieces of its excised heart continued to beat in a rhythmic fashion for some time. Foster's interest in the origin of the heartbeat continued unabated even after he transferred to Trinity College at Cambridge. While there he confirmed the myogenic basis for the heartbeat and created the experimental foundation for elaborate investigations into disorders of cardiac impulse formation and propagation. He was director of the laboratory of physiology at Cambridge between 1853 and 1903. During this long span of time he was responsible for spawning a number of intensive investigations and assigning them to a select group of brilliant men whose work was on the same level as that from the renowned Leipzig institute. The group included A. G. Dew-Smith, George Romanes and Walter H. Gaskell.

First of all, he and Dew-Smith advanced experimental proof that the 'fibers of the snail's heart were physiologically continuous; so that any change set up in any part of the ventricle can be propagated over the whole of it in the same way that a contraction wave, set going at any point in a striated fibre, is propagated along the whole length of the fibre'[50]. In the meanwhile Romanes had already begun his classical study into the mechanisms underlying the rhythmic contractions of the jellyfish, that graceful medusa of the seas. Gaskell, on the other hand, was continuing Foster's work on the origin of the heart beat in the snail.

A link between Gaskell's studies and the observations of Romanes was established when Romanes demonstrated that progressive sectioning of the bell portion of the medusa would eventually block progression of the contractile wave. Romanes outlined his perception of the link in a letter to his fellow worker and friend, Edward Schäfer. Schäfer was also destined to become a major figure of English physiologists. He, too, studied under Sharpey, and later became his successor to the chair of physiology at University College. In later life Edward Schäfer became Sir Edward Sharpey-Schäfer, the hyphenation being an expression of his high esteem for his former mentor. Romanes' link was expressed as an example of 'physiological continuity' and the following quotation is from that letter describing the relationship:

> … you no doubt remember that in the paper we heard Dr Foster read, he said that, the snail's heart had no nerves or ganglia, but nevertheless behaved like nervous tissue in responding to electrical stimulation. He hence concluded that in undifferentiated tissue of this kind, nerve and muscle were, so to speak amalgamated. Now it was principally with the view of testing this idea about 'physiological continuity' that I tried the mode of spiral and other sections mentioned in my last letter. The result of these sections, it seems to me, is to preclude on the one hand the supposition that the muscular tissue of medusae is merely muscular (for no muscle would respond to local stimulus throughout its substance when so severely cut), and on the other hand, the supposition of a nervous plexus (for this would require to be so very intricate, and the hypothesis of scattered cells is without microscopical evidence here or elsewhere). I think therefore, that we are driven to conclude that the muscular tissue of medusae, though more differentiated into fibres than is the contractile tissue of the snail's heart, is as much as the latter, an instance of 'physiological continuity'[51,52].

Returning again to Foster, it should be pointed out that his initial studies were focused primarily on the effects of electric current on the frog's heart. Although Foster was fully aware of the presence of ganglia in the frog's heart, and also aware of their probable motor function, he was convinced that these ganglia were not primarily responsible for initiating and maintaining the heart beat. His thoughts on the matter were concisely stated in his textbook published in 1878 when he wrote 'the muscular contractions which constitute the beat are caused by impulses which arise spontaneously in the heart itself'[53].

Foster was a strict 'myogenist' if such a word can be used. He had accumulated considerable evidence in favor of this view. One of the most important bits of evidence was his demonstration that the isolated apex of the frog's heart continued to beat on its own despite the fact that it had no ganglia in this region. He had already said in the second edition of his text that the beat of the heart was an automatic action with the impulses arising spontaneously within the heart itself[53]. The *in vivo* relationship between the autonomic nervous system (both vagal and sympathetic), the synaptic role of the cardiac ganglia, and the automaticity of the heart muscle itself were all, more or less, established by this time. Against this background it was natural for him to try to pinpoint the nature of the ultimate mechanism in the muscle itself in the belief that the autonomic nervous system played a modulating role rather than a primary one. The remaining and burning issue then was to uncover what in the heart muscle itself was responsible for its automaticity. Foster assigned the investigation of this critical point to Walter H. Gaskell, probably his most brilliant pupil.

Gaskell, like so many other young physiologists of the era, had also spent some time at the Leipzig institute under Ludwig. He graduated from Trinity College at Cambridge in 1865 and after studying at Leipzig he returned to the physiology laboratory of his alma mater in 1875[46].

In the early days of his studies, he thought that the initial stimulus for the heartbeat was provided by some, as yet, unidentified substance in the muscle itself, akin to the hormones secreted by the glands and that the vagal nerve controlled the rate of its formation[54]. A new technique and a new animal model were now called into service as he continued with his investigations. The tortoise replaced the frog, and he now recorded cardiac contractions with a new suspension method[55]. The role of the vagus nerve was delineated in more detail. He showed that vagal excitation decreased the rate of impulse initiation, retarded the velocity with which the impulse was conducted and also diminished the force of atrial contractions[45]. Gaskell never lost interest in the relationship between the autonomic nervous system and visceral function. A monograph on the subject was published posthumously in 1916. It was called *The Involuntary Nervous System*.

Over the course of time, especially between 1882 and 1887, Gaskell made several critical observations with his new techniques in the turtle. They could be summarized as follows:

(1) The turtle ventricle, unlike that of the frog, did not need any outside stimulus to maintain its beat;

(2) There were differences in degree of rhythmical power between the sinus and apical portions of the heart;

(3) There was a functional division of the atrium into a portion adjacent to the sinus which he called the 'sinus-auricle', and a 'ventricle-auricle' portion near the atrioventricular groove;

(4) The direction of contraction was from the 'sinus-auricle' to the 'ventricle-auricle', and from there to the ventricle;

(5) There was a temporary delay in the propagation of the impulse from the atria to the ventricles;

(6) The propagation of contraction between the atria and the ventricles could be permanently blocked by dividing the muscular bridge between them, with the result that any further contraction of the ventricle that did occur did so on an independent basis; and

(7) The basal part of the atrioventricular (AV) groove had the least share in the perpetuation of the sequence of atrial and ventricular beats.

In addition to the above, Gaskell also concluded from his experiments that cardiac beats depend on the rhythmic release of impulses by muscle cells in the large veins or sinus venosus and not ganglion cells; that other regions of the heart can generate impulses at slower rates, regardless of the presence of ganglion cells; and that the contraction wave spreads over atria and ventricles via muscular tissue at variable rates of speed depending on the region.

Gaskell produced a block between the atria and ventricles by mechanical compression. Robert Tigerstedt, while working in Ludwig's laboratory, extended Gaskell's observations on AV block and independent ventricular rhythmicity in mammalian hearts. He produced the block by crushing the border of the atrium with an atriotome[42].

Let us now turn our attention to the microscopic anatomy of the conduction system, an important element in solidifying the physiological observations on the origin of the heart beat and in establishing a structural basis for its propagation through the heart. Five men were involved. In chronological order they were Purkinje, His, Tawara, Keith and James. Purkinje's observations first appeared in 1839, and again in 1845[56,57]. After a long hiatus, an explosive surge of knowledge occurred in 1893 fueled by the contributions of His, Tawara and Keith. During the ensuing fourteen years virtually the entire anatomical basis for the conduction of impulses was established with unerring preciseness and detail. The microscope was the mainstay for these informative investigations.

Johannes Evangelista Purkinje was born in 1787. This son of Bohemian peasants was an accomplished linguist and poet but ironically a terrible lecturer. His ability to converse in so many languages reminds me of the linguistic gift that Pope John Paul II also possesses. Purkinje was a man of many talents and wide interests. They encompassed the elucidation of the physical principles underlying the spirometer, hearing aid and ophthalmoscope, the psychological nuances of dreams, and even dermatoglyphics. His niche in cardiac electrophysiology is secured by his description of the specialized fibers that are now known to be an integral part of the conduction system. Unfortunately he was able to find them only in ungulates and not in man. Nevertheless, it was an important discovery, and interestingly enough, made with a microscope paid for out of his own pocket. The university had denied him the $50 it cost.

Of the five men involved in the histological description of the conduction system, he was the only physiologist among them. Yet, by some strange quirk, he never bothered to explore the functional significance of the fibers. He was content merely to describe them without entertaining the slightest interest in their *raison d'être*. It was left to Tawara to allude to their role when he regarded these specialized fibers of Purkinje as the final ramifications of the His bundle.

I must point out, however, that even today, there is no definite agreement on the nature of the Purkinje fibers. Are they really fibers or actually cells? When Purkinje first described them in the ungulate, he restricted their location to the subendocardial region. It was much later before they were described as extending into the deeper layers of the myocardium. In 1931 Cardwell and Abramson showed that the Purkinje fibers were really a 3-dimensional network of fibers extending deeply into the ventricular myocardium[58]. Fibers similar to those of Purkinje and which appeared to connect the superior vena cava, sinoatrial (SA) node and inferior vena cava were described by Thorel in 1909[59]. A year later Mönckeberg reported that in his opinion, the fibers described by Thorel were pathological in origin rather than representative of a normal histological structure[60]. The matter remained unresolved until 1958 when Brian Hoffman and Paes de Carvalho of Columbia University presented both anatomical and physiological evidence for specialized intraatrial conducting paths[61]. They described the path as a distinct bundle between the SA node and AV node traversing in its course the caval edge of the crista terminalis. They obtained transmembrane electrical potentials from this bundle, a finding that

supports their belief that the bundle is made up of specialized conducting fibers. James described in 1963 cells of the Purkinje type in the human atria as well[62]. James also noted that these cells were to be found especially in those parts of the atria that are the sites of preferential conduction. This too represents an important anatomical linkage to conductivity. James published a paper in 1979 that attempted to delineate in a more precise manner the function of these cells[63]. In particular, he addressed the possibility that they might be the sites for automaticity. He brought out three points that effectively excluded them from this role.

> First, Purkinje cells seem specialized for rapid conduction whereas conduction in sites of normal automaticity (such as the sinus node) is always very slow. Second, the only normal automatic center and primary pacemaker in the heart, the sinus node, does contain specialized cells, but they are not Purkinje cells, differing markedly both by anatomic and physiologic definition. In fact, there are no Purkinje cells in the sinus node. Third, the cells in Purkinje strands, whether studied *in vitro* or *in vivo* are not spontaneously automatic under normal conditions, and induced automaticity differs significantly from that of the sinus node when biochemically defined[63].

The anatomical identification of the AV bundle and the delineation of its function are intimately interwoven with the efforts of Wilhelm His Jr. He was born in Basel, Switzerland, the son of an eminent anatomist. Not infrequently, the progeny of eminent people are overwhelmed by the parent's exalted position and either lead an unfulfilled or fruitless life. This was not so with young Wilhelm. He took advantage of every opportunity placed in his path and achieved eponymous immortality. His well-to-do father afforded him every educational advantage, both at home and in his formal schooling. His Sr personally instilled in his son a thorough knowledge of anatomy and techniques in embryology that were to benefit His Jr throughout his entire medical career. Young His also had the opportunity to study at Strassburg under Oswald Schmiedeberg, director of the world's first pharmacologic laboratory and discoverer of the sympathetic accelerator fibers in dogs[42].

Soon after receiving his doctorate in medicine at Leipzig, he was appointed an assistant at the Leipzig clinic which had just been taken over by Heinrich

Curschmann. The first assistant was Rudolph Krehl. His began his studies on the innervation of the heart and the transmission of impulses during these formative years at Leipzig. In 1893, just four years after his appointment he described the muscular bridge that connects the atrial and ventricular walls[64]. Very little interest was aroused by this paper, mainly because of its limited circulation. Much more attention was given to the more detailed paper that he wrote in 1933, just 18 months before his death, and 40 years after his initial description[65]. The article is really an apologia for his claims to priority. An excellent translation by Bost and Gardner appeared in the 1949 summer issue of the *Journal of the History of Medicine*[66].

K. A. Baer recounts an interesting anecdote about Bach and His Sr that is worth repeating[67]. It appears that the elder His was not only fond of music, but also interested in finding out all be could about Johann Sebastian Bach. In 1894 he was, in fact, responsible for locating and exhuming the reputed skeletal remains of the great Bach in the yard of old Johanniskirche. After satisfying himself that the remains were those of the composer, he had a plaster cast made of the skull which served as a model for a portrait-like bust. Seffner was the sculptor who executed this work, and it is said that the features resembled those of Bach. In addition, His Sr prevailed upon the Viennese otologist, Adam Politzer, to collaborate with him in conducting a detailed study of the skeletal make-up of the ear and its adjacent areas. They concluded that the unusual anatomical characteristics they encountered were related to Bach's perfect pitch and musical genius[67].

The burning question in the last decade of the 19th century was whether or not the cardiac ganglia were the centers for automaticity. Englemann, while at Utrecht, and Gaskell at Cambridge, repeatedly attempted to show that heart muscle was capable of initiating its own beat. Some of the difficulty could be ascribed to the conflicting observations that were being made regarding the locus of rhythm abnormalities during disease states. Were the abnormalities due to pathological changes in the heart ganglia or in the heart muscle or in both?

At that time His Jr was working on an embryological problem under the direction of his father. Since he was was well-versed in embryological techniques, he suggested to his co-workers, Krehl and Romberg, that they attempt to resolve the question based on an embryological approach. They agreed and each man was assigned a specific aspect of the problem. His Jr investigated the embryological development of the cardiac nervous system in all classes of vertebrates[68]. He was able to prove that the heart began to beat before the appearance of either the cerebrospinal nerves or the ganglia. Thus, intrinsic automaticity appeared to be a certainty.

The next question was how was the initiating stimulus propagated through the rest of the heart? Following the lead of Gaskell who had shown that in the frog and turtle the conduction passes through muscle substance, His searched for some sort of muscular bridge in both mammalian animals and in man. Again, by using serial sections at various stages of embryological development, His demonstrated that such a pathway did exist in both man and animals. This became known as the bundle of His, and as mentioned before, these findings were initially published in 1893[64]. The findings were not confirmed until 10 years later when Retzer and Bräuning fully substantiated them[65].

Tawara's contribution appeared in 1906, a full 16 years after the description by His[69]. Tawara showed that the fibers described by Purkinje were connected with the bundle of His to form the conduction system in the ventricles. The link-up with the atria was established by Keith and Flack in 1909 with their discovery of the sinus node (more about this later). J. Mall conducted a very exhaustive study of the system in man and reported his observations on its development in 1912[70]. Külbs expanded the study to the vertebrate series detailing the connection between the AV bundle and musculature of the ventricles[71].

Some controversy has arisen regarding priority in the discovery of the AV bundle. Three other men besides His are involved in the dispute. They are Kent and Gaskell of England, and Paladino of Italy.

His was not alone when he described the existence of the AV pathway. Kent's description appeared the same year as that of His in 1893[72]. Stanley Kent investigated many animals, and found that the higher the animal stands in the developmental series, the less developed the muscle bridges. But in his paper of 1893, his anatomical description of the conduction system is not very clear. According to His, again in his apologia of 1933, Kent probably saw only a part of the AV bundle. He identified its presence as it passed from the atrium to the ventricle but did not follow its course. This appears to be a valid point. The waters are muddied somewhat, however, when His goes on to say that Kent's description of the two broad muscle bands or the 'peculiar isolated cells' between the atria and the ventricles could not be verified by himself or other investigators. His himself is not clear on this point since Kent did describe an accessory pathway.

Since then the eponym His bundle has been used with reference to the primary conduction pathway and Kent's bundle to the accessory pathway. Later on other accessory pathways were described by Mahaim and James, and are now known by their respective eponyms.

Although Gaskell's studies did show that the impulse was propagated through muscle bridges, His still claimed priority on the ground that Gaskell's observations were confined to cold-blooded animals. I do not consider this a valid refutation for priority but despite my efforts I was unable to find in any of Gaskell's writings a description of the AV bundle similar to that of His.

Despite what His brought out in his article of 1933, there are still some who assert that the first description of the AV bundle must be attributed to Giovanni Paladino, professor of histology and general physiology at the University of Naples. On the other hand, Sonnino and Mawk did confuse the issue even more by referring to him as the 'true father of the accessory myocardial conduction pathways'[73].

In 1876, Paladino described muscle bridges in the atrioventricular valves in man. He described them as beginning in the atria and ending in the ventricles after passing through the valve cusps, chordae tendinae and papillary muscles. This was a good 17 years before His. Although the existence of these fibers in the AV valves was known since Reid and Kürschner described them in 1839 and 1840 respectively, their presence in man was in doubt. Paladino's work definitely laid this doubt to rest. His description appeared in *Il Movimento Medico-Chirurgico*[74]. In addition to humans, Paladino observed the bridges in other mammals and in the chicken and turtle.

The anatomist from Pisa, L. De Gaetani confirmed Paladino's findings in man and reported that the vascular bridges were to be found also in the cat, sheep and turkey cock[75]. Paladino, himself, claimed priority long after His' original description[76]. De Gaetani supported Paladino's claim in the following words:

And there is no doubt that the tribute and credit goes to Paladino for having first described the bundles uniting the auricle and ventricle, and to His for describing one of these bundles carefully, that is, a particular one of this system which is more completely illustrated by Paladino[75].

In his own defense, His Jr emphasized in his paper of 1933 that Paladino 'had not seen what we call the conduction system today'[77]. Moreover, as His rightfully points out, Paladino was totally wrong when he ascribed a mechanical function to the muscle fibers that he described rather than an electrophysiological one. Paladino did perform a series of experiments on isolated animal hearts in an attempt to identify their function. He erroneously concluded from these observations that the valvular component of the pathway was responsible for the movement of the AV valves. The valve musculature 'not only allows movement of the valves themselves, but also provides solidity to the union between atria and ventricles, and contributes in a special way to the general and total mechanisms of the cardiac pump'[78].

In my opinion there is a good deal of validity in what His had to say. Moreover, Paladino's description itself does not indicate that the muscle fibers he was describing were an integral part of a conduction pathway. In his words:

the muscle layer of the atria, arriving at the level of the atrioventricular ostia, loses the more external layers of circular fibers which stop here and combines with the longitudinal and intermediate circular fibers down to the internal aspect of the valve cusps. Of these fibers, the longitudinal ones end in the tendons of second and third order and some fascicles go directly to the ventricle wall where they become tendons in the midst of flattened muscle fibers which insert on the valve leaflets[79].

Also on the basis of this very description, I cannot see how Sonnino and Mawk could validate their view that Paladino should be considered the true father of the accessory myocardial conduction pathways. Their view is predicated purely on their interpretation of what he actually described, and they are merely confusing the issue all the more by their statement that 'the Paladino bundles, and not those of Kent, are therefore the 'original' accessory myocardial conduction pathways'[80].

THE ELECTROPHYSIOLOGIC CONTROL OF THE HEART

Sunao Tawara, born and educated in Japan, accomplished his monumental work on the conduction system during the three years he spent with Ludwig Aschoff in Marburg, Germany. He combined a superb native intelligence with an exacting attitude towards his work, a combination that was sure to carry him to great heights in his chosen field of medicine.

Tawara began his studies on the conduction system in 1903. His monograph on the subject appeared in 1906. It was called *Das Reitzleit-ungssystem des Saugetierherzens*. Tawara expanded the histologic descriptions of His. In doing so, he drew attention to the fact that the proximal end of the His bundle consisted of a compact meshwork of fibers resembling a knot or node, and that the Purkinje fibers making up the His bundle divided into a left and right branch.

There is no doubt that the compact node he described, and which is now called the AV node, was a great discovery. More importantly, however, was the insight he had to correctly interpret that the AV node together with the His bundle and Purkinje fibers were all part of a conduction system that allowed electrical impulses to spread from the atria to the ventricles. He thus synthesized the known anatomical findings into a coherent physiological scenario. The missing link was the SA node. This was to be supplied by Keith and Flack.

Just several months after Tawara's monograph appeared, Keith published his own descriptions of the conduction system in the human heart[81]. It appeared in *The Lancet*. The paper was a confirmation of Tawara's studies describing in detail the AV node, the His bundle and its branches and the Purkinje system.

James recounts how Keith went on to discover the SA node[82]. It begins with Keith vacationing during the summer in Kent when he heard from Sir James Mackenzie that the Japanese scientist, Tawara, had mapped out the AV conducting system. Of course, Keith already knew of this since his own paper on the AV bundle was an enthusiastic confirmation of Tawara's work. At any rate, Mackenzie's sole reason for alerting Keith was his desire for finding an anatomical basis for irregularities of cardiac rhythm. Keith had already established himself as a serious anatomist. Mackenzie prevailed upon him to explore the problem. In a very short time Mackenzie was sending to Keith hearts from individuals who during life had manifested cardiac arrhythmias. Flack was Keith's neighbor at the time and still a medical student.

Apparently Keith's vacation was a working one. He utilized the study in the house he was renting for his histologic investigations. Flack was assisting Keith in studying sections from a variety of mammalian hearts. One day during the course of this project, Keith, upon returning from an outing, was greeted by an excited Flack with the news that certain sections of a mole's heart revealed an unusual structure. Keith in looking over these sections noted that the structure that intrigued Flack bore a resemblance to a structure he had observed in the human hearts supplied by Mackenzie. A period of frenzied activity ensued. All sorts of animal hearts were examined as well as two from human embryos. The culmination was a paper co-authored by Keith and Flack on the form and nature of the muscular connections between the primary divisions of the vertebrate heart. It appeared in 1907[83]. They found that in the region of the sino-atrial junction in the human heart 'the fibers are striated, fusiform, with well-marked elongated nuclei, plexiform in arrangement, and embedded in densely packed connective tissue – in fact, of closely similar structure to the Knoten (node)'. This is their description of the SA node and the Knoten they were referring to was, of course, Tawara's AV node. This discovery rounded out the anatomical linkage of the conduction system between the atria and the ventricles.

Further work on the cellular level was now needed to gain even more insight into the electrophysiological phenomena of the heart. In time, it was to show that even though there is a myogenic basis for the initiation and propagation of the impulse *in vivo*, this activity is modulated through the autonomic nervous system orchestrated by an interplay of phosphates, enzymes, and ionic fluxes through receptors and hormones. The wheel was to make a complete circle with both myogenicists and neurogenicists actively participating in this symphony.

The electrocardiographic representation of impulse conduction depends upon the direction the wave of excitation takes as it spreads through the heart from its point of origin. Sir Thomas Lewis made many important contributions on the subject. His investigations were carried out primarily as a desire on his part to understand the mechanisms underlying the electrocardiographic patterns and the various types of rhythm disturbances that he encountered clinically. The science of electrocardiography was still in its infancy, at least in the clinical setting. Lewis developed his concept of the pathway of the excitation wave through his numerous experiments on the dog's heart. This was presented in a landmark paper published in conjunction with Rothschild in 1915[84]. Their studies showed that the wave of excitation followed the pathway of the conduction tissue rather than the muscle fibers. An *in vivo* anatomical correlation was thus established. They also demonstrated that the impulse traveled at a greater speed through the bundle of His and the Purkinje system than in the surrounding muscular tissue. Furthermore, they were able to show that the left side of the upper part of the interventricular septum was activated first followed by activation of the right side via a special branch from the left bundle, then coursed down the remainder of the septum equally on both sides and finally sped through both branches and ramifications of the bundle of His. Figure 4 is a diagram of the excitation process of the human ventricle as conceived by Lewis. The diagram was based on records obtained from multiple epicardial points on the dog's heart.

The third edition of his book describes in detail the manner in which the wave of excitation spreads through the atria as well as the ventricles[85]. These findings were later confirmed and amplified by Durrer (1955)[86], Puech (1956)[87], and De Carvalho and Hoffman (1958)[61].

In the 1950s improved instrumentation brought about a better understanding of how the excitation wave passed from the subendocardial region to the deeper layers of the myocardium. Cathode ray oscilloscopes, powerful amplifiers and penetrating electrodes were the technical tools that helped in these studies[88]. The experiments of Lewis and Rothschild gave us a peek but later observations revealed that the propagation of the wave of excitation is really a complex affair. It does not proceed in a straightforward manner as indicated by the simple diagram of Lewis. It is characterized rather by differences in rate and direction[89].

The current views are based on experimental studies of intraventricular block and on observations with direct epicardial leads as well as intracavitary electrocardiograms[88,90,91]. The initial studies with intracavitary electrocardiograms were conducted by Scher and his group in 1957. Sodi-Pollares of Mexico also used intracavitary electrodes during the same year to demonstrate the direction of the wave of excitation in the septum. Burchell's observations were obtained with the isolated interventricular septum just 6 years before and therefore not strictly comparable[92].

The current view on ventricular depolarization is that the left septal surface is the first to be activated, the impulse then traveling to the right and anteriorly. Up to this point, it is essentially no different from what Lewis presented. The concept now is that from this point of departure the wave of excitation spreads in an irregular manner through the Purkinje fibers. This results in activation of the entire ventricular myocardium from the endocardial to the epicardial regions as well as the central portion of the septum. During this phase the resultant forces are directed from base to apex, towards the left and posteriorly. The diaphragmatic portion of the left ventricle and the basal portions near the AV groove are the last to be activated. During this last phase the electrical forces are still directed posteriorly to the left but from apex to base.

In 1910 the German team of Eppinger and Rothberger reported the results of their studies with experimentally produced intraventricular block in the dog[93]. They created the block by injecting silver nitrate directly into the myocardium. There was no dispute about the resultant electrocardiographic pattern indicative of a block. Controversy arose, instead, regarding the validity of applying these observations in the dog to man. Indeed 20 years later Barker and Hirschfelder demonstrated rather dramatically that the standard lead patterns of intraventricular block in man were diametrically opposite to those of the dog[94]. Wilson sorted out most of the difficulties a year later[95]. This is not to say that the entire spectrum of intraventricular block has been resolved. Physiological questions and completely satisfactory histological correlations are still wanting. An example is arborization block, a term introduced by Oppenheimer and Rothschild in 1917[96]. Although these two men presented the view that the electrocardiographic pattern of this type of block is due to lesions in the finer ramifications of the conduction system there is no anatomical proof that this is actually so.

Köllicker and Müller were the first to point out in 1856 that recovery from excitation was also associated with electrical activity[97]. This was confirmed and amplified through the efforts of Meissner and Cohn in 1862, Donders in 1872,

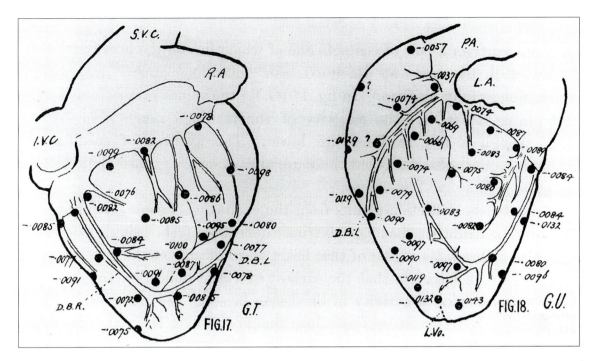

Figure 4 Lewis' diagram of the excitation process of the human ventricle. *Photo Source National Library of Medicine. Literary Source Lewis, T. and Rothschild, M.A. (1915). The excitatory process in the dog's heart. Part II. The ventricles. Phil. Trans. B, 206, 181. With permission*

Burdon-Sanderson and Page in 1878, and in this century through the classical studies of Wilson and Ashman[98].

Sir John Scott Burdon-Sanderson (1828–1905) was a brilliant experimenter and stands out as one of the great pioneers of cardiac electrophysiology. Hoffman and Cranefield acknowledged this when they wrote in their textbook on the electrophysiology of the heart:

> Many efforts have been made to relate the shape of the transmembrane potential to the shape of the electrogram. Little, however, has been added to the general idea advanced by Burdon-Sanderson and Page (1880–1884) that the electrogram is in some mathematical sense a derivative of the monophasic potential[99].

It should be emphasized that this work was done 70 years before anyone could even dream of measuring in a reproducible manner intracellular cardiac potentials[100]. Burdon-Sanderson was sometime Jodrell Professor of Human Physiology at Cambridge and later Regius Professor of Medicine at Oxford. He spent more than two decades investigating

potentials and current flow in the excited heart. His tools were the simple galvanometer and later the capillary electrometer. It was he who coined the term 'isoelectric interval'. He proved that as the temperature increased, the refractory period decreased. The electrophysiologic effects of changes in sequence of depolarization and repolarization were also explored by him[100,101].

The anatomical basis at the cellular level for the current views of impulse conduction evolved as a result of the electron microscope. Studies of the cardiac ultrastructure have shown that the myocardium consists of cells joined together by intercalated disks, and that double membranes enclose the sarcosomes (mitochondria), nucleus and intercalated disks[102]. Also, the ultrastructural relationship of the contractile elements with all the known histologic structures both within and outside the cell has been rather clearly outlined. The sum total of these revelations in conjunction with electrochemical studies have placed our current concepts of cardiac rhythm on a much firmer basis, while at the same time setting the stage for a proper therapeutic approach in dysfunctional situations.

Du Bois-Reymond pointed out in 1872 that changes in electrical activity occurred at the initiation of the excitatory process and that this process originated in the membrane of the muscle cells[88]. It was he, as I mentioned before, who coined the term 'action potential'. Much more needed to be known about this action potential and its chemical correlates. The first step in this direction was taken by Julius Bernstein, a protege of Du Bois-Reymond. Later, the introduction of a new animal model, the squid, and still later, the introduction of the microelectrode, all played a role in finalizing the current views.

Bernstein presented in 1910 a theory that, although flawed, represented an important advance because it served as a catalyst for the further investigation of bioelectric phenomena at the cellular level leading eventually to the current ionic hypothesis[103]. Bernstein's classical theory was based on assumptions that were not validated and proposed without any realization of the true complexity of the electrophysiologic reactions. The major error when he formulated his theory was his complete disregard for Englemann's observations on the 'overshoot' phenomenon published just six years after Du Bois-Reymond had described the action potential[104]. The giant axon of the squid provided the information that finally cast into oblivion Bernstein's classical theory. Its use as a model in neurophysiological experimentation was first suggested by Hodgkin and Huxley in 1933, and later promulgated by J. Z. Young in 1936, and Curtis and Cole in 1940[105–107]. The electrophysiologists at Cambridge, keenly aware of its potentialities, continued their observations with this 'meganerve' well into the 1950s[108,109]. These investigations were conducted under the aegis of Hodgkin, Huxley and Katz. Conductance, potential, resistance and capacitance were now being measured with ease.

Accurate quantitation of the slope and duration of the action potential was made possible with the introduction of transmembrane recording using the microelectrode devised by Ling and Gerard in 1949[110]. They used it to measure the changes in the sartorius fibers of the frog. As improvements in the microelectrode occurred, the initial investigations of the Cambridge group on the squid axon were expanded by others to heart muscle. Reports appeared by Woodbury, Hecht and Christopherson in 1951 on membrane resting and action potentials of single cardiac fibers from the frog ventricle[111].

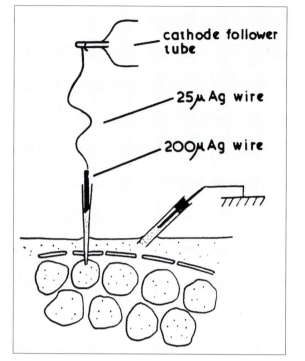

Figure 5 The 'riding' tungsten-wire glass capillary modification of the Ling–Gerard electrode. *Photo Source University of Central Florida. Literary Source Fishman, A.P. and Richards, D.W. (1957). Circulation of the blood, men and ideas. From Weidmann, S. (1957). Use of microelectrode for recording action potentials of cardiac muscle. Ann. NY Acad. Sci. With permission*

That same year Draper and Weidmann also described their recordings of the transmembrane potential in the isolated Purkinje fiber of the dog and kid heart[112].

The amazingly tiny electrode devised by Ling and Gerard aided by electron microscopy made possible the delineation of infinitesimal changes in electromotive force measured in terms of millivolts. The most recent modification of the Ling–Gerard electrode is the 'riding' tungsten wire glass capillary which leads off from a single fiber of the beating heart. The electrical changes are amplified by a cathode ray follower tube. Figure 5 is a diagrammatic representation of this latest modification.

The ionic hypothesis replaced Bernstein's theory as a result of these bioelectrical studies with the squid axon and the microelectrode technique. The ionic exchange is between sodium and potassium. Excitation of muscle on the basis of an exchange

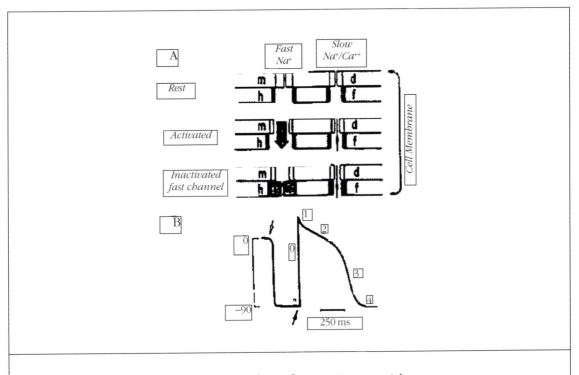

Relationship of ionic flux to action potential

Relationship of ionic flux to action potential

Depolarization

(1) Sequential propagation of electrical impulse depends on Na^+ ion flux through specialized membrane channels.

   (a) Called fast channels because of rapid movement of Na^+ through them.

   (b) Successive channels opened by electrical impulse in adjacent cells.

(2) Each channel has two gates.

   (a) M gate – moves rapidly to open channel.

   (b) H gate – moves more slowly to close channel.

(3) Extracellular Na+ move into cell through fast channel causing depolarization (phase 0)

   (a) The resultant electrical impulse, in turn, triggers another phase 0 in adjacent cells.

   (b) Rapidity of impulse propagation (conduction) depends upon intensity of this depolarizing current.

(4) Phase 1 begins with inactivation of fast Na channels and cessation of fast Na current.

Repolarization

(1) Brought about by outwardly directed K^+ currents

   (a) Until membrane potential returns to resting level (phases 1–3)

(2) As repolarization curve shows, rate of return slows immediately after phase 1.

   (a) Caused by another inward current by Na^+ and Ca^{++} through slow channels and thereby counter-acting repolarizing action of outwardly diffusing K^+.

   (b) Effect of this inward secondary current diminishes as cell gradually repolarizes – until phase 4 is reached.

   (c) Phase 4 is resting level.

(3) Threshold for activation of slow inward current is around -30 to -40 mV (compare with -60 to -70 mV for fast current).

Figure 6 Diagrammatic representation of ionic exchange as it correlates with the action potential. *Photo Source Author's lecture notes. Literary Source Personal lecture notes. No permission needed*

between sodium and potassium ions had already been suggested by Overton in 1902, and he could very well have brought his idea to fruition if he had had the squid axon and the microelectrode[113].

The ionic hypothesis states that the influx of sodium ions into the cells is responsible for depolarization which is represented on the action potential by a steep upward slope from the threshold level of stimulation. Repolarization is represented by the spike of the upward slope and the remaining portions of the curve as it declines to the threshold level again. The potassium ions move out of the cell during and after the plateau portion of the curve. The ionic components are restored to their previous levels and location during the resting intervals between each action potential. These changes are diagrammatically depicted in Figure 6.

When Draper and Weidmann reported their observations in 1951, they also described in the same paper certain differences in the action potential recorded from pacemaker and non-pacemaker tissues[112]. Weidmann elaborated on this in a paper which appeared in 1957[114]. He studied the pacemaker activity in the SA and AV nodes of mammals, fowls and amphibia. He showed that the action potential of pacemaker tissue is characterized by a slow depolarization component which is registered as a gradual upward convexity on the curve. It is also referred to as the 'prepotential', suggesting that it represents a gradual transition from rest to activity. It is now thought that when this prepotential component reaches a critical level, it initiates a propagated action potential[115].

Variations in the characteristics of the action potential have been described as being responsible for changes in the rate of impulse formation. Rather sophisticated experimentation has also brought out that changes in the action potential can be effected through stimulation of the known components of the sympathetic nervous system, changes in temperature, ionic concentration, oxygen levels, and especially with certain pharmaceutical agents such as digitalis and anti-arrhythmic agents. Indeed the pharmaceutical houses have expended a great deal of time and money in developing drugs targeted towards changing the characteristics of the action potential in an effort to find the ideal antiarrhythmic agent. Unfortunately, as of this writing, this desirable goal has yet to be realized. Nevertheless, there is no reason for

pessimism since the key to successful therapy may very well lie in the manipulation of the bioelectric processes behind impulse initiation and propagation. The foundation for understanding these mechanisms is already in place and further studies will, no doubt, help us in finding the 'holy grail'.

REFERENCES

1. *Encyclopaedia Britannica*, (1973), 15th edn., vol. 6, pp. 537–8
2. Amberson, W.R. (1958). The influence of fashion in the development of knowledge concerning electricity and magnetism. *Am. Sci.*, **46**, 33
3. Fleming, J.A. (1910). Electricity. *Encyclopaedia Britannica*, (11th edn.), vol. 9, 179
4. *Encyclopaedia Britannica*, (1973), 15th edn., vol. 6, p. 540
5. Bidwell, S. (1910). Magnetism. *Encyclopaedia Britannica*, 11th edn., **17**, 321
6. Gilbert, W. (1900). *On the Magnet, Magnetick Bodies also on the Great Magnet, the Earth*, tr. by S.P. Thompson. (London: Cheswick)
7. *Plato, I.O.N.* (1925). Tr. by W.R.M. Lamb. (Loeb Classical Library). (London: Heinemann)
8. Beasley, C. (1910). Alexander Neckam. *Encyclopaedia Britannica*, 11th edn., **19**, 336
9. Gilbert, W. (1600). *De Magnete, magneticisque corporibus, et de magno magnete tellure; physiologia nova, plurimis and argumentis and experimentis demonstrata.* (London: Short)
10. Brazier, M.A.B. (1958). The evolution of concepts relating to the electrical activity of the nervous system, 1600 to 1800. In *The Brain and its Functions*. (Springfield, Ill.: Thomas)
11. *Encyclopaedia Britannica*, (1973), 15th edn., vol. 6, p. 540
12. Guillemin, A.V. (1891). *Electricity and Magnetism*, tr. by S.P. Thompson. (London: Macmillan)
13. Cohen, I.B. (1954). Introduction. In Galvani, L. *Commentary on the Effects of Electricity on Muscular Motion*, tr. by M.G. Foley, Burndy Library, Norwalk, Conn.
14. Hall, A.R. (1954). *The Scientific Revolution, 1500–1800; the Formation of the Modern Scientific Attitude.* (New York: Longmans, Green)
15. Walsh, J. (1773–75). Of torpedoes found on the coast of England. *Phil. Trans.*, **64**, 464

16. Hunter, J. (1773). Anatomical observations on the torpedo. *Phil. Trans.*, **6**, 481

17. Fontana, F. (1936). Traité sur le vénin de la vipère, sur le poisons américains, sur le laurier-cerise, et sur quelques autres poisons végétaux. Florence, 1781. Cited by H.E. Hoff: Galvani and the pregalvanian electrophysiologists. *Ann. Sci.*, **1**, 157

18. Galvani, L. (1791). De viribus electricitatis in motu musculari commentarius. *De Bononiensi Scientarium et Artium Instituto atque Academia Commentarii*, **7**, 363–418

19. *Ibid.*

20. Volta, A. (1800). On the electricity excited by the mere contact of conducting substances of differenct kinds. *Phil. Trans.*, pt. 2, p. 405

21. Galvani, L. (1794). *Dell'uso e dell'attività dell'Arco conduttóre nelle contrazioni dei muscoli.* (Bologna: Tommaso d'Aquino)

22. von Humboldt, F.W.H.A. (1797). *Versuche über die gereizte Muskel und Nervenfaser nebst Vermuthungen über den chemischen Process des Lebens in der thier-und Pflanzenwelt*, vol. I. (Decker: Posen)

23. Schedlovsky, T. (1955). Introduction. In his *Electrochemistry in Biology and Medicine.* (New York: Wiley)

24. Amberson, W.R. (1958). The influence of fashion in the development of knowledge concerning electricity and magnetism. *Am. Sci.*, **46**, 33.

25. Oersted, C.H.C. (1820). Galvanic magnetism. *Phil. Mag.*, **56**, 394

26. Hoff, H.E. and Geddes, L.A. (1957). The rheotome and its pre-history: a study in the historical interrelation of electrophysiology and electromechanics. *Bull. Hist. Med.*, **3**, 212

27. Poggendorff, J.C. (1842). Ueber den Gebrauch der Galvanometer als Messwerkzeuge. *Ann. Phys. Lpz.*, **56**, 324

28. Poggendorff, J.C. (1860). *On the use of the galvanometer as a measuring instrument*, p. 396, tr. by J.D. Easter. (A.R. Smithson Inst.)

29. Matteucci, C. (1843). Sur le courant électrique des muscles des animaux vivant ou récemment tués. *C.R. Acad. Sci. (Paris)*, **16**, 197

30. Du Bois-Reymond, E. (1848–60). *Untersuchungen über thierische Elecktricität*, vols. I and II. (Berlin: Reimer)

31. Burdon-Sanderson, J. and Page, F.J.M. (1878). Experimental results relating to the rhythmical and excitatory motions of the ventricle of the heart of the frog, and of the electrical phenomena which accompany them. *Proc. R. Soc., B*, **27**, 410

32. Burdon-Sanderson, J. and Page, F.J.M. (1879–80). On the time-relations of the excitatory process in the ventricles of the heart of the frog. *J. Physiol. (London)*, **2**, 384

33. Singer, C. (1956). *Galen on anatomical procedures, translation of the surviving books with introduction and notes*, p. 184. (London: Oxford Univ. Press)

34. Siegel, R.A. (1968). *Galen's system of physiology and medicine: an analysis of his doctrines and observations of bloodflow, respiration, humors and internal diseases*, p. 45. (New York: S. Krager)

35. Harris, C.R.S. (1973). *The heart and vascular system in ancient Greek medicine from Alcmaeon to Galen.* (London: Oxford Univ. Press)

36. Singer, C. (1925). *The Evolution of Anatomy*, p. 149. (London: Kegan Paul, Trench, Trubner)

37. Curtis, J.G. (1915). *Harvey's views on the use of the circulation of the blood*, p. 82. (New York: Columbia Univ. Press)

38. Davis, A. (1973). *Circulatory physiology and medical chemistry in England 1650–1680.* (Lawrence, KS: Coronado Press)

39. Martin, E.G. (1905). The rise of the present conceptions as to the cause of the heart-beat. 1. Early ideas, and the neurogenic theory. *Johns Hopkins Hosp. Bull.*, **16**, 338

40. Howell, W. (1905–6). The cause of the heart beat. *Harvey Lect. Series*, p. 305

41. Hintzsche, E. (1972). (Victor) Albrecht von Haller. In Gillispie, C.C. (ed.) *Dictionary of Scientific Biography*, vol. 6, p. 61. (New York: Charles Scribner's Sons)

42. Wiggers, C.J. (1960). Some significant advances in cardiac physiology during the nineteenth century. *Bull. Hist. Med.*, **34**, 1–15

43. *Ibid.* p. 4

44. Hoff, H.E. (1940). The history of vagal inhibition. *Bull. Hist. Med.*, **8**, 461

45. Fye, W.B. (1987). The origin of the heart beat: a tale of frogs, jellyfish and turtles. *Circulation*, **76**, 493–500

46. Geison, G.L. (1978). *Michael Foster and the Cambridge School of Physiology: the Scientific Enterprise in Late Victorian Society*, p. 195. (Princeton: Princeton Univ. Press)

47. Riedo, P. (1970). Der Physiologe Moritz Schiff (1823–1896) und die Innervation des Herzens. *Züricher medizingeschichtliche Abhandlungen.* n.s. 85. (Zürich: Juris)

48. Hoff, H.E. (1942). The history of the refractory period: a neglected contribution of Felice Fontana. *Yale J. Biol Med.*, **14**, 635

49. Foster, M. (1859). On the beat of the snail's heart. *Rep. Br. Assoc. Adv. Sci.*, **29**, 160

50. Foster, M. and Dew-Smith, A.G. (1875). On the behavior of the hearts of mollusks under the influence of electric currents, *Proc. R. Soc. London*, **23**, 318

51. Romanes to Schäfer, 24 June 1875, Sharpey-Schäfer collection, *Contemporary Medical Archives*. (London: Wellcome Institute for the History of Medicine)

52. Romanes, E. (1896). *The Life and Letters of George John Romanes*, 2nd edn. (London: Longmans, Green and Co.)

53. Foster, M. (1878). *A Textbook of Physiology*, 2nd edn. (London: Macmillan and Co.)

54. Gaskell, W.H. (1882). On the rhythm of the heart of the frog, and on the nature of the action of the vagus nerve. *Philos. Trans. London*, **173**, 993

55. Gaskell, W.H. (1883). On the innervation of the heart, with special reference to the heart of the tortoise. *J. Physiol.*, **4**, 43

56. Purkinje, J.E. (1839). Nowe spostrzezenia i badania w przedmiocie fizyologi i drobnowidzowéj anatomii. Rocznik wydzialu lekarskiego w universitecie Jaqiellonskim Kraków; **2**, 44–67

57. Purkinje, J. (1845). Mikroskopischneurologische beobachtungen. *Arch. Anat. Physiol. Wissensch. Med.*, **11**, 281–95

58. Cardwell, J.C. and Abramson, D.I. (1931). The atrio-ventricular conduction system of the beef heart. *Am. J. Anat.*, **49**, 167

59. Thorel, C. (1909). Vorläufige Mitteilung über eine besondere muskelverbindung zwischen der Cava superior und dem Hisschen Bündel. *Münch. Med. Wschr.*, **56**, 2159

60. Mönckeberg, J.G. (1910). Zur Frage der besonderen muskulären Verbindung Zwischen Sinus und atrioventrikularknotien im Herzen. *Zbl. Herz. u. Gefasskr.*, **2**, 1

61. Paes de Carvalho, A. and Hoffman, B.H. (1958). Evidence for specialized intra-atrial conducting paths. *Fed. Proc.*, **17**, 120

62. James, T.N. (1963). The connecting pathways between the sinus node and A-V node and between the right and left atrium in the human heart. *Am. Heart J.*, **66**, 498–508

63. Katholi, R.E., Woods, W.T., Kawamura, K., Urthaler, F. and James, T.N. (1979). Dual dependence on both Ca++ and Mg++ for electrical stability in cells of canine false tendon. *J. Mol. Cell. Cardiol.*, **11**, 435–46

64. His, W. Jr. (1893). The activity of the embryonic human heart and its significance for the understanding of the heart movement in the adult. *Arb. Med. Klin. Leipzig*, 14–49

65. His, W. Jr. (1933). The story of the atrioventricular bundle with remarks concerning embryonic heart activity. *Klin. Wochenschr.*, **12**, 569–74

66. His, W. Jr. (1949). The story of the atrioventricular bundle with remarks concerning embryonic heart activity. Trans. by T.H. Bast and W.D. Gardner in *J. Hist. Med.*

67. Baer, K.A. (1951). Johann Sebastian Bach (1685–1750) in medical history. *Bull. Med. Libr. Assoc.*, **39**, 206–11

68. His, W. Jr. Abh. Math.-physik. KL. Sächs. *Ges. Wiss.*, **18**, Nr I.

69. Tawara, S. (1906). *Das Reizleitungssystem des Saugetierherzens*. (Jena: Fischer)

70. Mall, J. (1912). The Bundle of His. *Am. J. Anat.*, **3**, 13

71. Külbs (1914). Das Reizleitungssystem im Herzen. Handb. d. inn. Med. von Mohr-Staehelin 2, auch separat, Berlin 1913, dazu Lange. *Arch. mikrosk. Anat.*, **84**, 215

72. Kent, A.F.S. (1893). Researches on the structure and function of the mammalian heart. *J. Physiol.*, **14**, 233–52

73. Sonnino, R.E. and Mawk, J.R. (1988). Giovanni Paladino: true father of the accessory myocardial conduction pathways. *Chest*, **93**, 199–200

74. Paladino, G. (1876). Contribuzione all'anatomia, istologia e fisiologia del cuore. *Il Movimento Medico-Chirurgico (Napoli)*, **8**(28): 428–35; **8**(29): 451–70

75. de Gaetani, L. (1911). Atti della Soc. Toscana di sc. naturale **27**, 109 –*Anat. Anz.*, **39**, 209

76. Paladino (1909). *Rendiconti della R. Acad. delle scienze fisiche e matematiche di Napoli*, **15**, 268

77. His, W. Jr. (1933). *Op. cit.*, p. 323

78. Paladino, G. (1876). *Op. cit.*

79. *Ibid.*

80. Sonnino, R.E. and Mawk, J.R. (1988). *Op. cit.*

81. Keith, A. and Flack, M.W. (1906). The auriculo-ventricular bundle of the human heart. *Lancet*, **2**, 359–64

82. James, T.N. (1982). The development of ideas concerning the conduction system of the heart. *Ulster Med. J.*, **51**, 82–96

83. Keith, A. and Flack, M. (1907). The form and nature of the muscular connections between the primary divisions of the vertebrate heart. *J. Anat. Physiol.*, **41**, 172–89

84. Lewis, T. and Rothschild, M.A. (1915). The excitatory process in the dog's heart. Part II. The ventricles. *Phil. Trans. B.*, **206**, 181

85. Lewis, T. (1925). *The Mechanism and Graphic Registration of the Heart Beat*, 3rd edn. (London: Shaw)

86. Durrer, D. (1955). Electric activity of the sinus node, atrial myocardium and atrioventricular node. *Circulation*, **12**, 697

87. Puech, P. (1956). *L'activité électrique auriculaire normal et pathologique.* (Paris: Masson)

88. Scher, A.M. (1962). Excitation of the Heart. Chapter 12. In Hamilton, W.F. and Dow, P. (eds.) *Handbook of Physiology,* Section 2, p. 287. (Washington DC: Circulation. Am. Physiol. Soc.)

89. Kennamer, R., Bernstein, J.L., Maxwell, M.H., Prinzmetal, M. and Shaw, C.M. (1953). Studies on the mechanism of ventricular activity. V. Intramural depolarization potentials in the normal heart with a consideration of currents of injury in coronary artery disease. *Am. Heart J.*, **4**, 379

90. Scher, A.M. and Young, A.C. (1957). Ventricular depolarization and the genesis of QRS. *Ann. NY Acad. Sci.*, **6**, 768

91. Groedel, F.M. and Borchardt, P.R. (1958). *Direct Electrocardiography of the Human Heart and Intrathoracic Electrocardiography.* (New York: Brooklyn Medical Press)

92. Burchell, H.B., Pruitt, R.D. and Essex, H.E. (1951). Excitation of the isolated ventricular septum of the heart. *Proc. Soc. Exp. Biol. Med.*, **77**, 117

93. Eppinger, H. and Rothberger, C.J. (1910). Ueber die Folgen der Durchschneidung der Tawaraschen Schenkel des Reizleitungssystems. *Z. klin. Med.*, **70**, 1

94. Barker, L.F. and Hirschfelder, A.D. (1909). The effects of cutting the branch of the His bundle going to the left ventricle. *Arch. Intern. Med.*, **4**, 193

95. Wilson, F.N.A., Macleod, A.G. and Barker, P.S. (1931). The potential variations produced by the heart at the apices of Einthoven's triangle. *Am. Heart J.*, **7**, 207

96. Oppenheimer, B.S. and Rothschild, M.A. (1916). Abnormalities in the QRS group of the electrocardiogram associated with myocardial involvement. *Proc. Soc. Exp. Biol. Med.*, **14**, 57

97. Köllicker, A. and Müller, H. (1856). Zweiter Bericht über die im Jahr 1854/55 in der physiologischen Anstalt der Universität Würzburg angestellten Versuche. VII. Nachweis der negativen Schwankung des Muskelstroms am natürlich sich contrahirenden Muskel. *Verh. Phys.-Med. Ges. Würzb.*, **6**, 528

98. Katz, L.N. (1947). The genesis of the electrocardiogram. *Physiol. Rev.*, **27**, 398

99. Hoffman, B.F. and Cranefield, P.F. (1960). *The Electrophysiology of the Heart.* (New York: McGraw-Hill Book Co.)

100. Rogers, M.C. (1969). Sir John Scott Burdon-Sanderson (1828–1905). A pioneer in electrophysiology. *Circulation*, **40**, 1–2

101. Burdon-Sanderson, J.S. and Page, F.J.M. (1882). On the time relations of the excitatory process in the ventricle of the heart of the frog. *J. Physiol.*, **2**, 385

102. Muir, A.R. (1957). An electron microscope study of the embryology of the intercalated disk in the heart of the rabbit. *J. Biophys. Biochem. Cytol.*, **3**, 193

103. Bernstein, J. (1910). Die Thermoströme des Muskels und die 'Membrantheorie' der bioelektrischen Ströme. *Pflügers Arch. Ges. Physiol.*, **131**, 589

104. Englemann, T.W. (1878). Ueber das Verhalten des Thätigen Herzens. *Pflügers Arch. ges. Physiol.*, **17**, 68

105. Hodgkin, A.L. and Huxley, A.F. (1933). Action potentials recorded from inside a nerve fibre. *Nature (London)*, **144**, 710

106. Young, J.Z. (1936). Structure of nerve fibres and synapses in some invertebrates. *Cold Spr. Harb. Symp., Quant. Biol.*, **4**, 1

107. Curtis, H.J. and Cole, K.S. (1940). Membrane action potentials from the squid giant axon. *J. Cell. Comp. Physiol.*, **15**, 147

108. Hodgkin, A.L. and Katz, B. (1949). The effect of sodium ions on the electrical activity of the giant axon of the squid. *J. Physiol. (London)*, **108**, 37

109. Hodgkin, A.L., Huxley, A.F. and Katz, B. (1952). Measurement of current–voltage relations in the membrane of the giant axon of Loligo. *J. Physiol. (London)*, **116**, 424

110. Ling, G. and Gerard, R.W. (1949). The normal membrane potential. *J. Comp. Physiol.*, **34**, 383

111. Woodbury, L.A., Hecht, H.H. and Christopherson, A.R. (1951). Membrane

resting and action potentials of single cardiac muscle fibers of the frog ventricle. *Am. J. Physiol.*, **164**, 307

112. Draper, M.H. and Weidmann, S. (1951). Cardiac resting and action potentials recorded with an intracellular electrode. *J. Physiol. (London)*, **115**, 74

113. Overton, E. (1902). Beiträge zur allgemein Muskel-und Nervenphysiologie. *Pflügers Arch. Ges. Physiol.*, **92**, 346

114. Weidmann, S. (1957). Resting and action potentials of cardiac muscle. *Ann. NY Acad. Sci.*, **65**, 663

115. Brooks, C. McC., Hoffman, B.F., Suckling, E.E. and Orias, O. (1955). *Excitability of the Heart*. (New York: Grune and Stratton)

17   Regulation of blood pressure

Stephen Hales was the first to obtain measurements of blood pressure. His contribution does not reside in this fact alone, but rather in his understanding of an important mechanism at play. In particular, he pointed out the importance of blood volume in maintaining the pressure.

> I measured the blood as it run out of the artery, and after each quart of blood was run out, I refixed the glass tube to the artery to see how much the force of the blood was abated; this I repeated to the 8th quart, and then its force being much abated, I applied the glass tube after each pint had flowed out[1].

Hales' method and the evolution of other methods of measuring blood pressure are outlined in depth in Section 5.

In the course of time, it became quite evident that other parameters besides blood volume are involved in the regulation and maintenance of blood pressure. Homeostatic control is now known to be mediated through the vasomotor nerves, baroreceptive reflexes and hormonal agents channeled through bioelectric mechanisms at the cellular level in the heart and systemic vasculature.

Homeostasis is important because of the biological significance of blood pressure. This lies in the fundamental point that arterial pressure must be high enough to exceed the colloid osmotic pressure of plasma. If this were not so then diffusion of metabolites across the semipermeable membranes of the capillaries would not be possible, and the organism would soon die, since cellular metabolism is the basis of all life. Furthermore, the level at which the blood pressure is effective in maintaining the sanctity of the physical laws governing diffusion varies from species to species. Mammals manifest this variability to a marked degree, and it appears to be size-dependent. For example, blood pressure is much lower in the mouse than in the horse, elephant or giraffe. Warren illustrated this in 1957

when he found the blood pressure in a giraffe to range between 282/150 and 344/194 mmHg. Man's blood vessels would certainly burst at this level. A final but equally important point of biological significance is that homeostasis must include maintenance of blood pressure at proper levels in vital organs for effective nutrition during those periods when other areas of the body are undergoing hyperemia for one reason or another.

The tone of the peripheral arterioles is probably one of the most important variables in the regulation of blood pressure. Tone is a sate of vigor or tension within the vascular muscle that offers some resistance to passive elongation or stretch. It can be considered as a state of vascular readiness, a level of mildly sustained contraction from which a rapid response can ensue either in the form of dilatation or further contraction. It was first described by Lower in 1669 when, in describing the effect of venous dilatation on the heartbeat, he noted that an overdilated vein did not easily recover its tone[2]. The concept that tone also played a role in the arterial system was clearly put forth by Sénac in 1783[3]. He did not use the word tone as Lower did but he perceived that there was an inherent force in the muscular layer of the arteries that he thought made the arteries function in the same way as the heart. This is what he had to say:

> The arteries which are so active are true hearts in another guise; they have the same functions, the same movements ... These movements are alternate dilatations and contractions which succeed each other without pause ... The force inherent in the tissue of the arteries depends on the muscular fibers the very existence of which has been doubted ...[4].

The anatomical basis for such a view and the interrelationships with the nervous system had yet to be formulated. Henle was the first to describe and document the existence of smooth muscle in the peripheral arterioles[5]. It was already known that the walls of the blood vessels contained nerves, but it was left up to Stelling to delineate the presence of vasomotor fibers supplied through the sympathetic chain[6,7]. Apparently described but forgotten was Pourfois du Petit's report in 1727 that dilatation of the conjunctival vessels could be provoked by sectioning the ipsilateral cervical sympathetic nerves[8]. Stelling documented the existence of vasomotor fibers the same year that Henle described the smooth muscle in the peripheral arterioles. In fact, Stelling introduced into the physiological literature the term 'vasomotor' by which he meant that these nerves regulated the tone of both the arterial and venous walls.

This physiologic-anatomical description of the vasomotor nerves and their target, the muscle fibers of the blood vessels, was correct but devoid of any appreciation as to their actual role. Significant advances on this aspect had to await the initial studies of Claude Bernard, Charles Edouard Brown-Séquard, and Augustus Waller on the newly described 'nerfs vasomoteurs'.

Claude Bernard of Paris led the way with his experiments on ipsilateral temperature changes following section of the sympathetic chain or its connecting ganglia[9,10]. We have met and will continue to meet this great physiologist throughout this historical survey. His interests were wide and his contributions of the utmost importance in so many aspects of cardiology.

Brown-Séquard's observations on vasomotor activity were published in *The Medical Examiner and Record of Medical Science*[11]. He not only confirmed Bernard's observations but also added some of his own:

…if galvanism [direct electric current] is applied to the upper portion of the sympathetic nerve trunk after it has been cut in the neck [which in itself dilates blood vessels], the vessels of the face and of the ear after a certain time begin to contract; their contraction increases slowly, but at last it is evident that they resume their normal condition, if they are not even smaller. Then the temperature and the sensibility diminish in the face and the ear, and they become in the palsied side the same as in the sound side. When the galvanic current ceases to act, the vessels begin to dilate again, and all the phenomena discovered by Dr. Bernard reappear. I conclude,

that the only direct effect of the section [cutting across] of the cervical part of the sympathetic, is the paralysis and consequenly the dilatation of the blood vessels. Another evident conclusion is, that the cervical sympathetic sends motor nerve fibers to many of the blood vessels of the head'[11].

What is most intriguing was Brown-Séquard's ability to provoke constriction of the same blood vessels when he stimulated the peripheral end of their sectioned nerve[11,12]. The hyphenated name Brown-Séquard is derived from his American and French ancestry. His father was an American sailor named Brown. During one of his voyages, his ship stopped at the Island of Mauritius, at that time a French colony. While there Mr. Brown met and married a local girl named Séquard. Soon after impregnating his bride, the sailor went on another voyage but never returned because he and his ship were lost in the Pacific. Young Charles Edouard never met his father but this did not prevent him from acquiring an excellent education. A highly dedicated and motivated man, Brown-Séquard rose up the academic ladder to become successively, among his other appointments, professor of physiology at the Medical College of Virginia, then a professor of physiology and pathology at Harvard, and later, professor of experimental medicine at the University of Paris. Brown-Séquard crossed the Atlantic many times, dividing his time for variable periods between England, France, and America. He is remembered eponymously for his description of the syndrome produced by compression of the spinal cord.

Augustus Waller, the third member of this exciting trio, is remembered by generations of students of biology for the phenomenon known as 'Wallerian degeneration'. He discovered this in 1850. When a nerve is cut, those parts of the nerve fibers that are separated from their cells undergo rapid degeneration while the cells themselves remained intact. This proved that nerve fibers are anatomically and physiologically an extension of their nerve cells. He is of interest to us because he too showed that stimulation of the cervical sympathetic chain caused vasoconstriction of the recipient blood vessels.

These observations were but the tip of the iceberg. A search was now begun to determine how the sympathetic activity was controlled and where the control resided. Bernard's studies suggested that there were special centers in the brain that controlled vasoconstriction. Schiff, working independently, also came to the same conclusion[13], and in 1876 Owsjannikow confirmed the existence of 'tonischen und reflectorischen centren der gefässnerven'[14]. Owsjannikow's work stressed the reflex nature of sympathetic activity but how this came about was yet to be deciphered, although Thiry in 1864 did relate it to carbon dioxide levels[6]. Definite proof of the importance of carbon dioxide levels was provided four decades later by Henderson[15]. He showed that at the cellular level local concentrations of carbon dioxide were instrumental in regulating the threshold of excitability in the brain center and thus acted as a modulating influence on the reflex activity of the sympathetic system.

The concept that there was a neural basis for vasodilatation in addition to one for vasoconstriction also surfaced during the mid 1800s. Claude Bernard again was involved in demonstrating its existence, while, at the same time, showing that vasodilatation was a reflex reaction[16]. These findings were presented before the Academie des Sciences in 1858. 'In effect, if immediately after the exposure of the glandular vein and of the nerve in question (chorda tympani), a taste sensation is evoked in the tongue by instilling a little vinegar in the mouth, blood rapidly becomes ruddy in the vein because the taste sensation produced in the tongue is conducted to the nervous center and transmitted by reflex action, through the chorda tympani'[16]. Simultaneous and independent studies conducted by Schiff and the Florentine physiologist, Longet, also brought this out[17].

Research activity centering on reflex vasodilatation revealed the presence of a separate center in the brain and the fact that vasodilator fibers were ubiquitous in the body. Laffont discovered the brain center in 1880 when he demonstrated that destruction of the floor of the 4th ventricle or excision of portions of the medulla abolish reflex vasodilatation[18].

William Bayliss spent many years investigating the neural mechanism of vasomotor control. This led him to postulate an hypothesis that, though wrong, prevailed for at least half a century. His theory stated that all the vasodilator fibers were under the control of a specific center in the brain, and that reciprocal feedback mechanisms existed between the vasoconstrictor and vasodilator centers[19].

Bayliss' interest in electrophysiology was not restricted to cardiovascular innervation but extended also to innervation of the intestine, pancreas and salivary glands. His *Principles of General Physiology* was widely acclaimed and served as a standard text for many years. The monograph on the vasomotor system appeared in 1923, just one year before his death. It summarized all the knowledge of vasomotor control prevailing at the time.

Little did Lower realize how important vascular tone would prove to be in the regulation of blood pressure through its impact on peripheral resistance. As we have seen, most of the efforts since his description were directed towards finding the underlying anatomical pathways for vasoconstriction and vasodilatation. Having accomplished this the next step was to search for the determinants of vascular tone. Did these exist in the smooth muscle of the blood vessel itself? Were they of an automatic 'spontaneous' nature extrinsically controlled or did vascular tone depend on both myogenic and neural determinants? These were the very same questions confronting the students of cardiac rhythm.

Bayliss was of the opinion that the stimulus for maintaining vascular tone is mechanical in origin, arising as a reaction to the distention brought about by the force of the blood pressure itself. He advanced this opinion in 1902 without conclusive experimental documentation. Except for certain modifications, its basic principle is still considered valid.

A very important neural regulator of blood pressure is the reciprocal interplay that exists between the sympathetic vasodilator and vasoconstrictor fibers. This relationship is activated, for example, during exercise, when the sympathetic vasodilator fibers to skeletal muscle are stimulated to bring about the much needed increase in blood supply to them, while there is an intense activation of the accelerant fibers and of the constrictor fibers to other vascular beds. If this were not so there would be a marked decrease in blood pressure to vital organs, a factor incompatible with their preservation. Anatomically speaking, all vascular beds are supplied with vasoconstrictor fibers while vasodilator fibers are found in vascular beds that have a degree of basal tone to begin with (e.g. skeletal muscle). These facts were brought out by Folkow in 1955 and Uvnäs in 1954[20,21].

The veins constitute the capacitance segment of the circulatory system. They do not play any part in peripheral resistance but by acting as a blood supply pool, they can increase venous return, which in turn would increase cardiac output and therefore the systolic blood pressure. Mellander in 1960 demonstrated the interrelationship between the vasomotor fiber control of the pre- and post-capillary sections of the resistance vessels and of the capacitance vessels[22]. On the venous side (capacitance vessels) only vasoconstrictor fiber activity was noted. This means that the venous blood can be mobilized quite readily when needed.

An important breakthrough in our under-standing of the forces behind the regulation of blood pressure was the discovery of the baroreceptor reflexes from the aortic arch. Prior to this the very idea of a reflex regulator mechanism was first suggested by Cyon and Ludwig in 1866 when they discovered the depressor nerve in the rabbit[23]. This nerve runs alongside the cervical portion of the vagosympathetic trunks. They were able to provoke a marked drop in blood pressure and heart rate when they stimulated the central end of this nerve. The depressor nerve was also found in other mammals as well as in non-mammalian animals[7,24,25].

Cyon and Ludwig were in error in believing that the depressor nerve arose from within the heart itself. Its correct origin was demonstrated by Köster and Tschermak in 1902[26]. Using degeneration techniques they showed that it arose mainly from the aortic arch and in those areas of the arch where the great vessels originated. They also brought out that the cell bodies of the nerve were located in the jugular vagal ganglion. In a report published just one year later, Köster and Tschermak recorded action potentials when they distended the isolated aorta with saline[27]. A whole series of investigations then ensued from different centers regarding the reflex activity of this nerve.

In 1924 and again in 1925 Heymans and Ladon presented undeniable evidence that in dogs a reciprocal reflex relationship existed between the level of blood pressure and heart rate, and that this was mediated through the vagal nerves[28,29]. Also in 1925 Anrep and Starling demonstrated that a rise of pressure in the heart and aorta caused a reflex vasodilatation[30]. Anrep then, in conjunction with Segall, went on to confirm the findings described by Heymans and Ladon[31]. Segall was to return to Canada, his homeland, and achieve fame as an outstanding cardiologist and clinical investigator. At this point in time, the previously described

investigations left no doubt that the cardio-aortic nerves functioned in a vasoregulatory capacity.

Baroreceptor nerve endings were then found in the carotid sinus, the caval veins, the pulmonary circulation and within the heart, especially in the atria with their afferent fibers running in the vagal nerves.

The carotid and aortic bodies have receptors that are also sensitive to changes in the pH, and O_2 and CO_2 levels of the blood. Heymans discovered this in 1933[32]. The reflex reactions consist of hyperpnea, vasoconstriction, hypertension, and change in heart rate. The rise in blood pressure is mediated through the sympathetic vasoconstrictor fibers[32].

Ever since Tschermak in 1866 described his 'Vagusdruck-versuch' the role and mechanism of the carotid sinus reflex were the subject of much debate, experimentation and confusion. It was not until 1923 that an orderly concept began to emerge. This was primarily due to the efforts of H. E. Hering who was then professor of pathologic physiology at Cologne, the first to hold this chair[33]. He localized the origin of Tschermak's reflex to the carotid sinus. A year later he proved beyond the shadow of a doubt that when the carotid sinus wall of the dog was stimulated it induced a drop in blood pressure and bradycardia[34]. Hering's observations were confirmed and amplified by Koch[35], Heymans[36], and again by Heymans and Neil in 1958[37].

These findings, as confirmed, merely set the stage for answering the all-important question: what is the relationship between the baroreceptors and the blood pressure? Heymans and his group demonstrated in 1950 and again in 1952 that they were important in maintaining homeostasis of the blood pressure[38,39]. He showed that an increase in tension provokes a resetting of the baroreceptor mechanisms thereby adjusting the blood pressure to lower levels, whereas a decrease in tension resets the mechanism from normal to higher levels[40,41]. The possibility that this mechanism may play a role in the genesis of arterial hypertension was suggested by Matton in 1957[42]. Page's group also studied baroreceptor function in chronic renal hypertension and came to the conclusion that the baroreceptors are 'reset' in chronic hypertension to whatever the hypertensive pressure level is and that the buffer baroreceptive reflexes tend to maintain rather than prevent the chronic phase of renal hypertension.

The important role of the splanchnic nerves in the regulation of blood pressure was demonstrated initially by Ludwig and his associates in 1864 and outlined in depth by Bronk in his Harvey Lecture in 1933 [43,44].

Just prior to and alongside these findings on baroreceptor reflexes, other studies were demonstrating that vascular myogenic automaticity does exist and is equally important in the maintenance of vascular tone. Moreover, it also became apparent that, like heart muscle, myogenic activity is modulated by neurohormonal factors. Even more significant was the discovery that neural control is minimal in vital organs, and that the smallest precapillary vessels have the highest myogenic activity. This is important because it is these small vessels that account for the greatest degree of peripheral resistance.

The role and types of vasomotor fibers underwent intensive study by such investigators as Gaskell and Langley, then Cannon and Rosenblueth, followed by Elliott, Loewi and Dale. The concept that when the need arises, there is increased blood flow to a particular region, began to emerge as the 20th century approached. Each group of investigators contributed a portion to the currently accepted scenario. The autonomic pathway was sorted out by Gaskell and Langley; the discharge rate and vascular response by Cannon and his group; the neurochemical transmitter by Eliott, Loewi and Dale and the role of chemical vaso-dilating factors by Sir Thomas Lewis.

When Lewis in his later years turned away from his phenomenal work in electrocardiography, he focused his talents on investigating the blood vessels of the human skin and their responses [45]. As a result of his brilliantly conceived experiments he wrote in his monograph published in 1927 that there was a local vasodilating substance. He called it the 'H substance', because it resembled histamine in its action [46]. That this is so, was confirmed many times, but further experimentation by others revealed that this 'H substance' is but one of many chemical substances that can cause vasodilatation. Wood and his colleagues brought this out in 1955 when they attempted to unravel the mechanisms of limb segment reactive hyperemia in man [47].

Ever since Lewis published his views, several other mechanisms were advanced to account for the local vasodilatation. These have included hypoxia or hypercapnea, lactic acid, potassium ions, acetyl-choline, energy-rich phosphate bonds and so on [47-54]. Despite all these investigations not much more is known about the key substances involved in local hyperemia than the information provided by Sir Thomas Lewis in 1927. More work needs to be done in this area because maintenance of local blood flow, despite a drop in blood pressure, is important for the preservation of function in the vital organs.

The laboratory of Michael Foster at Cambridge provided the setting for unraveling the autonomic pathways, leading ultimately to a physiological classification of vasomotor control based on adrenergic and cholinergic activity. Gaskell and Langley were the chief investigators. We have already seen how Gaskell discovered the myogenic origin of the heartbeat. He was now lending his talents towards outlining the organization of the autonomic pathways [55]. Gaskell revealed how the sympathetic nerve cells were collected in ganglia running along each side of the vertebral column and Langley pinpointed which of these ganglia sent nerve fibers to specific blood vessels. Langley's efforts were based on a pharmacological as well as an anatomical approach.

To reiterate, Foster was blessed with a number of brilliant assistants as we have seen in that part of this Section dealing with the electrophysiologic mechanisms of the heart. Langley too was no slouch. He went on to succeed Foster as professor of physiology and as editor of the Journal of Physiology. In his presidential address to the British Association in 1899, his high standards in experimentation and observation were revealed when he said:

> The multitudinous facts presented by each corner of Nature form in large part the scientific man's burden today, and restrict him more and more, willy-nilly, to a narrower and narrower specialism. But that is not the whole of his burden. Much that he is forced to read consists of records of defective experiments, confused statement of results, wearisome description of detail, and unnecessarily protracted discussion of unnecessary hypotheses. The publication of such matter is a serious injury to the man of science; it absorbs the scanty funds of his libraries, and steals away his poor hours of leisure [56].

Langley used pilocarpine to study glandular secretions and nicotine to outline autonomic nerve control [57]. Gaskell used the crocodile in working out the anatomical arrangement of the vagus and sympathetic nerves to the heart. Figure 1 shows Gaskell and his assistant, Thomas Metcalfe, with almost boyish playfulness towards one of their crocodiles.

The role of humoral substances in vasomotor control was not fully realized until G. Oliver published his findings on the clinical effects of extracts obtained from the adrenal glands. This was in 1894[58]. Whether it was courage or insensitivity on his part, I do not know, but Oliver first observed the effects on his own child, and then in collaboration with F. A. Schäfer, he continued his studies in the dog. Sir Henry Dalle's account of this is quite revealing:

In March 1894, I was still a boy, so that the story as I know it, came to me some seven years later from those who … were in the laboratory of the University College, London, at the time. And the story … was remarkable enough … Dr. George Oliver, a physician of Harrogate (a summer resort) employed his winter leisure in experiments on his family, using apparatus of his own devising for clinical measurements. In one such experiment he was applying an instrument for measuring the thickness of the radial artery; and, having given his young son, who deserves a special memorial, an injection of an extract of the suprarenal adrenal gland, prepared from material supplied by the local butcher, Oliver thought that he detected a contraction or, according to some who have transmitted the story, an expansion of the radial artery. Whichever it was, he went up to London to tell Professor Schäfer what he thought he had observed, and found him engaged in an experiment in which the blood pressure of a dog was being recorded; found him, not unnaturally, incredulous about Oliver's story and very impatient at the interruption. But Oliver was in no hurry, and urged only that a dose of his suprarenal extract, which he produced from his pocket, should be injected into a vein when Schäfer's own experiment was finished. And so, just to convince Oliver that it was all nonsense, Schäfer gave the injection, expecting a triumphant demonstration of nothing, and found himself, like some watcher of the skies when a new planet swims into 'his ken' watching the mercury rise in the manometer with surprising rapidity and to an astounding height, until one wonders whether the float will be thrust right

out of the peripheral limb. So the discovery was made of the extraordinary active principle of the suprarenal gland, later found to come only from the medulla [the core] of the gland, and still later obtained as a pure, crystalline substance and variously named epinephrine or adrenalin.

Figure 2 illustrates the blood pressure in the dog rising from a basal level of 52 mmHg (A) to 208 mmHg at B after an injection of the extract[59]. The author's comments are also noteworthy. 'The blood pressure may mount up to a height of from 2 to 5 times or more that which it had originally; indeed, even although we have employed an exceptionally long manometer, in more than one instance the mercury has been entirely driven out from the open end of the tube'[59].

Cannon and Rosenblueth quantified the frequency-response characteristics of a number of autonomic neuroeffectors[60]. They found that a low discharge was all that was necessary to maintain normal vascular tone. These findings were also confirmed in man by B. Folkow in 1955[61]. Walter Cannon was one of America's outstanding physiologists. He held the chair at Harvard for many years, and is well-remembered for looking upon the sympathetic nervous system as a defense mechanism in the 'fight or flight' phenomenon. This concept was to form part of the acute alarm reaction and general adaptation syndrome developed by Hans Selye of Quebec over the ensuing years.

Cannon and his group were also responsible for developing the concept of sympathin E and sympathin I. Cannon believed that epinephrine was the mediating hormone in emergency situations, coordinating a number of reactions vital to survival. In an emergency it would be pumped directly into the bloodstream by the adrenal glands and quickly cause:

(1) Dilatation of the arterioles of the limbs for the necessary increase in blood supply;

(2) Relaxation of the bronchial muscles so as to allow an increased flow of fresh air to the lungs; and

(3) Shutting down of non-vital activities such as blood flow to the skin, gastrointestinal movement, and so on.

According to Cannon, the increase in heart rate was due to sympathin E while sympathin I, being

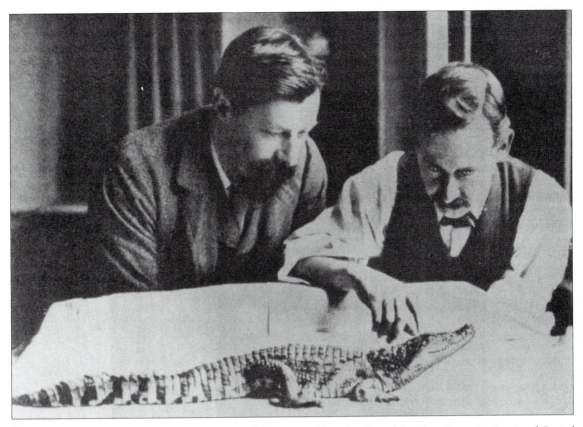

Figure 1 Gaskell and his assistant with one of their crocodile animal models. *Photo Source University of Central Florida. Literary source Fishman, A.P. and Richards, D.W. (1982). Circulation of the Blood, Men and Ideas. American Physiological Society, p.429. Taken from Franklin, K.J. (1953). Joseph Barcroft (Oxford: Blackwell). With permission*

inhibitory, was responsible for dilating the bronchi as well as the local blood vessels to the limbs. This concept was later rejected and proven wrong by Ahlquist. As we shall see in Section 6, Ahlquist was responsible for proving that epinephrine existed in only one form but that it exerted apparently paradoxical effects through its action on two different types of receptors which he called alpha and beta.

In the evolution of our knowledge concerning the humoral mechanisms of vasomotor control, three men emerge as important contributors. Two were from Cambridge. They are T. R. Elliott and Sir Henry Dale. The other is Otto Loewi, professor of pharmacology at Graz.

The initial studies were conducted by Thomas Elliott while he was a graduate student in the department of physiology. He was the first to suggest that the neurotransmitting element of sympathetic nerve stimulation was epinephrine or a substance related to it. This was expressed in his

paper 'On the action of adrenalin'[62]. Simply put, he demonstrated that no matter where in the body, the action of epinephrine was identical to that obtained by stimulating the sympathetic fibers to that part.

Was this a reactivation of the old Galenic teaching that the nerves were hollow and conducted through them a neurotransmitting agent arising from the brain? This was hardly likely, both on anatomical and physiological grounds. Structurally speaking the nerves are solid elements and not hollow. Moreover the rapidity of response after stimulation of the nerve is such that the humoral substance, in this instance, epinephrine, has to be present at the site, awaiting active transferral to the motor receptors. Proof of another humoral mechanism of this sort was finally provided by Loewi and Dale through their experiments on the parasympathetic system.

Loewi originally described his findings in 1921[63]. His experiments suggested that acetylcholine was the humoral neurotransmitter. Although he erred in

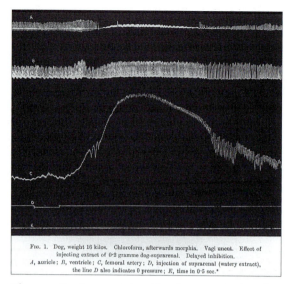

FIG. 1. Dog, weight 16 kilos. Chloroform, afterwards morphia. Vagi uncut. Effect of injecting extract of 0·2 gramme dog-suprarenal. Delayed inhibition.
A, auricle; *B*, ventricle; *C*, femoral artery; *D*, injection of suprarenal (watery extract), the line *D* also indicates 0 pressure; *E*, time in 0·5 sec.*

Figure 2 Increase in blood pressure in dog following injection with Oliver's adrenal extract. *Photo Source University of Central Florida. Literary Source Oliver, G. and Schafer, E.A. (1895). The physiological effect of extracts of the suprarenal capsules. J. Physiol., **18**, 230–76. With permission*

thinking that it was formed in the nerve terminals, he was right on all other counts. It is now known that acetylcholine is synthesized from acetate and choline and stored at the motor end plates waiting to be transferred to their appropriate receptors at a signal from the nerve impulse.

At the age of 80, Loewi published his autobiography wherein he describes how he arrived at his notion of a humoral agent, and how he went about proving that the notion was correct[64]. This was 40 years after his initial paper on the subject.

As far back as 1903, I discussed with Walter M. Fletcher from Cambridge England, then an associate in Marburg, the fact that certain drugs mimic the augmentary as well as the inhibitory effects of the stimulation of sympathetic and/or parasympathetic nerves on their effector organs. During this discussion, the idea occurred to me that the terminals of those nerves might contain chemicals, that stimulation might liberate them from the nerve terminals, and that these chemicals might in turn transmit the nervous impulse to the respective effector organs. At that time I did not see a way to prove the correctness of this hunch, and it entirely slipped my conscious memory until

it emerged again in 1920.

The night before Easter Sunday of that year I awoke, turned on the light, and jotted down a few notes on a tiny slip of thin paper. Then I fell asleep again. It occurred to me at six o'clock in the morning that during the night I had written down something most important, but I was unable to decipher the scrawl. The next night, at three o'clock, the idea returned. It was the design of an experiment to determine whether or not the hypothesis of chemical transmission that I had uttered seventeen years ago was correct. I got up immediately, went to the laboratory, and performed a simple experiment on a frog heart according to the nocturnal design. I have to describe briefly this experiment since its results became the foundation of the theory of chemical transmission of the nervous impulse.

The hearts of two frogs were isolated, the first with its nerves, the second without. Both hearts were attached to cannulas filled with a little Ringer [saline] solution. The vagus [parasympathetic] nerve of the first heart was stimulated for a few minutes. Then the solution that had been in the first heart during the stimulation of the vagus was transferred to the second heart. It slowed and its beats diminished. Similarly, when the [sympathetic] nerve was stimulated and the saline from this period transferred, the second heart speeded up and its beats increased. These results unequivocally proved that the nerves do not influence the heart directly but liberate from the terminals specific chemical substances which, in their turn, cause the well-known modifications of the function of the heart characteristic of the stimulation of its nerves.

The story of this discovery shows that an idea may sleep for decades in the unconscious mind and then suddenly return. Further, it indicates that we should sometimes trust a sudden intuition without too much skepticism. If carefully considered in the daytime, I would undoubtedly have rejected the kind of experiment I performed. It would have seemed likely that any transmitting agent released by a nervous impulse would be in an amount sufficient to influence the effector organ. It would seem improbable that an excess that could be detected would escape into the fluid which filled the heart. It was good fortune that at the moment of the hunch I did not think but acted immediately.

There was no bandwagon acceptance of Loewi's conclusions when he first reported this simple experiment in 1921. The scientific community had considerable reservations regarding the very existence of a humoral factor. Still convinced that he was right, Loewi returned 5 years later with more proof derived from another approach. This time, working with Navratil, he discovered an enzyme also occupying the same area as acetylcholine. In the course of his work he soon realized that this enzyme inactivated acetylcholine by splitting it into its components, acetate and choline. This led him to conclude that this enzyme had a modulating function, and because of its mode of action he labeled it cholinesterase. In essence, it prevented the acetylcholine from acting in an unbroken fashion. By immediately splitting the acetylcholine it allowed first, a succession of contractions to follow a succession of nerve impulses, and, second, it allowed the acetylcholine itself to undergo recycling as needed. His pharmacological orientation then led him to look for a substance that was capable of blocking the action of cholinesterase. This he found in a chemical substance derived from the calabar bean, an ordeal bean indigenous to northern Africa. It is called eserine (physostigmine). There was now at hand an agent that could prevent the inactivation of acetylcholine, therefore allowing it to accumulate in sufficient quantity so that its existence could be documented beyond the shadow of a doubt.

Otto Loewi shared with Dale the Nobel Prize in physiology in 1938 for their landmark work in electrophysiology. Their breakthrough ultimately led to finding the chemical means for modulating the activity of the autonomic nervous system. The pharmacological treatment of hypertension was a spinoff. It replaced surgical sympathectomy with pharmacological control.

Otto Loewi never intended to be a pharmacologist until he saw the frightful lack of therapeutic options in the management of patients with advanced tuberculosis while serving as an assistant in the City Hospital at Frankfurt. He began his career at the University of Marburg, and from here he went to Vienna before settling at Graz. Loewi was fortunate in that he had as his mentors such great men as Naunyn, Schmiedeberg, Meyer and Starling. He conducted his notable isolated frog heart experiment while he was professor of pharmacology at Graz[64].

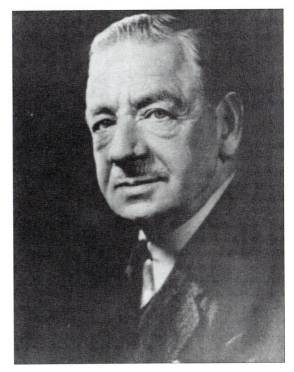

Figure 3 Portrait of Otto Loewi (1875–1962). *Photo Source University of Central Florida. Literary Source Fishman, A.P. and Richards, D.W. (1982). Circulation of the Blood, Men and Ideas. American Physiological Society, p.434. With permission*

America was fortunate when in 1940 he emigrated to New York where he became a professor at New York University. In 1938 he had been arrested by the Nazis, thrown into jail, later joined by his two sons, relieved of his Nobel Prize money and then deported. He managed to get to England. From there he went to Liége, Belgium, whence he departed for America[65]. Figure 3 is a portrait of Loewi revealing solidity of character and purpose in demeanor.

Henry Dale's research activities began under Gaskell and Langley. His greatest achievement lies in the way he outlined the role of both epinephrine and acetylcholine in neural mechanisms. The work was an extension of Elliott's theory of 'chemical transmission'. In his volume of selected papers, *Adventure in Physiology*, Dale recounts the historical background of this exciting breakthrough in the transmission of nerve impulses[66]. He was working at the time in the Wellcome Physiological Research Laboratory. This is how he said it:

About 1913, an accidental observation of the unusual activity of a particular extract of ergot [a fungus which occasionally replaces the grain in rye] quickened anew my interest in phenomena suggesting a chemical, pharmacodynamic transmission of excitation at the junctional contacts between nerve-endings and cells. What was supposed to be an ordinary liquid extract of ergot had been sent to me … for a routine control of its activity. When a conventional dose of this was injected into the vein of an anesthetized cat, it caused a profound inhibition of the heart-beat; I suspected, indeed, a fatal accident … till recovery set in, and successive repetitions of the injection then caused the same sequence at every trial. Tests of this extract on other biological reagents, such as isolated loops of intestine, confirmed the presence in it of an unusual constituent, with actions suggestively resembling those of muscarine poison from one species of mushrooms and muscarine, I thought, might perhaps turn up occasionally in a fungus like ergot. It was obviously impossible to pass an extract with such properties for therapeutic use, and I secured the whole batch of it for further investigation. My chemist colleague at that time, A. J. Ewins, succeeded thus in obtaining and purifying a few milligrammes of the abnormal active constituent, but it became clear that it could not be stable muscarine.

There seemed little hope then of further progress with minute amount in hand, till I recalled in conscious memory an observation made some 8 years earlier by my late friend Dr. Reid Hunt, then in Washington. Hunt and Taveau had found that when choline was acetylated its depressor activity was enormously intensified, the unstable ester, acetylcholine, being some ten-thousand times as active as the parent choline. When Ewins, accordingly, made me some acetylcholine, its identity with our substance from the ergot extract was immediately put beyond doubt. And when the actions of this came to be examined in detail, they showed as suggestive a correspondence to the effects of other nerves [the parasympathetic nerves] as those of adrenaline had shown to the effects of sympathetic nerves in particular. At that time there was no reason at all to believe that acetylcholine was a natural constituent of the animal and human body; but my late colleague, Dr. Dudley, and I found it there [in the spleen]

some 15 years later, again by accident, when we were looking for something else.

In the same volume Dale also wrote the following:

Elliott had there (in the *Journal of Physiology*, 1905 and 1907) set out arguments in favour of regarding the motor end-plates of striated muscle fibres as homologous with autonomic ganglion cells, not only on morphological grounds, but also on that of a kinship revealed by a common sensitiveness to nicotine and curare. I must have read this discussion, introduced by Elliott towards the end of a very big paper on the innervation of the bladder; but I cannot have had it in conscious memory when I wrote this one on the choline esters, though it may well have been subconsciously effective on my line of thought. Even more curious, however, is the fact, that, by this time both Elliott and I seem to have become shy of any open allusion to the 'chemical transmission' theory, which he had originated ten years earlier. I am sure that both of us had it still in the backs of our minds; and this paper, in fact, added points of real importance for its later detailed development. As I have elsewhere suggested, the stage was now set for it, and only a piece of direct evidence was needed to ring up the curtain; and, after a further gap of years due to the first World War, direct evidence of a very convincing kind was produced, in 1921 and the following years, by another friend of ours, Otto Loewi in Graz'[66].

Dale began his studies on acetylcholine in 1914, eight years after its discovery by Hunt and Taveau. This is when he first became aware of its parasympathetic activity. The difficulty of experimenting with the substance was due to its rapid destruction in the body by cholinesterase. This impediment was overcome in 1930 when Englehart, working in Loewi's laboratory, discovered that eserine was able to block the action of cholinesterase. Dale took advantage of this blocking action and devised experiments that were to prove that the parasympathetic nerve activity was mediated through acetylcholine as originally suggested by Loewi.

In 1934, during his Linacre lecture, Dale summarized the chemical transmission mechanisms in both the sympathetic and parasympathetic components of the autonomic nervous system. In essence, he stated that acetylcholine is the effector

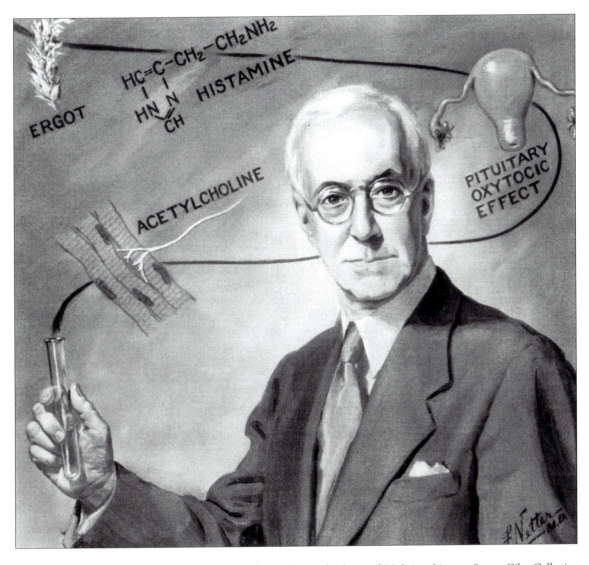

Figure 4 Portrait of Henry H. Dale. *Photo Source National Library of Medicine. Literary Source Ciba Collection of Medical Illustrations. Reprinted with permission from The Ciba Collection of Illustrations, illustrated by Frank H. Netter, M.D.*

substance in parasympathetic stimulation, whereas stimulation of the postganglionic sympathetic fibers liberated an adrenalin-like substance[66]. In 1936 Dale and Brown found that transmission of nerve impulses from motor nerve endings to skeletal muscle cells was also mediated through acetylcholine.

In 1947 and again in 1958, independent studies by Holtz and associates and Heymans with Neil added the final link in humoral transmission. They demonstrated that norepinephrine is liberated at the vasoconstrictive nerve endings while acetylcholine is the neurotransmitting substance for both sympathetic and parasympathetic vasodilator nerve fibers[67,68].

In Section 6, we will see how a good deal of this information was used in the development of the original antihypertensive agents that targeted vasomotor control through neural mechanisms.

REFERENCES

1. Hales, S. (1773). *Statical Essays: vol. 2, Containing Haemastaticks; or an Account of Some*

Hydraulick and Hydrostatical Experiments made on the Blood and Blood-vessels of animals. (London: Innys and Manby)

2. Lower, R. (1669). *Tractatus de Corde.* (London: Allestry)

3. Sénac, J. (1783). *Traité de la structure du coeur*, 2 éd. (Paris: Méquignon l âiné)

4. *Ibid.*

5. Henle, J. (1840). Ueber die Contractilität der Gefässe. *Wschr. Ges. Heilk.*, **21**, 329

6. Thiry, L. (1864). Ueber das Verhalten der Gefässnerven bei Störungen der Respiration. *Z. Med. Wiss.*, 722

7. Stelling, C. (1867). *Experimentelle Untersuchungen über den Einfluss des Nervus depressor aug die Herzthätigkeit und den Blutdruck.* (Dorpat: Laakmann)

8. Pourfois du Petit, F. (1727). Mémoire dans lequel il est demonstré que les nerfs intercostaux fournissent des rameaux qui portent des esprits dans les nerfs. *Hist. Acad. R. Sc., Paris*, **I**

9. Bernard, C. (1858). De l'influence de deux ordres de nerfs qui déterminent les variations de couleur du sang veineaux dans les organes glandulaires. *C.R. Acad. Sci. (Paris)*, **47**, 245

10. Bernard, C. (1858). *Leçons sur la physiologie et la pathologie du systéme nerveux.* (Paris: Bailliére)

11. Brown-Séquard, C.E. (1852). Experimental researches applied to physiology and pathology. *Med. Exam. (Philadelphia), N.S.*, **8**, 481

12. Brown-Séquard, C.E. (1854). Sur les résultats de la section et de la galvanisation du nerf grand sympathique au cou. *C.R. Acad. Sci., (Paris)*, **38**, 72

13. Schiff, M. (1853). Ueber den Einfluss der Nerven auf die Gefässe der Zunge. *Arch. Physiol. Heilk.*, **12**, 377

14. Owsjannikow, P.H. (1871). Die tonischen und reflectorischen Centren der Gefässnerven. *Ber. Säcks. Ges. (Akad.) Wiss.*, **23**, 135

15. Henderson, Y. (1907). Production of shock by loss of carbon dioxide, and relief by partial asphyxiation. *Am. J. Physiol.*, **19**, XIV

16. Bernard, C. (1858). *Op. Cit.*

17. Schiff, M. (1853). *Op. Cit.*

18. Laffont, M. (1880). De l'origine des nerfs vaso-dilateurs de la région buccolabiale. *C.R. Soc. Biol. (Paris)*, **32**, 297

19. Bayliss, W.M. (1923). *The Vaso-motor System.* (London: Longmans, Green)

20. Uvnäs, B. (1954). Sympathetic vasodilator outflow. *Physiol. Rev.*, **34**, 608

21. Folkow, B. (1955). Nervous control of the blood vessels. *Physiol Rev.*, **35**, 629

22. Mellander, S. (1960). Comparative studies on the adrenergic neurohormonal control of resistance and capacitance blood vessels in the cat. *Acta. Physiol. Scand. Suppl.*, **176**

23. De Cyon, E. and Ludwig, C. (1867). Die Reflexe eines der sensiblen Nerven des Herzens auf die motorischen-nerven der Blutgefässe. *Arb. Physiol. Anstalt Leipzig*, p. 128

24. François-Frank, C.A. (1899). Trajet cervical et cranien des filets sensibles du cordon cervical du sympathique. *J. Physiol. Path. Gén.*, **1**, 753

25. Bernhardt, E. (1868). Anatomische und physiologische Untersuchungen über den Nervus depressor bei der Katze. (Dorpat: Laakmann)

26. Köster, G. and Tschermak, A. (1902). Ueber Ursprung und Endigung des N. depressor und N. laryngeus superior beim Kaninchen. *Arch. Anat. Physiol. Anat. Abt., Suppl.*, p. 255

27. Köster, G. and Tschermak, A. (1903). Ueber den N. depressor als Reflexner der Aorta. *Pflügers Arch. Ges. Physiol.*, **93**, 24

28. Heymans, C. and Ladon, A. (1924). Sur le mécanisms de la bradycardie hypertensive et adrénalinique. *C.R. Soc. Biol. (Paris)*, **90**, 966

29. Heymans, C. and Ladon, A. (1925). Recherches physiologiques et pharmacologiques sur la tête isolée et le centre vague du chien. I. Anémie, asphyxie, hypertension, adrénaline, tonus pneumogastrique. *Arch. Int. Pharmacodyn.*, **30**, 145

30. Anrep, G.V. and Starling, E.H. (1925). Central and reflex regulation of the circulation. *Proc. R. Soc. B.*, **97**, 463

31. Anrep, G.V. and Segall, H.N. (1926). The central and reflex regulation of the heart rate. *J. Physiol. (London)*, **61**, 215

32. Heymans, C.J., Bouckaert, J. and Regniers, P. (1933). *Le sinus carotidien et la zone homoloque cardioaortique.* (Paris: Doin)

33. Hering, H.E. (1927). *Die Karotissinusreflexe auf Herz und Gefässe, vom normal physiologischen, pathologisch-physiologischen und klinischen Standpunkt.* (Dresden: Steinkopff)

34. *Ibid.*

35. Koch, E. (1931). *Die reflektorische Selbststeurung des Kreislaufes.* (Dresden: Steinkopff)

36. Heymans, C. (1929). *Le sinus carotidien et les autres zones vasosensibles réflexogènes.* (London: Lewis)

37. Heymans, C. and Neil, E. (1958). *Reflexogenic Areas of the Cardiovascular System.* (London: Churchill)

38. Heymans, C. and Van Den Heuvel-Heymans, G. (1950). Action of drugs on arterial way of carotid sinus and blood pressure. *Arch. Int. Pharmacodyn.*, **83**, 520

39. Mazzella, H., Wang, S.C., Heymans, C. and De Vleesch-Houwer, G.R. (1952). Mécanisme de l'action de la noradrénaline sur le sinus carotidien. *Arch. Int. Pharmacodyn.*, **89**, 122

40. Heymans, C. and Delaunois, A.L. (1953). Action of drugs on pressure-response and distensibility of carotid sinus arterial wall. *Arch. Int. Pharmacodyn.*, **96**, 99

41. Heymans, C., Delaunois, A.L. and Rovati, A.L. (1957). Action of drugs on pulsatory expansion of the carotid sinus and carotid artery. *Arch. Int. Pharmacodyn.*, **109**, 245

42. Matton, G. (1957). Pharmacological actions on the carotid sinus baroreceptors in arterial hypertension. *Arch. Int. Pharmacodyn.*, **110**, 474

43. Ludwig, C. and Thiry, L. (1864). Ueber den Einfluss des Halsmarkes auf den Blutstrom. *S.B. Akad. Wiss., Wien, Abt. 2*, **49**, 421

44. Bronk, D.W. (1933–34). The nervous mechanism of cardiovascular control. *Harvey Lect.*, **29**, 245

45. Lewis, T. (1927). *The Blood Vessels of the Human Skin and their Responses.* (London: Shaw)

46. *Ibid.*

47. Wood, J.E., Litter, J. and Wilkins, W.W. (1955). The mechanism of limb segment reactive hyperemia in man. *Circ. Res.*, **3**, 581

48. Dawes, G.S. (1941). The vasodilator action of potassium. *J. Physiol. (London)*, **99**, 224

49. Fleisch, A. and Weger, P. (1937). Die gefässerweiternde Wirkung der phosphoryl-ierten Stoffwechselprodukte. *Pflügers Arch. Ges. Physiol.*, **239**, 363

50. Fox, R.H. and Hilton, S.M. (1957). Sweat gland activity, bradykinin formation, and vasodilatation in human forearm skin. *J. Physiol. (London)*, **137**, 43P

51. Frey, E.K., Kraut, H. and Werle, E. (1950). *Kallikrein-Padutin.* (Stuttgart: Enke)

52. Hilton, S.M. and Lewis, G.P. (1955). The mechanism of the functional hyperaemia in the submandibular salivary gland. *J. Physiol. (London)*, **129**, 253

53. Kety, S.S. and Schmidt, C.F. (1948). The effects of altered arterial tensions of carbon dioxide and oxygen on cerebral blood flow and cerebral oxygen consumption of normal young men. *J. Clin. Invest.*, **27**, 484

54. Lundholm, L. (1958). The mechanism of the vasodilator effect of adrenaline. III. Influence of adrenaline, noradrenaline, lactic acid and sodium lactate on the blood pressure and cardiac output in unanesthetized rabbits. *Acta Physiol. Scand.*, **43**, 27

55. Gaskell, W.H. (1920). *The Involuntary Nervous System.* (London: Longmans, Green)

56. Comroe, J.H. (1983). *Exploring the Heart*, p. 225. (New York and London: W.W. Norton & Co.)

57. Langley, J.N. (1921). *The Autonomic Nervous System.* (London: Heffer)

58. Oliver, G. and Schäfer, E.A. (1894). On the physiological action of extract of the suprarenal capsules. *J. Physiol. (London)*, **16**, 1

59. Oliver, G. and Schäfer, E.A. (1895). The physiological effects of extracts of the suprarenal capsules. *J. Physiol.*, **18**, 230–76

60. Cannon, W.B. and Rosenblueth, A. (1949). *The Supersensitivity of Denervated Structures, a Law of Denervation.* (New York: Macmillan)

61. Folkow, B. (1955). Nervous control of the blood vessels. *Physiol. Rev.*, **35**, 629

62. Elliott, T.R. (1904). *On the action of adrenalin*, **32**, XX

63. Loewi, O. (1921). Über humorale Übertragbark heit der Herznerven-wirkung. I. Mitteilung. *Pflügers Arch. Ges. Physiol.*, **18**, 239

64. Loewi, O. (1953). *From the Workshop of Discoveries.* (Lawrence, Kansas: University of Kansas)

65. Comroe, J. (1983). *Op. Cit.*, p. 252

66. Dale, H.H. (1953). *Adventures in Physiology.* (London: Pergamon)

67. Holtz, P., Credner, P.K. and Kronberg, G. (1947). Über das sympathicomimetische pressorische prinzip des Harns ('Urosympathin'). *Arch. Exp. Path. Pharm.*, **204**, 228

68. Heymans, C. and, Neil, E. (1958). *Op. Cit.*

Section 4

Functional disturbances

18   Coronary artery disease

The earliest beginnings of knowledge regarding the syndrome that constitutes coronary artery disease originated from postmortem findings of arteriosclerosis but remained cloaked in ignorance regarding their significance for millennia. Coronary artery disease is inextricably linked with cardiac metabolism. This is a known fact but one only recently learned. In the evolution of our knowledge on the subject this was indeed the last aspect to be unraveled, though it is the ultimate basis for cardiac dysfunction in the presence of an impaired blood supply.

The normal anatomy of the coronary vessels had to be delineated first before any progress could be made. Clinicopathologic correlation followed and then in the 19th century, an era of physiological advances, investigations in the laboratory helped explain that an impaired blood supply was the key mechanism for the clinical spectrum ranging from angina pectoris to infarction along with their subsets of clinical manifestations and dysfunction.

Coronary artery disease is basically an arteriosclerotic process. The earliest references to this pathologic entity can be found in antiquity, but, as stated before, without any appreciation as to its clinical significance. Atherosclerosis is dealt with in Section 2, and in the chapter dealing with arterial lesions, the reader learned of Sir Marc Ruffer's contributions in his studies of Egyptian mummies[1]. Ruffer described the presence of coronary artery calcification and atheroma in his specimens of mummified Egyptians. The heart in his specimens was fortunately well preserved. In accordance with the embalming practices of the Egyptians at the time hearts were never removed as were the other organs. Religious beliefs at the time mandated that the heart remain with the dead man so as to safeguard him in afterlife.

These postmortem findings of calcification and atheroma must have been known to the physicians of that era but centuries had to pass before they were recognized as obstructive in behavior or even correlated with the clinical symptomatology that arises from an impaired blood supply.

During the Greek and Roman civilization the heart was considered to be the seat of consciousness and character. It was also inviolate and not subject to disease, a notion promulgated in particular by the great Aristotle. That it did have a functional role was also recognized by the ancients. Two of these functions received a good deal of attention. One was its role as the originator of the pulse and the other was its role in the formation of 'innate heat', the ancient counterpart of our modern concepts of metabolism. In the Aristotelian concept 'heat was a driving force and the heart was a kindling place of this animal heat'[2]. Aristotle expressed this concept when he said 'Animation and the possession of vitality are necessarily associated with heat... in the heart there is a continual accession of liquids from the nourishment; and their expansion by heat extending to the walls of the organ causes its pulsations'[3,4]. The concept that the heart was the source of animal heat prevailed well into the Renaissance. Mondino de Luzzi of Padua, in particular, adhered to this view[5].

Nothing further of true significance can be said until the anatomical makeup of the coronary vasculature was demonstrated by Andreas Vesalius. As pointed out in Section 1, the whole science of anatomy owes its very life to this man, whose remarkable achievements were accomplished within the unbelievably short span of seven years. In one fell swoop, he helped overturn Galenic authoritarianism and propelled the medical community into new frontiers.

Insofar as the coronary circulation is concerned, Figure 1 is representative of his contribution[6]. The drawing was executed by Jan Kalkar, his 'artist in residence'. It exemplifies how meticulous Vesalius was, relying on personal observation rather than on the erroneous descriptions of Galen. Vesalius, himself, actually dissected the human heart.

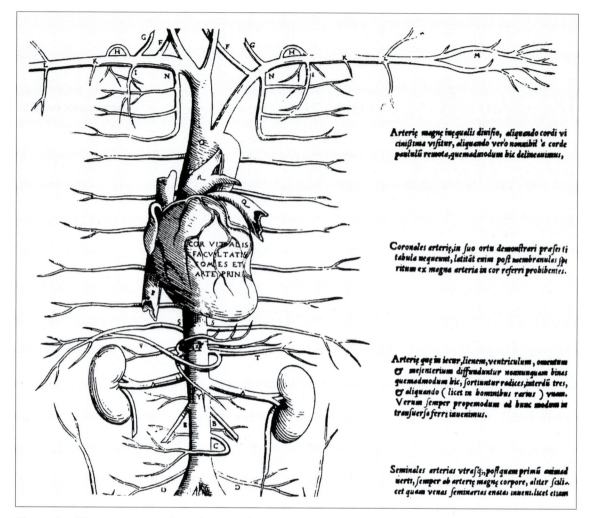

Figure 1 The coronary vessels, as drawn in the 'Six Tables' of Vesalius and Kalkar, from which Vesalius taught during his early years as professor of anatomy in Padua. *Photo Source National Library of Medicine. Literary source Vesalius, A. and Kalkar, J.S. (1538). Tabulae Anatomica, P.D. Bernardi, Venice. Courtesy of National Library of Medicine*

One of his students, a German by the name of Baldesar Heseler, in a series of notes, gave an eyewitness account of the master's method of teaching anatomy with actual dissection. These notes were discovered during this century in the Royal Library in Stockholm. We are indebted to Ruben Ericksson for their translation into English[7]. The highly charged atmosphere that existed at Bologna, because of Vesalius' iconoclastic references to the teachings of Galen, is brought to light by Heseler's detailed account of the acrimonious debate that ensued between Vesalius and Curtius. At that time, Matheus Curtius, an

arch-Galenist, held the chair of 'theoretical anatomy' at Bologna while Vesalius was presenting his 'lectures cum dissection' as a visiting professor. During one of these lectures, the arguments between these two men went back and forth like sparks. Each time Curtius would cite Galen as the authority. Vesalius would hit back with the actual dissection in hand.

Figure 1 shows the coronary vessels coursing over the epicardial surface and alongside them the description 'The coronary arteries at their origin cannot be demonstrated in the present table, because this origin is hidden behind the little membranes which prevent the spirits from flowing backward from the great artery into the heart'. The membranes refer to the valves and the great artery is the aorta.

Slightly more than a century was to elapse before another detailed description of the anatomy of the epicardial coronary vessels was to appear again. This was the contribution of Jean Riolan in 1648[8]. Riolan, however, like so many others before and after him, 'looked but did not see'. He had no conception whatsoever of the functional significance of his careful dissection. A Galenist to the core, Riolan still adhered to the Galenic view that blood passed through the invisible pores of the interventricular septum, and that the heart itself expelled only one or two drops of blood with each beat. Myocardial nutrition via the coronary arteries could not be part of this schema.

Further advances in the anatomy were made by actual dissection and by injection techniques. In 1669 Lower demonstrated the existence of intercoronary arterial anastomoses by injecting one artery from another. He regarded the presence of these anastomoses as a means of protecting the heart from any deficiency of 'vital heat and nourishment'[9]. Haller found extracoronary anastomoses with contiguous arteries in the mediastinum. These were confirmed by Hudson and his associates in 1932[10].

Raymond de Vieussens of Montpellier made several contributions on the coronary circulation. His most important one was his description of the intramural circulation. He injected the coronary arteries and veins with mercury and saffron dye, and noted that these materials passed directly into the cardiac chambers through small openings in the endocardium, thereby refuting Lower's assertion that the endocardium was an impervious lining. Figure 2 is a drawing of the heart as taken from his 'Traité nouveau de la structure et des causes du mouvement naturel du coeur'[11].

Thebesius confirmed the presence of these openings in 1708 utilizing the same injection technique of de Vieussens. These openings are now called the foramina of Thebesius, and the entire intramural vessels they drain is referred to as the Thebesian circulation. Vieussens held to the view that the endocardial openings were linked to the coronary arteries whereas Thebesius felt that they communicated instead with the veins[12].

The role played by the vessels described by Vieussens and Thebesius became the subject of numerous studies extending into the 20th century. These started in 1786 with Haller, who, while remarking on the difficulty of tracing their course by dissection, nevertheless gave a rather accurate account of their gross anatomical characteristics. He described 'still more and smaller veins in the heart, whose little trunks being very short cannot easily be traced by dissection and these open themselves by an infinite number of oblique small mouths, through all the numerous sinuosities observed on the surface of the right and left ventricle'[13]. In 1798 Abernethy used waxen injections to distend the Thebesian foramina[14]. Langer in 1880 was unable to demonstrate with his injection technique any communication in the ventricles between the Thebesian foramina and the coronary veins concluding that the Thebesian veins had their own capillary supply, separate and distinct from the coronary veins[15]. On the other hand Pratt did demonstrate just nine years later a direct communication between the coronary veins and the Thebesian vessels. He injected water, saline or defibrinated blood at constant pressure. Pratt was convinced that the Thebesian vessels were a source of nutrition for the heart[16]. Almost two centuries later (1929) Grant and Viko also utilized these foramina as their portal of entry for their injection technique. Using a dissection microscope they proved that Thebesius was right in claiming that they communicated directly with the coronary veins.

In 1928 Wearn reliably demonstrated, again with injection techniques, connections between the Thebesian vessels and the larger coronary arteries[17]. He also showed that the myocardial capillaries drained into the Thebesian veins. In a beautifully designed experiment Wearn showed how preservation of myocardial integrity was maintained through the Thebesian vessels during gradual closure of the orifices of the coronary arteries. Finally in 1933 Wearn and his group demonstrated the existence of direct channels between the coronary arteries and the heart chambers. They used celloidin for the injection, too thick to penetrate the capillaries. The channels were called arterioluminal and arteriosinusoidal vessels[18]. All these observations served to vindicate Vieussen's original premise that there are direct channels between the heart cavities and the myocardium. The anatomical spectrum of this portion of the intramural circulation was now complete. We can forgive Vieussens for this error in localizing the linkage.

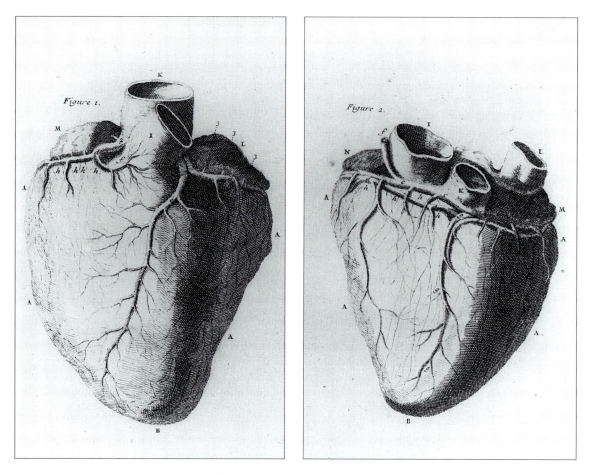

Figure 2   Two views of the heart as depicted by Vieussens. *Photo Source National Library of Medicine. Literary Source Vieussens, R. (1715). Traite Nouveau de la Structure et des Causes du Mouvement Naturel du Coeur. Toulouse. Courtesy of National Library of Medicine*

Vieussens was an outstanding anatomist; his position in the field made secure with the publication of his book *Neurographia Universalis*. It is too bad that he lost some of his well-earned reputation with his forays into chemistry, a discipline for which he was totally unprepared and in which he was woefully inadequate. During his Harveian Oration delivered to the Royal College of Physicians in 1968, D. Evan Bedford ventured the opinion that this might have been the underlying reason why Vieussens' book *Treatise on the Heart*, published the year of his death, did not receive the acclaim it merited[19].

In addition to the intramural circulation, Vieussens also presented a painstakingly detailed description of the epicardial coronary arteries and veins. In the process he discovered another coronary artery besides the usual left and right main trunks. He called it the adipose artery noting that after arising from the root of the aorta it crossed over the conus arteriosus to form an anastomotic ring which now bears his name. Schlesinger renamed it the conus artery in 1949 because of its course over the conus arteriosus[20]. This third coronary artery occurs as a normal accessory variant in 40–50% of cases. Gensini was able to selectively visualize it in 1967[21]. Of more importance is the curious fact that when present it is rarely the seat of an occlusive process.

Separate and distinct from de Vieussens' intramural circulation were the vexing questions concerning the existence of anastomoses between the coronary arteries and whether or not the coronary arteries functioned as 'end-arteries'. The actual existence of intercoronary anastomoses remained a bone of contention ever since Lower described them. Lower was initially supported by such luminaries as Haller, Thebesius and Sénac but as the 19th century progressed, further injection and experimental ligation studies served to renew the controversy. It was particularly important to find out if the coronary arteries were indeed 'end-arteries'. Experimental *in vivo* ligation of the coronary arteries had been carried out sporadically ever since Chirac performed the first one in dogs in 1698[22]. As the 19th century evolved, the experimental approach in pathology initiated by Rokitansky and Virchow began to assume an increasingly prominent role. This was to have an important bearing on the elucidation of the various pathophysiologic mechanisms in coronary artery disease, and on the morbid anatomical changes, both acute and chronic that ensued in the myocardium as a result of the obstructive process. These then went hand in hand with physiological as well as anatomical changes. The fabric that was finally woven came from pathologists, physiologists and clinicians. Many of the advances occurred concomitantly among these disciplines so that in tracing their evolution we will find ourselves at sometime or another in the deadhouse, the laboratory or the clinic; and at times in all three of them at once.

The transition from the purely anatomical description of the coronary arteries to the pathological one took place during the time of Harvey, Vieussens and Morgagni. Harvey was well aware of the role of the coronary arteries in nourishing the heart. He described this as part of his dissertation on the circulation[23]. Details of this are to be found in Section 2. At this point, I would like to emphasize that in refuting the existence of Galen's interventricular septal pores he wrote '... if the blood could permeate the substance of the septum, or could be imbibed from the ventricles, what use were there for the coronary artery and vein, branches of which proceed to the septum itself, to supply it with nourishments'[23]. This comment could serve then as the starting point for the future discoveries of the pathophysiology of coronary artery disease, for the deprivation of 'nourishments' is the fundamental change.

Morgagni's description of the pathologic changes that can involve the coronary arteries can be found in the 24th letter of his *De Sedibus*. The heart was that of a patient admitted to the hospital at Padua because of an incarcerated hernia. The description is as follows:

> As I examined the internal surfaces of the heart, the left coronary artery appeared to have been changed into a bony canal from its very origin to the extent of many fingers breadth, where it embraces the greater part of the basis. And part of that very long branch, also, which it sends down upon the anterior surface of the heart, was already bony to so great a space as could be covered by three fingers placed transversely[24].

The first anatomical correlation between myocardial changes and coronary artery disease was advanced by Sir Richard Quain in 1850[25]. He described two types of cardiomyopathy. They were fatty infiltration between the myocardial fibers and fatty degeneration of the muscle itself. He ascribed the latter finding to malnutrition, and obviously a result of diminished blood supply. 'I have seen the coronary arteries extremely ossified going directly to the only part of the heart affected ... This connection between fatty softened heart and obstructed arteries suggests an analogy with softening of the brain, in which a like condition of the vessel is known to exist'[25].

At the time Quain published his rather comprehensive review on 'fatty diseases of the heart' he was an attending physician at the Brompton Hospital, but he had become interested in the subject even before his appointment to the hospital. It was initiated by 'The sudden death of a gentleman, in whose body no sufficient explanation of that event could be found'[26]. A peculiar fatty condition of the heart was observed during the postmortem examination. The occurrence soon afterwards of two similar cases led him to conclude that the presence of this 'fatty matter in the heart's texture' bore some important relation to the structure and functions of the organ[26].

Quain was well qualified for pursuing this interest having studied under William Sharpey, the eminent physiologist at University Hospital, who was one of the first to use the microscope as a teaching tool in physiology. Quain capitalized on this background in microscopic investigation to identify this 'fatty degeneration' of the cardiac myocardial fibers and to correlate these changes with obstructive ossification of the coronary arteries.

Quain had before him the pathologic nuances of coronary artery disease from an ischemic process to a totally occlusive one. His review, however, was purely descriptive in nature pointing out the myocardial changes in the presence of coronary artery sclerosis with no insight as to the variable pathophysiologic scenario that could ensue. Descriptive studies of this kind were not unknown. What then was his contribution? He merits credit for being the first to describe the microscopic picture of the myocardial changes.

Subsequently, as the use of the microscope became more widespread, reports of a similar nature began to appear. Just nine years after the appearance of Quain's review, the Swedish pathologist, Duben, reported on the relationship between coronary occlusion and 'fatty degeneration' leading at times to rupture of the myocardium[27]. Rindfleisch in 1869 may have been the first to attribute fatty degeneration to a thrombus in the presence of atheromatous degeneration of the coronary arteries[28].

Fatty degeneration became a fashionable diagnosis during the latter part of the 19th century and the early decades of the 20th century. Austin Flint was one of the early American clinicians who was well aware of this pathologic entity and claimed that its antemortem diagnosis was not difficult, 'especially if the patient have passed the middle period of life, if his habits have been luxurious and indolent'[29]. Incidentally, he was one of the first to associate arcus senilis with coronary artery disease, a sign that without regret on my part has fallen by the wayside[29].

The works of Marshall Hall and John Erichsen contain the beginnings of the experimental approach in the morbid anatomy of coronary artery disease. Hall outlined in the Gulstonian lecture for 1842 the mutual relationships between anatomy, physiology, pathology and therapeutics, and, in doing so, presented his belief that sudden death was often caused by an obstructive process in the coronary circulation[30]. This was a rather advanced idea for the time. The solution revolved around the vexing question concerning the existence of intercoronary anastomoses and again whether or not the coronary arteries were anatomically and functionally 'end-arteries'. Hall suggested that the problem be addressed through animal experimentation. Pierre Chirac's observations on experimental ligation of the coronary arteries were buried in some dusty archive, awaiting rejuvenation. Hall's

suggestion was immediately taken up by John Erichsen. Before the year was out, Erichsen published his observations in the Medical Gazette in an article entitled *On the influence of the coronary circulation on the action of the heart*[31]. His experiments were conducted in the dog. Simple in design, they consisted of visual observation of changes in ventricular activity following ligation of the coronary arteries. He observed that the average duration of the ventricular action after the ligation of the coronary vessels was 23.5 minutes. This caused him to state 'Any circumstance that may interfere with the passage of the blood through the coronary arteries, either directly as in ossification of the coats of those vessels, or indirectly, by there being insufficient blood sent out of the left ventricle, as in cases of extreme obstruction or regurgitant disease of the aortic or mitral valves, may occasion the fatal event'[32].

It should be noted that while these experimental studies were going on, the clinicians were not remiss in presenting their own clinicopathologic correlates. One important description was that written by C. J. B. Williams (of stethoscope fame). He described in his text of 1840 a postmortem finding that he related to obstructive disease in the coronary vessels.

> A pallid yellowish appearance of the heart is not at all an uncommon accompaniment of other lesions of that organ, especially adhesions of the pericardium and accumulations of fat, but I should be inclined to refer this to an altered state of the nutrition of the organ, owing perhaps to partial obstructions in the coronary vessels, rather than to the immediate influence of inflammation[33].

A notable adherent of the experimental approach was Julius Conheim (1839–84), a pupil of Virchow. He and his two contemporaries, von Bezold and Panum, initiated the modern studies on perturbation of the coronary circulation.

Panum obstructed the coronary arteries with injections of powder, wax, oil or India ink[34]. Von Bezold ligated the coronary arteries and noted the effect on cardiac activity[35].

Conheim's contributions appeared during the same time period as those of Weigert. Both men were pupils of Virchow, from whom they inherited their interest in thrombosis. Weigert became Conheim's assistant and accompanied him to

Leipzig when they left the University of Breslau in 1878. Weigert's paper published in 1880 describes his findings in organ infarction. That part relating to the heart interests us here, especially his reasoning regarding coronary arterial occlusion and the usage of the term 'chronic myocarditis'[36]. This ill-chosen label was to survive well into the 1950s as a catch-all expression in coronary artery disease. During my early days in practice in New York City, it was used frequently as the basis for the so-called non-specific T wave changes. Weigert wrote:

... with atheromatous changes of the coronary arteries thrombotic or embolic occlusions of their branches not infrequently occur. If the closures result slowly, or, more important still, in such a way that collateral channels, even though insufficient for nourishment, exist, there ensues a slower atrophy with disappearance of the muscle fibers, but without injury to the connective tissue. These destroyed muscle fibers are then replaced by fibrous tissue, and the so-called chronic myocarditis is nothing else but such a process. If, however, a very sudden complete cutting off of the blood supply occurs in certain parts of the heart, yellow dry masses entirely similar to coagulated fibrin result. Here also, however, microscopic examination reveals almost no fibrous exudate, but often an apparently quite normal tissue (even the cross-striations of the muscle fibers often recognizable) but all muscle fibers and all connective tissue are devoid of nuclei. A reactive infiltration of round cells and spindle cells is present in the vicinity[36].

This landmark study by Weigert prompted the perception on the part of Carl Huber, a clinical colleague of Weigert, that angina pectoris and myocardial infarction were but different manifestations of an underlying disease involving the coronary arteries. A clinicopathologic link was being forged with this identification of two clinical subsets. Moreover, Conheim had already adopted the position that the fatty degeneration described by Quain was also a sequel of the same arteriosclerotic process.

In 1881 Conheim outlined his observations with ligation of the coronary vessels. He reported that ligation of the left coronary artery resulted in immediate stoppage of the heartbeat and death of the animal[37]. He also described collapse of the arterial pressure and the onset of ventricular

fibrillation. 'Extremely lively peristaltic fibrillary movements were noticed which persisted for 40 to 50 seconds or even longer; the atria meanwhile pulsated regularly'[37]. This form of cardiac arrest occurred within a minute after ligation. Moreover, he noted that the blood pressure did not rise during ventricular fibrillation. The blood pressures were determined by direct cannulation of the carotid or femoral arteries.

In the same paper Conheim tinkered with the possibility that hypoxia was the underlying metabolic defect. However, after commenting that lack of oxygen was an unlikely factor since oxygen deprivation of the whole animal provoked different abnormalities, he erroneously concluded that cardiac dysfunction following coronary occlusion was due to release of a poison within the heart muscle itself.

In 1882, Conheim went one step further, and this time, fortunately in the right direction. He showed that experimental ligation of the coronary artery need not be fatal. He expressed this, however, in an indirect manner by stating 'The occlusion of a coronary artery in case it does not prove fatal leads to destruction of the contractile substance of that portion of the heart which is fed by the affected artery, and afterwards by the formation there of so-called myocarditic indurations'[38]. I consider this observation as a landmark contribution. Segmental akinesia due to occlusion with replacement of necrotic myocardium by scar tissue can be, if large enough, a distressing and disabling sequel of coronary artery disease. It is an important component of the pathophysiologic spectrum in this disease. This aspect was quite unknown at the time, though we see it so often today because of our ventriculographic and nuclear imaging studies.

Ziegler also described a 'peculiar softening of the muscle of the heart, consequent on arterial anemia'[39]. He called this 'myomalacia cordis'. The term means softening of the heart. Although not as accurate as the currently accepted one of cardiomyopathy, it was at least a step in the right direction since it indicates what can happen to the myocardium as it is being deprived of an adequate blood supply. It is strange though that it never did achieve clinically the popularity of the ill-chosen 'chronic myocarditis'.

Ziegler should also be cited for two other important contributions. They involve the description of the histologic changes of myocardial infarction from the acute to the reparative stage and the prescient comment that 'When the destructive process has gone a certain length, and death does not ensue, processes of repair are set up'[40].

Collectively and individually, these observations kept refueling the controversy regarding the significance of the intercoronary anastomoses. Their very existence was being sporadically challenged. One of the most vocal was Hyrtle, a leading European anatomist of the late 19th century. He claimed that they existed only at the capillary level, basing this claim on an injection and corrosive technique[41]. The provocation of cardiac arrest following ligation was the main piece of evidence advanced by Conheim in support of his view that the coronary arteries were end-arteries. Some consider Pratt as being the first to introduce the concept of functional end-arteries. This was in 1898 when he also demonstrated a direct communication between the coronary veins and the Thebesian vessels. He claimed this mechanism prevailed when the resistance in the anastomotic channels exceeded the intracoronary filling pressure[42].

Except for the occasional clinician such as Huber, the experimental and postmortem observations had virtually no impact on clinical practice during the greater part of the 19th century. Huber's insight was unique and most clinicians did not differentiate between ischemic and totally occlusive episodes. Myocardial infarction never entered the mind of the clinician. If the patient had one and survived, the clinical manifestations were considered as being due to a prolonged episode of angina. As yet, the clinicians were not framing the pathologic specimens of the dead house within a broad pathophysiologic scenario. Little by little, however, and almost in a piecemeal fashion as older observations were reevaluated or confirmed, and newer ones were presented, the clinicians were gradually becoming alerted to the entire spectrum of coronary artery disease from the anginal phase to the totally occlusive one.

John Steven, a Scottish pathologist, and a former student of both Weigert and Huber, was one of the first to appreciate the spectrum. In his paper on the pathology of fibroid degeneration of the heart, he not only showed a connection between this and coronary artery disease, but also lamented the universal lack of recognition of such a connection[43]. Just three years before, Leyden had published a paper that classified coronary artery sclerosis into three clinical types[44]. This was his method of calling attention to the clinical subsets of the entire ischemic syndrome and was formulated on pathophysiologic grounds. Ernst Leyden had also commented on the frequent finding at postmortem of coronary artery narrowing, thrombotic occlusion or both in patients who during life had episodes of chest pain[44].

The occurrence of coronary thrombosis not due to coronary arteriosclerosis was not known to occur until Conheim's studies on thrombosis and embolism. Yet a case of coronary thrombosis diagnosed before death was reported in 1878, just before Conheim's observations were published. It was reported by Adam Hammer, a German physician practicing in St. Louis[45]. The obstruction of the coronary artery was actually caused by an aortic vegetation with an attached thrombus. In commenting on this paper Fye pointed out that Hammer had no idea of the underlying pathophysiologic process but he hoped that the paper he presented at a meeting of the German Medical Society of New York would stimulate further study on the matter[27].

One of the most outstanding figures to appear concerning the physiologic implications of coronary occlusion was William T. Porter. He began his experiments on ligation of the coronary arteries in May 1882, while pursuing postgraduate studies under Johannes Gad at the University of Berlin. Porter took up these experiments at the suggestion of his mentor, and continued them on his return to St. Louis Medical College[46]. The college was in the midst of a major transition. The year before, it had become the Medical Department of Washington University, and Porter was returning to a major new building replete with ultra-modern laboratories and facilities. What more could a young aspiring physician–scientist want? For several years he had been atwixt the horns of a dilemma, one that continues to confront many an enterprising medical graduate even today. This was expressed in a letter to his former teacher at St. Louis, Gustav Baumgarten, with whom Porter had cultivated a somewhat avuncular relationship.

> There can be no question that I can be more useful in St. Louis as a physiologist than as a practitioner. The making of a physiological institute in our community is worth living for. It is not possible to succeed in such an undertaking and

to succeed in practice at the same time. To practice medicine and experimental physiology is to be an amateur in two things. I must make a choice … Physiology means absolute poverty for some years, comparative poverty during life. Practice means giving up the best thing in sight for the sake of material comforts. These are the horns of the dilemma. I believe that I have chosen wisely'[47].

Fortunately for us, Porter chose wisely. Porter's experiments were quite fruitful. He noted that ligation of the left anterior descending artery or circumflex was most frequently associated with standstill of both ventricles. Fatal ventricular fibrillation was the most common arrhythmia, and was often preceded by extrasystoles. Porter had brought back with him the newly modified manometer of Karl Hürthle. Porter had already acquired some experience with it the year before while on a 'studenreise' at the University of Breslau in Hürthle's laboratory. Armed with this very sensitive instrument, Porter was able to obtain the first accurate measurements of intracardiac and intra-aortic pressures. He observed that ligation provoked an almost immediate but continuously gradual decrease in peak intraventricular pressure. After the onset of ventricular fibrillation a rise in left ventricular diastolic pressure was also noted. These observations, uniform and almost constant in their occurrence, led Porter to the obvious conclusion that ligation of the coronary arteries was fatal to the animal. Porter presented this work at the fifth annual meeting of the American Physiological Society in December, 1892[48].

Looking for greener pastures and an opportunity to devote himself exclusively to physiology, Porter transferred to Harvard where he was appointed assistant professor of physiology. He replaced William Howell who now assumed the chair of physiology at Johns Hopkins because of the forced resignation of his former teacher, H. Newell Martin. Unfortunately, Martin, America's leading physiologist, was suffering from the effects of alcoholism, a situation that managed to destroy a brilliant career and deprive us of his outstanding abilities[49]. We shall meet Martin, directly or otherwise, again and again throughout this text.

While still at St. Louis, and just prior to his departure, Porter was deeply involved with further experiments on ligation. In a whole series of observations he correlated the histopathologic features of myocardial infarction precipitated by ligation of the left anterior descending artery, expanding on the work first performed by Weigert in 1880[36,50]. Several years later, while at Harvard, Porter reported on the association between coronary artery ligation and decreased cardiac output, and the fact that rapid closure of the coronary artery resulted in death of the myocardial segment fed by that artery; an observation already known but worthy of confirmation[51]. In the same paper (presented as an updating of his research on closure of the coronaries) he expressed his notions on the functional significance of intercoronary anastomoses. He held the view that though anastomoses did, in fact, exist, they had no functional impact on the outcome of an acute occlusion of a major coronary artery.

The idea of terminal arteries is physiological, not anatomical. Terminal arteries differ from other arteries in that the peripheral resistance in the anastomosing vessels is too high to be overcome by the normal blood pressure in any of the arteries of which the communicating vessels are branches. Hence the rapid closure of any terminal artery cuts off the nutrition of its own capillary area because sufficient blood for the life of the area can not be sent through the communicating vessels on account of the high resistance in them. The resistance in the communicating vessels, and not their size, is the factor of first importance … I conclude, then, that the rapid closure of a coronary artery puts an end to the nutrition of the area which is supplied[51].

This is essentially what Pratt said two years later. If my dates are correct, and they should be since they are based on actual publication dates, Porter, rather than Pratt, appears to be the first in viewing the coronary arteries as functional end-arteries.

When Walter Baumgarten wrote his paper on myocardial infarction in 1899 it was a living expression of one of the greatest traditions in medicine, that part of the Hippocratic oath concerning fraternalism among physicians. Walter was the son of Porter's teacher and counselor, Gustav Baumgarten. Porter was paying back his debt by having his former mentor's son under his wing at Harvard. According to Fye, Walter's paper was 'the most comprehensive, and most insightful article on myocardial infarction written by an American in the 19th century'[49].

The 20th century saw a marked acceleration of interest on the question of coronary anastomoses. As better techniques were introduced it became evident that ligation need not be uniformly fatal. There had to be an anatomical reason for this. The advent of more sophisticated injection techniques in combination with radiography, stereoradiography and corrosion methods revealed the presence of numerous anastomoses between the coronary arteries at the precapillary levels; an anatomical finding that would have pleased Lower very much since he started the whole controversy. The most notable of these studies were conducted by Gross (1921)[52], Spaltehotz (1924)[53], Blumgart (1933)[54], James (1961)[55], and Fulton (1965)[56].

Injection techniques utilizing barium sulphate mixture and X-ray visualization were first introduced by Gross in 1921. Blumgart substituted lead phosphate agar[57]. This technique demonstrated that collateralization of the coronary vessels does occur and under a variety of conditions, especially in the presence of obstructive disease.

Let us retrace our steps for a moment and take up those studies concerning the physiology of the circulation since these too had an impact on our understanding of the entire spectrum of coronary artery disease.

The earliest efforts in unraveling the complexities of the coronary circulation were those of Giovanni Battista Scaramucci. He published in 1689 a monograph entitled *De Motu Cordis Mechanicum Theorema*, wherein he presented his concepts on the mechanisms of coronary blood flow. His views were very close to those currently held. Bedford brought this out when he quoted from Paul Wood's textbook published in 1968 the following remarks, that he felt 'were almost surely a paraphrase of Scaramucci's theorem': 'During systole ventricular contraction prevents blood flowing through the coronary vessels which penetrate the left ventricular muscle, and large arteries on the surface dilate to form an elastic reservoir which in recoil during diastole acts as an accessory pump forcing blood onwards'[19,58].

Scaramucci's monograph languished in dusty archives with hardly anyone giving it a second thought. The physiologists of the time, instead, riveted their attention on Stroem's hypothesis which appeared in print 18 years after that of Scaramucci. Stroem theorized that the coronary arteries filled only during diastole since blood was prevented from entering their ostia by the upward alignment of the aortic cusps during systole. The controversy continued until 1872 when Rebatel settled the issue. He was working in Chaveau's laboratory at the time assigned to investigating the coronary circulation in the horse and mule. Section 6 recounts how Chaveau and Marey had already introduced the technique of cardiac catheterization in unanesthetized horses. By measuring simultaneously the velocity of coronary flow and aortic and coronary arterial pressures, Rebatel was able to show that the coronary pulse was systolic in timing and that as systole progressed, the velocity of coronary blood flow decreased in concert with increasing intracoronary pressure. In his own words:

> In the very moment after the aortic valves have opened and the blood courses into the aorta, blood is ejected with violence into the opening of the coronary artery; this represents the first wave of blood entering the vessels. The elevation and the rapidity of both the spread and the rise of pressure demonstrate the rapidity of this wave and its coincidence with the aortic pulsation. Entrance of blood into the smaller vessels during systole is much more difficult. With diastole, the capillaries which have been empty of blood as a result of systolic compression, fill again from the larger coronary vessels. This represents the second weaker wave[59].

The experiments of H. Newell Martin and Sedgwick also suggested that blood enters the coronary arteries during diastole as well as during systole[60]. These observations have remained intact despite the refinements in technique introduced during the 20th century.

A landmark study of coronary blood flow was the one reported by Morawitz and Zahn in 1914[61]. They were able to determine the rate of coronary flow *in situ* by collecting blood from the coronary sinus via direct catheterization with a 'Tampon Kanule'. Anrep reviewed the whole subject in 1926[62]. In recent years accurate measurements of coronary blood flow have been made possible in humans through the pioneering efforts of André Cournand (see Section 6). The technique involves direct catheterization of the coronary sinus combined with the nitrous oxide method of blood flow measurement[63]. Bing and his group have also been the vanguard in these studies.

Proudfit suggested in his paper *Origin of concept of ischemic heart disease* that the clinical syndrome be called the 'British Disease' because Britain is where the pathophysiologic concept originated[64]. I suppose he said this with tongue in cheek and as a take-off of such appellations as the 'French disease', 'Montezuma's revenge', and so on. As far as priorities are concerned his suggestion may yet prove valid because the ischemic basis for angina pectoris was established by Heberden, Hunter, Black, Fothergill, Jenner, Parry and Burns; all from Great Britain.

Most historians begin the history of coronary artery disease in terms of clinical recognition with Heberden. Insofar as the description of the anginal state is concerned, Heberden deserves this recognition since his word-picture is unsurpassed and remains as one of the enduring classics of cardiology. Yet, an actual case of angina pectoris was described as early as 1632 in the memoirs of the Earl of Clarendon[65]. Morgagni presented a picture of the disease in 1707[66]. Several other accounts were also reported, including those of Fothergill, Home and one Dr Rougnon. But their descriptions lack the clarity and depth of Heberden's. Dr Rougnan wrote a letter to M. Larry describing the sudden death of a captain of cavalry during an attack of pain in the retrosternal region[67]. The captain had had similar episodes before, usually after exertion. The descriptions by Home and Fothergill will be presented shortly.

Whenever I read Heberden's account I call to mind Frank Netter's vivid drawing of a salesman outside a restaurant just after dinner and facing a snowstorm (Figure 3). The look of anguish on the man's face as he clutches his chest during an acute anginal episode is unforgettable. No one can deny how effective a Netter drawing can be in conveying a message. By comparing Heberden's account to Netter's vivid portrayal, I can offer no greater praise.

Heberden's paper was presented to the Royal College of Physicians in 1768. It appeared four years later in the transactions of the college as 'Some account of a disorder of the breast'[68]. It was reproduced 30 years later in Heberden's book *Commentaries on the History and Cure of Diseases*[69]. Figure 4 depicts the frontispiece of the book. Chapter 70 contains the account under the title 'Pectoris Dolor'.

Immediately after Heberden's account appeared in the transactions, it was completely reproduced in the March, 1772 issue of *Critical Review*, a popular

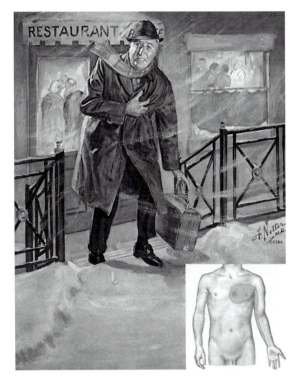

Figure 3 Netter's drawing of an acute episode of angina suggesting some of the various triggering mechanisms. *Photo Source Ciba Medical Education Division. Literary Source Ciba collection of medical illustrations. Plate 57, section V, vol. 5, p.223. Reprinted with permission from The Ciba Collection of Medical Illustrations, illustrated by Frank H. Netter, M.D.*

magazine of the time for the well-educated layman[70]. One of the readers of this article may have been a Dr John Haygarth, a distinguished physician in Chester[71,72] and supposedly the author of an interesting letter to Heberden. However, Proudfit presents enough evidence to indicate that he was not the 'unknown writer requesting that Heberden arrange for an autopsy on his body 'if it pleases God to take me away suddenly'[73]. This anonymous reader had been experiencing the very same symptoms that Heberden described and since the reader attributed the symptoms to either an 'obstruction of the circulation or a species of rheumatism', it was his wish that Heberden arrange for a postmortem correlation[74]. The wish was fulfilled only three weeks after Heberden received the letter.

Heberden had no idea of the relationship between the breast disorder and the heart. He

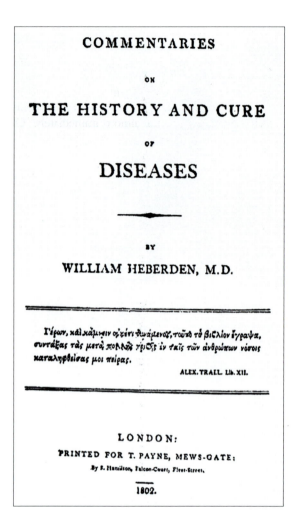

COMMENTARIES

ON

THE HISTORY AND CURE

OF

DISEASES

BY

WILLIAM HEBERDEN, M.D.

Γέρων, καὶ κάμνειν οὐκέτι δυνάμενος, ταύτα τὸ βιβλίον ἔγραψα, συντάξας τὰς μετὰ πολλῆς ἡμῖν ἐν ταῖς τῶν ἀνθρώπων νόσοις καταληφθείσας μοι πείρας.

ALEX. TRALL. Lib. XII.

LONDON:

PRINTED FOR T. PAYNE, MEWS-GATE;

By S. Hamilton, Falcon-Court, Fleet-Street.

1802.

Figure 4 Frontispiece of 'Commentaries on the History and Cure of Diseases' by Heberden. *Photo Source University of Central Florida. Literary Source Willius, F.A. and Keys, T.E. Cardiac Classics. The C.V. Mosby Co., St. Louis, MO. Courtesy of Mayo Clinic*

thought, erroneously, that it was some sort of spasmodic disorder with a nebulous foundation:

> The angina pectoris, as far as I have been able to investigate, belongs to the class of spasmodic, not of inflammatory complaints, For,
>
> In the 1st place, the access and the recess of the fit is sudden.
>
> 2dly, There are long intervals of perfect health.
>
> 3dly, Wine, and spirituous liquors, and opium, afford considerable relief.
>
> 4thly, It is increased by disturbance of the mind.

> 5thly, It continues many years without any other injury to the health.
>
> 6thly, In the beginning it is not brought on by riding on horseback, or in a carriage, as is usual in diseases arising from scirrhous, or inflammation.
>
> 7thly, During the fit the pulse is not quickened.
>
> Lastly, Its attacks are often after the first sleep; which is a circumstance common to many spasmodic disorders[69].

Heberden saw nearly a hundred people with this disorder. Most of his cases were in men near or past 50 years of age. He described it also in a boy 12 years old, and in three women. There is a report of only one autopsy, and it is of interest since 'a very skilful anatomist could discover no fault in the heart, in the valves, in the arteries or neighboring veins, excepting small rudiments of ossification in the aorta'. This last remark disturbs me. Did this patient's 'breast disorder' represent true angina pectoris or did he really die of something else? And yet, of interest is the description that after death, 'In this person, as it has happened to others who have died by the same disease, the blood continued fluid two or three days after death, not dividing itself into erassementum and serum, but thick, like cream'. Did the cream-like state indicate a hyperlipidemia? If so, it would seem incongruous that this man's coronaries did not bear the stigmata of obstructive disease.

Aside from these incongruities, how can anyone surpass the vibrant portrayal of the anginal syndrome as Heberden described it:

> But there is a disorder of the breast marked with strong and peculiar symptoms, considerable for the kind of danger belonging to it, and not extremely rare, which deserves to be mentioned more at length. The seat of it, and sense of strangling, and anxiety with which it is attended, may make it not improperly be called angina pectoris.
>
> They who are afflicted with it, are seized while they are walking, (more especially if it be up hill, and soon after eating) with a painful and most disagreeable sensation in the breast, which seems as if it would extinguish life, if it were to increase or to continue; but the moment they stand still, all this uneasiness vanishes.
>
> In all other respects, the patients are, at the beginning of this disorder, perfectly well, and in particular have no shortness of breath, from which

it is totally different. The pain is sometimes situated in the upper part, sometimes in the middle, sometimes at the bottom of the os sterni, and often more inclined to the left than to the right side. It likewise very frequently extends from the breast to the middle of the left arm. The pulse is, at least sometimes, not disturbed by this pain, as I have had opportunities of observing by feeling the pulse during the paroxysm. Males are most liable to this disease, especially such as have past their fiftieth year.

After it has continued a year or more, it will not cease so instantaneously upon standing still; and it will come on not only when the persons are walking, but when they are lying down, especially if they lie on the left side, and oblige them to rise up out of their beds. In some inveterate cases it has been brought on by the motion of a horse, or a carriage, and even by swallowing, coughing, going to stool, or speaking, or any disturbance of mind.

Such is the most usual appearance of this disease; but some varieties may be met with. Some have been seized while they were standing still, or sitting, also upon first waking out of sleep: and the pain sometimes reaches to the right arm, as well as to the left, and even down to the hands, but this is uncommon: in a very few instances the arm has at the same time been numbed and swelled. In one or two persons, the pain has lasted some hours, or even days; but this has happened when the complaint has been of long standing, and thoroughly rooted in the constitution: once only the very first attack continued the whole night[69].

Heberden also described a case of atypical angina which eventually seized the patient only while in bed.

A man in the sixtieth year of his life began to feel, while he was walking, an uneasy sensation in his left arm. He never perceived it while he was travelling in a carriage. After it continued ten years, it would come upon him two or three times a week at night, while he was in bed, and then he was obliged to sit up for an hour or two before it would abate so much as to suffer him to lie down. In all other respects he was very healthy, and had always been a remarkably strong man. The breast was never affected. This disorder, its seat excepted, perfectly resembled the angina pectoris, gradually increasing in the

same manner, and being both excited and relieved by all the same causes. He died suddenly without a groan at the age of seventy-five.

The termination of the angina pectoris is remarkable. For if no accident intervene, but the disease go on to its height, the patients all suddenly fall down, and perish almost immediately. Of which indeed their frequent faintness, and sensations as if all the powers of life were failing, afford no obscure intimation[69].

Heberden also brought out how the episodes could be aggravated by 'disturbances of the mind'. He uses the word 'spasmodic', but not in the sense of constriction of the arterial vessels. His spasmodic disorder refers instead to the clinical characteristic of episodic attacks with symptom-free intervals. Figure 5 is a portrait of Heberden.

Again, Heberden was not aware of any relationship between angina pectoris and coronary arteriosclerosis. John Fothergill on the other hand had the prescience to predict that future post-mortem studies would reveal 'the very substance of the heart to be affected'.

Although Fothergill's case reports appeared in 1776, his observations of one patient antedate those of Heberden by 12 years[75,76]. Two of his patients were subjected to a postmortem examination. In the first one the prosector was asked to pay particular attention to the heart. In doing so, he found a small white scar near the apical region about the size of a 'sixpence'. This may have represented a healed infarction. Fothergill's request that the heart be looked at would be but a natural consequence of his description of the syndrome when he wrote: 'I have very seldom met with this disease, but that it was attended with an irregular and intermitting pulse, but often when the patient was from pain and at rest'[75]. John Hunter performed the autopsy on Fothergill's second patient. It revealed severe coronary artery disease. 'The two coronary arteries from their origin to many of their ramifications upon the heart were become one piece of bone'[77].

John Wall of Worcester appears to have been the first to have outlined the natural history of angina pectoris and to have ascribed the cause to heart disease. In his letter to Heberden he described the necropsy findings in one of his '12 or 13 patients'. The most pertinent finding was stenosis of the aortic valve. Proudfit quoted him as saying with

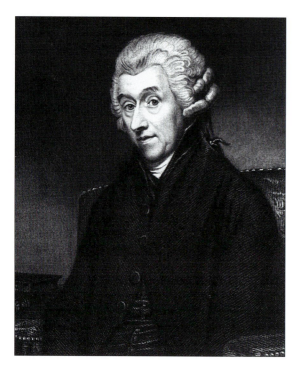

Figure 5 William Heberden (1710–1801). *Photo Source National Library of Medicine. Literary Source East, C.T. The Story of Heart Disease, plate 10. Courtesy of National Library of Medicine*

commendable caution: 'It is possible that this condition of the semilunar valves may not always be the cause of the disease, though it seems not improbable that some malformation of the heart or vessels, immediately proceeding from it, may do so'[78].

Lindgren depicted Wall's life as a 'profile in porcelain, painting and pectoral pain'[79]. This was a tribute to Wall's contribution in angina pectoris along with his ability as a painter and a worker in ceramics. Wall's avocation in ceramics became a vocation when he founded the Royal Worcester China Company.

There were three other small but pertinent papers published during this era. One was the rather well-known case report by J. Johnstone and the other two little-known papers by Samuel Black, both being case reports.

In 1787 J. Johnstone reported a case of angina pectoris from an 'unexpected disease of the heart'[80]. This was an excellent clinicopathologic correlate. He speculated that the symptoms of angina pectoris were manifestations of a 'defect of the power of the heart' and that the heart was 'unfit for its office of carrying on the circulation of the blood'. At autopsy this patient revealed a 'putrid' myocardium. I do not know exactly what he meant by 'putrid' but it could conceivably have been the softened area of a very recent myocardial infarction.

Very little is known about Samuel Black. A graduate of Edinburgh, he practiced in Newry, Northern Ireland, and for a while was a district health officer[81,82]. He did write a book on clinicopathologic correlation which had little or no impact on the medical community[83]. Nevertheless, it was representative of the emerging Parisian influence that clinical observations should be correlated and confirmed with postmortem findings.

Black's thoughts on the ischemic basis of angina pectoris were outlined in two letters to the Medical Society of London[84,85]. The first letter was published in the *Memoirs* of the Society in 1795. It is especially interesting because of his comments on the cause of angina pectoris, and why this cause was so often overlooked.

The primary and original cause of the disorder is, perhaps in every instance the ossification of the coronaries ... The coronaries are small vessels, and they do not lie altogether superficial, but are, in some degree, buried in the substance of the heart, for which reason, I think it very possible that their condition might pass unobserved, even by a very accurate dissector, if he were not particularly apprized of the necessity of attending minutely to that circumstance.

When Black's first letter was presented to the society he was still unaware of Parry's and Jenner's thoughts on the matter since they were yet to be published. Yet the detailed study of this case with postmortem correlation is truly reflective of how the patient himself is the best source for advances in knowledge. This was brought out all the more when Black published his book in 1819 on *Clinical and Pathologic Reports*[83–85]. It contained a summary of all his experience with angina pectoris. By this time, Black was well aware of the published works of Jenner and Parry and gave them full credit for their role while still presenting his own independent observations. He anticipated our current orientation on cardiac rehabilitation and prevention when he commented that those who engaged in exercise such as the foot soldier and the laborer seemed to be free of angina.

Edward Jenner was a 37 year old practitioner in the village of Berkeley, Gloucestershire, when he performed his oft quoted autopsy on a patient that had been under his care for angina pectoris. The findings in this and another autopsy performed on a patient of a surgeon friend of his convinced Jenner that obstructive disease of the coronary arteries was the cause of angina pectoris. These events were recounted in a letter that Jenner wrote to Parry, the details of which were revealed by Parry in his paper, *An inquiry into the symptoms and causes of syncope anginosa, commonly called angina pectoris*'[86]. Parry's paper appeared in 1799.

Two types of obstruction were noted. Jenner's patient had 'coronary ossification' with Jenner relating that as he cut into the heart he heard a grating noise that he initially attributed to falling plaster from the ceiling but soon realized that it was brought on by the hardness of the artery. The other obstruction was caused by a 'cartilaginous' substance that was removed by his surgeon friend, Thomas Paytherus, without difficulty, 'the intima separating as easily as a finger from a tight glove'[86].

When Jenner informed Heberden of his findings and conclusions, John Hunter, a mutual friend and Jenner's former mentor, was still alive and under the care of Heberden because of angina pectoris. Both men agreed to withhold this information from Hunter so as not to alarm him. Jenner was fully convinced of the ischemic nature of angina pectoris when in his letter to Heberden he stressed 'The importance of the coronary arteries and how much the heart must suffer from their not being able duly to perform their functions'[87]. He also ventured the opinion that 'all the symptoms may arise from this one circumstance'[87].

We have already met John Hunter, the noted anatomist, in Section 1. He was only 40 years of age when he began to experience recurrent episodes of angina. The description of the malady as it affected him was written by his brother-in-law, Everard Home, and is part of a short account of Hunter's life prefacing Hunter's treatise on the blood, inflammation and gunshot wounds[88]. Figure 6 is a reproduction of the title page from the first American edition of 1796. The following excerpts are from this account:

About the beginning of April, 1785 he was attacked with a spasmodic complaint, which at first was slight, but became afterwards very

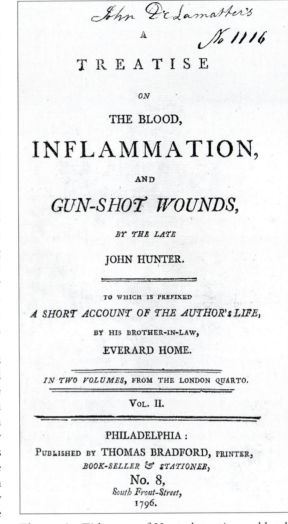

Figure 6 Title page of Hunter's treatise on blood, inflammation and gunshot wounds. *Photo Source National Library of Medicine. Literary Source Photo Archives. Courtesy of National Library of Medicine*

violent, and terminated in a fit of the gout in the ball of the great toe; this, like his other attacks, was brought on by anxiety of the mind; the first symptom was a sensation of the muscles of the nose being in action ... this sensation returned at intervals for about a fortnight, attended with an unpleasant sensation in the left side of the face, lower jaw and throat which seemed to extend into the head on that side and down the left arm, as low as the ball of the thumb, where it terminated all at once ... After they had continued for a fortnight they extended to the sternum, producing the same disagreeable sensations there, and giving the feel of the sternum being drawn backwards toward the spine. The relationship to exercise or an emotional disturbance is clearly brought out by the following passages:

> On Friday morning, the twentieth of May, between six and seven o'clock, he had a violent spasm, attended with most violent eructations of wind from the stomach for nearly a quarter of an hour. Dr. Pitcairn, who was sent for upon this occasion, asked him, if there was any distress upon his mind that had brought on this attack; and he confessed his mind to have been much harassed, in consequence of having opened the body of a person who died from the bite of a mad dog, about six weeks before, in doing which he had wounded his hand; and for the last fortnight his mind had been in continual suspense, conceiving it possible that he might be seized with symptoms of hydrophobia. This anxiety preying upon his mind for so long a time, there is every reason to believe was the cause of the present attack and probably had also brought on the former ones, which were all after the accident which had impressed his mind with this horrible idea... The exercise that generally brought it on was walking, especially on an ascent, either of stairs or rising ground, but never on going down either the one or the other; the affections of the mind that brought it were principally anxiety or anger: it was not the cause of the anxiety, but the quantity that most affected him; the anxiety about the hiving of a swarm of bees brought it on; the anxiety lest an animal should make its escape before he could get a gun to shoot it ...

Hunter had said that 'his life was in the hands of any rascal who chose to annoy or tease him'. As a matter of fact he died during an episode presumably precipitated by some unpleasantness at a board meeting of St. George's Hospital:

> On October the 16th, 1793, when in his usual state of health, he went to St. George's Hospital, and meeting with some things which irritated his mind, and not being perfectly master of the circumstances, he withheld his sentiments, in which state of restraint he went into the next room, and turning round to Dr. Robertson, one

of the physicians of the hospital, he gave a deep groan and dropt down dead.

At autopsy:

> The heart itself was very small ... upon the undersurface of the left auricle and ventricle, there were two spaces nearly an inch and a half square, which were of a white colour, with an opaque appearance, and entirely distinct from the general surface of the heart: these two spaces were covered by an exudation of coagulating lymph ... the muscular structure of the heart was paler and looser in its texture than the other muscles in the body ... the coronary arteries had their branches which ramify through the substance of the heart in the state of bony tubes, which were with difficulty divided by the knife, and their transverse sections did not collapse, but remained open.

A causal relationship with the heart was advanced by Home when he concluded this preface by remarking:

> From this account of the appearance observed after death, it is reasonable to attribute the principal symptoms of the disease to an organic affection of the heart ... the stoppage of the pulse arose from a spasm upon the heart, and in this state the nerves were probably pressed against the ossified arteries, which may account for the excruciating pain he felt at those times[88].

As mentioned before, Hunter's episodes had already been diagnosed by Jenner as being representative of angina pectoris. Also, Jenner was already convinced that the anginal syndrome described by Heberden was related to ossified coronary arteries. This opinion was communicated to the Fleece Medical Society. In full realization of Hunter's hyperreactivity to emotional stress, and not wishing to alarm Hunter, Heberden and Parry delayed spreading Jenner's view beyond the confines of the local society. Parry did not publish his *Inquiry into Syncope Anginosa* until 1799, six years after Hunter's death.

When Jenner diagnosed Hunter's episodes as angina pectoris, he advised the anatomist to avail himself of spa therapy at Bath. Hunter survived for 20 years following the initial episode that from its characteristics could have very well represented an acute myocardial infarction. At necropsy, Jenner's prediction that coronary artery disease would be found was confirmed. In addition the description of the myocardium, scanty as it is, could still be viewed as being consistent with another infarction. This certainly could have been the final blow with ventricular fibrillation being the immediate cause of death.

Friendly relationships carry with them the propensity for a free interchange of ideas. Parry enjoyed such a relationship with Jenner. This may have been the reason why Parry became fully supportive of angina pectoris. As early as 1778, just two years after Jenner's initial autopsy findings, Parry reported a similar clinicopathologic correlate in a minister who had been afflicted with angina for years. The autopsy revealed severe coronary artery disease, and Parry reported the case to the Fleece Medical Society[89]. Apparently the Fleece Society was a favorite forum for this tight circle of bright clinicians.

Parry's grasp of the pathophysiologic mechanisms in angina pectoris was truly remarkable. In his monumental monograph on the subject, he outlined how angina could occur in the presence of certain valvular defects, such as aortic stenosis, and during paroxysms of tachycardia. Parry paid more attention 'to the loss of strength of the heart muscle'. This is most interesting since his contention that myocardial contractility was impaired during an anginal episode was not fully appreciated until the 20th century with the advent of angiographic, echocardiographic and nuclear imaging techniques.

We have seen how important Allan Burns was in the survey dealing with arterial lesions in Section 2. He formed an important component of this cadre of English physicians with respect to coronary artery disease primarily because of his experimental approach. He strongly supported the obstructive process in the coronary arteries as the cause of angina pectoris. Burns' comments on angina pectoris are to be found in his book, *Observations on Some of the Most Frequent and Important Diseases of the Heart*[90]. The book contains a chapter devoted exclusively to 'syncope anginosa and disease of the coronary arteries'.

He relied very heavily on Parry's clinicopathologic descriptions, utilizing them for his exquisitely logical assessment of the underlying physiological disturbance; namely, impaired nutrition. The disparity between blood supply and demand is brought out in realistic detail in his analogy with a ligature around a limb:

The heart, like every other part, has particular vessels set apart for its nourishment. In health, when we excite the muscular system to more energetic action than usual, we increase the circulation in every part, so that to support this increased action, the heart and every part has its power augmented. If, however, we call into vigorous action a limb, around which we have with a moderate degree of tightness, applied a ligature, we find then that the member can only support its action for a very short time; for now its supply of energy and its expenditure do not balance each other; consequently, it soon, from a deficiency of nervous influence in arterial blood, fails and sinks into a state of quiescence. A heart, the coronary vessels of which are cartilaginous or ossified, is in nearly a similar condition; it can, like the limb, begirt with a moderately tight ligature, discharge its functions so long as its action is moderate and equal. Increase, however, the action of the whole body and along with the rest, that of the heart, and you will soon see exemplified the truth of what has been said; with this difference, that as there is no interruption to the action of the cardiac nerves, the heart will be able to hold out a little longer than the limb. If a person walks fast, ascends a steep hill or mounts a pair of stairs, the circulation in a state of health is hurried, and the heart is felt beating more frequently against the ribs than usual. If, however, a person with the nutrient arteries of the heart diseased in such a way as to impede the progress of the blood among them, attempts to do the same, he finds that the heart is sooner fatigued than the other parts are, which remain healthy ... By these exciting causes, applied to a person in whom nutrient arteries of the heart are diseased, an alarming fit of illness is induced. The heart is overpowered with blood accumulated in its cavities, it struggles with its load, but cannot free itself; the right ventricle ceases to propel the blood in due quantity into the pulmonary vessels, a sense of suffocation ensues, and an indescribable anxiety and oppression result from the accumulation of blood about the chest.

Despite the well thought out contributions by this elite group of British physicians, and the validity of their views, the clinical spectrum of coronary artery disease still remained unsettled for the remainder of the 19th century and well into the first half of the 20th century. Debate continued to center about the physiologic basis of angina. The various subsets of the clinical syndrome of ischemia and ischemic cardiomyopathy were not outlined until the introduction of cardiac catheterization, ventriculography, selective arteriography, and the whole gamut of technological instrumentation that is described in Section 6. Except again for this unique group of British physicians, the leading clinicians of the 19th century were too engrossed with the elements of physical diagnosis, the components of which did not lend themselves to many definitive observations regarding coronary artery disease. Pathologists were equally at fault. The reader is referred to Section 2 to find out how confusing the situation was when 'myocarditis' was the catch-all for disorders of the myocardium, when acute infarction was mistaken for fatty degeneration and when 'fatty heart' was the favored diagnosis. The very nature and natural history of myocardial infarction was unknown, a sad commentary on what is probably the most important complication of coronary artery disease.

That part of the clinical spectrum manifested by an acute infarction has a history all its own. Its cause, clinical manifestations and natural history were not truly worked out until the 20th century; and even then, in mid-century, confusion as to its cause arose once more. The introduction of the electrocardiogram was probably the most important modality that made its diagnosis *in vivo* possible. Prior to this it was a 'deadhouse' phenomenon, and for many years considered to be incompatible with life.

Although von Leyden's paper in 1884 and Rene Marie's thesis in 1896 were excellent summations of clinical thought on the subject up to this point in time, the clinical entity as such did not enjoy more widespread recognition until the American J. B. Herrick appeared on the scene.

Prior to him, and during the last two decades of the 19th century, three men figured prominently in the evolution of our knowledge concerning myocardial infarction. They were the pathologist, Ludwig Hektoen, and the internists, Sir William Osler and George Dock. Fye quotes a statement from an 1899 editorial *Infarction of the Heart* authored by Hektoen which reveals his understanding of the pathophysiology of coronary occlusion: 'While cardiac infarction may be caused by embolism, it is caused much more frequently by thrombosis, and thrombosis again is usually secondary to sclerotic changes in the coronaries'[91–93].

Sir William Osler was well aware that infarction was the result of total occlusion. In an unsigned editorial that appeared in Medical News in 1889, and attributed to him by Maude Abbott, he made the following statement: 'The local disturbances of nutrition caused by the blocking of a terminal branch of a coronary artery produce the condition known as infarct of the heart'[94]. In his lectures on angina pectoris Osler also brought out his belief that in virtually all cases, an acute myocardial infarction was fatal. He even referred to the left anterior descending artery as the artery of sudden death[95]. Words like this from such an eminent physician were bound to be accepted as 'ex cathedra' pronouncements. He did recognize, however, that death need not be sudden as witnessed by this remark: 'In a number of cases, death occurs suddenly, without any premonition; in other cases, precordial distress, pain in the left side, and signs of cardiac trouble have preceded the fatal illness for days or even weeks'[96].

The other internist was George Dock, first full-time professor of medicine at the University of Minnesota, and the father of the famous and outspoken William Dock (see Sections 2 and 5). George Dock was well grounded in pathology having pursued his postgraduate training under the tutelage of both Weigert and Leyden. In his *Notes on the coronary arteries*, which appeared in 1896, he attributed the growing awareness of coronary artery disease to the advances made in experimental pathology by his mentors and others of the Viennese school[97]. It was also in this very paper that Dock describes the antemortem diagnosis of myocardial infarction, one of the first clinicians to do so.

William Welch also recognized coronary thrombosis as an extremely important clinical event. He was a member of the original great four in the formative years of the Johns Hopkins Medical School. Halstead, Osler and Kelly were the other three. Welch enjoyed quite a reputation as one of the leading American pathologists. He too had studied under Conheim and Weigert. Despite his background and obvious capabilities, Welch was unfortunately, like so many of his contemporaries, still rather obscure on the pathophysiologic mechanisms of an acute myocardial infarction. To illustrate this Fye quoted Welch's comments from a paper Welch presented at a meeting of the

Pathological Society of Toronto in 1889[91]. Welch demonstrated a specimen 'in which a thrombus had formed in the apex of the left ventricle, a portion breaking off obstructed the left coronary artery completely, thus causing anemia of the wall, coagulation necrosis, and a white infarction'[98]. This is a rather confusing statement, and as Fye points out 'the pathologic observations were undoubtedly accurate, but the sequence of events described reveals a lack of understanding of the pathophysiology of myocardial infarction and its sequelae'[91].

The modern concept of coronary thrombosis and myocardial infarction was formulated by Herrick in a presentation before the Association of American Physicians in 1912[99]. The Association was started in 1886 as a protest against the manner in which the Section on Medicine of the American Medical Association was run. It was a perfect forum for Herrick since he too was a maverick when it came to outdated or poorly conceived ideas. Even in his day, the American Medical Association was considered to be a reactionary organization run, as Herrick put it, 'by a wire pulling, narrow-minded clique of old fogies'[100].

Emanuel Libman of New York was the only one who discussed Herrick's paper. Actually Libman, in his discussion, rambled on with his own observations on coronary artery disease rather than critiquing Herrick's paper, though later on Libman denied this when he told Means 'I was there when Herrick read his paper, and I was the only one present who had enough knowledge of this subject to discuss his paper'[101]. Means recounted this in his history of the Association of American Physicians. Means also recalled Herrick's disappointment at the lack of response on the part of the physicians the first time he presented the subject. This is how Herrick expressed his frustration:

> You know I've never understood it. In 1912 when I arose to read my paper at the Association I was elated, for I knew I had a substantial contribution to present. I read it, and it fell flat as a pancake. No one discussed it except Emanuel Libman, and he discussed every paper read there that day. I was sunk in disappointment'[101].

Herrick's paper on the subject was certainly the first of its kind on American soil. But, as Krikler rightfully points out, few realize that Herrick's diagnosis of coronary occlusion in the living patient was anticipated by two years by two physicians

from Kiev[102]. They were two Russians, Obrastzow and Straschesko. Their work was originally published in Russki Vrach, but republished in German almost at the same time[103]. Herrick was well aware of their work since he cited them when he presented his original paper in 1912.

Herrick, undaunted by the initial cold reception, presented an updated version in 1918 before the same society. This included rather concrete documentation in support of his conclusions. This consisted primarily of electrocardiograms taken on dogs and patients. This was the first time that electrocardiograms were used in the diagnosis of acute infarction. After Herrick had read his first paper, he suggested to his friend, Fred Smith, that he repeat Lewis' work on the effects of coronary ligation. Although Lewis had duly recorded the induction of a variety of arrhythmias on ligation, he failed to describe the now well-known ST-T changes. Was this omission an oversight on the part of Lewis? Not so, according to J. D. Howell. He advanced the opinion that although Lewis probably saw these changes he chose to ignore them since his interests lay in arrhythmias[104].

Thus it was that Fred Smith demonstrated the serial electrocardiographic changes in the dog following ligation of the coronary artery[105]. Two years after Herrick's second paper, Pardee published his observations on the electrocardiographic changes in acute myocardial infarction. The special characteristics of the T wave in its final inverted phase carried for a while the eponym, the Pardee T wave. In 1928, Bedford and Parkinson of England followed the evolution of acute myocardial infarction from onset to the healing stage with serial electrocardiograms.

When Herrick read his paper in 1918 there was no doubt about its acceptance. His description of an acute infarction rivals Heberden's description of angina pectoris:

> Most of the patients are middle-aged or elderly men. The heart and blood vessels in many show the evidences of arterial and cardiac sclerosis; the blood pressure may be high. In others no sign of such change is to be made out. In fact, in my 3 cases with autopsy the only significant vascular sclerosis was in the coronary arteries; the hearts were of normal size and there had been no hypertension during life. Previous attacks of

angina pectoris may or may not have been experienced. If so, the patient will describe the attack due to the coronary thrombosis as of unusual severity. Often there is no assignable cause for the attack, such as is commonly noted in the typical paroxysmal angina – walking, a heavy meal, undue excitement, etc., though in some cases these exciting factors seem to provoke the attack or at least greatly to aggravate it when it has started. The painful seizure is usually more enduring than in ordinary angina, the spell lasting many minutes or several hours or a status anginosus developing. The location of the pain, as in the classical angina, is commonly substernal with frequent radiation to the arms and neck. But in many of the thrombotic cases the pain is beneath the lower sternum or even in the upper epigastric region, and there may be no radiation to the arm or neck. This epigastric reference of the pain with the nausea and vomiting that frequently occur often suggests to patient and physician some abdominal accident such as acute pancreatitis, perforation of the gall bladder or of a gastric or duodenal ulcer. And these suspicions are strengthened by the fact that there are so frequently signs of shock and collapse – ashy hue of the face, clammy skin, small, rapid, feeble pulse.

The heart is commonly rapid even to 140 or more, though slow heart action has been recorded. There may be irregularities such as extra systoles or partial block. The pulse usually lacks in strength, may be almost imperceptible though in some cases the strength is wonderfully well preserved. Blood pressure is lowered and tends to grow lower in the unfavorable cases. The heart tones may be startlingly faint both because of the weakness of the heart's musculature as well as because of an acute emphysema that may develop and mask the heart sounds. Over the infarcted area a pericardial friction is sometimes heard. The heart may reveal evidence of dilatation by its increased area of dullness and its mitral systolic murmur, due to relative insufficiency of the valve. Rales in the bronchi with other evidence of pulmonary edema may be present. Passive congestion of the kidney may show in a trace of albumin being large in amount, the legs badly swollen and free fluid present in the abdominal cavity. The mind is commonly quite clear. I have been surprised at the preservation of bodily strength that is often manifested. Patients occasionally walk about within a few hours after such a seizure and within a few days may be out of doors trying to attend to business.

These symptoms will often enable one to make a reasonably certain diagnosis of acute obstruction of the coronary artery. As in so many other conditions the first essential is to think of this condition as a possibility and to rid the mind of the notion that such a diagnosis is only possible at autopsy.

If one were to depict Herrick's philosophy, there is no better source than his own autobiography which was published in 1949 under the title *Memoires of Eighty Years*[106]. He summarized it in one sentence: 'The true physician must possess a dual personality, the scientific toward disease, the human and humane toward the patient'[107]. This dualism was actually part of his life and not an empty phrase. For example, realizing that chemistry was becoming an important component in medical science and that he was sorely deficient in the field, he decided to rectify the situation at an age when most practitioners have already become mired in the demands of a busy practice. He was 43 years old when he matriculated at the University of Chicago for courses in biologic, physical and organic chemistry. This was while he was meeting the obligations of his practice. He pursued this interest in chemistry even further when he temporarily left his practice and went to Germany to study with the famous organic chemist, Emil Fischer.

His humanistic side was evident in his assessment of the role of the laboratory in clinical practice. He expressed it in the form of a remark by a patient who was about to undergo a physical examination. 'I hope you'll not be like the others; I want somebody who will examine me more and the x-ray films less'.

Herrick's work on infarction made a lasting impression. The term 'coronary thrombosis' became firmly entrenched in clinical practice. It was used synonymously with acute myocardial infarction since no one doubted the cause and effect relationship between thrombotic occlusion of a coronary artery and infarction of its recipient myocardial segment. The term was to prevail up until the first four decades of the 20th century.

A pivotal work appeared in 1939 that set into

motion a series of observations by several investigators that would eventually cast serious doubt on
this cause-and-effect relationship. Friedberg and
Horn presented evidence that myocardial infarction
was not uniformly attributable to an occlusive
thrombotic episode. A new clinical perspective was
about to evolve in light of their findings. They
suggested that the term coronary thrombosis be
abandoned in favor of the more generic one of
acute myocardial infarction[108].

In a 10 year span beginning in 1940, three
seminal papers were published by Blumgart and his
associates on the relationship between coronary
thrombosis and acute myocardial infarction. They
found that thrombotic occlusion could occur
without infarction when the collateral circulation
appeared adequate, and that, if an infarct did
develop it could usually be attributed to an
occlusive thrombus at a critical location in the
coronary tree[109–111].

In 1951 Miller and his co-workers pointed out
that subendocardial infarcts were rarely associated
with coronary thrombi whereas predominantly
transmural infarctions were frequently associated
with such thrombi[112]. Another study, this one by
Branwood and Montgomery, tentatively concluded
that thrombosis was the final event of an acute
myocardial infarction[113]. This extreme view was
sharply contested by Chapman[114], Harland[115], and
Sinapius of Germany[116].

In 1972 William Roberts of the National Heart
Institute added more fuel to the fire when he
suggested that coronary arterial thrombi are
consequences rather than causes of acute
myocardial infarction[117]. A suggestion of this sort
from such an eminent cardiac pathologist had the
force of an imprimatur, and represented a dramatic
turnaround from the deeply entrenched notion that
prevailed since the beginning of the 20th century.
Roberts advanced as evidence his own observations
as well as those of others[113,118–120].

In his study of 107 patients who came to
necropsy he found that only 54% of those with a
transmural infarction, and only 10% of those with
subendocardial necrosis, had a thrombus in the
infarct-related artery. An explanation for this was
sorely needed, and, as it turned out, the issue of
cause and effect was a crucial breakthrough in the
evolution of thrombolytic therapy (see Section 6).

Spain and Bradess had demonstrated that
coronary thrombi were more likely to be found in
those with longer intervals between the onset of
symptoms and death[118]. Hackel and his group as
well as that of De Sanctis from Boston also noted a
positive correlation between the presence of
coronary arterial thrombi in acute myocardial
infarction and the incidence of the power failure
syndrome[121–123]. They concluded that a patient
with a severely diminished cardiac output is much
more likely to have a thrombus at autopsy.

In an attempt to clarify the issue a workshop was
held on May 21, 1973 at the National Institutes of
Health under the joint sponsorship of the American
Heart Association and the National Institutes of
Health. The participants included among others,
Roberts, Chapman, Erhardt, Schwartz, Sinapius and
Spain; all of them respected for their contributions
on the subject matter. The incidence of coronary
thrombi with infarcted areas among these
participants ranged from a low of 54% (Roberts) to
a high of 96.5% (Sinapius). The frequency of
thrombosis in Roberts' cases was considerably lower
than that of the other reports. No satisfactory explanation emerged to account for this disparity.
Chapman, Schwartz, Sinapius and Spain all agreed
that there was a causal relationship between
thrombus and infarction. Erhardt was of the opinion
that the coronary thrombus may be a secondary
event. Roberts stated that the coronary thrombus
follows rather than precipitates the acute myocardial
infarction[124]. Roberts, in addition, questioned the
ischemic effect of thrombosis occurring in coronary
arteries already severely narrowed by arteriosclerosis.
Schwartz presented data showing that thrombi
decline in frequency as infarcts become older,
whereas atherosclerotic plaques increase in number.
This brought up the question of spontaneous lysis of
the thrombi and the possibility that incompletely
lysed thrombi are transformed into atherosclerotic
plaques as they are organized and incorporated into
the arterial wall[125–127].

In his study, Roberts divided the patients into
two groups, those with antemortem clots and those
without. Forty-two patients had antemortem clots.
In this group the interval between death and
autopsy ranged from 2–23 hours. In those without
antemortem clots (65 patients), this interval ranged
from 2–26 hours. These findings indicated that the
interval between death and the performance of the
autopsy had really no bearing on the presence or
absence of antemortem clots. But other questions
remained; one was why an acute myocardial

infarction occurred in the absence of an acute occlusion. Inadequate postmortem examination of the coronary arteries was possible but hardly likely, especially in Roberts' study. He was quite meticulous and detailed in his methodology.

Could infarction occur without a thrombus? The answer was to be found in at least one of three possible mechanisms: spasm of the coronary artery, acute decrease in blood supply brought about by a decrease in perfusion pressure, and an acute increase in oxygen demand as in tachycardia.

All of the postmortem studies lacked one crucial point – what was the status of the coronary arteries in terms of thrombotic occlusion between the onset of symptoms and the remainder of the postinfarction period? The essential factor in establishing a precise relationship between coronary thrombosis and acute myocardial infarction is the time course of thrombus formation in relation to the onset of the infarction. Histological criteria proved to be too unreliable in estimating the age of coronary thrombi in infarction[128–130]. Spontaneous lysis of antemortem clots was a real possibility and could easily explain the lack of thrombi in all cases of infarction. Schwartz gave an indication that this could be so when he showed a decline in the incidence of demonstrable thrombi as infarcts became older[128–130]. Obviously, *in vivo* studies within the clinical setting were needed to resolve the issue.

The role of thrombosis in acute myocardial infarction became firmly established in 1980 when DeWood and his associates described the prevalence of total coronary occlusion during the early hours of transmural myocardial infarction by means of coronary arteriography[131]. This was a very courageous and highly aggressive feat on their part. Contrast visualization of the coronary arteries was anathema in acute myocardial infarction. Their successful breakthrough, however, soon encouraged others to perform such studies during the acute phase of infarction. These led Forrester and his coworkers to conduct coronary angioscopy during episodes of unstable angina (pre-infarction syndrome)[132–134]. They were able to document by direct visualization the presence of thrombi in the formative stages of an infarction. Finally there was repeated demonstration of fresh thrombi in the majority of patients undergoing emergency coronary artery bypass surgery[131].

Thus, the data supplied from these three sources provided convincing clinical evidence for a cause-and-effect relationship between thrombotic occlusion and acute myocardial infarction. The efforts of Forssmann and Cournand in the development of cardiac catheterization bore fruit in still another component of the clinical spectrum of ischemic heart disease.

Until now this narrative has outlined just one aspect of the evolution of thought regarding the ischemic basis for angina. It is that the disparity between blood supply and demand is basically due to a fixed obstruction. That such a situation exists is quite evident in so-called effort angina. What about that part of the clinical spectrum wherein the ischemic episode occurs at rest or is induced by emotional factors? This too, has emerged as an important component of the syndrome. In fact, recent clinical investigators have shown that frank spasm of the major coronary arteries does indeed occur and that in a significant number of cases it plays an important role in the precipitation of acute myocardial infarction. There is also good reason to believe that sudden death due to cardiac arrhythmia may also be provoked by spasm of the coronary vessels.

In the light of this current knowledge it would be interesting to trace the successive events that led to our present perception of vasomotion. An excellent and comprehensive review was published by Rex MacAlpin in 1980, and I owe him a debt of gratitude for his depth of information and bibliographic sources[135].

We have already seen how Heberden described angina at rest or even upon 'first awakening from sleep'. We now feel that the latter may be a part of the circadian rhythm representing a response to increased secretion of catecholamines. But this is 20th century thought and certainly did not enter the minds of those British clinicians who contributed so much towards the concepts of ischemic heart disease. Heberden, as we know, had no idea of the underlying mechanism. Neither did William Harvey, a century before, when he described the ischemic scenario of Sir Robert D'Arcy: '... When he had reached to about the middle period of life, made frequent complaint of a certain distressing pain in the chest, especially in the night season; so that dreading at one time syncope, at another suffocation in his attacks, he led an unquiet and anxious life'[136].

One of the cases that Parry described also had anginal episodes that occurred only at rest. This 66-

year-old minister had no difficulty at all when exerting himself and yet he was subject to frequent episodes of angina at rest, arising spontaneously and for no apparent reason. Syncope anginosa formed part of the title in Parry's paper. The syncope no doubt refers to the loss of consciousness that occurred at times with the spontaneous episodes that afflicted this patient. We now know that syncope is not at all uncommon in that variant of angina that carries the eponym, Prinzmetal's angina. The consensus of opinion today is that Prinzmetal's angina is due to transient episodes of coronary arterial spasm.

John Blackall wrote a monograph in 1813 on the nature and cure of dropsy[137]. It contains an appendix devoted to a description of several cases of angina pectoris. The part that is most pertinent to us at this time is his comment that muscular spasm could be the cause of certain episodes of angina and his recounting of the conjecture advanced by a Dr Parr that the spasm involves the musculature of the aortic arch or the arteries that go to the arm. This was an ill-conceived attempt to explain why at times the chest discomfort radiated to the left arm. Latham on the other hand took a different tack, ascribing the entire episode of angina at rest to a spasm of the myocardium[138]. The postmortem examination of this patient failed to reveal any abnormalities of the coronary arteries.

Erroneous beliefs as to the locus of the spasm persisted well into the latter part of the 19th century. John Fothergill placed the locus in the systemic arterioles reasoning that the angina was brought on by distention of the heart as it attempted to overcome the increased peripheral resistance induced by the arteriolar spasm[139]. He did say though that angina could also be provoked if spasm of the coronary vessels were to occur as part of the generalized systemic arteriolar constriction.

Henri Houchard's comments in 1889 showed a remarkable insight that anticipated current documentation with our highly technological modalities. He suggested that paroxysmal spontaneous episodes of angina could be explained on the basis of spasm superimposed on fixed obstructive lesions[140]. Equally interesting was his speculation that coronary arterial spasm could be induced by the nicotine in tobacco. Ever since Huchard made this comment, severe tobacco addiction was thought to be an all-important factor in the perpetuation of anginal episodes. Proof that

this could be so was supplied in 1941 by Wilson and Johnston[141]. They described characteristic electrocardiographic changes of ischemia in a patient after smoking. 'The patient was asked to smoke two cigarettes ... This caused a slight burning sensation on the lateral aspect of the left upper arm ... the electrocardiogram showed slight downward displacement of the RS-T junction in Lead I and pronounced upward displacement of this junction in Leads II and III'. Ten minutes later the electrocardiogram was normal. When compared to the control measurements, no significant change in blood pressure or heart rate was noted. The patient incidentally was obese and smoked about 20 cigarettes daily.

William Osler also held to the view that spasm played an important role in the anginal syndrome. In his Lumleian lectures on angina pectoris he stated 'Spasm, or narrowing of the coronary artery or even one branch, may so modify the action of a section of the heart that it works with disturbed tension, and there are stretching or strain sufficient to arouse painful sensations'[142].

In one of these lectures he described the case of a 26-year-old man whose anginal episodes were triggered by cold or exertion. Some of these episodes were associated with syncope. No organic lesions of the coronary vessels were noted at autopsy. We know now that exposure to cold induces systemic arteriolar constriction. It is quite possible, though speculative on my part, that there was spasm of the coronary arteries in Osler's patient as part of the vasomotion response to cold.

In hindsight many of the cases of angina at rest described by Louis Gallavardin appear to be examples of the circadian rhythm[143]. Several of these cases were also found to have normal coronary arteries at autopsy. He brought out, however, that in his experience the vast majority of patients had angina on effort as well as at rest[144]. He tried to explain this dual presentation on a variety of spasm-inducing factors superimposed on fixed obstruction. This was a restatement of Huchard's suggestions first proposed in 1889. Gallavardin compared these transient episodes of spasm to those seen in Raynaud's disease, especially because of the aggravating influence of cold and emotions. This was also not a new idea since in 1884 both Duroziez and Constantine Paul independently made the same comparison[144]. In all fairness Gallavardin did credit Duroziez with this analogy.

The very idea that spasm could occur in rigid arteriosclerotic arteries was not universally accepted. Its very possibility was rejected by many clinicians. Two views emerged from various centers throughout Europe and America. In America Chester Keefer and William Resnik argued that spasm played no role in the creation of ischemia in an arteriosclerotic vessel[145]. This was in 1928 and meanwhile electrocardiographic studies were being reported that showed ST segment depression during acute anginal episodes. The earliest observations were those of A. Clerc (1927) and the team of Siegel and Feil (1928)[146,147]. A short time later Siegel and Feil also noted ST segment elevation in some cases of spontaneous angina[148].

In 1933 Hausner and Scherf described ST elevation during experimental ligation of the coronary artery in the dog[149]. They supported the concept that these changes had to be due to spasm since there was no change in heart rate or blood pressure to indicate an increase in myocardial metabolic requirements. Wilson and Johnston also supported this concept. In 1941 they described several cases of spontaneous angina in which there was also no change in heart rate or blood pressure. Their cases, however, did have characteristics of a variant type of angina that Prinzmetal was to describe in detail in 1959[141].

It seems to be the prevailing opinion that the substernal discomfort and transient electrocardiographic changes which occur in anginal paroxysms are dependent upon myocardial ischemia brought about by an increase in the work of the heart, rather than by a change in the caliber of the coronary arteries affected. When, as in Case 5, pronounced electrocardiographic changes of the kind produced by temporary occlusion of a large coronary artery appear, disappear, and reappear without any material increase in heart rate or in blood pressure, this view is clearly untenable. It must, we think, be admitted that in some instances anginal paroxysms are precipitated by contraction of the coronary arteries involved. Whether contraction of the larger coronary arteries takes place, or whether it is the caliber of the arterioles that changes, it is not possible to say. The character of the electrocardiographic changes suggests the change in arterial or arteriolar caliber is local, not general[141].

Prinzmetal and his associates carefully delineated the clinical features of this syndrome in 1959[150,151]. They stressed the transient electrocardiographic changes that simulated those of myocardial infarction. It was their belief that the entire syndrome was due to increased coronary artery tonus and that this occurred even in patients with fixed obstructive lesions. The concept that spasm could occur in rigid arteriosclerotic vessels was still not universally accepted. Prinzmetal went out of his way to avoid using the word spasm. For a while he called this syndrome angina pectoris inversa. He and his group finally decided to label it as a variant form of angina, a designation that became incorporated into the eponym 'Prinzmetal's variant angina'[151]. Proof that spasm could indeed occur, came in 1973 when Oliva and his associates demonstrated it during episodes of Prinzmetal's angina. Despite the evident arteriosclerotic lesions, coronary arteriography documented spasm as the underlying mechanism[152].

Two other men should be cited for demonstrating *in vivo* that spasm of the arteriosclerotic coronary arteries does occur during an anginal episode. They are G. Arnulf and G. Gensini. Both men were prime movers in the development of coronary arteriography (see Section 5). In 1959 Arnulf and then in 1962, Gensini visualized through arteriography actual spasm during an anginal paroxysm[153,154]. Arnulf reversed the spasm with intravenous administration of nicotinic acid and papaverine. Gensini relieved the spasm with sublingual isosorbide dinitrate. In the dog, Gensini was able to induce marked coronary vasoconstriction, with intracoronary injection of pitressin[154]. The angiographic demonstration of spasm by these two men assumes the dimensions of a remarkable feat when one recalls that they visualized the coronary arteries by flooding the aortic root during acetylcholine-induced cardiac arrest and with rather primitive radiographic equipment. Such was not the case in 1973, when Oliva demonstrated coronary spasm in Prinzmetal's angina. By this time Sone's method of selective coronary arteriography was well established and radiographic equipment had already undergone marked improvement[155]. In their well-documented case report consisting of five separate observations Oliva's group was able to subject the patient to coronary arteriography while simultaneously recording elevation of the ST segments.

Since 1973 the avalanche of angiographic studies relating to both variant and spontaneous angina was truly phenomenal. Attilio Maseri and his group at Pisa were probably the most daring if not the most productive. They documented in 1975 and 1978 that ST segment changes in either direction were due to coronary arterial spasm arising *de novo* or superimposed on fixed obstructive lesions[156,157]. Coronary vasomotion was now acknowledged to be an important component of the clinical spectrum of coronary artery disease. Maseri became the Sir John McMichael Professor of Cardiology at Hammersmith Hospital, and when he left Pisa he took along with him a sizeable number of assistants. While there, this group made a number of important contributions on silent ischemia, a newly appreciated component of the ever-expanding clinical spectrum of coronary artery disease. Also in 1977, Oliva and Breckenridge showed conclusively that at times spasm was an actually operative mechanism in precipitating an acute myocardial infarction[158].

Pharmacological provocation of coronary spasm was an experimental approach that also yielded fruitful observations. A clinical report appeared in 1929, written by M. Labbé and co-workers, that described the precipitation of angina pectoris following the administration of ergotamine[159]. We have already seen how Gensini in 1962 provoked marked constriction with the intracoronary injection of pitressin in the dog. In 1953, Stein and Weinstein described an 'unusual reaction to ergonovine maleate in coronary insufficiency'[160]. Their patient developed classical symptoms of angina with simultaneous elevation of the ST segments.

Although ergonovine provocation was entertained by several investigators during the 1950s it never did gain any degree of acceptance until Proudfit and his group began their studies in 1972. The work was done at the Cleveland clinic. The results were not reported until 1975. The paper bore the title, *The ergonovine maleate test for the diagnosis of coronary artery spasm*, with F. A. Huepler Jr as the leading author[161].

I was well aware that my good friend and colleague, Dr R. Charles Curry Jr, spent a great deal of time during his tenure at the University of Florida on ergonovine and coronary vasospasm. In view of this, I prevailed upon him to describe to me his experiences with ergonovine provocation. This he did in a delightfully anecdotal letter. I reproduce it with his permission and without editing, since it represents, as is, Charles' intellectual ability and his firm grasp of an important part of the pathophysiologic spectrum of coronary artery disease.

Dear Lou:

It is with great pleasure that I respond to your request to elaborate on the historic development of coronary vasospasm, particularly as it concerns the University of Florida and my involvement.

When first asked to elaborate on coronary vasospasm, we have to set the stage. Coronary vasospasm was first discussed as a mechanism of acute myocardial ischemia in the early 1970s. At that time, patients with acute myocardial infarction, with rest pain and ST segment elevation, were being hospitalized in the coronary care unit. They were treated with several days of bed rest, morphine, xylocaine for arrhythmias and, if necessary, hemodynamic monitoring while being treated for congestive heart failure. Patients were not invaded who had acute myocardial infarction and no thrombolytic agents were being given. In fact, the use of nitroglycerin and digoxin in the mid-1970s was controversial. There was a doctor working at the University of Colorado who published a paper about 1974 or 1975 who was bold enough to take 6 patients to the catheterization laboratory during the acute phase of myocardial infarction. I am sure I can come up with the name of that doctor, if necessary. The purpose of his study, as I recall, was to test the hypothesis as to whether or not patients with chest pain at rest and ST segment elevation may in fact have vasospasm of the coronary artery, leading to acute myocardial infarction. He found in this rather bold study, for the time, that two of six patients had some vasospasm as identified by significant change in a major epicardial coronary artery following challenge with either sublingual or intracoronary nitroglycerin. It was that study, along with several other studies, that led us to be much more aggressive in the evaluation and treatment of patients with coronary vasospasm. I would suggest to you that it was the search for the mechanism of acute ischemia, that is whether or not it was thrombosis or critical narrowing of the coronary artery, or vasospasm, which heralded the present era of thrombolysis and acute intervention for myocardial infarction. Prior to that time, things had evolved from the arm chair treatment of myocardial infarction to the coronary care unit to hemodynamic monitoring and, of course, recognition and treatment of cardiac arrhythmias and resuscitation.

The second major influence on our interest came from the work of Dr. Fred Huepler who published an abstract in the early 1970's from the Cleveland Clinic on a new provocative test using ergonovine to bring on coronary vasospasm and, thereby, producing an attack of chest pain at rest with ST segment elevation in a sub-group of patients with ischemic heart disease. Thus, the stage was set, at least for me, in 1975, when I first became interested in vasospastic angina, having a test for trying to identify patients with vasospasm as a mechanism. The next part of the puzzle was the patient.

I should mention that in the 1970s we always referred to the pathophysiology of myocardial ischemia as being analogous to a see saw with factors leading to myocardial demand on one side and factors having to do with supply on the other side. That was our concept and early in the 1970s coronary vasospasm was definitely not accepted as a mechanism for acute ischemic pain. It was felt to be related simply to increasing one's myocardial oxygen demand versus decreasing the supply with acute thrombosis or critical narrowing.

I should also mention that a number of names immediately come to mind outside the University of Florida when talking about the whole spectrum of investigators active in setting coronary vasospasm as a mechanism for ischemic pain. I have mentioned Dr. Fred Huepler at the Cleveland Clinic. We should mention Dr. Prinzmetal who originally described vasospastic angina in the 40s. It fell upon deaf ears for many years until it was rekindled in the 1970s. Dr. Attilio Maseri and his assistant, whom you know, were also probably the leading proponents of coronary vasospasm. Other investigators included Dr. John Schroeder at Stanford University, Dr. Rex McAlpin at the University of California at Los Angeles, Dr. Michele Bertrand, at Lile, France, Dr. Robert Cachine who was working out of the University of Texas in Houston at that time, along with Dr. Raznier who still remains at the University of Texas. Dr.

David Waters and Dr. Henry Mascalo at Montreal Heart Institute were also active in the field. Dr. Spencer King even had an early paper on coronary vasospasm and with whom we communicated early in our experience when we had a particular drug called perhexiline. Dr. David Hilis, along with Dr. Eugene Braunwald, published one of the landmark articles in the New England Journal of Medicine which established them as the investigators with significant interest and expertise in coronary vasospasm. At the University of Florida, I was the first to develop an interest in vasospastic angina, but the work was in collaboration with Drs. Conti, Pepine, and Robert Vellman.

As mentioned above, the availability of a test for coronary vasospasm, along with a budding interest in being more invasive in patients with acute myocardial ischemia, a willing patient, plus perhaps a prepared mind, led to our interest at the University of Florida which now has spanned some 17 years of experience up to date.

In 1975, I was an assistant professor at the University of Florida and was, as I recall, on the coronary care unit rotation. We received a patient from Tampa by helicopter. The patient had had a near syncopal episode. He was said to have chest discomfort which occurred at rest and had episodes of tachyarrhythmia. Once he arrived at the Veterans' Administration Hospital in Gainesville, he was pain-free. There was no evidence of myocardial infarction. On rounds we talked about the patient, especially in regard to the diagnosis. As I recall, he underwent cardiac catheterization and had evidence of mild coronary artery disease, particularly in the anterior descending branch and in the right coronary arteries. He was a cigarette smoker and was on no anti-anginal treatment at that time. Thus, we had a clinical problem in that we had a gentleman who had evidence of ischemia from his clinical history, but with a normal electrocardiogram and catheterization data showing mild coronary artery disease. Did he have ischemic heart disease or not? I felt that giving him ergonovine would be important to see if this man with chest pain at rest and perhaps an ischemia-related arrhythmia would in fact be provoked by this agent.

The first ergonovine test was performed in the coronary care unit while the patient was undergoing electrocardiographic monitoring. Ergonovine 0.2 mg was administered. Within 1-½ to 2 minutes he developed profound ST segment elevation followed by ventricular tachycardia and ventricular flutter. He was administered sublingual nitroglycerin and given also an intravenous bolus of lidocaine followed by a maintenance drip. His blood pressure dropped and he became transiently unresponsive, only to regain full consciousness in less than a minute. Needless to say, we were mortified at the events that we had created. I felt that we had almost done Mr. 'C' in. He had the most profound electrocardiographic changes that I had ever seen up until that time in a gentleman with mild coronary artery disease and no evidence of exertional chest discomfort. When asked after the stress study, how this attack compared to other attacks, Mr. 'C' told me that this was a relatively mild attack. He had had repeated episodes similar to this one which had occurred out of the hospital, many of which had led to syncope. He had previously been a truck driver and had had an accident at one time. I don't believe he was having black out spells at that time, although one never knows.

Next, I showed the electrocardiograms to Drs. Conti and Pepine who were also rather surprised at the profound changes brought about by the ergonovine. We wondered how many of our patients that were being seen for other reasons may have had, in fact, coronary vasospasm as an etiologic mechanism for their chest pain. I should mention that this was an important question because there was just beginning to arrive on the clinical horizon new classes of drugs called calcium channel blockers which were felt to possibly be specific for coronary vasospasm. Thus, it was a combination of many things which happened to fall into place at the right time, including a method of provoking spasm, a sincere interest based on the profound changes in one patient, as well as the hope for specific treatment for this problem.

I next embarked upon a project where virtually any patient who came in to our cardiology clinic or to the cath laboratory, who had a history of chest pain, received ergonovine. As I recall, we did 300–400 intravenous ergonovine studies, looking for people who might have a response similar to that of Mr. 'C'.

These studies were performed in the stress test lab, in the coronary care unit, or in the catheterization laboratory. We developed a protocol of dose titration where depending upon our clinical suspicion of the presence of vasospastic angina, we would give initially 0.05 mg of ergonovine followed by a 2nd 0.05 mg dose, then followed by 0.1 mg; all usually over a 5–10 minute period while the electrocardiogram, blood pressure and symptoms were monitored. In a patient in whom there was a low index of suspicion, we would give the entire 0.2 mg of ergonovine and make our observations over a period of 5 minutes. At the end of each examination, we would give 0.4 mg sublingual nitroglycerin. Care was taken before each study to make sure that the patient had not received any long acting medications that might interfere with the study. Our findings, which we reported subsequently, indicated that, in a random group of veterans being treated for ischemic heart disease, less than 10% developed chest pain and ST segment elevation.

The next step was to take the patients to the catheterization laboratory where, after the completion of the routine diagnostic study, the patients would again receive ergonovine using the same criteria as outlined. We again found and selected patients with a history of rest pain and associated ST segment elevation capable of being reversed with sublingual nitroglycerin. At that time, we were not administering intracoronary drugs of any type. Although some responses were dramatic, for example, with ST elevation in the anterior precordial leads accompanied by hypotension and marked ischemia, sublingual nitroglycerin 0.4 mg would in each case relieve the symptoms within 30 seconds to a minute and a half. Again, it was sometimes hairy because of the profound changes which we would observe. However, we felt justified in doing this because in essence, we were provoking the same symptoms which the patients (like Mr. 'C') had when they were not under medical observation. This is no different from the patient who had stress induced angina on the basis of a treadmill exercise study.

We next wanted to compare the results of ergonovine provoked coronary vasospasm as it might compare with spontaneously induced coronary vasospasm and ischemia. It was Dr.

Pepine's idea that the patients not be given any pre-medication, such as nitroglycerin or atropine, so that if in fact the patient had chest discomfort, we would immediately inject both right and left coronary arteries before giving nitroglycerin. By performing cardiac catheterization in this fashion, we were able to make observations on a number of patients with chest pain at rest, which occurred spontaneously during the stress of cardiac catheterization and later on after that episode was relieved, usually with either a tensor of time or carotid massage. We would then challenge the patient with ergonovine. Then, those responders gave us a cohort of patients in whom we had an opportunity to observe, both spontaneous and ergonovine induced coronary vasospastic attacks. This was a subject of one of our reports. What we found was that the spontaneous attacks in regard to the electrocardiographic leads, ST segment changes, the coronary artery involved, as well as the actual morphologic changes in the coronary arteries were extremely similar. Thus, in my mind, this clinched the ergonovine stress study as being a very valid study for trying to determine who had vasospastic angina.

Next, calcium channel blockers were just being evaluated experimentally. One of the questions that we had was whether or not patients who were receiving calcium channel blockers with vasospastic angina could be provoked again. Those patients taking calcium channel blockers were again challenged with our standard ergonovine protocol and we found a variable response. Some seemed to be inducible, some were not, and I was never able to fully understand the meaning of this, except that calcium channel blockers clearly were not a cure-all. There was clinical evidence of breakthrough attacks, so that the treatment with calcium channel blockers was not an all-or-none phenomenon. This could be verified, either based on their clinical response or based on their response to ergonovine stress testing.

Another question had to do with the mechanism of vasospasm. It was extremely rare to find a patient without coronary artery disease who had vasospasm, although there were a few. This may have had to do with our population being mostly veterans who have a high incidence of ischemic heart disease to begin with.

However, at the University hospital, we did have some ladies with the problem. We were never able to figure out the exact mechanism. We were able to identify a group of patients who had rather profound diffuse coronary constriction, but without ST segment changes, in whom we were able to reproduce their pain. We took this one step further with our gastroenterology colleagues and found a high percentage of esophageal spasm which we could provoke in patients with normal coronary arteries with chest pain without ST segment changes following the challenge of ergonovine. This was the subject of another communication.

Finally, I think to understand some of the mysteries of vasospastic angina, we have to go back to Mr. 'C'. His problem remained an enigma to multiple doctors who saw him and treated him until his premature death in the early 1980s. His autopsy, along with several other patients, was the subject of another communication. Because Mr. 'C' lived out of our immediate Ketchman area at the VA Hospital in Gainesville, he frequently would have attacks that would cause him to wind up in an emergency room or in the intensive care unit. Perhaps he would be cathed. At least one time at the VA Hospital in Tampa he received a permanent pacemaker thinking that his problem was in fact transient Stokes-Adams attacks because his black outs were such a prominent feature of his illness. No doubt these were due to the vasospasm of the left anterior descending artery bringing on profound left ventricular ischemia and the documented ischemia-induced ventricular arrhythmia. I had explained to him on multiple occasions that, in fact, his problem was vasospasm, but other doctors just didn't quite understand that problem. In fact, even in death at the VA Hospital in Tampa, an autopsy was performed with detailed sectioning of the coronary arteries, thinking that his problem was severe coronary atherosclerosis which incidentally was not found. I presume that he died as a result of one of his attacks of vasospasm. He did have evidence of progressive atherosclerosis, but it was not critical and he never had bypass surgery. I was very moved by his family who, after his death, requested that I receive the heart from the autopsy to perform further studies in hopes that it would help other people. Clearly Mr. 'C', both during his lifetime and after death, had made a profound effect on myself as well as on our institution in showing us that coronary vasospasm was a mechanism of myocardial ischemia which had not before that time been appreciated. I should mention that although he was improved with various agents, he was never totally relieved of his attacks. They would follow a cyclic pattern and he would have months without any attacks and then have one or two. Calcium channel blockers were clearly life-saving for him, but I do not recall exactly the circumstances around his fatal illness, although I do think that he was not on calcium channel blockers.

I hope this will be of help to you. I must admit I rather enjoyed going over the stories again and remembering a lot of the feelings which we all had during the period between 1974 and 1979, as this important segment of patients with ischemic cardiac pain were further elucidated, better understood, and the mechanism of coronary vasospasm became established.
Sincerely,
R. Charles Curry, Jr., M.D.

Exercise tests in the diagnosis of coronary artery disease did not come into being until the 1940s. The response of humans to exercise, though, was not a newly introduced approach. It had already been a subject for investigation for millennia. Endurance capability was the initial objective because of the need for fast long-distance runners in the transmission of messages. Physiological interest in exercise did not begin, however, until the end of the 19th century. At this time, heart rate and respiratory activity were the main parameters evaluated. The introduction of technological methods for measuring respiratory gas exchange and the increasing use of the electrocardiogram were the main reasons for an acceleration of interest in the field. The main spurt of research with increasing attention towards the effects on the heart occurred between 1930 and 1960[162,163].

The term 'physiologic hypertrophy' entered the literature but was soon replaced by 'athlete's heart'. For a while the increase in heart muscle mass was cloaked in the mythical belief that it created a better pump. There was not a shred of scientific data to support this view. Wyatt and Mitchell, and later Stone found that exercise not only increased ventricular mass but also resulted in an increase in the end-diastolic volume[164,165].

Froelicher in 1977 presented anecdotal evidence that one of the benefits of exercise training was an increase in the size of the coronary vascular bed[166]. The logical implication was that this would result in an increase in coronary reserve capacity and a reduction in coronary blood flow at any cardiac workload. Restorff also suggested that myocardial oxygen consumption was less in the trained state than in the untrained state[167]. The physiologic basis for this was outlined by Stone[168]. He showed that oxygen consumption was reduced because of alterations in heart rate, myocardial wall tension, and the contractile state of the myocardium. Stone also demonstrated that exercise training alters the structural components or size of the coronary resistance vessels while bringing about an increase in the coronary collateral blood flow and an alteration in the neural control of the coronary vascular bed. These advances in exercise physiology formed the basis for the exercise component of the cardiac rehabilitation and prevention programs that sprang up during the 1970s and 1980s.

It is quite probable that Einthoven himself may have been the first to have recorded an exercise electrocardiogram. He reproduced in 1908 two tracings, one with the patient at rest and the other after the patient ran up a flight of stairs. The only difference between the two was an increase in heart rate. No abnormalities were noted[169].

Nothing further was reported until the 1930s when there was a reactivation of interest in exercise as a means of testing the functional status of the heart. By this time the electrocardiogram had become a fairly well-established clinical tool and it seemed appropriate to determine if it could be used as a parameter.

In America three Philadelphian physicians were the first to suggest the recording of a postexercise electrocardiogram as a means of determining whether chest pain was cardiac or non-cardiac in origin. They were Francis Wood, Mary Livesey, and Charles Wolferth[170]. They stressed that the procedure should be done only in the face of an uncertain diagnosis since it was potentially dangerous. Four years later Scherf began his work on exercise electrocardiography. He did not concern himself with any standardized protocol. His approach was a purely individualistic one insisting only that the patient repeat the effect that brought on his pain[171]. This, of course, left much to be desired since effort angina can be precipitated by a wide range of physical activity, both in degree and type. Investigations were also carried out by L. Katz and H. Landt, and M. Missal[172,173]. They used a standardized protocol.

For the most part, though, clinical application of these investigations became a rather haphazard affair. Varying exercise protocols were used without regard to age, sex, height and weight. The variety of effort was limited only by the doctor's imagination. Thus, some would be told to hop, use dumbbells, do pushups, stoop, raise their hands above the head up and down, and countless other maneuvers. Master and his colleague, Oppenheimer, the English physiologist, thought that this was chaos personified, and felt that, at the least, the exercise should be standardized according to age, sex, weight and height. After much discussion of permutations and various combinations, they decided on two steps, each 9 inches high, with the walks up and down performed in exactly 1.5 minutes. The time was later changed to 3 minutes because this longer interval gave more precise results. Blood pressure and pulse rate were recorded (see Figure 7). A table of trips was then constructed for them by a member of the mathematics department at Columbia University. The final table was constructed so that it correlated the number of trips performed within 3 minutes with the patient's age, sex and weight. It was found that the height of the patient was irrelevant and it therefore was not included in the final module. Cardiac efficiency was measured in foot-pounds per minute. Foot-pounds were derived by multiplying the number of trips performed by the patients' weight. In the late 1930s they began using the electrocardiogram since it was more stable and did not vary with emotion or excitement[174]. In the 1940s Master began recording the electrocardiogram during the exercise itself[175,176]. He found this to be very important in detecting arrhythmias. At first, ST segment changes were interpreted with such vague expressions as 'possibly innocuous', 'possibly abnormal' or 'definitely abnormal'. In 1958, Paul Wood of London clarified the interpretation by describing the ischemic depression of the ST segment[177].

Master was convinced of the infallibility of the two-step test. He thought it was a sure way of uncovering latent coronary artery disease. Baye's theorem had yet to be formulated. He was also

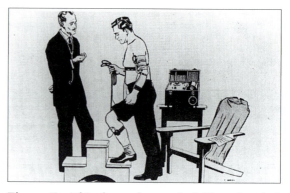

Figure 7   This shows the standard '2-step' each 9 inches high and an electrocardiograph machine with 'instomatic' action. Also shown are an Adirondack chair with wide arms (as made in the mountains of that name), technician or physician with stop watch in hand, person to be tested with electrodes strapped on and blood pressure cuff and gauge bound around arm. *Photo Source National Library of Medicine. Literary Source Master, A.M. Reminiscences of fifty years in cardiology at Mount Sinai with special reference to the two-step test. Mount Sinai Journal of Medicine, vol.39, Sept.–Oct., 1972. With permission*

strongly opposed to the more strenuous types of exercise tests currently in vogue, feeling that the two-step test was adequate and not inherently dangerous as was the more strenuous one.

In time exercise physiologists from around the globe became interested in the matter and developed treadmill or bicycle stress testing to bring out the disparity between blood supply and demand for a given level of exercise. Numerous protocols were introduced, each one known by the name of its formulator, but all designed to provide a graded stress with time for physiologic equilibration within particular stages. In time the exercise protocols became incorporated into the nuclear imaging diagnostic techniques (see Section 5). Besides serving in a diagnostic capacity these graded tests also became useful as a means of formulating an exercise prescription for each patient.

The therapy of angina pectoris has had a rather speckled history. It is characterized by surgical and pharmacological approaches with the details of each approach dependent upon the prevailing view regarding its etiology.

Prussic acid was the earliest therapeutic agent specifically utilized for relief of angina pectoris. Two men in particular reported their experience with this product in separate and independent case reports. They were Elliotson in 1829 and Schlessier of Pietz in 1841[178,179]. T. P. Teale, a contemporary of Elliotson, believed in the neural origin of angina, and for this reason resorted to topical applications to the cervical and dorsal vertebrae[180]. Angina as a form of neuralgia was a widely prevailing notion throughout Europe for a good part of the first half of the 19th century. Duchenne also shared Teale's view but he suggested electrical stimulation over the chest during an anginal paroxysm[181,182]. This form of therapy was quite popular in France for all types of neuralgia. Even Laénnec considered it appropriate for angina.

The historical background of nitrite and nitroglycerine therapy is presented in Section 6. Despite the well-known relief that these agents provided, an occasional practitioner still favored his own remedy. As late as 1924 L. F. Bishop and L. T. Thorne reported their experience with these alternative methods. Bishop was convinced that the pain in angina originated in the myocardium, that it was transmitted through the sympathetic system, and that it was influenced by gastrointestinal factors[183]. His castor oil therapy was based on this premise stating that 'no matter how severe a condition of chronic anginal pain may be, one can often count up to 24 hours of increased comfort following a dose of castor oil'[183]. Thorne took a balneological approach, claiming that he was able to effect a 'cure' with one or more courses of Nauheim baths[184]. He believed that the cutaneous vasodilatation induced by the baths brought relief with the concomitant drop in blood pressure and reversal of spasm in the remaining vessels.

Induced hypothyroidism was a popular remedy between 1935 and 1955. Its alleged beneficial effects were ascribed by some to a decreased work load on the heart as a result of the decrease in metabolic activity. Others entertained the notion that lack of thyroid hormone decreased the sensitivity of the myocardium to the hypoxic effects of epinephrine. Blumgart, Freedberg and Kurland collected the largest series of patients treated in this manner, reporting their results in 1950[185]. They claimed that 75% of their total of 720 patients demonstrated significant improvement. This is rather strange in view of the marked hyper-cholesterolemia associated with the hypothyroid state. They were well aware, however, that the therapy was purely a palliative one. Raab reported his experience in 1945, 10 years after Blumgart's original paper on this form of therapy[186,187]. He had abandoned X-ray treatment of the adrenal glands in favor of thiouracil ablation of thyroid function[188]. The secondary elevation of blood cholesterol in hypothyroidism did suggest to Raab an unfavorable impact on coronary artery sclerosis, a remarkable bit of insight at a time when our knowledge concerning the relationship of cholesterol to arteriosclerosis was still in its formative stages.

The first half of the 20th century also saw the introduction and rapid demise of a host of pharmacological approaches, many of which had neither rhyme nor reason or were based on ill-conceived pharmacological principles. Each one had its day in the limelight only to be replaced by another agent with credentials just as dubious. Among them were insulin, glucose, pancreatic extract, theophylline calcium salicylate, cobra venom, papaverine, theophylline aminoisobutanol, testosterone propionate, alcohol and visammin (khellin). The length of this list above is a testament to their lack of efficacy[189–200].

Fortunately, by the mid 20th century, a more rational approach was initiated. The efficacy of existing drugs as well as newer ones were now subjected to careful evaluation by means of objective measurements, and controlled double-blind studies[201–203]. The electrocardiogram became an increasingly important tool, especially in determining the prevention or reversal of ischemic changes as manifested through deviations in the ST segments. Riseman studied patients over a 15 year period evaluating almost 100 drugs[202]. This was, indeed, an outstanding contribution. Antimalarials, sedatives, purines and nitrites were but a few of the many categories of pharmaceutical agents subjected to evaluation. Nitrites emerged by far as the most effective.

Russek, Zohman and Dorset evaluated drugs that were specially designed to dilate the coronary arteries[203]. This was in 1955. They used as an objective parameter for efficacy the ability to modify the electrocardiographic response to graded levels of exercise. This protocol is still in use today for the clinical trials of each newly introduced agent.

The historical background of the surgical procedures as well as the more recently developed interventional techniques may be found in Section 6. In the final analysis, all these approaches, whether surgical or pharmacological, are purely palliative in nature. The cure for angina pectoris will be realized only when we find the means to prevent or delay the development of arteriosclerosis for this is the major cause of it all.

REFERENCES

1. Ruffer, M.A. (1911). On arterial lesions found in Egyptian mummies (1580 BC–AD 525). *J. Path. Bact.*, **15**, 453

2. Bing, R.J. (1982). Coronary circulation and cardiac metabolism. In Fishman, A.P. and Richards, D.W. (eds.) *Circulation of the Blood, Men and Ideas*, p. 202. (Baltimore, Md.: Waverly Press, Inc.)

3. Aristotle (1874–89). *Opera omnia. Graece et Latine, cum indice nominum et rerum absolutissimo.* (Paris: Firmin-Didot)

4. Dalton, J.C. (1884). *Doctrines of the Circulation; A History of Physiological Opinion and Discovery, in Regard to the Circulation of the Blood.* (Philadelphia: Lea)

5. Singer, C. (1925). The Fasciculo de Medicina, Venice, 1493. In Sigerist, H.E. (ed.) *Monumenta Medica*, vol. II. (Florence: Lier)

6. Vesalius, A. and Kalkar, J.S. (1538). *Tabulae anatomicae.* (Venice: D. Bernardi)

7. Heseler, B. (1959). *Andreas Vesalius' First Public Anatomy at Bologna, 1540; an Eyewitness Report.* Tr. by R. Ericksson. (Upsala: Almqvist & Wiksells)

8. Riolan, J. (1648). *Encheiridium anatomicum et pathologicum.* (Paris: Meturas)

9. Lower R. (1932). De corde. In Gunther, R.T. *Early Science in Oxford*, v. IX. Tr. by K.J. Franklin. (Oxford)

10. Hudson, C.L., Moritz, A.R. and Wearn, J.T. (1932). *J. Exp. Med.*, **56**, 19

11. Vieussens, R. (1715). *Traité Nouveau de la Structure et des Causes du Mouvement Naturel du Coeur.* (Toulouse)

12. Thebesius, A.C. (1716). *De Circulo Sanguinis in Corde.* Leyden. Revised edition

13. von Haller, A. (1786). *First Lines of Physiology*, **1**, 75, tr. from the Correct Latin Edition. (Edinburgh: Elliot)

14. Abernethy, J. (1798). Observations on the foramina Thebesü of the heart. *Phil. Trans.*, p. 103

15. Langer, L.J. (1880). Die Foramina Thebesii im Herzen des Menschen. S.B. Ahad. Wiss., Wien. *Math-Naturw. Kl.*, 3. Abt., **82**, 25

16. Pratt, F.H. (1898). The nutrition of the heart through the vessels of Thebesius and the coronary veins. *Am. J. Physiol.*, **1**, 86

17. Wearn, J.T. (1928). The role of the Thebesian vessels in the circulation of the heart. *J. Exp. Med.*, **47**, 293

18. Wearn, J.T., Mettier, S.R., Klumpp, T.G. and Zschiesche, L.J. (1933). *Am. Heart J.*, **9**, 143

19. Bedford, D.E. (1968). Harvey's Third Circulation. De Circulo Sanguinis in Corde. *Br. Med. J.*, **4**, 273–7

20. Schlesinger, M.J., Zoll, P.M. and Wessler, S. (1949). *Am. Heart J.*, **38**, 823

21. Gensini, G.G., Bounanno, C. and Palacio, A. (1967). *Dis. Chest*, **52**, 125

22. Chirac, P. (1698). *De motu cordis adversaria analytica.* (Montspelü: Martel)

23. Harvey, W. (1928). *Exercitatio anatomica de motu cordis et sanguinis in animalibus.* Tr. by C.D. Leake. (Springfield, Ill.: Thomas)

24. Morgagni, G.B. (1761). *De sedibus et causus morborum per anatomen indagatis.* (Venice: Ex Typographia Remondiniana)

25. Quain, R. (1850). On fatty diseases of the heart. *Med. Chir. Trans.*, **33**, 120

26. *Ibid*

27. Fye, W.B. (1985). The delayed diagnosis of myocardial infarction: it took half a century. *Circulation*, **72**, 262–71

28. Rindfleisch, E. (1872). *A Manual of Pathological Histology to Serve as an Introduction to the Study of Morbid Anatomy* (trans. by E.B. Baxter). (London: New Sydenham Society)

29. Flint, A. (1870). *A Practical Treatise on the Diagnosis, Pathology and Treatment of Diseases of the Heart*, 2nd edn. (Philadelphia: Henry C. Lea)

30. Hall, M. (1842). On the mutual relations between anatomy, physiology, pathology, and therapeutics, and the practice of medicine. *The Gulstonian Lectures for 1842.* (London: Baillière)

31. Erichsen, J.E. (1842). On the influence of the coronary circulation on the action of the heart. *Med. Gazette*, n.s. **30**, 561

32. *Ibid.*

33. Williams, C.J.B. (1840). *Pathology and Diagnoses of Diseases of the Chest*, 4th edn. (London: Churchill)

34. Panum, P.L. (1862). Experimentelle Beiträge zur Lehre von der Emboli. *Virchows Arch. Path. Anat.*, **25**, 308

35. von Bezold, A. and Breyman, E. (1867). Veränderungen des Herzschlages nach dem Verschlusse der Coronarnerven. Untersuch-

ungen physiol. *Lab. Würzburg. I. Heft*, **288**

36. Weigert, C. (1880). Ueber die Pathologischen Gerinnungsvorgänge. *Arch. Path. Anat. (Virchow)*, **79**, 87

37. Conheim, J. and von Schultheiss-Rechberg, A. (1881). Ueber die Folgen der Kranzarterien-verschliessung für das Herz. *Virchows Arch. Path. Anat.*, **85**, 503

38. Conheim, J. (1889). *Lectures on General Pathology*, 2nd edn., (trans. from the German by A.B. McKee). (London: New Sydenham Society)

39. Ziegler, E. (1881). *Lehrbuch der allgemeinen und speciellen pathologischen Anatomie für Arzte*. (Jena: Fischer)

40. *Ibid.*

41. Hyrtl, J. (1873). *Die Corrosions-Anatomie und ihrer Ergebnisse*. (Vienna)

42. Pratt, F.H. (1898). *Op. cit.*

43. Steven, J.L. (1887). Lectures on fibroid degeneration and allied lesions of the heart, and their association with diseases of the coronary arteries. *Lancet*, **2**, 1153

44. Leyden, E. (1884). Ueber die Sclerose der Coronar-Arterien und die davon Abhängigen Krankheitszustände. *Z. Klin. Med.*, **7**, 459

45. Hammer, A. (1878). Thrombosis of one of the coronary arteries of the heart diagnosed during life (trans. by J. Workman). *Can. J. Med. Sci.*, **3**, 353

46. Porter to Baumgarten (1892). *Baumgarten Papers*

47. Porter to Baumgarten (1890). *Baumgarten Papers*

48. Porter, W.T. (1893). On the results of ligation of the coronary arteries. *J. Physiol.*, **15**, 121

49. Fye, W.B. (1985). Acute coronary occlusion always results in death-or does it? The observations of William T. Porter. *Circulation*, **71**, 4–10

50. Porter, W.T. (1893). Über die Frage eines Coordinations centrum im Herzventrikel. *Arch. Ges. Physiol. (Bonn)*, **55**, 366

51. Porter, W.T. (1896). Further researches on the closure of the coronary arteries. *J. Exp. Med.*, **1**, 46

52. Gross, L. (1921). *The Blood Supply to the Heart; in Its Anatomical and Clinical Aspects*. (New York: Hoeber)

53. Spalteholz, K.W. (1924). *Die Arterien der Herwand*. (Leipzig)

54. Blumgart, H.L, Levine, S.A. and Berlin, D.D. (1933). *Arch. Int. Med.*, **51**, 866

55. James, T.N. (1961). *The Anatomy of the Coronary Arteries*. (New York)

56. Fulton, W.F.M. (1965). *The Coronary Arteries*. (Springfield, Ill.)

57. Blumgart, H.L., Zoll, P.M., Freedberg, A.S. and Gilligan, D.R. (1950). The experimental production of intercoronary arterial anastomoses and their functional significance. *Circulation*, **1**, 10

58. Wood, P. (1968). *Diseases of the Heart and Circulation*, 3rd edn. (London)

59. Rebatel, F. (1872). *Recerches expérimentales sur la circulation dans les artères coronaires*, Thése no. 288. (Paris)

60. Martin, N.H. and Sedgwick, W.J. (1882). Observations on the mean pressure and the characters of the pulse-wave in the coronary arteries of the heart. *J. Physiol. (London)*, **3**, 165

61. Morawitz, P. and Zahn, A. (1914). Untersuchungen über den Coronarkreislauf. *Dtsch. Arch. Klin. Med.*, **116**, 364

62. Anrep, G.V. (1926). *Physiol. Rev.*, **6**, 596

63. Bing, R.J., Hammond, M.M., Handelsman, J.C. *et al.* (1949). The measurement of coronary blood flow, oxygen consumption and efficiency of the left ventricle in man. *Am. Heart J.*, **38**, 1

64. Proudfit, W.L. (1983). Origin of concept of ischaemic heart disease. *Br. Heart J.*, **50**, 209–12

65. (1759). *Earl of Clarendon, his life. Case of Henry Hyde, 1632*, p. 9. (Oxford)

66. Morgagni, J.B. (1761). *Op. cit.*, p. 282

67. Rougnon de Magny, N.F. (1768). Lettre Æ M. Lorry, touchant les causes de la mort de feu Monsieur Charles, ancien capitaine de cavalerie, arrivée Æ Besançon le 23 février, 55 pp.

68. Heberden, W. (1772). Some account of a disorder of the breast. *Medical Transactions*, **2**, 59–67. (London: Royal College of Physicians)

69. Heberden, W. (1802). *Commentaries on the History and Cure of Diseases*. (London)

70. Anonymous (1772). *Medical Transactions, Critical Review*, **II**, 203–4

71. Kligfield, P. (1981). The frustated benevolence of 'Dr. Anonymous'. *Am. J. Cardiol.*, **47**, 185–7

72. Elliott, J. (1913). A medical pioneer. John Haygarth of Chester. *Br. Med. J.*, **i**, 235–42

73. Proudfit, L. (1983). *Op. cit.*, p. 209

74. Heberden, W. (1785). A letter to Dr. Heberden, concerning the angina pectoris; and Dr. Heberden's account of the dissection of one, who had been troubled with that disorder. *Medical Transactions*, **III**, 1–11. (London: Royal College of Physicians)

75. Fothergill, J. (1776). Case of an angina pectoris, with remarks. *Medical Observations and Inquiries*

by a Society of Physicians in London, **5**, 233–51

76. Fothergill, J. (1776). Farther account of the angina pectoris. *Medical Observations and Inquiries by a Society of Physicians in London*, **5**, 252–8

77. Fothergill, J. (1782). *A Complete Collection of the Medical and Philosophical Works, with … Life and … Notes*, ed. by Elliot, J. (London: Robinson)

78. Proudfit, L. (1983). *Op. cit.*, p. 209

79. Lindgren, K.M. (1979). Dr. John Wall: a profile in porcelain, painting and pectoral pain. *J.A.M.A.*, **242**, 1053–5

80. Johnstone, J. (1787). Case of angina pectoris, from an unexpected disease in the heart. *Memoirs of the Medical Society of London*, **1**, 376–88

81. Records of the University of Edinburgh Medical School

82. Records of the Royal College of Physicians of Ireland

83. Black, S. (1819). *Clinical and Pathological Reports.* (Newry: Alexander Wilkinson)

84. Black, S. (1795). Case of angina pectoris, with remarks. *Memoirs of the Medical Society of London*, **4**, 261–79

85. Black, S. (1805). A case of angina pectoris, with a dissection. *Memoirs of the Medical Society of London*, **6**, 41–9

86. Parry, C.H. (1799). *An Inquiry into the Symptoms and Causes of the Syncope Anginosa, Commonly Called Angina Pectoris.* (Bath: R. Crutwell)

87. Baron, J. (1838). *The Life of Edward Jenner, MD.* (London: Henry Colburn)

88. Hunter, J. (1794). *A Treatise on the Blood, Inflammation and Gun-shot Wounds*, to which is prefixed a short account of the author's life, by his brother-in-law, Everard Home. (London: Richardson)

89. Proudfit, L. (1983). *Op. cit.* p. 209

90. Burns, A. (1809). *Observations on some of the most frequent and important diseases of the heart*, **136**. (Edinburgh: Thomas Bryce)

91. Fye, W.B. (1985). The delayed diagnosis of myocardial infarction. It took half a century! *Circulation*, **72**, 262–71

92. Infarction of the Heart (1899). *J. Am. Med. Assoc.*, **33**, 919

93. Hektoen, L. (1892). Embolism of the left coronary artery; sudden death. *Med. News*, **61**, 210

94. Osler, W. (1889). Rupture of the heart. (This unsigned editorial is attributed to Osler by his bibliographer Maude Abbott). *Med. News*,

54, 129

95. Osler, W. (1897). *Lectures on Angina Pectoris and Allied States.* (New York: D. Appleton & Co.)

96. Osler, W. (1892). *The Principles and Practice of Medicine.* (New York: D. Appleton & Co.)

97. Dock, G. (1896). Notes on the Coronary Arteries. (Ann Arbor, Michigan: Inland Press)

98. Welch, W. (1889). Diseases of the coronary arteries and alterations in the muscular walls of the heart. *Proc. Trans. Pathol. Soc. Toronto*, **1**, 8

99. Herrick, J.B. (1912). Certain clinical features of sudden obstruction of the coronary arteries. *Trans. Assoc. Am. Phys.*, **27**, 100

100. Ross, R.S. (1983). A parlous state of storm and stress. The life and times of James B. Herrick. *Circulation*, **67**, 955–9

101. Means, J.H. (1961). *The Association of American Physicians. Its First Seventy-five Years*, p. 108. (New York: McGraw-Hill)

102. Krikler, D.M. (1987). The search for Samojloff: a Russian physiologist in times of change. *Br. Med. J.*, **295**, 1624–7

103. Obrastzow, W.P. and Straschesko, N.D. (1910). Zur Kenntnis der Thrombose der Koronarterien des Herzens. *Zeitschrift für Klinische Medizin.*, **71**, 116–32

104. Howell, J.D. (1984). Early perceptions of the electrocardiogram from arrhythmias to infarction. *Bull. Hist. Med.*, **58**, 183–98

105. Smith, F.M. (1918). The ligation of coronary arteries with electrocardiographic study. *Arch. Int. Med.*, **22**, 8–27

106. Herrick, J.B. (1949). *Memoires of Eighty Years.* (Chicago: Univ. of Chicago Press)

107. *Ibid.* p. 84.

108. Friedberg, C.K. and Horn, H. (1939). Acute myocardial infarction not due to coronary artery occlusion. *J. Am. Med. Assoc.*, **112**, 1675–9

109. Blumgart, H.L., Schlesinger, M.J. and Davis, D. (1940). Studies on the relation of the clinical manifestations of angina pectoris, coronary thrombosis, and myocardial infarction to the pathologic findings. *Am. Heart J.*, **19**, 1–91

110. Blumgart, H.L., Schlesinger, J.M. and Zoll, P.M. (1941). Angina pectoris, coronary failure and acute myocardial infarction. *J. Am. Med. Assoc.*, **116**, 91–6

111. Blumgart, H.L., Zoll, P.M. and Wessler, S. (1950). Angina pectoris. Clinical pathologic study of 177 cases. *Trans. Assoc. Am. Physicians*, **63**, 262–7

112. Miller, R.D., Burchell, H.B. and Edwards, J.E.

(1951). Myocardial infarction with and without acute coronary occlusion. *Arch. Intern. Med.*, **88**, 597–604

113. Branwood, A.W. and Montgomery, G.L. (1956). Observations on the morbid anatomy of coronary artery disease. *Scott. Med. J.*, **1**, 367–75

114. Chapman I. (1968). Relationships of recent coronary artery occlusion and acute myocardial infarction. *J. Mt. Sinai Hosp.*, **35**, 149–54

115. Harland, W.A. (1969). The pathogenesis of myocardial infarct and coronary thrombosis. In Sherry, S., Brinkhous, K.M., Genton, E. *et al.* (eds.) *Thrombosis* pp. 126–31. (Washington DC: National Academy of Sciences)

116. Sinapius, D. (1972). Beziehungen zwischen Koronarthrombosen und Myokardinfarkten. *Dtsch. Med. Wochenschr.*, **97**, 443–8

117. Roberts, W.C. and Buja, L.M. (1972). The frequency and significance of coronary arterial thrombi and other observations in fatal acute myocardial infarction. *Am. J. Med.*, **52**, 425–43

118. Spain, D.M. and Bradess, V.A. (1960). Relationship of coronary thrombosis to coronary atherosclerosis and ischemic heart disease. A necropsy study covering a period of 25 years. *Am. J. Med. Sci.*, **240**, 701–10

119. Ehrlich, J.C. and Shinohara, Y. (1964). Low incidence of coronary thrombosis in myocardial infarction. A restudy by serial block technique. *Arch. Path. (Chicago)*, **78**, 432–45

120. Meadows, R. (1965). Coronary thrombosis and myocardial infarction. *Med. J. Aust.*, **2**, 409–11

121. Hackel, D.B., Estes, E.H., Walston, A., Koff, S. and Day, E. (1969). Some problems concerning coronary artery occlusion and acute myocardial infarction. *Circulation* **39** and **40**, (suppl. IV), IV-31ùIV-35

122. Walston, A., Hackel, D.B. and Estes, E.H. (1970). Acute coronary occlusion and the 'power failure' syndrome. *Am. Heart J.*, **79**, 613–19

123. Page, D.L., Caulfield, J.B., Kastor, J.A., DeSanctis, R.W. and Sanders, C.A. (1971). Myocardial changes associated with cardiogenic shock. *N. Engl. J. Med.*, **285**, 133–7

124. Coronary Thrombosis in Myocardial Infarction. Report of a Workshop on the Role of Coronary Thrombosis in the Pathogenesis of Acute Myocardial Infarction. *Am. J. Cardiol.*, **34**, 823–32

125. Mitchell, J.R.A. and Schwartz, C.J. (1965). *Arterial Disease*, pp. 107–14. (Oxford: Blackwell Scientific Publications)

126. Mitchell, J.R.A. and Schwartz, C.J. (1963). The relation between myocardial lesions and coronary artery disease. II. A selected group of patients with massive cardiac necrosis or scarring. *Br. Heart J.*, **25**, 1–25

127. Schwartz, C.J. and Mitchell, J.R.A. (1962). The relation between myocardial lesions and coronary artery disease. I. An unselected necropsy study. *Br. Heart J.*, **24**, 761–86

128. Roberts, W.C. (1976). The coronary arteries in fatal coronary events. In Chung, E.K. (ed.) *Controversies in Cardiology*, p. 1. (New York, Springer-Verlag)

129. Chandler, A.B. (1975). Relationship of coronary thrombosis to myocardial infarction. *Mod. Concepts Cardiovasc. Dis.*, **44**, 1

130. Barold, G. (1978). Pathological anatomy of myocardial infarction. In Wilhelmsen, L. and Hjalmarson, A. (eds.) *Acute and Long-Term Medical Management of Myocardial Ischemia*, p. 41. (Sweden: Mölndal)

131. DeWood, M.A., Spores, J., Notske, R., Mouser, L.T., Burroughs, R., Golden, M.S. and Lang, H.T. (1980). Prevalence of total coronary occlusion during the early hours of transmural myocardial infarction. *N. Engl. J. Med.*, **303**, 897

132. Forrester, J.S., Litvack, F., Grundfest, W. and Hickey, A. (1987). A perspective of coronary disease seen through the arteries of a living man. *Circulation*, **75**, 505

133. Wilson, R.F., Holida, M.D. and White, C.W. (1986). Quantitative angiographic morphology of coronary stenoses leading to myocardial infarction or unstable angina. *Circulation*, **73**, 286

134. Sherman, C.T., Litvack, F., Grundfest, W., Lee, M., Hickey, A., Chaux, A., Kass, R., Blanche, C., Matloff, J., Morgenstern, L., Ganz, W., Swan, H.J.C. and Forrester, J. (1986). Coronary angioscopy in patients with unstable angina pectoris. *N. Engl. J. Med.*, **315**, 913

135. MacAlpin, R.N. (1980). Coronary arterial spasm: a historical perspective. *J. Hist. Med. Allied Sci.*, **35**, 288–311

136. *Ibid.*, p. 289.

137. Blackall, J. (1813). On the nature and cure of dropsies ... to which is added an appendix, containing several cases of angina pectoris with dissections, etc., p. 244. (London)

138. Latham, P.M. (1876–78). *Collected works*, 2 vols., **1**, 461. (London)

139. Fothergill, J.M. (1879). *The Heart and its Diseases with their Treatment*, 2nd edn., p. 263. (Philadelphia)

140. Huchard, H. (1889). *Traité des Maladies du Coeur et des Vaisseaux, Artériosclérose, Aortities, Cardiopathies Arterielles, Angines de Poitrine*, p. 466. (Paris)

141. Wilson, F.N. and Johnston, F.D. (1941). The occurrence in angina pectoris of electrocardiographic changes similar in magnitude and in kind to those produced by myocardial infarction. *Am. Heart J.*, **22**, 64–74

142. Osler, W. (1910). The Lumleian lectures on angina pectoris II. *Lancet*, **1**, 839–44

143. Gallavardin, L. (1925). *Les Angines de Poitrine*. (Paris)

144. Paul, C. (1884). *Diagnosis and Treatment of Diseases of the Heart*, p. 207 (tr. from the French). (New York)

145. Keefer, C.S. and Resnik, W.H. (1928). Angina pectoris: a syndrome caused by anoxemia of the myocardium. *Arch. Intern. Med.*, **41**, 769–807

146. Clerc, A. (1927). 'Anomalies electrocardiographiques au cours de l'oblitération coronarienne,' *Presse Méd.*, **35**, 499–502

147. Feil, H. and Siegel, M.L. (1928). Electrocardiographic changes during attacks of angina pectoris. *Am. J. Med. Sci.*, **175**, 255–60

148. Siegel, M.L. and Feil, H. (1931). Electrocardiographic studies during attacks of angina pectoris and of other paroxysmal pain. *J. Clin. Invest.*, **10**, 795–806

149. Hausner, E. and Scherf, D. (1933). Über angina pectoris – Probleme. *Z. Klin. Med.*, **126**, 166–93

150. Prinzmetal, M. *et al.* (1959). Angina pectoris, I. a variant form of angina pectoris. *Am. J. Med.*, **27**, 375–88

151. Prinzmetal, M. *et al.* (1960). Variant form of angina pectoris: previously undelineated syndrome. *J. Am. Med. Assoc.*, **174**, 102–8

152. Hurst, J.W. (1986). Coronary spasm as viewed by Wilson and Johnston. *Am. J. Cardiol.*, **57**, 1000–1

153. Arnulf, G. (1959). Étude artériographique de la vasomotricité coronnarienne chez l'animal et chez l'homme. *Presse Med.*, **67**, 2055–7

154. Gensini, G. *et al.* (1962). Arteriographic demonstration of coronary artery spasm and its release after the use of a vasodilator in a case of angina pectoris and in the experimental animal. *Angiology*, **13**, 550–3

155. Oliva, P.B., Potts, D.E. and Pluss, R.G. (1973). Coronary arterial spasm in Prinzmetal angina: documentation by coronary arteriography. *N. Engl. J. Med.*, **288**, 745–50

156. Maseri, A. *et al.* (1975). Coronary artery spasm as a cause of acute myocardial ischemia in man. *Chest*, **68**, 625–33

157. Maseri, A. *et al.* (1978). 'Variant' angina: one aspect of a continuous spectrum of vasospastic myocardial ischemia. *Am. J. Cardiol.*, **42**, 1019–35

158. Oliva, P.B. and Breckenridge, J.C. (1977). Arteriographic evidence of coronary arterial spasm in acute myocardial infarction. *Circulation*, **56**, 366–74

159. Labbé, M. *et al.* (1929). L'angine de poitrine ergotaminique. *Presse Méd.*, **37**, 1069

160. Stein, I. and Weinstein, J. (1953). Unusual reaction to ergonovine maleate in a case of coronary insufficiency. *N.Y. J. Med.*, **53**, 1454–5

161. Huepler, F.A. Jr. *et al.* (1975). The ergonovine maleate test for the diagnosis of coronary artery spasm. *Circulation*, Suppl. II, **52**, 11

162. Clausen, J.P. (1977). Effect of physical training on cardiovascular adjustments to exercise in man. *Physiol. Rev.*, **57**, 779–815

163. Scheuer, J. and Tipton, C.M. (1977). Cardiovascular adaptations to physical training. *Annu. Rev. Physiol.*, **39**, 221–51

164. Wyatt, H.L. and Mitchell, J.H. (1974). Influences of physical training on the heart of dogs. *Circ. Res.*, **35**, 883–9

165. Stone, H.L. (1977). The unanesthetized instrumented animal preparation. *Med. Sci. Sports*, **9**, 253–61

166. Froelicher, V.F. (1977). Does exercise conditioning delay progression of myocardial ischemia in coronary atherosclerotic heart disease. *Cardiovasc. Clin.*, **8** No. 1, 11–31

167. von Restorff, W., Holtz, J. and Bassenge, E. (1977). Exercise induced augmentation of myocardial oxygen extraction in spite of normal coronary dilatory capacity in dogs. *Pflugers Arch.*, **372**, 181–5

168. Stone, H.L. (1977). Cardiac function and exercise training in conscious dogs. *J. Appl. Physiol.*, **42**, 824–32

169. Einthoven, W. (1908). Weiteres über das Elektrokardiogramm. *Archiv für Physiologie*, **122**, 317

170. Wood, F.C., Wolferth, C.C. and Livesey, M.M. (1931). Angina Pectoris I. The clinical and electrocardiographic phenomena of the attack and their comparison with the effects of experimental temporary occlusion. *Arch. Intern. Med.*, **47**, 220

171. Scherf, D. and Goldhammer, S. (1933). Zur Fruhdiagnose der Angina Pectoris mit. Helfe

des Elektrokardiograms. *Ztschr. J. Klin. Med.*, **124**, 111

172. Katz, L. and Landt, H. (1935). The effect of standardized exercise in the four lead electrocardiogram. *Am. J. Med. Sci.*, **189**, 346

173. Missal, M.E. (1938). Exercise test and the electrocardiograph in the study of angina pectoris. *Ann. Intern. Med.*, **11**, 2018

174. Master, A.M., Friedman, R. and Dack, S. (1942). The electrocardiogram after standard exercise as a functional test of the heart. *Am. Heart J.*, **24**, 777–93

175. Rosenfeld, I., Master, A.M. and Rosenfeld, C. (1964). Recording the electrocardiogram during the performance of the Master two-step test. I. *Circulation*, **29**, 201

176. Rosenfeld, I. and Master, A.M. (1964). Recording the electrocardiogram during the performance of the Master two-step test. II. *Circulation*, **29**, 212

177. Wood, P., McGregor, M., Magidson, O. and Whittaker, W. (1958). Effort test in angina pectoris. *Br. Heart J.*, **12**, 363

178. Elliotson (1829–30). Clinical Lecture. *Lancet*, **2**, 408

179. Schlessier (1841). Efficacy of hydrocyanic acid in angina pectoris. *Lancet*, 618

180. Teale, T.P. (1829). A treatise on neuralgic diseases, dependent on irritation of the spinal marrow, and the ganglia of the sympathetic nerve. *Lancet*, 325

181. Jennings, S.A. (1966). A history of the therapy of angina pectoris. *J. Arkansas Med. Soc.*, **62**, 407–11

182. Jarcho, S. (1960). The treatment of angina pectoris by electricity (Duchenne, 1855). *Am. J. Cardiol.*, **6**, 338–43

183. Bishop, L.F. (1925). Castor oil as a remedy in angina pectoris. *Therap. Gaz. XIIX*, **313**, 1925.

184. Thorne, L.T. (1924). The balneological treatment of angina pectoris. *Practitioner*, **112**, 375–9

185. Blumgart, H.L., Freedberg, A.S. and Kurland, G.S. (1950). Hypothyroidism produced by radioactive iodine in the treatment of euthyroid patients with angina pectoris and congestive heart failure. *Circulation*, **1**, 1105–41

186. Raab, W. (1945). Thiouracil treatment of angina pectoris. *J. Am. Med. Assoc.*, **128**, 249–56

187. Blumgart, H.L., Berlin, Davis, Riseman and Weinstein (1935). Total ablation of the thyroid in angina pectoris and congestive failure. *J. Am.*

Med. Assoc., **104**, 17–26

188. Raab, W. (1940). Roentgen treatment of the adrenal glands in angina pectoris. *Ann. Intern. Med.*, **14**, 688–710

189. Coogan, T.J. (1934). Some clinical observations on the uses of theophyllin calcium salicylate. *Trans. Am. Therap. Soc.*, **34**, 137–45

190. Dembo, D.H. and Antlitz, A.M. (1964). Chlordiazepoxide therapy in angina pectoris. *Angiology*, **15**, 207–9

191. Halprin, H. (1960). An amine oxidase inhibitor in angina. *Angiology*, **11**, 348–55

192. Parsonnet, A.E. and Bernstein, A. (1940). Cobra Venom: its use in stenocardia. *Am. J. Med. Sc.*, **200**, 581–6

193. Freedberg, A.S. and Riseman, J.E.F. (1945). Cobra Venom in the treatment of angina pectoris. *N. Engl. J. Med.*, **233**, 462–6

194. Russek, H.I., Naegele, C.F. and Regan, F.D. (1950). Alcohol in the treatment of angina pectoris. *J. Am. Med. Assoc.*, **143**, 355–7

195. Rosenman, R.H., Fishman, A.P., Kaplan, S.R., Levin, H.G. and Katz, L.N. (1950). Observations on the clinical use of Visammin (Khellin). *J. Am. Med. Assoc.*, **143**, 160–5

196. Gray, W., Riseman, J.E.F. and Stearnes, S. (1945). Papaverine in the treatment of coronary artery disease. *N. Engl. J. Med.*, **232**, 389–94

197. Waldman, S. (1945). The treatment of angina pectoris with testosterone propionate. *J. Clin. Endocrinol.*, **5**, 305–17

198. Schwartzman, M.S. (1930). Muscle extract in the treatment of angina pectoris and intermittent claudication. *Br. Med. J.*, **I**, 855–6

199. Smith, K.S. (1933). Insulin and glucose in the treatment of heart disease. *Br. Med. J.*, **1**, 693

200. Steinburg, F. and Jensen, J. (1945). On the use of theophylline aminoisobutanol in angina pectoris. *J. Lab. Clin. Med.*, **30**, 769–73

201. Greiner, T. (1950). A method for the evaluation of the effects of drugs on cardiac pain in patients with angina of effort. *Am. J. Med.*, **9**, 143–55

202. Riseman, J.E.F. (1959). The treatment of angina pectoris. *N. Engl. J. Med.* **261**, 1017–20, 1126–9, 1236–9

203. Russek, H.I., Zohman, B.L. and Dorset, V.J. (1955). Objective evaluation of coronary vasodilator drugs. *Am. J. Med. Sc.*, **229**, 46–54

19 Hypertension

The story of hypertension begins with Richard Bright. This astute physician practiced during the first half of the 19th century, a time when the physical examination was an important element of bedside diagnosis, and when the findings in life were correlated with the pathological changes seen at postmortem. Bright was one of those physicians who religiously observed this practice, adding his own contributions to those of his contemporaries such as Addison and Hodgkin at the prestigious Guy's Hospital.

Bright's interests were directed primarily towards renal dysfunction. Twelve years of clinical experience correlated with observations at autopsies performed by him on his own patients were summarized in his meticulously detailed monograph that appeared in 1827[1]. In 1836 he published a report concerned with the 'morbid appearances in 100 cases connected with albuminous urine'[2]. His description of the anatomical changes in the kidneys and heart in these two publications constitute the first analytical correlation between 'dropsy with coagulable urine' and the cardiorenal changes. Although he was describing primarily a chronic form of kidney disease which we now know to be associated with hypertension, he did bring out that the hypertrophy of the heart may have been related to

> ... some less local cause, for the unusual efforts to which the heart has been impelled; and the two most ready solutions appear to be, either that the altered quality of the blood affords irregular and unwanted stimulus to the organ immediately; or, that it so affects the minute and capillary circulation, as to render greater action necessary to force the blood through the distant sub-divisions of the vascular system[2].

Although not couched in current terms, this passage is a perfect description of increased peripheral resistance. It should also be emphasized that Bright was talking about the vascular system in

general and not merely that portion serving the kidneys. Richard Bright is depicted during the prime of his life in Figure 1.

Bright's disease, as it came to be known, occupied the attention of several outstanding physicians over the succeeding decades. Their studies were seminal because they brought out important changes in the arterial system. The first of these important studies were those of George Johnson. In 1868 he described the presence of muscular hypertrophy in the smaller arteries of many organs in the body besides the kidney[3]. He postulated that the cause of the left ventricular hypertrophy in Bright's disease was to be found in the smaller arteries throughout the body.

> We must look for the cause of this hypertrophy rather in the fact that the blood, in consequence of degeneration of the kidney, being contaminated by urinary excreta and otherwise deteriorated, is impeded in its transit through the minute arteries throughout the body.'

Bright suggested it but this is the first time that anyone unequivocally mentioned increased peripheral resistance as the fundamental basis for left ventricular hypertrophy. Furthermore, he correlated this increased peripheral resistance as manifested by 'the full, hard, throbbing pulse, which is a very common phenomenon in the advanced stage of chronic Bright's disease' with an elevated arterial pressure. He was referring to Burdon-Sanderson's recently published *Handbook of the Sphygmograph* wherein the comment is made that 'in case of chronic Bright's disease with hypertrophy of the left ventricle, the sphygmograph affords decided evidence of increased arterial pressure'[3]. The sphygmograph, despite the relatively primitive stage of its evolution at the time, was fast becoming an integral part of the physical examination. Johnson then went on to say 'Still more conclusive evidence of an impediment to the circulation is afforded by

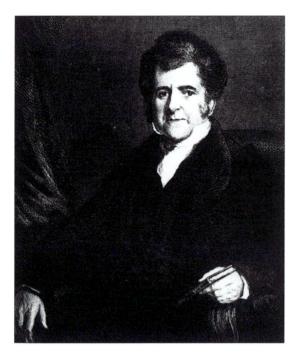

Figure 1 Richard Bright (1789–1858). *Photo Source National Library of Medicine. Literary Source Photo Archives. Courtesy of National Library of Medicine*

the existence of hypertrophy of the muscular walls of the arteries in various tissues and organs'[3].

Further clinicopathologic studies on Bright's disease were conducted by Sir William Gull of Guy's Hospital and H. G. Sutton of the London Hospital. In 1872 they described three forms of the disease based on postmortem correlates in the kidneys:

(1) marked contraction of the kidneys,

(2) slight contraction of the kidneys, and

(3) healthy appearing kidneys.

All forms of the disease manifested 'a heart much hypertrophied', and 'minute arteries and capillaries thickened by hyaline-fibroid substance'[4]. The vascular changes were different from those described by Johnson ... 'this alteration is due to a hyaline-fibroid formation in the walls of the minute arteries, and a hyaline-granular change in the corresponding capillaries ... this change occurs chiefly outside the muscular layer, but also in the tunica intima of some arterioles'[4]. In anatomical terms, Bright described two types of chronic kidney disease. These were based on gross

descriptions only. Although he began to use the microscope 14 years after he began his studies, he left no published reports with this method[5]. The hard contracted variety was often present without symptoms; the other, usually associated with generalized edema, was very large and white. A good 50 years after Bright's original description, an attempt was made by Bartels to classify these two types on etiologic grounds[6]. He proposed that the large white kidney was due to chronic parenchymatous nephritis while the small contracted kidney was the result of chronic interstitial nephritis. Later observations proved that both varieties represented end-stages of renal disease with different pathogenic pathways.

While the English were expanding on Bright's original descriptions, the Germans were also carrying on their studies, focusing particularly on the association between kidney disease and cardiovascular changes; and the notable elevation of blood pressure. In addition to Bartels, they included Ewald, Jores, Traube, Leyden, Lewinski, and the team of Grawitz and Israel. Four of them (Ewald, Jores, Traube and Leyden) were primarily clinical investigators. The remainder initiated the period of experimental hypertension. What they were looking for was finally delineated by Harry Goldblatt of America and later elaborated upon through the renin–angiotensin metabolic pathway.

Ewald's attention was focused primarily on the small vessels of the pia mater[7]. His observations were no different from those of Johnson. Jores reported the presence of a 'fatty-hyalin' thickening in the intima of the arteries of all organs except (strangely) in the heart and skeletal muscle[8].

The latter half of the 19th century was a time when physiological experimentation under the bright star of Karl Ludwig was a dominant force throughout the academic world. Although not an experimentalist in the strict sense of the word, Leyden expressed very nicely the underlying philosophy prevalent at the time when he said: 'Since we live today in a period of Medicine, in which the facts observed daily at the sick bed are only considered to be proven, when they can be experimentally reproduced, so clinical facts would be cast in doubt, so long as experimental confirmation is lacking'[9,10]. Thus, another element was added to the still popular postmortem correlation.

Leyden (1832–1910) was a distinguished clinical investigator. He championed the view that high blood pressure was part and parcel of Bright's disease. More significantly, he had the foresight to suspect that reduced renal blood flow played a major role in the clinical manifestations[10].

It was Traube, however, who set the stage for physiological experimentation with his clinico-pathological investigations. He attempted to explain the mechanisms on the structural changes that he saw. His paper published in 1856, long before Leyden's and Bartel's, was specifically directed towards an elucidation of the mechanisms responsible for left ventricular hypertrophy in the presence of kidney disease. The steps that he outlined in his hypothesis[11] came to be known as Traube's theory.

Traube attributed the increase in the arterial pressure to two factors arising primarily from the contracted state of the kidney.

> The shrinking of the renal parenchyma has, therefore, two-fold consequences. It will act, first, by decreasing the blood volume which flows out in a given time from the arterial system into the venous system. It will, secondly, act by decreasing the amount of liquid which at the same time is removed from the arterial system as urinary secretion. As a result of both these conditions, particularly because of the latter, as is clear from what has just been stated, the mean pressure of the arterial system must increase. Consequently again, an increase in resistance is produced which oppose the emptying of the left ventricle[12].

It is apparent from this reasoning that both factors induced a hypervolemic state and that this was responsible for the hypertensive state. At least this is my interpretation of this paragraph. On the other hand, his last statement is even more intriguing. He acknowledges an increase in resistance that the left ventricle has to face; but at this point he fails to mention how this increased resistance comes about on an anatomical basis. As one reads his paper further, he does mention the existence of narrowed blood vessels in the kidneys, and the perception arises that Traube really regarded the sustained elevation of blood pressure as a compensatory phenomenon to combat the impedance produced by these narrowed vessels. The heart had to become hypertrophied in order to increase blood pressure more effectively so that more blood could be pushed through the kidneys despite the narrowed vessels.

Julius Conheim, the eminent German patholo-gist, was in full support of this erroneous concept. He lent the weight of his esteem and authority when he expressed this view in his text on pathology in 1877[13]. Naturally, adherence to this view meant only one thing as far as the clinician was concerned. Do not meddle with the blood pressure! Lowering it would remove nature's way of coping with the decreased blood flow that prevailed in Bright's disease.

Fortunately, in terms of impact on the natural course of the disease, no adverse affects could have resulted from this point of view. Even if one wanted to lower the blood pressure, effective anti-hypertensive therapy did not exist at the time. Much more detailed physiological experimentation was needed before such therapy could be realized.

Traube's view regarding the compensatory mechanism was really cast into oblivion when Gull, Sutton and Mahomed described their clinico-pathologic observations. However, this did not prevent the German team of Grawitz and Israel from subjecting the several elements of Traube's theory to animal experimentation. In essence, they produced in their rabbits temporary episodes of renal ischemia. After what they considered a suitable period of time they sacrificed the animals to determine the effect, if any, on heart mass.

They did not find any sustained rise in blood pressure. They did find (what they considered to be) an increased incidence of cardiac hypertrophy. But their methodology was seriously flawed and cast considerable doubt on the validity of their observations as well as conclusions. They did not realize at the time, that blood pressure does not rise by merely removing one kidney or by damaging one kidney with a temporary period of ischemia. Moreover, although their investigations were conducted primarily to determine the incidence of cardiac hypertrophy in this setting, their method for determining hypertrophy was also flawed. Therefore, when they concluded that cardiac hypertrophy did occur but not through elevation of blood pressure, they were obviously in error on both points, and Traube's theory, though challenged, was not refuted by them.

A year later Lewinski described his observations 'On the relation between contracted kidney disease and cardiac hypertrophy'[14]. He did not fall into the same trap as Grawitz and Israel. He compromised the renal function in the dog by narrowing both renal arteries rather than completely occluding one. This was a step in the right direction but careful analysis of his paper reveals again a markedly flawed methodology and therefore his paper did not contribute in any way towards elucidating the relationship to cardiac hypertrophy or hypertension.

Up until now we have seen how hypertension had come to be regarded as an integral part of chronic kidney disease without a firm understanding of the underlying mechanism. As time went on, it became increasingly obvious to some observers that certain pathologic changes in the kidney were the result of longstanding hypertension and not the cause of it as initially believed. It became evident that in addition to the heart, the kidneys could also be looked upon as a target organ in sustained elevation of blood pressure. In addition, as blood pressure measurements became part and parcel of the trappings of the physical examination, it became apparent that a large number of people had chronically elevated blood pressure with either no apparent etiologic factor or secondary to some systemic disturbance other than the kidney. The presence of hypertension without an overtly known cause took on the designation, primary or idiopathic. As more of the natural history of this syndrome became known, it brought forth the knowledge that it would eventually lead to a disabling or lethal involvement of the heart, brain or kidney, singly or in combination. This type of hypertension constituted, by far, the vast majority of cases. It became known as the silent killer because it can exert its pathogenic effect on the target organs without obvious clinical manifestations. In its quiet relentless way, many years would elapse before overt clinical signs of target organ damage become demonstrable. Knowledge regarding the secondary types of hypertension evolved in concert with newer insights into metabolism, neurophysiology, valvular and vascular abnormalities. This survey will be limited to the essential type.

One of the first to systematically incorporate the measurement of the blood pressure as part of the clinical evaluation was an English physician of Indian parentage by the name of Frederick Mahomed. He was so enthralled with blood pressure measurements that he introduced his own improved modification of the sphygmograph available at the time. This was at least 24 years before Riva-Rocci's model made its appearance in 1896. Mahomed's instrument was really a

modification of Marey's device (see Chapter 24). It was rather clumsy as one can see from Figure 2. It actually measured the tension of the pulse rather than the blood pressure itself[15]. Mahomed had an early interest in sphygmology. He modified Marey's device while still a student at Guy's Hospital, for which he was awarded the Pupils' Physical Society Prize of 1870[16].

Concurrently with the Germans, Mahomed was making many valuable contributions towards the clinical spectrum of Bright's disease. He described its evolution as occurring in three phases. The first was characterized by an elevated blood pressure without structural changes either in the kidney or blood vessels. 'Arteriocapillary fibrosis' was the predominant structural change in the second phase but still without albuminuria. The final phase was the full blown picture with nephritis dominating the clinical scenario.

Mahomed should be credited with being the first to realize that acute nephritis is associated with an increase in arterial pressure. This was reported in his paper *The etiology of Bright's disease and the prealbuminuric stage*, published in 1874, only two years after qualifying as a medical practitioner. This was followed by a series of papers dealing with 'arteriocapillary fibrosis' and the various clinical manifestations of Bright's disease. He combined for the first time estimates of arterial tension, measured in troy ounces, with clinical and pathological observations.

Mahomed died prematurely of typhoid fever at the age of 35. I wonder what he could have accomplished if he had lived for at least another two or three decades. Although priority for recognition of primary hypertension is generally ascribed to Huchard, von Basch, and Albutt, his description of 'arteriocapillary fibrosis' and other observations have been advanced as evidence that he too recognized the presence of hypertension not causally related to kidney disease. In his paper on the sphygmographic evidence of 'arteriocapillary fibrosis' he commented on how he observed people with no overt evidence of kidney disease, either in the urine or otherwise, and yet, who manifested 'high arterial tension'[17]. Even in his collection of postmortem studies on the kidneys, he describes patients with 'red contracted kidneys' with symptoms of heart disease or cerebral hemorrhage who had 'signs of high arterial tension taken together with the absence of albuminuria'[18].

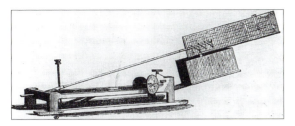

Figure 2 Mahomed's modification of Marey's sphygmograph. *Photo Source National Library of Medicine. Literary Source Shaw, Batty A. Guy's Hospital Report, 1952. With permission*

The following comments from his writings underscore the fact that he recognized the existence of high blood pressure without obvious cause or antecedent kidney disease.

> My first contention is that high pressure is a constant condition in the circulation of some individuals and that this condition is a symptom of a certain constitution or diathesis … These persons appear to pass on through life pretty much as others do and generally do not suffer from their high blood pressures, except in their petty ailments upon which it imprints itself … As age advances the enemy gains accession of strength … the individual has now passed forty years, perhaps fifty years, of age, his lungs begin to degenerate, he has a cough in the winter time, but by his pulse you will know him … Alternatively headache, vertigo, epistaxis, a passing paralysis, a more severe apoplectic seizure, and then the final blow … Of this I feel sure, that the clinical symptoms and the pathological changes resulting from high arterial pressure are frequently seen in cases in which very slight, if any disease is discoverable in the kidney. The observations provide strong evidence of Gull and Sutton's work. It appears to me that these clinical, and their pathological, observations must stand or fall together; that one is the pathological, the other the clinical aspect of the same condition [18,19].

Ten years later, Huchard of Paris recognized quite clearly that hypertension can occur without antecedent kidney disease. Mahomed wrote that 'the clinical symptoms and the pathological changes resulting from high arterial pressure are frequently seen in cases in which very slight, if any disease is discoverable in the kidneys'. Huchard did not equivocate at all when he wrote in his *Maladies du Coeur et des Vaisseaux*: 'It has been wrongly assumed that chronic hypertension only appears following interstitial nephritis. The opposite is true; arterial hypertension is the cause of arteriosclerosis; it precedes by a varying time interval the evolution of different diseases (heart disease and arterial nephritis, etc.) which are in turn secondary to vascular sclerosis' [20].

I have described in Chapter 23 the contributions of von Basch in the development of the sphygmomanometer. During the course of his observations with his version of the device, he established (what he considered to be) the normal range of systolic blood pressure. His critical level for abnormality was 150 mmHg, not far from our currently accepted values. The reader must be warned however, that our current values for normal blood pressure should not be considered as final. The introduction of 24-hour ambulatory monitoring and the recent perception that the older population may have normally higher systolic levels than currently accepted, may very well result in different values. At any rate, aside from his presentation of normal values, von Basch was of the view that arteriosclerosis caused the high blood pressure [21].

Mahomed's observations of hypertension in the absence of albuminuria were also noted by Albutt of Cambridge. They were made on a very small series consisting of only five patients. Albutt's report appeared in 1895 [22]. Much more important was his proposed classification of arterial disease which appeared 20 years later [23]. One type which he labeled decrescent arteriosclerosis was a form of arterial degeneration and not accompanied usually by a rise in blood pressure. The other two types had in common an elevated blood pressure, one with Bright's disease and the other without. Hyperpiesis was the name he gave to the latter: 'A malady in which at or towards middle life blood pressures rise excessively, a malady having a course of its own and deserving the name of a disease' [23].

As the 20th century unfolded, it became generally accepted that hypertension could exist without renal disease or even be caused by it. As more people were identified with what came to be known as essential hypertension, knowledge of its natural history began to be pieced together. The vascular complications of hypertension, whether on the heart or on other components of the vascular system, were clearly recognized by Janeway of

Columbia University. He is responsible for introducing the term hypertensive cardiovascular disease.

Theodore Janeway began his studies on
hypertension in 1903. His observations were clinical
in nature and derived from a large private practice
that he shared with his father. Between the years
1903 and 1912, he recorded the systolic pressure in
every one of their patients, 7872 in all[13]. Initially, he
recorded only the systolic level. When Korotkoff's
auscultatory method became known in 1905, he
also measured the diastolic level. But, at the time,
there was so much confusion and variability in
assessing what was normal or abnormal regarding
the diastolic level, he reported only the systolic
measurements, and regarded a level greater than
160 mmHg as being indicative of hypertension.

Janeway regarded hypertension as a disease of the
circulatory system, and it is for this reason that he
chose the unifying designation of the syndrome as
hypertensive cardiovascular disease. This is how he
phrased it: 'The most prominent symptoms
associated with high blood pressure are circulatory
rather than renal. The disease underlying high
arterial pressure is predominantly a disease of the
circulatory system, and is best designated hypertensive cardiovascular disease'[24].

An important element in the natural history of
the disease was the discovery that there were those
in whom the condition remained overtly
unchanged but in whom the relentless effects of
sustained hypertension took their toll on the heart
and brain and another subset characterized by a
malignant course with renal involvement. Volhard
recognized this quite well, and in 1931, he
described the two forms as red and white
hypertension[25]. Red hypertension was characterized by a long duration and no demonstrable renal
involvement. He ascribed its etiology to an elastosis
of the pre-arterioles, a natural accompaniment of
age. It is now well known that the vast majority of
hypertensives seemingly tolerate their elevated
blood pressure with minimal or no symptoms for
many years. This is why it was given the sobriquet
'the silent killer'. It is only when manifestations of
target organ damage appear that the course of the
disease assumes a rapidly progressive downhill path.
Comroe recounts how Janeway himself wrote of
one patient with a systolic blood pressure of 280 for
more than 10 years. Even more illuminating is
Comroe's paraphrase of David Reisman's report
(also in 1931) that 'Though high blood pressure is

not conducive to longevity and on the whole is no
blessing, he cared for a patient from age 72 to 97
years whose blood pressure ranged between 220
and 274'[26].

Volhard's 'Bösartige Sklerosis' was the white form
of hypertension, and the one that was characterized
by renal disease and rapidly leading to uremia and
death. He noted that those with renal disease would
have retinal changes and abnormal urinary findings.
The retinal changes are now called hypertensive
retinopathy and are clinically divided into four
stages, beginning with arteriovenous nicking, and, if
progressive, manifested by retinal hemorrhages and
exudates, and in the most malignant form by
papilledema. Retinal changes in hypertension
associated with kidney dysfunction were first
described by von Graefe in 1854[27]. It was called
'retinitis albuminurica' by Liebreich in 1859[28].

Fahr had demonstrated in 1914 that the white
(or malignant) form was associated with arteriolar
necrosis in the kidneys[29]. Volhard seized upon this
pathological abnormality to present a view that
anticipated Goldblatt's work as well as the renin-
angiotensin formulation. Volhard postulated that
the pale form of hypertension was caused by a renal
pressor substance released through renal ischemia.
The renal ischemia could be precipitated by two
mechanisms. Those with established kidney disease
such as nephritis would be subjected to ischemia by
virtue of the fixed obstruction in the renal pre-
arterioles, made worse by superimposed spasm.
People with red hypertension could be transformed
into the pale type by repeated episodes of spasm.
Either way, a vicious circle would be created
involving progressive ischemia and increasing levels
of liberated pressor substance.

There was no longer any doubt that the kidney
played an important role in certain subsets of
hypertension. This was demonstrated time and
again. Despite all this progress in differentiating the
hypertensive syndromes, much work still remained
regarding the elucidation of the basic cause or
causes of the essential or idiopathic variety. In
pursuing this objective many experimental
methods and several animal models were
introduced. The lines of investigation were still
focused on the possible role of the kidney but, in
addition, a neural basis for vasomotor control was
now an item of considerable interest.

As the reader has seen in Chapter 17, much of
the knowledge concerning the mechanisms for the

regulation of blood pressure has stemmed from investigations into vasomotor control. The first inkling that vasomotor dysfunction could be the underlying mechanism for the hypertensive state came from the studies of Koch and Mies in 1929[30]. They were pupils of Hering and their experiments were based on their mentor's demonstration of the importance of baroreceptors in regulating blood pressure. Koch and Mies were able to induce a prolonged hypertensive state by sectioning the nerves involved in the baroreceptor reflex. They used rabbits, cats and dogs as their subjects. Their work was quickly confirmed and amplified by Heymans and Bouckaert[31]. There seemed to be no doubt that elimination of the baroreceptor reflex was, if not the only, then at least, an important factor in causing hypertension.

This view was shattered by two teams of investigators working independently of each other. They were Gammon and the group headed by Pickering[32,33]. These two groups found that in patients with essential hypertension, the carotid sinus reflex was intact and functioning normally. This is another example of how observations derived from animal experiments are not, *ipso facto*, applicable to humans.

Goldblatt and his group approached the problem through the old standby, the kidney itself. Using dogs they found that when both renal arteries were constricted, hypertension would ensue. The same sequence was observed even if only one renal artery was constricted provided that the other kidney had been removed. This was a remarkable breakthrough but pointing once again to diminution in renal blood flow as being the initiating mechanism. His group expanded their findings with further experimentation[34,35]. They were able to show that when renal arterial flow was markedly reduced, cardiac hypertrophy and the retinal and arteriolar changes of malignant hypertension were more likely to occur[34].

A great controversy now arose. Were they correct in their observations and interpretation? Goldblatt always maintained that essential hypertension in man was also due to renal ischemia no matter how it was produced. He went on record with this view in his paper published in 1947 bearing the title *The renal origin of hypertension*[35]. Examples of the Goldblatt kidney are seen quite regularly in clinical practice, due mainly to the increasing use of angiography. These cases manifest variable degrees of renal arterial stenosis, but by no means do they account for the vast majority of hypertensive patients. When stenosis is found and the hypertension is moderated by removal of the blockage, the condition is currently referred to as renovascular hypertension.

Goldblatt's view was supported by Moritz and Oldt. In 1937 they described an association in advancing age between arterial sclerotic changes in the kidneys and the presence of a hypertensive state. No one can deny that these changes are indeed present. They were there for all to see but the crucial question still remained unanswered. Were these changes the cause of the hypertension in that individual or were they the result of a prolonged hypertensive state?

E.T. Bell kept the controversy going when he expressed the view in 1951 that the vascular changes were the result rather that the cause of high blood pressure[36]. He based this assertion primarily on the evidence that early cases of hypertension are not necessarily accompanied by vascular changes in the kidney. Wasn't all this brought out by the English clinicians of the late 19th century?

Goldblatt's work was seminal in alerting the physiologists once more to the true role of the kidney in essential hypertension. But his observations covered only the tip of the iceberg. Deep down in the kidneys, at the cellular level, humoral mechanisms were waiting to be discovered.

In 1937 Blalock and Levy opened the door to these mechanisms[37]. They were able to obtain a rise in blood pressure in animals with a heterotopically transplanted kidney if the renal artery of that kidney were constricted. They were able to reverse this rise by removing the constriction. In their experiments the kidney was transplanted to the neck and devoid of all neural connections. The same alterations in blood pressure were produced by Heymans, Alpert and Page[38–40] even with the kidney *in situ* when renal artery constriction was carried out in combination with bilateral paravertebral ganglionectomy. These investigators pointed to the possibility that the renal mechanism involved a humoral substance of some kind, and independent of the nervous system. It was definitely not epinephrine. This was brought out by Pickering and Kissin in 1936[41].

Since the kidney was involved in all these previous experiments, it was logical to assume that the pressor substance was supplied by the kidney itself. This very thought occurred to Pickering and also to Landis[42]. Pickering and Landis pursued the thought with a vengeance and persistence that finally culminated in the emergence of renin as a factor. After some difficulty in preparing consistently effective renal extracts, Pickering's group finally achieved success with saline extracts of alcohol-dried kidney in unanesthetized rabbits. The group led by Landis was able to get an even more purified form by heating the saline extracts to 56° C and discarding the precipitate[42].

The pressor response obtained with these extracts finally vindicated the claims of Robert Tigerstedt and his co-worker Bergmann when they reported from Stockholm as far back as 1894 the presence of a pressor substance in the kidney which they named renin[43]. For years its very existence was doubted. Prior to Pickering and Landis only one group had been successful in repeating the work of Tigerstedt and Bergman. This was the German group headed by Bingel. Their reports were published in 1909[43,44]. In commemoration of Tigerstedt's achievement, the American Society of Hypertension established an annual award and lectureship.

George Pickering's role in understanding the nature of hypertension merits special consideration. We might have gained more if he had lived longer, but 78 years is not too short a span for human life. Pickering's contributions on the subject of hypertension were of such importance that he was knighted by the Queen.

Two years after Pickering's death, W. S. Peart, one of his more famous students, wrote a highly vivid word picture of the famous professor. Peart recalled his initial encounter with Pickering at Harefield Hospital and described him as 'a small man with hair blown in the wind, piercing blue eyes, talking over the side of a battered Morris Minor Tourer'. Later, Peart was impressed with Pickering's bedside teaching. His was 'a true spirit of critical scientific inquiry … combined with qualities of a great physician … and his consuming interest in the use of English and the precision of mind required for its mastery'[45].

Pickering was initially interested in agriculture but fortunately for medicine he was persuaded to pursue a degree in biochemistry or physiology. After obtaining a sound foundation in the basic sciences while on a scholarship at Pembroke College, Cambridge, he received his medical training as a clinical fellow at St. Thomas' Hospital. Peart adds

the interesting note that after qualification, Pickering temporarily served as house physician to Sir Maurice Cassidy who is remembered as being the first one to point out the relationship between carcinoidosis and right-sided valvular heart lesions[45].

Pickering's background in basic sciences and his interest in clinical medicine propelled him to seek scientific work in physiology. One of his teachers at Cambridge was responsible for his appointment as an assistant to Thomas Lewis at University College Medical School. Elliott, the proposer of the adrenalin hypothesis in sympathetic transmission, was chair of the department of medicine at the time. Despite the acerbic personality of Lewis, Pickering managed to stay with him long enough to realize the importance of accurate observation and the 'simplest possible type of experimentation'[45].

Pickering's early work was concerned with the mechanism of vasodilatation and vasoconstriction in the hands. This was no doubt due to the fact that Lewis was studying vascular changes in the skin at the time Pickering was associated with him. Later, Pickering showed that in most forms of arterial hypertension increased vascular resistance in the hand was not due to excessive sympathetic activity. In collaboration with Wayne he described the angina and intermittent claudication that was associated and therefore reversible. He was able to show that the headache following an injection of histamine was due to vasodilatation. The headache of high blood pressure was shown by him to be correlated with a high cerebrospinal fluid pressure only in the malignant phase of hypertension. Pickering's greatest achievement was probably his rediscovery of renin together with the American, Prinzmetal. This stimulated others to finally outline the renin–angiotensin–aldosterone concept that seems to be the key determinant in the development and maintenance of high blood pressure in most hypertensives.

In 1956 Pickering was appointed to the Regius chair of Oxford. During his tenure there, the department of medicine was oriented towards clinical research. His book on *High Blood Pressure* was the epitome of all knowledge on the subject up to that point in time.

Peart ends his testimonial to George Pickering with the words 'His most important contribution … was his ability to attract the young by his infectious enthusiasm'[45]. Isn't this true of all the great men, no matter what their discipline?

During the same year that Pickering and Landis reported their findings, and in the year immediately following, several centers reported their observations with renin, the rediscovered pressor substance. In 1938 Hessel proved with his method of preparation that renin actually existed[46]. The following year was notable in that independent workers from various parts of the globe were able to show that renin itself was only part of a more complex system that ultimately produced the active pressor principle which was finally identified and labeled angiotensin II.

In 1939, the Buenos Aires group led by Braun-Menendez, and Irwin Page with his team, independently showed that renin actually acted as an enzyme and that the substrate on which it acted was a plasma protein. This substrate was later identified and given the name angiotensinogen. Braun-Menendez called the resultant pressor substance produced from this reaction hypertensin while Page referred to it as angiotonin[47,48].

Irwin H. Page was an interesting personality to say the least. He was quite outspoken, often self-deprecating and endowed with a brilliant intellect who was able to keep in check any arrogance that was likely to surface from a brilliant mind by a unique, self-directed sense of humor. We owe a vivid sketch of his personality and a treasure trove of anecdotes about him to Nancy Hoffman. Her article appeared in the *Journal of the American Medical Association* in 1980[49].

Page began his work on hypertension while he was associated with the great van Slyke at the Rockefeller Institute. Page was assigned the task of studying kidney blood flow as part of van Slyke's studies in Bright's disease. How Page managed to become associated with van Slyke is, in itself, an interesting bit of trivia. Page was already well-known for his work in brain chemistry. It all started in 1928 when he was invited by the University of Munich to organize a new department in brain chemistry. In the process he managed to marry Beatrice Allen, a beautiful dancer.

It was while he was in Munich that Page's desire to meet van Slyke was suddenly realized. While visiting in Munich, van Slyke's daughter came down with an infected finger. Van Slyke prevailed upon Page to attend to this ailment. In Page's words, the telephone rang and this is what transpired:

A diffident voice said 'This is Donald van Slyke'.

For once in my life, I listened instead of talking. 'My daughter has an infection in her finger. I understand that you're the only resident American doctor here. I'd appreciate it if you'd come down to the hotel and take care of her finger'. Page said 'I can tell you this: no finger ever got better care. And that girl's finger is why we could go back to New York with a job, why I went to the Rockefeller Institute and the Rockefeller Hospital, why I went into cardiovascular disease'[50].

The year 1937 was a pivotal one for Page. He left van Slyke to become director of the Lilly Laboratory for Clinical Research at The Indianapolis City Hospital. His book on brain chemistry was published, only the second book on the subject since 1884. And lastly, in that year, he announced the first reversal of malignant hypertension. Three years later, Page announced with Helmer the discovery of angiotonin (later called angiotensin). Before several years passed, he also announced the discovery of serotonin in collaboration with Rupert and Green; and in a cooperative effort with McCubbin he demonstrated the role of the neuroendocrine system in producing hypertension.

In 1945, Page moved to Cleveland to become director of research at the Cleveland Clinic. All his efforts remained focused on the etiology of hypertension in the hope of finding a cure. Unfortunately, proper therapy was still an elusive goal. Later when reserpine was introduced as an antihypertensive agent this is what he had to say:

For instance, when reserpine came out, it seemed such a great antihypertensive that some wanted to provide it free to everybody who needed it. I argued, 'My Lord, you don't even know what reserpine can do to people'. At that time, we were prescribing 10 mg of reserpine and we were wondering why our patients were becoming parkinsonian. Now, the dose is 0.1 mg. If we had dosed the American public with 10 mg of reserpine, we would have had a bunch of zombies[51].

What is more important is the book he published at the age of 79 that outlines in depth his mosaic theory of hypertension. He began to conceptualize the theory during the fourth year of his tenure at the Cleveland Clinic. This is how he explained his mosaic theory to Nancy Hoffman:

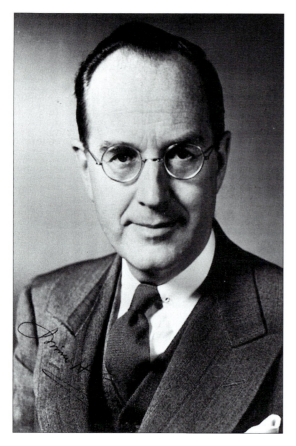

Figure 3 Irwin H. Page. *Photo Source National Library of Medicine. Literary Source Photo Archives. Courtesy of National Library of Medicine*

Gibb's Phase Rule states that, in any solution of mixed salts, if you increase the concentration of one salt, another salt changes its concentration. It's an equilibrated system ... I decided that the same rule applied to the body, that regulation of the blood perfusion system is equilibrated. You cannot alter any one of the regulatory mechanisms without affecting another ... I first talked about the mosaic theory in 1949. But people are reluctant to yield the comfortable notion of a single cause for anything[52].

Page's discovery of angiotonin excited the interest of two groups of workers. One was the group in his own backyard at Cleveland and the other consisted of Pickering and Peart from England. Skeggs, Kahn and Shumway, the Cleveland team, demonstrated that there were two types of 'hypertensin' (angiotensin) which they labeled I and II. This was in 1954[53]. Two years later, Peart, working in Pickering's laboratory at St. Mary's Hospital, also isolated two forms of 'hypertensin'[54]. Both groups demonstrated that 'hypertensin II' (angiotensin II) was the active principle and that it was derived from the inactive hypertensin I through an enzymatic reaction. The enzyme in this reaction is now known as angiotensin converting enzyme.

Further studies revealed that angiotensin is the most powerful pressor substance known, far exceeding the capability of epinephrine as a vasoconstrictor. It is this action that is responsible for its ability to raise the diastolic pressure more than the systolic. Angiotensin was also found to have several other physiological properties in man. It was found to decrease blood flow through the kidneys, lower the glomerular filtration rate, and act as a marked antidiuretic with a significant fall in output of sodium chloride. Figure 3 is a photograph of Page in his prime.

Two other outstanding figures remain to be considered in this historical background of hypertension. They are Harry Goldblatt (Figure 4) and John Laragh. These two played an important role in developing renin–angiotensin blockade as a mode of therapy in hypertension, and more recently in congestive heart failure.

We have already seen Goldblatt's significant contributions regarding reduced renal blood and the development of hypertension. Goldblatt attributed the rise in blood pressure in the experimental animal to excessive secretion of renin.

Most of us were brought up in the school that every disease has to have a cause, and that cause is single, not multiple. Well within 20 years of its beginnings, around 1930, hypertension research was a shambles. One school blamed the kidney. Others indicted the adrenals. Somebody else said, 'No, it's the brain'. The more I thought about it, the more it seemed to me that while we all were looking for a single cause, the body isn't as stupid as we were. The function of blood pressure is to distribute blood equitably throughout the whole body, responding fairly to each organ's demands ... It occurred to me that the body has a variety of mechanisms that regulate these functions. To perform properly, each mechanism has to be in synchrony with all the others. Otherwise, it's like a big communication system with no Central ...

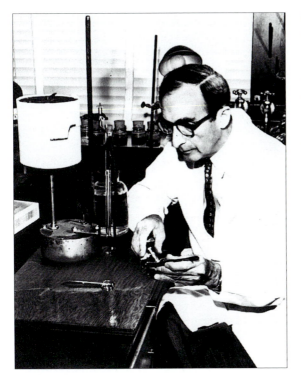

Figure 4 Harry Goldblatt. *Photo Source National Library of Medicine. Literary Source Photo Archives. Courtesy of National Library of Medicine*

He felt that the same mechanism prevailed in human essential hypertension; the ischemia brought about through many micro-occlusions of the arteriolar vessels secondary to nephrosclerosis. In his view, then, the kidney was always the initiating factor[55].

Goldblatt spent most of his later career pursuing this idea. At one point he attempted to treat essential hypertension by nullifying the metabolic activity of renin with antibodies induced by passive immunization. This approach fell into disfavor because of variable results and inability on the part of others to confirm his findings[56]. Specific anti-renin therapy also lost its allure until more knowledge was gained regarding the renin–angiotensin system. The immune approach was recently resurrected at the meeting of the American Society of Hypertension in New York City during the summer of 1990. A report was presented by Dr R. S. Tuttle, bolstered by considerable experimental evidence, suggesting that the immune system figures in the etiology and/or prevention of hypertension. He suggested further that the basic link between the immune system and hypertension may involve the beta receptor.

In 1972, John Laragh and his group at Cornell were able to show that sustained elevation of blood pressure required an interplay among renin, angiotensin and aldosterone[57]. Laragh's group then found that patients with malignant hypertension were saddled with markedly high levels of aldosterone and that this was secondary to marked oversecretion of renin[57–62]. These observations created a reawakening of interest in the role of renin and the possibility was again entertained that the blocking of renin secretion could form the basis for an effective therapeutic approach[63].

The study by Laragh's group with propranolol (a beta-adrenergic blocking agent) demonstrated that this drug does lower plasma renin levels in normal subjects. This finding appeared to support the view that in some cases, renin did indeed play an important role. They went on to show that the blood pressure was effectively lowered in those individuals that manifested high or moderately increased levels of renin in their blood stream. In 1976, Laragh's group showed that beta-blockers do not lower the blood pressure in animals or humans without kidneys[64]. In fact, many times they raised the blood pressure.

These findings, of course, did not resolve the issue as to renin's role in all cases of essential hypertension. Other pathways had to be found to explain the elevated blood pressure in the low-renin form of essential hypertension. John Laragh expressed it well when he commented on 'The basic heterogeneity of so-called essential hypertension'. This is similar to Page's mosaic theory, but, in reality, Laragh still thought that renin was an all-important factor.

In order to verify the importance of renin as suggested by the beta blockade, Laragh's group realized that 'a pharmacologic probe was needed with an unchallenged anti-renin action but also without agonist properties that might dilute the results'[65]. This path would eventually lead to a major breakthrough in the treatment of hypertension – the converting enzyme inhibitor.

Snake venom was the unlikely source for this inhibitor. Sergio Ferreira was the first to isolate a mixture of peptides from the venom of a Brazilian snake, *Bothrops jararaca*, in 1965[66]. Two years later he and Vane showed that some of the peptides could inhibit the pulmonary enzyme that normally

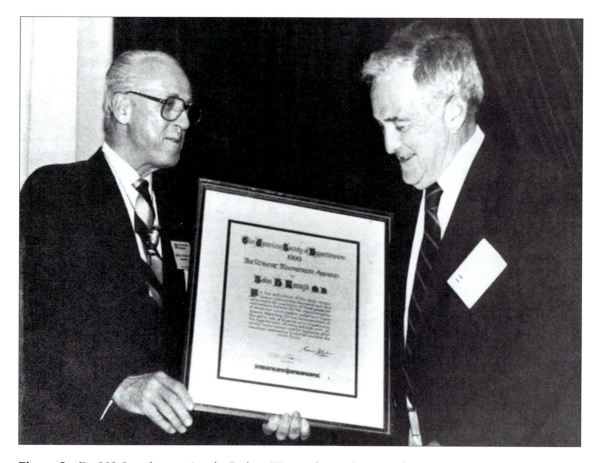

Figure 5 Dr. J.H. Laragh accepting the Robert Tigerstedt award citation from Dr. E.G. Biglieri, President of the American Society of Hypertension. *Photo Source American Society of Hypertension. Literary Source ASH News, vol. 4, no. 2, summer, 1990. With permission from American Society of Hypertension*

degrades bradykinin[67]. That same year Vane, now working with Ng, was able to report that these same peptides from snake venom would also block the conversion of angiotensin I to angiotensin II[68]. This opportunity could not be ignored. Laragh and his associates began an intensive investigation with this product in 89 patients that took all of three years. These investigations, along with evidence already obtained with beta-blockers and saralasin (also a renin system antagonist) led Laragh to state 'the three converging lines of evidence made it virtually incontrovertible that renin activity plays a major sustaining role in the hypertension of most patients with essential hypertension'[65].

Encouraged by these clinical trials, Cushman and Ondetti, two scientist working at the Squibb Institute, lent their talents to developing an orally active converting enzyme inhibitor based on these snake venom peptides. This they did with their successful synthesis of captopril[69,70]. The value of this drug lies both in its specificity of action and in its practical attributes. It prevents the formation of angiotensin II. If the patient's blood pressure does not fall then the attending physician can deduce that he is dealing with a low-renin sodium–volume form of hypertension. On the other hand, if a marked drop in blood pressure occurs the physician is alerted to the presence of a renin factor with the implication that he should now look for a curable renovascular disease. Moreover, the added clinical value of this type of agent lies in its ability to lower blood pressure while at the same time increasing blood flow to the heart, brain and kidneys, an extremely important consideration[71].

John Laragh was the recipient of the Robert Tigerstedt Award from the American Society of Hypertension in 1990 (see Figure 5). The Award cited him 'for his definition of the renin–angiotensin–aldosterone hormonal axis as a servocontrol for regulation of blood pressure (BP) and sodium balance, for his characterization of renin system patterns in hypertensive disorders, for his demonstration of the active participation of plasma renin in many patients with essential hypertension and for developing pharmacologic approaches, i.e. beta blockers and angiotensin converting-enzyme (ACE) inhibitors to identify and treat the renin factor.'

In his Award Lecture, Dr Laragh reviewed the discovery and evolution of the renin–angiotensin–aldosterone axis as a key determinant in the causation and maintenance of high blood pressure in most hypertensives.

Renin profiling, Dr Laragh pointed out, 'reveals two long-term mechanisms of arteriolar vasoconstriction'. One is directly related to plasma renin level; the other, which is induced by sodium retention, is inversely related to plasma renin. At one extreme, high renin vasoconstriction entails malignant hypertension, which leads to renal, cardiac and cerebrovascular disease and early death. At the opposite end of the spectrum, low renin vasoconstriction is typified by primary aldosteronism, which is a benign condition with few vascular complications.

Identification of these renin related patterns, Dr Laragh noted, led to the study of the possible relationship between renin and ischemic vascular damage in hypertension. These studies showed, he said, that 'low renin patients, despite higher pressures and greater age, were impressively protected from stroke and heart attack'[72].

John Laragh graduated from Cornell Medical College. After completing his postgraduate work at Columbia Presbyterian, he remained there to become chief of the Nephrology Division and Hypertension-Nephritis Clinic, and director of the Clinic Research Center. He returned to his alma mater in 1975 as chief of the division of cardiology and director of the Cardiovascular Center. Laragh was the first president of the American Society of Hypertension. At this writing he is editor-in-chief of the *American Journal of Hypertension*.

How do all these findings in experimental hypertension and clinical research fit in with the mechanisms of high blood pressure in man? Is the kidney really responsible all the time or does it play a major role only in some cases? One thing appears to be certain, namely, that increased total peripheral resistance due to vascular narrowing is a major mechanism for elevating the blood pressure in essential hypertension. The various pathways of how this can come about have been outlined in this brief historical survey. It is now evident that in persistent hypertension the ordinary nervous control of the distribution of blood is superimposed on a fairly general increase in vascular resistance.

Pickering suggested that in man the mechanisms that could be responsible in acute nephritis involve a pressor substance and that in chronic nephritis or essential hypertension there is evidence of vascular narrowing of non-nervous origin. The concepts that led to the formulation of the renin–angiotensin–aldosterone have certainly clarified matters a great deal. But this is not the final answer. Probably, the mosaic theory of Page will prevail as further studies uncover other pathways. An important factor to be considered is the genetic one. The first epidemiological studies on this aspect were conducted by Wilhelm Weitz from Tübingen. His report appeared in 1923[73]. Although small in numbers, it was a carefully controlled study limited to local inhabitants. In his series, inheritance appeared as the only identifiable factor.

REFERENCES

1. Bright, R. (1827). *Reports of Medical Cases Selected with a View of Illustrating the Symptoms and Cure of Diseases by a Reference to Morbid Anatomy*, 2 vols. (London: Longman)

2. Bright, R. (1836). Tabular view of the morbid appearances in 100 cases of hypertension connected with albuminous urine. With observations. *Guy's Hosp. Rep.*, **1**, 380

3. Johnson, G. (1868). I. On certain points in the anatomy and pathology of Bright's disease of the kidney. II. On the influence of the minute blood vessels upon the circulation. *Med-Chir. Trans.*, **51**, 57

4. Gull, W.W. and Sutton, H.G. (1872). On the pathology of the morbid state commonly called chronic Bright's disease with contracted kidney ('Arterio-capillary fibrosis') *Med-Chir. Trans.*, **55**, 273

5. Hale-White, W. (1921). Richard Bright and his

discovery of the disease bearing his name. *Guy's Hosp. Rep.*, **1**, 1

6. Bartels, C. (1877). Structural diseases of the kidney and the general symptoms of renal infection. In von Ziemssen, H. (ed.) *Cyclopaedia of the Practice of Medicine*, tr. by R. Southey and R. Bertolet, vol. 15, p. 3. (London: Sampson Low)

7. Ewald, C.A. (1877). Ueber die Veränderungen kleiner Gefässe bei Morbus Brightii und die darauf bezüchen Theorien. *Virchows Arch. Path. Anat.*, **71**, 453

8. Jores, L. (1904). Ueber die Arteriosklerose der kleinen Organarterien und ihre Beziehungen zur Nephritis. *Virchows Arch. Path. Anat.*, **178**, 367

9. Gordon, D.B. (1970). Some early investigations of experimental hypertension. *Texas Rep. Biol. Med.*, **28**, 3

10. Leyden, E. (1881). Klinische Untersuchugen über Morbus Brightii. Ueber Nierenschrumpfung und Nierensklerose. *Z. Klin. Med.*, **2**, 133–71

11. Traube, L. (1871). Ueber den Zusammenhang von Herz-und Nieren-Krankheiten. In Gesammelte Beitraege zur Pathologie und Physiologie (Collected Contributions to Pathology and Physiology) vol. II: Part 1, *Clinical Investigations*, pp. 290–353. (Berlin: A. Hirschwald)

12. *Ibid.*

13. Comroe, J.H. Jr. (1983). *Exploring the Heart: Discoveries in Heart Disease and High Blood Pressure*, p. 229. (New York: W.W. Norton & Co.)

14. Lewinski, L. (1880). Ueber den Zusammenhang zwischen Nierenschrumpfung und Herzhypertrophie. *Z. Klin. Med.*, **1**, 561–582

15. Mahomed, F.A. (1872). The physiology and clinical use of the sphygmograph. *Med. Times & Gaz.*, **1**, 62

16. Pickering, G. (1982). Systemic arterial hypertension. In Fishman, A.P and Richards, D.W. (eds.) *Circulation of the Blood, Men and Ideas*, p. 499. (Baltimore Md.: Waverly Press, Inc.)

17. Mahomed, F.A. (1877). 3. On the sphygmographic evidence of arteriocapillary fibrosis. *Trans. Path. Soc.*, **28**, 394

18. Mahomed, F.A. (1879). On chronic Bright's disease, and its essential symptoms. *Lancet*, **I**, 46

19. Mahomed, F.A. (1879). Some of the clinical aspects of chronic Bright's disease. *Guy's Hosp. Rep.*, 3rd. ser., **24**, 363

20. Huchard, H. (1889). *Maladies du Coeur et des Vaisseaux*. (Paris: Doin)

21. von Basch, S. (1893). *Ueber latente Arteriosklerose und deren Beziehung zu Fettleibigkeit, Herzerkrankungen und anderen Begleiterscheinungen.* (Vienna: Urban and Schwartzenberg)

22. Albutt, T.C. (1895). Senile plethora or high arterial pressure in elderly persons. *Abstr. Trans. Hunter. Soc.*, **77**, 38

23. Albutt, T.C. (1915). *Diseases of the Arteries Including Angina Pectoris.* (London: Macmillan)

24. Janeway, T.C. (1913). A clinical study of hypertensive cardiovascular disease. *Arch. Intern. Med.*, **12**, 755

25. Volhard, P. (1931). Nieren und ableitende Harnwege. In von Bergmann, G. and Staehelin, R. (eds.) *Handbuch der innerin Medizin*, vol. 6, part 1. (Berlin: Springer)

26. Comroe, J. (1983). *Op. cit.*, p. 230

27. von Graefe, A. (1854–55). Nachträgliche Bemerhung über Sclerotico-chorioideitis posterior. *Albrecht V. Graefes Arch. Ophthal.*, **1** (2. Abt.), 307

28. Liebreich, R. (1859). Ophthalmoskopischer Befund bei Morbus Brightii V. *Graefes Arch. Ophthalm.*, **5**, 265

29. Volhard, F. and Fahr, T. (1914). Die Brightsche Nierenkrankheit. *Klinik, Pathologie und Atlas.* (Berlin: Springer)

30. Koch, E. and Mies, H. (1929). Chronischer arterieller Hochdruck durch experimentelle Dauer ausschaltung der Blutdruckzügler. *Krankheitsforschung*, **7**, 241

31. Heymans, C. and Bouckaert, J.J. (1934). Modifications de la pression artérielle après section des quatre nerfs frénateurs chez le chien. *C.R. Soc. Biol.(Paris)*, **117**, 252

32. Gammon, G.D. (1936). The carotid sinus reflex in patients with hypertension. *J. Clin. Invest.*, **15**, 153

33. Pickering, G.W., Kissin, M. and Rothschild, P. (1936). The relationship of the carotid sinus mechanism in persistent high blood pressure in man. *Clin. Sci.*, **2**, 193

34. Pickering, G.W. (1942). The relationship of benign and malignant hypertension. *J. Mt. Sinai Hosp.*, **8**, 916

35. Goldblatt, H. (1947). The renal origin of hypertension. *Physiol. Rev.*, **27**, 120

36. Moritz, A.R. and Oldt, M.R. (1937). Arteriolar sclerosis in hypertensive and non-hypertensive individuals. *Am. J. Pathol.*, **13**, 679

37. Blalock, A. and Levy, S.E. (1937). Studies on the etiology of renal hypertension. *Ann. Surg.*, **106**, 826

38. Heymans, C., Bouchaert, J.J., Elaut, L., Bayless, F. and Samaan, A. (1937). Hypertension artérielle chronique par ischémie rénale chez le chien totalement sympathectomisé. *C.R. Biol. (Paris)*, **126**, 434

39. Alpert, L.K., Alving, A.S. and Grimson, K.S. (1937). Effect of total sympathectomy on experimental renal hypertension in dogs. *Proc. Soc. Exp. Biol.*, **37**, 1

40. Freeman, N.E. and Page, I.H. (1937). Hypertension produced by constriction of the renal artery in sympathectomized dogs. *Am. Heart J.*, **14**, 405

41. Pickering, G.W. and Kissin, M. (1936). The effects of adrenaline and of cold on the blood pressure in human hypertension. *Clin. Sci.*, **2**, 201

42. Landis, E.M., Montgomery, H. and Sparkman, D. (1938). The effects of pressor drugs and of saline kidney extracts on blood pressure and skin temperature. *J. Clin. Invest.*, **17**, 189

43. Bingel, A. and Claus, R. (1910). Weitere Untersuchungen über die blutdrucksteigernde Substanz der Niere. *Dtsch. Arch. Klin. Med.*, **100**, 412

44. Bingel, A. and Strauss, E. (1909). Ueber die blutdrucksteigende Substanz der Niere. *Dtsch. Arch. Klin. Med.*, **96**, 476

45. Peart, W.S. (1984). Sir George Pickering (1904–1982). *Clin. Sci.*, **67**, 15–8

46. Hessel, G. (1938). Über Renin. *Klin. Wschr.*, **17**, 843

47. Braun-Menendez, E., Fasciolo, J.C., Leloir, L.F. and Muñoz, J.M. (1939). La substancia hipertensora de la sangre del rinon isquemiado. *Rev. Soc. Argent. Biol.*, **15**, 420

48. Page, I.H. and Helmer, O.M. (1940). A crystalline pressor substance (angiotonin) resulting from the reaction between renin and renin-activator. *J. Exp. Med.*, **71**, 29

49. Hoffman, N., Irvin, H. and Page, M.D. (1980). Not one man, but many. *J. Am. Med. Assoc.*, **244**, 1765

50. *Ibid.*, p. 1766

51. *Ibid.*, p. 1766

52. *Ibid.*, pp. 1766–7

53. Skeggs, L. Jr, Marsh, W.H., Kahn, J.R. and Shumway, N.P. (1954). The existence of two forms of hypertensin. *J. Exp. Med.*, **99**, 275

54. Peart, W.S. (1956). The isolation of a hypertensin. *Biochem. J.*, **62**, 520

55. Goldblatt, H.J., Lunch, R.F., Hanzal, R.F. *et al.* (1934). Studies on experimental hypertension. Production of persistent elevation of systolic blood pressure by means of renal ischemia. *J. Exp. Med.*, **49**, 347–79

56. Page, I.H. and McCubbin, J.W. (1968). *Renal Hypertension.* (Chicago: Year Book Medical Publishers)

57. Laragh, J.H., Baer, L., Brunner, H.R., Bühler, F.R., Sealey, J.E. and Vaughan, E.D. Jr (1972). Renin, angiotensin and aldosterone system in pathogenesis and management of hypertensive vascular disease. *Am. J. Med.*, **52**, 644–52

58. Laragh, J.H., Ulick, S., Januszewicz, V., Deming, Q.B., Kelly, W.G. and Lieberman, S. (1960). Aldosterone secretion and primary and malignant hypertension. *J. Clin. Invest.*, **39**, 1091–106

59. Laragh, J.H., Angers, M., Kelley, W.G. and Lieberman, S.L. (1960). Hypotensive agents and pressor substances. The effect of epinephrine, norepinephrine, angiotensin II and others on the secretory rate of aldosterone in man. *J. Am. Med. Assoc.*, **174**, 234–40

60. Laragh, J.H. (1960). The role of aldosterone in man: evidence for regulation of electrolyte balance and arterial pressure by renal-adrenal system which may be involved in malignant hypertension. *J. Am. Med. Assoc.*, **174**, 293–5

61. Vaughan, E.D. Jr, Bühler, F.R., Laragh, J.H., Sealey, J.E., Baer, L. and Bard, R.H. (1973). Renovascular hypertension; renin measurements to indicate hypersecretion and contralateral suppression, estimate renal plasma flow and score for surgical curability. *Am. J. Med.*, **55**, 402–14

62. Sealey, J.E., Bühler, F.R., Laragh, J.H. and Vaughan, E.D. Jr (1973). The physiology of renin secretion in essential hypertension: estimation of renin secretion rate and renal plasma flow from peripheral and renal vein renin levels. *Am. J. Med.*, **55**, 391–401

63. Bühler, F.R., Laragh, J.H., Baer, L., Vaughan, E.D. Jr and Brunner, H.R. (1972). Propranolol inhibition of renin secretion. A specific approach to diagnosis and treatment of renin-dependent hypertensive diseases. *N. Engl. J. Med.*, **287**, 1209–14

64. Drayer, J.I.M., Keim, J.H., Weber, M.A., Case, D.B. and Laragh, J.H. (1976). Unexpected pressor responses to propranolol in essential hypertension. *Am. J. Med.*, **60**, 897–903

65. Laragh, J.H. (1984). Concept of anti-renin system therapy. Historic perspective. *Am. J. Med.*, pp. 1–6 (Aug. 20)

66. Ferreira, S.H. (1965). A bradykinin-

potentiating factor (BPF) present in the venom of Bothrops jararaca. *Br. J. Pharmacol. Chemother.*, **24**, 164–9

67. Ferreira, S.H. and Vane, J.R. (1967). The disappearance of bradykinin and eledoisin in the circulation and vascular beds of the cat. *Br. J. Chemother.*, **30**, 417–24

68. Ng, K.K.F. and Vane, J.R. (1967). Conversion of angiotensin I to angiotensin II. *Nature (London)*, **215**, 762–6

69. Ondetti, M.S., Williams, N.J., Sabo, E.F., Pluscec, J., Weaver, E.R. and Kocy, O. (1971). Angiotensin-converting enzyme inhibitors from the venom of Bothrops jararaca: isolation, elucidation of structure and synthesis. *Biochemistry*, **10**, 4033–9

70. Ondetti, M.A., Rubin, B. and Cushman, D.W. (1977). Design of specific inhibitors of angiotensin-converting enzyme. New class of orally effective antihypertensive agents. *Science*, **196**, 441–4

71. Rajagopalen, B., Raine, A.E.G., Cooper, R. and Ledingham, J.G.G. (1984). Changes in cerebral blood flow in patients with severe congestive cardiac failure before and after captopril treatment. *Am. J. Med.*, **76**(5B), 86–91

72. *American Society of Hypertension News*, vol. 4, no. 2, p. 3, summer 1990

73. Weitz, W. (1923). Zur Äteliogie der genuinen oder vasculären Hypertension. *Z. klin. Med.*, **96**, 151

20   Electrophysiologic disturbances

The earliest observations of disturbances of cardiac rhythm were made by feeling the pulse and much later by observing the heart beat with the naked eye. Section 5 deals with the evolution of sphygmology and its impact on the detection of arrhythmia; an impact which was minimal in our understanding of electrophysiologic disturbances.

There are two generic terms that indicate a disturbance in rhythm. The oldest one is 'arrhythmia' and the most recent is 'dysrhythmia'. Rudolph Heidenhain introduced arrhythmia as the designation for any disturbance of cardiac rhythm in 1872[1]. Dysrhythmia was introduced as a synonymous term for changes in either rate or rhythm, but the word arrhythmia seems to be more firmly entrenched.

Currently, electrophysiologic disturbances deal essentially with abnormalities of rate, rhythm and conduction of impulses. The introduction of the electrocardiogram was the technological innovation that initiated the development of our knowledge concerning arrhythmias and conduction disturbances. The advent of cardiac electrophysiological techniques proved to be a singularly instrumental factor in broadening our knowledge of the underlying electrophysiologic mechanisms for rhythm and conduction aberrations. The evolution of the bioelectric mechanisms was presented in Section 3.

Sir Thomas Lewis was at the forefront in defining most of the arrhythmias on a clinical level. His electrocardiographic observations were extensive and definitive[2,3]. The importance of his contribution in the clinical identification and classification of arrhythmias cannot be overemphasized. It was monumental to say the least. The electrophysiologic basis for these arrhythmias was a different matter, evolving in the hands of a number of investigators. Among the earliest were Alfred Cushny and Alfred Goodman Levy. Cushny was engaged in the experimental production of arrhythmia while Levy was involved in devising a chloroform inhaler so as to minimize chloroform's

arrhythmogenic potentialities[4]. All these individuals were members of the staff at University College Hospital with each one benefiting from the mutual intellectual stimulation and a free interchange of ideas. An example of this was the collaborative effort of Lewis and Levy on disturbances of rhythm induced by chloroform[5]. In the belief that chloroform induced ventricular tachycardia and that fibrillation was dose dependent, it was this work that led Levy to devise an inhaler that reduced the amount of chloroform delivered while maintaining an adequate level of anesthesia. University College was enjoying a rather prestigious image at the time due to the productivity and brilliance of so many of its faculty.

The meticulous and analytical approach of Lewis helped put the electrocardiographic interpretation of a number of arrhythmias on a rather firm basis and resulted in stimulating interest in this modality from various parts of the world. Many of the more notable American cardiologists of the era came under his tutelage. Among them were Alfred Einstein Cohn, Paul D. White, and Francis R. Fraser, a triumvirate of master teachers who left behind them a whole cadre of great cardiologists. Cohn brought the first string galvanometer to the United States[6]. White's impact on American cardiology left a lasting impression, and we shall meet with his numerous contributions throughout this text. Fraser did much of his early work on digitalis. He collaborated with Cohn not only on this but also in publishing a seminal paper on paroxysmal tachycardia and vagal stimulation[7]. Although they did not know it at the time they were the first to describe a patient with paroxysmal episodes of supraventricular tachycardia due to pre-excitation[8].

It can be said with a definite degree of certainty, and, as we shall see later, with even more assurance, that Britain set the stage by defining the clinical spectrum of the major arrhythmias. Her physiologists also acted as catalysts by stimulating her American counterparts in unraveling many of the electro-physiologic mechanisms. Lewis, Mackenzie, Cushny, Levy and Gaskell are but a few of the giants that led the way. In America Louis Nelson Katz, aided by European emigrés, including Richard Langendorf and Alfred Pick, made significant fundamental advances.

The introduction of cardiac electrophysiologic studies was the spark that produced even more important advances, not only in a better under-standing of the mechanisms but also in providing the means for interventional therapeutic techniques. Intracardiac electrophysiologic techniques began when Lenègre and Maurice first reported the recording of electrical activity from the cardiac chambers in man[9]. Their work was carried out during World War II but was not reported until 1945. It was strictly an experimental exercise on their part. Little did they realize what an avalanche of clinical studies it would create; so much so that, in its evolution over the next five decades, cardiac electrophysiology would acquire the status of a discipline within modern cardiology. Several technical difficulties had to be surmounted, however, before this technique could be made available to clinicians. Battro and Bidoggia, Sodi-Pollares, and Hecht helped in this regard by modifying and refining the original method, all within three years of the original report[10–12]. At first the technique was limited to the right heart. Subsequently Levine, Sodi-Pollares, and Sealy's group extended its application to recordings from the coronary sinus and left cardiac chambers[13,14]. Complex cardiac rhythm disturbances were then subjected to scrutiny. Kossman and his co-workers obtained electrograms in atrial flutter, atrial tachycardia, and atrial fibrillation[15]. During the same time, Torner Soler's group also studied in man the electrophysiologic nature of atrial fibrillation[16]. The electrical activity of the His bundle was recorded for the first time by Alanis, Gonzalez and Lopez in 1958[17]. The isolated heart of the dog was their model. The first attempt to record His bundle activity in man occurred in 1959. Brian Hoffman and his group localized the bundle of His with a surface electrode during cardiotomy[18]. Giraud, Puech, and Latour were the first to use an electrode catheter in man[19]. The pioneering efforts of Scherlag were responsible, however, for popul-arizing the method which in a short span of time led to its widespread acceptance and use[20].

Benjamin Scherlag was a postdoctoral fellow in Hoffman's laboratory at Columbia University when he started his epic journey that led to the development of the His bundle recording technique. He was assigned a project that required the induction of permanent heart block in the anesthetized dog. In an effort to overcome the limited time window for blocking the His bundle area by incision or injection of formalin, Scherlag used the approach devised by Pruitt and Essex[21]. This utilized the AV node as a guide, and after much trial and error he succeeded in developing a technique for formaldehyde injection of the His bundle area through the atrial wall without an atriotomy[22].

Scherlag continued to be interested on the subject when he transferred to Anthony Damato's laboratory at the Staten Island Public Health Service Hospital. Damato gave young Scherlag his unstinting support and provided him with a dog laboratory all his own. Scherlag now abandoned the formaldehyde injection in favor of what he termed the plunge wire technique. He impaled the His bundle area with two teflon coated stainless steel wires to obtain his recordings. The idea came to him from reading the reports of Scher, Alanis, and Sodi-Pollares[17,23,24]. After some practice he was able to get consistently good results. Two things were accomplished with this technique. He was able to record the His bundle activity, and at the same time perform ventricular pacing from the same site with a normal ventricular activation pattern. The electrical activity of the His bundle could now be mapped contrary to the pessimism of Wilhelm His Jr who did not believe that cardiac catheterization could be the means for doing so[25].

The plunge wire electrode was replaced with a 12 pole electrode catheter designed by John Lister, Scherlag's colleague at the hospital. Lister originally used it for exploring the right heart. In time, this catheter minus many of its 12 rings, provided Scherlag with consistently good recordings of the His bundle merely by placing it at the AV junction in the right heart[26]. Richard Helfant, a clinical colleague, suggested to Scherlag that the standard NBIH 5–7 French electrode might work even better than Lister's device. This proved to be an excellent suggestion and with a little bit of practice Scherlag found he could place the catheter tip at the AV junction with the utmost ease. Scherlag used the femoral vein approach, advancing the electrode tip without the aid of fluoroscopy, relying solely on the electrographic recordings for guidance. The word soon got around at the hospital that Scherlag was on to something 'hot', and in short order, several colleagues translated their interest into collaborative research projects.

The femoral approach was apparently critical in obtaining favorable recordings. Entry through the antecubital vein made it rather difficult to position the catheter at the AV junction. According to Scherlag this was probably why Watson and his group failed to obtain consistently good recordings[22].

The collaborative efforts of Scherlag and his colleagues at the Staten Island facility were focused on characterizing AV nodal and His–Purkinje function during atrial pacing in all forms of heart block and in the Wolff–Parkinson–White (WPW) syndrome. Scherlag recounts in his historical survey how three papers resulted from these studies and how Howard Burchell (at that time, editor of *Circulation*), apologetically overrode the highly critical and negative comments of his reviewers and accepted two of the three manuscripts for publication. One was not accepted because it was more of a case report rather than a true research project and therefore did not meet the criteria for publication in *Circulation*. In Scherlag's words: 'Dr. Burchell prophetically indicated that, contrary to the several reviewers' comments, he believed the paper describing the His bundle recording technique would become a 'standard reference'[23].

Indeed, His bundle recording was a major impetus in the maturation of clinical cardiac electrophysiology. The significance and mechanism of AV conduction disturbances were clarified because of the ease and accuracy in obtaining His bundle electrograms. These brought to light such physiologic phenomena as concealed conduction, concealed His bundle depolarization, concealed transseptal activation and the pre-excitation syndromes.

Scherlag's group was also instrumental in furthering the clinical use of this new method for studying arrhythmias[27]. Independent studies of arrhythmias with the technique were also conducted by Coumel and Puech[28,29]. The technique was then expanded to record electrical activity from the sinus node and accessory AV pathways[30–32]. In 1980 Reiffel and his associates used a transvenous catheter technique to record sinus node electrograms and compared directly measured and indirectly estimated sinoatrial conduction time in adults[30]. By using direct endocardial recordings they localized the site of the block, evaluated the effect of anti-arrhythmic drugs, and also attempted a cure with non-surgical ablation. This was a rather imposing feat.

The disturbed electrical activity in areas of myocardial infarction was another accomplishment. Led by Josephson and Horowitz, the group from Philadelphia was looking for a mechanism of recurrent ventricular tachycardia following a myocardial infarction[33]. Invasive electrophysiologic studies have confirmed much of what was learned about arrhythmias from deductive analysis[34].

Another major impetus in the development of clinical cardiac electrophysiology was the introduction of programmed electrical stimulation. A means was now at hand for testing the concepts of automaticity and re-entry, and also for the management of several types of disturbed rhythm. We are indebted to the genius of Dirk Durrer for this significant breakthrough in methodology.

Dirk Durrer should be considered as one of the major founders of modern electrocardiology. He has also been labeled as the godfather of Dutch cardiology. He was mainly responsible for making Amsterdam a mecca of study and research in cardiology. His creation of the Netherlands Interuniversity Institute of Cardiology was one of the highlights of his amazingly productive career.

Durrer's zest and enthusiasm were contagious. His ideas were described by Meijler, one of his pupils, as 'unexpected and full of brand-new logic and beauty'[35]. He could be imperious and caustic when the quality of work was not up to his standards. Others accused him of arriving at judgements too rapidly[36]. But how can anyone fault him when it is realized that he helped shape modern electrocardiology with his work on total excitation of the human heart, the calcium paradox, postextrasystolic potentiation, epicardial and intramural excitation in acute and old myocardial infarction in the dog, and the jewel of them all, programmed electrical stimulation.

Durrer believed firmly in the multidisciplinary approach. His collaborators included surgeons, pathologists, engineers, medical physicists, cell biologists, and a host of other specialists from different disciplines. 'If you don't have the brains yourselves, hire them'[37]. He was fortunate, especially, in having established early in his career a close working relationship with Prof. L.H. van der Tweel of the Department of Medical Physics.

Durrer's earliest work was on the spread of activation in the left ventricular wall of the dog. His collaborator was Prof. van der Tweel. The results were published in 1953[38]. The two of them devised a multi-terminal intramural needle that transformed empirical electrocardiography into a 'quantitative and predictive clinical discipline'[39]. The needle had two small electrodes in close proximity to each other. When the needle is inserted into the epicardial or intramural portion of the ventricle, an electrical signal from the closely spatially related electrodes results in a differential spike that occurs at the beginning of the fast portion of the intrinsic deflection of the unipolar lead. This is proof of the fact that the intrinsic deflection in unipolar leads is due to the passage of the excitation front under that particular lead. Knowledge obtained with the aid of this multi-electrode needle, and observations over a period of 18 years enabled him to publish the classic paper on the total excitation of the isolated revived human heart[40]. In addition, the Durrer needle, as it came to be known, was pressed into service during the 1950s as a stimulating device. Several important papers resulted from its use in this role[41,42]. Conduction velocity and duration of refractory period are the two key elements for the initiation and perpetuation of re-entry, and the Durrer needle had the capacity to unravel this activation sequence. It is still used today during operations on patients with intractable tachycardia to document spread of activation in the ventricular wall when pre-excitation is the culprit. The activation map then serves as a landmark for the surgeon in ablating the anomalous atrioventricular pathway.

The Wilhelmina Gasthuis in Amsterdam became a beehive of research in electrocardiology during the 1960s. The whole range of impulse formation and conduction came under investigation, all under the direction of Dirk Durrer.

A number of studies were begun on re-entry and ventricular arrhythmias in local ischemia and infarction in the intact dog heart[43]. Durrer's group was able repeatedly to reproduce ventricular fibrillation by applying two premature stimuli to the surviving tissue within the infarct. They found that the induction of fibrillation depended on the site of stimulation and the coupling intervals of the premature stimuli. Once the fibrillation was

established, in order to prove that re-entry was the perpetuating mechanism, they needed simultaneous recordings from as many sites as possible. This led them to develop multiplexing systems so that as many as 128 sites could be recorded simultaneously. The conclusion derived from observations with this technique was that re-entry was indeed responsible for ventricular tachycardia and fibrillation, occurring spontaneously during the first 10 minutes of myocardial ischemia[44]. Janse was the leading author of the paper documenting this conclusion.

A well-known pathologist was also smitten during his formative years with Durrer's obsession for elucidating the mechanisms of the pre-excitation syndrome. He was Anton Becker. He provided the anatomical support along with Anderson of England for a clinicopathologic correlation in seven patients with the WPW syndrome. The other two collaborators were Durrer and Wellens; another example of Durrer's multidisciplinary approach. These four men proved unequivocally that the anatomical accessory pathways were functionally significant[45]. Sealy and Gallagher of Duke University were also delineating at the same time the gross anatomy of the Kent bundle with the purpose of developing a surgical approach for ablation of the accessory pathway[46,47]. Becker then, in collaboration with the British pathologist, Anderson, focused his attention on the anatomical features of the AV node and His bundle and their relationship to pre-excitation[48]. Both men proposed on the basis of this work a new nomenclature for the various anatomical substrates[49]. Becker, incidentally, brought out in his *Salute to Dirk Durrer* that his mentor had quite an outspoken view on one of the substrates, the 'Mahaim fibers'. Durrer quite flatly said that the Mahaim fibers had no functional significance[50].

The continuing collaboration between Durrer and the medical physics faculty resulted in the development of an apparatus capable of stimulating the heart and recording the resultant electrical activity. It was built by Mr Leo Schoo of the Department of Medical Physics. Durrer began to work with it in 1966. The apparatus was capable of delivering three electrical impulses, separately or combined, and varying in strength and duration. The interval between impulses could also be chosen within an accuracy of 1 ms.

The first studies were done on patients with WPW syndrome. De Boer and Holzman, and

Scherf had already developed the concept of a re-entry mechanism for the recurrent tachyarrhythmias of this syndrome, reasoning that reentry was possible because of an accessory pathway of conduction with a different conduction time from the normal pathway. The chance to prove this presented itself in 1966. The patient was undergoing surgery for an atrial septal defect. He also had the WPW syndrome. Durrer demonstrated with epicardial mapping that the accessory AV pathway was responsible for early activation of the right ventricle. Through programmed electrical stimulation Durrer was then able to show differences in conduction time between the normal and accessory AV pathways[51,52].

That same year Wellens and another young cardiologist used the same approach in another patient with WPW syndrome, proving again that the two AV pathways had different electrophysiologic properties. Wellens, at that time an assistant in Durrer's laboratory, was to mature later into one of the brighter stars of Durrer's firmament.

> ... Dr. Reinier Schuilenburg and myself [Wellens] positioned a stimulating catheter in the right atrium and started to give atrial premature beats ... On increasing the prematurity of the test pulse a gradual widening of the QRS complex was observed demonstrating that an increasing area of the ventricle was activated by way of the accessory pathway ... Suddenly, on reaching a critical value for the atrial premature beat, a narrow QRS complex followed indicating that the refractory period of the accessory pathway was reached and exclusive AV conduction occurred over the AV nodal–His pathway[53].

Over the next several months it was shown that in those patients who were experiencing recurrent paroxysms of tachycardia, programmed stimulation demonstrated the requirements for induction of circus movement tachycardia, with the circuit consisting of both the accessory pathway and the normal AV nodal–His pathway. They were also able to terminate a paroxysm with an appropriately timed premature atrial or ventricular beat. The premature beat, so timed, would break up the circus movement by rendering the tachycardia circuit refractory. These observations were published in a landmark paper in 1967[52]. It sparked a world-wide interest in the use of programmed electrical stimulation for the study and treatment of various cardiac arrhythmias.

Dirk Durrer died in April of 1984. That same year an entire issue of the *International Journal of Cardiology* was dedicated to his memory. It was a fitting tribute in many ways. The progenitor of this journal was the European Journal of Cardiology which he helped establish in 1974. The small memorial section written by his now famous former pupils relived in very expressive words the many contributions of this titan of cardiology (Figure 1).

Programmed electrical stimulation was also used by Coumel for the study of tachyarrhythmias[54–56]. Barold, Goldreyer, Gallagher and Damato were also partial to this method in their studies on supraventricular arrhythmias[57–59]. In 1972 Wellens applied the technique for the study of ventricular tachycardia[60]. This work was done in collaboration with Schuilenburg and under the guidance of Durrer. Diagnostic application was expanded to include assessment of sinus nodal, AV nodal and the His–Purkinje system.

Let us look now at some of the arrhythmias *per se*, including intraventricular block, and those that cause cardiac arrest and sudden death. After we have done that we can explore the exciting therapeutic approaches that cardiac electrocardiology has spawned. These include the defibrillator, and the interventional modalities using ablation techniques and implantable devices for the control of cardiac rhythm. Intraventricular block will be dealt with first.

INTRAVENTRICULAR CONDUCTION DEFECTS

Knowledge concerning intraventricular conduction was made possible through the unique ability of the electrocardiogram to record abnormalities in ventricular excitation. When Einthoven recorded a human electrocardiogram in 1894 with Lippman's capillary electrometer that demonstrated a wide QRS, it was probably the first recording of its kind in a human. In 1924 Einthoven presented this recording in his Nobel lecture and compared it to another one from the same patient taken 31 years later. The second tracing was taken with the string galvanometer. Figure 2 illustrates the two tracings one above the other documenting the existence of an intraventricular block[61]. Einthoven did not realize when he recorded the first tracing that he was

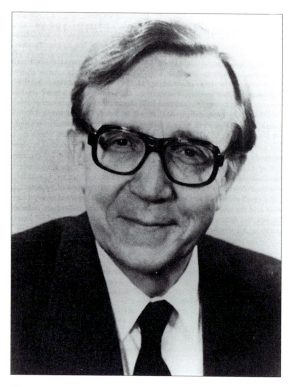

Figure 1 Dirk Durrer. *Photo Source National Library of Medicine. Literary Source International Journal of Cardioliology, **6**, 750, 1984. With permission*

dealing with delay of impulse transmission. The physiological basis was known to him by the time he gave his Nobel lecture in 1924, but only as a result of the observations of others engaged in research on the subject.

Although the current concepts of intraventricular block owe their formulation mostly to the efforts of Mauricio Rosenbaum and his colleagues, Marcello Elizari and Julio Lazzari, the groundwork was laid by the various investigators who preceded them. Rosenbaum and co-workers were the prime movers who put together the cumulative experimental and clinical data that led to the creation of a comprehensive concept so that now we think in terms of hemiblocks and trifascicular block[62–64].

The beginnings of the concept date back to 1909 when Eppinger and Rothberger injected silver nitrate into both the interventricular septum and the free ventricular wall of the dog[65]. Injection into the interventricular septum caused electrocardiographic changes that they ascribed to injury of the major branches of the His bundle[66]. This was

the earliest experimental demonstration of bundle branch block. The QRS pattern varied according to whether a left- or right-sided injection was given. Clinical studies were then reported in the following year. Eppinger and Stoerck found that in their clinical cases, the electrocardiographic changes were similar to those produced in the dog[67]. In 1910 Eppinger and Rothberger cut both branches of the His bundle and noticed the precipitation of complete heart block. This was obviously due to loss of infranodal impulse transmission[66,68].

In 1912 Lewis proposed 'aberration of the supraventricular impulse' to describe those wide QRS complexes that were seen at times following premature atrial beats[69]. He noticed this in a patient afflicted with recurrent paroxysms of tachycardia. Thirteen years later when he published his monograph on the mechanism and graphic registration of the heartbeat he stated: 'I term the resultant beats aberrant, for they are caused by impulses which have gone astray'[70]. In 1914 Lewis and the American, Cohn, described a patient in whom 'unusual curves were obtained, which permitted the suggestion that even though no injury to the main stem of the conduction system was present, a defect in conduction from the auricles to a single ventricle existed, due possibly to a lesion of the bundle branch to this ventricle or to one of its subdivisions[71]. In an attempt to understand what exactly was causing these changes in the human, and apparently not content with the studies of Eppinger and Rothberger, Lewis devised his own technique for producing intraventricular block. He devised a special form of clamp to squeeze the septum in a stepwise manner until he produced the typical electrocardiogram (ECG) patterns that he had observed in the patients. Moreover he could also manipulate the clamp so that he could alternately squeeze either the left or right bundle branch. This technique did not satisfy him either simply because he could not obtain accurate histological correlation. He then adopted the tenotomy knife technique of Eppinger and Rothberger and went on to consistently produce wide QRS complexes when the corresponding bundle division was cut. When the left bundle was divided, initial activation was confined to the right ventricle. He termed the resultant electrocardiogram a dextrocardiogram. Division of the right bundle produced a levocardiogram, again because

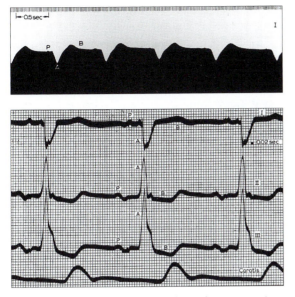

Figure 2 Electrocardiograms from the same patient taken by Einthoven (above) in 1894 with capillary electrometer (lead I), and (below) in 1925 with a string galvanometer (leads I, II, and III and carotid pulse tracing). *Photo Source University of Central Florida. Literary Source Einthoven, W. (1965). The string galvanometer and the measurement of the action currents of the heart. Nobel Lectures: Physiology of Medicine, 1992–44, p.110. (Amsterdam: Elsevier). With permission*

now the initial activation was confined to the left ventricle. He also noted that a left axis deviation occurred when the right bundle was cut, while cutting the left bundle resulted in deviation of the axis to the right[71].

The tracings from these animal experiments were then compared to the human tracings. Two main patterns were identified in the human. One was characterized by a tall R wave in lead I and a deep S_3. The reverse characterized the second group. The human tracing with a deep S_3 and left axis deviation had its counterpart in the dog when the right bundle was cut. The human tracings with a broad S_1 had no counterpart in the dog. This latter finding puzzled Lewis and acting on the possibility that this might be a species characteristic he repeated his experiments on a rhesus monkey. However, he divided the right, not the left bundle and calculated the dextrocardiogram from the levocardiogram and bicardiogram. This error resulted in an apparent confirmation of the extrapolation made from the dog. He concluded there was no

species difference and therefore continued to mislabel the QRS complexes in relation to the culprit bundle. Even Eppinger and Stoerck were in error when they correlated in 1910 the electrocardiographic changes with the postmortem gross and microscopic findings of the conducting tissue[67]. Their findings seemingly confirmed their erroneous conclusions drawn from their previous animal work.

In a detailed critique on the matter, Hollman brings out convincing evidence attesting to the error of their interpretations[72]. All told, Lewis was satisfied that his interpretation of the QRS patterns was correct with regard to the location of the bundle branch block.

In 1917, Rothberger and Winterberg also correlated the electrocardiographic changes with experimentally produced intraventricular conduction disturbances. It was a pioneering effort that went a long way towards elucidating peripheral conduction defects. The study was well-designed, involving the cutting of the dog's left anterior and posterior conduction fibers, interruption of the left and right main stem bundles, and interruption of the right and portions of the left bundle[73,74]. That same year Oppenheimer and Rothschild described electrocardiographic changes that they attributed to conduction delay in the finer ramifications of the His bundle Purkinje system. They introduced the term 'arborization block'[73]. Then in 1920, Oppenheimer in collaboration with Pardee published a study on the site of the cardiac lesion in two instances of intraventricular block[75]. Their ECG criteria for left or right bundle branch block were at complete variance with those of Lewis. Although rather cautious in their conclusions, they nevertheless suggested that other studies be done to explore the possibility of revising the criteria advocated by Lewis. Fahr also published in 1920 a paper that describes the current (and correct) interpretation of human QRS bundle branch block patterns. Fahr had done exactly what Lewis did but both came to different conclusions[76]. This is what Fahr wrote:

A high RI and deep SIII means left bundle branch block, for the vectors show that the right heart is negative first and that as the left heart becomes negative the right sided preponderance is neutralized and the resultant approaches zero. Vice versa, a high RIII and deep SI in bundle branch block indicates right bundle lesion for the construction of the direction of the potential difference in the heart shows that the left side is negative first and the vector is swung toward the right about 0.05 or 0.06 seconds after the beginning of the electrocardiogram. The diagnosis of right and left bundle branch lesion as commonly made is probably wrong.

Obviously not everyone was at ease with the criteria established by Lewis. Despite all this, Lewis refused to budge. Indeed in the third edition of his book on the mechanism and graphic registration of the heart beat, published five years after the reports by Fahr, Oppenheimer and Pardee, there is no mention at all of their work. Lewis did list Fahr's paper in the bibliography but without comment in the text.

In 1931, Mann utilized his monocardiograph studies (see Section 5) correlated with postmortem observations to cause him to say that 'they seemed sufficiently conclusive to justify routinely reporting the localization of bundle branch block in a manner opposite to the published interpretation of Lewis'[77]. Hollman rightfully points out, however, that Mann, too, was in error. Although Mann arrived at the right answer from his clinico-pathologic investigations, he was totally wrong in interpreting the monocardiograms[78].

The issue was finally resolved in 1932 with the publication of the definitive paper by Wilson and co-workers[79]. Two important innovations accounted for the validity of their work. Multiple precordial recordings were made as well as direct observations. After producing a bundle branch block in the dog, the exploring electrode was placed in various positions over the heart whose surface had been covered with a pad of gauze soaked in saline. The exploring electrode was called a semidirect lead since all recordings were obtained through this and another lead attached to the left leg. The recordings in man were obtained from several copper disks strategically placed on the chest wall so as to simulate the exploring technique in the exposed heart of the dog. Eight years later further confirmatory observations were made by Wilson's group when the excitatory process was observed in the exposed human heart[80]. Just three years prior to this, William Kountz was able to make direct observations in revived human hearts[81]. This was a remarkable approach. Although not always successful he was able in at least a third of his attempts to revive hearts

and with coronary perfusion keep them beating regularly for two hours or more. In some of them he cut the left or right bundle branch and recorded the resultant electrocardiogram from the limb leads of the cadaver. These experiments also supported the interpretations of Oppenheimer and Pardee, Fahr, and Wilson's group.

Wilson also introduced the term 'incomplete bundle branch block'. By this he meant that the QRS complexes were transitional in duration between normal and frank block. His group also suggested as early as 1934 that deep S waves in leads II and III could be due to a lesion of the anterior fascicle of the left bundle[82].

Grant's studies on intraventricular block began in 1950. These were reviewed by him in his monograph on clinical electrocardiography published in 1957[83]. He pointed out that blocks could involve independently either of the two fascicles of the left bundle and that such lesions were associated with unusual electrocardiographic patterns. He also described in 1954 perinfarction block, and later went on to say that there were two clinically predominant types, anterior and diaphragmatic[84,85].

The delineation of the detailed anatomy was helped significantly with the introduction of macroscopic staining techniques. In 1960 Uhley and Riokin used Lugol's solution to stain the endocardial surface of the heart[86]. As a result they were able to outline in particular detail the peripheral ramifications of both bundle branches. This was a significant histological breakthrough. It was now possible to verify with exactitude the site of an experimentally produced lesion and correlate it with the changes on the electrocardiogram. Over the next four years Uhley and Rivkin, with the aid of cardiopulmonary bypass, conducted direct visual observations and simultaneous ECG recordings to demonstrate the effect of lesions in either fascicle of the left bundle as well as in the peripheral branches of the right ventricular conduction system[87,88]. Watt and his associates produced experimental arborization block in dogs in 1965[89]. They used a sawing ligature technique enabling them to record small but definite electrocardiographic changes.

It was the peculiar changes in the electro-cardiograms of a patient that aroused the interest of Rosenbaum and his colleagues in intraventricular block. The patient at first manifested a right bundle branch block with a QRS axis of -75°. Several weeks later the QRS axis alternated between

+110° and -75° with the right bundle branch block remaining unchanged. They reasoned that the changes in axis occur only because of a block in either the anterior or posterior fascicle of the left bundle. They turned to the laboratory for proof with their initial experiments on the dog's heart, having as their objective the production of a block in the various divisions of the His bundle with electrocardiographic correlation[63].

Subsequent studies by them revealed that cardiomyopathy and coronary artery disease were the two most common cardiac abnormalities associated with right bundle branch block and left anterior hemiblock[63]. Rosenbaum's group also investigated aberrancy of ventricular conduction in the presence of premature supraventricular beats. They found that in this setting the aberrancy is most often due to the creation of physiologic right bundle branch block, and that it was more frequently associated with left anterior hemiblock rather than left posterior hemiblock.

These definitive studies as well as a review of all preceding ones were summarized and conceptualized as trifascicular intraventricular conduction disturbances in their book published in 1968[62]. It was originally in Spanish and became available on a global basis when it was translated into English two years later[63]. The concept acted as a catalyst for further investigation by anatomists, pathologists, and electrophysiologists[90–101].

HEART BLOCK

In electrocardiographic terms, three stages of heart block are recognized. They are classified as first degree when the PR interval is prolonged, second degree manifested by either a Mobitz I or II pattern, and third degree or complete heart block when there is complete dissociation between atrial and ventricular beats. The historical background of complete heart block is by far the most interesting of the three, and I will treat it at some length.

William Harvey described several examples of atrioventricular block. He observed prolongation of the interval between atrial and ventricular contraction and also noted how, at times, the ventricles would contract only after several atrial beats. His Jr also relied on visual observation to demonstrate prolongation of the interval between atrial and ventricular contraction when he

experimentally injured the bundle he described just two years previously[102].

Edward Shapiro called the electrocardiogram the Rosetta stone of arrhythmias[103]. This is quite true but it does not mean that mechanical devices were not used before the introduction of the electrocardiogram for the identification of various forms of arrhythmia. It is also true that the electrocardiogram launched the clinicians into a whole new world by enabling them to identify the P waves and QRS complexes, and their relationship to each other. But, the ink-writing polygraph of Mackenzie gave for the most part practically the same information. The only difference was that the polygraph, through its registration of the a and v waves, was recording the mechanical contraction of the atria and ventricles rather than electrical activity *per se*. The polygraph tracings were considered so reliable that for years they served as the standard frame of reference against which the electrocardiographic interpretation of arrhythmias was compared. During the early years of electrocardiography, interpretation of arrhythmias based on this modality lacked the exactitude that it currently enjoys[103].

The laddergram used so often today as an aid in the interpretation of arrhythmias was originally devised by Engelmann in 1896 for the interpretation of polygraph tracings[104]. Wenkebach described the type of heart block that carries his name also with the aid of the polygraph. This was in 1899. The tracings were obtained by recording the radial pulse.

Luciani had described in 1872 a peculiar rhythm in the isolated ventricle of a frog after it had been supplied with serum. The contractions were irregular and occurred in distinct groups, with pauses of varying lengths between the groups. Wenkebach's polygraph tracings revealed a pulse that varied in a manner similar to the contractions observed by Luciani, and for this reason, he called the pauses 'Luciani periods'. His book *Die Arrhythmie, als Ausdruck bestimmter Funktionsstörungen des Herzens* was based entirely on recordings made with Mackenzie's polygraph.

Ritchie wrote in the introduction to his book on *Auricular Flutter* (1914) that Wenkebach's 'critical analysis of the sphygmographic tracings demonstrated that each form of cardiac irregularity represented a disorder of one or other of the functional activities of the heart, namely, of stimulus production, excitation, contractility, and conductivity'[105]. This interpretation of the cardiac arrhythmias had been adopted and amplified by Mackenzie in 1908[106].

The electrophysiological principles underlying conduction and refractoriness were established before the introduction of the string galvanometer as a clinical tool. These were to prove all-important in understanding and appreciating the various forms of heart block. Some of the historical background has already been presented in that part of Chapter 16 dealing with electrophysiologic mechanisms. I should like to mention at this time that the existence of the refractory period in cardiac muscle was established by Marey in 1896[107]. In 1906, A. J. Carlson, working with the invertebrate heart, described the excitability of the heart during the different phases of the heartbeat. On the basis of this work he expanded Marey's refractory period into an 'absolute and relative frequency period'[108]. Wiggers noted in his historical account of cardiac physiology that many of the electrophysiologic properties of heart muscle such as automaticity and refractory period had been well formulated through the efforts of Engelmann, Wenkebach and Bowditch[109]. Most of this background can also be found in Chapter 16.

Erlanger, another American giant of physiology, provided the best experimental proof that partial or complete heart block depended on lesions within the bundle of His. He also used a mechanical recording method. He did this in 1905 by varying the pressure on the His bundle while graphically recording the varying degrees of heart block[110].

The earliest clinical descriptions of complete heart block are to be found in writings pertaining to the pulse. Description of the cardiac findings on auscultation had to wait for the invention of the stethoscope by Laénnec.

There is an account on page 23 of *Appendix ad Ephemeridem Academiae Caesaro-Leopoldino-Carolinae Naturae Curiosorum in Germania, 1719, Centuriae VII et VIII* which reads as follows:

> … More unusual moreover I observed this in two patients about the pulse: truly that one of them a melancholy hypochondriac indeed had commonly when well a pulse so slow, that before a subsequent pulse followed the preceding one, three pulsations would have certainly passed in another healthy person; who moreover after the passing of August fell into a malignant fever, had on the contrary a frequent pulse, and through all the different ills of varying kinds, such as I had never observed. Therefore afterwards as the commencement of the disease and until now I had predicted a bad termination of the illness. Such remarkable departure from nature, from the healthy state did not seem possible and only the worse fate was predicted. The man at other times was robust, exact in his movements, but is now slow, often seized with dizziness, and from time to time subject to slight epileptic attacks[111].

Its author was Marcus Gerbezius also known as Verbez of Laibach. Figure 3 shows Gerbezius' text. This appears to be the first reference to an association between a slow pulse and fainting episodes, accompanied at times by convulsive seizures. The Slovene name is Marko Gerbec. He was born at Sentvid in Carmola, at that time part of the Austrian Empire, and now Slovenia. Gerbezius received his doctorate in medicine from Bologna, but also studied for a short time at Padua. He must have made a very favorable impression at Padua because, despite his short stay there, his portrait hangs in the Sala dei Quaranta (Hall of the Forty). Gerbezius' original description was published again in 1731 as part of the encyclopedic work of J. J. Manget, a pathologist from Geneva, Switzerland, entitled *Bibliotheca scriptorum medicorum veterum et recentorium*.

Fourteen years after Gerbezius' publication, George Cheyne wrote a treatise on the *English Malady or nervous diseases of all kinds*[112]. In it, the malady afflicting the Honorable Colonel Townshend has him experiencing episodes of unconsciousness associated with slowing or actual absence of pulse. No convulsive seizures are described. Except for an enlarged heart, no other cardiac abnormalities were noted at autopsy.

When Morgagni described the syndrome in 1761 he too listed it under a neurological disturbance. It is to be found in his ninth letter which deals with epilepsy[113]. This is the first time that convulsive seizures are mentioned in association with a slow pulse. It is true that Gerbezius did describe 'from time to time slight epileptic attacks' but it was never related to a slow pulse. Morgagni was quite aware of the many contributions that Gerbezius made. He surely must have read some of the nine books that Gerbezius wrote. Morgagni did

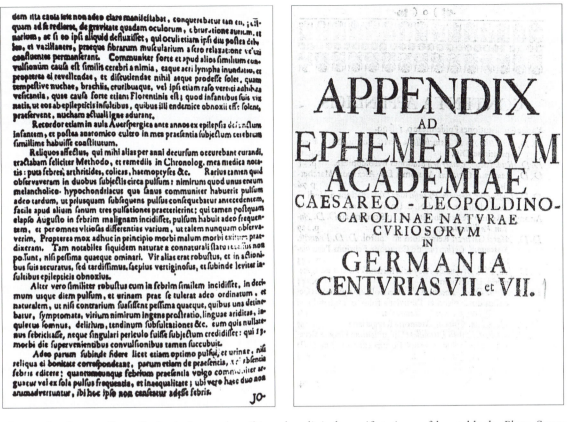

Figure 3 A page from Gerbezius' text describing the clinical manifestations of heart block. *Photo Source National Library of Medicine. Literary Source Appendix ad Ephemeridem Academiae Caesoro-Leopoldino-Carolinae Naturae Curiosum in Germania, 1719, Centuriae VII et VIII, p.24. Courtesy of National Library of Medicine*

mention the observations of Gerbezius but the stress was on the neurological manifestations rather that the pulse. In addition to this citation, Gerbezius' other observations are cited by Morgagni on ten other occasions. There is some doubt really as to whether the patient described by Gerbezius actually had complete heart block. The details are not specific enough. He could have had a sick sinus syndrome with episodes of marked bradycardia.

In 1793 Thomas Spens of Edinburgh described a scenario in a 54 year old male characterized by recurrent episodes of loss of consciousness, and in whom the pulse rate was only 24 beats per minute. During one episode the pulse rate was a mere 10 beats per minute with the patient having convulsive seizures. The patient's entire illness lasted but four days. Just prior to death he developed aphasia and a right hemiplegia. Spens too did not recognize the

cardiac basis for the neurological picture but at the same time he did not believe it was primarily a nervous affliction[114].

A case report appeared in 1824 written by William Burnett but read before the Medical and Chirugical Transactions of London by Dr James Johnson[115]. It described in detail a

> case of epilepsy attended with remarkable slowness of the pulse … on examining his pulse I found it to beat 36 to the minute, but it was regular and small. On the following morning the pulse was only beating twenty in the minute, but in the evening it got up to 32, and from time to time till the 6th of May, it varied from 28 to 56, but was generally under the latter number though without any return of the paroxysms[115].

Although the abnormal pulse is described in detail, Burnett did not consider a cardiac arrhythmia

345

as part of the mechanism. He may have been swayed too much by Morgagni's commentary and his own perception of the similarity between his case and that of Morgagni. Burnett's report did not appear until 1827.

Robert Adams' report also appeared in 1827, but his differed from all the others in that he was the first to realize that the seizures were cardiac in origin[116]. This is how he described it:

An officer in the revenue, aged 68 years, of a full habit of body, had for a long time been incapable of any exertion, as he was subject to oppression of his breathing and continued cough. In May, 1819, in conjunction with his ordinary medical attendant, Mr. Duggan, I saw this gentleman: he was just recovering from the effects of an apoplectic attack, which had suddenly seized him three days before. He was well enough to be about his house, and even to go out. But he was oppressed by stupor, having a constant disposition to sleep, and still a very troublesome cough. What most attracted my attention was, the irregularity of his breathing, and remarkable slowness of his pulse, which generally ranged at the rate of 30 in a minute. Mr. Duggan informed me that he had been in almost continual attendance on this gentleman for the last seven years; and that during this period he had seen him, he is quite certain, in not less than twenty apoplectic attacks. Before each of them he was observed, for a day or two, heavy and lethargic, with loss of memory. He would then fall down in a state of complete insensibility and was on several occasions hurt by the fall. When they attacked him, his pulse would become even slower than usual; his breathing loudly stertorous. He was bled without loss of time and the most active purgative medicines were exhibited … He recovered from these attacks without any paralysis. Oedema of the feet and ankles came on early in December; his cough became more urgent, and his breathing more oppressed; his faculties too become weaker.

The autopsy revealed marked 'fatty degeneration' of the myocardium, a finding in conjunction with the abnormal pulse that led Adams to base the entire illness on a cardiac disturbance.

William Stokes was the one who very clearly and accurately described all the cardiac findings that form the basic component of the disturbance that

now carries the eponym Stokes–Adams syndrome. Some misguided chauvinists have insisted that Morgagni should be included in the eponym. No matter how one twists and turns Morgagni's description of the fat priest, Anastasio Poggi with the florid complexion, it must be recalled that at no time did Morgagni suggest a disturbance of cardiac rhythm as the causative factor for the entire picture.

It was not until 1889 that the eponym Stokes-Adams first appeared. Huchard used it in his book *Maladies du Coeur et des Vaisseaux*. Why he gave Stokes first place is at first not easily explained since he acknowledges that Adams preceded Stokes in describing the clinical syndrome[117]. Although this is true, it was really Stokes who was the first to render in no uncertain terms all the cardiac findings that form the basic components of complete heart block.

Stokes' description appeared in 1846. It combines the tactile and auscultatory elements of the physical examination. This is how he put it:

The impulse of the heart is extremely slow, and of a dull prolonged, heaving character, giving the idea of feeble as well as of slow action. The first sound is accompanied by a soft bruit de soufflet, which is prolonged until the commencement of the second sound, and is heard very distinctly up along the sternum and even into the carotid arteries. The second sound is also imperfect, though very slightly so; the imperfection being much more evident after some beats than after others. Pulse 28 in the minute, of a prolonged sluggish character; the arteries pulsate vividly all over the body, but no bruit is audible in them[118].

At the time, physical diagnosis was enjoying its heyday as part of the Parisian influence of bedside clinical diagnosis. Stokes learned his lessons well because he later described 'a very remarkable pulsation in the right jugular vein … about every third pulsation is very strong and sudden … the remaining waves are much less distinct … These may possibly correspond with those imperfect contractions which have already been noticed in the heart'[118].

Thirty years elapsed before this syndrome was given the clinical importance that it deserved. This occurred with the publication of George Balfour's text on diseases of the heart and aorta in 1876[119]. In the chapter devoted to intermittency and irregularity of the pulse he described a case that had all the earmarks of the syndrome.

An old lady … had been suddenly seized while shopping with what seemed to be an epileptic attack. These attacks continued to recur when she made the slightest exertion … They were associated with flatulent dyspepsia and an extremely slow pulse, averaging about 20 in the minute … I found that her heart acted with perfect regularity, but with unequal force, so that the apparently abnormal slowness of the pulse was simply due to the fact that only about every third beat reached the periphery. It was not difficult to connect this defective cardiac action with diminished arterial pressure, generally sufficient to produce all the phenomena of cerebral anemia on the one hand, and among these epileptic seizures, and also defective secretion generally, and as one of the results of the flatulent dyspepsia[119].

Balfour, of course, was still unaware of the conduction disturbance that was responsible for the intermittency and slowness of the pulse. This was yet to come. But, he appreciated the gravity of the situation when he commented that 'such cases are always more serious than those of simple irregularity of the cardiac action, and are not always so simply to be remedied, considerable degeneration of the cardiac muscle being only too frequently concomitant'[119].

The first graphic recording of complete heart block was obtained by Galabin in 1875[120]. It was an apexcardiogram. Gaskell originated the term heart block in 1883, ten years before the conduction system was discovered[121]. In 1885 Chauveau was following a patient with a pulse rate of 24 beats per minute, and who had repeated episodes of vertigo and syncope. He demonstrated with venous tracings that the atria and ventricles were beating independently of each other and at different rates. He attempted to correlate the dissociation with hyperactivity of the vagus nerve based upon his observations in the horse that on vagal stimulation the atria beat faster than the ventricles. Of course, this hypothesis was wrong but Chauveau should be credited for being the first to investigate the dissociation in the physiology laboratory[122].

The underlying conduction disturbance was finally delineated by His in 1895 when he experimentally produced heart block, and on the basis of his observations, he suggested that a lesion of the AV bundle was responsible for blocking the conduction of impulses from the atria to the ventricles. His was fortunate enough to document this in 1899 in a patient who had heart block associated with syncope[123]. The recording was made with Mackenzie's polygraph. Mackenzie himself had the opportunity to record the polygraphic abnormalities in a patient with a similar history in 1902[124].

When Joseph Erlanger complied with Osler's request for a bedside physiological evaluation in a patient whose clinical manifestations puzzled the great clinician, Erlanger did not need much persuasion to do so. He had already published, the year before, his studies on the physiology of heart block in mammals[125]. He and Blackman created chronic heart block in dogs by using adjustable clamps until they induced Stokes–Adams episodes. At the bedside Erlanger recorded the patient's radial pulse with his own sphygmomanometer and the patient's apex impulse with Marey's cardiograph[126]. The findings were included in a paper he wrote describing the physiology of heart block in mammals with 'especial reference to the causation of Stokes–Adams disease'[126].

The introduction of the electrocardiogram finally gave graphic proof that the underlying electro-physiologic disturbance was dissociation between atrial and ventricular impulses. Einthoven was the first in 1906 to record the dissociation with an electrocardiogram. Four years later Lewis did the same and two years after, he and Cohn described the electrocardiographic and necropsy findings in a patient who died of complete heart block[127]. They were not the only ones to show a correlation between disease of the AV bundle and clinical evidence of AV block. In 1905 Hay also described his findings at postmortem in a patient with AV block[128].

Yater (1935), Lev (1958) and Lenegre (1963) outlined mechanogenic and degenerative lesions as non-ischemic causes[103]. Ischemia and the non-ischemic causes just mentioned count for the vast majority of the cases. Many other causes have been incriminated however during the past 50 years. They include toxic, inflammatory, infectious, carcinogenic and granulomatous processes.

EXTRASYSTOLES

Extrasystoles as such were not recognized until the advent of the stethoscope. Prior to this, reference to ventricular ectopy was made through palpation of the pulse. Herophilus described in the 2nd century BC abnormalities of the pulse that could be consistent with extrasystoles[129]. Galen wrote extensively on the pulse and in Section 5 the reader will find among the descriptions, reference to the 'intermittent pulse' which no doubt was also a reflection of extrasystoles. This Galenic label persisted well into the 19th century when physiological experimentation began to lay the groundwork for the electrophysiologic observations of the 20th century[130].

Theodore Engelmann coined the word extrasystole when he visually observed the extra beats in the animal heart[131,132]. He explained the compensatory pause by saying that the next atrial impulse fell during the refractory period set up by the premature ventricular contraction, making the ventricle await the next atrial stimulus[133]. This was not a new concept. He merely confirmed by visual observation of the frog's heart what Marey and Knoll had previously enunciated. In 1876 Marey demonstrated that the ventricle was excitable by artificial stimuli only during diastole[107]. Knoll, four years earlier, had shown the compensatory pause following a premature ventricular beat was exactly twice the original cardiac cycle; this without benefit of electrocardiography[134]. In 1899 both Wenkebach and Cushny independently arrived at the opinion that the intermittent pulse was caused by extrasystoles[135,136]. Both men also noted atrial extrasystoles in humans. In a short span of four years the experimental studies of Hering[137], Pan[138], and Trendelenburg[139] provided additional support for the view that extrasystoles caused the intermittent pulse. In 1903 Wenckebach collated these studies and in a landmark paper he defined in unequivocal terms the intermittent pulse as a manifestation of cardiac origin[140].

The electrocardiogram now made its entry into clinical practice, and for the first time there was clinical documentation of extra beats arising from the heart[141]. Kraus and Nicolai introduced an erroneous concept in 1908[142]. They called it hemisystole. By this they meant that the premature beat was caused by contraction of a single ventricle. Even Mackenzie subscribed to this view. Lewis proved the concept wrong when he recorded simultaneously the electro-cardiogram and tracings of the venous pulse[3].

The cardiac origin of extrasystoles was now established beyond the shadow of a doubt but their significance was to remain a bone of contention well into current times. Such luminaries as Lewis, Mackenzie and Osler felt that extrasystoles were essentially benign, especially in the absence of other signs of cardiac disease. As electrocardiography became more firmly established in the clinical setting, it became obvious that there were different kinds of extrasystoles in terms of cause, frequency and sites of origin. At one time or another these differences were advanced to answer the ever burning question: when does ventricular ectopy portend a sudden fatal outcome? Despite attempts at risk stratification, the most notable of which is Lown's classification, the answer still eludes us.

In 1969 the well-known epidemiological study of Tecumseh, Michigan was published[143]. The leading author was B. Chiang and when initially interpreted the data appeared to indicate that sudden death occurred most commonly in those who had ventricular extra beats. This was in sharp contrast to the views espoused by Mackenzie, Lewis and Osler. However, when the data were subjected to reanalysis another concept emerged, one which prevails even today. This is that the Tecumseh group consisted of different subsets, some with and others without associated heart disease; and that the prognosis of ventricular ectopy was linked to the subset, and not to the group as a whole. The damage, however, had already been done. Anecdotal experiences now began to play an important role in the eyes of individual practitioners. Depending on the circumstances in their own practice some clinicians were more pessimistic than others on the outlook while there was a substantial number at the opposite end of the spectrum. The significance of ventricular ectopy was rendered even more obscure by the publication of several studies conducted in the coronary care unit and post-discharge[144–146]. Further epidemiologic studies pointed out once more that prognosis depended on the presence of heart disease rather than on the ectopy itself. It also became obvious that no definitive conclusion could be reached when the statistical studies attempted to analyze other factors besides the underlying heart disease.

Prior to these statistical studies which were really a 20th century tool, efforts had been directed towards analyzing the electrocardiographic patterns of extrasystoles, their site of origin and the correlation of their occurrence with various stimuli, mechanical, electrical and otherwise. Kountz recorded four different types of extrasystoles by electrical stimulation of various regions of the ventricles. These were part of his experiments on bundle branch block in revived human hearts[81]. Rothberger and Winterberg, and Lewis as well, noted that an extrasystole originating from the right ventricle with its late activation of the left ventricle gave the same pattern as left bundle branch block and *vice versa*[68]. Hoffmann in 1914 was the first to produce extrasystoles experimentally in man[147]. Since the patient had undergone rib resection, Hoffmann was able to stimulate the left ventricle with a directly applied galvanic current to the overlying soft tissues. He was also able to induce an extrasystole by mechanically tapping the precordial area with a percussion hammer. Patients with a similar easy accessibility to the heart were seen by Einthoven and later by Oppenheimer and Stewart. In Einthoven's patient the sternum had been surgically removed. The patient of Oppenheimer and Stewart earned his livelihood by billing himself as the 'Human Heart Wonder'[148].

TACHYARRHYTHMIAS

As electrocardiographic studies uncovered in a more accurate fashion the basic mechanisms of tachyarrhythmias the nomenclature and classification of these arrhythmias has also undergone revision. Traditionally, two broad categories were recognized according to site of origin, namely supraventricular and ventricular[149,150].

Intracardiac recordings helped clarify the various mechanisms, and in doing so, a classification based on these mechanisms was proposed. Still another classification was proposed using descriptive characteristics such as onset, duration rate and morphology. A whole plethora of new terms arose from this approach. Each classification had its own advantages and disadvantages.

Cotton in 1867 and again in 1869 described the first few cases of supraventricular tachycardia[151]. In 1888 Bristowe described nine cases. Although his report carried the title *On recurrent palpitations of extreme rapidity in persons otherwise apparently healthy*, some of them did have serious heart disease[152]. One year later Bouveret gave the arrhythmia the name 'la tachycardie essentielle paroxystique'[153]. A monograph based on 135 cases was published by Augustus Hoffman in 1900[154]. He called the arrhythmia paroxysmal tachycardia.

Winternitz was the first to show that supraventricular tachycardia really consisted of a series of atrial extrasystoles. He brought this out with pulse tracings obtained with the polygraph[155]. We will see throughout this section how many arrhythmias were accurately diagnosed with this wonderful invention of Mackenzie, long before the electrocardiogram became established. In 1909 Lewis was able to experimentally produce paroxysmal tachycardia and observe the effects of ligation of the coronary arteries on the arrhythmia[156]. He did not subscribe to the circus movement as the underlying mechanism. This view was based on his perception that the atrium was too small to accommodate a circus wave of sufficient speed. Moreover, he believed the slower rate of supraventricular tachycardia when compared to that seen in atrial fibrillation also argued against the possibility of a circus movement. In 1928 Schmidt and Erlanger did present rather convincing evidence for reentry as a valid mechanism[157]. David Scherf in 1947 and Prinzmetal several years later both expressed a belief in the focal atrial origin of supraventricular tachycardia[158,159]. Lown made an important contribution in 1959 when he emphasized that paroxysmal atrial tachycardia was a sign of either digitalis toxicity or hypokalemia[160].

In 1983 Reddy and Surawicz, in a reevaluation of these approaches, suggested a revamping of the entire classification guided by the new knowledge derived from modern electrophysiologic studies and clinical application[161]. In the process, old terms were rejected, retained or modified, while new ones were introduced[162,163].

The term supraventricular tachycardia is inherently too broad and imprecise in the light of current knowledge. Such rhythms may originate from anywhere above the bundle of His. The rhythm may be regular or irregular with the underlying mechanism being reentry or triggered automaticity. Some attempts were made in the past to localize the site of origin in a more precise manner. In 1910 Lewis produced ectopic atrial complexes with a negative P wave in lead II by stimulating the left atrial appendage or the region of the inlet of the pulmonary veins[164]. Many years later Abramson also studied the electrical activity of the left atrium with electrocardiographic recordings. He stimulated the left atrium of the dog with mechanical or electrical means[165]. The ectopic atrial rhythm had upright P waves in leads II and III and inverted ones in lead I. The advent of cardiac catheterization afforded another opportunity for mechanically stimulating the left atrium. All these studies, including the most recent ones, failed to establish reliable criteria for localizing the site of origin of ectopic impulse formation within the atria[166–168]. It is for this reason that Reddy and Surawicz suggested abandoning the terms left or right atrial in favor of ectopic atrial rhythms.

Experimental observations to test the hypothesis that ectopic rhythms could originate in the coronary sinus were initiated by Erlanger and Blackman in 1907[169], followed by Eyster and Meek in 1922[170] and Scherf in 1944[171]. Experimental and clinical studies were then conducted by Giraud[172], Puech[173], Lancaster[174], Lau[175], Moore[176] Waldo[177], and Massumi and Tawakkol[178]. These studies were recorded with surface and esophageal electrocardiograms along with intracardiac electrograms. Despite all the time and effort, it is still not possible to make the diagnosis of coronary sinus rhythm with any degree of certainty. Reddy and Surawicz suggested that this term also be abandoned and substituted with the broader label of atrial rhythm.

The evaluation of supraventricular tachycardias was an interesting phase in the development of electrophysiologic techniques. It began in 1967 when Durrer demonstrated that he could precipitate and terminate this arrhythmia in patients with the WPW syndrome by inducing appropriately timed atrial and ventricular premature beats[179]. But this is a special situation and differs from the ectopic atrial completely, though it is now known that ectopic atrial tachycardia is associated with a reentrant mechanism or enhanced automaticity.

JUNCTIONAL RHYTHM

A series of studies conducted by Zahn in 1912 and 1913 led to the concept of upper, middle and lower AV nodal rhythms[180,181]. Zahn's conclusions were accepted quite readily and uncritically by electrocardiographers despite the fact that his data were obtained with crudely estimated placement of his specially designed thermode onto tiny anatomical structures that are difficult to locate in an empty heart, let alone in a beating blood-filled one[182]. Even Lewis made ambiguous statements about Zahn's work, which in the light of his reputation, only served to keep the concept alive.

He stated that although Zahn's statements were 'scarcely convincing … there seems no reason to doubt the more general conclusions'[183]. In 1913 Meek and Eyster attempted to examine Zahn's concept with more careful electrical studies, but they too were not successful in their technical approach[184]. In fact Spach, Goodman and Hoffman independently demonstrated that the electrocardiograms of Meek and Eyster were actually recorded from atrial muscle and not from the AV node[185–188]. Waldo and James, commenting on the inaccuracies of the work carried out by Zahn and then by Meek and Eyster, made the statement that 'Sixty years after Zahn's experiments, we are still at the beginning of understanding of AV junctional rhythms'[182].

ATRIAL FLUTTER

When MacWilliam saw the fluttering atria in a dog with his naked eye he was the first to describe this rather common arrhythmia. This was in 1887[189]. He wrote that the current 'sets the auricle with a rapid flutter'. There is an electrocardiographic recording in Einthoven's paper Le Télécardiogramme which shows an atrial flutter with 2 : 1 block[141]. Einthoven did not recognize it as such. The patient was a mile away at the Academic Hospital with the recording obtained by the legendary underground cable (see Chapter 24). The honor of being the first to recognize atrial flutter in man belongs to William Ritchie[190]. The patient had a complete block and this is probably why Ritchie was able to recognize it with the polygraph in 1905. Four years later he and Jolly had the opportunity to restudy the same patient. This time the recording was made with the electrocardiogram[191]. In another four years Lewis outlined the electrocardiographic diagnostic criteria[192]. In 1921 Lewis showed that the underlying mechanism was a circus movement[193,194]. This was confirmed in 1947 by Cabrera and Sodi-Pollares using the Lewis bipolar electrogram method[195]. Further confirmation came from Rytand in 1966[196]. He accomplished this by direct exploratory activation-mapping of an exposed heart during surgery. Unfortunately, several years later Wellens could not find a circus movement in the exposed heart[197]. His paper on epicardial excitation of the atria in a patient with atrial flutter, and Prinzmetal's studies showing a normal P wave axis in at least 15% of flutter, raised the question of reentry or circuits involving the right internodal tracts, but not a circus movement[159]. Guiraudon's group in 1986 finally demonstrated that atrial flutter is associated with a reentrant circuit made up of an excitable gap and a critical area of slow conduction in the region of the coronary sinus orifice[198]. This was an extremely important observation especially in the light of recently introduced ablative techniques based on cardiac mapping.

ATRIAL FIBRILLATION

Total irregularity of the pulse was known to ancient physicians. The subject of debate was not its existence but rather its relationship to the heartbeat. The stethoscope put the debate to rest because of its ability to synchronize the audible cardiac rhythm with palpation of the pulse.

Adams was probably the first to recognize it clinically. He considered it as a sure sign of mitral stenosis[199]. Hope's contribution was in the same vein, emphasizing that mitral stenosis was often associated with a totally irregular pulse[200]. In addition, he pointed out that it was different from intermittent pulse in that exercise would worsen the total irregularity whereas it would abolish the intermittent pulse. Bouillaud described another clinical aspect. He observed that digitalis reduced the rate dramatically even though the irregularity was still present. He described this action with the words: 'Ce grand modérateur, cette sorte d'opium du couer'[201]. Marey in 1863 published a pulse tracing of atrial fibrillation from a patient with mitral stenosis[202].

Vulpian is said by some authors to be the first to have visually observed atrial fibrillation *in vivo*. Like atrial flutter, this too was seen in the dog. In his report published in 1874, he noticed the chaotic rhythm of the atria while carrying on experiments with direct 'faradization' in the intact heart of the animal[203]. He called it 'mouvement fibrillaire'. However, in Chapter 4 of Harvey's *De Motu Cordis*, the following remarks seem to indicate that he, rather than Vulpian, was the first to observe with the naked eye the arrhythmia *in vivo*: 'But I … have noticed, that after the heart proper, and even the right auricle were ceasing to beat and appeared on the point of death, an obscure movement,

undulation/palpation had clearly continued in the right auricular blood itself for as long as the blood was perceptibly imbued with warmth and spirit.' Granted, the description is not as specific as that of Vulpian but it should be remembered that when Harvey wrote these words in the early part of the 17th century, 'delirium cordis' was a totally unknown phenomenon while Vulpian had the advantage of clinical precedent and cardiac auscultation.

In 1894 two studies appeared. One was by Mackenzie and the other by Engelmann. The latter theorized that atrial fibrillation was caused by multiple foci in the atria[204]. Mackenzie's paper described his observations with the polygraph[205]. I will deal with Mackenzie in more depth shortly. Meanwhile, let me mention that in 1903, H.E. Hering referred to atrial fibrillation as 'pulsus irregularis perpetuus'[206]. Five years later he demonstrated two electrocardiograms that were obvious examples of atrial fibrillation, but for some strange reason he described them as failing to show any evidence of atrial activity[207].

Lewis first described atrial fibrillation in man in 1909, two years before the recognition of atrial flutter[208]. Lewis pointed out that it was a common clinical condition. He was the first to use the letter 'f' as a designation for the flutter waves. It was also at this time when he expressed the view that digitalis decreased the ventricular rate in atrial fibrillation by enhancing a previously existing atrioventricular block; a view that he held to the exclusion of all else, and that was to prove to be a sore point between him and Mackenzie. The German team of Rothenberger and Winterberg also published in 1909 a clinical description of atrial fibrillation. They used two terms to describe it. One was 'arrhythmia perpetua' and the other 'fibrillation of the auricles' (Vorhofflimmern)[209].

In 1911 Lewis published a classic visual description of atrial fibrillation in a horse that begs for reproduction:

This horse was a gelding, aged 16, in height 15½ hands. It was seen through the kindness of General Smith and Colonel L. Blenkinsop of Salisbury … The symptoms had been present for 7 months. It [the horse] had been under observation for 7 years, and was not known to have suffered from strangles or any other illness. The symptomatology consisted of very irregular and tumultuous action of the heart, marked breathlessness, epistaxis, faltering and occasionally falling, upon moderate exertion ... The horse was examined on Bulford Plain on June the 25th, 1910. The heart was absolutely irregular, long pauses of 2 seconds were frequent and short runs of rapid beats were noted from time to time. The rate was from 40 to 60 beats per minute while resting. Upon exertion the rate showed increase, and a welling pulsation, not marked but distinct, appeared at the root of the neck. Breathlessness was fairly conspicuous after the animal had cantered a few times round a small paddock. The heart sounds were clear, there were no murmurs. The heart beats were more numerous than the arterial pulsations ... The horse was thrown in a covered yard and was chloroformed. It was then shot in the head, in compliance with the regulations, and the windpipe was opened. A good deal of blood poured from the trachea; the shot had broken the base of the skull. As a consequence, artificial respiration was not free. The chest was opened by an incision on the right side and the removal of two ribs, and an excellent view of the beating heart was obtained. The ventricular movements were forcible and the spacing of the beats corresponded with what had been heard at the previous examination. For the horse they were rapid, and the irregularity was extreme. The ventricle showed no distention. At first no intrinsic movements could be seen in the auricle, it appeared to lie still except for the tugging transmitted from the ventricle. There was certainly no general shortening of its fibers. Closer inspection of the musculature revealed the presence of fibrillary movements. The epicardium covering the right auricle in the horse is comparatively thick and opaque and fibrillary movements are not readily seen in the underlying muscle. Close inspection of the ridges and, more especially, attention to the light reflection on its surface, particularly in the neighborhood of the appendix, were conclusive. The independent movements of the several light reflections and the activity of the tissues generally was well displayed and was demonstrated to and recognized by the bystanders, including Colonel Blenkinsop. They were watched for several minutes, the ventricle continuing its active coordinate but irregular movements during the whole of this time. A hand was then placed under the ventricle, which was commencing to dilate, and in lifting it out of the pericardium it fibrillated. The auricle continued to fibrillate as before; the two chambers were watched until all movements ceased in them'[210].

A short biography of Lewis as well as his other contributions to electrocardiography will be found in Chapter 24.

At this point let us look a bit more closely at Mackenzie and his role in atrial fibrillation. However, to begin with, although Mackenzie's fame rests on his contributions to cardiology, especially in the realm of arrhythmias and his polygraph, it should be emphasized that his interests encompassed all of medicine. He was proud of the fact that he was a general practitioner, and, except for a short interlude as a Harley street consultant in cardiology, his entire career was spent in general practice.

He had a restless, inquisitive mind. He was also highly observant and meticulous in recording his observations. Mackenzie turned to the study of pulsations in 1889, and finally published his observations in his classical monograph *The Study of the Pulse* which appeared in 1902[211]. By this time he was already well-known and respected because of his numerous lectures and publications on the subject. Polygraph tracings of the pulse were obtained from any accessible site. These included venous, abdominal, peripheral and apical impulses of the heart.

It was he who noted that when atrial fibrillation was present the jugular vein lost its atrial contraction wave, and the presystolic murmur of mitral stenosis. Both are due to atrial contraction and he was fully aware that no effective contractions occurred when the atria were fibrillating. In fact he looked upon atrial fibrillation as functional paralysis of the atria.

He was initially wrong in believing that the total irregularity of the heartbeat was due to nodal rhythm. This was based on his perception that because the sinus origin of the heartbeat no longer prevailed, the origin of the heartbeat was taken over by the AV node. Mackenzie changed his mind after Cushny showed him in 1906 the electrocardiographic tracings from a dog with atrial fibrillation. But Mackenzie waited five years before he publicly acknowledged acceptance of Cushny's interpretation. It was during his Schorstein lecture at the London Hospital in 1911. The correct interpretation also finally appeared in the revised editions of his book. This change in interpretation, however, did not include any acceptance on Mackenzie's part of the underlying mechanism that Lewis proposed in 1921. Mackenzie had grave doubts about the validity of the circus movement that Lewis espoused in his Oliver-Sharpey lectures. In reality, Mackenzie had an antipathy towards the electrocardiogram, and, in time, his relationship with Lewis also deteriorated. Protection of one's 'turf' may have been the motivating factor for Mackenzie's view that the electrocardiogram could not be used as a standard of reference in any arrhythmia, let alone atrial fibrillation.

Mackenzie's relationship with Lewis took a turn for the worse not only because of their divergent views on atrial fibrillation but, probably, also because of the acerbic, rigid and authoritarian personality of Lewis. The whole matter came to a boil when Lewis, as editor, rejected Mackenzie's manuscript for publication in *Heart*. Sir John McMichael brought this out in detail in his historical account of Mackenzie and atrial fibrillation in 1981[212]. The argument revolved around whether or not digitalis reduced the ventricular rate in atrial fibrillation through the vagus nerve. Lewis' letter of rejection to Mackenzie is reproduced in Figure 4 and Mackenzie's response is shown in Figure 5. It so happened that eventually Mackenzie was proven to be right, and it also turned out that Lewis had misquoted Cushny when refuting Mackenzie's hypothesis[213].

Regarding the mechanism of atrial fibrillation itself, Lewis could not be budged from his view that it was due to an irregular circus movement. On the other hand, Englemann and Scherf both subscribed to the belief that high-frequency heterotopic foci were responsible rather than circus movement[214]. In 1948, Scherf injected aconitine into the head of the sinus node to induce atrial fibrillation that could be reversed by local cooling[215]. This was his method for clarifying the mechanism. Prinzmetal also could not find any circus movement when he visualized the fibrillating atria with high-speed cinematography and later viewed them in slow motion[216]. He described 'hetero-rhythmic large and small waves occurring simultaneously at rapid and irregular rates'. Söderström found in 1970 that the ventricular response was found to be related to exit block[217]. Even the computer was drafted to help delineate

My, dear Mackenzie,
I have read your letter with close attention. May be I am wrong, may be not, on this matter of digitalis and its action on the vagus. My position is that the pure action through the vagus is not proved; and that it can be contended that the main action in fibrillation is a direct one on the muscle. I am not dogmatic about it; but say simply that the mode of action is subject to contention still, and that such being the case it does not sufficiently support your main thesis. It is not a clear example . . .

. . . What I want you to consider is whether the present illustration will not in the long run damage rather than help your general hypothesis.
It is because I think that it will that I am unwilling to send your M.S. to press.

Figure 4 Lewis' letter to Mackenzie, 21 February 1921; opening and concluding paragraphs (Lewis–Mackenzie Correspondence, 1909–1925, letter 465). *Photo Source Wellcome Institute Library. Literary Source Lewis–Mackenzie correspondence, 1909–1925, letter 465. By courtesy of the Wellcome Trustees*

the mechanism. Bootsma analyzed the R-R intervals with the computer and came to the conclusion that the totally irregular response of the ventricles was due to 'the effect of randomly spaced atrial impulses of random strength reaching the AV node from random directions'[218]. Current belief is that atrial fibrillation is due to continuous activation of the atria by multiple wavelets whose perpetuation requires a critical surface area[219,220].

SICK SINUS SYNDROME

The term 'sick sinus syndrome' was coined by Lown in 1967 when he recognized that at times the sinus node failed to function adequately after cardioversion for atrial fibrillation[221]. It is now known that the syndrome can exhibit itself in a variety of arrhythmias which at one time were thought to be unrelated to each other. Thus the sinoatrial block described by Mackenzie in 1904 during an influenza epidemic was thought at first to be a benign dysfunction of the vagus nerve[222]. It is now considered to be part of the sick sinus syndrome. Another example is the case report by Cohn and Lewis in 1912 of a patient who had

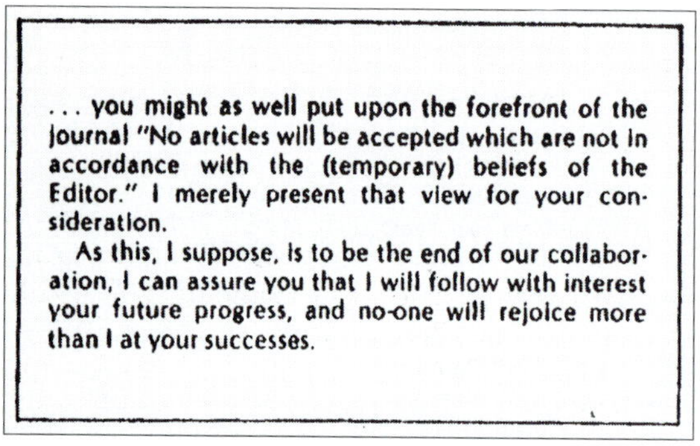

> ... you might as well put upon the forefront of the journal "No articles will be accepted which are not in accordance with the (temporary) beliefs of the Editor." I merely present that view for your consideration.
>
> As this, I suppose, is to be the end of our collaboration, I can assure you that I will follow with interest your future progress, and no-one will rejoice more than I at your successes.

Figure 5 Mackenzie's letter to Lewis, 10 March 1921; extract from concluding remarks (Lewis–Mackenzie Correspondence, 1909–1925, letter 466). *Photo Source Wellcome Institute Library. Literary Source Lewis–Mackenzie correspondence, 1909–1925, letter 466. By courtesy of the Wellcome Trustees*

paroxysms of atrial fibrillation, and who at one time became transiently unconscious because of an episode of sudden asystole[223]. Four years later Samuel Levine described four patients with paroxysmal atrial fibrillation complicated by sinoatrial arrest following termination of the paroxysm[224]. Pick, Langendorf and Katz attempted to tie all this together when they suggested in 1951 that cardiac pacemakers could be depressed by premature impulses[225]. Actually, it was Short who conceptualized the sick sinus syndrome leaving it to Lown to give it its name. In 1954 he wrote a paper describing a syndrome of alternating bradycardia and tachycardia[226]. For the first time such varied arrhythmias as paroxysmal atrial fibrillation, sinus bradycardia, sinoatrial exit block, and sinoatrial arrest were shown to have a common denominator – a dysfunctional sinus node. Both Short and Lown felt that atrial fibrillation was nature's method of dealing with a disturbed sinus node, and that in such instances it was best not to attempt restoration to a regular rhythm. M. Irene Ferrer, sister of the famous actor Jose Ferrer, played an important role in informing the medical community on the various presentations of the sick sinus syndrome[227]. She did not, however, include the tachycardia-bradycardia scenario.

In the section dealing with electrophysiologic control I outlined Gaskell's role in delineating some of the physiological mechanisms in impulse initiation. It was during these studies that Gaskel demonstrated how repetitive stimuli could suppress these pacemaker cells[228]. This was in 1883. In 1971, almost a century later, Rosen, while studying cardiac conduction in patients with sinus node disease, made the same observations. He was able to suppress the sinus node by overdriving it with atrial pacing. His objective was to determine the presence of a malfunctioning sinus node. In doing so he suggested using as a parameter of sinus node function, the length of time it took for the sinus node to recover after having been suppressed with rapid atrial pacing. This was expressed as the sinus node recovery time. It has since been accepted as a standard for assessing sinus node function. Reiffel refined the method by directly measuring sinoatrial conduction time with the sinus node electrogram[229,230].

ATRIAL STANDSTILL

In atrial standstill the atria do not move at all. They neither fibrillate nor contract. Regular rhythm is maintained by the ventricles. Most of the cases are transient occurring in association with digitalis or quinidine toxicity, hypoxia, hyperkalemia or myocardial infarction. Persistent atrial standstill is rare with only a few cases reported.

Cushny was the first to describe the arrhythmia in 1897, noting that it occurred during his experiments with the effects of high-dose digitalis in animals[231]. When Cushny reported his findings he commented that Knoll also observed it in animals after receiving helleborein. Hyperactivity of the vagus nerve was also cited as a precipitating mechanism by Laslett in 1908[232]. The other mechanisms were uncovered by subsequent investigators.

Lewis, White and Meekin produced it in cats during the preterminal stages of asphyxia, reporting this in 1913[233]. Several years later Greene and Gilbert demonstrated 'changes in the pacemaker and in the conduction during extreme oxygen want, as shown in the electrocardiogram'[234]. The first ones to demonstrate the ability of quinidine to provoke it were Boden and Neukirck. They added quinidine to isolated perfused rabbit's and fetal hearts. The atrial standstill was reversed with a perfusion of Tyrode's solution[235]. Korns confirmed that quinidine could do the same thing in living animals two years later[236].

Subsequent investigators not only reconfirmed the quinidine effect but also added several other drugs capable of causing atrial standstill. These included Haskell's work with quinidine in dogs (1927)[237], Wolff and Paul D. White's experience with the drug in humans (1929)[238,239], and the ability of benadryl, procainamide and strophanthin to induce standstill of the atria[240-247]. In 1927 Borman and McMillan were able to produce it in animals by destroying the sinoatrial tissue with radon seed implantation and cooling of the SA node region[248].

In addition to drugs Marzahn reported its occurrence with infective endocarditis[242], and also with rheumatic pancarditis[243]. Sir Thomas Lewis described it in two cases of myocarditis[241]. In 1961 James described it as a complication of myocardial infarction[249], and in 1963 Surawicz mentioned its association with electrolyte disturbances, notably hyperkalemia[250]. Its relationship to facioscapulohumeral dystrophy was brought out in 1968 by Caponnetto and his colleagues (see Section 2)[251].

Rosen and his group conducted a correlative electrophysiologic postmortem study in 1971[229]. Although their report dealt with only two patients, one with transient and the other with persistent atrial standstill, their contribution was significant because of their meticulous attention to detail. It is an excellent example of Mackenzie's dictum of careful observation. In the light of such studies one does not need to resort to complex statistical analyses. The patient with the transient atrial standstill had a total occlusion of the left circumflex artery proximal to the sinoatrial nodal artery takeoff, sinoatrial nodal arteriolosclerosis without infarction, and leftsided cardiac skeletal sclerosis disrupting the penetrating portion of the His bundle and the left bundle branch. Postmortem examination of the patient with persistent atrial standstill revealed a 'previously undescribed atrial disease characterized by arteriolosclerosis, fibroelastosis, fatty infiltration, and vacuolar degeneration with only moderate SA and AV nodal involvement'. Left sided cardiac skeletal sclerosis was also present, disrupting the branching portion of the His bundle[229].

WOLFF–PARKINSON–WHITE SYNDROME

The Wolff–Parkinson–White syndrome is the eponym for what we now know is a manifestation of preexcitation. Wolff was an assistant to White,

and it was he who originally 'worked up' the patient at the request of his mentor. Sir John Parkinson was apparently the only European who became interested in the syndrome after White described it to him. Earlier examples of what the trio described may be found in earlier reports by Frank N. Wilson in 1915, Wedd in 1921, and separately by Bach and Hamburger in 1929. The report by Wolff, Parkinson and White appeared in 1930[252].

When Wilson published his report he described it as 'a case in which the vagus influenced the form of the ventricular complex of the electrocardiogram'[253]. Four distinct rhythms were described and at least three types of ventricular complexes. When the *Selected Papers of Dr. Frank N. Wilson* appeared in 1954, one of its editors and a former associate, Johnston, revealed how Wilson went back to his 1915 paper after having read about the 'new syndrome' described by Wolff, Parkinson and White[254]. He was quick to note that his fourth figure was an exact replica of the WPW electrocardiogram.

Wedd reproduced his tracings as examples of paroxysmal tachycardia. He also discussed the role of intrinsic cardiac nerves[255]. Bach's report dealt with a case of paroxysmal tachycardia of 48 years' duration and with evidence of right bundle branch block, with a commentary on their unusual clinical features[256].

The case that aroused Paul Dudley White's interest was that of a 35 year old instructor of calisthenics who was referred to him because of unexplained bouts of atrial fibrillation and atrial tachycardia[257]. A resting electrocardiogram revealed a short PR interval and a wide QRS complex resembling a bundle branch block. Since the patient told White that the paroxysms were brought on, at times, by exercise, the young man was asked to run up and down four flights of stairs. He and Wolff were surprised when an electrocardiogram taken immediately after this exercise showed not only an expected heart rate of 120 but also an unexpected normal PR interval along with a QRS complex of normal duration. When the heart returned to the patient's usual resting level, the electrocardiogram again showed the previously noted abnormalities. Atropine was given and the electrocardiogram again reverted to a normal pattern. Another time, in the face of a normal tracing, the abnormality was brought out again with carotid massage.

White found six similar patterns in his files. He took them all with him on a trip to Europe, hoping to find an explanation. The Viennese expert, Dr Scherf, assured him that the electrocardiograms were examples of atrioventricular nodal rhythm with aberrant ventricular conduction. This was not an unreasonable interpretation but White was not satisfied. Several other cardiologists on the continent were simply not interested. While in London, White showed the tracings to his former mentor, Lewis, but he too showed no interest. White managed to ignite an enthusiastic response from Sir John Parkinson, who then searched his own files for similar examples. Parkinson found five and mailed the tracings to White, who, by this time, had returned to Boston[257,258].

Holzmann and Scherf were the first to propose that the syndrome was due to an accessory pathway between the atria and ventricles[259]. Apparently Scherf reconsidered his originally erroneous interpretation and within two years of the original publication by Wolff, Parkinson and White, he set his sights upon unraveling the underlying electrophysiologic mechanism. A year later Wolferth and Wood proposed that the pathway was the accessory bundle that Kent had described in 1893 (see Section 3)[260]. Butterworth and Poindexter confirmed this in 1942[261]. Using the cat as a model they transmitted greatly amplified action currents from the SA node to the ventricle. This was, in essence, an electromechanical bypass simulating the anatomical one. The resultant electrocardiograms resembled those of the WPW syndrome. They also reversed the conduction pathway by sending impulses from the ventricle to the atrium. This resulted in bursts of tachycardia. A year later Wood, Wolferth and Geckler confirmed at autopsy the presence of muscular bridges between the right atrium and right ventricle in a patient suspected of having anomalous atrioventricular conduction. The patient was a boy who died during one of his episodes of tachycardia[262]. Within the year the same findings were described by Ohnell in another patient with evidence of preexcitation[263]. In 1945 Wilson and his group studied a patient with normal and alternating anomalous conduction, recording the potential variations of the thorax and esophagus during excitement of the anomalous atrioventricular pathway[264].

M. Irene Ferrer presented in 1967 new concepts relating to what was now recognized as a preexcitation syndrome[265]. She described the syndrome as basically consisting of variants of preexcitation depending upon the anatomical anomaly; the bundle of Kent, Mahaim's fibers, and the anomalous pathway of the Lown–Ganong–Levine syndrome. The French group, headed by Lenègre, demonstrated that certain patients had multiple tracts, sometimes latent, and sometimes severally active[266].

The group at Duke University led by Gallagher, Sealy and Svenson provided significant breakthroughs in the development of techniques for the evaluation of accessory pathways and the supraventricular tachyarrhythmias that characterize the WPW syndrome[267].

VENTRICULAR TACHYCARDIA

Panum produced ventricular tachycardia in 1862 by injecting tallow into the coronary arteries[268]. Lewis also observed its occurrence with coronary artery ligation[269]. These experiments conducted in 1909 formed the basis for his views on the underlying mechanism. The first electrocardiographic recording of ventricular tachycardia in man was made by Robinson and Herrmann in 1921[270]. The patient had an acute myocardial infarction so that this tracing represented a clinical example of coronary artery occlusion. Subsequently, it was also noted that heart disease need not be present. In 1932 Wilson documented its occurrence as a result of exertion, even in the absence of heart disease[271]. Four years before, Katz had brought out his concept of the vulnerable period[272]. This could easily have explained Wilson's findings, since it is not at all unusual to develop premature ventricular beats during exercise with the possibility of them falling on the T wave and precipitating ventricular tachycardia.

TORSADE DE POINTES

Torsade de pointes means twisting of the points. It is a form of ventricular tachycardia wherein the QRS complexes show alternating polarity and changing amplitude in an undulating pattern. It is strictly an electrocardiographic finding. The term was introduced by Dessertenne in 1966[273], but its electrocardiographic features were initially described by Gallavardin in 1922[274], then by MacWilliam a year later[275], and again by Wiggers in 1929[276].

Its clinical features and its association with bradycardia and ventricular fibrillation were described by Schwartz in 1949[277]. In 1981 Horowitz and co-workers pointed out that it was closely related to recurrent sustained ventricular tachycardia and a precursor of ventricular fibrillation. His conclusion that it is due to a rapid reentry mechanism was based on electrophysiologic studies[278]. Reddy and Surawicz suggested in 1983 that the term torsade de pointes be restricted only to those cases associated with a prolonged QT interval[279].

VENTRICULAR FIBRILLATION

There is a passage in the Ebers Papyrus that, according to Lyman Brewer, may be a description of ventricular fibrillation[280]. Written around 3500 BC, the words are: 'When the heart is diseased, its work is imperfectly performed: the vessels proceeding from the heart become inactive, so that you cannot feel them … If the heart trembles, has little power and sinks, the disease is advancing and death is near'[281]. The key words are the trembling of the heart and the lack of pulsation. I agree with Brewer that these signs are key features of ventricular fibrillation. However, in terms of clinical significance I find nothing in this passage that can be construed as important in the formulation of our knowledge concerning ventricular fibrillation. Vesalius, several millennia later, also described 'worm-like' movements of the heart during his vivisections of animals. These too could have been and probably were episodes of ventricular fibrillation just before death. But, again, Vesalius merely described and did not conceptualize these events in terms of physiological aberrations or impact.

Ventricular fibrillation, as we know it today, was probably first described by Erichsen in 1842. He noted it following ligation of the coronary artery[282]. Ludwig and Hoffa were able to induce it with a faradic current in 1850[283]. Vulpain labeled it 'mouvement fibrillaire' when he described it in 1874[203]. This was the same designation he gave to atrial fibrillation. MacWilliam made an outstanding contribution when in 1887, without benefit of electrocardiography, he delineated many of the features of this lethal arrhythmia[284].

August Hoffmann published the earliest electrocardiogram of ventricular fibrillation in man[285]. Lewis' contribution regarding his concept of the circus movement has already been mentioned. Kerr and Bender presented in 1922 the first electrocardiographic documentation of ventricular tachycardia evolving into ventricular fibrillation[286]. The reentry mechanism was also advocated by De Boer[287]. He also demonstrated how a single electric shock delivered late in systole to the frog's ventricle precipitated fibrillation of that chamber. Louis Katz was the first in 1928 to bring out the danger of PVCs falling on the T wave. This was later termed the vulnerable period by Wiggers and Wegria in 1940[288]. They confirmed De Boer's work when they induced ventricular fibrillation with a single localized induction and condensor shock applied during this phase of systole. A year later, Wigger's group, now including Gordon Moe, compared the vulnerable period and fibrillation thresholds of normal and idioventricular beats. At this time they found that the vulnerable period was of longer duration in premature ventricular beats[289].

CARDIAC ARREST AND RESUSCITATION

Sudden death may be due to either cardiac asystole or ventricular fibrillation. In terms of cardiac rhythm total absence of the pulse may indicate either asystole or ventricular fibrillation. The ancients could not tell the difference but it really did not matter. Although 'asphyxia' in the original Greek was the word used to describe absence of pulse, whatever efforts were exerted for revival centered about restoration of respiration rather than cardiac rhythm. This is probably why the connotation of the word changed over the centuries. At any rate, mouth-to-mouth respiration was the method of choice in the treatment of asphyxia until the third decade of the 16th century. No doubt it was practiced widely since breathing is the visible *sine qua non* of life.

[32]When Elisha reached the house, there was the boy lying dead on his couch. [33]He went in, shut the door on the two of them and prayed to the Lord. [34]Then he got on the bed and lay upon the boy, mouth to mouth, eyes to eyes, hands

to hands. As he stretched himself out upon him, the boy's body grew warm. [35]Elisha turned away and walked back and forth in the room and then got on the bed and stretched out upon him once more. The boy sneezed seven times and opened his eyes.

[36]Elisha summoned Gehazi and said, 'Call the Shunammite'. And he did. When she came, he said, 'Take your son'. [37]She came in, fell at his feet and bowed to the ground. Then she took her son and went out.

Except for this biblical reference (II Kings, Chapter 4, Verse 34–37) there is no written history on cardiorespiratory resuscitation until the 16th century. Accordingly then, the prophet Elisha may have been the first to resuscitate a victim of asphyxia (cardiac stoppage) in 850 BC.

Tracheostomies were performed as early as the 12th century but these were reserved for cases with obvious obstruction in the upper respiratory tract. Meanwhile mouth-to-mouth resuscitation was the only method for victims of true asphyxia until 1530 when Paracelsus substituted the ubiquitous fireside bellows as a means of insufflating the lungs with air. The precursor of the modern endotracheal tube was introduced by Smellie in 1763[290]. It was a long flexible tube that was inserted under direct vision into the trachea and the operator would insufflate the lungs by blowing through it. Mucus from the victim was collected by suction into a glass tube attached to the middle of the flexible one.

In 1776 John Hunter read a paper before the Royal Society of London entitled *Proposals for the recovery of people apparently drowned*[291]. Despite the excellent correlation between laboratory and clinical observations, it fell on deaf ears. He stressed that death from drowning resulted from inability to ventilate the lungs. We know today that intense laryngospasm is the key mechanism and that the cardiac irregularities are secondary to the profound deprivation of oxygen. The relationship between oxygen want and the failing heart was demonstrated by the following experiment:

A pair of double bellows were provided, constructed in such a manner as by one action to throw fresh air into the lungs, and by another to suck out again the air which had been thrown in by the former, without mixing them together. The muzzle of these bellows was fixed into the trachea of a dog, and by working them he was kept perfectly alive. While this artificial breathing was going on I took off the sternum of the dog, and exposed the lungs and heart; the heart continued to act as before, only the frequency of its action was considerably increased. I then stopped the motion of the bellows and the heart became gradually weaker, and less frequent in its contraction, till it left off moving altogether. By renewing my operation, the heart again began to move, at first very faintly, and with long intermissions, but by continuing the artificial breathing, the motion of the heart became again as frequent and as strong as before. This process I repeated upon the same dog ten times, sometimes stopping for five, eight, or ten minutes. I observed that every time I left off working the bellows, the heart became extremely turgid with blood, and the blood in the left side became as dark as that in the right, which was not the case when the bellows were working. These situations of the animal appear to me exactly similar to drowning.

The last sentence of his description was the reason he advocated the application of the method to victims of drowning. The apparatus he contrived for artificial respiration was rather cumbersome but logical when viewed on the basis of his reasoning.

A proper apparatus is also essentially necessary to the institution: a description of which I here annex. First, a pair of bellows, so contrived with two separate cavities, that by opening them, when applied to the nostrils or mouth of a patient, one cavity will be filled with the common air, and the other with air sucked out from the lungs; and by shutting them again, the common air will be thrown into the lungs, and that sucked out of the lungs discharged into the room. The pipe of these should be flexible, in length a foot or a foot and a half, and at least three eights of an inch in width: by this the artificial breathing may be continued while the other operations … are going on; which cannot conveniently be done if the nozzle of the bellows be introduced into the nose. The end next the nose should be double, and applied to both nostrils … When assistance is called soon after the immersion, perhaps blowing air into the lungs may be sufficient to effect a recovery.

He even thought of using pure oxygen previously preserved for such emergencies when he wrote: 'Perhaps the dephlogisticated air described by

Dr. Priestley may prove more efficacious than common air. It is easily procured and may be preserved in bottles or bladders'[291].

Several years later Hunter added a very prescient footnote in a revised version of his original manuscript. 'Electricity has been known to be of service and should be tried when other methods have failed. It is probably the only method we have of immediately stimulating the heart'[292]. During the interval he had apparently become aware of the potentialities of galvanic stimulation. His original statement was more cautiously worded: 'How far electricity may be of service, I know not; but it may however be tried, when every other method has failed'[291].

This is the way matters stood for some time. Resuscitation methods still focused on the respiratory component rather than the cardiac, and for the most part there was little investigative interest on the entire subject. Sporadic reports were appearing but there was no concentrated effort. When interest was aroused the methodology of cardiac resuscitation evolved along three fronts: cardiac massage and electrical stimulation for the asystolic state, and electric shock for the fibrillating heart. In the process cardiac pacing was born, first as a therapeutic modality for the emergency state, then as a diagnostic tool (as we have already seen), and finally in its present form for long term control of various cardiac arrhythmias. The historical background is rather complex because it involves an evolution of knowledge regarding the identification and understanding of the mechanisms of cardiac arrest itself, the role it plays in sudden death, and the differentiation on clinical grounds between asystole and ventricular fibrillation. If, at times, the discourse seems to ramble, it is only because of the difficulty in tying all the loose ends together.

According to Fye there were two major stimuli for the renewal of interest in resuscitation that occurred during the latter part of the 19th century. These were the increasing use of chloroform anesthesia and the electrification of cities and towns that brought with it the attendant risk of accidental electrocution.

There was a great deal of opposition initially to anesthesia, especially in the British Isles, and especially in childbirth. The controversy was primarily a religious one with the clergy pitted against the medical profession regarding the propriety of anesthesia in childbirth. James Simpson

of Edinburgh had introduced chloroform anesthesia in childbirth in 1847. Aside from the religious controversy which was soon settled with the aid of biblical passages, his reputation hovered between that of innovator and charlatan because of repeated instances of cardiac standstill while under the anesthesia. Continuing reports of catastrophic events with chloroform anesthesia served to put the medical profession on alert.

An outstanding example was the death of a 15 year old while being subjected to the banal removal of her toenail in 1848. Eighteen months later Bleeck was in the process of performing a mastectomy under chloroform anesthesia. The patient suddenly had cardiac arrest. He revived her with mouth-to-mouth resuscitation, and proceeded to complete the mastectomy without anesthesia, oblivious to the 'cries of the patient'. Mouth-to-mouth resuscitation was also performed by J. Metcalf in 1850 to counteract the cardiac standstill induced again by chloroform. In his report to the New York Academy of Medicine he described these fateful moments as mouth-to-mouth resuscitation brought back to life an individual who was for all intents and purposes gone from this world.

Schiff was a leader in demonstrating that asphyxia could be reversed by artificial respiration while chloroform-induced cardiac arrest was correctable by direct massage of the heart[293]. His views on the physiological mechanisms responsible for recovery were resurrected in the mid 1900s. He opined that cardiac massage maintained nutrition to the myocardium due to filling of the coronary arteries. He also pointed out that blood could be diverted to the heart and brain during cardiac arrest by compressing the abdominal aorta. Many of Schiff's animals were able to be revived even when the heart was in asystole for up to 11½ minutes.

CARDIAC MASSAGE

Schiff's work ushered in the era of cardiac massage as a viable mechanical approach for restoring the heartbeat in asystole. Langenbuch performed the first cardiac massage in patients in 1887[294,295]. He was unsuccessful and so were the attempts of Niehaus of Berne in 1889[296], and the French surgeon, Tuffier, in 1898[297]. In 1900 Maag's patient lived for 11 hours after restoration of cardiac rhythm by direct cardiac massage[298]. Starling and Lane were the first to report a successful attempt in 1902. They massaged the heart through a trans-diaphragmatic approach and combined the procedure with artificial respiration[299]. The patient was undergoing an appendectomy when the cardiac arrest occurred. The first one to actually achieve a successful recovery was Inglesburd. His report appeared, however, in 1904, three years after it actually took place[299,300]. These two reports, however, failed to overcome the negative perception of the previously reported unsuccessful attempts.

Resurgence of interest in direct cardiac massage came about only after Claude Beck's proseletyzing crusade. The groundwork for this was laid as far back as 1906 when Crile and Dolley of The Cleveland Clinic published their work on the resuscitation of dogs[301]. Two years before, Crile had been successful in resuscitating a 12 year old during surgery. He had initiated treatment with perfusion of adrenaline under pressure into the brachial artery. Crile was one of the first to appreciate that the most important obstacle to success was anemia of the brain rather than the heart. Shortly after the turn of the 20th century Ringer, Kuliabo and Sollman showed that the excised heart could be made to beat again even after fairly long periods of asystole[302].

Let us leave cardiac massage for a moment and look into the events that led to the use of electrical means in resuscitation. As the story unfolds we shall see how the lessons learned with mechanical methods of revival were coupled with new knowledge regarding electrical methods, especially in the induction and termination of ventricular fibrillation, and how this knowledge was employed clinically, first through thoracotomy and then with closed chest methods.

The first written record of cardiac resuscitation in a human by electrical means dates back to 1774. According to Schechter this coincided with the inauguration of the Royal Humane Society of London, a body organized specifically for the support of efforts in resuscitation from any cause[303,304]. The description of this first successful electroresuscitation was published in the *Register of the Royal Humane Society of London* and is as follows:

Sophia Greenhill, on Thursday last, fell out of a one-pair-of-stairs window, and was taken up by a man to all appearance dead. The surgeons at the Middlesex Hospital, and an apothecary, declared that nothing could be done for the child. Mr. Squires (of Soho) tried the effects of electricity. Twenty minutes elapsed before he could apply the shock, which he gave to various parts of the body in vain;-but, upon transmitting a few shocks through the thorax, he perceived a small pulsation; in a few minutes the child began to breathe with great difficulty, and after some time she vomited. A kind of stupor, occasioned by the depression of the cranium, remained for several days, but, by the proper means being used, her health was restored[305].

Figure 6 is a reproduction of a portion of this description.

The registers contain several accounts of revival with electrical means that attest to the efficacy of the method whether apparent death was caused by falling, lightning or even drowning. The same source also reveals suggestions regarding the differentiation between life and apparent death by application of electric shock. An interesting account is the essay on electricity by Adams that includes a personal letter to him by John Birch, a surgeon. Birch describes in the letter how he prolonged the life of a woman for 8 months with repeated electric shock despite her moribund state[306].

The Royal Humane Society was but one of many such societies. The first one was established in Amsterdam and the second one in London. Many of them were then founded throughout Europe and finally in the USA[307]. Drowning or near-drowning accidents were just as prevalent in the 1700s as they are today[308]. There was a marked interest in reviving these victims since to do otherwise meant premature death in otherwise healthy people. Though not known at the time, there is some recent evidence that survival is possible even after submersion for as long as 40 minutes[309]. The societies were founded to foster support of methods and research in the resuscitation of such victims. In addition, they were also concerned with other causes of sudden death. They spread the 'gospel', as it were, by educational lectures and materials; procurement, maintenance, and loan of necessary equipment; stimulation of research through prizes and grants; and a host of many ancillary activities. In essence, they operated in much the same way as the current American Heart Association and similar organizations throughout the world.

Mr. SQUIRES, OF SOHO, COMMUNICATED TO THE Rev. Mr. SOWDEN and Dr. HAWES.

ELECTRICITY RESTORED VITALITY.

ONE PART OF OUR BENEVOLENT DESIGN IS TO MANIFEST THE POSSIBILITY OF RECOVERY IN THE VARIOUS INSTANCES OF SUDDEN DEATH, WHERE THE VITAL POWERS ARE SUSPENDED, WITHOUT ANY ESSENTIAL INJURY TO THE FRAME. THIS EXTRAORDINARY RELATION OF RESUSCITATION ALSO MANIFESTS THE ADMIRABLE POWERS OF THE ELECTRICAL SHOCK; WHICH WE WOULD EARNESTLY RECOMMEND IN ALL CASES OF SUSPENDED ANIMATION.

SOPHIA GREENHILL, on Thursday last, fell out of a one-pair-of stairs window, and was taken up by a man to all appearance dead. The surgeons at the Middlesex Hospital, and an APOTHECARY, declared that nothing could be done for the child.—Mr. SQUIRES, tried the effects of electricity.—Twenty minutes elapsed before he could apply the shock, which he gave to various parts of the body in vain;—but, upon transmitting a few shocks through the THORAX, he perceived a *small pulsation*; in a few minutes the child began to breathe with great difficulty, and after some time she vomited.—A kind of stupor, occasioned by the depression of the cranium, remained for several days, but, by the proper means being used, her health was restored.

The first successful reversal of apparent death by electroshock took place in 1774. This singular incident secured for the resuscitationist, Mr. Squires, a niche in the archives of medical history. However, he was never heard from again after that brief moment of glory.

Figure 6 Reproduction of a portion of the description of the first successful electroshock. *Photo Source University of Central Florida. Literary Source Schecter, D.C. (1971). Early experience with rescuscitation by means of electricity. Surgery, 69, 363, (Fig. 1). Taken from Registers of the Royal Humane Society of London, Nichols & Sons, London, 1774–1784. With permission*

In 1774 the concept of closed chest cardiac massage had yet to be formulated. It was for this reason that the Royal Humane Society, at this time, was interested in gathering and spreading information on electricity and resuscitation. Although Mr Squires, despite his innovative effort, has remained in almost total obscurity, the Society's sponsorship and interest in resuscitation continued to play a leading role in establishing the foundation for future progress. In later years the Humane Society of New York was quite convinced of the efficacy of electricity in such circumstances. It made available detailed instructions on how the shock was to be delivered, spelling out, in particular, the nuances in the strength of the shocks, and detailed instructions in number and site. They are quite similar to the recommendations outlined by Zoll in 1952 for restoring the heartbeat in ventricular standstill[309,310].

Aldini favored artificial respiration in combination with 'the application of the galvanic power externally to the diaphragm, and to the region of the heart, and afterwards to various parts of the muscular system'[311]. He was careful to delineate the differences between syncope, apoplexy and the heart, as indicated by the characteristics of the pulse and respiration. He was very well aware that the integrity of respiration was an important factor in successful reanimation.

In the case of persons apparently drowned, recourse should immediately be had to an inflation of the lungs, at the same time that the galvanic application is made. This stimulant has the power of exciting the contractions of the heart, and of causing the blood to flow through the lungs. The latter can only be accomplished when the lungs are distended, and when it is assisted by their subsequent subsidence. Every contraction of the heart, excited by too powerful an impulse, and at the improper time, lessens the small remains of vital power. Therefore, moderate shocks, cautiously and gradually increased, and passed through the chest in different directions, are attended with the best effects. These cannot fail, when galvanism is combined in such a manner with the aid of artificial respiration, that the action of the one keeps in perfect unison with the action of the other, and in no respect interferes with it … The success attending the application of electricity, as well as in galvanism, must materially depend upon the mode in which it is employed. According to the strength and direction of the electrical current, it may be made to produce different or even opposite effects'[311].

Notice how he stressed caution in the strength of the shocks, and how the increments in strength should be gradual. Figure 7 is an illustration in Aldini's book depicting his experiments on corpses regarding the feasibility of resuscitation by means of galvanic stimulation.

Aldini was Galvani's nephew, and, no doubt, his interest in 'Galvanism' stemmed from this relationship. His public demonstrations with dead animals and his flair for sensationalism brought him a mixture of fame and notoriety. On one occasion (February 16, 1803), the *London Morning Post* described how 'the head of an ox, recently decapitated, exhibited astonishing effects; for the tongue, being drawn out by a hook fixed into it, on applying the exciters, in spite of the strength of the assistant, was retracted, so as to detach itself by tearing itself from the hook; at the same time a loud noise issued from the mouth, attended by violent contortions of the whole head and eyes'. Haggard quotes a satirical verse which describes this very demonstration before many dignitaries in Dr Pearson's lecture room. To wit:

He cut off a bullock's head, I ween,
Sheer off, as if by guillotine;
Then (Satan aiding the adventure)
He made it bellow like a Stentor!
And this most comical magician
Will soon in public exhibition,
Perform a feat he's often boasted,
And animate a dead pig-roasted.

With powers of these metallic tractors,
He can revive dead malefactors;
And is re-animating daily,
Rogues that were hung once, at Old Bailey![312]

Although such public demonstrations were but a reflection of Aldini's desire for recognition, animal experimentation with galvanism (as we have already seen in Chapter 16) was not new. The possibilities of galvanism had intrigued many investigators since the invention of the voltaic pile. Eugenio Valli, for one, demonstrated how he was able to revive fowl and frogs with a galvanic current[313]. Richard Fowler may have been the first to prove experimentally that reanimation was possible long after death. He reported in 1796 his observations on a frog whose heart, despite being in asystole for one hour, was restored to normal rhythm by applying a galvanic current to the vagus and sympathetic nerves[314]. That same year Alexander von Humboldt temporarily revived a linnet that he found lying on the ground in his garden, and, who, for all intents, was apparently dead. His method for doing so was imaginative, to say the least. He created the electric shock by connecting a wire between a sliver of silver

in its rectum and a small blade of zinc in its back. Humboldt described 'very vivid flashes before the eyes' when he set up the same type of circuit between his own mouth and anus[315]. Humboldt's method in modified form was later used on humans. It was said to be a more effective method of total electrification then insufflating tobacco smoke into the rectum, a method that Schechter said was prevalent at the time[316]. Some other methods were quite outrageous and even dangerous. Some of them required equipment that because of their size and mode of construction precluded their use in emergency situations. An example of this was a bathtub made of alternate sheets of different metals and filled with brine or dilute vinegar. The victim was immersed in this and electrified with chains wrapped around his body[317]. Schechter also describes how some doctors, always ready for an emergency, were rumored to have carried with them walking canes containing all the necessary materials for creating an electric current on the spot[318,319].

R. Reece published in 1824 *A medical guide for the use of the clergy, heads of families, and junior practitioners in medicine and surgery*[320]. In it he describes the 'Pensile Galvanic Pile', uniquely conceived, and an example of one of the earliest batteries. It was designed by Dr De Sanctis. All the parts necessary for making the pile at the emergency site were carried in a small case, and it took but a few minutes to create this source of energy.

As galvanotherapy became better known, its application in humans was tentatively recommended at first as an adjunct procedure. This was particularly so in the many cases of asphyxiation from coal-gas fumes; the industrial revolution being responsible for its increasing prevalence.

Some enlightenment can be obtained on the resuscitative protocol during this period from Good's description in his textbook of medicine published in 1836[321]. 'If insensible, cold water should be dashed on his face; strong vinegar, and especially aromatic vinegar, be rubbed about his nostrils, and held under them, and stimulating clysters (enemas) be injected, as recommended under the first variety. The lungs should be inflated with the warm breath of a healthy man, or which is better, with oxygen gas'.

It seems as though clysters were the first line of intervention followed by mouth-to-mouth resuscitation and then, as the following paragraph indicates, galvanotherapy, but only as an adjunct

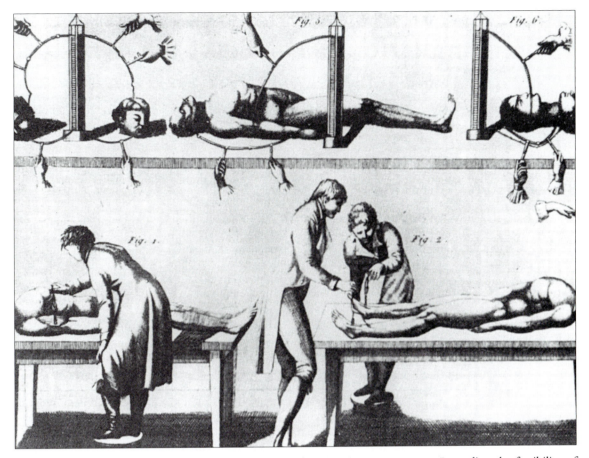

Figure 7 Illustration in John Aldini's book depicting his experiments on corpses regarding the feasibility of rescuscitation by means of galvanic stimulation. *Photo Source University of Central Florida. Literary Source Aldini, J. (1804). Essai Theorique et Experimental pour le Galvanisme. (Paris: Fournier fils). With permission*

measure. 'A proper use of voltaic electricity is also in many instances found highly serviceable. No advantage, however, is likely to accrue from passing the electric aura across the chest, directly through the heart and lungs, which is a common practice. The fluid should be transmitted along the channel of the nerve, from the seat of the diaphragm, or that of the par vagum immediately under the sterno-mastoid muscles, and that of the great sympathetic nerve, which sends forth branches to the heart'[321].

All these methods, whether crude, bizarre or refined, serve to indicate that there must have been a great deal of enthusiasm behind reanimation by electrification during the first half of the 19th century. Unfortunately, no living wills were in force then, and many individuals were subjected to the prevailing modes of resuscitation – against their wishes, if they had only been able to express themselves. How reflective this is of today's hell-bent measures for 'saving lives', no matter what.

This widespread interest in electricity continued unabated throughout the remainder of the 19th century. At the same time investigators also focused their attention on the arrhythmogenic properties of electricity, with more and more reports appearing as the 20th century began to unfold, while continuing to explore the therapeutic potentialities of this modality as well.

Thus, in 1850 Ludwig and Hoffa were able to provoke ventricular fibrillation in the animal by applying a 'faradic' current to the heart[322]. At the same time, the recurrent reports of sudden death due to chloroform anesthesia remained a powerful factor in adherence to electrical measures as a means of resuscitation[323], so much so that in 1851, a paper was presented before the French Academy of Sciences urging that operating rooms be equipped with the electrical means, then in vogue, for reanimation. This was two years before Snow's bold delivery of Queen Victoria under chloroform anesthesia. The same year that Queen Victoria exposed herself to possible death, Jobert de Lamballe placed his imprimatur on electroresuscitation by presenting a protocol before the same society that included electropuncture and shocks to the buccal and rectal mucosa, and electrification through moistened sponges placed directly on the thorax[324].

Not many years later, T. Green, a surgeon, installed a galvanic battery as standard equipment in his operating room. In his paper published in the *British Medical Journal* in 1872 he reported successful revival in six out of seven cases of cardiorespiratory arrest due to chloroform anesthesia[325]. It was not uncommon in the ensuing years to use a galvanic stimulus of over 300 volts from batteries made up of more than 200 cells. When faradic current became popular, it was also used with good results.

Von Ziemssen was a leader in applying electricity as a therapeutic agent within the clinical setting. He reported in 1882 that he could alter the heart rate and rhythm by applying electricity either directly to the heart or by passing a direct current through the chest wall[326,327]. Catherina Serafin was the patient whose heart was directly stimulated with this modality. Access to the heart was made possible because of the presence of a thoracic 'window' produced by removal of several ribs during the removal of a malignancy of the chest wall[327].

John A. MacWilliam, a young physiologist who had the benefit of training under Ludwig, Stirling and Schäfer, began to explore cardiac electro-physiologic phenomena early in his career[328]. When he assumed the professorship of physiology at Aberdeen in 1886, he extended his research from cold-blooded animals to mammals. Ventricular fibrillation occupied his attention for several years. His visual description of this arrhythmia in the intact mammalian heart rivals that of Erichsen: 'The ventricular muscle is thrown into a state of irregular arrhythmic [sic] contraction, whilst there is a great fall in the arterial blood pressure, the ventricles become dilated with blood as the rapid quivering movement of their walls is insufficient to expel their contents; the muscular action partakes of the nature of a rapid incoordinated twitching of the muscular tissue'[329].

MacWilliam's knowledge of ventricular fibrillation became quite profound and extensive. His experimental observations included hemodynamic monitoring with the obvious loss of cardiac output and all its consequences. I have always admired the British physicians in their mastery of the language. MacWilliam is no exception. How vivid is his word picture on the loss of cardiac output: 'The cardiac pump is thrown out of gear, and the last of its vital energy is dissipated in the violent and prolonged turmoil of fruitless activity in the ventricular walls'[330].

MacWilliam showed how ventricular fibrillation could be terminated by applying a series of induction shocks 'through the heart, one electrode being applied over the apex of the heart and the other over the sixth or seventh dorsal vertebra, the electrodes to be of large extent. The shocks ought to be about the normal rate of the heart beat'[331]. This was presented before the International Medical Congress held in Washington DC in 1887. In the same paper MacWilliam stressed the clinical importance of abolishing ventricular fibrillation, especially when it occurred during anesthesia … 'In the clinical aspect it specially concerns the cardiac failure which is so grave a possibility among the results of the action of anesthetic agents'[332]. He was also aware that sudden death due to ventricular fibrillation could occur in hearts with 'atheromatous, calcareous, or sclerotic' coronary arteries. In addition, he also described such predisposing factors as 'degenerative changes of a fatty or fibroid nature of the muscular walls, aortic regurgitant disease with its more or less effective compensatory changes in the organ', and in some cases, 'a flabby condition of the muscular tissue'[330]. In 1889 he described his experiences with electrical stimulation of the heart in man[333].

Many years had to elapse before MacWilliam's work and its relationship to resuscitation were fully appreciated. He had even pointed out how cardiac arrest could be due to asystole as well as ventricular fibrillation. A good part of the difficulty lay in the fact that ventricular fibrillation or asystole were such acutely catastrophic events that electrocardiographic documentation was not possible until the advent of monitoring devices. Sir Thomas Lewis was well aware of and troubled by this lack of documentation in man. In his collected *Lectures on the heart* published in 1915 he remarked 'Why is fibrillation of the ventricles so uncommon an experience? For a good reason: fibrillation of the ventricles is incompatible with existence ... If it occurs in man, it is responsible for unexpected and sudden death'[334]. In 1911, he and Levy did present, however, electro-cardiographic evidence that when cardiac arrest occurred during chloroform anesthesia, it was due to ventricular fibrillation, and that frequently this terminal arrhythmia was preceded by the appearance of multiform ventricular extrasystoles or ventricular tachycardia[335].

In 1923 MacWilliam published a review of ventricular fibrillation and sudden death. By this time the electrocardiograph had become firmly established as an experimental and clinical tool. The pathophysiology of coronary artery disease was still undergoing the pangs of clarification, yet, he was fully convinced that a fatal outcome in coronary obstruction could be due to ischemic-induced ventricular fibrillation[336].

Numerous observations show that in the presence of the defective blood supply following ligation the abnormal conditions that develop in the anaemic areas can only predispose and lead up – often after months – to fibrillation, either during muscular exercise or during rest, but that the abrupt onset of fatal fibrillation may come without preceding signs of cardiac failure, as tested by exercise, or without premonitory evidences of cardiac disturbance in the shape of extrasystolic irregularities, tachycardia, etc. Thus fibrillation can occur without apparent exciting cause and quite apart form the sequence commonly observed – extrasystoles, tachycardia and fibrillation – when death suddenly comes as an early event after coronary ligation[336].

Cardiac arrest due to accidental electrocution was recognized as early as 1882. In a Gulstonian lecture, later published in 1913, A. J. Jex-Blake described how he had observed many years before that cardiac arrest was the cause of death in a man electrocuted by a 250 volt alternating current[337]. In the last year of the 19th century Prevost and Battelli, two physiologists at the University of Geneva, were able to identify what amount of voltage and current were necessary to precipitate ventricular fibrillation in the dog[338]. During this study they made the remarkable discovery that it was also possible to convert ventricular fibrillation to regular sinus rhythm by shocking the heart with a strong electrical current. This finding was emphasized by Jex-Blake during the Gulstonian

lecture as heralding possibly a new approach in the resuscitation of people accidentally electrocuted[339]. This was a new twist on the homeopathic principle of 'similae simila curantur'. The idea was sound but technology had not yet reached the stage to make it possible.

The increasing numbers of accidental deaths due to electrocution brought about a collaborative effort in 1920 between academia and the electrical utilities to find ways of managing this lethal potentiality of electricity. The Bell Telephone scientists also became involved, working primarily with the faculty at Columbia University. The Columbia team under the direction of L. P. Ferris utilized as a base the work reported by R. H. Cunningham in 1899[340].

Aided by a grant from Con Edison of New York five committees were formed to investigate the various aspects of the problem. One of the committees was under a mandate to investigate the physiological phenomena surrounding electro-cution. It was chaired by John Howell and included three other members from the Johns Hopkins faculty: R. D. Hooker, another physiologist, O. R. Langworthy, a neurologist, and B. Kouwenhoven, an electrical engineer. Howell also asked Wiggers to become involved. Wiggers pursued the problem at Western Reserve University in Cleveland. Howell's invitation to Wiggers was more than appropriate because there had already existed at Western Reserve a marked interest in cardiac resuscitation since the beginning of the 20th century. It was initiated by Charles Guthrie, presumably because his brother had been accidentally electro-cuted back in 1902[341,342]. At any rate the studies initiated by Guthrie, and later conducted by Crile, Sollman and Stewart, were continued and expanded further by Wiggers when he assumed the chair of physiology in 1918.

William Kouwenhoven was to play a major role in the evolution of electrical modalities in the management of sudden death. He became noted for three landmark contributions. They were the confirmation that electric shock could indeed reverse ventricular fibrillation, the development of defibrillating devices, and introduction of the technique of external cardiac massage. His interest in cardiovascular physiology began in 1928 when he focused his attention on the effects of electric current on the heart. Most of his early experiments were concerned with the induction and termination of ventricular fibrillation in dogs by electrical means. In 1933 he and his colleagues proved beyond the shadow of a doubt that Prevost and Battelli were right – an electric shock could restore a fibrillating heart to normal rhythm[343,344]. The Albert and Mary Lasker Award for Clinical Medical Research was given to him in 1973. His co-recipient was Paul M. Zoll.

Hooker's early work was also involved with defibrillation. Prior to his collaboration with Kouwenhoven on the effect of alternating currents, Hooker had been successful in defibrillating the dog's heart with an arterial perfusion of a solution of calcium, sodium and potassium ions[345,346]. This was obviously not a practical approach to the problem for out-of-hospital resuscitation.

Wiggers' research was initially an amplification of Crile's pharmacological approaches to cardiac resuscitation but soon included direct cardiac massage[341]. It was only after Kouwenhoven and Hooker confirmed the observations of Prevost and Battelli that Wiggers became interested in the electric approach. He admitted many years later that prior to this he was not convinced of the validity of the experiments conducted by the French team. 'I did not deem a reinvestigation of their claims worthy of the time, effort or expense it would involve'[347]. However, Wiggers' meticulous attention to detail was enough to provide a sound experimental basis for the entire technique of direct electric defibrillation. Wiggers added manual cardiac compression in an effort to increase his success rate. The results of his experiments were presented at a meeting of The American Physiological Society in 1936[348]. Four years after this presentation he and Wegria reported that ventricular fibrillation could be induced by applying an alternating current shock directly to the exposed heart, during the vulnerable period, and then terminated by a second, stronger shock[349]. This is why they called the second jolt of electricity, countershock.

This observation was the outcome of numerous experiments regarding the effects of electrical stimulation of varying intensity and duration, and at varying intervals after a preceding beat. This approach enabled them to delineate the phases of cardiac excitability and allowed them to identify an interval that they called the 'vulnerable phase'. This phase is an interval during the relative refractory period during which a long and strong stimulus well above the threshold for a single response may produce multiple or repetitive beats that could evolve into ventricular fibrillation. The stimuli that provoked this response during the vulnerable period had a duration of 10 ms. This was an extremely important finding since it was to form the basis that regulated the duration of stimuli in the pacemakers that were to come. Stimulus duration in these pacemakers was limited to 3 ms or less in order to avoid the complications of the vulnerable period.

In 1946 two Russian workers, Gurvich and Yuniev reported in the American Review of Soviet Medicine the successful restoration of regular rhythm in the fibrillating mammalian heart with capacitor discharges applied externally across the closed chest[350].

Claude Beck was the first to successfully apply Wigger's countershock method for terminating intraoperative ventricular fibrillation[351]. He performed an emergency thoracotomy, applied the alternating current countershock to the exposed heart and followed through with direct cardiac massage. This protocol formed the basis for his widely accepted seminars on cardiac resuscitation. The one great impediment that prevented its implementation under all circumstances was the necessity to open the chest.

Beck's initial report appeared in 1947 but his interest in treating ventricular fibrillation dated back to 1937 when he commented favorably on 'the splendid work of Hooker and Wiggers and of their respective associates'[352,353]. At that time he had been conducting his experiments on coronary occlusion. Since clamping of the aorta would frequently induce ventricular fibrillation, it was obviously an impediment to any prolonged in vivo study of the heart. It took him, however, 22 years before he applied what he learned about resuscitation in the laboratory to an actual occurrence on the operating table[354]. He improved his success rate when he reduced the surface irritability of the heart and decreased myocardial hyperirritability by adding procaine to the emergency protocol[355].

Beck waited until 1950 before he established, in conjunction with Rand and Hosler, an educational program for the prevention and treatment of cardiac arrest. It was designed for surgeons, anesthetists, dentists and nurses[356,357]. The Cleveland Area Heart Society sponsored it. The course was immensely popular and attracted many participants from all over the USA and many foreign countries, every time it was offered. This course was probably the most important single factor in plucking cardiac resuscitation from an abyss of ignorance and fatalism to an enthusiastic and successful approach. Today's basic cardiopulmonary resuscitation (CPR) and advanced cardiac life support (ACLS) courses sponsored by the American Heart Association are the current versions of the Cleveland Clinic's courses. Innumerable lives have been saved in the process.

Interest in cardiac resuscitation was also quite pronounced in Russia. The Russians created the special Institute of Resuscitation in Moscow for basic research on the subject. Hosler found on his visit to Russia in 1958 that every hospital in Russia had a department of resuscitation whose specially trained members acted in a standby capacity during major surgery[358].

As time went on it became quite obvious that circumstances surrounding out-of-hospital cardiac resuscitation mandated the need for closed chest methods. The electrical utilities especially were aware of the pressing need every time an electrocution occurred some distance from the nearest hospital. What was needed was a portable defibrillator that could work anywhere on a patient without opening his chest. In 1951 the Edison Electric Institute asked Kouwenhoven to meet this need. He was on the original committee when Howell was chairman. By this time Howell had died and Langworth had a busy psychiatric practice. Alfred Blalock now offered Kouwenhoven space in the department of surgery laboratory. Kouwenhoven's initial experiments were with dogs and by 1957 he had developed an AC type of defibrillator that could be used in humans. In the meantime, Paul Zoll in Boston had developed his own AC defibrillator for external use. He reported this a year before Kouwenhoven[359]. Zoll played a major role in advancing our knowledge concerning electrical control of cardiac rhythm. We shall meet him again shortly.

The next advance in resuscitation was remarkable because of its utter simplicity and ease of performance. The technique was called closed-chest cardiac massage when it was introduced by Kouwenhoven in 1960[360]. The word massage is a misnomer. No one actually handles the heart as in the open-chest protocol of Beck. The heart is resuscitated by rhythmic mechanical compression of the thorax as it transmits a mechanical stimulus to the ventricle which, in turn, keeps the circulation going. It is in essence a stop-gap measure to assure adequate blood supply to the vital organs while other measures are brought into play. When Kouwenhoven first introduced it the intent was to keep the patient alive until an external defibrillator could be deployed. It is now a standard part of the cardiopulmonary resuscitation protocol and with the advent of portable monitoring devices one can easily determine if the heart is in asystole or fibrillating so that prompt corrective measures can be instituted.

Many hours were spent in the morgue by Kouwenhoven and his colleagues practicing and exploring the maneuver on cadavers before rigor mortis set in. Refinements were adopted as their experience grew. They learned how to compress the heart between the lower sternum and vertebrae without damaging the chest or abdominal structures.

The concept was not original with Kouwenhoven. Several others had tried it before without creating any enthusiasm or acceptance. But the time was ripe for its ready acceptance when Kouwenhoven reintroduced it. The technique was first used clinically by John Hill, a British dentist, in 1868[361]. Boehm described its use in cats in 1878[362]. Another clinical report appeared by Koenig in 1883. Maas of Gottingen described it in 1892[363] during chloroform anesthesia, and in 1904, the innovative American surgeon, George Crile was also successful with his attempt[364].

When Kouwenhoven's report appeared in 1960 it was soon followed by an avalanche of papers on the subject. Many of them were concerned with the efficacy of closed chest massage versus the open chest direct method. The closed chest method has withstood all the objections and continues to remain a safe, simple, and effective emergency measure in cardiac arrest. The standards and principles for cardiopulmonary resuscitation were firmly established in 1967 and 1974, and, as mentioned previously, the American Heart Association has been responsible for training lay and medical personnel.

Although most cases of cardiac arrest are due to ventricular fibrillation, mechanical stimulation of the heart in asystole was also found to be effective in reestablishing a normal beat. The simple procedure of thumping the precordium in such cases was first described by Schott in 1920, and reactivated by Scherf and Bornemann in 1960[365,366].

Calcium chloride or adrenaline were suggested as alternative means of reactivating an asystolic heart when precordial thumping did not restore a normal beat. Calcium chloride injection was introduced by Kay and Blalock in 1951[367].

CORONARY CARE UNIT

The emergence of the coronary care unit has probably been one of the most beneficial advances in the management of cardiac disturbances. As technological and pharmacological improvements were being made in cardiac resuscitation, it was only logical to apply the lessons learned to circumstances surrounding other types of cardiac dysfunction. The feasibility of creating an environment capable of dealing with acute and potentially lethal cardiac emergencies required the availability of monitoring and therapeutic modalities, and skilled personnel trained specifically for managing such emergencies.

The beginnings of the coronary care unit were the mobile 'crash cart', ever ready to respond to 'code blue'. The term arose out of the fact that patients in need of cardiac resuscitation were often cyanotic. By this time cardiopulmonary resuscitation with mouth-to-mouth respiration and electrical cardioversion of ventricular fibrillation were proving to be effective modes of therapy. Unfortunately, the most pressing need could not be met with the mobile crash cart alone. The equipment was there but trained personnel to utilize it properly were not.

Hughes Day was instrumental in the establishment of the mobile crash cart concept at his institution, the Bethany Medical Center in Kansas City. But in just 3 months he realized only too well that lack of trained personnel could never allow the mobile crash cart to function optimally. He met with his chief, Dr E. Grey Dimond, in the hope of creating a special environment for those cardiac patients most likely to develop emergency situations requiring resuscitation. Dr Dimond gave his full support for the creation of a special area that was to be designated as the 'coronary care unit'.

An 11 bed unit was opened on May 20, 1962. It was built with the support of a grant from the Hartford Foundation of New York City. The unit was prepared to admit only patients with a diagnosis of acute myocardial infarction. Constant and close supervision was provided by a highly trained nursing staff well-versed in the diagnosis and management of acute cardiac emergencies, especially the arrhythmias.

The early results of the concept were presented at a meeting of the American College of Chest Physicians in Los Angeles in November of 1962. Day recounts how very few physicians remained to hear the presentation, but that, fortunately, this had no bearing on the outcome since the chairman, Eliot Corday, became quite interested[368]. It was through his efforts that The American College of Cardiology threw its weight behind the concept and helped formulate the coronary care nursing program.

The second unit to open was limited to two beds at the Presbyterian Hospital in Philadelphia. The third unit was at the Miami Heart Institute. It was under the direction of Paul Unger and had the support of the American Heart Association. Several months later William Grace began operating a specially constructed unit at St. Vincent's Hospital in New York City. It boasted the latest in monitoring devices.

It did not take long for the coronary care unit concept to be implemented around the world. In the process much was learned about arrhythmias associated with myocardial infarction. Also, hemodynamic dysfunction was delineated even more precisely when the Swan–Gans flow guided catheter was introduced to the coronary care unit. It proved to be a boon in the management of the various subsets of patients with myocardial infarction.

The coronary care unit concept was first presented in England to the British Thoracic Society in July, 1961. Malcolm White and Gaston Bauer were so impressed they immediately set into motion the mechanisms for creating a coronary care unit at Sidney Hospital. The unit was in operation in less than a year. When these innovators submitted their first manuscript on their experiences with this new concept to the British Medical Journal, it was rejected because 'it was irresponsible to suggest that all patients with acute myocardial infarction should be admitted to wards in which they can receive intensive care'[369]. This was to prove to be the ultimate in editorial arrogance and ignorance.

At this writing the value of the coronary care unit has been proven again and again. An immediate and significant reduction in mortality from an acute myocardial infarction was realized. Previously unrecognized and potentially lethal arrhythmias were instantly recognized and aborted. This was, perhaps, the most important reason for the reduction in mortality.

CARDIAC PACING

The development of electric control of cardiac rhythm is one of the major triumphs of modern technology. It is a fascinating chapter that bore fruit only after multiple contributions throughout the centuries, with the earlier contributions being purely sporadic. The intensive and focused research of the 20th century resulted in the astonishing capacity of current devices.

Two factors were responsible for the current level of sophistication in cardiac pacing. The first is the great strides in electronics that occurred in the first half of the 20th century and the second represents the fruits of a close collaboration between medical scientists and electronic engineers.

The first capacitor as we have seen was the Leyden jar. The forerunner of the battery was the Voltaic pile. Then came the vacuum tube triode. This was invented by Lee De Forest in 1906. Oscillators which perform a key function in pacemaker circuits were developed between 1910 and 1915. No one man can claim credit for their development. Several workers contributed towards their design, all working independently of each other. It was the growth of radio that stimulated the production of small batteries in the 1920s and 1930s. Perhaps the most important technical development in the field of cardiac pacing was the introduction of the semiconductor transistor in 1948. It was the brain child of three Bell laboratory scientists. They were William Schockley, John Bardeen and Walter Brattain[370–373]. All three were to receive the Nobel Prize in 1956. It was this technological breakthrough that made possible the development of an implantable artificial pacemaker. The subsequent refinements in semiconductor electronics coupled with advances in battery and lead technologies led to the modern micro-processor pacemakers of today.

We have seen how in 1774 Aldini successfully resuscitated a child with intermittent precordial stimulation: Nysten published his experiences with a decapitated man in 1802[374]. Specifically it was the second month of the calendar of the first French Republic (le 14 Brumaire). Actually I am surprised that Nysten described his experiments with only one corpse. Heads were falling off with such profusion during this period of the French revolution that one would think they would be as abundant as acorns on the ground during a windstorm. Be that as it may, Nysten showed that different regions of the heart varied in their ability to be reactivated. The left ventricle was the first to lose this ability, followed by the right ventricle, then the left atrium, and last the right atrium and lower part of the superior vena cava.

In 1862, in his treatise on the heart and great vessels, Walshe advocated electrostimulation for cardiac arrest, but this too went unnoticed[375], except for Duchenne who, ten years later, described his success with electrostimulation in a child with diphtheria[376]. His technique was similar to the one used by Aldini almost a hundred years before. An indifferent electrode was applied to the skin while the stimulating electrode was applied to the precordium in a repetitive and rhythmic fashion.

Von Ziemssen's patient had practically an exposed heart. Only skin covered the precordial area; the ribs having been removed because of a tumor involving them. While stimulating various portions of the precordium he noted that the area overlying the atrioventricular groove was very sensitive[377]. This coincided with later descriptions by Kent and His on the location of the conduction pathways of the AV node and bundle of His. Von Ziemssen also made another important discovery in this and subsequent patients. He noted that intermittent rhythmic stimulation by a sufficiently intense current, at a rate above the spontaneous rate of the heart would now drive the heart at the faster rate, while slower stimulation rates would compete with the spontaneous rate and result in erratic, and, at times, slower heart rate.

Schechter pointed out that during the early experiments with electrostimulation, it was soon observed that a better contraction of the heart was obtained with direct cardiac stimulation than with attempts to activate via nervous pathways[378].

MacWilliam brought cardiac stimulation into the 20th century. His research efforts began in the early 1900s and continued well into the last days of World War I[379]. His technique in cardiac arrest consisted of applying rhythmic stimulation at 60 or 70 impulses per minute. Each stimulus was applied either directly to the myocardium or transthoracically via large saline-moistened paddles over the back and precordium[379].

Marmorstein also deserves credit for his work in 1927. He used endocardial unipolar, bipolar or tripolar electrodes to stimulate the SA node and either ventricle in dogs[380]. Entry was gained through the venous or arterial route.

Albert Hyman is credited as being the originator of the artificial cardiac pacemaker. His paper appeared in the Archives of Internal Medicine in 1932[381]. He was a physician at the Beth David Hospital in New York City who became interested in developing an effective means of stimulating the heart in ventricular standstill. After experimenting with rabbits, he was able to resuscitate several patients using periodic voltage impulses applied to the right atrium via a transthoracic needle electrode powered by an apparatus of his own design. It was a magneto-like device with a spring mechanism that had to be rewound every six minutes. He referred to it as an artificial pacemaker and the term has become part of our medical vocabulary. The apparatus is illustrated in Figure 8.

Two years before the publication of his paper, Hyman had described personally to Schechter the detailed specifications of this portable apparatus, and though quite primitive and crude, it did, in principle, presage our current ones. The pulse generator in Hyman's words and as Schechter quoted them was 'small enough to fit into a doctor's bag', and had as its current source 'a common flashlight battery'[382]. The contemplated design also included timing and current regulating devices and an interrupter mechanism. Although designed primarily for use in animals, it was later successfully used by Hyman in humans on a number of occasions[383].

Hyman's classic paper refers to a number of similar and previous attempts at electrostimulation in animals, and more importantly to an Australian by the name of Gould who, three years earlier, had developed, successfully used, and published information on a similar piece of apparatus. For years, though, Gould's role seemed to have been forgotten. He was never mentioned in any of the subsequent publications on the subject. This seemed rather strange since Hyman's own milestone contribution was acknowledged time and again.

In 1982, a paper appeared by Harry Mond and his associates that went very far in unraveling the reasons for lack of recognition or knowledge on the role Gould played in the development of the first artificial pacemaker[384]. The fact of the matter is that

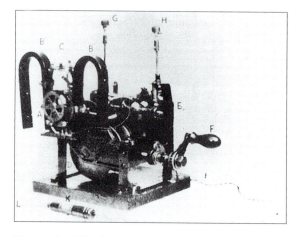

Figure 8   The first pacemaker as designed by Albert Hyman. *Photo Source University of Central Florida. Literary Source Gold, R.D. Cardiac pacing – from then to now. Medical Instrumentation, vol.18, no.1, Jan–Feb.1984. (Fig.1). With permission*

Gould never existed. The actual inventor was Mark C. Lidwill. When describing the Australian contribution Hyman wrote the following: 'In 1929 at the Medical Congress held in Sydney, Australia, Gould demonstrated an electric device for stimulating the heart; this apparatus consisted of a neutral plate and a positive needle electrode which was inserted into the heart. Gould reported the case of a baby who was resuscitated by such electrical stimulations of this organ'. Mond and his associates searched the transactions of the Third Session of the Australasian Medical Congress (British Medical Association) held in Sydney, Australia from September 2nd to 7th, 1929. There was no record of a paper having been presented by an author called Gould. On the other hand the search did reveal a paper presented by Mark C. Lidwill with the relevant data on the invention of a pacemaker given in an appendix to that paper. Figure 9 illustrates the front page of the transactions on the left while the right panel shows the first page of Lidwill's paper.

The following excerpts from the appendix describes the invention. Major Booth's help in designing the machine is acknowledged.

… if this fails to respond, one can supply an artificial impulse. With this in view, I designed some time ago a machine by means of which direct stimulation to the heart's muscle may be applied. It was unknown, at first, what voltage

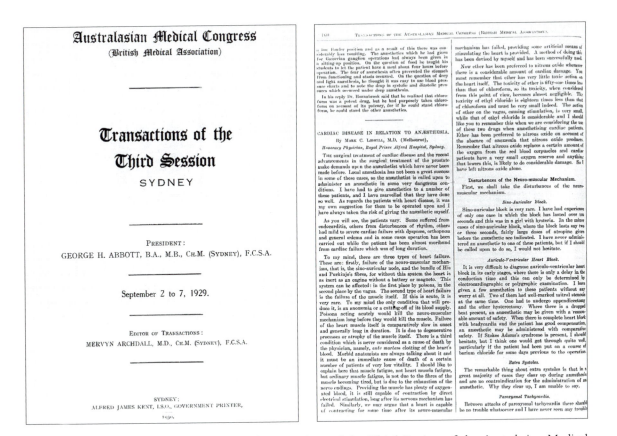

Figure 9 Illustration of the front page of Transactions of the Third Session of the Australasian Medical Congress in Sidney, 1929. On the right, the first page of Lidwill's paper. *Photo Source National Library of Medicine. Literary Source Mond, H.G.,Sloman, J.G. and Edwards, R.H. (1982). The first pacemaker. Pace, **5**, 279–82 (Fig.1). With permission*

was required. Dr. Briggs who was at the Crown-street Women's Hospital, carried out experiments for me in stillborn infants. Voltage was used from 1.5 up to 120 and it was found that somewhere about 16 volts was the pressure required. The method was tried in two or three cases and was completely successful in the case of a stillborn infant, when everything else had been done to revive the child, artificial respiration, injections of 'Pituitrin' and adrenalin injected into the heart itself. After this had failed, the needle of the machine was plunged into the auricle and various voltages were tried with no result. The needle was then plunged into the ventricle, and the heart responded to each impulse. At the end of ten minutes the current was stopped and it was found that the heart would beat of its own accord. The child recovered completely and is now living and quite healthy. After Dr. Briggs left the Women's

Hospital the work was not carried on, as the machine was so complicated that it was very difficult to understand. I now demonstrate to you a portable and simplified form of this machine. The rate of impulses can be varied from about eighty to one hundred and twenty. This method of cardiac revival is applicable to the following types of cases: (i) Cardiac failure during anæsthesia, (ii) cases of drowning, if combined with intratracheal insufflation, (iii) certain types of gas poisoning, (iv) sudden death during the incidence of acute disease, for example diphtheria, (v) possibly, sudden death during cardiac disease.

The machine, as shown, requires only to be plugged into a lighting point and its use does not require very much intelligence. One pole is applied to a pad on the skin, say the left arm, and is saturated with strong salt solution. The other pole which consists of a needle insulated except at its point, is plunged into the ventricle and the machine is started. It may be necessary to alter the polarity of the poles and there is a switch for doing this. When the current is applied to the apparently dead body, the whole thorax and arm contract. I think if this machine were used, it would often save lives. There may be many failures, but one life in fifty or even a hundred, is a big advancement where there is no hope at all.

For his help in the design of this new machine, I should like to thank Major Booth, of the Physics Department, University of Sydney[385].

The next important paper appeared in 1950. It was the work of Wilfred Bigelow, John Callaghan and Jack Hopps[386]. Callaghan was a research fellow in Bigelow's laboratory at the Banting Institute in Toronto. Hopps, the engineer, had been working on the radio-frequency pasteurization of beer when he was asked to join Bigelow in 1949[387]. Hypothermia as an aid in cardiac surgery was the focus of their research (see Chapter 29). The pacemaker was developed as a result of their efforts to overcome the occurrence of cardiac standstill when the experimental animal was subjected to hypothermia. The first commercial pacemaker was built to their design by Smith and Stone Ltd. More than twenty units of this design were then supplied to centers in Canada, the USA and Europe[387].

Banting recalled how it all started in a short paper published in Pace. These are his words:

One morning, a standard experiment was planned. As I entered the laboratory, an anesthetized dog was already being cooled in refrigeration blankets with ice bags. At a body temperature of 22°C, with regular heart action and adequate blood pressure, the cooling was discontinued, the top blanket removed, and the chest opened. Cardiac arrest was not expected to occur until 20°C, so the pericardium was opened. We were now ready to make certain physiologic observations regarding hypothermia, after which the pericardium and chest would be closed and the animal rewarmed.

Just as we were about to begin these tests, the heart unexpectedly stopped and lay quietly in standstill. Cardiac massage did not restart it. In some frustration and desperation, since the experiment would have to be postponed, I gave the left ventricle a good poke with the forceps I was holding. There was an immediate and strong

contraction that involved all chambers – and then it returned to standstill. I did it again with the same result and marvelled at the unexpected observation. I poked it regularly every second. It resembled a normal beating heart. The technician/anesthetist said, 'Hey, I am getting a blood pressure here'. Not only were these real contractions that I induced, but the heart was forcibly expelling blood into the circulation. Our experimental animal was successfully resuscitated by maintaining heart action in this manner and with manual cardiac massage while it was being rewarmed, and it later recovered completely.

We had now found a project to be pursued with vigor. The heart had stopped while it appeared to be perfectly capable of continued function. Perhaps an electrical impulse had the same effect as a mechanical poke. We had read reports of research indicating that in laboratory animals, and presumably humans, nerve impulses were not conducted along the nerve below body temperatures of 9–10° C, while in hibernators, conduction was not affected down to body temperatures of 2–3° C. In an atmosphere of excitement and anticipation, John Callaghan and I discussed the prospects of an electrical stimulator or pacemaker for the heart. ... We were in need of help from electrical engineering.

Bigelow assigned the project to Callaghan and Hopps. Initial studies were carried out in the turtle. They then progressed to controlled stimulation of the heart beat in dogs. Transvenous leads were designed by Hopps and made by the National Research Council of Canada. Unfortunately, they limited themselves to transvenous pacing of the SA node and right atrium. Escher commented in his review that had they advanced the electrode into the right ventricle, they might have arrived at the 'pacing' treatment of Stokes–Adams syndrome a decade earlier[388].

When Callaghan presented the results of their animal experimentation at the American College of Surgeons meeting in Boston on October 23, 1950, it turned out to be one of the highlights of the session. The newspapers were eager to spread the information. Even the usually staid New York Times carried the story under a rather eye-catching headline and written by the well-respected science reporter, William L. Laurence. Figure 10 is a photograph of the beginning of the article.

Paul M. Zoll was one of the attenders at the meeting. According to Callaghan, Zoll wrote to him in the space of a week asking for more data and the details of the circuitry. Callaghan complied and sent Zoll all the experimental data and a diagram of the circuitry as developed by Hopps. Unfortunately when Zoll published his article in 1952, he forgot to indicate the source of the electric circuit diagram that he used in his pacemaker[389]. In 1972, when Zoll traced the historical development of cardiac pacemakers in an article written specifically for publication in *Progress in Cardiovascular Diseases*, he stated: 'I found that he [Callaghan] used a standard physiologic pacemaker made by the Grass Instrument Co. in Quincy, Mass., and I managed to borrow one from Otto Krayer, head of the Pharmacology Department at the Harvard Medical School'[390].

In 1987 he wrote a letter to the editor of Pace commenting on Bigelow's historical review of the pacemaker story. This time he said,

> After his lecture in Boston in 1950, William Callaghan told me he had used the commercially available Grass Physiological Stimulator, which we then acquired and used successfully in experimental and clinical applications with proper identifications of the instrument. I have publicly acknowledged Callaghan's assistance for this many times. We did not copy the Canadian instrument devised by Jack Hopps as Professor Bigelow implies; the output shown on its panel would have been too low for noninvasive transcutaneous stimulation. My engineer, Alan Belgard, went on independently to design and manufacture a commercially successful pulse generator as well as related instruments, such as implantable cardiac pacemakers, the cardiac monitor, and external (noninvasive) defibrillator[391].

All of this does not detract from the importance of Zoll's paper in 1952. He made a quantum leap whether or not he applied the circuitry of Hopps as an external method of cardiac electrostimulation[392]. His early experiments were carried out in dogs. 'With a long wire electrode in the esophagus and the second electrode over the precordium in a dog, we were able to demonstrate that an electric stimulus would indeed arouse atrial or ventricular electrical responses and effective myocardial contractions with which cardiac arrest could be reversed and the circulation maintained'[392].

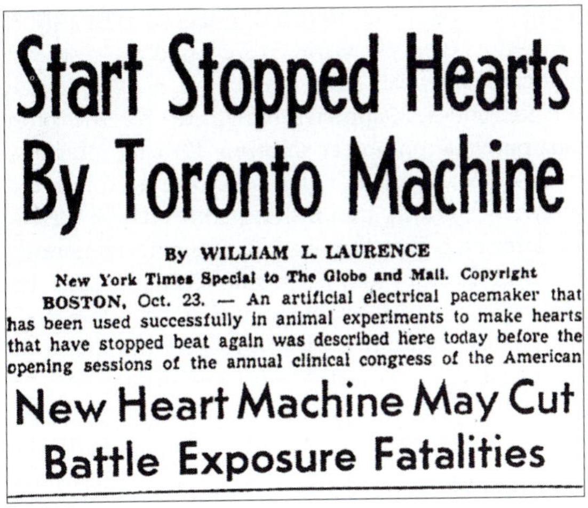

Start Stopped Hearts By Toronto Machine

By WILLIAM L. LAURENCE
New York Times Special to The Globe and Mail. Copyright
BOSTON, Oct. 23. — An artificial electrical pacemaker that has been used successfully in animal experiments to make hearts that have stopped beat again was described here today before the opening sessions of the annual clinical congress of the American

New Heart Machine May Cut Battle Exposure Fatalities

Figure 10 New York Times article by William L. Laurence. *Photo Source University of Central Florida. Literary Source Bigelow, W. (1987). The pacemaker story: a cold heart spinoff. Pace, **10**, 142–51 (Fig.8). With permission of the New York Times*

Zoll decided to try the esophageal rather than the transvenous approach of Callaghan because of the close anatomical relationship of the esophagus and the heart. Although not truly external, the technique offered promise because it avoided thoracotomy. Further investigations were then conducted to refine and simplify the procedure, identify and eliminate hazardous complications, and define its clinical indications and limitations. The method was tried for the first time in man just before the publication of his paper. The patient had complete heart block. He applied 2 ms stimulus pulses of 75–150 volts via two metal paddles on the anterior chest wall. Zoll's breakthrough did not impress many people, least of all the US Public Health Service – they turned down his request for a $5000 grant to pursue his studies[393]. Undaunted, Zoll continued with his studies. At times, patients could be maintained on this form of stimulation for days but really long-term usage was out of the question. There were several drawbacks to Zoll's method: skin burns; at times, almost intolerable pain because of mass muscle contraction; and erratic results in thick-walled or emphysematous individuals[394,395]. The problems were overcome by Weirich but his solution involved insertion directly into the myocardium of temporary wires that could be removed later by a slight tug[396]. Initially, one wire was inserted into the myocardium, with the indifferent electrode attached to the skin. In a short time the Weirich wires were used as a direct myocardial bipolar lead. There was no doubt that the method was effective but it was for the most part purely a temporary solution. Usually, after two weeks, the increasing myocardial threshold resulted in a continuously diminishing ability to be paced. Zoll realized that this was due to a foreign body reaction to the minute sterile contaminants on the electrode surface. He solved it by using inert metals for the active electrode and boiling it in soap flakes[397].

Furman's solution was the transvenous endocardial approach. He became increasingly disenchanted with the Zoll and Weirich techniques because of their obvious drawbacks, and set about to design his own equipment. Furman was not only interested in resuscitation; he was seeking a method that could be used for sustained pacing and the endocardial approach seemed quite feasible to him. He was unaware of the efforts of Bigelow, Callaghan and Hopps.

Preliminary experiments were conducted on dogs. His initial electrode was a diagnostic Cournand cardiac catheter. A steel wire acted as the conductor. It was soldered distally to tinfoil wrapped around the tip of the catheter and proximally to the steel hub of the catheter. These studies led to several important considerations, all of which were to prove useful with cumulative experience. The myocardium could be stimulated with a threshold as low as 0.5 A. Faster rates could be induced in the subject's heart so long as the applied stimulus was at a rate above that of the inherent rhythm. Rapid pacing was able to suppress idiorhythmicity; abrupt withdrawal then of the pacing stimuli would result in resumption of intrinsic rhythm after a long pause. Most importantly, missed beats and competitive pacing were not likely to provoke ventricular fibrillation.

Furman's first patient was an elderly man with an 11 year history of Stokes–Adams seizures due to complete heart block. It was to be purely a precautionary measure while the patient was undergoing surgery for a non-related condition. All went without a hitch until the moment came to stop the pacing postoperatively. Doing so abruptly resulted in asystole. The patient was finally able to revert to his preoperative idioventricular rhythm by gradually reducing the pacing rate to a level just below his own[398,399].

This initial success was soon followed by others, but not without difficulties and complications, foreseen or unexpected. Clotting and infection were two major concerns. Others were durability of the electrode and stabilization of its site of placement. Nobody had any idea regarding the possibility or even the feasibility of long term pacing. Source of power was an extremely important consideration. Furman's second patient exemplified the elaborate setup that was required. He was placed on an alternating current-powered Electrodyne Pacemaker Monitor with an asystolic alarm to activate pacing. The patient could not walk very far. He was tethered to the power source and monitor, both of which were perched on a rolling cart and attached by a 50 foot cord to a wall outlet[400].

Furman's original electrode was made by the US Catheter and Instrument Corp. It consisted of a steel ball embedded in the tip of a Cournand no.6 diagnostic catheter and connected to a proximal metal pin by a copper wire within the lumen. The steel ball was later replaced by a platinum tip ensuring permanent durability[401]. In 1962 Parsonnet and Zucker introduced the bipolar electrode thereby eliminating the indifferent skin electrode and the pain it caused while at the same time allowing the use of higher pacing currents.

The interest that pacing aroused was amazing. European, British and American centers soon established their own programs and within a span of just a few years, further refinements appeared.

Glenn demonstrated in 1959 that a radio frequency coupled pacer was feasible[402]. He used a vacuum tube transmitter circuit. A tuned coil of wire was implanted subcutaneously and connected through a detector diode to a myocardial electrode. Another coil of wire was cemented to the skin directly over the implanted coil. This was the prototype for many small portable transmitters that achieved some degree of popularity for several years. The patient had to carry the external transmitter strapped or taped to the skin. Batteries had to be replaced on a weekly or monthly basis depending on the size of the unit. The Italian, Camilli, developed his version in 1964[403]. In the same year Abrams and Norman of England introduced direct coupling of the stimulating pulse without benefit of an RF carrier frequency[404].

The totally implantable pulse generator became a reality with the invention at first of the point contact transistor by the Bell laboratory scientists in 1948, followed two years later by their junction transistor. The first ones to apply the benefits of technological miniaturization clinically were the Swedes, Ake Senning and Rune Elmqvist. Their considerably down-sized pulse generator was implanted in 1958[405,406]. A thoracotomy was needed to suture the two electrodes into the left ventricular myocardium. The transistorized pacemaker with a rechargeable nickel–cadmium battery was implanted in the abdominal wall. Elmqvist, an engineer, was responsible for designing the electronic components. Unfortunately, the pacer functioned for only three hours. The replacement lasted for only eight days. Gold recounts how the patient, also an engineer, had to wait three years before an adequately functioning replacement was available. The patient, in fact, collaborated with Elmqvist and Senning in redesigning the replacement[407]. He had complete heart block and was subject to recurrent Stokes–Adams seizures. The collaboration paid off since he was still alive and well more than 20 years and 2 dozen implants later.

In the USA the electronic engineer responsible for the development of another version of an implantable pacemaker was Wilson Greatbatch. He worked with William Chardack and Andrew Gage. The pacemaker contained only eight circuit components including two transistors. Ten mercury–zinc cells provided the power source. All the components were enclosed in an epoxy resin with an outer coating of silicone rubber. This type of encapsulation remained in vogue until the 1970s[408]. Their bipolar myocardial disk electrode was a modified version of the type designed by Hunter and Roth[409,410]. The pacer was asynchronous. It delivered a periodic stimulus to the ventricle regardless of the underlying ventricular rhythm of the moment.

Actually Samuel Hunter was the first to achieve long term pacing in complete heart block with the bipolar myocardial electrode[411]. The obvious disadvantage was that myocardial implantation required a thoracotomy. Despite this, several series of studies were conducted with this method resulting in the accumulation of enough evidence to regard this type of pacemaker–electrode system as being adequate for the long-term management of the Stokes–Adams syndrome. Working independently, the investigators involved were, besides Chardack, Paul Zoll and A. Kantrowitz[412,413].

The feasibility of implanted pacemakers was now an established fact, and accelerated technological improvements and widening clinical applications. Completely implantable units were developed by Zoll in 1961 and Kantrowitz in 1962[412,413].

Close cooperation among manufacturers, engineers and cardiac electrophysiologists resulted in such an explosive growth that cardiac pacing soon achieved the status of a subspecialty within the field of cardiology. No doubt a profit-motive existed, but, despite this, the involved corporations should be acclaimed for their research, integrity and dedication to perfection.

Advances were made in circuitry, batteries, electrodes and leads, and pacer cases. Various pacing modes were introduced as the clinical indications expanded far beyond the original Stokes–Adams syndrome. They now include, among so many, the sick sinus syndrome, recurrent tachyarrhythmias, and pre-excitation syndromes. Programming, telemetry and instrumentation reached a high degree of sophistication. The leaders in the industry were Medtronics Corp. and Cordis.

This reminds me of what Brother Alfred loved to say in his philosophy class during my undergraduate days at Manhattan College. 'Philosophers get to know less and less about more and more, while scientists get to know more and more about less and less'.

Subsequent developments in semiconductor microelectronics contributed to increased pacer longevity and broader clinical indications. R. N. Noyce was responsible for inventing the planar silicon integrated circuit[414]. The other important invention was the complementary metal oxide semiconductor (CMOS) field-effect integrated circuit. Ted Cuddy implanted one of the first pacers containing an integrated circuit in 1971[415]. It was also the first electronically controlled, noninvasive programmable pacer to be implanted.

Semiconductor microprocessors had made their appearance by the end of the 1970s. An early Sequicor made by Cordis was the first such device to be implanted. It was designed and developed by Peter Tarjan, Michael Leckrome, and Vincent Cutolo. It was the first programmable universal DDD pacer to be implanted. V. Parsonnet was responsible for its initial implantation in the summer of 1980[416].

The mercury–zinc cell was developed by Friedman and McCauley in 1947[417]. Greatbatch, as we have seen, was the first to incorporate it as the pacemaker power source in 1960[418]. It rapidly supplanted the nickel–cadmium rechargeable cell because of its longer life, which was, in reality, about 2 years, far less than the theoretical one of 5–7 years. It was also plagued with many premature failures because of its corrosive liquid electrolyte. Despite these faults, and because the competitive weekly rechargeable nickel–cadmium cell was inconvenient, the mercury–zinc remained as the favored power source until a better one could be found.

Biomechanical and bioelectric approaches were also studied. Parsonnet and co-workers reported on their experience with two biomechanical power sources in 1964[419]. On the other hand, the problems associated with the use of body fluids to form a galvanic cell (bioelectric approach) were too formidable and were subsequently abandoned[420,421]. Nuclear batteries were then proposed. They have an estimated pacer life of 25–30 years. The first such power source was implanted in France in 1970[422]. Although such pacemakers show the highest cumulative survival rate of all current power sources, inherent disadvantages have limited their acceptance. They have two major drawbacks: possible radiation injury to both patient and others and possible contamination of the environment if the hermetically sealed cases were to rupture.

The more recently introduced lithium based cells appear to have resolved many of the problems associated with the previous ones. The Italians were the first to implant this type of power source in 1972. It was a lithium–iodide cell developed by Greatbatch[423]. Cardiac Pacemakers Inc. were the first to incorporate them in their pacemakers with the first American implant taking place several months after the Italians'. Today lithium is in virtually all implants. The highest survival rate has been found in the lithium–cupric–sulfide system[424]. Gabano had introduced this system as far back as the late 1960s[425].

The implantation of electrodes via the transvenous route was introduced primarily to circumvent the necessity of a thoracotomy with the myocardial approach. However, the early difficulties encountered with the transvenous method made it difficult for a while to choose between the two approaches. Wound infection, electrode perforation of the heart, dislodgement of electrodes and leads, wire fracture, inadvertent muscle and diaphragmatic stimulation were some of the more important complications with the transvenous approach. A good number of these disadvantages were overcome or minimized by such improvements as:

(1) multifilar and carbon filament leads,

(2) replacement of silicone elastomer with polyurethane as a lead insulator, and

(3) the lead introducer by Philip Littleford which allows two leads to be placed in the subclavian vein more easily than with the silicone leads[426].

Lead durability was also increased. The incidence of lead dislodgement was markedly reduced with the introduction of fins or tines as well as porous-tipped and porous-surfaced electrodes. Some of the newer leads also have a screw-in tip that may be non-retractable or retractable, an important consideration.

Stimulation thresholds were also brought down with the reduction in electrode areas. The changes in material, size, shape and weight of the pacer case itself also brought about significant improvements. Titanium coupled with the use of hermetically sealed batteries helped eliminate the seepage of body fluids and battery electrolytes into the electronic circuit compartment.

The introduction of various pacing modes constitutes one of the greatest advances in the field. The first devices, as we have seen, were asynchronous and rather limited in their application. In 1962, D. A. Nathan and S. Center implanted the first AV synchronous pacer in a patient[427]. It was manufactured by Cordis Corp. and marketed under the name Atricor[428]. Keller was the electronic engineer responsible for its development. This was a major breakthrough in terms of simulating a true 'physiologic state'. P-wave synchronous pacemakers evolved through the efforts of Folkman and Watkins[429], Stephenson[430], and Kahn[431]. They utilized a portable battery-powered, exteriorized and transistorized P-wave pulse generator. As improvements were made in leads and integrated circuitry the AV sequential pacing mode was followed by the dual-chamber ones. In the single chamber mode, demand, standby or R-wave inhibited pacers emerged. Leatham had thought of such pacers in 1956[432]. Nicks' group described their devices in 1962[433]. They were much simpler; a preset period of asystole initiated an output pulse that continued until the output was deactivated manually. Berkovits designed the modern inhibited pacer. Clinical experience with it was reported first by Lemberg in 1965, and over the next two years by Parsonnet and Furman[434–436].

Other types of pacing modes were developed. The R-wave synchronous mode called the Ectocor was introduced by Cordis Corp. in 1966[437]. Parsonnet presented a coding method in 1974 to help identify and describe the ever increasing proliferation of pacing methods[438]. These are under constant revision as new modes keep emerging.

Technological refinements opened the door to a virtually unlimited number of programmable pacing parameter combinations. The first non-invasive electronically controlled programmable pacing system was introduced by Cordis in 1972. The inventors were Terry and Davies, working under the guidance of William Murphy Jr and Keller[439,440].

An important achievement in our endless pursuit of methods to prolong life was the invention of the AICD. This implantable defibrillator is a self-contained diagnostic-therapeutic system that provides automatic detection and correction of malignant ventricular tachyarrhythmias. It is now common knowledge that many instances of sudden death are due to some derangement in the heart's electrical stability. In the vast majority of such cases the catastrophic arrhythmia is ventricular fibrillation. About 20% have a lethal bradyarrhythmia.

The AICD was meant to abort the ventricular fibrillation at its onset thus averting the inevitably fatal outcome. It was largely the brain-child of Michael Murowski and his co-workers at Sinai Hospital in Baltimore. The Intec Systems of Pittsburgh was the industrial collaborator. The result was another example of the fruits to be realized from such cooperation.

Some of the seeds for the concept can be traced to Zoll and Lown. When Zoll introduced his external method of pacing in complete heart block, he soon observed that there was an ancillary and important benefit. This was the ability of the stimulator to suppress recurrent episodes of multifocal ventricular beats and ventricular fibrillation. This led to the concept that 'overdrive' could effectively suppress competing rhythmic foci[441]. This important observation was put to practical use by Sowton in 1964[442].

In 1954 Zoll developed a technique for external electric countershock defibrillation in the dog and pig[443]. Guyton had already outlined the factors concerned in electrical defibrillation of the heart through the unopened chest[444]. Zoll used a 60 cycle A–C discharge of 0.15 second duration with a voltage up to 750. This technique was found effective in atrial tachycardia, atrial fibrillation, ventricular tachycardia and ventricular fibrillation. In essence, his laboratory experiments indicated that the method could terminate any type of tachyarrhythmia. This ability was later to be confirmed time and again in clinical trials[445].

In 1961 Lown suggested a method of applying external direct current shocks so that the stimulus would fall immediately after the R wave so as to avoid the vulnerable phase[446]. Lown called his method synchronized cardioversion. It is routinely used today being especially effective in eliminating the hazard of precipitating ventricular fibrillation when trying to convert other types of tachyarrhythmia.

More than a decade of research went into the design of the original automatic implantable cardiac defibrillator. It automatically sensed the onset of ventricular fibrillation, and within 15–20 seconds it delivered an electric countershock for conversion to normal sinus rhythm. An improved version then had the capability of identifying and correcting ventricular tachycardia; often a forerunner of ventricular fibrillation. These second generation devices should actually be called implantable cardioverters.

Mirowski was 44 years old when he settled permanently in America. He was fortunate in that although he was affiliated with a community hospital, it had a dog laboratory, Morton Mower, a colleague with an interest in an implantable defibrillator equal to his own, and a bioengineering laboratory directed by William Staewen. In August, 1969, and in less than a month of collaboration, the trio launched their research efforts with a plate from a broken defibrillator paddle and an electrode made up of several catheters soldered together for insertion into the dogs' superior vena cava. Eleven years were to elapse before they received their first patient[447].

Their work began amid much skepticism that it would ever become a clinical reality. The technical problems that had to be overcome included miniaturization of the electronic components, a reliable system for sensing the ventricular fibrillation, and the development of a method for automatically charging and discharging the defibrillator.

Further dog experiments established that defibrillation could be consistently achieved with low energy levels if the shock were applied directly to the heart. This was found to be in the range between 30 and 50 J. Similar experiments were conducted by J. C. Schuder and colleagues at the University of Missouri. The results were about the same[448].

Mirowski and associates published their initial observations in 1970 in the *Archives of Internal Medicine*[449]. The paper provoked much criticism. Many cardiologists were skeptical of its value and feasibility. Bernard Lown wrote an editorial that was particularly distressing because of his influence in the field of arrhythmias and sudden death. Lown's reservations about the new device were summarized in the following words: 'The very rare patient who has frequent bouts of ventricular fibrillation is best treated in a coronary care unit and is better served by an effective anti-arrhythmic program or surgical correction of inadequate coronary flow or ventricular malfunction. In fact, the implanted defibrillator system represents an imperfect solution in search of a plausible and practical application[450]. The objections, many of them valid on technical grounds, stimulated Mirowski and co-workers to greater efforts. They were not even daunted by the inability to get research grants.

Early on they did arrange a collaborative effort with a pacemaker company but this was short-lived. Mirowski and Mower then allied themselves with Dr Stephen Heilman who had founded Medrad, a small company but an important supplier of angiographic injectors. This proved to be a mutually beneficial relationship. In two years' time they developed sensing circuits that were able to identify ventricular fibrillation on the basis of a mathematical formula called Probability Density Function (PDF). They also managed to make several electrode improvements[448].

After intensive trials with 25 dogs over a period of several years, the team was ready to try it on a patient. This occurred in February, 1980 at the Johns Hopkins Hospital[451,452]. It was successful and during the next five years the device was installed in 800 patients in several centers[453].

Upon completion of the clinical trials and with FDA approval in hand, the demand for the units exceeded Medrad's ability to manufacture them. CPI, the pacemaker subsidiary of Eli Lilly, was assigned all of Medrad's rights. By 1988 over 5000 patients were implanted with the now markedly improved device.

To date more than 25 000 AICDs have been implanted, and an ever increasing number of implanting and referral centers are following these patients. Third generation devices have incorporated such improvements as programmability, incorporation of a pacemaker, antitachycardia pacing, improved sensing capabilities, and the ability to deliver programmed electrical stimulation. The first Ventrak P programmable AICD automatic implantable cardioverter defibrillator is shown in Figure 11.

Figure 12 shows a multi-programmable tachyarrhythmia control system with non-thoracotomy and epicardial leads. It was designed to detect a rapid heart rate and to stop it in one of three ways: pacing, cardioversion and defibrillation. The system was also designed to regulate the heart rate if there should be marked bradycardia. There is no end in sight.

ABLATION TECHNIQUES

Ablation in electrophysiology is a term that refers to the use of physical agents capable of modifying or destroying conduction in a restricted area of the myocardium for treating or preventing cardiac arrhythmias. The technique may involve surgical excision or destruction with high-energy direct current electric shocks, radiofrequency, and more recently the laser beam.

The rationale for ablation rests upon the presence of either a discrete or diffuse electrophysiologic substrate. The discrete substrate may or may not be associated with a localized and definitive anatomical structure (e.g. an accessory pathway). An example of a diffuse substrate would be that associated with atrial fibrillation. This too may or may not involve diffuse pathologic changes.

Discrete arrhythmogenic anatomical substrates can be neutralized by the ablation techniques previously mentioned. Diffuse arrhythmogenic substrates are much more difficult to handle. A prerequisite for successful ablation is cardiac mapping. Simple point by point mapping has proven adequate for routine ablation in the WPW syndrome. The more sophisticated computerized mapping systems are reserved for complex ventricular arrhythmias.

Direct surgery for management of incapacitating tachyarrhythmias in the WPW syndrome was pioneered by W. C. Sealy and his colleagues in 1968. Since then definite guidelines were established for the selection of the proper surgical approach in every variety of tachyarrhythmia. Surgical therapy for ventricular arrhythmias evolved initially through indirect approaches and then by direct ablative techniques. The indirect approaches were those related to the surgical management of coronary artery disease, which, of course, is the most common predisposing factor in the development of ventricular tachyarrhythmia. The procedures included dorsal sympathectomy, aortocoronary bypass, ventricular aneurysmectomy, infarctectomy or resection of fibrotic myocardium. They offered the hope that removal of the underlying pathophysiologic condition would eliminate the conditions responsible for the perpetuation of the arrhythmia. Unfortunately, clinical experience proved otherwise. The cure rate varied markedly, and for this reason the direct surgical approach was adopted. The hope now was that this would open the door for a higher and more consistent rate of cure.

ARRHYTHMIA SURGERY

In 1968 a 32 year old fisherman was admitted to Duke Hospital for relief of an uncontrollable fast pulse. He had the WPW syndrome with reentrant tachycardia. Sealy and his colleagues successfully identified the Kent bundle, destroyed it, and by interrupting the circus movement permanently relieved him of his fast pulse. This was the beginning of arrhythmia surgery.

Will C. Sealy recounted the background and subsequent scenario in the *North Carolina Medical Journal* in 1983[454]. He called it the case of the fisherman with the fast pulse and the beginning of arrhythmia surgery.

When division was begun, the Kent bundle, as our studies of the few observations made on the anatomy had warned us, was neither visible nor palpable. The decision was made that its narrowest point had to be where it crossed the ring that supported the tricuspid valve. Thus the valve ring was uncovered from the outside of the heart, and a long incision was made dividing the connection of the right ventricle into the valve ring. To do this, the patient had to be placed on

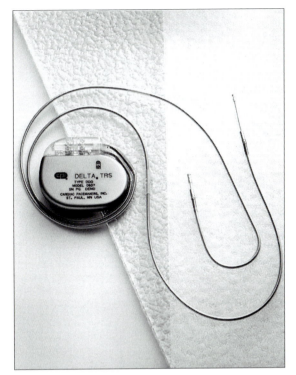

Figure 11 The first Ventrak P programmable AICD automatic implantable cardioverter defibrillator. *Photo Source Cardiac Pacemakers, Inc. Literary Source Cardiac Pacemakers, Inc. Courtesy of Cardiac Pacemakers, Inc.*

the heart lung machine. After repairing the heart, the patient recovered, the Kent bundle had been divided, and the signs and symptoms of the WPW syndrome including the ones on his electrocardiogram disappeared. The patient was able to return to his job as a commercial fisherman[454].

Sealy and his associates were new to the field of clinical cardioelectrophysiology. They were introduced to it by Henry Wallace who, in turn, was trained in it while a fellow at the National Heart Institute. Localization of the accessory bundle was accomplished with Durrer's technique of epicardial activation mapping. At surgery John Boineau conducted the electrophysiologic exploration. He 'was able to show that an impulse originating in the sinus node first entered the right ventricle at the right lateral wall at its connection to the atrium'[454].

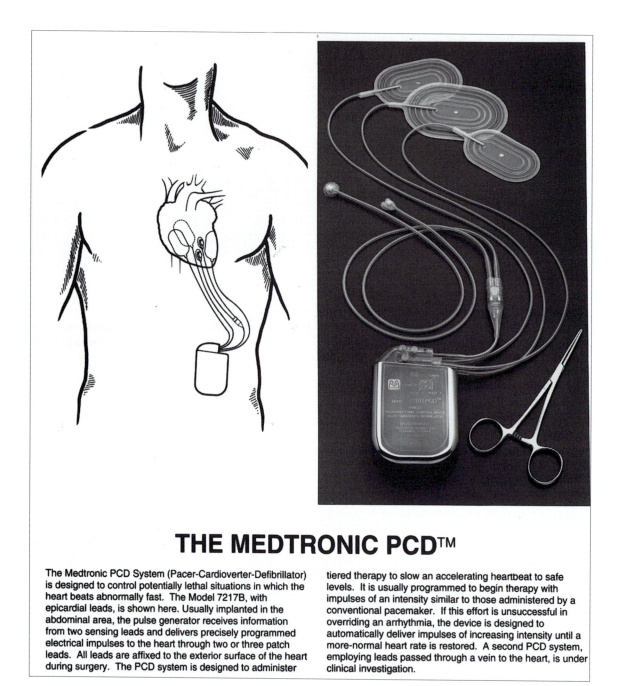

THE MEDTRONIC PCD™

The Medtronic PCD System (Pacer-Cardioverter-Defibrillator) is designed to control potentially lethal situations in which the heart beats abnormally fast. The Model 7217B, with epicardial leads, is shown here. Usually implanted in the abdominal area, the pulse generator receives information from two sensing leads and delivers precisely programmed electrical impulses to the heart through two or three patch leads. All leads are affixed to the exterior surface of the heart during surgery. The PCD system is designed to administer tiered therapy to slow an accelerating heartbeat to safe levels. It is usually programmed to begin therapy with impulses of an intensity similar to those administered by a conventional pacemaker. If this effort is unsuccessful in overriding an arrhythmia, the device is designed to automatically deliver impulses of increasing intensity until a more-normal heart rate is restored. A second PCD system, employing leads passed through a vein to the heart, is under clinical investigation.

Figure 12   The Medtronic PCD – the latest refinement of Mirowski's original device. *Photo Source Medtronic, Inc. Literary Source Medtronic, Inc. Used with permission from Medtronic, Inc. Copyright, Medtronic, Inc. 1992*

Sealy concluded his account with the statement that 'The case of the lucky fisherman with the fast pulse served to whet the interest of the surgeon in rhythm problems of the heart, spurred the heart specialist into searching for other patients with arrhythmias, and thus was the beginning of the encroachment on the last frontier of heart surgery: arrhythmia surgery'[454].

Since that historic event, Sealy and then Cox improved the technique by adopting an endocardial approach[455,456]. The French group led by Guiraudon introduced in 1989 an alternative technique using an epicardial approach on the normothermic beating heart[457]. It was based on the observation that most accessory pathways course within the coronary sulcus. The structures within the atrioventricular groove are dissected first and then the atrioventricular junction is cryoablated. This approach eliminated the need for cardiopulmonary bypass, and at the same time allowed continuous electrophysiological monitoring during the cryoablation of the exposed AV junction[458-461].

In AV nodal reentrant tachycardia the electrophysiologic substrate is a dual A-V nodal pathway[462,463]. This was demonstrated by Mendez and Moe in 1966[462]. Because the actual route of the pathways cannot be mapped, His bundle ablation was the only surgical intervention possible until the landmark report by D. Ross and D. Johnson in 1987[464]. In 1990 Guiraudon described an anatomically guided dissection of the AV node[465,466]. The AV nodal skeletonization is aimed at debulking the AV nodal area by ablation of perinodal atrial myocardium, and posterior and superficial atrial input. That same year Cox and his group introduced cryoablation[467].

Moe introduced the multiple wavelet hypothesis as the prevailing mechanism in atrial fibrillation in 1962[468]. This hypothesis is still accepted. This means then that the perpetuation of atrial fibrillation requires a critical surface area. Cox described a surgical procedure for management of this arrhythmia utilizing multiple atriotomies[469]. It is called the Maze operation. Guiraudon designed the corridor operation or sinus node–AV node insulation procedure that restores the chronotropic function of the sinus node, in 1986[470,471]. The sinus node and AV node are isolated from the rest of the atria by constructing a strip of atrial tissue (corridor). He advised that the operation be limited to those with normal heart anatomy and normal sinus node function.

Also in 1986, Guiraudon's group demonstrated macroreentry and the feasibility of operative therapy in atrial flutter[472]. They showed that the reentrant circuit is made up of an excitable gap and a critical area of slow conduction in the region of the coronary sinus orifice. Their operative intervention involves cryoablation of the area of slow conduction guided by cardiac mapping.

As we have seen, Sealy and his co-workers in the USA and Guiraudon's group in France demonstrated repeatedly the feasibility of interrupting the reentrant circuit in the WPW syndrome. It was only natural to assume that this concept could also be applied in the treatment of drug resistant ventricular tachycardia occurring within the clinical spectrum of coronary artery disease. We have seen how unpredictably successful the indirect approaches were. Extrapolation of the concept led to the development of simple ventriculotomy[473-475]. It seemed to be quite the right thing to do since late post-infarction ventricular tachyarrhythmia is dependent upon a reentry circuit. But simple ventriculotomy also did not prove to be uniformly successful. A new approach was introduced by Guiraudon in 1978[476]. He called it encircling endocardial ventriculotomy. It is a transmural ventriculotomy performed perpendicular to the wall and extended completely around the limits of endocardial fibrosis associated with previous infarction. The rationale for the procedure was based on the belief that the culprit reentrant circuits are located along the border zone with the ischemic subendocardial layers participating in the process.

When Guiraudon presented his findings at the 14th Annual Meeting of the Society of Thoracic Surgeons, he was asked by Dr John Moran, an attender, about the possibility that the scar resulting from the incision could also bring about delayed conduction and reentry. Guiraudon responded that since only fibrous tissue made up the scar, it did not have the same morphologic makeup of a healed myocardial infarction which consists of fibrosis and mixed normal and ischemic muscle. In order for reentry to occur a zone of delayed conduction must be in close proximity to a zone of normal or rapid conduction. Thus, the likelihood of inducing further episodes of ventricular tachycardia was probably a remote one[476].

In 1979 Josephson and his associates reported their experience with endocardial excision as a means of treating medically refractive ventricular tachycardia secondary to ischemic heart disease[477]. They had a series of 12 patients, all with ventricular aneurysm. In all instances intraoperative mapping localized the tachycardia to the border of the aneurysm, a site not routinely resected during aneurysmectomy. Resection of endocardium in the area of origin up to normal muscle was performed. Ten survived and remained free of sustained ventricular tachycardia during a follow-up period of 9–20 months. Despite the difference in technique, their results were similar to those of Guiraudon.

Although for a while it appeared that these innovative direct approaches had a marked therapeutic value, by the time the 1990s arrived, many physicians were growing increasingly disenchanted with them. A number of factors accounted for this change in attitude. Chief among them were the complexity of mapping the reentry circuits, criteria for selection of patients, unpredictable anti-arrhythmic effects and high mortality rates. Probably the most important factor was the efficacy of the automatic implantable cardiac defibrillator with its ease of deployment and increasing sophistication as later generations of the device appeared.

ELECTRODE CATHETER ABLATION

Electrode catheter ablation was first described by R. Gonzalez and co-workers in 1981. They used direct current energy for ablating the His bundle in dogs[478]. Within a year's time the same group and another team consisting of Gallagher, Svenson and Kasell applied the technique to humans in the treatment of refractory supraventricular tachy-cardias[479,480]. They created complete heart block via direct current energy transmitted between one or more poles of a standard electrode catheter (the cathode) positioned across the tricuspid valve, and a posterior, subscapular dermal plate or patch acting as the anode. His bundle activity was recorded through the cathode. The direct current energy was delivered via a standard external cardioverter defibrillator.

Morady and Scheinman described the use of a transvenous catheter technique for delivery of a high-energy direct current electrical shock to a posteroseptal accessory pathway in a patient with the WPW syndrome in 1984[481]. They were successful in ablating the pathway. Other reports by the group followed, and because of the relatively high success rate (about 70%) and low incidence of complications, the procedure seemed like a reasonable alternative to surgery[482]. However, more than 60% of accessory pathways are located in the left free wall, and the high complication rate with this technique in such cases rendered it unsuitable.

Three separate groups of investigators proposed then that ablation be accomplished with radio-frequency current. It lacked barotrauma and electrical arcing[483–485]. Huang and associates had demonstrated its feasibility in dogs in 1987[486]. Its many advantages over direct current energy soon established it as a superior source of energy. It is performed with a standard electrosurgical coagulator using energy with a frequency range of 350–750 kHz. Numerous investigators have repeatedly confirmed the use-fulness of this modality both in the USA and abroad[487–489].

J. Richard Spears and his group were the first to explore the possibility of ablating accessory pathways with laser. Spears had already developed a laser balloon catheter in 1987[490]. Their preliminary results in dogs reported in 1990 suggested that percutaneous laser balloon ablation of left-sided accessory pathways from the coronary sinus is feasible, and free of immediate major complications[491].

REFERENCES

1. Heidenhain, R. (1872). Über arrhythmische Herzhätigkeit. *Pflügers Arch. Ges. Physiol.*, **5**, 143–53

2. Lewis, T. (1911). *The Mechanism of the Heart Beat*. (London: Shaw)

3. Lewis, T. (1924). *The Mechanism and Graphic Registration of the Heart Beat*, 3rd. edn. (London: Shaw)

4. Krickler, D.M. (1969). Alfred Goodman Levy – Bulawayo's first doctor. *Centr. Afr. J. Med.*, **15**, 97–9

5. Levy, A.G. and Lewis, T. (1911). Heart irregularities, resulting from the inhalation of low percentages of chloroform vapour and their relationship to ventricular fibrillation. *Heart*, **3**, 99–112

6. Burch, G.E. and De Pasquale, N.P. (1964). *A History of Electrocardiography*, pp. 86–8. (Chicago: Year Book Medical)

7. Cohn, A.E. and Fraser, F.R. (1913). Paroxysmal tachycardia and the effect of stimulation of the vagus nerves by pressure. *Heart*, **4**, 93–105

8. Krickler, D.M. (1985). The development of the understanding of arrhythmias during the last 100 years. In *Medical History*, suppl. no. 5, p. 80, 1985. In *The Emergence of Modern Cardiology*, edited by W.F. Bynum, C. Lawrence, and V. Nutton. (London: Wellcome Inst. for Hist Med.)

9. Lenègre, J. and Maurice, P. (1945). De quelques resultats obtenus par la dérivation directe intracavitaire des courants électriques de l'oreillette et du ventricule droit. *Arch. Mal. Coeur*, **38**, 298–302

10. Battro, A. and Bidoggia, H. (1947). Endocardiac electrocardiogram obtained by heart catheterization in man. *Am. Heart J.*, **33**, 604–32

11. Sodi-Pollares, D., Vizcaino, M., Soberon, J. *et al.* (1947). Comparative study of the intracavity potential in man and in dog. *Am. Heart J.*, **33**, 819–48

12. Hecht, H.H. (1948). Potential variations of the right auricular and ventricular cavities in man. *Am. Heart J.*, **32**, 39–51

13. Levine, H.D. and Goodale, W.T. (1950). Studies in intracardiac electrography in man: IV. The potential variations in the coronary venous system. *Circulation*, **2**, 48–59

14. Sodi-Pollares, D., Estandia, A., Soberon, J. *et al.* (1950). The left intra-ventricular potential of the human heart. II. Criteria for diagnosis of incomplete bundle branch block. *Am. Heart J.*, **40**, 655–69

15. Kossman, C.E., Rader, B., Berger, A. *et al.* (1950). Electrograms in atrial flutter, atrial tachycardia and atrial fibrillation. *Premier Congrès Mondial de Cardiologie*. (Paris: Bailliere)

16. Torner Soler, M., Gilbert Queralto, J., Paravisini Para, J. *et al.* (1950). La fibrillation auriculaire dans l'électrocardiographie intracardiaque droit. *Premier Congrès Mondial de Cardiologie*. (Paris: Bailliere)

17. Alanis, J., Gonzales, H. and Lopez, E. (1958). The electrical activity of the bundle of His. *J. Physiol.*, **142**, 127–40

18. Stuckey, J.H., Hoffman, B.F., Amer, N.S. *et al.* (1959). Localization of the bundle of His with a surface electrode during cardiotomy. *Surg. Forum*, **10**, 551–4

19. Giraud, G., Puech, P., Latour, H. *et al.* (1960). Variations de potentiel liées a l'activité du système de conduction auriculo-ventriculaire chez l'homme. *Arch. Mal. Coeur*, **53**, 757–76

20. Scherlag, B., Lau, S., Helfant, R. *et al.* (1969). Catheter technique for recording His bundle activity in man. *Circulation*, **39**, 13–18

21. Pruitt, R.D. and Essex, H.D. (1960). Potential changes attending the excitation process in the AV conduction system of bovine and canine hearts. *Circ. Res.*, **8**, 149

22. Scherlag, B.J. (1979). The development of the His bundle recording technique. *Pace*, **2**, 230–3

23. Scher, A.M., Rodrigues, M.I., Liikane, J. and Young, A.C. (1955). Direct recording from the AV conducting system in the dog and monkey. *Science*, **121**, 398

24. Sodi-Pollares, D., Medrano, G.A., Bisteni, A. and DeMichelli, A. (1959). Electrograms of the conductive tissue in the normal dog's heart, *Am. J. Cardiol.*, **4**, 459

25. Forssman, W. (1974). Experiments on myself. *Memoirs of a Surgeon in Germany*, p. 87. (London: St. James Press)

26. Scherlag, B.J., Kosowsky, B.D. and Damato, A.N. (1967). Technique for ventricular pacing from the His bundle of the intact heart. *J. Appl. Physiol.*, **22**, 584

27. Narula, O.S., Scherlag, B.J. and Samet, P. (1970). Pervenous pacing of the specialized conducting system in man: His bundle and AV nodal stimulation. *Circulation*, **41**, 77–87

28. Coumel, P., Waynberger, M., Slama, R. *et al.* (1970). L'enregistrement de l'activité électrique du faisceau de His. Étude preliminaire: Application à l'étude des blocs auriculo-ventriculaires. *Presse Med.*, **78**, 365–9

29. Puech, P., Latour, H., Grolleau, R. *et al.* (1970). L'activité électrique du tissu de conduction auriculo-ventriculaire en electrocardiographie endocavitaire. *Arch. Mal. Coeur*, **63**, 500–20

30. Reiffel, J.A., Gang, E., Gliklich, J. *et al.* (1980). The human sinus node electrogram: a transvenous catheter technique and a comparison of directly measured and indirectly estimated sinoatrial conduction time in adults. *Circulation*, **62**, 1324–34

31. Jackman, W.M., Friday, K.J., Scherlag, B.J. *et al.* (1983). Direct endocardial recording from an accessory atrioventricular pathway: Localization of the site of block, effect of antiarrhythmic drugs, and attempt at nonsurgical ablation. *Circulation*, **68**, 906–16

32. Prystowsky, E.N., Browne, K.F. and Zipes, D.P. (1983). Intracardiac recording by catheter electrode of accessory pathway depolarization. *J. Am. Coll. Cardiol.*, **1**, 468–70

33. Josephson, M.E., Horowitz, L.N. and Farshidi, A. (1978). Continuous local electrical activity: a mechanism of recurrent ventricular tachycardia. *Circulation*, **57**, 659–65

34. Fisch, C. (1983). Electrocardiography of arrhythmias: from deductive analysis to laboratory confirmation – twenty-five years of progress. *J. Am. Coll. Cardiol.*, **1**, 306–16

35. Meijler, F.S. (1984). Prof. Dirk Durrer,

godfather of Dutch cardiology. A personal note. *Int. J. Cardiol.*, **6**, 750–3

36. Burchell, H.B. (1984). Dirk Durrer, M.D. A personal American tribute. *Int. J. Cardiol.*, **6**, 755–6

37. Janse, M.J. (1984). Dirk Durrer and experimental cardiology. *Int. J. Cardiol.*, **6**, 763–6

38. Durrer, D. and Van der Tweel, L.H. (1953). Spread of activation in the left ventricular wall of the dog (I). *Am. Heart J.*, **46**, 683–91

39. Meijler, F.L. (1984). Historical notes on Professor Dirk Durrer. *Eur. Heart J.*, **5**, 607

40. Durrer, D., van Dam, R.T., Freud, G.E., Janse, M.J., Meijler, F.L. and Arzbaecher, R.C. (1970). Total excitation of the isolated human heart. *Circulation*, **41**, 895–912

41. Van Dam, R.T.H., Durrer, D., Strackee, J. and Van der Tweel, L.H. (1955). The excitability for cathodal and anodal stimulation of the dog's ventricle during the cardiac cycle. *Proc. K. Ned. Akad. Wet. Ser.*, C58 No. 4, 421–7

42. Van Dam, R.T.H., Durrer, D., Strackee, J. and Van der Tweel, L.H. (1956). The excitability cycle of the dog's left ventricle, determined by anodal, cathodal and bipolar stimulation. *Circ. Res.*, **4**, 196–204

43. Durrer, D., Van Dam, R.T., Freud, G.E. and Janse, M.J. (1971). Re-entry and ventricular arrhythmias in local ischemia and infarction of the intact dog heart. *Proc. K. Ned. Akad. Wet. Ser.*, C74 No. 4, 321–34

44. Janse, M.J., Van Capelle, F.J.L., Morsink, H., Kléber, A.G., Wilms-Schopman, F., Cardinal, R., Naumann d'Alnoncourt, C. and Durrer, D. (1980). Flow of 'injury' current and patterns of excitation during early ventricular arrhythmias in acute regional myocardial ischemia in isolated porcine and canine hearts. Evidence for 2 different arrhythmogenic mechanisms. *Circ. Res.*, **47**, 151–63

45. Becker, A.E., Anderson, R.H., Durrer, D. and Wellens, H.J.J. (1978). The anatomical substrates of Wolff-Parkinson-White syndrome: a clinico-pathologic correlation in seven patients. *Circulation*, **57**, 870–9

46. Sealy, W.C., Gallagher, J.J. and Pritchett, E.L.C. (1978). The surgical anatomy of Kent bundles based on electrophysiological mapping and surgical exploration. *J. Thorac. Cardiovasc. Surg.*, **76**, 804–15

47. Sealy, W.C. and Gallagher, J.J. (1980). The surgical approach to the septal area of the heart based on experience with 45 patients with Kent bundles. *J. Thorac. Cardiovasc. Surg.*, **79**, 542–51

48. Anderson, R.H., Becker, A.E., Brechenmacher, C., Davies, M.J. and Rossi, L. (1975). The human atrioventricular junctional area. A morphologic study of the AV node and bundle. *Eur. J. Cardiol.*, **3**, 11–25

49. Anderson, R.H., Becker, A.E., Brechenmacher, C., Davies, M.J. and Rossi, L. (1975). Ventricular preexcitation. A proposed nomenclature for its substrates. *Eur. J. Cardiol.* **3**, 27–36

50. Becker, A.E. (1984). A salute to Dirk Durrer. *Int. J. Cardiol.*, **6**, 767–9

51. Durrer, D. and Ross, J.P. (1967). Epicardial excitation of the ventricle in a patient with the Wolff-Parkinson-White syndrome. *Circulation*, **35**, 15

52. Durrer, D., Schoo, L., Schuilenburg, R.M. and Wellens, H.J. (1967). The role of premature beats in the initiation and the termination of supraventricular tachycardias in the Wolff-Parkinson-White syndrome. *Circulation*, **36**, 644

53. Wellens, H.J. (1984). Durrer and programmed electrical stimulation of the heart. *Int. J. Cardiol.*, **6**, 759–61

54. Coumel, P. (1975). Supraventricular tachycardias. In Krickler, D.M. and Goodwin, J.F. (eds.) *Cardiac Arrhythmias. The Modern Electrophysiologic Approach*, pp. 116–43. (London: W.B. Saunders, Ltd.)

55. Coumel, P. and Attuel, P. (1974). Reciprocating tachycardia in overt and latent preexcitation: influence of functional bundle branch block on the rate of the tachycardia. *Eur. J. Cardiol.*, **1**, 423–36

56. Coumel, P., Cabrol, C., Fabiato, A. *et al.* (1967). Tachycardie permanente par rhythm réciproque. I. Preuves du diagnostic par stimulation auriculaire et ventriculaire. II. Traitement par l'implementation intra-corporelle d'un stimulateur cardiaque avec entrainement simultané de l'oreillette et du ventricule. *Arch. Mal. Coeur*, **60**, 1830–64

57. Barold, S.S., Linhart, J.W., Samet, P. *et al.* (1969). Supraventricular tachycardia initiated and terminated by a single electrical stimulus. *Am. J. Cardiol.*, **24**, 37–41

58. Goldreyer, B.N. and Bigger, J.T. (1969). Spontaneous and induced re-entrant tachycardia. *Ann. Intern. Med.*, **70**, 87–98

59. Goldreyer, B.N., Gallagher, J.J. and Damato, A.N. (1973). The electrophysiological demonstration of atrial ectopic tachycardia in man. *Am. Heart J.*, **85**, 205–15

60. Wellens, H.J.J., Schuilenburg, R.M. and Durrer, D. (1972). Electrical stimulation of the heart in patients with ventricular tachycardia. *Circulation*, **46**, 216–26

61. Einthoven, W. (1965).The string galvanometer and the measurement of the action currents of the heart. *Nobel Lectures: Physiology of Medicine 1922–41*, p. 110. (Amsterdam: Elsevier)

62. Rosenbaum, M.B., Elizari, M.V. and Lazzari, J.O. (1968). *Los Hemibloqueos*. (Buenos Aires: Ed Paidos)

63. Rosenbaum, M.B., Elizari, M.V. and Lazzari, J.O. (1970). *The Hemiblocks. New Concepts of Intraventricular Conduction Based on Human Anatomical, Physiological and Clinical Studies.* (Oldsmar, Fl, Tampa Tracings)

64. Rosenbaum, M.B., Elizari, M.V., Lazzari, J.O., Nau, G.J., Halperns, M.S. and Levi, R.J. (1972). The differential electrocardiographic manifestations of hemiblocks, bilateral bundle branch block and trifascicular blocks. In Schlant, R.C. and Hurst, J.W. (eds.) *Advances in Electrocardiography*, pp. 145–82. (New York: Grune & Stratton)

65. Eppinger, H. and Rothberger, C.J. (1909). Zur Analyse des Elektrokardiogramms. *Wien. Klin. Wochenschr.*, **22**, 1091–8

66. Eppinger, H. and Rothberger, F.J. (1910). Über die Folgen der Durchschneidung der Tawaraschen Schenkel des Reizleitungssystems. *Z. Klin. Med.*, **70**, 1–20

67. Eppinger, H. and Stoerck, O. (1910). Zur Klinik des Elektrokardiogramms. *Klin. Med.*, **71**, 157–64

68. Rothberger, C.J. and Winterberg, H. (1917). Experimentelle Beitrage zur Kenntniss der Reizleitungsstörungen in den Kammern des Saugetierherzens. *Z. Gesamte. Exp. Med.*, **5**, 264–320

69. Lewis, T. (1912). Observations upon disorders of the heart's action. *Heart*, **3**, 279–300

70. Lewis, T. *Op. cit.*, ref. 3

71. Cohn, A.E. and Lewis, T. (1914). The pathology of bundle branch lesions of the heart. Proc. *NY Path. Soc.*, **14**, 207–16

72. Hollman, A. (1985). The history of bundle-branch block. In *Medical History,* suppl. no. 5, p. 92, 1985. In *The Emergence of Modern Cardiology*, edited by W.F. Bynum, C. Lawrence, and V. Nutton. (London: Wellcome Institute for Hist. Med.)

73. Uhley, H.N. (1979). The concept of trifascicular intraventricular conduction: historical aspects and influence on contemporary cardiology. *Am. J. Cardiol.*, **43**, 643–6

74. Rosenman, R.H., Pick, A. and Katz, L.N. (1950). Intraventricular block. Review of the literature. *Arch. Intern. Med.*, **86**, 196–232

75. Oppenheimer, B.S. and Pardee, H.E.B. (1920). The site of cardiac lesion in two instances of intraventricular heart block. *Proc. Soc. Exp. Biol. Med.*, **17**, 177–9

76. Fahr, G. (1920). An analysis of the spread of the excitation wave in the human ventricle. *Arch. Intern. Med.*, **25**, 146

77. Mann, H. (1931). Interpretation of bundle-branch block by means of the mono-cardiograph. *Am. Heart J.*, **6**, 447–57

78. Hollman, A. (1985). *Op. cit.* (ref. 72)

79. Wilson, F.N., MacLeod, A.G. and Barker, P.S. (1932). The order of ventricular excitation in human bundle branch block. *Am. Heart J.*, **7**, 305–30

80. Barker, P.S., MacLeod, A.G. and Alexander, J. (1940). The excitatory process observed in the exposed human heart. *Am. Heart J.*, **5**, 720–42

81. Kountz, W.B. (1937). Revival of human hearts. *Ann. Intern. Med.*, **10**, 330–6

82. Wilson, F.N., Johnson, F.D. and Barker, P.S. (1934). Electrocardiograms of the unusual type in right bundle branch block. *Am. Heart J.*, **9**, 472–9

83. Grant, R.P. (1957). *Clinical Electrocardiography*, p. 110. (New York: McGraw-Hill)

84. Grant, R.P. and Murray, R.H. (1954). QRS complex deformity of myocardial infarction in the human subject. *Am. J. Med.*, **17**, 587–609

85. Grant, R.P. (1959). Periinfarction block. *Prog. Cardiovasc. Dis.*, **2**, 237–47

86. Uhley, H.N. and Rivkin, L.M. (1960). Peripheral distribution of the canine atrioventricular conduction system. Observations on gross morphology. *Am. J. Cardiol.*, **5**, 688–91

87. Uhley, H.N. and Rivkin, L.M. (1961). Electrocardiographic patterns following interruption of the main and peripheral branches of the canine bundle of His. *Am. J. Cardiol.*, **7**, 810–16

88. Uhley, H.N. and Rivkin, L.M. (1964). Electrocardiographic patterns following interruption of main and peripheral branches of the canine left bundle of His. *Am. J. Cardiol.*, **13**, 41–7

89. Watt, T.B. Jr., Murao, S. and Pruitt, R.D. (1965). Left axis deviation induced experimentally in a primate heart. *Am. Heart J.*, **70**, 381–9

90. Hecht, H.H., Kossmann, C.E., Childers, R.W., Langendorf, R., Lev, M., Rosen, K.M., Pruitt, R.D., Truex, R.C., Uhley, H.N. and Watt, T.B. Jr. (1973). Atrio-ventricular and intraventricular conduction. Revised nomenclature and concepts. *Am. J. Cardiol.*, **31**, 232–44

91. Lev, M., Unger, P.N., Rosen, K.M. and Bharati, S. (1974). The anatomic substrate of complete left bundle branch block. *Circulation* **50**, 479–86

92. Lev, M. and Bharatii, S. (1975). Atrioventricular and intraventricular conduction disease. *Arch. Intern. Med.*, **135**, 405–40

93. Rossi, L. (1976). Histopathology of conducting system in left anterior hemiblock. *Br. Heart J.*, **38**, 1304–11

94. Strickland, A.W., Horan, L.G. and Flowers, N.C. (1972). Gross anatomy associated with patterns called left posterior hemiblock. *Circulation*, **46**, 276–82

95. Demoulin, J.C., Simar, L.J. and Kulbertus, H.E. (1975). Quantitative study of left bundle branch fibrosis in left anterior hemiblock: a stereologic approach. *Am. J. Cardiol.*, **36**, 751–6

96. Rizzon, P., Rossi, L., Baissus, C., Demoulin, J.C. and DiBlase, M. (1975). Left posterior hemiblock in acute myocardial infarction. *Br. Heart J.*, **37**, 711–20

97. Krongard, E., Bharati, S., Steinfield, L. and Lev, M. (1977). Histologic observations of the cardiac conduction system in a patient with postoperative bilateral bundle branch block. *Am. J. Cardiol.*, **40**, 635–40

98. Bharati, S., Lev, M., Dhingra, R., Wu, D., Aruguete, J., Mir, J. and Rosen, K.M. (1976). Pathologic correlations in three cases of bilateral bundle branch disease with unusual electrophysiologic manifestations in two cases. *Am. J. Cardiol.*, **38**, 508–18

99. Rosen, K.M., Rahimtoola, S.H., Bharati, S. and Lev, M. (1973). Bundle branch block with intact atrioventricular conduction. Electrophysiologic and pathologic correlation in three cases. *Am. J. Cardiol.*, **32**, 783–93

100. Steiner, C., Lau, S.H., Stein, E., Wit, A.L., Weiss, M.B., Damato, A.W., Haft, J.I., Weinstock, M. and Gupta, P. (1971). Electrophysiologic documentation of trifasicular block as the common cause of complete heart block. *Am. J. Cardiol.*, **28**, 436–41

101. Castellanos, A. Jr., Agha, A.S., Befeler, B., Castillo, C.A. and Berkovitz, B.V. (1973). A study of arrival of excitation of selected ventricular sites during human bundle branch block using close bipolar catheter electrodes. *Chest*, **63**, 208–13

102. Hollman, A. (1985). *Op. cit.* (ref. 72)

103. Shapiro, E. (1980). The electrocardiogram and the arrhythmias: historical insights. In William J. Mandel: *Cardiac Arrhythmias, Their Mechanisms, Diagnosis and Management*, 2nd edn. (Phil.: J.B. Lippincot Co.)

104. Shapiro, E. (1977). Engelmann and his laddergram. *Am. J. Cardiol.*, **39**, 464

105. Ritchie, W.T. (1914). *Auricular Flutter*, p. 2. (New York: Paul B. Hoeber)

106. Mackenzie, J. (1908). *Diseases of the Heart.* (London)

107. Marey, E.J. (1876). Des excitations électriques du coeur. In *Physiologie Experimentale. Travaux de Laboratorie de M Marey*, vol. 2, p. 63. (Paris: Masson)

108. Carlson, A.J. (1906). Comparative physiology of the invertebrate heart. VI. The excitability of the heart during the different phases of the heart beat. *Am. J. Physiol.*, **16**, 67

109. Wiggers, C.J. (1957). Cardiac physiology of 50 years ago. *Circ. Res.*, **5**, 121

110. Erlanger, J. (1905). On the physiology of heart block in mammals, with especial reference to the causation of Stokes–Adams disease. *J. Exp. Med.*, **7**, 676

111. Musis, D., Rakovec, P., Jagodic, A. and Cibic, B. (1984). The first description of syncopal attacks in heart block. *Pace*, **7**, 301–3

112. Cheyne, G. (1733). *The English Malady or a Treatise of Nervous Diseases of All Kinds*, p. 307. (London: Strahan & Leake)

113. Morgagni, J.B. (1769). *The Seats and Causes of Disease*, **1**, 192. (Trans. by B. Alexander) London

114. Spens, T. (1793). Sect. II. Medical observations. I. History of a case in which there took place a remarkable slowness of the pulse; communicated to Dr. Duncan by Dr. T. Spens. *Medical Commentaries*, **7**, 463

115. Burnett, W. (1827). Case of epilepsy, attended with remarkable slowness of the pulse; (communicated by Dr. James Johnson, and Read, April 13, 1824). *Med. Chir. Trans.*, **13**, 202

116. Adams, R. (1827). Cases of diseases of the heart, accompanied with pathological observations. *Dublin Hosp. Rep.*, **4**, 396

117. Huchard, H. (1889). Maladies du Coeur et des Vaisseaux, p. 255. (Paris: Octave Dion)

118. Stokes, W. (1846). Observations on some cases of permanently slow pulse. *Dublin J. Med. Sci.*, **2**, 73

119. Balfour, G.W. (1876). *Diseases of the Heart and Aorta*, p. 243. (Philadelphia: Lindsay & Blakiston)

120. Galabin, A.L. (1875). On the interpretation of cardiographic tracings and the evidence they afford as to the murmurs attendant upon mitral stenosis. *Guy's Hosp. Rep.*, **20**, 261

121. Gaskell, W.H. (1883). On the innervation of the heart, with especial reference to the heart of the tortoise. *J. Physiol.*, **4**, 43

122. Chauveau, A. (1885). De la dissociation du rhythme auricularie et du rhythme ventriculaire, *Rév. Méd.*, **5**, 161

123. His, W. Jr. (1899). Ein Fall von Adams-Stokes'scher Krankheit mit ungleichzeitigen Schlagen der Vorhöfe und Herzkammern (Herzblok). *Dtsch. Arch. Klin. Med.*, **64**, 316

124. Mackenzie, J. (1902). *The Study of the Pulse*, pp. 136, 279–282. (Edinburgh and London: Pentland)

125. Erlanger, J. and Blackman, J.R. (1904). Further studies on the physiology of heart-block in mammals. *Heart*, **1**, 117

126. Erlanger, J. (1905). On the physiology of heart block in mammals, with especial reference to the causation of Stokes–Adams disease. *J. Exp. Med.*, **7**, 676

127. Cohn, A.E. and Lewis, T. (1912–1913). A description of a case of complete heart-block; including the postmortem examination. *Heart*, **4**, 7

128. Hay, J. (1905). The pathology of bradycardia. *Br. Med. J.*, **2**, 1034

129. Arcieri, G.P. (1945). *The Circulation of the Blood and Andrea Cesalpino of Arezzo*. (New York: S.F. Vanni)

130. Shugoll, G.I., Bowen, P.H., Moore, J.P. *et al.* (1972). Follow-up observations and prognosis in primary myocardial disease. *Arch. Intern. Med.*, **129**, 62–72

131. Engleman, T.W. (1894). Beobachtungen und Versuche am suspendirten Herzen. Zweite Abhandlung. Über die Leitung der Bewegungsreize im Herzen. *Pflügers Arch. Ges. Physiol.*, **56**, 149–202

132. Fisch, C. (1983). Aberration: seventy-five years after Sir Thomas Lewis. *Br. Heart J.*, **50**, 297–302

133. Engelmann, T.W. (1896–97). Ueber den Ursprung der Herzbewegung und die physiologischen Eigenschaften der grossen Herznerven des Frosches. *Arch. Ges. Physiol.*, **65**, 109

134. Knoll, P. (1872). Ueber die Veränderung des Herschlages bei reflectorischer Erregnung des vasomotorischen Nervensystems. *Wiener Sitzungberichte der deutschen Akadamie der Wissenschafter*, **66**, 195

135. Wenkebach, K.F. (1900). Zur Analyse des unregelmässigen Pulses. *Z. Klin. Med.*, **39**, 293

136. Cushny, A.R. (1899). On the interpretation of pulse tracings. *J. Exp. Med.*, **4**, 327

137. Hering, H.E. (1900). Zur experimentellen Analyse der unregelmassigkeiten des Heerzschlages. *Arch. Ges. Physiol.*, **82**, 1

138. Pan, O. (1903). Klinische Beobachtung über ventrikulare Extrasystolen ohne kompensatorische Pause. *Dtsch. Arch. Klin. Med.*, **78**, 128

139. Trendelenburg, W. (1903). Ueber den Wegfall der compensatorischen Ruhe am spontan schlagenden Froschherzen. *Arch. Anat. Physiol.*, p. 311

140. Wenckebach, K.F. (1903). *Die Arhythmie als Ausdruck bestimmter Funktionsstorungen des Herzens.* (Leipzig, Germany: Engelmann)

141. Einthoven, W. (1906). Le telecardiogramme. *Arch. Int. Physiol.*, **4**, 132

142. Kraus, F. and Nicolai, G.F. (1908). Ueber des Elektrokardiogramm unter normalen und pathologischen Verhältnissen. *Berl. Klin. Wchnschr.*, **34**, 1

143. Chiang, B., Perlman, L., Ostrander, L. *et al.* (1969). Relationship of premature systoles to coronary heart disease and sudden death in the Tecumseh epidemiological study. *Ann. Intern. Med.*, **70**, 1159–66

144. The Coronary Drug Project Research Group (1973). Prognostic importance of premature beats following myocardial infarction: Experience in the Coronary Drug Project. *J. Am. Med. Assoc.*, 223–116–1124

145. Kotler, M.N., Tabatznik, B., Mower, M.M. *et al.* (1973). Prognostic significance of ventricular ectopic beats with respect to sudden death in the late post-infarction period. *Circulation*, **47**, 959–66

146. Ruberman, W., Weinblatt, E., Goldberg, J. *et al.* (1977). Ventricular premature beats and mortality after myocardial infarction. *N. Engl. J. Med.*, **297**, 750–7

147. Hoffman, A. (1914). *Die Elektrographie als Untersuchungen des Herzens und ikre Ergebnisse.* (Wiesbaden: J.F. Bergmann)

148. Oppenheimer, B.S. and Stewart, H.J. (1926). Dependence of the form of the electrocardiogram upon the site of mechanical stimulation of the human ventricles. *J. Clin. Invest.*, **3**, 593–612

149. Katz, L.N. and Pick, A. (1956). *Clinical

Electrocardiography. Part I. The Arrhythmias. (Philadelphia: Lea & Febiger)

150. Zipes, D.P. (1975). Tachycardia. In Conn, H.F. (ed.) *Current Therapy.* (Philadelphia: W.B. Saunders Co)

151. Cotton, P. (1867). Notes and observations upon a case of unusually rapid action of the heart. *Br. Med. J.,* **1**, 629

152. Bristowe, J.S. (1888). On recurrent palpitations of extreme rapidity in persons otherwise apparently healthy. *Brain*, **10**, 164

153. Bouveret, L. (1889). De la tachycardie essentielle paroxystique. *Rév. Méd.,* **9**, 753

154. Hoffman, A. (1900). *Die paroxysmale Tachycardie.* (Wiesbaden: Bergmann)

155. Winternitz, W. (1883). Ein Beitrag zu den Motilitätsneurosen des Herzens. *Berl. klin. Wchnschr.,* **20**, 93, 112

156. Lewis, T. (1909). The experimental production of paroxysmal tachycardia and the effect of ligation of the coronary arteries. *Heart*, **1**, 98

157. Schmidt, F.O. and Erlanger, J. (1928–29). Directional differences in the conduction of the impulse through heart muscle and their possible relation to extrasystolic and fibrillary contractions. *Am. J. Physiol.,* **87**, 326

158. Scherf, D. (1947). Studies on auricular tachycardia caused by aconitine administration. *Proc. Soc. Exp. Biol. Med.,* **64**, 233

159. Prinzmetal, M., Corday, E., Bill, C. *et al.* (1952). *The Auricular Arrhythmias*, p. 189. (Springfield, Ill., Charles C. Thomas)

160. Lown, B., Marcus, F. and Levine, H.D. (1959). Digitalis and the atrial tachycardias with block. *N. Engl. J. Med.,* **260**, 301

161. Reddy, C.P. and Surawicz, B. (1983). Terminology of tachycardias: historical background and evolution. *Pace*, **6**, 1123–42

162. Surawicz, B., Uhley, H., Borun, R., *et al.* (1978). Bethesda conference report: optimal electrocardiography task force I: standardization of terminology and interpretation. *Am. J. Cardiol.,* **41**, 130

163. New York Heart Association (1979). *Nomenclature and Criteria for Diagnosis of Diseases of the Heart and Great Vessels.* (Boston, Little, Brown and Co.)

164. Lewis, T. (1910). Galvanometric curves yielded by cardiac beats generated in various areas of the auricular musculature: The pacemaker of the heart. *Heart*, **2**, 23

165. Abramson, D.I., Fenichel, N.M. and Schookhoff, C. (1938). A study of electrical activity in the auricles. *Am. Heart J.,* **15**, 417

166. MacLean, W.A.H., Karp, R.B., Kouchokos, N.T. *et al.* (1975). P waves during ectopic atrial rhythms in man. A study utilizing atrial pacing with fixed electrodes. *Circulation*, **52**, 426

167. El-Sherif, N. (1971). AV junctional versus left atrial rhythm. *Br. Heart J.,* **33**, 358

168. Jomain, S.L., Moore, E.N., Stuckey, J.H. *et al.* (1962). Unreliability of P wave polarity in diagnosing ectopic rhythms arising from atrioventricular (AV) nodal region. *Circulation*, (Abstract), **26**, 738

169. Erlanger, J. and Blackman, J.R. (1907). A study of relative rhythmicity and conductivity in various regions of the auricles of the mammalian heart. *Am. J. Physiol.,* **19**, 125

170. Eyster, J.A.E. and Meek, W.J. (1922). Studies on the origin and conduction of the cardiac impulse. *Am. J. Physiol.,* **61**, 117

171. Scherf, D. (1944). Upper auriculo-ventricular rhythm (coronary sinus rhythm) experimentally produced. *Proc. Soc. Exp. Biol. Med.,* **56**, 22

172. Giraud, G., Latour, H. and Puech, P. (1954). L'electrocardiographie du sinus coronaire. II. étude electrocardiographie endocavitaire des dysrythmies du sinus coronaire chez l'homme. *Arch. Mal. Coeur.,* **47**, 1008

173. Puech, P. (1956). *L'Activite Electrique Auriculaire, Normal et Pathologique.* (Paris: Masson)

174. Lancaster, J.F., Leonard, J.J., Leon, D.F. *et al.* (1970). The experimental production of coronary sinus rhythm in man. *Am. Heart J.,* **70**, 89

175. Lau, S.H., Cohen, S.I., Stein, E. *et al.* (1970). P waves and P loops in coronary sinus and left atrial rhythms. *Am. Heart J.,* **79**, 201

176. Moore, E.N., Jomain, S.L., Stuckey, J.H. *et al.* (1967). Studies on ectopic atrial rhythms in dogs. *Am. J. Cardiol.,* **19**, 676

177. Waldo, A.L., Witikainen, K.J., Kaiser, G.A. *et al.* (1970). The P wave and P-R interval. Effects of the site of origin of atrial depolarization. *Circulation*, **42**, 653

178. Massumi, R. and Tawakkol, A.A. (1967). Direct study of left atrial P waves. *Am. J. Cardiol.,* **20**, 331

179. Durrer, D., Schoo, L., Schuilenburg, R.M. *et al.* (1967). The role of premature beats in the initiation and the termination of supraventricular tachycardia in the Wolff-Parkinson-White syndrome. *Circulation*, **36**, 644–62

180. Zahn, A. (1912). Experimentelle Untersuchungen über Reizbildung im Atrioventrikularknoten

und Sinus Coronarius. *Zbl. Physiol.*, **26**, 495

181. Zahn, A. (1913). Experimentelle Untersuchungen über Reizbildung und Reizleitung im Atrioventrikularknoten. *Arch. Ges. Physiol.*, **151**, 247

182. Waldo, A.L. and James, T.N. (1973). A retrospective look at AV nodal rhythm. *Circulation*, **17**, 222–3

183. Lewis, T. (1925). *Op. cit.*, ref. 72

184. Meek, W.J. and Eyster, J.A.E. (1913). Experiments on the origin and propagation of the impulse on the heart: III. The effect of vagal stimulation on the location of the pacemaker in auriculo-ventricular rhythm, and the effect of vagal stimulation on this rhythm. *Heart*, **5**, 227

185. Spach, M.S., Kong, T.D., Barr, R.C., Boaz, D.E., Morrow, M.N. and Herman-Giddens, S. (1969). Electrical potential distribution surrounding the atria during depolarization and repolarization in the dog. *Circ. Res.*, **24**, 857

186. Goodman, D., van der Steen, A.B.M. and van Dam, R.T. (1971). Endocardial and epicardial activation pathways of the canine right atrium. *Am. J. Physiol.*, **220**, 1

187. Spach, M.D., Lieberman, M., Scott, J.G., Barr, R.C., Johnson, E.A. and Kootsey, J.M. (1971). Excitation sequences of the atrial septum and the AV node on isolated hearts of the dog and rabbit. *Circ. Res.*, **29**, 156

188. Vitikainen, K.J., Waldo, A.L. and Hoffman, B.F. (1972). Observations on the retrograde P wave. *Circulation*, **46** (suppl. II), 11–24

189. MacWilliam, J.A. (1887). Fibrillar contraction of the heart. *J. Physiol.*, **8**, 296

190. Ritchie, W. (1905). Complete heart block with dissociation of the action of the auricles and ventricles. *Proc. R. Soc. Edinburgh*, **25**, 1085

191. Jolly, W.A. and Ritchie, W.T. (1910–11). Auricular flutter and fibrillation. *Heart*, **2**, 177

192. Lewis, T. (1913). Observations upon a curious and not uncommon form of extreme acceleration of the auricle: 'Auricular flutter'. *Heart*, **4**, 171

193. Lewis, T., Feil, H.S. and Stroud, W.D. (1920). Observations upon flutter and fibrillation. Some effects of rhythmic stimulation of the auricle. *Heart*, **7**, 247

194. Lewis, T., Drury, A.N. and Iliescu, C.C. (1921). A demonstration of circus movement in clinical flutter of the auricles. *Heart*, **8**, 341

195. Cabrera, C.E. and Sodi-Pollares, D. (1947). Discussion del movimiento circular y prueba directa de su existencia en el flutter auricular

clinico. *Arch. Inst. Cardiol. Mex.*, **17**, 850

196. Rytand, D. (1966). The circus movement entrapped. Circus wave hypothesis and atrial flutter. *Ann. Intern. Med.*, **65**, 125

197. Wellens, H.J.J., Janse, M.J., Van Dam, R.T. *et al.* (1971). Epicardial excitation of the atria in a patient with atrial flutter. *Br. Heart J.*, **33**, 233

198. Klein, G.J., Guiraudon, G.M., Sharma, A.D. and Milstein, S. (1986). Demonstration of macroreentry and feasibility of operative therapy in the common type of atrial flutter. *Am. J. Cardiol.*, **8**, 587–91

199. Adams, R. (1827). Cases of diseases of heart accompanied with pathological observations. *Dublin Hosp. Rep.*, **4**, 353

200. Hope, J. (1839). *A Treatise on the Diseases of the Heart and Great Vessels*, 3rd. (London: Churchill)

201. Bouillaud, J.B. (1935). *Traite Clinique des Maladies du Couer*, 2 vols. (Paris: J.B. Bailliére)

202. Marey, E.J. (1863). *Physiologie Médicale de la Circulation du Sang*, p. 525. (Paris: Delahaye)

203. Vulpian, A. (1874). Notes sur les éffets de la faradisation directe des ventricules du coeur chez le chien. *Arch. Physiol. Norm. Path.*, **6**, 975

204. Engelmann, T.W. (1894–95). Refractäre Phase and kompensatorische Ruhe in ihrer Bedeutung für den Herzrhythmus. *Arch. Ges. Physiol.*, **59**, 309

205. Mackenzie, J. (1894). The venous and liver pulses, and the arrhythmic contraction of the cardiac cavities. *J. Pathol. Bacteriol.*, **2**, 84–154

206. Hering, H.E. (1903). Analyse des Pulses irregularis perpetuus. *Prager Med. Wchnschr.*, **38**, 377

207. Hering, H.E. (1908). Das Elektrocardiogram des Pulsus irregularis perpetuus. *Dtsch. Arch. klin. Med.*, **94**, 205

208. Lewis, T. (1909). Auricular fibrillation: a common clinical condition. *Br. Med. J.*, **2**, 1528

209. Rothenberger, C.J. and Winterberg, H. (1909). Vorhoffimmern und Arrhythmia perpetuus. *Wien. Klin. Wchnschr.*, **22**, 839

210. Lewis, T. (1911). *Heart*, **9**, 161

211. Mackenzie, J. (1902). *Op. cit.*, ref. 124

212. McMichael, J. (1981). Sir James Mackenzie and atrial fibrillation: a new perspective. *J. R. College Gen. Practitioners*, **31**, 402–6

213. Harrison, D.C., Mason, J.W., Schroeder, J.S. *et al.* (1978). Effects of cardiac denervation on cardiac arrhythmias and electrophysiology. In Prevention of Arrhythmias. *Br. Heart J.*, Suppl., 17–23

214. Scherf, D. (1928). Versuche zur Theorie des

Vorhofflatterns und Vorhofflimmerns. *Z. Ges. Exp. Med.*, **61**, 30

215. Scherf, D., Romano, F.J. and Terranova, R. (1948). Experimental studies on auricular flutter and auricular fibrillation. *Am. Heart J.*, **6**, 241

216. Prinzmetal, M., Oblath, R., Corday, E. *et al.* (1951). Auricular fibrillation. *J. Am. Med. Assoc.*, **146**, 1275

217. Södorström, N. (1970). What is the reason for the ventricular arrhythmia in cases of atrial fibrillation. *Am. Heart J.*, **40**, 212

218. Bootsma, B.K., Hoelen, A.J., Strackee, J. *et al.* (1970). Analysis of R-R intervals in patients with atrial fibrillation at rest and during exercise. *Circulation*, **41**, 783

219. Moe, G.K. (1962). On the multiple wavelet hypothesis of atrial fibrillation. *Arch. Int. Pharmacodyn.*, **CXL**, 183–8

220. Allessie, M.A., Bonke, F.I.M. and Schopman, F.J.G. (1977). Circus movement in rabbit atrial muscle as a mechanism of tachycardia. III. The 'leading circle' concept: a new model of circus movement in cardiac tissue without the involvement of an anatomic obstacle. *Circ. Res.* **41**, 9–18

221. Lown, B. (1967). Electrical reversion of cardiac arrhythmias. *Br. Heart J.*, **29**, 469

222. Mackenzie, J. (1902). The cause of heart irregularity in influenza. *Br. Med. J.*, **2**, 1411

223. Cohn, A.E. and Lewis, T. (1912–13). Auricular fibrillation and complete heart block. A description of a case of Adams-Stokes syndrome, including the postmortem examination. *Heart*, **4**, 15

224. Levine, S. (1916). Observations on sino-auricular heart block. *Arch. Intern. Med.*, **17**, 153

225. Pick, A., Langendorf, R. and Katz, L.N. (1951). Depression of cardiac pacemakers by premature impulses. *Am. Heart J.*, **41**, 49

226. Short, D.S. (1954). The syndrome of alternating bradycardia and tachycardia. *Br. Heart J.*, **16**, 208

227. Ferrer, M.I. (1968). The sick sinus syndrome in atrial disease. *J. Am. Med. Assoc.*, **206**, 645

228. Gaskell, W.H. (1883). On the innervation of the heart with especial reference to the heart of the tortoise. *J. Physiol. (Lond.)*, **4**, 43–127

229. Rosen, K.M., Rahimtoola, S.H., Gunnar, R.M., and Lev, M. (1971). Transient and persistent atrial standstill with His bundle lesions. *Circulation*, **44**, 220–36

230. Rosen, K.M., Loeb, H.S., Sinno, M.Z. *et al.* (1971). Cardiac conduction in patients with symptomatic sinus node disease. *Circulation*, **43**, 836–44

231. Cushny, A.R. (1897). Atrial Standstill. *J. Exp. Med.*, **2**, 232

232. Laslett (1908). *Quart. J. Med.*, **11**, 347

233. Lewis, T., White, P.D. and Meekin, J. (1913). *Heart*, **5**, 289

234. Greene, C.W. and Gilbert, N.C. (1921). Studies on the responses of the circulation to low oxygen tension. III. Changes in the pacemaker and in the conduction during extreme oxygen want, as shown in the human electro-cardiogram. *Arch. Intern. Med.*, **27**, 517

235. Boden, E. and Neukirck, P. (1921). *Deutsches Arch. klin. Med.*, **136**, 181

236. Korns, H.M. (1923). *Arch. Intern. Med.*, **31**, 15

237. Haskell, C.C. (1927). *J. Pharmacol. Exp. Ther.*, **32**, 233

238. Wolff, L. and White, P.D. (1929). Auricular standstill during quinidine therapy. *Heart*, **14**, 295

239. Wolff, L. and White, P.D. (1929). Auricular fibrillation. Results of seven year's experience with quinidine sulphate therapy (1921–1928). *Arch. Intern. Med.*, **43**, 653

240. Lewis, T., Drury, A.N. and Iliescu, C.C. (1921). *Heart*, **9**, 21

241. Lewis, T. (1913). *Q. J. Med.*, **6**, 221

242. Marzahn, H. (1925). *Ztschr. Klin. Med.*, **128**, 270

243. Marzahn, H. (1935). *Deutsches Arch. Klin Med.*, **178**, 50

244. White, P.D. (1916). *Boston Med. Surg. J.*, **175**, 233

245. Wilson, F.N. and Wishart, S.W. (1926). *Tr. A. Am. Phys.*, **41**, 55

246. Buckley, J.J. and Jackson, J.A. (1961). *Anesthesiology*, **22**, 723

247. Linenthal, A.S., Winer, B.M. and Klayman, M.I. (1953). *Am. Heart J.*, **46**, 443

248. Borman, M.C. and McMillan, T.A. (1927). *Am. Heart J.*, **3**, 208

249. James, T.N. (1961). Myocardial infarction and atrial arrhythmias. *Circulation*, **24**, 761

250. Surawicz, B. (1963). Electrolytes and the electrocardiogram. *Am. J. Cardiol.*, **12**, 656

251. Caponnetto, S., Pastorini, C. and Tirelli, G. (1968). Persistent atrial standstill in a patient affected with facioscapulohumeral dystrophy. *Cardiologia*, **53**, 341

252. Wolff, L., Parkinson, J. and White, P.D. (1930). Bundle branch block with short PR interval in healthy young people prone to paroxysmal tachycardia. *Am. Heart J.*, **5**, 685

253. Wilson, F.N. (1915). A case in which the vagus influenced the form of the ventricular complex

of the electrocardiogram. *Arch. Intern. Med.*, **16**, 1008

254. Johnston, F.D. and Lepeschkin, E. (eds.) (1954). *Selected Papers of Dr. Frank N. Wilson.* (Ann Arbor, Mich.: J.W. Edwards)

255. Wedd, A.M. (1921). Paroxysmal tachycardia with reference to normotropic tachycardia and the role of the intrinsic cardiac nerves. *Arch. Intern. Med.*, **27**, 571

256. Bach, F. (1929). Paroxysmal tachycardia of forty-eight years duration and right bundle branch block. *Proc. R. Soc. Med.*, **22**, 412

257. Wolff, L. (1965). The Wolff-Parkinson-White syndrome. *Am. J. Cardiol.*, **15**(4), 553

258. Hamburger, W.W. (1929). Bundle branch block. Four cases of intraventricular block showing interesting and unusual clinical features. *Med. Clin. North Am.*, **13**, 343

259. Holzmann, M. and Scherf, D. (1932). Ueber Electrokardiogramme mit verkwezter Vorhof-Kammer-Distanz und positiven P-Zacken. *Ztschr. Klin. Med.*, **121**, 404

260. Wolferth, C.C. and Wood, F.C. (1933). The mechanism of production of short PR intervals and prolonged QRS complexes in patients with presumably undamaged hearts: Hypothesis of an accessory pathway of auriculo-ventricular conduction (bundle of Kent). *Am. Heart J.*, **8**, 297

261. Butterworth, J.C. and Poindexter, C.A. (1942). Short PR interval associated with a prolonged QRS complex. A clinical and experimental study. *Arch. Intern. Med.*, **69**, 437

262. Wood, F.C., Wolferth, C.C. and Geckler, G.D. (1943). Histological demonstration of accessory muscular connections between auricle and ventricle in a case of short PR interval and prolonged QRS complex. *Am. Heart J.*, **25**, 454

263. Ohnell, R.F. (1944). Pre-excitation, a cardiac abnormality. *Acta Med. Scand. (Suppl.)*, **152**, 74

264. Rosenbaum, F.F., Hecht, H.H., Wilson, F.N. and Johnson, F.D. (1945). The potential variations of the thorax and the esophagus in anomalous atrioventricular excitement (Wolff-Parkinson-White syndrome). *Am. Heart J.*, **29**, 281

265. Ferrer, M.I. (1967). New concepts relating to the preexcitation syndrome. *J. Am. Med. Assoc.*, **201**, 162

266. Brechenmacher, C., Laham, J., Iris, L. *et al.* (1974). Etude histologique des voies anormales de conduction dans un syndrome de Wolff-Parkinson-White et dans un syndrome de Lown-Ganong-Levine. *Arch. Mal. Coeur*, **67**, 507

267. Gallagher, J.J., Gilbert, M., Svenson, R.H. *et al.* (1975). Wolff-Parkinson-White syndrome. The problem, evaluation and surgical correction. *Circulation*, **51**, 767–83

268. Panum, P.L. (1862). Experimentale Beiträge zur Lehre der Emboli. *Arch. Pathol. Anat.*, **25**, 308

269. Lewis, T. (1909). The experimental production of paroxysmal tachycardia and the effect of ligation of the coronary arteries. *Heart*, **1**, 98

270. Robinson, G. and Herrmann, G. (1921). Paroxysmal tachycardia of ventricular origin and its relation to coronary occlusion. *Heart*, **8**, 59

271. Wilson, F.N., Wishart, S.W., Mcloed, A.C. *et al.* (1932). A clinical type of paroxysmal tachycardia of ventricular origin in which paroxysms are induced by exertion. *Am. Heart J.*, **7**, 155

272. Katz, L.N. (1928). The significance of the T wave in the electrogram and the electrocardiogram. *Physiol. Rev.*, **8**, 447

273. Dessertenne, F. (1966). La tachycardie ventriculaire a deux foyers opposes variables. *Arch. Mal. Coeur.*, **59**, 263

274. Gallavardin, L. (1922). Extra-systolie ventriculaire à paroxysmes tachycardiques prolonges. *Arch. Mal. Coeur.*, **15**, 209

275. MacWilliam, J.A. (1923). Applications of physiology to medicine. Ventricular fibrillation and sudden death. *Br. Med. J.*, **2**, 215

276. Wiggers, C.J. (1929). Studies of ventricular fibrillation caused by electric shock. *Am. Heart J.*, **5**, 351

277. Schwartz, S.P., Orloff, J. and Fox, C. (1949). Transient ventricular fibrillation. *Am. Heart J.*, **37**, 21

278. Horowitz, L.N., Greenspan, A.M., Spielman, S.R. *et al.* (1981). Torsades de pointes: electrophysiologic studies in patients without transient pharmacologic or metabolic abnormalities. *Circulation*, **63**, 1120

279. Reddy, C.P. and Surawicz, B. (1983). *Op. cit.*, ref. 161

280. Brewer, L.A. (1983). Sphygmology through the centuries. Historical notes. *Am. J. Surg.*, **145**, 696–702

281. *Ibid.*

282. Erichsen, J.E. (1842). On the influence of the coronary circulation on the action of the heart. *London Med. Gaz.*, **2**, 561

283. Hoffa, M. and Ludwig, C. (1850). Ein neue Versuche über Herzbewegung. *Z. Rat. Med.*, **9**, 107

284. MacWilliam, J.A. (1887). *Op. cit.*, ref. 189

285. Hoffman, A. (1912). Fibrillation of ventricles

at the end of an attack of paroxysmal tachycardia in man. *Heart*, **3**, 213

286. Kerr, W.J. and Bender, W.L. (1922). Paroxysmal ventricular fibrillation with cardiac recovery in a case of auricular fibrillation and complete heart block while under quinidine sulfate therapy. *Heart*, **9**, 269

287. De Boer, S. (1923). Die Physiologie und Pharmakologie des Flimmers. *Ergeb. Physiol.*, **21**, 1

288. Wiggers, C.J. and Wegria, R. (1940). Ventricular fibrillation due to single localized induction and condenser shocks applied during the vulnerable phase of ventricular systole. *Am. J. Physiol.*, **128**, 500,

289. Wegria, R., Moe, G.K. and Wiggers, C.J. (1941). Comparison of the vulnerable period and fibrillation thresholds of normal and idioventricular beats. *Am. J. Physiol.*, **133**, 651

290. Hosler, R.M. (1959). Historical notes on cardiorespiratory resuscitation. *Am. J. Cardiol.*, **3**, 416–19

291. Hunter, J. (1776). Proposals for the recovery of people apparently drowned. *The Philosophical Transactions*, **66**, 412

292. Hunter, J. (1840). *Observations on Certain Parts of the Animal Oeconomy.* (Philadelphia: Haswell, Barrington, and Haswell)

293. Schiff, M. (1882). Ueber die direkte reizing der herzoberflacke. *Arch. Ges. Physiol.*, **28**, 200

294. Langenbuch (1887) Cited by Kulebyakin (1913) From Nevogskü, V.A. (1960)

295. Nevogskü, V.A. *Resuscitation and Artificial Hypothermia.* (Moscow: Medgiz) (English Translation, Pitman Medical Publishing Co. Ltd. London)

296. Niehaus (1889) cited by Zesas (1903). Über massage des freigelegton herzens beim chloroformkollaps. *Zbl. Chir.*, **22**, 588

297. Tuffier, T. and Hallion, L. (1898). De la compression rhythmee du coeur dans la syncope cardiaque par embolie. *Bull. Mém. Soc. Chir.*, **24**, 937

298. Maag (1900) Cited by Barber, R.F. and Madden, J.L. (1945). Historical aspects of cardiac resuscitation. *Am. J. Surg.*, **5**, 70

299. Starling, E. and Lane, W.A. (1902). Report of Society of Anesthetists. *Lancet*, **2**, 1397

300. Inglesburd (1945). *Op. cit.*, ref. 298

301. Crile, G. and Dolley, D. (1906). Experimental research into the resuscitation of dogs. *J. Exp. Med.*, **8**, 713

302. Sollman, T. (1905). Revival of the excised

mammalian heart. *Am. J. Physiol.*, **15**, 121

303. Schechter, D.C. (1971). Early experience with resuscitation by means of electricity. *Surgery*, **69**, 360–72

304. Schechter, D.C. (1969). Role of the Humane Societies in the history of resuscitation. *Surg. Gynec. Obstet.*, **129**, 811

305. Registers of the Royal Humane Society of London (1774–84). (London: Nichols & Sons)

306. Birch, J. (1792). In: Adams G: An essay on electricity ... to which is now added a letter to the author, from Mr. John Birch, Surgeon, on the subject of medical electricity, 4th edn. (London: R. Hindmarsh)

307. Bartecchi, C.E. (1980). Cardiopulmonary resuscitation: an element of sophistication in the 18th century. *Am. Heart J.*, **100**, 580–1

308. Editorial (1978). Near-drowning. *Lancet*, **11**, 194

309. Margotta, R. (1968). *The Story of Medicine.* (New York: Golden Press)

310. Zoll, P.M. (1952). Resuscitation of the heart in ventricular standstill by external electrical stimulation. *N. Engl. J. Med.*, **247**, 768

311. Aldini, J. (1804). *Essai Théorique et Experimental pour le Galvanisme.* (Paris: Fournier fils)

312. Haggard, H.W. (1936). The first published attack on Perkinism: an anonymous eighteenth century poetical satire. *Yale J. Biol. Med.*, **9**, 137

313. Valli, E. (1793). *Experiments on Animal Electricity.* (London: J. Johnson)

314. Fowler, R. (1786). Experiments and observations relative to the influence lately discovered by Mr. Galvani, and commonly called animal electricity. *Bibl. Br.*, **11**, (1)

315. von Humboldt, F.W.H.A. (1797). Versuche ueber die gereizte Muskel- und Nervenfaser nebst Vermuthungen ueber den chemischen Process des Lebens in der Thier- und Pflazenwelt, Posen, 1797, Decker. Also: Lettre de Humboldt à Loder sur les applications du Galvanisme, *Bibl. germanique 4*, **301**, 1797. Also: Lettre de Humboldt à Blumenbach, *Ann. de Chimie, Paris*, **64**, 1

316. Schechter, D.C. (1971). *Op cit.*, ref. 303

317. *Ibid.*

318. *Ibid.*

319. Haynes, C.M. (1887). *Elementary Principles of Electro-therapeutics*, edn. 4. (Chicago: W. T. Keener)

320. Reece, R. (1824). *Medical Guide for the Use of the Clergy, Heads of Families, and Junior Practitioners in Medicine and Surgery*, edn. 14. (London: Longman, Hurst & Co.)

321. Good, J. (1936). *The Study of Medicine.* (New York: Harper & Bros.)

322. Hoffa, M. and Ludwig, C. (1850). Einige neue Versuche über Herzbewegung. *Z. Rationale Med.*, **9**, 107

323. Colwell, H.A. (1922). *An Essay on the History of Electrotherapy and Diagnosis.* (London: William Heinemann)

324. de Lamballe, J. (1873). Cited by Althaus, J: *A Treatise on Medical Electricity*, edn. 3. (London: Longmans, Green & Company)

325. Green, T. (1872). On death from chloroform: its prevention by galvanism. *Br. Med. J.*, **1**, 551–3

326. Von Ziemssen, H. (1857). *Die Electricität in der Medicin.* (Berlin: August Herschwald)

327. Von Ziemssen, H. (1882). Studien über die Bewegungsvorgänge am menschlichen Herzen, sowie über die mechanische und elektrische Erregbarkeit des Herzens und des Nervus Phrenicus, angestellt an dem freiliegenden Herzen der Catharina Serafin. *Dtsch. Arch. Clin. Med.*, **30**, 270

328. MacWilliam, J.A. (1885). On the structure and rhythm of the heart in fishes, with especial reference to the heart of the eel. *J. Physiol.*, **6**, 192

329. MacWilliam, J.A. (1887). Fibrillar contraction of the heart. *J. Physiol.*, **8**, 296

330. MacWilliam, J.A. (1889). Cardiac failure and sudden death. *Br. Med. J.*, **1**, 6

331. MacWilliam, J.A. (1887). On electrical stimulation of the mammalian heart. *Trans. Int. Med. Congress, 9th session. Washington*, vol. III. p. 253

332. *Ibid.*

333. MacWilliam, J.A. (1889). Electrical stimulation of the heart in man. *Br. Med. J.*, **1**, 348

334. Lewis, T. (1915). *Lectures on the Heart.* (New York: Paul B. Hoeber)

335. Levy, A.G. and Lewis, T. (1911). Heart irregularities, resulting from the inhalation of low percentages of chloroform vapour, and their relationship to ventricular fibrillation. *Heart*, **3**, 99

336. MacWilliam, J.A. (1923). Some applications of physiology to medicine: II. Ventricular fibrillation and sudden death. *Br. Med. J.*, **2**, 215

337. Jex-Blake, A.J. (1913). The Goulstonian lectures on death by electric currents and by lightning. *Br. Med. J.*, **1**, 425, 492, 548, 601

338. Prevost, J-L. and Battelli, F. (1899). La mort par les courants électriques: courant alternatif a bas voltage. *J. Physiol. Path. Gen.*, **1**, 399

339. *Ibid.*

340. Cunningham, R.H. (1899). The cause of death from industrial electric current. *NY Med. J.*, **70**, 581, 615

341. English, P.C. (1980). *Shock, Physiological Surgery, and George Washington Crile: Medical Innovation in the Progressive Era.* (Westport, CT: Greenwood Press)

342. Stephenson, H.E. (1981). Charles Claude Guthrie's contribution to cardiac resuscitation. *Crit. Care. Med.*, **9**, 428

343. Ferris, L.P., Spence, P.W., King, B.G. and Williams, H.B. (1936). Effect of electric shock on the heart. *Electrical Eng.*, **55**, 498

344. Kouwenhoven, W.B. (1969). The development of the defibrillator. *Ann. Intern. Med.*, **71**, 449

345. Hooker, D.R., Kouwenhoven, W.B. and Langworthy, O.R. (1933). The effect of alternating electrical currents on the heart. *Am. J. Physiol.*, **103**, 444

346. Hooker, D.R. (1929). On the recovery of the heart in electric shock. *Am. J. Physiol.*, **91**, 305

347. Wiggers, C.J. (1958). *Reminiscences and Adventures in Circulation Research.* (New York: Grune & Stratton)

348. Wiggers, C.J. (1936). Cardiac massage followed by countershock in revival of mammalian ventricles from fibrillation due to coronary occlusion. *Am. J. Physiol.*, **116**, 161

349. Wiggers, C.J. and Wégria, R. (1940). Ventricular fibrillation due to single, localized induction and condenser shocks applied during the vulnerable phase of ventricular systole. *Am. J. Physiol.*, **128**, 500–5

350. Gurvich, N.L. and Yuniev, G.S. (1946). Restoration of a regular rhythm in the mammalian fibrillating heart. *Am. Rev. Soviet Med.*, **3**, 236–9

351. Beck, C.S., Pritchard, W.H. and Feil, H.S. (1947). Ventricular fibrillation of long duration abolished by electric shock. *J. Am. Med. Assoc.*, **135**, 985–6

352. Beck, C.S. and Mautz, F.R. (1937). The control of the heart beat by the surgeon: with special reference to ventricular fibrillation occurring during operation. *Ann. Surg.*, **106**, 525

353. Beck, C.S. (1941). Resuscitation for cardiac standstill and ventricular fibrillation occurring during operation. *Am. J. Surg.*, **54**, 273

354. Beck, C., Weckesser, E. and Barry, F. (1956). Fatal heart attack: successful resuscitation. *J. Am. Med. Assoc.*, **16**, 434

355. Beck, C.S. and Mautz, F.R. (1937). The control of the heart beat by the surgeon. *Ann. Surg.*, **106**, 525

356. Geddes, L.A. and Hamlin, R. (1983). The first human heart defibrillation. *Am. J. Cardiol.*, **52**, 403

357. Beck, C.S. (1970). Reminiscences of cardiac resuscitation. *Rev. Surg.*, **27**, 76

358. Hosler, R.M. (1959). *Op. cit.*, ref. 290

359. Zoll, P.M., Linenthal, A.J., Gibson, W., Paul, M.H. and Norman, L.R. (1956). Termination of ventricular fibrillation in man by externally applied electric countershock. *N. Engl. J. Med.*, **254**, 727

360. Kouwenhoven, W.B., Jude, J.R. and Knickerbocker, G.G. (1960). Closed chest cardiac massage. *J. Am. Med. Assoc.*, **173**, 1064

361. Hill, J. (1868). *Br. J. Dent. Sci.*, **11**, 355

362. Boehm, R. (1878). V. Arbeiten aus dem pharmakologischen. Institute der Universitat Dorpat. 13. Über weiderbelegung nach vergifteingen und asphyxie. *Arch. Exp. Path. Pharmak.*, **8**, 68

363. Maas (1892). Die Methode der Weiderbelebung bei Herztod nach Chloroformeinathmung. *Berl. Klin. Wschr.*, **12**, 265

364. Crile, G. (1904). Cited by Keen, W.W. *Therap. Gaz. (Detroit)*, **20**, 217

365. Schott, E. (1920). Ueber Ventrikelstillstand (Adams-Stokes'sche Anfaelle) nebst Bemerkungen ueber andersartige Arrhythmien passager. *Natur., Dtsch. Arch. Klin. Med.*, **131**, 211

366. Scherf, D. and Bornemann, C. (1960). Thumping the precordium in ventricular standstill. *Am. J. Cardiol.*, **5**, 30

367. Kay, J.H. and Blalock, A. (1951). The use of calcium chloride in the treatment of cardiac arrest in patients. *Surgery, Gynec., Obstet.*, **93**, 97

368. Day, H.W. (1972). History of coronary care units. *Am. J. Cardiol.*, **30**, 405–7

369. Julian, D.G. (1987). The history of coronary care units. *Br. Heart J.*, **57**, 497–502

370. Thalen, H.J. (1977). History of cardiac pacing. In Harthorne, J.W. and Thalen, H.J.T. (eds.) *Boston Colloqium on Cardiac Pacing*, pp. 1–22. (The Hague: Martinus Nijhoff Medical Division)

371. Bardeen, J. and Brattain, W.H. (1948). The transistor, a semiconductor triode. *Phys. Rev.*, **74**, 230

372. Bardeen, J. and Brattain, W.H. (1949). Physical principles involved in transistor action. *Phys. Rev.*, **75**, 203

373. Schockley, W. (1949). The theory of p-n junctions in semiconductors and p-n junction transistors. *Bell Sys. Tech., J.*, **28**, 435

374. Nysten, P.H. (1802). *Experiences sur le Coeur et les Autres Parties d'un Homme Decapite le 14 Brumaire, Au XI.* (Paris: Levkault)

375. Walshe, W.H. (1862). *A Practical Treatise on Diseases of the Heart and Great Vessels.* (Philadelphia: Blanchard & Lee)

376. Duchenne de Boulogne (1872). *De L'électrisation Localise et son Application a la Pathologique et a la Therapeutique.* (Paris: Baillière)

377. Von Ziemssen, H. (1882). *Op. cit.*, ref.327

378. Schechter, D.C. (1971). Background of clinical cardiac electrostimulation, 1. Responsiveness of quiescent, bare heart to electricity. *NY State J. Med.*, **71**, 2575

379. Schechter, D.C. (1972). Background of clinical cardiac electrostimulation. IV. Early studies on the feasibility of accelerating heart rate by means of electricity. *NY State J. Med.*, **72**, 395

380. Marmorstein, M. (1927). Contribution à l'étude des excitations électriques localisées sur le coeur en rapport avec la topographie de l'innervation du coeur chez le chien. *J. Physiol. Pathol.*, **24**, 40

381. Hyman, S. (1932). Resuscitation of the stopped heart by intracardiac therapy. *Arch. Intern. Med.*, **50**, 283

382. Schechter, D.C. (1972). Background of clinical cardiac electrostimulation. V. Direct electro-stimulation of heart without thoracotomy. *NY State J. Med.*, **72**, 605

383. Schechter, D.C. (1972). Background of clinical cardiac electro-stimulation. VI. Precursor apparatus and events to the electrical treatment of complete heart block. *NY State J. Med.*, **72**, 953

384. Mond, H.G., Sloman, J.G. and Edwards, R.H. (1982). The first pacemaker. *Pace*, **5**, 279–82

385. Lidwill, M.C. (1929). Cardiac disease in relation to anaesthesia. In *Transactions of the Third Session. Australasian Medical Congress (British Medical Association)*, Sydney, Australia, September 2 to 7, p. 160

386. Bigelow, W.G., Callaghan, J.C. and Hopps, J.A. (1950). General hypothermia for experimental intracardiac surgery. The use of electrophrenic respirations, an artificial pacemaker for cardiac standstill, and radio-frequency rewarming in general hypothermia. *Ann. Surg.*, **132**, 531

387. Hopps, J.A. (1981). The development of the pacemaker. *Pace*, **4**, 106–8

388. Escher, D.J.W. (1980). Historical aspects of cardiac pacing. In Samet, P. and El-Sherif, N. (eds.) *Cardiac Pacing*, 2nd edn., p. 634. (Grune & Stratton)

389. Bigelow, W.G. (1987). The pacemaker story: a cold heart spinoff. *Pace*, **10**, 142–51

390. Zoll, P.M. (1972). Historical development of cardiac pacemakers. *Progress in Cardiovascular Diseases*, vol. XIV, No. 5, p. 423

391. Zoll, P.M. (1987). Letter to Editor. *Pace*, **10**, 1388

392. Zoll, P.M. (1952). Resuscitation of the heart in ventricular standstill by external electric stimulation. *N. Engl. J. Med.*, **247**, 768

393. Thalen, H.J.T. (1977). *Op. cit.,* ref. 370

394. Thalen, H.J.T., van den Berg, J.W., van der Heide, J.N. *et al.* (1969). *The Artificial Cardiac Pacemaker*, chapter 3. (Assen, The Netherlands: Royal Vangorcum)

395. Furman, S. and Escher, D.J.W. (1970). *Principles and Techniques of Cardiac Pacing*, chapter 5. (New York: Harper & Row)

396. Weirich, W.L., Gott, V.L. and Lillehei, C.W. (1957). The treatment of complete heart block by the combined use of a myocardial electrode and an artificial pacemaker. *Surg. Forum*, **8**, 360

397. Zoll, P.M. (1973). Development of electric control of cardiac rhythm. *J. Am. Med. Assoc.*, **226**, 881–6

398. Furman, S. and Robinson, G. (1958). The use of an intracardiac pacemaker in the correction of total heart block. *Surg. Forum*, **9**, 245

399. Furman, S. and Schwedel, J.B. (1959). An intracardiac pacemaker for Stokes-Adams seizures. *N. Engl. J. Med.*, **261**, 943

400. Schwedel, J.B., Furman, S. and Escher, D.J.W. (1960). Use of an intracardiac pacemaker in the treatment of Stokes-Adams seizures. *Prog. Cardiovasc. Dis.*, **3**, 170

401. Schwedel, J.B. and Escher, D.J.W. (1964). Transvenous electrical stimulation of the heart. *Ann. NY Acad. Sci.*, **111**, 972

402. Glenn, W.W.L., Mauro, A., Longo, E. *et al.* (1959). Remote stimulation of the heart by radiofrequency transmission: clinical application to a patient with Stokes-Adams syndrome. *N. Engl. J. Med.*, **261**, 948

403. Camilli, L. *et al.* (1964). Radio-frequency pacemaker with receiver coil implanted on the heart. *Ann. NY Acad. Sci.*, **111**, 1007

404. Abrams, L.D. and Norman, L. (1964). Experience with inductive coupled cardiac pacemakers. *Ann. NY Acad. Sci.*, **111**, 1030–40

405. Elmqvist, R. *et al.* (1963). Artificial pacemaker for treatment of Adams-Stokes syndrome and slow heart rate. *Am. Heart J.*, **65**, 731

406. Senning, A. (1959). Discussion of a paper by Stephenson *et al.* Physiologic P-wave cardiac stimulator. *J. Thorac. Surg.*, **38**, 369

407. Gold, R.D. (1984). Cardiac pacing from then to now. *Medical Instrumentation*, vol. 18, no. 1

408. *Ibid.*

409. Chardack, W.M., Gage, A.D. and Greatbach, W. (1960). A transistorized self-contained, implantable pacemaker for the long-term correction of heart block. *Surgery*, **48**, 643

410. Hunter, S.W., Roth, N.A., Bernardez, D. *et al.* (1959). A bipolar myocardial electrode for complete heart block. *Lancet*, **70**, 506

411. Hunter, S.W. *et al.* (1959). A bipolar myocardial electrode for complete heart block. *Lancet*, **79**, 506–8

412. Zoll, P.M., Frank, H.A., Zarsky, L.R.N. *et al.* (1961). Long-term electrical stimulation of the heart for Stokes-Adams disease. *Ann. Surg.*, **154**, 330

413. Kantrowitz, A., Cohen, R., Raillard, H. *et al.* (1962). The treatment of complete heart block with an implanted controllable pacemaker. *Surg. Gynecol. Obstet.*, **115**, 415

414. Noyce, R.N. Semiconductor device-and-lead structure. U.S. Patent 2, 981,877, filed July 30, 1959; patented April 25, 1961

415. Gold, R.D. (1984). *Op. cit.*, ref. 407

416. Parsonnet, V. *et al.* (1981). A revised code for pacemaker identification. *Pace*, **4**, 396

417. Friedman, M. and McCauley, C.E. (1947). The Ruben cell, a new alkaline dry cell battery. *Trans. Electrochem. Soc.*, **92**, 195

418. Chardack, W.M. *et al.* (1960). A transistorized, self-contained, implantable pacemaker for the long term correction of complete heart block. *Surgery*, **48**, 643

419. Parsonnet, V. *et al.* (1964). The potentiality of the use of biologic energy as a power source for implantable pacemakers. *Ann. NY Acad. Sci.*, **11**, 915

420. Schaldach, M. (1971). Implantable electro-chemical energy sources. In *Proc. 9th. International Conference on Medical and Biological Engineering*, Melbourne, M-8, 18

421. Cywinski, J.K. *et al.* (1973). Biogalvanic power sources. In Thalen, H.J.T. (ed.) *Cardiac Pacing, Proc. IVth International Congress on Cardiac Pacing*, pp. 216–20. (Assen, The Netherlands: Van Gorcum & Co.)

422. Sowton, E. (1977). Energy Sources for pacemakers. In Watanabe, Y. (ed.) *Cardiac Pacing, Proc. Vth. International Congress on Pacing*, pp. 438–46. (Amsterdam: Excerpta Medica)

423. Greatbatch, W. (1973). Chemical power

supplies for implantable cardiac pacemakers. In Thalen, H.J.T. (ed.) *Cardiac Pacing, Proc. IVth. International Congress on Cardiac Pacing,* pp. 188–91. (Assen, The Netherlands: Van Gorcum & Co.)

424. Gold, R.D. (1983). The state of the art in pacer technology. *Cardiol. Prod. News,* **3**, 6

425. Gabano, J.P. (1983). *Lithium Batteries,* p. 137. (New York: Academic Press)

426. Littleford, P.O. and Spector, D. (1979). Method for the rapid atraumatic insertion of permanent endocardial pacemaker electrodes through the subclavian vein. *Am. J. Cardiol.,* **43**, 980

427. Nathan, D.A. and Center, S. (1963). An implantable synchronous pacemaker for the long term correction of complete heart block. *Circulation,* **27**, 682

428. Center, S. *et al.* (1983). The implantable synchronous pacemaker in the treatment of complete heart block. *J. Thorac. Cardiovasc. Surg.,* **46**, 744

429. Folkman, J.M. and Watkins, E. (1957). An artificial conduction system for the management of experimental heart block. *Surg. Forum,* **8**, 331

430. Stephenson, S.E. Jr., Edwards, W.H., Jolly, P.C. *et al.* (1959). Physiologic P-wave cardiac stimulator. *J. Thorac. Cardiovasc. Surg.,* **38**, 604

431. Kahn, M., Senderoff, E., Shapiro, J. *et al.* (1969). Bridging of interrupted AV conduction in experimental chronic complete heart block by electronic means. *Am. Heart J.,* **59**, 548

432. Leatham, A. *et al.* (1956). External electric stimulator for treatment of ventricular standstill. *Lancet,* **2**, 1185

433. Nicks, R. *et al.* (1962). Some observations on the treatment of heart block in degenerative heart disease. *Med. J. Austral.,* **2**, 857

434. Lemberg, L. *et al.* (1965). Pacing on demand in A-V block. *J. Am. Med. Assoc.,* **191**, 12

435. Parsonnet, V. *et al.* (1966). Clinical use of an implantable standby pacemaker. *J. Am. Med. Assoc.,* **196**, 784

436. Furman, S. *et al.* (1967). Electrocardiographic manifestation of standby pacing. *J. Thorac. Cardiovasc. Surg.,* **54**, 723

437. Neville, J. *et al.* (1966). An implantable demand pacemaker. *Clin. Res.,* **14**, 256

438. Parsonnet, V. *et al.* (1974). Implantable pacemakers: status report and resource guideline. Pacemaker study group (ICHD). *Circulation,* **50**, A21

439. Terry, R.S. and Davies, G.L. Implantable cardiac pacemaker having adjustable operating parameters. U.S. Patent No. 3, 805, 796.

440. Tarjan, P. (1978). History of cardiac pacing. *Am. J. Cardiol.,* **41**, 614

441. Zoll, P.M. (1973). *Op. cit.,* ref. 397

442. Sowton, E., Leatham, A. and Carson, P. (1964). Suppression of arrhythmias by artificial pace-making. *Lancet,* **2**, 1098–100

443. Zoll, P.M. *et al.* (1956). Effects of external electric currents on the heart: control of cardiac rhythm and induction and termination of cardiac arrhythmias. *Circulation,* **14**, 745–56

444. Guyton, A.C. and Satterfield, J. (1951). Factors concerned in electrical defibrillation of heart particularly through unopened chest. *Am. J. Physiol.,* **167**, 81–7

445. Zoll, P.M., Linenthal, A.J. and Zarsky, L.R. (1960). Ventricular fibrillation: treatment and prevention by external electric currents. *N. Engl. J. Med.,* **262**, 105–12

446. Lown, B., Amarasingham, R. and Neuman, J. (1962). New method for terminating cardiac arrhythmias: use of synchronized capacitor discharge. *J. Am. Med. Assoc.,* **182**, 548–55

447. Kastor, J.A. (1989). Michel Mirowski and the automatic implantable defibrillator. *Am. J. Cardiol.,* **63**, 1121–6

448. Winkle, R.A. (1983). The implantable defibrillator in ventricular arrhythmias. *Hosp. Pract.,* **18**, 149–65

449. Mirowski, M., Mower, M.M., Staewen, W.S., Tabatznik, B. and Mendeloff, A.I. (1970). Standby automatic defibrillator. An approach to prevention of sudden coronary death. *Arch. Intern. Med.,* **126**, 158–61

450. Lown, B. and Axelrod, P. (1972). Implanted standby defibrillators. *Circulation,* **46**, 637–9

451. Mirowski, M., Reid, P.R., Mower, M.M., Watkins, L., Gott, V.L., Schauble, J.F., Langer, A., Heilman, M.S., Kolenik, S.A., Fischell, R.E. and Weisfeldt, M.L. (1980). Termination of malignant ventricular arrhythmias with an implanted automatic defibrillator in human beings. *N. Engl. J. Med.,* **303**, 322–4

452. Watkins, L., Mirowski, M., Mower, M.M., Reid, P.R., Griffith, L.S.C., Vlay, S.C., Weisfeldt, M.L. and Gott, V.L. (1981). Automatic defibrillation in man. The initial surgical experience. *J. Thorac. Cardiovasc. Surg.,* **82**, 492–500

453. Mirowski, M. and Mower, M.M. (1987). The automatic implantable defibrillator: some historical notes. In Brugada, P. and Wellens, H.J.J. (eds.) *Cardiac Arrhythmias: Where to Go*

from Here, 655–62. (Mount Kisco, New York: Futura Publishing)

454. Sealy, W.C. (1983). The case of the fisherman with the fast pulse and the beginning of arrhythmia surgery. *NCMJ*, **44**, 489–90

455. Sealy, W.C., Gallagher, J.J. and Pritchett, E.L.C. (1978). The surgical anatomy of Kent bundles based on electrophysiological mapping and surgical exploration. *J. Thorac. Cardiovasc. Surg.*, **76**, 804–15

456. Cox, J.L., Gallagher, J.J., Caine, M.E., *et al.* (1985). Experience with 118 consecutive patients undergoing operation for the Wolff-Parkinson-White syndrome. *J. Thorac. Cardiovasc. Surg.*, **90**, 490–501

457. Guiraudon, G.M., Klein, F.J., Sharma, A.D. *et al.* (1989). Surgery for the Wolff-Parkinson-White syndrome: the epicardial approach. *Sem. Thorac. Cardiovasc. Surg.*, **1**, 21–33

458. Klein, G.J., Guiraudon, G.M., Perkins, D.G. *et al.* (1984). Surgical correction of the Wolff-Parkinson-White syndrome in the closed heart using cryosurgery: a simplified approach. *JACC*, **3,2,1**, 405–9

459. Guiraudon, G.M., Klein, G.J., Gulamhusein, S. *et al.* (1984). Surgical repair of Wolff-Parkinson-White: a new closed-heart technique. *Ann. Thorac. Surg.*, **37**(1), 67–71

460. Guiraudon, G.M., Klein, G.J. and Sharma. A.D. (1986). Closed-heart technique for Wolff-Parkinson-White syndrome: further experience and potential limitations. *Ann. Thorac. Surg.*, **42**, 651–7

461. Guiraudon, G.M., Klein, G.J., Sharma, A.D. and Yee, R. (1989). Left ventricular free wall accessory pathways do not require cardiopulmonary bypass when using the 'direct' epicardial approach (abstr). *Circulation*, **80**(4), II–222

462. Mendez, C. and Moe, G. (1966). Demonstration of dual AV nodal conduction system in the isolated rabbit heart. *Circ. Res.*, **19**, 378–93

463. Sharma, A.D., Yee, R., Guiraudon, G.M. and Klein, G.J. (1988). AV nodal reentry. *Current Concepts and Surgical Treatment; Progress in Cardiology*, pp. 129–45. (Philadelphia: Lea & Febiger)

464. Johnson, D.C., Nunn, G.R., Richards, D.A. *et al.* (1987). Surgical therapy for supraventricular tachycardia, a potentially curable disorder. *J. Thorac. Cardiovasc. Surg.*, **93**, 913–18

465. Guiraudon, G.M., Klein, G.J., Sharma, A.D. *et al.* (1990). Skeletonization of the atrio-ventricular node surgical alternative for AV nodal reentrant tachycardia experience with 32 patients. *Ann. Thorac. Surg.*, **49** (4), 565–73

466. Guiraudon, G.M., Klein, G.J., Van Hemel, N. *et al.* (1990). Anatomically guided surgery to the AV node: AV nodal skeletonization: experience in 46 patients with AV nodal reentrant tachycardia. *Eur. J. Cardiothorac. Surg.*, **4** (9), 461–5

467. Cox, J.L., Ferguson, G., Lindsay, B.D. and Cain, M.E. (1990). Perinodal cryosurgery for atrioventricular node reentry tachycardia in 23 patients. *J. Thorac. Cardiovasc. Surg.*, **99**, 440–50

468. Moe, G.K. (1962). On the multiple wavelet hypothesis of atrial fibrillation. *Arch. Int. Pharmacodyn.*, **CXL**, 183–8

469. Cox, J.L., Schuessler, R.B., Cain, M.E. *et al.* (1989). Surgery for atrial fibrillation. *Sem. Thorac. Cardiovasc. Surg.*, **1** (1), 67–73

470. Guiraudon, G.M., Klein, G.J., Sharma, A.D. *et al.* (1986). Surgical treatment of supraventricular tachycardia: a five year experience. *Pace*, **9**, 1376–80

471. Guiraudon, G.M., Klein, G.J. and Yee, R. (1990). Surgery for cardiac tachyarrhythmias. *The Heart House Learning Center Highlights*, 6, 5, 9

472. Klein, G.J., Guiraudon, G.M., Sharma, A.D. and Milstein, S. (1986). Demonstration of macroreentry and feasibility of operative therapy in the common type of atrial flutter. *Am. J. Cardiol.*, **57** (8), 587–91

473. Spurrell, R.A.J. (1975). Surgery for ventricular tachycardia. In Krickler, D.M. and Goodwin, J.F. (eds.) *Cardiac Arrhythmias*, pp. 195–207. (Philadelphia: WB Saunders)

474. Spurrell, R.A.J., Yates, S.K., Thornburn, C.W., Sowton, G.E. and Deuchar, D.C. (1975). Surgical treatment of ventricular tachycardia after epicardial mapping studies. *Br. Heart J.*, **37**, 155

475. Gallagher, J.J. (1978). Surgical treatment of arrhythmias, current status and future directions. *Am. J. Cardiol.*, **41**, 1035

476. Guiraudon, G., Fontaine, G., Frank, R., Escande, G. *et al.* (1978). Encircling endocardial ventriculotomy: a new surgical treatment for life threatening ventricular tachycardias resistant to medical treatment following myocardial infarction. *Ann. Thorac. Surg.*, **26**, 438–44

477. Josephson, M.E., Harken, A.H. and Horowitz, L.N. (1979). Endocardial excision: a new surgical technique for the treatment of recurrent ventricular tachycardia. *Circulation*, **60**, 1430–8

478. Gonzalez, R., Scheinman, M., Margaretten, W. and Rubinstein, M. (1981). Closed-chest-catheter technique for His' bundle ablation in dogs. *Am. J. Physiol.*, **241**, H283–7

479. Gallagher, J.J., Svenson, R.H., Kasell, J.H. *et al.* (1982). Catheter technique for closed chest ablation of the atrioventricular conduction system: a therapeutic alternative for the treatment of refractory supraventricular tachycardia. *N. Engl. J. Med.*, **306**, 194–200

480. Scheinman, M.M., Morady, F., Hess, D.S. and Gonzalez, R. (1982). Catheter induced ablation of the atrioventricular junction to control refractory supraventricular arrhythmias. *J. Am. Med. Assoc.*, **284**, 851–5

481. Morady, F. and Scheinman, M.M. (1984). Transvenous catheter ablation of a posteroseptal accessory pathway in a patient with the Wolff-Parkinson-White syndrome. *N. Engl. J. Med.*, **310**, 705–7

482. Morady, F., Scheinmann, M.M., Kou, W.H., Griffin, J.C., Dick, M., Herre, J., Kadish, A.H. and Langberg, J. (1989). Long term results of catheter ablation of a posteroseptal accessory atrioventricular connection in 48 patients. *Circulation*, **79**, 1160–70

483. Huang, S.K., Graham, A.R., Bharati, S., Lee, M.A., Gorman, G. and Lev, M. (1988). Short and long term effects of transcatheter ablation of the coronary sinus by radiofrequency energy. *Circulation*, **78**, 416–27

484. Jackman, W.M., Kuck, K.H., Naccarelli, G.V., Carmen, L. and Pitha, J. (1988). Radiofrequency current directed across the mitral annulus with a bipolar epicardial–endocardial catheter electrode configuration in dogs. *Circulation*, **78**, 1288–98

485. Langberg, J., Griffin, J.C., Herre, J.M., Chin, M.C., Lev, M., Bharati, S. and Scheinman, M.M. (1989). Catheter ablation of accessory pathways using radiofrequency energy in the canine coronary sinus. *Eur. J. Cardiol.*, **13**, 491–6

486. Huang, S.K., Bharati, S., Graham, A.R. *et al.* (1987). Close chest catheter desiccation of the atrioventricular junction using radio-frequency energy: a new method of catheter ablation. *J. Am. Coll. Cardiol.*, **9**, 349–58

487. Evans, G.T., Scheinman, M.M., Zipes, D.P. *et al.* (1988). The percutaneous cardiac mapping and ablation registry: final summary of results. *Pace*, **11**, 1621–6

488. Levy, S. and Bru, P. (1986). Percutaneous electric interruption of normal auriculoventricular conduction: analysis of French cases. *Arch. Mal. Coeur*, **79**, 1145–50

489. Marchese, A.C., Pressley, J.C., Sintetos, A.L. *et al.* (1987). Cryosurgical versus catheter ablation of the atrioventricular junction. *Am. J. Cardiol.*, **59**, 870–3

490. Spears, J.R. (1987). PTCA restenosis: potential prevention with laser balloon angioplasty. *Am. J. Cardiol.*, **60**, 61–4B

491. Schuger, C.D., Steinman, R.T., Lehmann, M.H. *et al.* (1990). Percutaneous transcatheter laser balloon ablation from the canine coronary sinus: implications for the Wolff-Parkinson-White syndrome. *Lasers in Surgery and Medicine*, **10**, 140–8. (Wiley-Liss, Inc.)

21   Genetics and cardiovascular disease

Although genetics is a relatively new discipline in the biological sciences, it has already made a dramatic impact on medical practice and will continue to do so in ever increasing magnitude. The importance of genetics in medicine was emphatically underscored by Paul Berg in 1981 during his Nobel lecture on dissections and reconstructions of genes and chromosomes. His remarks were prescient. They are as follows:

> Just as our present practice of medicine relies on the sophisticated knowledge of human anatomy, physiology and biochemistry, so will dealing with genetic disease in the future demand a detailed understanding of the molecular anatomy, physiology and biochemistry of the human genome. We shall have to have physicians who are as conversant with the molecular anatomy and physiology of the chromosomes and genes as the cardiac surgeon is with the structure and workings of the heart and circulatory tree'[1].

The father of genetics was Johann Gregor Mendel. He was born in 1822 in a town that was originally part of Austria. The exigencies of war have changed the name from Heinzendorf, Austria to Hyncia Czechoslovakia. As a child, Mendel showed exceptional intellectual abilities, and in an effort to exploit these qualities, he was initially enrolled in the Piarist secondary school at Leipnik and then at the gymnasium in Troppan.

His diploma from the gymnasium was inscribed with the words 'primae classis eminentia', a testament to his industriousness and intellectual achievements.

After a lapse of several months due to an illness brought on by the necessity to augment the meagre family income through private tutoring, young Mendel continued his studies so that he could be enrolled at the University of Olmütz. The dire financial straits of his family and another absence from his studies due to illness slowed his educational progress but did not stop him in his relentless pursuit of knowledge. He was able to complete the program at the University rendering him familiar with philosophy, physics and mathematics. He also studied at this time under Professor Fux from whom he learned the principles of combinatorial operations, and which he later employed, with great success, in his research.

Again, because of financial necessity and not out of response to a 'vocational call', Mendel entered the Augustinian order of monks taking the name Gregor. This was the best possible solution for continuing his education and pursuing his research. Within the tranquil ambience of the monastery and with the financial security (though modest) of the monastic order, Brother Gregor was now able to give his undivided attention to intellectual activities. The monastery was a center for learning and scientific endeavor, and many of its members were teachers at the gymnasium or at the Philosophical Institute.

Upon entering the order, Mendel came under the tutelage and supervision of Mathew Kläcel, a botanist of repute who was already investigating variations, heredity and evolution in plants. Kläcel soon put Mendel in charge of the experimental garden. Simultaneously with this obligation, Mendel pursued his theological studies, as well as attending courses in agriculture, pomology and viticulture given by the celebrated F. Diebl.

Upon the completion of his theological studies, Brother Gregor was assigned to minister to the spiritual needs of the patients in the neighboring hospital. The abbott, aware of Mendel's inability to cope with the travails of the hospitalized faithful, sympathetically relieved him of these duties and transferred him to the grammar school at Znojmo in southern Moravia where Mendel now began to enjoy and excel in his new role as teacher.

In order to overcome some obvious deficiencies in his educational background, Brother Gregor was then ordered to attend the University of Vienna as a student where he obtained a thorough background in botany, experimental physics, zoology and chemistry. It was during his tenure as a student that Mendel first became thoroughly acquainted with the principles of propagation and hybridization. The text that he used is still preserved in the Mendelianium. It contains notations made by Mendel himself on 'Pisum' characteristics, and marked pages where pea hybrids are mentioned.

Mendel suffered another nervous breakdown while attempting to take for the second time the university examinations for teacher of natural sciences. He made no further attempts and remained a substitute teacher at Brno until 1868 when he was elected abbott. He now became heavily involved with the political, financial and spiritual problems of the monastery.

Mendel's first experiments in artificial plant hybridization began in 1857. After 8 years of work, he presented his findings for the first time at a meeting of the Natural Sciences Society of Brno. This presentation was published a year later (1866) in the Society's *Verhandlungen*. Except for local recognition by the fruit growers of the region and his co-members in the society, Mendel's work went completely unnoticed until 1900. At that time, three papers appeared by independent authors from Amsterdam, Vienna and Tübingen. Each one of them stated that just before completing his work, he learned of the unknown monk's antecedent research. Overnight, Mendel's labors of 8 years received the acclaim they deserved. Rescued from obscurity, Mendel's presentation before the local society of confreres is now acknowledged as the basis for the increasingly important science of genetics.

Brother Gregor Mendel, son of peasants, later abbot, industrious experimenter, died of chronic renal failure in 1884 – unknown at his death, acclaimed posthumously[2]. His portrait is shown in Figure 1, and the title page of a translation of his original paper, in Figure 2.

When Mendel first postulated his theory of inheritance in 1865, he used the term 'factor' for the particle carrying the genetic information. The choice of word was wise in that it was noncommittal regarding its nature or composition. At that time neither chromosomes nor their behavior in gametogenesis had yet been discovered. It was Walter Flemming of Kiel, Germany who first described chromosomes. This was in 1877, a good twelve years after Mendel's landmark presentation[3]. Flemming was also the first to picture

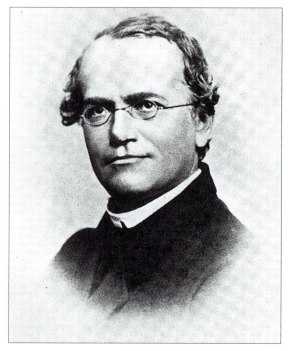

Figure 1 Gregor Mendel. *Photo Source National Library of Medicine. Literary Source Photo Archives. Courtesy National Library of Medicine*

human chromosomes in an article which appeared in 1882[4]. The process of 'reduction division' (meiosis) was not recognized until the 1880s and 1890s. At that time considerable evidence was accumulating supporting the thesis that Mendel's 'factors' were to be found in the chromosomes and that these 'factors' were transmitted via the reduction division process. E. B. Wilson collated all the available evidence in favor of this position and published the data in 1896. Further supporting evidence was supplied in 1902 by Walter S. Sutton while he was a graduate student at Columbia University. Nine years later Thomas Hunt Morgan, also of Columbia University, described and clarified the exact manner of alignment of the genes before they separated during meiosis for ultimate transmission to each daughter cell. By this time, Johannsen of Copenhagen had already designated Mendel's 'factors' as genes. E. B. Wilson was also the first to identify a gene in a human chromosome. This was in 1911 and the gene was responsible for color blindness[5]. X-linked traits were then identified by characteristic pedigree patterns over the succeeding years.

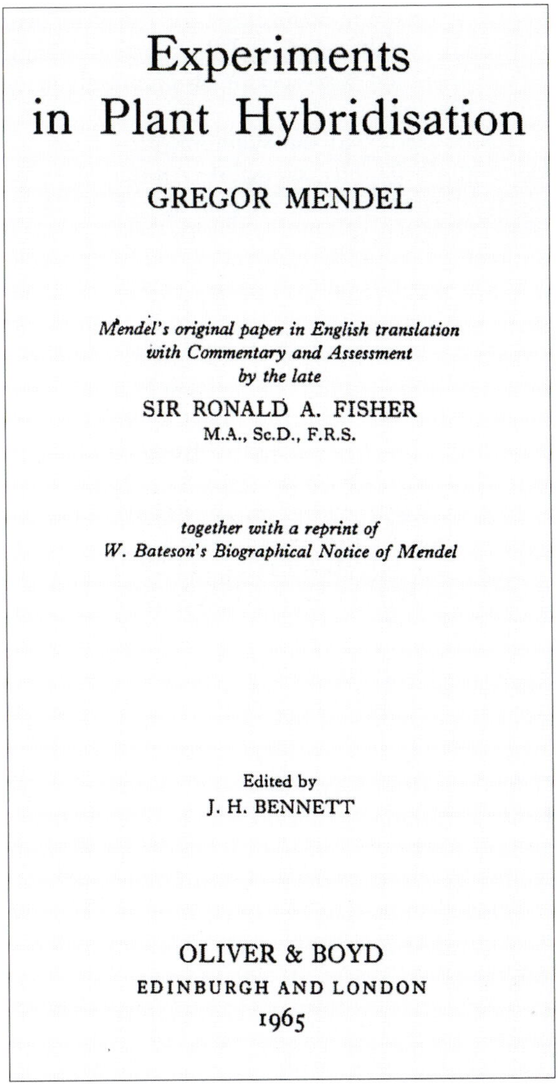

Experiments in Plant Hybridisation

GREGOR MENDEL

Mendel's original paper in English translation with Commentary and Assessment by the late

SIR RONALD A. FISHER
M.A., Sc.D., F.R.S.

together with a reprint of
W. Bateson's Biographical Notice of Mendel

Edited by
J. H. BENNETT

OLIVER & BOYD
EDINBURGH AND LONDON
1965

Figure 2 Title-page of 'Experiments in Plant Hybridisation' by Gregor Mendel. *Photo Source National Library of Medicine. Literary Source Mendel, Gregor: Experiments with Plant Hybrids. Edited by J.H. Bennet. Oliver & Boyd, Tweeddale Court, Edinburgh, Scotland. With permission*

A total of 57 years elapsed before Donahue and his colleagues at Johns Hopkins University successfully assigned a gene to an autosomal chromosome utilizing the linkage method[6]. The principles underlying linkage mapping had already been formulated by E.B. Wilson back in 1911. An alternative mapping method for autosomal assignment of genes had been introduced by Weiss and

Green just one year before Donahue's publication[7]. They used the somatic cell hybridization (SCH) method. It was Edwards who in 1956 was the first to suggest that prenatal diagnosis of genetic disease in the fetus could be accomplished by aspiration and study of amniotic fluid.

The 1970s saw the initiation of a flood of information on human gene mapping utilizing the method introduced by Weiss and Green and reinforced by family linkage studies. Research in this area was aided in no small measure by the techniques developed by Caspersson and his associates in identifying each chromosome through its unique banding pattern[8-10]. During the same decade, further progress in molecular genetics was also made possible through the discovery of restriction enzymes. These are produced by bacteria and are capable of breaking down foreign DNA. In McKusick's words: 'These enzymes became the scalpel for dissecting the human genome'[11]. The technology of recombinant DNA was now about to open the floodgates to an almost unbelievable amount of information. 'Fingerprinting' through DNA was now possible. To illustrate the astounding level of ultrastructural identification that was now at hand, mention must be made of the publication in 1981 by Sanger's group regarding the complete nucleotide sequence of the human mitochondrial genome[12].

In the 1980s, recombinant DNA technology was fortified with the addition of immunofluorescent techniques for the direct identification of genes. Even more astounding is the recent ability to map segments of DNA down to the level of individual nucleotides utilizing recombinant DNA, restriction endonucleases, and DNA sequencing[13].

This is the level of methodology that geneticists have reached today. Changes are occurring so rapidly, though, that by the time these words appear in print someone will be sure to point out (and correctly) how incomplete this historical background is. Be that as it may, this brief historical survey should help us appreciate and understand more fully the various nuances in the evolution of current knowledge regarding genetic factors in the pathogenesis of many diseases of the heart.

The genetic basis for those diseases of the heart generated in this manner can be found in chromosomal abnormalities, single-gene disorders, or in a multifactorial setting. The multifactorial dependent disorders would be the result of an interaction between multiple genes and various exogenous or environmental factors. Examples of chromosomal disorders would be the Down and Turner syndromes. The Noonan, LEOPARD and Kartagener syndromes would be illustrative of single gene disorders. Most of the more common diseases of the heart such as coronary artery disease and congenital heart disease fit best in the multifactorial category.

In the midst of all this, it must be emphasized that genetic mutation is an important hereditary mechanism in the causation of cardiac abnormalities. This could manifest itself clinically in a wide variety of disturbances encompassing congenital malformations, derangement of the vascular and connective tissue components of the heart, cardiac tumors, pericardial lesions, arrhythmias, the cardiomyopathies, and last, but decidedly not least, coronary artery disease. Delineation of the basic genetic defect in each of these aberrations should provide the necessary structural and biochemical information responsible for the clinical picture.

Archibald Garrod was the first to suggest that a single mutant gene can disturb a biochemical pathway in the body's milieu [14]. He described this in 1901 in a patient with black urine. Forty years later, the 'one-gene, one-enzyme' concept was introduced by Beadle and Tatum [15,16]. Linus Pauling was instrumental in demonstrating that mutant genes alter the amino acid sequence of proteins [17].

CHROMOSOMAL DISORDERS

The association between Down's syndrome and congenital cardiac abnormalities was first recognized by A. E. Garrod of London in 1894 [18]. The presence of atrioventricular canal malformation in the disorder was brought out by Maude Abbott in 1924 [19]. The specimen was a new accession in her expanding museum of cardiac anomalies. It is now known that a wide variety of congenital cardiac malformations may be represented in Down's syndrome. The most extensive series statistically validating this association were provided by three teams of investigators working independently of each other. These were Berg and associates in 1960 [20], Rowe and his co-worker in 1961 [21], and the team of Tandon and Edwards in 1973 [22]. In a review of 55 specimens, Tandon and Edwards observed that the leading types of major anomalies were

persistent common atrioventricular canal, isolated ventricular septal defect and Tetralogy of Fallot, either alone or with persistent common atrioventricular canal.

Turner described the syndrome that bears his name in 1938 [23]. His original description included the triad of infantilism, congenital webbed neck, and cubitus valgus. Ullrich had described a similar syndrome in 1930 [24]. Since then, the grouping of patients on a clinical basis and the changing cytogenic methodology make it quite difficult to remain on course when attempting to trace the historical background. The major stumbling block in all of this has been the initial confusion with Noonan's syndrome, until it became quite evident that Noonan's syndrome is due to a single gene disturbance in contrast to the aneuploidy of the sex chromosomes in Turner's syndrome.

The first detailed chromosomal studies in Turner's syndrome were conducted by Ford and his associates in 1959. Three years before, the same group, with Polani as the leading author, had already demonstrated a negative X chromatin (XO) pattern from buccal smears in many of their patients [25]. Ten years after Polani's findings, van den Berghe also found various structural abnormalities in the remaining X chromosome [26]. This definitely proved that the chromosomal disorder in Turner's syndrome was structural as well as numerical.

Subsequent years saw the publication of numerous reports describing both female and male patients with a Turner phenotype but a normal karyotype. Different terms were introduced to designate these patients such as 'male Turner's syndrome' and 'Turner's syndrome with 46 XX karyotype'. In 1963, Noonan and Ehmke described what they claimed was a syndrome distinct and different from Turner's [27]. Noonan later elaborated on this in another paper published five years later [28]. Six males and three females were described in the first paper, all of whom had in common, similar facies, multiple extracardiac anomalies, and pulmonic valvular stenosis. In addition, all had a normal karyotype. Noonan suggested that the syndrome occurred in a familial manner; a finding that was later confirmed by Nora and Sinha whose work also indicated that the disturbance was genetically transmitted via an autosomal dominant trait [29]. This latter work definitely put Noonan's syndrome into the category of a single gene disturbance. Despite this, there was still opposition to Noonan's view that the syndrome she described was distinct from that of Turner. Again, a confusion of definitions and genetic designations continued to muddy the waters. For example, Siggers and Polani in 1972 applied Turner's eponym to male patients with hypogonadism and a normal XY karyotype[30]. They also categorized patients of both genders who had the somatic features of Turner's syndrome but normal sexual development and normal karyotype as examples of Ullrich's syndrome. Ehlers and his group advanced in the same year another classification based entirely on the genotypic makeup of the patient[31]. They distinguished between Turner's syndrome and Turner's phenotype of either the 46XY or 46XX variety. In 1972 and again in 1974, Nora and co-workers proposed the eponym Ullrich-Noonan for those patients who had Turner's phenotype but normal genotypes[32].

It is now definitely established that Turner's and Noonan's syndromes are separate and distinct disorders. Turner's is a chromosomal disorder with a karyotype of XO whereas Noonan's is a disorder due to a single mutant gene inherited as an autosomal dominant trait. The unraveling of the genetic differences rests on firm ground due to the research efforts of Nora and Sinha[29]. Historically, the two syndromes have been intertwined primarily because of the similarity in the somatic clinical features. As further observations continued to be reported, it became obvious that the other major differences between the two syndromes lay in the location of the predominant cardiovascular abnormalities and in the fact that Turner's syndrome affects only females while Noonan's may involve males as well as females.

Most of the studies that have appeared over the years since Turner's original report point to a predominance of left-sided cardiovascular lesions when congenital abnormalities are present. These were described in greater detail by Haddad and Wilkins in 1959[33], and again by Rainier-Pope and colleagues in 1964[34]. Most had coarctation of the aorta. A high incidence of aortic stenosis was found in Vernant's series in 1966[35]. In 1970, Nora and colleagues provided hemodynamic and chromosomal evidence to indicate that coarctation of the aorta is the typical congenital cardiovascular abnormality in the 'XO Turner syndrome while pulmonic stenosis is the typical heart lesion of the XX and XY phenotype'[36]. This was two years before Nora's group proved that a single mutant gene was responsible for the XX and XY phenotypes and therefore not a variant of Turner's syndrome[29].

The other cardiac abnormalities that have been described in Turner's syndrome include bicuspid aortic valve (which is responsible probably for the high incidence of aortic stenosis in Vernant's series); hypertrophic obstructive cardiomyopathy, mitral valve prolapse, and dextrocardia[36]. At least ten cases of aortic dissection have also been reported in Turner's syndrome, beginning with Salgado's initial description in 1962[37] up to Price's addition to the list in 1983[38]. In at least six of the cases, cystic medial necrosis was the basic histologic lesion.

SINGLE GENE DISORDERS

Cardiac abnormalities

There are at least three important syndromes with cardiac abnormalities that can be ascribed to single gene disorders. These are Noonan's syndrome, the LEOPARD syndrome, and Kartagener's syndrome. We have already seen how Noonan's syndrome, originally regarded as a variant of Turner's, finally emerged as a distinct entity. At this point I should like to develop in more depth the historical background of this interesting disorder.

Noonan's syndrome

The first published illustration of the Noonan syndrome appears to be that by Kobylinski in 1883 while he was a medical student at the Russian/Estonian University of Dorpat[39]. It was reproduced by Opitz and Pallister in 1979[40] (Figure 3). It depicts a 20-year-old Jewish man with a webbed neck (pterygium colli), and other somatic features compatible with the current clinical description of Noonan's syndrome.

The peculiar characteristic of a webbed neck became the subject of many early publications following Kobylinski's description. Among them, there began to emerge descriptions of still another syndrome having in common the same peculiar webbed neck. A photograph illustrating this syndrome appeared in a surgical journal in 1902[41]. The author was a surgeon called Funke. This photograph was also reproduced by Opitz and

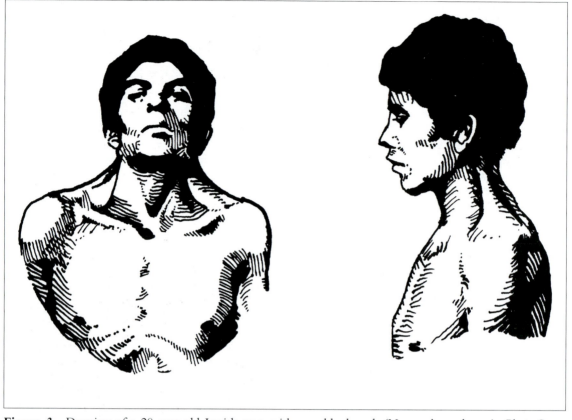

Figure 3 Drawing of a 20-year-old Jewish man with a webbed neck (Noonan's syndrome). *Photo Source University of Central Florida. Literary Source Opitz, J.M. and Pallister, D.P. (1979). Brief historical note: The concept of 'gonadal dysgenesis'. Am. J. Med. Genet., **4**, 333–43. With Permission*

Pallister in the same paper that had the photo of Kobylinski's patient. Opitz and Pallister commented that Funke's patient, as illustrated, represented the phenotype of the Ullrich-Turner syndrome. It will be recalled that Ullrich described his patient eight years before Turner's report. The somatic similarities between both patients led many subsequent observers to categorize such patients under the combined eponym Ullrich-Turner syndrome. The confusion was compounded even further by another surgeon in 1943. Flavell in that year published a case report, the subject of which had features similar to those of the Ullrich-Turner syndrome[42]. But he preferred to call his description the 'male Turner syndrome'.

We have seen how in 1963, Noonan and Ehmke described a series of boys and girls with congenital heart disease who were similar in appearance to those with the Turner's (XO) syndrome but with a normal karyotype. By this time, cytogenetic studies had already demonstrated a chromosomal abnormality in the Ullrich-Turner syndrome. None was found in the avalanche of studies that appeared during the 1960s in the 'male Turner syndrome'. Two things were also becoming apparent during this decade. Noonan's description fitted the 'male Turner syndrome' and some females with normal chromosomes previously diagnosed as having the Ullrich-Turner syndrome were in fact females with the 'male Turner syndrome'. Indeed, Noonan's description was the first time that females were included in the 'male Turner syndrome'. In order to clarify the issue, Opitz proposed that the 'male Turner syndrome' eponym be dropped in favor of the 'Noonan syndrome'[43]. This was in 1965. It took several years before this eponym was accepted, even in the face of efforts on the part of Nora and his group in 1972 and again in 1975 to hyphenate it with Ullrich.

Noonan's second report on the syndrome appeared in 1968[28]. This time she described 19 cases, 12 males and 7 females. Pulmonic stenosis was present in 17 of these patients while 2 had patent ductus arteriosus. It was in the same year that Nora and Sinha reported their study of a family spanning 3 generations with a mother to offspring mode of transmission[44]. At that time, they proposed an X-linked dominant inheritance of either a single mutant gene or a submicroscopic deletion. In 1969, Abdel-Salem and Tentamy reported 2 affected siblings from a first-cousin marriage[45]. They suggested autosomal recessive inheritance. Baird and DeJong in 1972 described 7 cases in 3 generations. One affected woman had 5 affected children out of 6 with 2 different husbands[46]. A particularly convincing pedigree for autosomal dominant inheritance was reported by Bolton and colleagues in 1974[47]. They found the condition in a man and 4 sons. All but one had pulmonic stenosis.

D.W. Smith in 1970 stated in his monograph on recognizable patterns of human malformations that congenital heart disease was present in at least 48% of patients with Noonan's syndrome[48]. In 1977, Pearl collected 204 cases from the world literature[49]. He added two of his own. Since Noonan's original description, a host of cardiovascular abnormalities have been reported in this syndrome. By far the vast majority of the malformations have been pulmonary valvar and branch stenosis with or without dysplasia of the valve[49]. Abnormalities of the left heart are uncommon but eccentric left ventricular hypertrophy was described by Ehlers and associates in 1972[50]. In 1973, Phornphutkul and his co-workers extended the observations of Ehlers with 3 more case reports[51]. They described both the obstructive and non-obstructive type of cardiomyopathy.

An interesting historical perspective of Noonan's syndrome was provided by Roger Cole in a short paper he wrote which appeared in *Pediatrics* in 1980[52]. Rather than try to paraphrase Cole's inimitable presentation, I believe the following excerpts from his paper would be better appreciated. He starts off by saying that pediatrics and fine art do not often cross paths, 'but such an example seems to have occurred with Noonan's syndrome and a famous painting by Ivan Le Lorraine Albright'.

Some 40 years before Noonan's description was published, Albright, best known for his work *The Picture of Dorian Gray*, had painted another

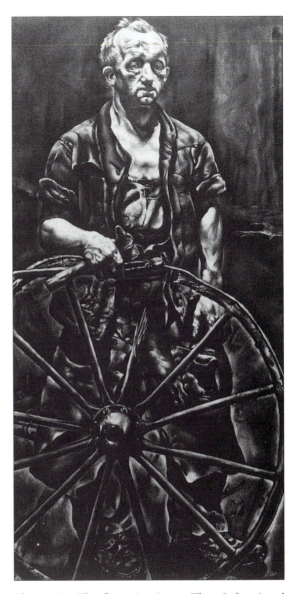

Figure 4 The figure in *Among Those Left*, painted by Albright, shows features suggestive of Noonan's syndrome. *Photo Source University of Central Florida. Literary Source Cole, R. (1980). Noonan's syndrome: a historical perspective. Pediatrics, **66**, 468–9 (Fig. 1). Permission from the Museum of Art, Carnegie Institute, Pittsburgh*

portrait entitled *Among Those Left* (Figure 4) in Warrenville, Illinois, during the summers of 1928 and 1929. The local blacksmith, H.K., was the model, and his facial features, low-set ears, short stature, and probable pectus deformity would strongly suggest Noonan's syndrome … H.K.

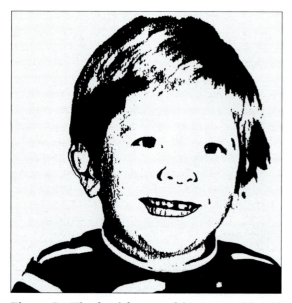

Figure 5 The facial features of this 3-year-old child suggest the presence of Noonan's syndrome. *Photo Source University of Central Florida. Literary Source Cole, R. (1980). Noonan's syndrome: a historical perspective. Pediatrics, 66, 468–9 (Fig.2). Permission for Fig.2 from the publisher*

was the maternal great-grandfather of patient E.S., who underwent cardiac catheterization studies at The Children's Memorial Hospital at 3 years of age. E.S. had facial features suggestive of Noonan's syndrome (Figure 5), and a mild pectus deformity. His height and weight were in the low range of normal and his mental development was also within normal range. A heart murmur was first heard at three weeks of age and he was considered to have pulmonic stenosis and insufficiency … Cardiac catheterization studies at 3 years of age confirmed the presence of a 32-mm peak systolic gradient across the pulmonary valve and the angiographic appearance suggested a dysplastic pulmonary valve. The architecture of the left ventricle was abnormal, consistent with those abnormalities of left ventricular musculature noted in Noonan's syndrome. … Since familial recurrences of Noonan's syndrome have been reported, a detailed family history was obtained and family photographs were reviewed. No other living members of the family, male or female, bore a likeness to E.S. It was during this photographic investigation that the mother indicated E.S.'s resemblance to the great-

grandfather whose portrait by Albright was owned by the Museum of Art, Carnegie Institute, Pittsburgh. The maternal great-grandfather died in old age, apparently of natural causes, and autopsy was not performed. E.S. has remained asymptomatic, on no cardiac medications, and no surgery has been recommended to date … Ivan Le Lorraine Albright had been a recognized medical illustrator early in his career, but the canvas of the local blacksmith may well have unknowingly been his most prestigious medical contribution. In addition to corroborating the family history in this case, it serves as the pictorial record of a syndrome described by Noonan in the medical literature some 40 years later.

LEOPARD syndrome

LEOPARD is a mnemonic suggested by Gorlin and his co-workers for a rare single-gene determined complex of congenital abnormalities[53]. L stands for lentigines which is the most distinctive and striking feature of the syndrome. Cardiac abnormalities are commonly seen in the disorder; the E stands for electrocardiographic conduction defects and the P for pulmonic valve stenosis. The other letters in the mnemonic represent ocular hypertelorism (O), genital abnormalities (A), retardation of growth (R), and deafness (D). Other structural abnormalities of the heart have been reported such as hypertrophic cardiomyopathy, aortic stenosis and endocardial fibroelastosis[54].

In 1957, Lamy and colleagues analyzed 1188 cases of congenital heart disease in children[55]. Among them were found cases of abnormal pigmentation and deafness in addition to the cardiac findings. This seems to be one of the earliest reports I could find on the association of familial cardiac disorders with abnormalities of cutaneous pigmentation.

Moynahan in 1962 described what he believed was the first male case of a new syndrome[56]. Three unrelated patients were described, two females and one male. All three had multiple symmetrical moles and stunted growth. The boy had hypospadia and undescended testes and one girl had an absent ovary with the other being hypoplastic. The cardiac abnormalities that he described may have been endocardial fibroelastosis but there was no documentation of this. In 1966, Forney and his group also described a syndrome that appeared to be genetic in origin and which was characterized by deafness, heart disease, and abnormal pigmentation[57]. The cardiac abnormality in their description was mitral insufficiency. The affected individuals of the kindred they studied also had multiple osseous defects. The possibility of a new syndrome was also raised by the authors of the paper. During the same year a report appeared by Walther and his co-workers on electrocardiographic abnormalities in a family with generalized lentigo[58]. The mother, son and daughter were affected. Although they were all asymptomatic as far as the heart was concerned, on cardiac catheterization the mother was found to have mild pulmonary stenosis and the son's electrocardiogram was suggestive of a previous myocardial infarction. A year later, Watson published his studies of three families in which two generations contained individuals with cafe-au-lait spots. In all, 14 persons were affected and many of these had pulmonary valve stenosis. Although deafness was not reported, dull intelligence among them was noted.

Lentigo in association with electrocardiographic changes was described by Mathews in 1968[59]. He also described the presence of murmurs. His subjects consisted of a mother and two half-sibling children. Various electrocardiographic abnormalities continued to be reported over the succeeding years by a number of different observers. These ranged in significance from being totally asymptomatic as Walther had noted in 1966, to being well tolerated as reported by Mathews in 1968, to being capable of causing sudden death as emphasized by Cronje and Feinberg in 1973[60].

Gorlin and associates substantiated the thesis that the disorder was inherited as an autosomal dominant trait with variable expressivity[61]. This was in 1971. The following year Polani and Moynahan confirmed that it was of neuroecto-dermal origin[62]. Its pleiotropic effects on tissues and organs of mesodermic origin were demonstrated by Norlund's group in 1973[63].

The presence and severity of myocardial and endocardial abnormalities have varied considerably. This was brought out by Moynahan in his original description in 1962 when he noted the lack of any cardiac abnormality as well as the presence of endomyocardial fibroelastosis in his three patients[56]. So-called functional murmurs without evidence of organic heart disease were described by McKusick and Capute in the cases they presented at the first conference on the clinical delineation of birth defects in 1968[64]. The majority of the murmurs that have been described, however, were definitely organic in origin. Most of them have been shown to be due to pulmonary valve stenosis as reported by Mathews in 1968[59], Gorlin in 1969[53], and Pickering in 1971[65]. Pickering also described occasional involvement of the mitral valve.

The first autopsy findings of the syndrome were published by Moynahan in 1970[66]. At this time, Moynahan described in detail the progressive cardiomyopathy that can be seen in lentiginosis. It should be obvious to us by now that Moynahan has emerged as an outstanding authority on this disease and that we are in his debt for his valuable contributions in delineating its clinical spectrum and pathogenesis.

In 1972, Somerville and Bonham-Carter suggested that any patient with lentigo and heart murmurs should undergo a cardiac evaluation and should be monitored very closely[67]. On the basis of the three patients that they studied, two of whom underwent an autopsy, they admonished that cardiomyopathy should be the first diagnosis to be considered even when initially there is no evidence of cardiac abnormalities. The Mayo clinic group headed by St. John Sutton in 1981 added eleven more patients to the growing list of those with hypertrophic obstructive cardiomyopathy and lentiginosis[68]. All of their 11 cases were sporadic, and 10 of them were male.

Kartagener's syndrome

The first definite case report of bronchiectasis associated with situs inversus was probably that of Siewert in 1904[69]. However, it was Kartagener who presented a detailed study of 11 cases in 1933, describing the triad of clinical signs and implicating a common pathogenic predisposition[70]. Two years later, he called attention to the high incidence of sinusitis[71]. Infertility in affected males was not noted as part of the syndrome until a much later date. A. M. Olsen of the Mayo clinic added in 1943 another 14 cases of bronchiectasis associated with dextrocardia[72]. In attempting to address the etiology of the bronchiectasis, he advanced the view that patients with situs inversus had a predisposition to bronchiectasis and sinusitis because of inherited defects of the respiratory tract. He had already described two years earlier bronchiectasis and absent frontal sinuses in identical twins[73].

The surgical team, Mayo and Rice, also from the Mayo clinic, published in 1949 a statistical review of total situs inversus involving 76 cases[74]. There were 17 patients in this review with combined situs inversus and bronchiectasis; 14 of these 17 patients had already been cited by Olsen; the remaining three were new ones added to the growing list. Sinus involvement in the form of hyperplasia of one or more sinuses, polyposis or simple infections was described as part of the syndrome by Safian and Mandeville in 1959[75]. These two observers also reported the occurrence of the syndrome in identical male twins and a female sibling. A year before, Overholt and Bauman had described phenotypic variants of Kartagener's syndrome[76]. They felt that these variations were probably due to a single genetic abnormality. Knox and his associates supported this view with data derived from the linkage method[77]. In 1962, Kartagener in collaboration with Stucki presented the evidence that had accumulated since his initial description in support of the contention that the genetic abnormality is inherited as an autosomal recessive trait[78]. In tracing this aspect of the historical background, it seems to me that the foundation for these evolving views on the genetic characteristics of the syndrome can be dated as far back as 1938 when E. A. Cockayne wrote about the genetics of transposition of the viscera[79].

The Mayo clinic continued its contributions towards an understanding of the syndrome with a study of another 19 patients conducted by Miller and Divertie in 1972[80]. Although their conclusions on the pathogenesis were purely speculative, they did point out that the disease is not incompatible with a long life. The oldest patient in their series was a 72 year old woman.

Concerning the pathogenesis of the syndrome, Miller and Divertie are but one example in the many that were engaged in this exercise. Throughout the years, none of the proposed modes merited acceptance until the appearance of the landmark studies of Björn Afzelius[81]. His paper, published in 1976, established through electron microscopic studies of ciliated bronchial mucosal biopsies as well as sperm ejaculate that the primary defect is a mutant gene. The motility of cilia and sperm is dependent upon dynein arms. These are protein structures that normally form temporary

cross bridges between adjacent microtubules in cilia and sperm tails. They are analogous to myosin in muscle in that they allow the microtubules to slide upon each other so as to generate movements of the tail or cilia. Any morphologic abnormality of the dynein arms would result then in immotility of the cilia and sperm. A mutant gene is responsible for the synthesis of the abnormal dynein arm.

The evidence supporting Afzelius' conclusions is quite convincing regarding the sinopulmonary and infertility components of the syndrome. However, as yet there is no satisfactory explanation regarding the molecular basis for the malrotation of the heart and viscera. Afzelius assumed that 'chance alone will determine whether the viscera will take up the normal or the reversed position during embryogenesis'[81].

Hereditary disorders of connective tissue

At least 17 different hereditary connective tissue disorders are recognized with cardiovascular involvement as a prominent feature. A single-gene mechanism is also responsible in all of them. Seven of them are known to cause premature coronary artery disease. In nine of the others, mitral and or aortic regurgitation are significant consequences of the disorder. One (cutis laxa) may be complicated by arterial aneurysms or peripheral pulmonic stenosis while its counterpart (Ehlers–Danlos syndrome) is often accompanied by rupture of the aorta and large arteries.

Among these connective tissue disorders, Marfan's syndrome and mitral valve prolapse stand out because they are relatively common. The others are quite rare. Not all of them will be discussed. Purely on an arbitrary basis, we will start with two syndromes recognizable by their cutaneous manifestations. These are the Ehlers–Danlos syndrome and cutis laxa.

Ehlers–Danlos syndrome and cutis laxa

The nosography of the Ehlers–Danlos syndrome and cutis laxa has been punctuated historically by repeated episodes of semantic and clinical confusion. In fact, the eponym 'Ehlers–Danlos' was proposed on the basis of the original and independent case reports from these two observers in which the subjects of the reports were presented, instead, as examples of cutis laxa[82,83].

In cutis laxa, the skin hangs in loose folds, especially in those areas where the skin is slightly loose to begin with. McKusick uses the word 'bloodhound' to describe the sagging jowls of the face[84]. Several synonyms have been introduced to describe the cutaneous manifestations of cutis laxa. Among them are dermatochalasia and chalasoderma. These were suggested by H. Fittke in 1942 on the basis of the relaxed or loose appearance of the skin[85]. The pendulous appearance of the skin also caused it to be confused with neurofibromatosis as indicated by the erroneous case reports of Mott in 1854 and Alibert a year later[86,87].

The clinical differences between cutis laxa and the Ehlers–Danlos syndrome were clearly spelled out by F. Parkes Weber in 1923[88]. The semantic aspects were finally clarified to a great degree by Francesco Ronchese in 1936 and again in 1958[89,90].

Goltz and his associates were responsible for delineating the systemic manifestations of cutis laxa[91,92]. Their histologic and electron microscopic studies indicated that the elastin in the skin is abnormal. This view was supported by the investigations of Graham and Beighton in 1971[93]. As yet, the biochemical defect in the abnormal elastin is still unknown.

In still another paper a year later, Beighton brought out that the genetically determined cutis laxa is transmitted by either an autosomal recessive or autosomal dominant gene[94]. This hypothesis was based upon careful analysis of the pedigrees in his cases as well as in those of the many case reports that appeared, beginning with Graf in 1936 and Siegmund in 1938. Furthermore, he noted that in the recessive type of cutis laxa, the skin changes are severe and pulmonary and cardiovascular involvement is common. The cardiovascular lesions are peripheral pulmonic stenosis and arterial aneurysms.

Currently, the Ehlers–Danlos eponym is applied to those patients with hyperelasticity of the skin. These patients also have hypermobility of the joints and fragile tissues with a bleeding diathesis. The most striking characteristic is the skin which appears quite firm but is so easily and markedly stretchable that it acts like a rubber band.

It is quite possible that the famous Italian violinist, Nicoló Paganini may have been a victim of the syndrome. This suggestion was put forth by Smith and Worthington in 1967[95]. The

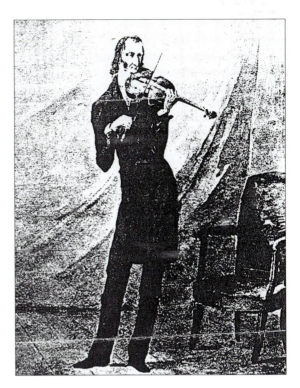

Figure 6 Drawing of Paganini playing the violin. *Photo Source University of Central Florida. Literary Source Weissmann, A. (1918). Der Virtuose, p.46. (Berlin: Paul Cassirer). With permission*

hypermobility of the virtuoso's fingers, the laxity of his joints, and his slender physique were advanced by these authors as indications of this possibility. This is their hypothetical solution to the riddle of what made Paganini so unique and unbeatable among violinists, past, present and future. Figure 6 is a drawing of Paganini playing the violin. It appears in *Der Virtuose*[96].

Dr Francesco Bennati of Paris, was the most durable of the countless physicians that Paganini retained throughout the years for his innumerable and varied afflictions. His observations of the virtuoso were published in the *Revue de Paris* in 1831[97]. They are so descriptively precise that it would be recreant on our part not to present them verbatim.

Paganini is pale and thin, and of medium height. Although he is only 47 years old, his leanness and lack of teeth, which causes his mouth to be drawn in and leaves his chin more salient, give his countenance the expression of more advanced age. At first glance his bulky head, which is supported by a long slender neck, offers a rather marked disproportion with his fragile limbs … His chest is narrow and rounded; his left side being slightly less ample than the right side and slightly depressed in the superior part. Breathing is equal and easy, though the right side distends more than the left … Let one but remark the manner in which he grasps and places his violin, or the position in which he sometimes places his arm, and then tell me of an artist who can imitate him. For example, who else, to produce certain effects, would be able to cross his elbows almost one on top of the other before his chest? … Where else, except in Paganini would we find that natural arrangement which prodigiously facilitates his playing: the left shoulder being more that an inch higher that the other–which, when he stands with his arms hanging down, makes the right seem much longer that the left? And the extensibility of the capsular ligaments of both shoulders, the slackness of the ligaments which connect the wrists to the forearm, the carpals to the metacarpals and the phalanges – who else will have these and thus have the ability to do what he does? … His hand is not of disproportionate size, but, he doubles its reach by the extensibility achieved in all the parts. For example, he can impart to the first phalanges of the fingers of his left hand … an extraordinary flexing motion which, without the hand moving, bears them in a direction lateral to their natural flexion – and this with ease, precision, and speed … Nature must have bestowed upon him the organic disposition which practice perfected …[97].

The historical background of the Ehlers–Danlos syndrome dates back to 1682[98]. Job van Meekeren, a Dutch surgeon, described a peculiar stretchability of the skin in a 23-year-old Spaniard. 'The skin was so elastic and stretchable that the subject, on request, could pull the skin over the right pectoral area, for example, all the way to the left ear, and on letting go, it would retract promptly to its original location without any telltale signs of having been subjected to this maneuver'. Figure 7 illustrates this extraordinary phenomenon.

McKusick's description of van Meekeren's illustration was translated from the original Latin by Dr Owsei Temkin. It is as follows:

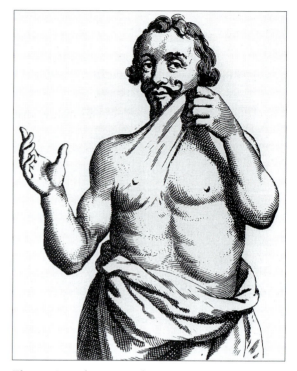

Figure 7 Job van Meekeren's case of the Spaniard with the stretchable skin. *Photo Source National Library of Medicine. Literary Source McKusick, V.A. Heritable Disorders of the Connective Tissue. 4th ed. C.V. Mosby Co., St. Louis, Missouri, Fig. 6–1, p.293. Taken from Van Meekeren, J.A. (1682). De dilatabilitate extraordinaria cutis, chap.32, Observations medicochirugicae, Amsterdam. Public domain*

In the year 1657, in the presence of the very distinguished John van Horne and Francis Sylvius, professors of medicine in the famous Academy of Leyden, as well as of William Piso and Francis vander Schagen, practitioners of Amsterdam, we saw in our hospital a certain young Spaniard, 23 years of age, by the name of George Albes, who with his left hand grasped the skin over his humerus and right breast and stretched it till it was quite close to his mouth. With each hand he first pulled the skin of his chin downward like a beard to his chest, hence he lifted it upwards to the vertex of his head so as to cover each eye with it. As soon as he removed his hand the skin contracted to reassume its proper smoothness. In the same way he pulled the skin of his right knee upwards or downwards, to the length of half an ell; then it easily returned to its natural position. It was worthwhile noting that the skin which covered the forementioned parts on the left side could not be extended since it firmly adhered to them. It has, thus far, not been possible to learn the cause [of this anomaly?].

The scattered reports of the abnormality that subsequently appeared were mainly from dermatologists because of the striking behavior of the skin. Many of the subjects in the case reports were the 'India rubber men' of the side shows. I, too, remember seeing them with delight and awe when my father took me along with the rest of his brood to the annual circus at the old Madison Square Garden in New York City.

Kopp's description of a father and son in 1888 is often cited as the first example of hereditary transmission of the syndrome[99]. But, as McKusick aptly points out, Kopp's cases should be more accurately categorized as being illustrative of cutis laxa in accordance with Kopp's original designation.

Tschernogobow in 1891, presented two cases at a meeting of the Moscow Dermatologic and Venerologic Society[100]. This appears to be the first detailed description of the syndrome. Tschernogobow recognized at the time that the defect in both cases was to be found in the connective tissue. To illustrate how ill-defined the syndrome was at the time, Tschernogobow presented his cases as examples of cutis laxa. In retrospect, and on the basis of current definitions and knowledge, the clinical features of his two patients fit more precisely with the Ehlers–Danlos syndrome. Jansen also suggested in 1954 that the defect was to be found in the collagen tissue[101]. It was in the same paper, that Jansen gave Tschernogobow credit not only for first suggesting this possibility but also for being the first to give a detailed description of the Ehlers–Danlos syndrome. Jansen also wrote two other papers; one concerned itself with the mode of transmission, and the other with the structure of the connective tissue as an explanation for symptoms of the Ehlers–Danlos syndrome[102,103].

An autosomal dominant inheritance was demonstrated by Johnson and Falls in 1949[104]. Their conclusion was derived from a study of a large kindred involving 32 affected persons. McKusick suggested a heterogeneous genetic mechanism in the second edition of his *Heritable*

Disorders of Connective Tissue. Over the years, it became apparent that there were several clinical varieties of the disorder, some transmitted by an autosomal dominant trait, and others by an autosomal recessive or X-linked recessive trait. Beighton recognized in 1970 at least five distinct clinical forms, one of which was transmitted via an X-linked recessive trait[105]. Krane, Pinnell and Erbe identified a sixth form in 1972, and at the same time determined its molecular defect[106]. It was found to be a deficient synthesis of type III collagen and transmitted via an autosomal recessive mutant gene. Lichtenstein and his group confirmed this within the same year[107].

Unna and his co-workers, DuMesnil and Williams, attempted to delineate the histopathologic basis of the disorder. Their contributions were published during the last decade of the 19th century[108–110]. They were unable to interpret with any degree of certainty the non-specific histologic changes. During the same decade, Ehlers pointed out the proneness of these patients towards subcutaneous hemorrhages and laxity of the joints[111].

One of the two patients that Tschernogobow described was a 50 year old woman with the so-called 'Molluscoid pseudotumors' in the vicinity of the hip, knee and elbow joints[112]. Danlos in 1908 also described the development of tumefactions in various subcutaneous sites, and included these growths as part of the syndrome[113]. Incidentally, both he and Tschernogobow were still describing the syndrome under the erroneous label of cutis laxa.

Among the many case reports that began to appear over the succeeding decades, a few of them referred to the presence of cardiovascular abnormalities[114]. Many of these were descriptions of systolic murmurs. Some described the presence of mitral valvular disease, while others described aortic insufficiency. Even congenital defects were found such as a right-sided aortic arch or septal defects. The most important descriptions were probably those that referred to the occurrence of arterial rupture or the presence of intracranial vascular malformations[114].

In 1966, McKusick was still uncertain as to the significance of these cardiovascular abnormalities within the context of the Ehlers–Danlos syndrome[115]. He was not sure whether they were part and parcel of the syndrome or whether they represented a purely coincidental association. Beighton, too, addressed this question prior to leaving St. Thomas' Hospital in London for his new post at Johns Hopkins with McKusick. He surveyed 100 patients in southern England with the syndrome. In addition, he searched for cardiovascular abnormalities in the more than 300 case reports that had been previously published on the Ehlers–Danlos syndrome. In his paper, which appeared in 1969, he concluded that there was no consistent pattern of cardiac abnormality among these patients except for those with evidence of arterial bleeding or intracranial vascular malformations. Apart from these last two phenomena, he regarded the finding of structural cardiac lesions as 'chance or very rare concomitants of the syndrome'[114].

Shortly after the publication of this paper, Beighton recognized that the vascular abnormalities were not a chance occurrence in the type IV variety of the Ehlers–Danlos syndrome. It is now known that more than 95% of the individuals with Type IV have cardiovascular abnormalities, the major manifestation of which is rupture of the aorta or other large arteries[116].

Marfan's syndrome

Cardiac abnormalities occur in at least 60% of those afflicted with this generalized disorder of connective tissue. Marfan's syndrome is inherited as an autosomal dominant trait[117]. The sporadic cases that occur (15%) probably represent new mutations in the germ cells of one of the parents[118].

We have already referred to the association between annuloaortic ectasia and Marfan's syndrome with the predisposition of the ectasia towards the development of aortic dissection or aortic regurgitation. The basic biochemical defect leading to weakening of the aortic wall is still unknown but histologic studies have revealed marked loss of elastic tissue fibers in the medial layer of the wall. These are similar to those described by Erdheim in cystic medial necrosis. Mitral regurgitation can also occur, and when it does it is usually because of redundant cusps and chordae tendineae. Massive calcification of the mitral annulus can, though rarely, be responsible for the mitral regurgitation[117,119]. Superimposed bacterial endocarditis has also been reported[117].

Antoine Bernard Jean Marfan first described the syndrome that bears his name in a 5½ year old child in 1896[120]. Marfan, at the time, was a renowned professor of pediatrics at the University of Paris. Because the child had long thin extremities which were an expression of the gross skeletal abnormalities that originally attracted his attention, Marfan suggested the name 'dolichostenomelia'. Six years later, the child was described again by Méry and Babonneix[121]. They preferred the term 'hyperchondroplasia' meaning excessive growth at the cartilaginous level. During the same year (1902) and in the same issue of the same journal, Achard, obviously in an attempt to extrapolate Marfan's original simile of 'spider legs', decided to rename the condition 'arachnodactyly' because of the spider-like appearance of the long tapering fingers[122]. For no apparent reason that I can find, Achard's designation has persisted as the preferred term for this stigma of Marfan's syndrome.

A case report was published by Salle in 1912 describing an infant who had abnormalities of the extremities that were highly suggestive of Marfan's syndrome. The child had cardiac symptoms during her very brief life (2½ months), and at autopsy there was evidence of a dilated heart, patent foramen ovale and changes in the mitral leaflets[123]. This is the first reference to a possible association of a cardiovascular abnormality in the syndrome. Börger in 1914 reported two cases of congenital heart disease in association with arachnodactyly[124]. Piper and Irvine-Jones also reported on this association in a paper which appeared in 1926[125]. This paper, incidentally, has the distinction of being the first case report of Marfan's syndrome in the American literature. Most of the early reports describing the cardiovascular abnormalities in the Marfan syndrome or arachnodactyly were based on clinical findings in infants and children. Especially prominent were the descriptions of cardiac murmurs in association with cardiac enlargement. This may have been the reason why so many of the early reviews of the syndrome suggested that the cardiovascular lesions in Marfan's syndrome were congenital in origin. In fact, in 1940, Ellis in his discussion of ectopia lentis and arachnodactyly in a father and daughter suggested that congenital cardiovascular disease occurred in about one third of the cases[126]. This erroneous impression was not corrected until the publication of the definitive studies by Taussig's group in 1943[127]. Theirs was the first detailed description of the occurrence of aortic dilatation and dissection in this syndrome. During the same year, Etter and Glover presented their findings of arachnodactyly complicated by rupture of a dissecting aneurysm of the aorta[128]. Their work, too, was a definitive study. Probably the earliest report, however, on the aortic complications of the syndrome can be found in a paper by Bronson and Sutherland, published in 1918 and entitled *Ruptured aortic aneurysms in childhood*[129]. Although the authors presented a detailed review of reports of aortic aneurysms in children with many of the cases manifesting the external characteristics of Marfan's syndrome, their paper did not have the impact generated by the publications of Taussig's group and the team of Etter and Glover.

The poor prognosis in the syndrome is due primarily to the aortic complications. Emphasizing this factor was the major contribution by Etter and Glover and Taussig's group. Prior to them, the aortic complications were not fully appreciated; most of the emphasis being placed instead on the congenital abnormalities, especially the septal defects[130]. Further observations have repeatedly confirmed the trail-blazing work of these individuals. They are to be found in the papers by Goyette and Palmer in 1953[131], McKusick in 1955[132]. Hirst and his group in 1958[133], and Bowers in 1959[134]. McKusick's paper, in particular, presented the most complete description up to then of the various cardiovascular abnormalities in Marfan's syndrome.

The reader will find in Chapter 22 reference to the so-called 'Lincoln-Brooks' sign as a physical diagnostic indicator of the presence of aortic regurgitation. This was advanced by Schwartz in 1964 as part of the evidence pointing to the view that Abraham Lincoln was a victim of Marfan's syndrome. Two years earlier, Gordon had already expressed the opinion that Lincoln, indeed, did have the syndrome[135].

Murdoch and associates evaluated the life expectancy and causes of death in 1972[136]. Among their various conclusions was the one that pregnancy poses a serious threat to the life of the patient with the Marfan syndrome because it greatly increases the risk of aortic dissection. In 1965, Donaldson and Alvarez had already gone on record that therapeutic abortion should be recommended in women with Marfan's disorder who showed evidence of aortic disease prior to the age of 30[137].

Bacterial endocarditis caused two deaths in Murdoch's series. In one, the disease developed during pregnancy, and in the other seven years after an aortic graft[136]. When McKusick wrote his classic paper in 1955, he was able to find only three cases, including one of his own[132]. The problem of bacterial endocarditis in the Marfan syndrome was explored further by Bowers and Lim in 1962[138], and then, three years later by Wunsch and his associates[139].

In addition to the well-known aortic complications, many reports appeared since 1954 stressing the frequency with which the Marfan syndrome may be complicated by mitral insufficiency. The most usual cause for the regurgitation has been the redundant cusps and chordae tendineae (as part of the connective tissue disturbance). Several reports were also published attributing the leakage instead to a calcified mitral valve annulus. Miller and Pearson described such an individual in 1959[140]. McKusick described a case of calcified mitral annulus associated with a floppy mitral valve and severe mitral insufficiency in the third edition of his text on heritable disorders of connective tissue[141]. Two years later, Grossman and his colleagues described what they believed to be the youngest Marfan victim with mitral annulus calcification and the second in whom the calcification was uncomplicated by inflammation[142].

The first clear demonstration that the Marfan syndrome is hereditary was made by Weve in 1931[143]. He was able to document the genetic transmission on the basis of a dominant trait. Furthermore, he was convinced that the abnormality resided in a defect of the mesenchymal tissues and for this reason he suggested the term 'dystrophia mesodermalis congenital typus Marfanis'. McKusick reviewed 50 kinships in his landmark paper[143]. Hirst and Gore in their review of the Marfan syndrome (1973) stated that 'the disease is transmitted as a dominant trait, often with incomplete penetrance of the gene, resulting in a variable phenotype'[144].

It was Gore in 1953 who postulated that a biochemical or metabolic defect was responsible for the premature degeneration of the connective tissues in the disease[145]. Evidence in support of this view was supplied by Sjoerdsma in 1958, and again by Jones and his colleagues in 1964[146,147]. They demonstrated an increased renal excretion of an amino acid called hydroxyproline which is derived from collagen. The increased urinary excretion of this acid was interpreted by them as being the result of an accelerated breakdown of collagen. A year earlier, Berenson and Geer noted in their cases of arachnodactyly, a marked increase in the urine of mucopolysaccharide, especially chondroitin A or C[148].

The term 'forme fruste', although imprecise, is currently accepted as valid for describing those patients with the Marfan syndrome that do not manifest all the classical features. The most common cardiovascular manifestation in this subtype is aortic insufficiency with or without dilatation or dissection of the ascending aorta[149]. This was brought out by Emanuel and his group in 1977, in their study of 18 patients. They also noted that the 'forme fruste' variety has the same mode of inheritance as the classical syndrome in keeping with the generally held belief of incomplete penetrance and variability in phenotype.

Mitral valve prolapse

Mitral valve prolapse is a condition of the mitral valve wherein one or both leaflets slip back into the left atrium during ventricular systole. It has been called the floppy valve denoting the lack of tautness of the leaflets in closing, and the balloon valve to describe how the cusps billow into the atrium during closure. The types of auscultatory phenomena that have been observed in the syndrome account for such designations as 'midsystolic click-late systolic murmur syndrome, midsystolic click syndrome or late systolic murmur syndrome'.

It is a heterogeneous disorder with many causes, some of which are heritable and some of which are not. It can be seen as an idiopathic or familial type; as part of other heritable disorders such as Marfan's, Ehlers–Danlos, and Turner's syndromes; or as secondary to a variety of abnormalities involving the mitral leaflets, chordae tendineae, papillary muscles or mitral annulus.

The majority of the cases are idiopathic and in many of these a familial pattern has been observed apparently with an autosomal dominant inheritance. Since so many of the patients with the idiopathic or familial form of prolapse have thoracic or other features consistent with the Marfan syndrome, it has been suggested by some observers that they represent a 'forme fruste' of Marfan's syndrome.

The basic pathologic defect in the idiopathic or familial type is myxomatous degeneration[150,151]. The degeneration is characterized by replacement of the central fibrous tissue with metachromatically staining loose myxomatous material accompanied by fibroelastic thickening of the overlying endocardium[150]. There is a possibility that there may be two types of the idiopathic variety showing in common a basic myxomatous element. One is the true familial type which is heritable and manifests itself at an early age, and the other is the so-called 'senile variety' in which the myxomatous degeneration occurs with increasing age. Davies and his associates reported this latter phenomenon in a large series of necropsy studies in 1978[152].

It should be emphasized that the idiopathic or familial type is a benign condition. The vast majority suffer no appreciable consequences from their floppy valves. Rarely, however, serious complications may arise from potentially lethal arrhythmias, severe mitral regurgitation, bacterial endocarditis or cerebral events.

The earliest clinical description of the idiopathic type was based on certain auscultatory findings without any knowledge of their true origin, pathogenesis and significance. It dates back to the report of 'a bruit de galop mesosystolique' by Cuffer and Barbillon in 1887[153]. In 1892, Griffith described and commented on the presence and significance of midsystolic and late systolic murmurs. He attributed them to mitral valve dysfunction[154]. This was followed by Hall's paper in 1903 on late systolic murmurs. He also opined that the murmurs were due to mitral valve dysfunction[155].

The prestige of Gallavardin seemed to settle the issue on the origin of the clicks when he wrote in 1913 that they were due to pleuro-pericardial lesions[156]. He appeared to cement this opinion even further in another paper on the subject in 1932[157]. Apparently Paul D. White's prestige was not of sufficient magnitude to counteract Gallavardin's pronouncements. In his text, published just a year before Gallavardin's second paper, White attributed the click and or late systolic murmur to mitral valve dysfunction, an opinion in accord with the previously mentioned views of Griffith and Hall. Another three decades had to elapse before Reid postulated the true mechanisms for the click and murmur[158]. He ascribed the click to sudden tautening of previously lax chordae. This would be analogous to the snapping noise produced by a parachute on opening fully when the rip cord is pulled. Reid felt that when the late systolic murmur was present, it was due to leakage between the improperly coapting mitral cusps. The presence of mitral regurgitation in the 'click–murmur' syndrome was demonstrated by Barlow and his associates 2 years later using angiographic techniques[159].

Barlow and his group became leaders in the field, contributing not only to advancement of knowledge concerning its etiology and clinical spectrum but also by acting as a catalyst for further studies throughout the world. They published one of the earliest comprehensive reviews on the subject in 1966[160]. As a matter of fact, Barlow's contributions have been so extensive that many times the idiopathic type of mitral valve prolapse has been eponymously referred to as 'Barlow's syndrome'. In that same review he suggested that the combination of a late systolic murmur with a non-ejection systolic click is highly indicative of mitral valve prolapse. This has come to be regarded as a specific sign of prolapse when present.

Further studies by Barlow, Hancock and Cohn[161] (1966), Stannard and associates[162] (1967), and Jeresaty[163] (1973), have shown that the posterior leaflet is affected in the majority of cases in the idiopathic form, and that this form occurs predominantly in females, and at virtually any age. Hancock, Cohn and Jeresaty also noted that palpitations, syncope and presyncope can usually be attributed to atrial or ventricular arrhythmias. Sudden death, presumably due to ventricular arrhythmias, was also recorded by Barlow and then confirmed by Shappell and his group in 1973 as well as by several other observers[164]. Gulotta and his associates (1974) recognized the occurrence of left ventricular dysfunction in some cases[165]. A year earlier, Ranganathan described the same complication due to severe mitral regurgitation[166]. It was the first such study documented by angiographic-morphologic correlation. The occurrence of neurologic deficits was reported by Barlow and Bosman in 1966[167] but the truly definitive studies on the neurologic complications are attributable to Pomerance in 1969 and to Barnett and his associates in 1975[168,169]. Pomerance described the presence of thrombi on the mitral leaflets. Barnett's group delineated the occurrence of cerebral ischemic episodes on the basis of a thrombo-embolic mechanism.

Barlow and Bosman were the first to document a family aggregation. They identified a kindred in 1966 in which 6 of 17 relatives were affected[167]. Three years later, Hunt and Sloman suggested an autosomal dominant mode of inheritance based on their study of one family with 11 affected members[170]. These subjects represented half the children of affected parents and were made up of both sexes. A total of 53 relatives of 17 propositi were examined by Weiss and co-workers in 1975[171]. Utilizing auscultation, echocardiography and phonocardiography, they found 47% of the first degree relatives were affected. This, too, is certainly consistent with an autosomal dominant mode of inheritance. In 1893, Strahan and colleagues reported their findings in the families of 12 propositi who had mitral valve prolapse of the idiopathic type[172]. Of the progeny, 47% were affected in comparison to 30% of the parents. Out of 26 sibs, 10 (38%) were affected. Their genetic analysis included a discussion of a three-compartmental penetrance model to help explain the variation in expression with age that they encountered. The model was divided into a latent stage where no signs were present, an affected stage with overt signs, and a stage wherein the subjects were withdrawn because of treatment, regression or death. Although their results were based on small numbers, they did tend to point to an age-dependent onset with a decline in signs with increasing age.

This brief historical survey illustrates the remarkable advances made in the recognition of this syndrome. It also highlights how no one person has been responsible for adding to the fund of knowledge. The voluminous literature that has accumulated over the past three decades from myriad observers attests to this. We have learned to distinguish the idiopathic form from that due to coronary artery disease or that variety of prolapse found in association with other connective tissue disorders such as Marfan's and Turner's. Despite all this, the syndrome still remains an enigma. The knowledge that has accumulated since the original observations is purely descriptive. What is the nature of and the basis for the myxomatous degeneration? An autosomal dominant form of inheritance has been well documented but where is the mutant gene and what biochemical defect exists because of the mutation? Moreover, what is the cause of the chest pain or the arrhythmias? How does one explain many of the associated psychosomatic complaints? Is there such a thing as an associated hyperadrenergic state? Questions, questions and more questions!

Mucopolysaccharidoses

The mucopolysaccharidoses (MPS) are a group of metabolic disorders due to incomplete breakdown of the parent mucopolysaccharide. The resultant metabolite of this abnormal breakdown (a simpler form of MPS), accumulates within the cells and becomes directly responsible for disturbed cellular function. Mutant genes are responsible for the disorder since they are unable to produce the specific enzymes for the metabolic degradation of the parent mucopolysaccharide. Various syndromes are produced depending upon which enzyme is deficient. To date, at least 7 different types are recognized with the type II (Hunter) divided into mild and severe forms. The various types are also labeled with eponyms representing, not always, however, the original describer. For example, type IV is also known as the Morquio syndrome. It was originally described by Brailsford of England in 1929[173,174].

There appear to be only two modes of inheritance. The two forms of the Hunter syndrome (type II) are X-linked while the remaining types are transmitted by an autosomal recessive trait. Although he did not comment on sex-linkage, Wolff in 1942 was the first to describe the pedigree in Hunter's syndrome clearly indicating an X-linked inheritance[175]. Four years later Nja of Norway documented and proposed an X-linked mode of transmission for the Hunter syndrome[176].

Again, the one gene–one enzyme concept of Beadle and Tatum governs the metabolically disturbed pathway. For example in type I-H (Hunter's syndrome), the mutant autosomal recessive gene fails to produce α-L-iduronidase, thereby disturbing the metabolic breakdown of those mucopolysaccharides dependent upon this enzyme. The resultant mucopolysaccharide metabolites that accumulate are dermatan sulfate and heparan sulfate.

The entire group of disorders has been saddled at various times with various descriptive terms that failed to indicate the basic biochemical defect of the disease. The term 'gargoylism' was favored by Cockayne[177] and Ellis[178]. Husler suggested the term 'dysostosis multiplex'[179]. McKusick castigates the term 'lipochondrodystrophy' as being a misnomer[180]. Washington suggested it in 1937, mistakenly believing the disorder was the result of a disturbance in lipid metabolism[181]. McKusick also criticizes the term 'gargoylism' citing it as being 'unnecessarily

cruel in view of the facts that the intellect may be little impaired and that survival to adulthood is not infrequent'[173].

Despite the fanciful nature of some of the names given to so many syndromes in medicine, I am afraid that the practice is difficult to eliminate. A case in point is the euphemism suggested by W. L. Donohue to describe a rare familial disorder. In 1948 he described a syndrome in a female infant with hirsutism, elfinlike facies and multiple endocrine abnormalities[182]. He originally gave it the name 'dysendocrinism' to emphasize the endocrine involvement. However, he became disenchanted with the impersonal tone of 'dysendocrinism' and in a subsequent paper published in 1954, he suggested the substitution of 'leprechaunism'[183]. In Irish folklore, leprechauns are little hairy sprites. Some maintain they are also male and green. His apologia for the usage of leprechaunism is as follows: 'Although it may be argued that our cases do not fulfill all the suggested descriptive requirements of a leprechaun, with a little imagination the term can be as suitably applied to the syndrome encountered in these two infants as the terms gargoylism, cretinism (little Christian) and mongolism, which are common usage'.

All of the types currently recognized are complicated by cardiovascular lesions. Aortic and mitral regurgitation are the two most common ill effects. Coronary artery disease is also seen in the Hurler and Hunter syndromes. Type I-H (Hurler) has been associated with cardiomyopathy. The altered collagenous material resulting from the incomplete breakdown of the parent mucopolysaccharides accumulates in the fibroelastic cells of the cardiovascular system. This was the view advanced by Lindsay in 1950[184]. When deposited in the mitral and aortic valves, regurgitation in these damaged valves is the usual pathophysiologic disturbance.

The cardiovascular manifestations of the mucopolysaccharidoses were described by Ellis (1936)[185], Krovetz and co-workers in 1968[186], McKusick in 1972[187], Krovetz again in the same year[188] and by Schieken and his group in 1975[189]. The occurrence of heart failure in patients with type I-MPS was first described by Ellis and Payne in 1936. They found no evidence of valvular abnormalities in these patients. In 1960, mitral stenosis was the predominant lesion in the case report by Vance and his co-workers[190]. This was the first time that a stenotic process was described in gargoylism.

At autopsy the mitral valve was found to be thickened and distorted with the connective tissue showing the usual abnormalities of the collagen fibers. McKusick pointed out in a paper on the genetic mucopolysaccharidoses which appeared in 1965[191] that a pseudo-atherosclerotic picture is produced if the abnormal metabolites are deposited in the intima of the coronary arteries, aorta or pulmonary artery.

In 1975, Schieken and associates presented their findings derived from a systematic clinical study of nine children with various types of MPS using the non-invasive technique of echophono-cardiography[189]. No postmortem studies were done. They had two brothers in their series with the I H/S type. Both had evidence of calcified mitral stenosis, and represent two more unusual cases manifesting stenosis rather that regurgitation of the mitral valve. In addition, one patient with type VI A MPS had both aortic and mitral involvement with stenosis being the dominant lesion in the mitral valve. Their type IIA patients, though without symptoms, had echocardiographic evidence of myocardial dysfunction. The authors attributed this last finding to deposition of the metabolites (dermatan sulfate and heparan sulfate), either in the myocardium or coronary arteries without, however, any histopathologic or biochemical confirmation.

The historical background of this rare but interesting group of disorders begins with John Thompson of Edinburgh. He is said to have described the clinical characteristics of what may have been the Hurler variety between the years 1900 and 1913[192]. During the same period of time the German clinician, Berkham, described two cases of 'Skaphokephalia' which also had the clinical features of Hurler's syndrome[193]. However, the first definitive report on the Hurler type did not appear until 1917. It was written by Charles H. Hunter and it was published in the *Proceedings of the Royal Society of Medicine*[194]. Two brothers are described, both in their childhood. The older brother had an enlarged heart and two distinct murmurs. The systolic murmur was heard best at the apex while the diastolic murmur was audible close to the sternum in the left third and fourth interspaces. McKusick was able to obtain follow-up information on them, and in the 4th edition of his text on heritable disorders of connective tissue he was able to state that the brothers had the type of mucopolysac-charidosis now known as MPS II which is due to a deficiency of sulfoid uronate sulfatase transmitted by an X-linked recessive mutant gene.

Gertrud Hurler of Munich described what is now classified as the MPS I type in 1919[195]. This type now also carries her eponym. The mutant gene is an autosomal recessive one and causes a deficiency of α-L-iduronidase (I-H allele). Her chief, Meinhard von Pfaundler, also presented two infants with the same type of clinical manifestations at a pediatric society meeting during the same year[196]. This explains why this variety of MPS carries the hyphenated eponym, Hurler-Pfaundler.

In 1952, Brante isolated dermatan sulfate from the liver of two patients with the Hurler syndrome[197]. The excessive hepatic accumulation of this byproduct from the incomplete breakdown of mucopolysaccharides was the basis of his suggestion that Hurler's syndrome should be designated as a 'mucopolysaccharidosis'. His paper carried the title *Gargoylism: a mucopolysaccharidosis*. Five years later, D. H. Brown published his studies on the tissue storage of mucopolysaccharides in what was sometimes eponymously called Hurler-Pfaundler's disease[198]. It was at this time that he isolated from the liver of such a patient another byproduct of incomplete MPS breakdown. It is heparan sulfate. The final link in this metabolic pathway was forged by the investigations of Dorfman and Lorincz in 1957[199], and those of Meyer's group a year later[200]. Both teams documented the presence of excessive amounts of sulfated mucopolysaccharides in the urine of patients with gargoylism (Hurler's syndrome).

Danes and Bearn in 1965 demonstrated that they could study the Hurler syndrome in detail utilizing the fibroblast culture technique[201]. In a series of papers published between 1968 and 1969, Fratantoni and associates, also utilizing fibroblast culture techniques, were able to outline the biochemical characteristics of both the Hurler and Hunter syndromes[202-205]. They were not only able to identify the specific biochemical defect in both syndromes, but they were also able to demonstrate correction of this metabolic defect *in vitro* by the usage of a diffusible factor produced by normal cells or by cells from a different variety of mucopolysac-charidosis. Morphologic identification of the abnormal cell of the syndrome, i.e. the gargoyle cell, was demonstrated by the electron microscopic studies of Van Hoof and Hers several years earlier[206]. These studies suggested that the ultrastructural characteristics of the cells were consistent with lysosomal disorders and that because of this the mucopolysaccharidoses should be classified as such.

Cardiomyopathies

Among the various forms of cardiomyopathy, at least nine are currently recognized as being single-gene determined. These are Pompe's disease, familial hypertrophic obstructive cardiomyopathy, familial cardiomyopathy, idiopathic hemochromatosis, familial amyloidosis, myotonic dystrophy, Duchenne muscular dystrophy, Friedreich's ataxia, and endocardial fibroelastosis. As the names imply, some are part of the neurologic disorder with which they are associated, some are part of a generalized metabolic disease, while others are dominated primarily by the myocardial involvement.

Pompe's disease

This is a very rare disorder inherited as an autosomal recessive trait. The defective gene, carried on chromosome 17, is unable to produce the enzyme α-1,4-glucosidase. This results in inability to break down glycogen which then accumulates in all the tissues of the body including the heart. Massive enlargement of the heart occurs with progressive decrease in pumping ability culminating in heart failure and death.

Glycogen storage disease of the myocardium is only one of a group of disorders exhibiting glycogenosis of one or more organs or tissues. In 1960, Stetten and Stetten classified the group into six basic types based on what enzyme was demonstrably lacking or the natural history of the disease or both[207]. Pompe's disease was his type II or cardiac type.

The first case of glycogen storage disease of the myocardium was reported by Pompe in 1932[208]. Scattered case reports then began to appear throughout the world literature. Di Sant' Agnese and his group conducted a critical analysis of these reports in 1950 and they came to the conclusion that only 14 of them could be accepted as being certifiably accurate[209]. In 1959, di Sant' Agnese modified his criteria to require the demonstration of a normal structure of the deposited glycogen as well as preserved glycogenolysis in liver and striated muscle[210].

Ehlers and her group from Cornell University described in 1962 the first case of glycogen storage disease of the myocardium with obstruction to the outflow tract of the left ventricle. This unique case represented at that time one of the few instances of left ventricular outflow obstruction with a proven etiology, namely glycogen storage disease. It had both functional and anatomic evidence of muscular subaortic stenosis[211]. Ehler's paper represented the 54th well-documented case of Pompe's disease meeting all the criteria established by di Sant' Agnese, who had, by this time, emerged as the leading American authority on glycogen storage disease.

Familial hypertrophic obstructive cardiomyopathy

The most characteristic and constant feature of this disease is an asymmetric septal hypertrophy (ASH), often without obstruction of the left ventricular outflow tract[212]. Many large genetic pedigrees have been reported. In the majority of them an autosomal dominant trait has been found. The most impressive one is that published by Paré and his group in 1961.

In the historical background of hypertrophic obstructive cardiomyopathy that was presented in Chapter 6, the reader will recall that the first published description of what is now known as idiopathic hypertrophic subaortic stenosis (IHSS) was the report by Schmincke of Würzburg, Germany. In his paper which appeared in 1907, he described the presence of a diffuse hyperplasia of the muscle mass constituting the wall of the left ventricular outflow tract in two adult women at necropsy[213]. These women were unrelated to each other, and Schmincke made no mention of a familial occurrence. Almost fifty years had to elapse before Davies described a family in which many members had heart disease[214]. Only one member of that family was subjected to a postmortem examination, but that one member did have changes in the heart consistent with those of idiopathic hypertrophic subaortic stenosis. Braunwald recounts how this member died immediately after an injection of a drug given for the relief of an acute asthmatic episode. In his words, 'although the nature of the drug is unknown, it now seems likely that this event represents the first example of the intensification of obstruction by a pharmacologic agent which stimulates the myocardium such as epinephrine'[215].

It must be realized that the full-blown case of IHSS develops only when the asymmetrical septal hypertrophy progresses to the point where it produces obstruction of the left ventricular outflow tract at the subaortic level. This is what both Schmincke and Davies described, and this is what makes it so difficult at times to trace the historical background of the genetics of familial obstructive cardiomyopathy. The earlier reports failed to emphasize asymmetrical septal hypertrophy as the pathognomonic feature, and the cases that were described or analyzed would now come under the heading of hypertrophic cardiomyopathy without obstruction. Familial merely means that the cardiomyopathy is recurrent within a kinship, and idiopathic hypertrophic obstructive cardiomyopathy is but one example of a broad clinical spectrum ranging from the asymptomatic to the full-blown variety.

Bearing this in mind then, the first reference of this sort in a family would be the paper by Addarii and his group[216]. In 1946, he and his associates described the presence of bundle branch block and heart failure in two brothers. Their mother had died of an unknown type of heart disease at the age of 34. At necropsy, the heart of one of the brothers revealed hypertrophy and diffuse fibrosis of the myocardium. Hypoplasia of the aorta was also present. Evans in 1949 described a degenerative disease of the myocardium that occurred in the same family[217]. He gave it the name familial cardiomegaly. He described in all a group of 10 patients, five of whom were members of separate families. One of them was a 16 year old boy who showed considerable enlargement of 'the base of the left ventricle' at autopsy.

Two features were common to the various reports that appeared between the time of publication of Evans' paper in 1949 and that of Paré in 1961[218–240]. These were a familial occurrence, at times, traceable over several generations, and the invariable presence of myocardial fibrosis and hypertrophy at autopsy. The reports emanated from various European and American centers and were presented for the most part under the designation of familial cardiomegaly. Some emphasized the obstructive manifestations while others, the non-inflammatory or non-vascular origin of their cases.

Up until the publication of the study conducted by Paré and his group, not enough cases were involved to delineate a specific genetic pattern. Their paper was entitled *Hereditary cardiovascular dysplasia*, taking into account that some patients failed to show cardiac enlargement or that hypoplasia of the aorta was seen in their autopsied cases[241]. Only three autopsies were performed, and in two of them, an 'unusual localized hypertrophy of the interventricular septum was found in which the hypertrophied myocardial fibers possessed a bizarre, haphazard architectural arrangement'.

Theirs was the first comprehensive genetic study, involving 77 members of a family in which a total of 30 members were affected. They were able to conduct a genealogical survey of French-Canadian marriages in the lower St Lawrence region[242]. This information plus data derived from their own detailed histories of the 77 members, enabled the authors to draw a rather complete family tree dating back to the original immigrant from France in the early 1600s. This man who was married in the province of Quebec in 1650 was, himself, the offspring of a marriage between two cousins, once removed. He had three brothers and three sisters, who all married and left many descendants.

It is interesting to note that much of the genealogical information dating back to the first identifiable case, an uncle who died in 1860, was supplied by a 95 year old man who, the authors claimed, had an excellent memory. On the basis of this genealogic survey, Paré's group concluded that 'the pattern of occurrence over the five generations since the death (in 1860) of the man who is believed to have had the first case of heart disease in the family clearly indicates a dominant non-sex-linked mode of transmission'.

The National Institutes of Health entered the picture with a paper by Braunwald and his co-workers in 1964[215]. They studied in detail 64 patients with idiopathic hypertrophic stenosis and found multiple cases in 11 families. Two years later, Horlick and his associates reported their findings in a family spanning 4 generations[243]. Their observations were derived from clinical, hemodynamic and pathologic features of IHSS. In 1967, Nasser and his group pointed out that left ventricular outflow tract obstruction was not necessarily present in all the affected members of the same family[244]. A year after, Jorgensen saw an association between sporadic cases and elevated paternal age[245]. He expressed the view that the sporadic cases may have represented fresh mutations.

Further contributions were made by the group of investigators from the National Institutes of Health. Henry, Clark and Epstein published two landmark papers in the same issue of *Circulation* in 1973. One focused on observations regarding the pathogenesis, pathophysiology and course of IHSS. In it, they considered ASH as the unifying link in the IHSS disease spectrum[246]. The other, with Henry again as the leading author, advanced the view that the echocardiographic identification of ASH should be considered a pathognomonic sign of IHSS[247]. This was based on the observations previously made in the companion paper that ASH is present in every patient falling within the spectrum of IHSS regardless of whether or not an obstructive process is in effect.

In still another paper during the same year but with Clark now as the leading author, the group demonstrated a high familial prevalence of IHSS utilizing the echocardiographic identification of ASH as the *sine qua non* for the disease[248]. In the 30 families that came under their scrutiny, almost half of all the first-degree relatives had ASH. Furthermore since there was an equal prevalence in males and females, with affected males often having affected fathers, X and Y linkage as modes of transmission were eliminated. This suggested that the disease is inherited via an autosomal dominant trait.

In 1974, the National Institutes of Health was responsible for yet another study. This was headed by B. J. Maron, and concerned itself with the findings in 4 infants who died with ASH at some time during the first 5 months of life[249]. One was stillborn. ASH was demonstrated in one first-degree relative of each infant. In 1976, Maron headed another study that analyzed the clinical picture of 46 children with ASH[250].

In 1979, Darsee and his associates differentiated two forms of hypertrophic cardiomyopathy based on human leukocyte antigen (HLA) linkage[251]. They found a lod score of 77 for linkage between ASH and HLA. They concluded that in addition to the hereditary form linked to HLA, there is a sporadic unlinked form which is associated with severe systemic hypertension. White patients with ASH were B12; black patients were B5. McKusick considered this a superb example of linkage, demonstrating genetic heterogeneity[252].

Familial cardiomyopathy

This is an ill-defined heterogeneous group sharing in common, enlargement of the heart due to an anatomical derangement of heart muscle resulting in congestive cardiomyopathy and occurring in families. The histology reveals diffuse fibrosis with severe hypertrophy of the surviving muscle fibers. The hypertrophy of the muscle fibers in this syndrome probably represents a compensatory phenomenon to overcome the ineffectual contractility of the fibrotic elements.

The reader should be aware that all the disorders classified as familial cardiomyopathy are not necessarily the same. As we said previously, familial merely means that the cardiomyopathy is recurrent within a kinship.

The very heterogeneity of familial cardiomyopathy with its ill-defined diagnostic criteria make any attempt at outlining its historical background a difficult task to say the least. Until a more precise classification can be formulated based on histopathologic changes consonant with a specific biochemical defect, the historical details will continue to remain hazy.

To emphasize the point, three types of pathological changes have been described in the various case reports that were published over the years as being representative of familial cardiomyopathy. To illustrate, Boyd and his group cite as examples the case reports and analyses of Hollman and associates (1960), Paré's group (1961) and Teare's classical paper[253]. In accordance with the current definition, these are properly examples of hypertrophic cardiomyopathy and not familial cardiomyopathy. In the papers written by Evans (1949)[217], Brigden (1957)[254], Garrett (1959)[255], Bishop (1962)[256], and Barry (1962)[257], the histologic changes consist of myocardial fibrosis and hypertrophy of the surviving muscle fibers. These are more in keeping with the currently accepted description of the histopathologic changes of familial cardiomyopathy. The third pathologic process is that described by Battersby in 1961[258]. He noted the deposition of a non-metachromatic, diastase-resistant, PAS-positive polysaccharide in the myocardium suggesting a metabolic defect. This appears to be a step in the right direction.

Perhaps I, too, am guilty of adding to the confusion by my unbridled efforts to sort out the semantics. At any rate, it might be better from the genetic point of view to include all the cardiomyopathies with a familial recurrence under the genetic designation of familial cardiomyopathy. Since they all appear to be single gene disorders, further subtyping can proceed under the mutant gene with its specific biochemical defect.

Until then, Addarii may have been historically the first to have described a case that meets the current histopathologic criteria of familial cardiomyopathy with diffuse fibrosis and hypertrophy. I have already alluded to this possibility while attempting to trace the historical background of hypertrophic cardiomyopathy. Evans too, may have included in his study examples other than those of hypertrophic cardiomyopathy. Aside from the 16 year old boy who had 'considerable enlargement of the base of the left ventricle', there are three cases in Evans' paper that had the clinical manifestations of a dilated cardiomyopathy, and since familial transmission was proven they too would fall under the same category. Paré's group reported the autopsy findings in only three subjects. It is true that the findings in these three correspond to what one would expect in hypertrophic cardiomyopathy. However, the rest are assumed to have had hypertrophic cardiomyopathy by extrapolation and not by histopathologic confirmation. It can be said with a greater degree of certainty that the case reports by Brigden, Garrett, Bishop, Barry and Battersby fit in more with the ill-defined group of cardiomyopathy. These last mentioned papers then would, in my opinion, form the historical links in the evolution of knowledge concerning the genetic mechanisms of familial cardiomyopathy.

If this be so, the mode of inheritance would be less uncertain as W. J. Taylor contended in his monograph on the genetic aspects of the cardiomyopathies[259]. There is no doubt that in those families in which vertical transmission is documented, autosomal dominant inheritance is likely, including male to male transmission, through two or more generations[259]. Yamaguchi and Toshima pointed out an autosomal recessive pattern in their genetic analysis of idiopathic cardiomyopathies in Japan[260]. It must be emphasized, however, that their statements are derived from studies of cardiomyopathic states that lack consistent histologic support as to the type of pathologic changes involved.

Such is not the case with the studies of Berko and Swift that appeared in 1987[261]. They described a large kindred in which 11 young male members had definite or possible evidence of idiopathic dilated cardiomyopathy. Three mothers of the affected males had been diagnosed as having late onset dilated cardiomyopathy. Two other mothers were labeled with the possibility of having had the disorder. Autopsies were done on 4 of the affected males. These revealed widespread patchy fibrosis of the myocardium. One other male had undergone an endomyocardial biopsy which showed minimal interstitial fibrosis. The pattern of consistent early expression and rapid progression of cardiomyopathy in their male subjects, later onset and slower progression in the mothers, and no male to male transmission suggests an X-linked mode of inheritance[261].

In 1976, just 11 years before the genetic analysis of Berko and Swift, the team of Csanady and Szasz presented their findings in 8 patients of a kindred spanning 3 generations. Their paper carried the title *Familial Cardiomyopathy*[262]. The clinical picture in 6 of the 8 patients did indeed correspond to the syndrome of congestive cardiomyopathy.

An autosomal dominant pattern of inheritance was documented. However, this paper illustrates again, how careful one must be in tracing the historical background. There is no doubt that the authors were aware that familial congestive cardiomyopathy is not a completely uniform disease yet their histopathologic description is meagre and limited to 2 patients. In a sentence they note the presence of diffuse myocardial fibrosis and hypertrophy. This may be all good and well until we come to another paragraph where in their own words 'According to the pathologist, our cases can be considered as familial endocardial fibrosis'. Is it or isn't it?

Idiopathic hemochromatosis

Primary or idiopathic hemochromatosis is a rare illness due to excessive deposition of iron in the tissues. It has a long latent period that may span 40 years or more. Its chief clinical manifestations are skin pigmentation, cirrhosis, diabetes and cardiac disorders. There is general agreement today that it is an inherited disorder, but the genetic mechanisms have been a bone of contention ever since Sheldon first suggested that it was an inherited disorder in 1934[263].

Sheldon also published a book on the subject which appeared in 1935[264]. It contained a review of 311 cases reported before 1934. Most of the cases were diagnosed at postmortem, and Sheldon's analysis of the necropsy findings in these reports led him to conclude that the cases differed significantly in the 'target organs' involved. He also noted that at least 10% of the cases failed to show any accumulation of iron in the myocardium. Sheldon recognized 15 instances of recurrence within families which led him to suggest that the disease was hereditary. We must give him credit for his astuteness in advancing the view that the idiopathic or primary form of the disorder is due to an inborn error of metabolism. This view was not generally accepted for many years. Even as late as 1966, McDonald contended that the cirrhosis was caused by alcohol, not iron[265]. Also for years, a debate swirled around the role of excessive iron in food and drink.

During this time, several investigators, having already accepted a genetic basis for the malady, now proposed differing mechanisms for the mode of transmission. As early as 1954, Neel and Schull stated in their book on human heredity that the culprit was an autosomal dominant gene with a variable degree of penetrance or expressivity[266]. This opinion was shared by Finch and Finch in their comprehensive and esteemed review on hemochromatosis which appeared in 1955[267]. Several other papers appeared in support of this mode of inheritance. These were by Johnson and Frey in 1962[268], Balcerzak and his group in 1966[269], and Sinniah in 1969[270].

Unspecified hereditary factors were considered by Schapira (1962)[271], Mendel (1964)[272], Powell (1965)[273] and Charlton and co-workers in 1967[274]. In 1977, Crosby suggested a diversity of genetic lesions to account for the diversity of target organs that Sheldon observed[275]. He also observed in 1966 that when hemochromatosis was found in identical twins, the target organs were identical[276]. Sinniah[270] and Saddi and Feingold[277] independently suggested the disorder was due to a recessive gene with variable manifestations in heterozygotes. In a very stimulating article on the genetics of primary hemochromatosis, Scheinberg in 1973 cited a very important and fundamental fact that lends credence to the currently accepted view of an autosomal recessive mode of inheritance. This is that 'phenotypic manifestations may occur in an individual heterozygous for a mutant recessive gene

even though frank disease is seen only in abnormal homozygotes'[278]. This statement was made by H. Harris in 1970, and is to be found in his book *The Principles of Human Biochemical Genetics*[279]. This implies that a mutant gene may fail to synthesize the specific enzyme in question, or if it does, the enzyme is so structurally altered that it has defective properties. Thus, a heterozygous individual produces enough normal enzyme via the normal gene to meet the metabolic needs of the body but at the same time may be producing enough abnormal enzyme through the mutant gene to cause disease. This would result in a less than fully developed syndrome; a concept that was elaborated upon by both Williams and his co-workers in 1962[280], and Mendel in 1964[272].

Bothwell and his associates presented this hypothesis as being the most reasonable in their chapter on idiopathic hemochromatosis in Stanbury's *Metabolic Basis of Inherited Disease* published in 1983[281].

Scheinberg in the same paper that I previously mentioned belabors the usage of 'dominant' and 'recessive' in describing a gene. He feels that these terms have 'obscured rather than clarified the pathogenesis of hemochromatosis'. He goes on to say that 'it may be more useful to consider a gene in terms of its capacity to modify qualitatively or quantitavely the synthesis of a protein'[278]. Scheinberg's point appears to be quite valid. Of course, the validity of this proposal will be secured only when the biochemical defect in idiopathic hemochromatosis has been identified. Until then, it can be said with a virtual degree of certainty that the mutant gene is an autosomal recessive. This was confirmed by studies of the HLA genotype in affected individuals and their relatives by Simon and his colleagues in 1976, 1977 and again in 1980[282].

Familial amyloidosis

Amyloid is a fibrous protein that has an amorphous, hyaline-like appearance under the light microscope. Congo Red is widely used for staining, but it stains collagen and elastic tissue as well. Schleiden coined the word 'amyloid'[283]. He used it to describe a normal starchy component of plants. Virchow noted the presence of this material in certain histologic sections, and erroneously named it amyloid. He mistook it for starch rather than protein.

Bonet may have been the first to describe amyloidosis though he did not realize it[283]. It was in a patient who had marked enlargement of the spleen in association with a liver abscess. The spleen was studded with white stones and may, very well, have been the sago spleen of amyloidosis. Two centuries later, Rokitansky described a waxy liver with 'lardaceous degeneration' in people dying with such chronic illnesses as tuberculosis, syphilis and rickets[283]. Lardaceous is a term that was repeatedly seen as a synonym for amyloid since grossly the organs do look as though they are heavily laden with fat. It was Budd who later suggested that the waxy appearance of the liver was not due to 'lardaceous degeneration' but was rather the result of infiltration with an albuminous substance[283]. Friedreich and Kehulé agreed with Budd, describing amyloid as an 'albuminoid' material. But, despite its proteinaceous nature, these authors felt that the term amyloid should be retained.

Meckel, a member of that eminent family noted for its contributions to pathologic anatomy, must be credited with emphasizing the propensity for amyloid to be deposited in a widespread manner. He described its deposition not only in the liver and spleen but also in the kidneys, intestinal wall and in the arterial system[283].

The classification of amyloidosis has undergone repeated revisions ever since Reimann and his associates introduced their simple one of primary and secondary forms in 1935[284]. Most patients with cardiac amyloidosis have the secondary variety. That is, it is found in association with a chronic illness such as tuberculosis, chronic osteomyelitis, or multiple myeloma. There is a form of amyloidosis that is localized exclusively to the heart. It is called senile cardiac amyloidosis. The one we are interested in at the moment is the dominantly inherited form of primary systemic amyloidosis. Although it is systemic, its major clinical picture centers around the heart. Characteristically, this familial disorder manifests itself as a restrictive cardiomyopathy producing congestive heart failure and death within three to six years after the onset of symptoms, the first signs usually appearing during the fifth decade of life. The cardiac dysfunction is due to deposition of amyloid within the myocardium and the walls of the coronary arteries[285]. Deposits have also been found within the cardiac valves.

Wilks described a 51 year old man with 'lardaceous viscera' in 1856[286]. The changes were found in the absence of any chronic disease. It appears to have had all the criteria for acceptance as an example of primary amyloidosis. Despite this, Wild's case report in 1886 is generally credited with being the first to describe the systemic form of the disorder[287].

Ostertag was the first to draw attention to the familial form of primary systemic amyloidosis. He described on two occasions, six members of a family spanning three generations[288,289]. All had died of renal failure. Postmortem examination revealed widespread deposition of amyloid. Ostertag's first paper appeared in 1932. His second paper, which was much more detailed, appeared in 1950.

Four years after Ostertag's initial paper, Maxwell and Kimbell reported widespread deposition of amyloid in three brothers, all of whom had no evidence of any other illness[290]. Congestive heart failure was instrumental in the death of one brother. In 1952, Andrade presented a large series from Portugal[291]. Twelve families were involved. Da Silva Horta reported the pathologic findings in a number of Andrade's cases, confirming the diagnosis of primary systemic amyloidosis and drawing attention to the extensive myocardial deposits[292].

An extremely important paper appeared in 1956. The leading author was J.G. Rukavina[293]. It was an experimental, genetic and clinical study of 29 cases. Its greatest value lay in its comprehensive review of the subject; the first of its kind in that order of magnitude. In addition to their own cases, they analyzed another 154 cases culled from the literature. Another comprehensive review, concerned primarily with the genetic aspects, appeared in 1969[294]. It originated from McKusick's department, no doubt one of the foremost centers of medical genetics in America and the world. The leading author was Mahloudji.

Several studies have concerned themselves with the electrocardiographic and hemodynamic alterations in amyloid involvement of the heart. Low voltage, alterations of the PR interval, right bundle branch block and left ventricular hypertrophy have been described. Chronologically, these electrocardiographic changes were reported by Eisen in 1946[295], Lindsay[296], Wessler and Freedberg[297], all in 1948, Josselson and Pruitt[298] in 1953, and Bernreiter[299] in 1958.

Hemodynamic findings have been described in only a few cases. Fisher and his group were the first in 1950 to subject a patient to right heart catheterization[300]. Measurements were not included in their paper but they did report that there was no increase in cardiac output or stroke volume after increasing blood volume with an intravenous infusion of human serum albumin. This suggested to them that there was mechanical limitation of diastolic filling and systolic ejection. The second case to undergo cardiac catheterization was a subject in heart failure. The most important hemodynamic finding in this report by Hetzel and co-workers in 1953, was the 'dip-plateau' pressure curve in the right ventricle[301]. This is considered today as a characteristic sign of impaired diastolic filling of the ventricle. Gunner's group presented their catheterization findings in 1955[302] and Himbert in 1959[303].

One of the most outstanding contributions on familial amyloid heart disease is the paper by Frederiksen and co-workers which was published in 1962[304]. They described five cases. The predominant clinical feature was cardiac involvement. Hemodynamic studies were performed in all five patients. They confirmed the previously reported findings and in addition, presented a rather extensive discussion and review of the clinical, pathologic and pathophysiologic features of the syndrome.

Myotonic dystrophy

The manifestations of cardiac dysfunction in this inherited disorder may vary from electrocardiographic abnormalities to overt rhythm disturbances. It is transmitted via an autosomal dominant trait. It was Hawley and his group in 1983 who initiated the suggestion that the tendency to have arrhythmia or conduction disturbances such as heart block is a familial characteristic with myotonic dystrophy[305]. Inherent with this suggestion was the implication that there were two forms of myotonic dystrophy, with and without cardiac involvement. They studied 18 families and found heart block in 4.

Myotonic dystrophy was the first disease model for demonstrating genetic linkage in man; an approach that carries great diagnostic and predictive potentiality for identifying subjects at risk for inheriting genetically determined diseases. Mohr used the model in 1954 in Danish families afflicted with the disease, and who had been

previously studied and reported by Thomasen in 1948[306,307]. Mohr suggested that the linkage was between the Lutheran and Lewis blood groups. Although Mohr did also suspect a linkage between the secretor gene and myotonic dystrophy, proof of this had to wait for the studies reported by Renwick and his group in 1971[308], those by McKusick's group in 1971[308], and those by McKusick's group again a year later[309]. The secretor gene determines the secretion of the ABO blood group substances into body fluids. This includes saliva and amniotic fluid. Thus, knowledge of the existence of such a linkage would provide the foundation for predicting the possible inheritance of the mutant gene for myotonic dystrophy by determining the secretor status of the fetus as obtained through amniocentesis.

It is of interest to note that all the early work on the linkage relation was carried out without any knowledge of the chromosomal location of the mutant gene. This did not come about until it was shown that there was a linkage among the secretor gene, the Lutheran blood group and complement component 3 (C3). This was demonstrated by Mohr and his group in 1983[310]. Whitehead and his associates had already shown a year earlier with hybrid cells that the C3 gene was located on chromosome 19[311].

The localization of the mutant gene of myotonic dystrophy to chromosome 19 opens the way for the isolation and characterization of the gene itself, and hopefully for the identification of the biochemical defect that it causes. Utilizing a different technique, that of skin fibroblast cultures, Swift and Finegold did find in 1969, very large amounts of material that had the staining properties of acid mucopolysaccharides[312].

Duchenne muscular dystrophy

This genetically determined disorder is transmitted via an X-linked recessive gene. The chief cardiac manifestations are to be found in the electrocardiogram and in the rhythm disturbances that complicate the disease.

Although not invariably present, the electrocardiographic changes, when seen, are quite characteristic. They consist of abnormally tall right precordial R waves and abnormally deep limb lead and/or lateral precordial Q waves. The diagnostic significance of the electrocardiographic pattern was initially reported by Schott and associates in 1955[313]. Further observations with repeated confirmations of the abnormalities were reported by a number of investigators beginning with S. Gailani in 1958[314], followed by Manning and Cropp in the same year[315], Skiring and McKusick in 1961[316], and Gilroy and colleagues along with Welsh and his group in 1963[317,318]. In 1966, and again in 1967, Perloff and his associates revisited the subject[319,320]. In 1967, they published their findings of an electrocardiographic pathologic correlative study in two patients. On the basis of this study, they advanced the view that the 'posterobasal location of myocardial fibrosis [in Duchenne's dystrophy] provides an acceptable explanation for the anterior shift of the QRS complex'[320]. This view was not entirely new since the QRS changes in progressive muscular dystrophy have repeatedly been considered a reflection of the fibrotic process that is so characteristically localized in this disease. What was new was the necropsy evidence that this could actually be the basis.

Insofar as the rhythm disturbances are concerned, two pathologic features have been implicated as possibly being responsible. These were the findings of James in 1962[321], and those of Rossi and James in 1964[322], in which the probable predisposing causes were listed as being the degeneration of the nodal fibers and the narrowing of the intramural coronary arteries. In the first of Perloff's two cases, the intramural coronary arteries in the atria were thick-walled with marked narrowing of the lumen, especially the small arteries feeding the sinus and AV nodes[320]. The other case showed essentially no abnormalities.

Friedreich's ataxia

Friedreich's account of this heritable disorder appeared in 1863[323]. Although he did mention the presence of cardiac lesions, this aspect of the syndrome was not emphasized until many years later. The first report to do so was that by Pitt which appeared in 1886[324]. The second report by Saury appeared in 1905[325]. Another 24 years had to elapse before attention was focused again on the cardiac disturbances in Friedreich's ataxia. Mollaret at this time described the electrocardiographic abnormalities in the disorder[326]. The many reports

that followed were summarized in 1938 in the same paper wherein he advanced the catecholamine hypothesis in the pathogenesis of the cardiomyopathy[327]. Subsequent reports have described not only the electrocardiographic findings but the occurrence of cardiomegaly, cardiac murmurs, heart failure, myocarditis, and myocardial fibrosis[328–336].

Russell appears to be the first to propose that both the neurologic and cardiac manifestations are the result of a genetically determined biochemical defect with a metabolic pathway that affects several organs[335]. This is known as pleiotropy. At one point a deficiency of lipoamide dehydrogenase was designated as the biochemical defect. This was disputed by Robinson and his group in a letter to the *New England Journal of Medicine*[337].

McKusick's clinic saw 27 kindreds between 1935 and 1957 at the Johns Hopkins Hospital[338]. In three families, a dominant form of inheritance was noted: 'affected individuals in each of the remaining 24 families were confined to single sibships, and in 18 of these limited to a single patient'[338]. This study published in 1962 demonstrated the relative infrequency of an obviously dominant mode of inheritance. In 1939, two independent teams had also commented on the relative infrequency of a dominant mode of inheritance. These were Bell and Carmichael from England and Leers and Scholz from Germany[339,340].

Hewer in 1968 found that almost 75% of the patients with Friedreich's ataxia had evidence of cardiac dysfunction during life, and that at least half of the 82 fatal cases they analyzed died of heart failure[341]. Elias reported on the association of muscular subaortic stenosis in 1972[342]. Ackroyd and coworkers reported the cardiac findings in 12 children in 1984[343]. All had echocardiographic abnormalities consisting of symmetric, concentric, hypertrophic cardiomyopathy. Ten of the 12 children also had electrocardiographic abnormalities. Winter and his group found about twice as many first-cousin marriages among the parents of affected sibships as was expected. Their interpretation of this was genetic heterogeneity[344].

Unlike myotonic dystrophy, the locus of the abnormal gene is still unknown. Chamberlain and co-workers excluded chromosome 19 as the locus in 1987[345].

Primary endocardial fibroelastosis

The disorder is known by several names. These are primary endocardial fibroelastosis, subendocardial fibroelastosis, endocardial sclerosis, ventricular fibroelastosis, and endocardial fibrosis. The name endocardial fibroelastosis is the currently favored one. It was introduced by Weinberg and Himelfarb in 1943[346].

Gowing in 1953 defined endocardial fibroelastosis as a 'congenital condition of unknown etiology in which there occurs a diffuse thickening up of the mural endocardium associated in most cases with myocardial hypertrophy and leading to early death'[347]. Actually, it has a diverse etiology. Most cases have a multifactorial basis, and many of them may occur on a non-genetic basis.

Andersen and Kelly proposed in 1956 that the disorder be differentiated into primary and secondary forms[348]. The primary variety, which is more common, is associated with other congenital cardiac abnormalities while the secondary form has no associated anomalies of the heart.

Numerous reports and studies have appeared suggesting three modes of inheritance. For the most part they have shown an autosomal recessive mode while some have demonstrated an X-linked recessive trait. One group suggested an autosomal dominant mode. Among the earliest case reports describing the occurrence of the disorder among siblings are those by Dordick in 1951[349] and Axtrup in 1954[350] followed three years later by that of Tulczynska of Poland[351]. Nadas mentions in his text on pediatric cardiology that he had seen two cases in each of two sibships[352]. Winter and associates in 1960 added two more affected sibs and collected nine other cases from the literature[353]. Vestermark described two more cases in each of two sibships in 1962[354].

When Andersen and Kelly presented their classification in 1956, they reported at the same time a 23% familial incidence in the primary group. A sizable series of 72 cases was studied by Forfar and his associates in 1964, and they reported practically the same percentage of familial recurrence[355]. Similar findings were noted during the same year by Sellers, Keith and Manning[356]. The only ones to suggest an autosomal dominant inheritance were Hunter and Keay. Their study which appeared in 1973 described a family in which two sisters had five affected children by different husbands[357].

Westwood and co-workers reviewed heredity in primary endocardial fibroelastosis in 1975 and suggested that familial cases may result from a genetically transmitted abnormality affecting cardiac metabolism[358]. Impairment of aerobic metabolism was suggested by Olsen in 1975[359] and again by Peters and his group in 1977[360]. In one form of autosomal recessive inheritance, the biochemical basis was found to be a severe deficiency of plasma and tissue carnitine[361]. This was discovered in a family in which the cardiomyopathy was found in four of five children. The study was conducted by M. Tripp and her associates from the University of Wisconsin. It was published in 1981. Three of the affected four children died suddenly and at postmortem, endocardial fibroelastosis was found. Carnitine deficiency in humans was first described by Engel and Angelini in 1973[362]. The disease affecting this family is unique among reported cases of systemic carnitine deficiency.

Constrictive pericarditis

A genetic cause of constrictive pericarditis is a rare autosomal recessive disorder called mulibrey nanism. It was first described by J. Perheentupa and co-workers in 1970[363]. Since then, this group from Finland has continued to be the major contributors on the subject[364,365].

The basic defect is unknown. The changes do seem to be restricted to cells of mesodermal origin, and the search for the basic defect is being directed to fibroblasts. The term 'mulibrey' was coined by the group in its original communication. It stands for muscle, liver, brain and eyes since all these organs are affected. Nanism, of course, is from the Greek word for dwarf. 'Cardiopathy is a constant and grave part of the syndrome; pericardial constriction seems to be its most regular component'[364]. The same group suggested that the disorder is transmitted by an autosomal recessive gene[364]. Histologic studies conducted by Voorhees and colleagues in 1973 showed a thickened pericardium with calcium deposits as a prominent feature, but with no evidence of active inflammation[366].

Cardiac tumors

The two most common primary tumors of the heart can occur with or without familial involvement. These are the myxomas and rhabdomyomas.

Most of the cardiac myxomas occur as sporadic cases. Since 1971, however, at least five families have been reported with multiple affected members. The first report was by Krause and his colleagues[367]. It concerned a 34 year old patient with a myxoma of the pulmonic valve complicated by bacterial endocarditis. The patient had a brother who died at the age of 25 with a left atrial myxoma. Two years later Heydorn's group reported two teenage brothers with atrial myxomas[368]. During the same year, Kleid and his group also described two teenage brothers with a myxoma. The myxoma was located in the left atrium in the younger brother, and in the right atrium in the older brother[369]. A sister and brother were involved in Farah's report in 1975[370]. The following year, Siltanen and associates described its occurrence in a mother and her three sons[371], while Powers' group described its presence in a father and daughter[372]. Despite all these reports, the pattern of genetic disturbance has not been determined as yet.

At least 50% of patients with a single rhabdomyoma, and probably all patients with multiple rhabdomyoma have simultaneously tuberous sclerosis[373,374]. Adenoma sebaceum and epiloia have both been used as synonyms. Adenoma sebaceum does not accurately describe the dermal lesions. Facial angiofibroma would be more specific. McKusick was told by Gorlin that epiloia is an acronym for epilepsy, low intelligence and adenoma sebaceum[375]. Actually, the term was introduced by Sherlock in 1911[376].

Von Recklinghausen's description in 1862 appears to be the first reference to this disorder[377]. He had found at necropsy numerous rhabdomyomas of the heart in association with sclerotic changes in the brain of a stillborn infant. His description of the cerebral lesions are quite characteristic of those now known to occur in tuberous sclerosis. Two years after von Recklinghausen's report, Virchow also described a child who had cerebral tuberous sclerosis and rhabdomyoma of the heart whose sister died of a cerebral tumor[378]. This was the first inkling of the familial nature of the disease.

The term 'sclerose tuberoeuse' was introduced by Bourneville in 1880 when he presented the first detailed account of the clinical and pathologic features of the disease[379].

A number of etiologic mechanisms were proposed as being responsible until it was definitely established that the various lesions and mental disturbances are pleiotropic effects of an autosomal dominant gene. Bourneville attempted to implicate fetal encephalitis as a causative factor[380], while a neoplastic mechanism was postulated by Hartdegen in 1881 and again by Vogt in 1908[381,382], and Bielschowsky and Gallus in 1913[383].

The fact that both the skin and nervous system are involved caused Alzheimer in 1907 and Bouwdijk-Bastiaanse 15 years later to classify the disorder under the congenital neuroectodermal dysplasias[384,385]. Feriz in 1930 expressed the view that the disease was due to an exaggerated proliferation of atypical germinal and supporting tissue in the midst of and replacing functioning tissue[386].

Clear recognition of the heredo-familial nature of the disorder was provided by Berg in 1913[387]. He described three cases in three successive generations in one family. Genetic mechanisms were then traced by Gunther and Penrose in 1935[388], Penrose in 1954[389], and Marshall, Saul and Sachs in 1959[390]. The paper by Marshall and his associates describes a family in which 13 of the 45 members in 4 successive generations had inherited the disease.

In 1979, Sybert and Hall pointed out that expression is highly variable, and involvement may be missed in the mildly affected individual[391]. An excellent review of the subject was presented by Gomez in 1979[392]. It was based on the cumulative experience of the Mayo clinic between the years 1935 and 1979.

Kandt and his associates reported the occurrence of cerebral embolization from a cardiac rhabdomyoma in 1985[393]. McKusick recounts how Journel's group recorded 'the curious experience' of making the diagnosis of familial tuberous sclerosis by finding intracardiac tumors (rhabdomyoma) by routine ultrasonography[375]. In investigating the family, they uncovered a maternal aunt with the clinical characteristics of tuberous sclerosis[394]. Smith (1987) pointed to the great variability of tuberous sclerosis observed in a single family and to the fact that a substantial number of obligate heterozygotes have no clinical manifestations[395].

427

Coronary artery disease

The evidence for the importance of genetic factors in the pathogenesis of coronary artery disease has been derived almost entirely from long-term epidemiologic studies (a relatively new research tool in medicine), postmortem observations and animal experiments. Most patients with coronary artery disease have inherited multiple predisposing genes that in combination with several environmental factors result in arteriosclerosis which is the underlying lesion. In some patients only a single abnormal gene is responsible for the arteriosclerotic process. At least thirteen different mutant genes have been identified so far. Among them, the most common are those single-gene disorders that cause hyperlipidemia. These include familial hypercholesterolemia, familial hypertrigceridemia, multiple lipoprotein-type hyperlipidemia and familial dysbetalipoproteinemia[396]. The mutant genes in these disorders cause inborn errors of metabolism that affect the synthesis, degradation or structure of a plasma lipoprotein; all of which predispose to atherosclerosis.

The remaining monogenic disorders are associated with mutant genes that are responsible for other types of inborn errors of metabolism, and which can involve the coronary arteries by virtue of the biochemical defect. An example of this would be the accumulation of glycolipids in the walls of the coronary arteries in Fabry's disease. This is an X-linked disorder wherein there is a deficiency of α-galactosidase A[397,398].

Familial hypercholesterolemia

This is an outstanding example of a single mutant gene which because of its inability to produce low density lipoprotein (LDL) receptors results in deposition of excessive amounts of circulating blood cholesterol in the arterial walls with consequent atherosclerosis. The gene is transmitted in an autosomal dominant manner with heterozygotes occurring quite often (1 in 500)[399,400]. The disorder is a very important one in the pathogenesis of premature coronary artery disease[401,402]. The homozygous variety is very rare with a frequency rate of about one in a million. Those afflicted usually die before the age of 30 with generalized atherosclerosis being the principal pathologic

manifestation[400]. Aortic stenosis as a result of cholesterol deposition has been described[400,403,404]. Endocardial thickening with xanthomatous plaques has also been reported[400,403]. Involvement of the mitral endocardial surface may explain why, at times, clinical signs of mitral stenosis and insufficiency may be present[403,404]. Diffuse xanthomatous infiltration of the myocardium was described by Goldstein in 1972[403].

The earliest descriptions of xanthomas in tendons associated with atheromatous arterial lesions are to be found in a number of reports dating back to the late 19th century. One of the earliest that I could find was the one written by C. H. Fogge entitled *General xanthelasma or vitiligoidea*. It appeared in 1872 in the *Transactions of the Pathological Society of London*[405]. A case of multiple xanthelasma was reported in *The Lancet* in 1879 by T. C. Fox[406]. Two more case reports then appeared in the German literature. The first one was by A. Poensgen in 1883[407], and the other by Lehzen and Knauss in 1889[408]. Muller[409,410] and Thannhauser[411,412] separately suggested a genetic basis when they recognized a familial clustering of patients exhibiting xanthomas, hypercholesterolemia and premature coronary artery disease. This was confirmed by a number of subsequent studies from different centers during the 1940s and 1950s. Notable among these were the papers by Wilkinson[413,414], Adlersberg[415], Bloom[416] and the Epstein group[417]. The studies of Kachadurian from Lebanon in the early 1960s incriminated a single gene mutation as the genetic basis for the disorder[418]. He also delineated and clarified the clinical and genetic differences between heterozygotes and homozygotes.

By the mid 1950s, the technique of analytical ultracentrifugation was quite well established. Lipoproteins of different densities were now recognized. It was at this time that Gofman and his co-workers demonstrated with this technique that the plasma concentration of low-density lipoprotein (LDL) was elevated in familial hypercholesterolemia[419,420]. During the next decade, the concept was advanced by Frederickson and Levy that the disorder in familial hypercholesterolemia was a metabolic one involving both the apoprotein and cholesterol components of LDL[421]. It was the brilliant work of Brown and Goldstein in the 1970s that defined the basic biochemical defect. These two workers discovered the existence of a receptor on the cell surface of LDL and uncovered the fact that in familial hypercholesterolemia, this receptor was either reduced in number or completely lacking due to malfunction of an inherited mutant gene. They received the Nobel Prize in 1986 for this extraordinary bit of investigation. Their concept of a receptor-mediated pathway for cholesterol homeostasis stems from research beginning in 1972 which attempted to learn more about a human genetic disease called familial hypercholesterolemia (FH)[399]. They applied the techniques of cell culture utilizing skin fibroblasts. Studies in the 1960s by Bailey[422] and Rothblat[423] had already demonstrated that several types of cultured animal cells could be utilized for the synthesis of cholesterol. This led Brown and Goldstein to reason that the defect associated with familial hypercholesterolemia could be studied in cultured skin fibroblasts. In addition to the seminal work of Bailey and Rothblat regarding this technique, a classic paper had been published by Neufeld and Fratantoni in 1970 which definitely showed that cultured skin fibroblasts could be used for delineating complex cellular metabolic pathways[424].

The studies of Brown and Goldstein led to the discovery that the transport protein for cholesterol known as LDL had a receptor on the surface of its cells which bound plasma cholesterol during transit in the bloodstream, and which was also responsible for mediating feedback control of cholesterol synthesis[425,426]. In the words of Brown and Goldstein, ...

FH was shown to be caused by inherited defects in the gene encoding the LDL receptor, these defects disrupt the normal control of cholesterol metabolism. Study of the LDL receptor in turn led to an understanding of receptor-mediated endocytosis, a general process by which cells communicate with each other through internalization of regulatory and nutritional molecules. Receptor-mediated endocytosis differs from previously described biochemical pathways because it depends on the continuous and highly controlled movement of membrane-embedded proteins from one cell organelle to another in a process termed receptor recycling. Many of the mutations in the LDL receptor that occur in FH patients disrupt the movement of the receptor between organelles. These mutations define a

new type of cellular defect that has broad implications for normal and deranged human physiology ... Two properties of the receptor, its high affinity for LDL and its ability to cycle multiple times in and out of the cell, allow large amounts of cholesterol to be delivered to body tissues, while at the same time keeping the concentration of LDL in blood low enough to avoid the buildup of atherosclerotic plaques. When LDL receptor function is inappropriately diminished as a result of genetic defects or in response to regulatory signals, the protective mechanism is lost, cholesterol builds up in plasma, and atherosclerosis ensues.

The existence of the LDL receptor was confirmed when LDL was radiolabeled with ^{125}I and incubated with normal and FH homozygous fibroblasts[427].

These studies attest to Carl Müller's astuteness when he described familial hypercholesterolemia in 1938 as an inborn error of metabolism[428], and had concluded that it was transmitted as an autosomal dominant trait prior to Kachadurian's delineation of the genetic basis.

Goldstein and Brown also studied the fibroblasts from 110 patients with the clinical phenotype of homozygous familial hypercholesterolemia. They found four major classes of genetic defects in the LDL receptor. On a structural basis, the genetic defect in FH seems quite clear but it still did not reveal how LDL generated the signal that suppressed human menopausal gonadotropin coenzyme A reductase in the feedback control. Goldstein and Brown also asked this question by studying the fate of the surface-bound LDL[425].

Familial hypertriglyceridemia

This common autosomal dominant disorder, and in particular, its genetic aspects, have been described by several investigators. Among them are Neufeld and Goldbourt[429], Havel[430], Chait and Brunzell[431], Namboordiri[432], and, of course, Goldstein[433]. Its relationship to atherosclerosis is still uncertain since many patients have concomitant diabetes, obesity and hypertension; all factors which can predispose to atherosclerosis in and of themselves.

In 1973, Goldstein and associates analyzed the pedigree of affected persons who had survived an episode of myocardial infarction. They found that the relatives of these affected persons had normal cholesterol distribution and biomodal triglyceride distribution[433]. Evidence for diabetes mellitus and genetic forms of hypertriglyceridemia as independent entities was supplied by Brunzell and his group in 1975[434]. Frederickson and Levy placed the phenotype under type IV of their classification of the hyperlipoproteinemias[435]. Namboordiri and co-workers analyzed the segregation and linkage data of a large pedigree with hypertriglyceridemia and a high frequency of cardiac disturbance[432]. They observed that triglycerides showed a 75% of the variance accountable by genetic transmission and that it was only 52% for cholesterol.

In 1978, Breckenridge and colleagues described a 59 year old man with markedly elevated blood triglyceride level in association with a deficiency of apolipoprotein C-II[436]. They were able to reduce the triglyceride level temporarily with a transfusion of one unit of plasma.

Karathanasis and associates (1983) demonstrated a linkage between APOA 1 gene and the APAC 3 gene[437]. Rees demonstrated in the same year a DNA polymorphism adjacent to the human apoprotein A-1 gene[438]. Karathanasis suggested that the association of the DNA polymorphism with hypertriglyceridemia may be due to a single base pair substitution in the 3' noncoding region of APO C-III MRNA[437].

Familial combined hyperlipidemia

This is the most common genetic form of hyperlipidemia. It was described as a new inherited disorder by Goldstein and his group in 1973[418]. The original paper was the same one that described familial hypertriglyceridemia. It concerned itself with a genetic analysis of lipid levels in 176 families which had among them survivors of a myocardial infarction with demonstrably increased blood levels of cholesterol and triglycerides. These investigators also demonstrated a predisposition of affected individuals towards myocardial infarction and that the mode of inheritance was via an autosomal dominant trait.

Familial dysbetalipoproteinemia

This disorder is also transmitted by a single gene mechanism. The defective gene cannot encode a

plasma apolipoprotein (Apo E). Again, the genetic aspects and association with coronary artery disease were primarily the work of the same group of investigators led by Goldstein and Brown.

The clinical characteristics of the disorder were described by Goldstein, Brown, Frederickson, Levy, Havel and Brunzell; all members of the original group at one time or another. The most important descriptions are to be found in two texts. They are *Diseases of Metabolism* published in 1980 with Havel as the leading author of the chapter and in the *Metabolic Basis of Inherited Disease* with Brown now as the leading author of the chapter dealing with the disorder[439,440].

In 1975, Morganroth, Levy and Fredrickson described in detail the biochemical, clinical and genetic features. In particular, they drew attention to the marked generalized atherosclerosis that occurs with this condition[441].

REFERENCES

1. Berg, P. (1981). Dissections and reconstructions of genes and chromosomes (Nobel lecture). *Science*, **213**, 296–303
2. Gillespie, C.C. (1974). Editor-in-chief. *Dictionary of Scientific Biography*, vol. IX, pp. 277–9. (New York: Charles Scribner's Sons)
3. McKusick, V.A. (1986). The morbid anatomy of the human genome: a review of gene mapping in clinical medicine. *Medicine*, **65**, 1–33
4. *Ibid.*, p. 2
5. Wilson, E. B. (1911). The sex chromosomes. *Arch. Mikrosk. Anat. Entwicklungsmech.*, **77**, 249–71
6. Donahue, R.P., Bias, W.B., Renwick, J.H. and McKusick, V.A. (1968). Probable assignment of the Duffy blood group locus to chromosome 1 in man. *Proc. Natl. Acad. Sci.*, **61**, 949–55
7. Weiss, M. and Green, H. (1967). Human-mouse hybrid cell lines containing partial complements of human chromosomes and functioning human genes. *Proc. Natl. Acad. Sci.*, **58**, 1104–11
8. Caspersson, T., Zech, L. and Johansson, C. (1970). Differential banding of alkylating fluorochromes in human chromosomes. *Exp. Cell. Res.*, **60**, 316–19
9. Caspersson, T., Zech, L., Johansson, C. and Modest, E.J. (1970). Quinacrine mustard fluorescent banding. *Chromosoma*, **30**, 215–27

10. Caspersson, T., Lomakka, C. and Zech, L. (1971). Fluorescent banding. *Hereditas*, **67**, 89–102

11. McKusick, V.A. (1986). *Op. cit.*, p. 4

12. Anderson, S., Bankier, A.T., Barrell, B.O., deBruijn, M.H.L., Coulson, A.R., Drouin, J., Eperson, I.C., Nierlich, D.P., Roe, B.A., Sanger, F., Schreier, P.H., Smith, A.J.R., Staden, R. and Young, I.G. (1981). Sequence and organization of the human mitochrondrial genome. *Nature (London)*, **200**, 457–65

13. McKusick, V.A. (1986). *Op. cit.*, p.4

14. Garrod, A.E. (1923). *Inborn Errors of Metabolism*, pp. 1–216. (London: Oxford University Press)

15. Beadle, G.W. (1959). Inborn errors of metabolism. *Science*, **129**, 1715

16. Tatum, E.L. *Ibid.*, p. 171

17. Pauling, L.A., Itano, H.A., Singer, S.J. and Wells, I.C. (1949). *Ibid.*, **110**, 543

18. Garrod A.E. (1894). On the association of cardiac malformations with other congenital defects. *St. Bartholomew's Hosp. Rep.*, (London), **30**, 53

19. Abbott, M.E. (1924). New accessions in cardiac anomalies: pulmonary atresia of inflammatory orgin; persistent ostium primum with mongolian idiocy. *Int. A M Museums Bull.*, **10**, 111

20. Berg, J.M., Crome, L. and France, N.E. (1960). Congenital cardiac malformations in mongolism. *Br. Heart J.*, **22**, 331

21. Rowe, R.D. and Uchida, I.A. (1961). Cardiac malformation in mongolism. *Am. J. Med.*, **83**, 76

22. Tandon, R. and Edwards, J. (1973). Cardiac malformations associated with Down's syndrome. *Circulation*, **47**, 1349–55

23. Turner H.H. (1938). A syndrome of infantilism, congenital webbed neck, and cubitus valgus. *Endocrinology*, **23**, 566

24. Ullrich, O. (1930). Über typische Kombinations bilder multipler Abartungen. *Zeitschrift für Kinderheilkunde*, **49**, 271–6

25. Ford, C.E., Jones, K.W., Polani, P.E., de Almeida, J.C. and Briggs, J.H. (1959). A sex-chromosome anomaly in a case of gonadal dysgenesis (Turner's syndrome). *Lancet*, **1**, 711–13

26. Van den Berghe, H. (1966). *Het zogenaamde Syndroom van Turner*. (Antwerpen: Thesis Leuven. Standaard Wetenschappelijke Uitgeverij)

27. Noonan, J.A. and Ehmke, D.A. (1963). Associated non-cardiac malformations in children with congenital heart disease (abstract). *J. Ped.*, **63**, 468–70

28. Noonan, J.A. (1968). Hypertelorism with Turner phenotype: a new syndrome with associated congenital heart disease. *Am. J. Dis. Child.*, **116**, 373–80

29. Nora, J.J., Sinha, A.K. and Nora, A.H. (1972). Dominant inheritance of the Noonan syndrome. *Birth Defects*, **8**, 118–21

30. Siggers, D.C. and Polani, P.E. (1972). Congenital heart disease in male and female subjects with somatic features of Turner's syndrome and normal sex chromosomes (Ullrich's and related syndromes). *Br. Heart J.*, **34**, 41–6

31. Ehlers, K.H., Engle, M.A., Levin, A.R. and Deely, W.J. (1972). Eccentric ventricular hypertrophy in familial and sporadic instances of 46 XX, XY Turner phenotype. *Circulation*, **45**, 639–52

32. Nora, J.J., Nora, A.H., Sinha, A.K., Spangler, R.D. and Lubs, H.A. (1974). The Ullrich-Noonan syndrome (Turner phenotype). *Am. J. Dis. Child.*, **127**, 48

33. Haddad, H.M. and Wilkins, L. (1959). Congenital anomalies associated with gonadal aplasia: review of 55 cases. *Pediatrics*, **23**, 885–902

34. Rainier-Pope, C.R., Cunningham, R.D., Madas, A.S. and Crigler, J.F. (1964). Cardiovascular malformations in Turner's syndrome. *Pediatrics*, **33**, 919

35. Vernant, P., Corone, P., Grouchy, J., Gennes, J.L. and Emerit, I. (1966). Le coeur dans le syndrome de Turner-Ullrich. *Archives des Maladies du Coeur et des Vaisseaux*, **59**, 850–75

36. Van der Hauwaert, L.J., Fryns, J.P., Dumoulin, M. and Logghe, N. (1978). Cardiovascular malformations in Turner's and Noonan's syndrome. *Br. Heart J.*, **40**, 500–9

37. Salgado, C.R. (1961). Sindrome de Turner. Communicacion de un caso asociado con aneurisma disecante de la aorta. *Rev. Fac. Clienc. Med. Cordoba*, **19**, 193–204

38. Price, W.H. and Wilson, J. (1983). Dissection of the aorta in Turner's syndrome. *J. Med. Genet.*, **20**, 61–3

39. Kobylinski, O. (1883). Über eine flughautähnliche Ausbreitung am Halse. *Arch. Anthropol.*, **14**, 342–8

40. Opitz, J.M. and Pallister, D.P. (1979). Brief historical note: the concept of 'gonadal dysgenesis.' *Am. J. Med. Genet.*, **4**, 333–43

41. Funke, O. (1902). Pterygium colli. *Dtsch. Zeitschr. Chir.*, **63**, 162–7

42. Flavell, G. (1943). Webbing of the neck with Turner's syndrome in the male. *Br. J. Surg.*, **31**, 150–3

43. Opitz, J.M., Summitt, R.L. and Sarto, G.E.

(1965). Noonan's syndrome in girls: a genocopy of the Ullrich-Turner syndrome. *J. Pediatr.*, **67**, 968

44. Nora, J.J. and Sinha, A.K. (1968). Direct familial transmission of the Turner phenotype. *Am. J. Dis. Child.*, **116**, 343–50

45. Abdel-Salem, E. and Tentamy, S.A. (1969). Familial Turner phenotype. *J. Pediatr.*, **74**, 67–72

46. Baird, P.A. and De Jong, B.P. (1972). Noonan's syndrome (XX and XY Turner phenotype) in three generations of a family. *J.Pediatr.*, **80**, 110–14

47. Bolton, M.R., Pugh, D.M., Mattioli, L. *et al.* (1974). The Noonan syndrome: a family study, *Ann. Intern. Med.*, **80**, 626–9

48. Smith, D.W. (1970). *Recognizable Patterns of Human Malformation.* (Philadelphia: W.B. Saunders)

49. Pearl, W. (1977). Cardiovascular anomalies in Noonan's syndrome. *Chest*, **7**, 677–9

50. Ehlers, K.H., Engle, M.A., Levin, A.R. *et al.* (1972). Eccentric ventricular hypertrophy in familial and sporadic instances of 46 XX, XY phenotype. *Circulation*, **45**, 639–52

51. Phornphutkul, G., Rosenthal, A. and Nadas, A.S. (1973). Cardiomyopathy in Noonan's syndrome. Report of 3 cases. *Br. Heart J.*, **35**, 99–102

52. Cole, R.B. (1980). Noonan's syndrome: a historical perspective. *Pediatrics*, **66**, 468–9

53. Gorlin, R.J., Anderson, R.C. and Blau, M. (1969). Multiple lentigens syndrome. *Am. J. Dis. Child.*, **117**, 652

54. Seunaez, H., Màne-Garzon, F. and Kolski, R. Cardio-cutaneous syndrome (the 'LEOPARD' syndrome). Cited by Gorlin in reference 53.

55. Lamy, M.J., De Grouchy, P. and Schweisguth, O. (1957). Genetic and non-genetic factors in the etiology of congenital heart disease. A study of 1188 cases. *Am. J. Hum. Genet.*, **9**, 17–41

56. Moynahan, E.J. (1962). Multiple symmetrical moles, with psychic and somatic infantilism and genital hypoplasia: first male case of a new syndrome. *Proc. R. Soc. Med.*, **55**, 959–60

57. Forney, W.R., Robinson, S.J. and Pascoe, D.J. (1966). Congenital heart disease, deafness and skeletal malformations. A new syndrome? *J. Pediatr.*, **68**, 14–28

58. Walther, R.J., Polansky, B. and Grots, I.A. (1966). Electrocardiographic abnormalities in a family with generalized lentigo. *N. Engl. J. Med.*, **275**, 1220–5

59. Mathews, N.L. (1968). Lentigo and electrocardiographic changes. *N. Engl. J. Med.*, **278**, 780–1

60. Cronje, R.E. and Feinberg, A. (1973). Lentiginosis, deafness and cardiac abnormalities. *S. Afr. Med. J.*, **47**, 15–17

61. Gorlin, R.J., Anderson, R.C. and Moller, J.H. (1971). The Leopard (multiple lentigines) syndrome revisited. *Birth Defects: Original Article Series VII*, No. 4, 110–15

62. Polani, P.E. and Moynahan, E.J. (1972). Progressive cardiomyopathic lentiginosis. *Q. J. Med.*, **41**, 205–25

63. Norlund, J.J., Lerner, A.B., Braverman, I.M. and McGuire, J.S. (1973). The multiple lentigines syndrome. *Arch. Dermatol.*, **107**, 259–61

64. McKusick, V.A. and Capute, A.J. (1968). Congenital deafness with multiple lentigines in mother and daughter. Read before the *First Conference on the Clinical Delineation of Birth Defects.* (Baltimore: Johns Hopkins Hospital)

65. Pickering, D., Laski, B., MacMillan, D.C. and Rose, V. (1971). 'Little Leopard' syndrome. Description of three cases and review of 24. *Arch. Dis. Child.*, **46**, 85–90

66. Moynahan, E.J. (1970). Progressive cardio-myopathic lentiginosis: first report of autopsy findings in a recently recognized inheritable disorder (autosomal dominant). *Proc. R. Soc. Med.*, **63**, 448–51

67. Somerville, Bonham-Carter, R.E. (1972). The heart in lentiginosis. *Br. Heart J.*, **34**, 58–66

68. St. John Sutton, M.G., Tajik, A.J., Giuliano, E.R., Gordon, H. and Su, W.P.D. (1981). Hypertrophic obstructive cardiomyopathy and lentiginosis: a little known neural ectodermal syndrome. *Am. J. Cardiol.*, **47**, 214–17

69. Siewert, A.K. (1904). Ueber einen Fall von Bronchiectasis bei einem: putienten mit situs inversus viscerum. *Berlin München Tieraerztl Wachr*, **2**, 139–41

70. Kartagener, M. (1933). Zur pathogenese der Bronchiektasien. I. Mitteilung: bronchiektasien bei situs viscerum inversus. *Beltr. Klin. Erforsch. Tuberk. Lungenkr.*, **83**, 489–501

71. Kartagener, M. and Horlacher, A. (1935). Bronchiektasien bei situs viscerum inversus. *Schweiz. Med. Wschr.*, **65**, 782–4

72. Olsen, A.M. (1943). Bronchiectasis and dextrocardic observations on the aetiology of bronchiectasis. *Am. Rev. Tuberc.*, **47**, 435–9

73. Pastore, P.N. and Olsen, A.M. (1941). Absence of frontal sinuses and bronchiectasis in identical twins. *Proc. Staff Meet. Mayo Clin.*, **16**, 593–9

74. Mayo, C.W. and Rice, R.E. (1949). Situs inversus totalis: a statistical review of data on seventy-six cases with special reference to disease of the biliary tract. *Arch. Surg.*, **58**, 724–30

75. Safian, L.A. and Mandeville, F.B. (1959). Kartagener's syndrome in identical male twins and a female sibling: report of cases, with comments on pathology and familial manifestations. *J. Florida Med. Assoc.*, **45**, 1143–8

76. Overholt, E.L. and Bauman, D.F. (1958). Variants of Kartagener's syndrome in the same family. *Ann. Intern. Med.*, **48**, 574–9

77. Knox, G., Murray, S. and Strang, L. (1960). A family with Kartagener's syndrome: linkage data. *Ann. Hum. Genet.*, **24**, 137–40

78. Kartagener, M. and Stucki, P. (1962). Bronchiectasis with situs inversus. *Arch. Pediatr.*, **79**, 193–207

79. Cockayne, E.A. (1938). The genetics of transposition of the viscera. *Q. J. Med.*, **7**, 479–93

80. Miller, R.D. and Divertie, M.B. (1972). Kartagener's syndrome. *Chest*, **62**, 130–5

81. Afzelius, B.A. (1976). A human syndrome caused by immotile cilia. *Science*, **193**, 317

82. Danlos, M. (1908). Un cas de cutis laxa avec tumeurs par contusion chronique des coudes et des genoux (xanthome juvenile pseudo-diabetique de M.M. Hallopeau et Mace de Lépinay). *Bull. Soc. Franc. Derm. Syph.*, **19**, 70

83. Ehlers, E. (1901). Cutis laxa, Neigung zu Hämorrhagien in der Haut, Lockerung mehrerer Artikulationen. *Derm. Wschr.*, **8**, 173

84. McKusick, V.A. (1972). *Heritable Disorders of Connective Tissue*, 4th edn., p. 372. (St. Louis: C.V. Mosby Co.)

85. Fittke, H. (1942). Ueber eine ungewöhnliche Form 'multipler Erbabartung' (Chalodermie und Dysostose). *Z. Kinderheilk.*, **63**, 510

86. Mott, V. (1884). Remarks on a peculiar form of tumour of the skin denominated pachydermatocele. *London Med. Chirurg. Trans.*, **37**, 155

87. Alibert, J.L. (1855). Histoire d'un berger des environs de Gisors (dermatose hypermorphe). *Monogr. Derm.*, **2**, 719

88. Weber, F.P. (1923). Chalasodermia or 'loose skin,' and its relationship to subcutaneous fibroids or calcareous nodules. *Urol. Cutan. Rev.*, **27**, 407

89. Ronchese, F. (1936). Dermatorrhexis, with dermatochalasis and arthrochalasis (the so-called Ehlers–Danlos syndrome). *Am. J. Dis. Child.*, **51**, 1403

90. Ronchese, F. (1958). Dermatomegaly. *Arch. Derm.*, **76**, 666

91. Goltz, R.W. and Hult, A.M. (1965). Generalized elastolysis (cutis laxa) and Ehlers–Danlos syndrome (cutis hyperelactica); a comparative clinical and laboratory study. *Southern Med. J.*, **58**, 848

92. Goltz, R.W., Hult, A.M., Goldfarb, M. and Gorlin, R.J. (1965). Cutis laxa; a manifestation of generalized elastolysis. *Arch. Derm.*, **92**, 373

93. Graham, R. and Beighton, P. (1971). The physical properties of skin in cutis laxa. *Br. J. Dermatol.*, **84**, 326–9

94. Beighton, P. (1972). The dominant and recessive forms of cutis laxa. *J. Med. Genet.*, **9**, 216–20

95. Smith, R.D. and Worthington, J.W. (1967). Paganini; the riddle and connective tissue. *J. Am. Med. Assoc.*, **199**, 820

96. Weissmann, A. (1918). *Der Virtuose*, p. 46. (Berlin: Paul Cassirer)

97. Bennati, F. (1831). Notice physiologue sur Paganini. *Revue de Paris*, **11**, 52–60

98. van Meekeren, J.A. (1682). De dilatabilitate extraordinaria cutis, chap. 32. *Observations Medico-chirugicae*, Amsterdam

99. Kopp, W. (1888). Demonstration zweier Fälle von 'Cutis laxa.' *München, Med. Wschr.*, **35**, 259

100. Tschernogobow, A. (1892). Cutis laxa (Presentation at first meeting of Moscow Dermatologic and Venereologic Society, Nov. 13, 1891). *Mhft. Prakt. Derm.*, **14**, 76

101. Jansen, L.H. (1954). *De Ziekte van Ehlers en Danlos.* (Gravenhage: Uitgeverij Excelsor's)

102. Jansen, L.H. (1955). Le mode de transmission de la maladie d'Ehlers–Danlos. *J. Genet. Hum.*, **4**, 204

103. Jansen, L.H. (1955). The structure of the connective tissue, an explanation of the symptoms of the Ehlers–Danlos syndrome. *Dermatologica*, **110**, 108

104. Johnson, S.A.M. and Falls, H.F. (1949). Ehlers–Danlos syndrome; a clinical and genetic study. *Arch. Derm. Syph.*, **60**, 82

105. Beighton, P. (1970). Ehlers–Danlos syndrome. *Ann. Rheum. Dis.*, **29**, 332

106. Krane, S.M., Pinnell, S.R. and Erbe, R.W. (1972). Decreased lysyl-protocollagen hydroxylase activity in fibroblasts from a family with a newly recognized disorder. hydroxylysine-deficient collagen. *J. Clin. Invest.*, **51**, 52a

107. Lichtenstein, J., Nigra, T.P., Sussman, M.D., Martin, G.R. and McKusick, V.A. (1972). Molecular defect in a form of the Ehlers–Danlos syndrome: hydroxylysine deficient collagen (abstract). (Philadelphia: Am. Soc. Hum. Genet.)

108. Unna, P.G. (1896). *The Histopathology of the Diseases of the Skin*, pp. 984–8. Translated from the German by N. Walker with the assistance of the author. (New York: The Macmillan Co.)

109. DuMesnil. (1880). *Beitrag zur Anatomie und Aetiologie bestimmter Hautkrankheiten*, Dissertation, Würzburg, cited by Unna

110. Williams, A.W. (1892). Cutis laxa. *Monatsschr. Prakt. Derm.*, **14**, 490

111. Ehlers, E. (1901). Cutis laxa, Neigung zu Haemorrhagien in der Haut, Lockerung mehrerer Artikulationen. *Derm. Zschr.*, **8**, 173

112. Tschernogobow, A. (1892). Ein Fall von Cutis laxa. Protokoly Moskowskawo wenerologitscheskawo i dermatologitscheskawo Obtschestwa, vol. 1. Quoted in *Jahresb. Ges. Med.*, **27**, 562

113. Danlos, M. (1908). Un cas de cutis laxa avec tumeurs par contusion chronique des coudes et des genoux (xanthome juvenile pseudodiabetique de M.M. Hallopeau et Mace de Lépinay). *Bull. Soc. Franc. Derm. Syph.*, **19**, 70

114. Beighton, P. (1969). Cardiac abnormalities in the Ehlers–Danlos syndrome. *Br. Heart J.*, **31**, 227–31

115. McKusick, V.A. (1966). *Heritable Disorders of Connective Tissue*, pp. 179–229, 3rd edn. (St. Louis: C.V. Mosby)

116. McKusick, V.A. (1972). *Op. cit.*

117. McKusick, V.A. (1972). *Op. cit.*

118. Murdock, J.L., Walker, B.A. and McKusick, V.A. (1972). Parental age effects on the occurence of new mutations for the Marfan syndrome. *Ann. Hum. Genet.*, **35**, 331

119. Pan, C.W., Chen, C.C., Wang, S.P. *et al.* (1985). Echocardiographic study of cardiac abnormalities in families of patients with Marfan's syndrome. *J. Am. Coll. Cardiol.*, **6**, 1016

120. Marfan, A.B. (1896). Un cas de déformation congénitale des quatre membres plus prononcée aux extrémités charactérisée par l'allongement des os avec un certain degré d'amincissement, *Bull. Mém. Soc. Méd. Hôp., Paris*, **13**, 220

121. Méry, H. and Babonneix, L. (1902). Un cas de déformation congénitale des quatre membres. hyperchondroplasie. *Bull. Mém. Soc. Méd. Hôp. Paris*, **19**, 671

122. Achard, C. (1902). Arachnodactylie. *Bull. Mém. Soc. Méd. Hôp., Paris*, **19**, 831

123. Salle, V. (1912). Ueber einen Fall von angeborener abnormen Grosse der Extremiteten mit einen an Akronemegalia erinnerden Symptomenkomplex. *Jahrb. Kinderheilk.*, **75**, 540

124. Börger, F. (1914). Über zwei Falle von Arachnodaktylie. *Z.F. Kinderheilkd.*, **12**, 161–84

125. Piper, R.K. and Irvine-Jones, E. (1926). Arachnodactylia and its association with congenital heart disease. *Am. J. Dis. Child.*, **31**, 832–9

126. Ellis, R.W.B. (1940). Arachnodactyly and ectopia lentis in a father and daughter. *Arch. Dis. Child.*, **15**, 267–73

127. Baer, R.W., Taussig, H.B. and Oppenheimer, E.H. (1943). Congenital aneurysmal dilatation of aorta associated with arachnodactyly. *Bull. Johns Hopkins Hosp.*, **72**, 309–31

128. Etter, L.E. and Glover, L.P. (1943). Arachnodactyly complicated by dislocated lens and death from rupture of dissecting aneurysm of aorta. *J. Am. Med. Assoc.*, **123**, 88–9

129. Bronson, E. and Sutherland, G.A. (1918). Ruptured aortic aneurysms in childhood. *Br. J. Child. Dis.*, **15**, 241

130. Piper, R.K. and Irvine-Jones, E. (1926). Archachnodactylia and its association with congenital heart disease: report of a case and review of the literature. *Am. J. Dis. Child.*, **31**, 832–9

131. Goyette, E.M. and Palmer, P.W. (1953). Cardiovascular lesions in arachnodactyly. *Circulation*, **7**, 372–9

132. McKusick, V.A. (1955). The cardiovascular aspects of Marfan's syndrome: a heritable disorder of connective tissue. *Circulation*, **11**, 321–42

133. Hirst, A.E. Jr, Johns, V.J. Jr, Kime and S.W. Jr (1958). Dissecting aneurysm of the aorta: a review of 505 cases. *Medicine (Baltimore)*, **37**, 217–79

134. Bowers, D. (1959). Marfan's syndrome and the Weill-Marchesan syndrome in the S. family. *Ann. Intern. Med.*, **51**, 1049–70

135. Gordon, A.M. (1962). Abraham Lincoln − a medical appraisal. *J. Kentucky Med. Assoc.*, **60**, 249

136. Murdoch, J.L., Walker, B.A., Halpern, B.L., Kuzma, J.W. and McKusick, V.A. (1972). Life expectancy and causes of death in the Marfan syndrome. *N. Engl. J. Med.*, **286**, 804–8

137. Donaldson, L.B. and De Alvarez, R.R. (1965). The Marfan syndrome and pregnancy. *Am. J. Obstet. Gynecol.*, **92**, 629–41

138. Bowers, D. and Lim, D.W. (1962). Subacute bacterial endocarditis and Marfan's syndrome. *Can. Med. Assoc. J.*, **86**, 455–8

139. Wunsch, C.M., Steinmetz, E.F. and Fisch, C. (1965). Marfan's syndrome and subacute bacterial endocarditis. *Am. J. Cardiol.*, **15**, 102–6

140. Miller, R. Jr and Pearson, R.J. Jr (1959). Mitral insufficiency simulating aortic stenosis: report of

an unusual manifestation of Marfan's syndrome. *N. Engl. J. Med.*, **260**, 1210–13

141. McKusick, V.A. (1966). *Heritable Disorders of Connective Tissue*, edn. 3. (St. Louis: C. V. Mosby Co.)

142. Grossman, M., Knott, A.P. and Jacoby, W.J. (1968). Calcified annulus fibrosus with mitral insufficiency in the Marfan syndrome. *Arch. Intern. Med.*, **121**, 561–3

143. Weve, H. (1931). Ueber Arachnodaktylie (Dystrophia mesodermalis congenita, typus Marfanis). *Arch. Augenheilk.*, **104**, 1

144. Hirst, A.E. Jr and Gore, I. (1973). Marfan's syndrome: a review. *Progress in Cardiovascular Diseases*, vol XVI, no.2, p. 187

145. Gore, I. (1953). Dissecting aneurysms of aorta in persons under forty years of age. *A.M.A. Arch. Path.*, **55**, 1–13

146. Sjoerdsma, A., Davidson, J.D., Udenfriend, S. and Mitoma, C. (1958). Increased excretion of hydroxyproline in Marfan's syndrome. *Lancet*, **2**, 994

147. Jones, C.R., Bergman, M.W., Kittner, P.J. *et al.* (1964). Urinary hydroxyproline excretion in Marfan's syndrome as compared with age matched control. *Proc. Soc. Exp. Biol. Med.*, **116**, 931–3

148. Berenson, G.S. and Geer, J.C. (1963). Heart disease in the Hurler and Marfan syndromes. *Arch. Intern. Med.*, **111**, 58–69

149. Emanuel, R., Ng, R.A.L., Marcomichelakis, J., Moores, E.C. *et al.* (1977). Formes frustes of Marfan's syndrome presenting with severe aortic regurgitation. *Br. Heart J.*, **39**, 190–7

150. Wigle, E.D., Rakocoski, H., Ranganathan, N. and Silver, M.D. (1976). Mitral valve prolapse. *Annu. Rev. Med.*, **27**, 165–80

151. Strahan, N.V., Murphy, E.A., Fortuin, N.J., Come, P.C. and Humphries, J.O. (1983). Inheritance of the mitral valve prolapse syndrome. Discussion of a three-dimensional penetrance model. *Am. J. Med.*, **74**, 967–72

152. Davies, M.J., Moore, B.P. and Braimbridge, M.V. (1978). The floppy mitral valve. Study of incidence, pathology and complications in surgical, necropsy and forensic material. *Br. Heart J.*, **40**, 468–81

153. Cuffer, Barbillon (1887). Nouvelles recerches sur le bruit de galop. *Arch. Med. Gen. Trop.*, **1**, 131–49, 301–20

154. Griffith, J.P.C. (1892). Mid-systolic and late systolic mitral murmurs. *Am. J. Med. Sci.*, **104**, 285–94

155. Hall, J.N. (1903). Late systolic mitral murmurs. *Am. J. Med. Sci.*, **125**, 663

156. Gallivardin, L. (1913). Pseudodoublement du deuxieme bruit de coeur simulant le redoublement mitral par bruit extra cardiaque telesystolique surajoute. *Lyon Med.*, **121**, 409

157. Gallavardin, L. (1932). Nouveble observation avec autopsie d'un pseudodoublement du il bruit de coeur simulant le redoublement mitral. *Prat. Med. Fr.*, **13**, 19

158. Reid, J.V.O. (1961). Mid-systolic clicks. *S. Afr. Med. J.*, **35**, 353–5

159. Barlow, J.B., Pocock, W.A., Marchand, P. and Denny, M. (1963). The significance of late systolic murmurs. *Am. Heart J.*, **66**, 443–52

160. Barlow, J.P., Bosman, C.K., Pocock, W.A., Marchand, P. (1966). Late systolic murmurs and non-ejection ('mid-late') systolic clicks. *Br. Heart J.*, **30**, 203

161. Hancock, E.W. and Cohn, K. (1966). The syndrome associated with mid-systolic click and late systolic murmur. *Am. J. Med.*, **41**, 183–96

162. Stannard, M., Sloman, J.G., Hare, W.S.C. and Goble, A.J. (1967). Prolapse of the posterior leaflet of the mitral valve: a clinical, familial, and cineangiographic study. *Br. Med. J.*, **3**, 71–4

163. Jeresaty, R.M. (1973). Mitral valve prolapse-click syndrome. *Prog. Cardiovasc. Dis.*, **15**, 623–52

164. Shappell, S.D., Marshall, C.E., Brown, R.E. and Bruce, T.A. (1973). Sudden death and familial occurrence of mid-systolic click, late systolic murmur syndrome. *Circulation*, **48**, 1128–34

165. Gulotta, S.J., Gulco, L., Padmanaohan, V. and Miller, S. (1974). The syndrome of systolic click, murmur, and mitral valve prolapse – a cardiomyopathy? *Circulation*, **49**, 717–28

166. Ranganathan, N. *et al.* (1973). Angiographic-morphologic correlation in patients with severe mitral regurgitation due to prolapse of the posterior mitral valve leaflet. *Circulation*, **48**, 514–18

167. Barlow, J.B. and Bosman, C.K. (1966). Aneurysmal protrusion of the posterior leaflet of the mitral valve. *Am. Heart J.*, **71**, 166–78

168. Pomerance, A. (1969). Ballooning deformity (mucoid degeneration) of atrio-ventricular valves. *Br. Heart J.*, **31**, 343–51

169. Barnett, H.J.M., Jones, M.W. and Boughner, D. (1975). Cerebral ischemic events associated with prolapsing mitral valve. *Arch. Neurol.*, **32**, 352–3 (Abstr.)

170. Hunt, D. and Sloman, G. (1969). Prolapse of the posterior leaflet of the mitral valve occuring in

eleven members of a family. *Am. Heart J.*, **78**, 149–53

171. Weiss, A.N., Mimbs, J.W., Ludbrook, P.A. and Sobel, B.E. (1975). Echocardiographic detection of MVP. *Circulation*, **52**, 1091–6

172. Strahan, S., Murphy, E.A., Fortuin, N.J., Come, P.C. and Humphries, J.O. (1983). Inheritance of the mitral valve prolapse syndrome: discussion of a three-dimensional model. *Am. J. Med.*, **74**, 967–72

173. McKusick, V.A. (1972). *Op. cit.*, p.523

174. Brailsford, J.F. (1953). Chondro-osteo-dystrophy, roentgenographic and clinical features of child with dislocation of vertebrae. *Am. J. Surg.*, **7**, 404, 1929. *The Radiology of Bones and Joints*, edn. 5. (Baltimore: The Williams & Wilkins Co)

175. Wolff, D. (1942). Microscopic study of temporal bones in dysostosis multiplex (gargoylism). *Laryngoscope*, **52**, 218

176. Nja, A. (1946). A sex-linked type of gargoylism. *Acta Paediatr.*, **33**, 267

177. Cockayne, E.A. (1936). Gargoylism (chondro-osteodystrophy, hepatosplenomegaly, deafness in two brothers). *Proc. R. Soc. Med.*, **30**, 104

178. Ellis, R.W.B. (1936). Gargoylism (chondro-osteodystrophy, corneal opacities, hepatosplenomegaly and mental deficiency). *Proc. R. Soc. Med.*, **30**, 158

179. Husler, J. *Handbuch der Kinderheilhunde*, 4th edn. vol. 1, p.651

180. McKusick, V.A. (1972). *Op. cit.*, p. 524

181. Washington, J.A. (1937). Lipochondrodys-trophy. In Brennemann's *Practice of Pediatrics*, vol. 4, chap. 30. (Hagerstown, MD.: W.F. Prior Co., Inc.)

182. Donohue, W.L. (1948). Clinicopathologic Conference at The Hospital for Sick Children. Dysendocrinism. *J. Pediatr.*, **32**, 739

183. Donohue, W.L. and Uchida, I. (1954). Leprechaunism. A euphemism for a rare familial disorder. *J. Pediatr.*, **45**, 505–19

184. Lindsay, S. (1950). The cardiovascular system in gargoylism. *Br. Heart J.*, **12**, 17

185. Ellis, R.W.B. and Payne, W.P. (1936). Glycogen disease. *Q. J. Med.*, **29**, 31

186. Krovetz, L.J., Lorinez, A.E. and Schiebler, G.L. (1968). Cardiovascular manifestations of the Hunter-Hurler syndrome. In Moss, A.J. and Adams, F.H. (eds.) *Heart Disease in Infants, Children and Adolescents*, chap. 41 (Baltimore: Williams and Wilkins Co.)

187. McKusick, V.A. (1972). *Op. cit.*, p. 525

188. Krovetz, L.J. and Schiebler, G.L. (1972). Cardiovascular manifestations of the genetic mucopolysaccharidoses. *Birth Defects*, **8**, 192

189. Schieken, R.M., Kerber, R.E., Ionasescu, V.V. and Zellweger, H. (1975). Cardiac manifestations of the mucopolysaccharidoses. *Circulation*, **52**, 700–5

190. Vance, P.W., Friedman, S. and Wagner, B.M. (1960). Mitral stenosis in an atypical case of gargoylism. *Circulation*, **21**, 80

191. McKusick, V.A. (1965). The genetic muco-polysaccharidoses. *Circulation*, **31**, 1

192. Henderson, J.L. (1910). Gargoylism; review of principal features with report of five cases. *Arch. Dis. Child.*, **15**, 215

193. Berkham, O. (1907). Zwei Fälle von Skapho-kephalie. *Arch. Anthrop.*, **34**, 8

194. Hunter, C. (1917). A rare disease in two brothers. *Proc. R. Soc. Med.*, **10**, 104

195. Hurler, G. (1919). Ueber einen Typ multipler Abartungen, vorwiegend am Skelettsystem. *Z. Kinderheilk.*, **24**, 220

196. Pfaundler, M. (1920). Demonstrationen über einen Typus kindlieher Dysostose. *Jahrb. Kinderheilk.*, **92**, 420

197. Brante, G. (1952). Gargoylism: a mucopolysac-charidosis. *Scand. J. Clin. Lab. Invest.*, **4**, 43

198. Brown, D.H. (1957). Tissue storage of mucopolysaccharides in Hurler-Pfaundler's disease. *Proc. Natl. Acad. Sci. USA*, **43**, 783

199. Dorfman, A. and Lorincz, A.E. (1957). Occurrence of urinary acid mucopolysac-charides in the Hurler syndrome. *Proc. Natl. Acad. Sci. USA*, **43**, 443

200. Meyer, K., Grumbach, M.M., Linker, A. and Hoffman, P. (1958). Excretion of sulfated mucopolsaccharides in gargoylism (Hurler's syndrome). *Proc. Soc. Exp. Biol. Med.*, **97**, 275

201. Danes, B.A. and Bearn, A.G. (1965). Hurler's syndrome; demonstration of an inherited disorder of connective tissue in cell culture. *Science*, **149**, 987

202. Fratantoni, J.C., Hall, C.W. and Neufeld, E.F. (1969). The defect in Hurler's and Hunter's syndromes. II. Deficiency of specific factors involved in mucopolysaccharide degradation. *Proc. Natl. Acad. Sci. USA*, **64**, 360

203. Fratantoni, J.C., Hall, C.W. and Neufeld, E.F. (1968). The defect in Hurler's and Hunter's syndromes; faulty degradation of mucopolysac-charide. *Proc. Natl. Acad. Sci. USA*, **60**, 699

204. Fratantoni, J.C., Hall, C.W. and Neufeld, E.F. (1968). Hurler and Hunter syndromes; mutual

correction of the defect in cultured fibroblasts. *Science*, **162**, 570

205. Fratantoni, J.C., Neufeld, E.F., Uhlendorf, B.W. and Jacobson, C.B. (1969). Intrauterine diagnosis of the Hurler and Hunter syndromes. *N. Engl. J. Med.*, **280**, 686

206. Van Hoof, F. and Hers, H.G. (1964). L'ultra-structure des cellules hépatiques dans la maladie de Hurler (gargoylisme). *C.R. Acad. Sci.*, **259**, 1281

207. Stetten, D. Jr and Stetten, M.R. (1960). Glycogen metabolism. *Physiol. Rev.*, **4**, 505

208. Pompe, J.C. (1932). Over idiopatische hyper-trophy van het hart. *Nederl. Tijdschr. Geneesk.*, **76**, 304

209. Di Sant'Agnese, P.A., Andersen, D.H. and Mason, H.H. (1950). Glycogen storage disease of the heart. II. Critical review of the literature. *Pediatrics*, **6**, 607

210. Di Sant'Agnese, P.A. (1959). Diseases of glycogen storage with special reference to cardiac type of generalized glycogenesis. *Ann. NY Acad. Sci.*, **72**, 439

211. Ehlers, K.H., Hagstrom, J.W.C., Lukas, D.S., Redo, S.F. and Engle, M.A. (1952). Glycogen-storage disease of the myocardium with obstruction to left ventricular outflow. *Circulation*, **25**, 96–109

212. Maron, B.J., Nichols, P.F. III, Pickle, L.W., Wesley, Y.E. and Mulvihill, J.J. (1984). Patterns of inheritance of hypertrophic cardiomyopathy. Assessment by M-mode and two-dimensional echocardiography. *Am. J. Cardiol.*, **53**, 1087

213. Schmincke, A. (1907). Über linkseitige musk-ulose Conusstenosen. *Deutsche med. Wchnschr.*, **33**, 2082

214. Davies, L.G. (1952). A familial heart disease. *Br. Heart J.*, **14**, 206

215. Braunwald, E., Lambrew, C.T., Rockoff, S.D., Ross, J. Jr and Morrow, A.G. (1964). Idiopathic hypertrophic subaortic stenosis. I A description of the disease based upon an analysis of 64 patients. *Circulation*, Suppl. IV to vols. XXIX and XXX, pp. IV–3 to IV–207

216. Addarii, F., Martini, L., Mahaim, I. and Winston, M. (1946–7). Nouvelles recherches sur le 'bloc bilateral manque.' *Cardiologia*, **11**, 36

217. Evans, W. (1949). Familial cardiomegaly. *Br. Heart J.*, **11**, 68

218. Davies, R.R., Marvel, B.J. and Genovese, P.D. (1951). Heart disease of unknown etiology. *Am. Heart J.*, **42**, 546

219. Elster, S.K., Horn, H. and Tuchman, L.R. (1955). Cardiac hypertrophy and insufficiency of unknown etiology. *Am. J. Med.*, **18**, 900

220. Serbin, R.A. and Chojnacki, B. (1955). Idiopathic cardiac hypertrophy. *N. Engl. J. Med.*, **252**, 10

221. Paulley, J.W., Jones, R., Green, W.F.D. and Kane, E.P. (1956). Myocardial toxoplasmosis. *Br. Heart J.*, **18**, 55

222. Sommers, B. (1956). Problems in the clinical diagnosis and classification of ventricular hyper-trophy in adults. III. Familial cardiomyopathy. *Minnesota Med.*, **39**, 153

223. Nikkila, E.A. and Pelkonen, R. (1959). Isolated (Fiedler's) myocarditis and idiopathic cardiac hypertrophy. *Acta Med. Scand.*, **165**, 421

224. Shah, P.M. (1957). Familial cardiomegaly: case reports with review of literature. *Indian J. Med. Sci.*, **11**, 818

225. Soulie, P., DiMatteo, J., Abaza, A., Nouaille, J. and Thibert, M.H. (1957). Cardiomegalie familiale. *Arch. Mal. Coeur*, **50**, 22

226. Kremer, R. and Delchevalerie, J. (1957). Cardiomegalie familiale avec blocs de branche. *Cardiologica*, **12**, 527

227. Facquet, J., Alhomme, P., Welth, J.J., Bonnet, J.L. and Tinturier, J. (1958). Cardiomegalie familiale apparemment benigne affectant plusiers enfants d'une nombreuse famille. *Bull. Mém. Soc. Méd. Hôp. Paris*, **74**, 80

228. Soulie, P., DiMatteo, J. and Nouaille, J. (1957). Cardiomegalie familiale. *Bull. Mém. Soc. Méd. Hôp. Paris*, **73**, 1091

229. Faivre, G., Debray, G., Gilgenkantz, J.M., Panthu, J.J. and Schwartz, G. (1958). Cardio-megalie familiale. *Rev. Méd. Nancy*, **83**, 1075–93

230. Brigden, W. (1957). Uncommon myocardial diseases – the non-coronary cardiomyopathies. *Lancet*, **273**, 1179, 1243

231. Teare, D. (1958). Asymmetrical hypertrophy of the heart in young adults. *Br. Heart J.*, **20**, 1

232. Bercu, B.A., Diettert, G.A., Danforth, W.H., Pund, E.E., Ahlvin, R.C. and Belliveau, R. (1958). Pseudoaortic stenosis produced by ventricular hypertyrophy. *Am. J. Med.*, **25**, 814

233. Brent, L.B., Fisher, D.L. and Taylor, W.J. (1959). Familial muscular subaortic stenosis. (Abst.) *Circulation*, **20**, 676

234. Brachfeld, N. and Gorlin, R. (1959). Subaortic stenosis: a revised concept of the disease, *Medicine*, **38**, 415, 32 & 33 (old 21 & 22)

235. Braunwald, E., Morrow, A.C., Cornell, W.F., Avgen, M.M. and Kilbish, T.F. (1960). Idiopathic hypertrophic subaortic stenosis;

clinical, hemodynamic and angiographic manifestations. *Am. J. Med.*, **29**, 924

236. Morrow, A.G. and Braunwald, E. (1959). Functional aortic stenosis; a malformation characterized by resistance to left ventricular outflow without anatomic obstruction. *Circulation*, **20**, 181

237. Goodwin, J.F., Hollman, A., Cleland, W.P. and Teare, D. (1960). Obstructive cardiomyopathy simulating aortic stenosis. *Br. Heart J.*, **22**, 403

238. Brock, R.C. (1957). Functional obstruction of the left ventricle. *Guy's Hosp. Rep.*, **106**, 221

239. Greenberg, J. and Simon, M.A. (1949). Subaortic stenosis in an adult. *Can. M.A.J.*, **61**, 50

240. Averill, J.H., Randall, R.V., Joffe, E. and White, P.D. (1957). Heart disease of unknown cause in siblings. *Ann. Intern. Med.*, **47**, 49

241. Paré, J.A.P., Fraser, R.G., Pirozynski, W.J., Shanks, J.A. and Stubington, D. (1961). Hereditary cardiovascular dysplasia. *Am. J. Med.*, **31**, 37–61

242. Frere Eloi-Gerard (1949). *Genealogies des Familles de Beauce, Dorchester et Frontenae*, vol. 1, Beauceville, Quebec, L'Eclaireur

243. Horlick, L., Petkovich, N.J. and Bolton, C.F. (1966). Idiopathic hypertrophic subvalvular stenosis. A study of a family involving four generations. Clinical, hemodynamic and pathologic observations. *Am. J. Cardiol.*, **17**, 411–18

244. Nasser, W.K., Williams, J.F., Mishkin, M.E., Childress, R.H., Helmen, C., Merritt, A.D. and Genovese, P.D. (1967). Familial myocardial disease with and without obstruction to left ventricular outflow: clinical, hemodynamic and angiographic findings. *Circulation*, **35**, 638–52

245. Jorgensen, G. (1968). Genetische Untersuchungen bei funktionell-obstruktiver subvalvulaerer Aortenstenose (irregulaer hypertrophische Kardiomyopathie). *Humangenetik*, **6**, 13–28

246. Henry, W.L., Clark, C.E. and Epstein, S.E. (1973). Asymmetric septal hypertrophy (ASH): the unifying link in the IHSS disease spectrum – observations regarding its pathogenesis, pathophysiology and course. *Circulation*, **47**, 827–32

247. Henry, W.L., Clark, C.E. and Epstein, S.E. (1973). Asymmetric septal hypertrophy; echocardiographic identification of the pathognomonic anatomic abnormality of IHSS. *Circulation*, **47**, 225–33

248. Clark, C.E., Henry, W.L. and Epstein, S.E. (1973). Familial prevalance and genetic transmission of idiopathic hypertrophic subaortic stenosis. *N. Engl. J. Med.*, **289**, 709–14

249. Maron, B.J., Edwards, J.E., Henry, W.L., Clark, C.E., Bingle, G.J. and Epstein, S.E. (1974). Asymmetric septal hypertrophy (ASH) in infancy. *Circulation*, **50**, 809–20

250. Maron, B.J., Henry, W.L., Clark, C.E., Redwood, D.R., Roberts, W.C. and Epstein, S.E. (1976). Asymmetric septal hypertrophy in childhood. *Circulation*, **53**, 9–19

251. Darsee, J.R., Heymsfield, S.B. and Nutter, D.O. (1979). Hypertrophic cardiomyopathy and human leukocyte antigen linkage: differentiation of two forms of hypertrophic cardiomyopathy. *N. Engl. J. Med.*, **300**, 877–82

252. McKusick, V.A. (1972). *Op. cit.*, p. 531

253. Boyd, D.L., Mishkin, M.E., Feigenbaum, H. and Genovese, P.D. (1965). Three families with familial cardiomyopathy. *Ann. Intern. Med.*, **63**, 386–401

254. Brigden, W. (1957). Uncommon myocardial disease: the non-coronary cardiomyopathies. *Lancet*, **2**, 1243

255. Garrett, G., Hay, W.J. and Rickards, A.G. (1959). Familial cardiomegaly. *J. Clin. Path.*, **12**, 355

256. Bishop, J.M., Campbell, M. and Jones, E.W. (1962). Cardiomyopathy in four members of a family. *Br. Heart J.*, **24**, 715

257. Barry, M. and Hall, M. Familial cardiomyopathy. *Ibid.*, p. 613

258. Battersby, E.J. and Glenner, G.G. (1961). Familial cardiomyopathy. *Am. J. Med.*, **30**, 382

259. Taylor, W.J. (1983). Genetic aspects of the cardiomyopathies. *Prog. Med. Genet.*, **5**, 163–89

260. Yamaguchi, M. and Toshima, H. (1980). A genetic analysis of idiopathic cardiomyopathies in Japan. In Sekiguchi, M. and Olsen, E.G.J. (eds.) *Cardiomyopathy: Clinical, Pathological, and Theoretical Aspects*, pp. 421–8. (Baltimore: University Park Press)

261. Berko, B.A. and Swift, M. (1987). X-linked dilated cardiomyopathy. *N. Engl. J. Med.*, **316**, 1186–91

262. Csanady, S. and Szasz, K. (1976). Familial cardiomyopathy. *Cardiology*, **61**, 122–30

263. Sheldon, J.H. (1934). Haemochromatosis. *Lancet*, **2**, 1031

264. Sheldon, J.H. (1935). *Haemochromatosis.* (London: Oxford Univ. Press)

265. MacDonald, R.A. (1966). Idiopathic hemochromatosis. Acquired or inherited? In Ingelfinger, E.J., Relman, A.S, and Finland, M. (eds.) *Controversy in Internal Medicine*, pp.271–84. (Philadelphia: Saunders)

266. Neel, J.V. and Schull, W.J. (1954). Human

Heredity, p.164. (Chicago: Univ. of Chicago Press)

267. Finch, S.C. and Finch, C.A. (1955). Idiopathic hemochromatosis, an iron storage disease. *Medicine* (Baltimore), **34**, 381–430

268. Johnson, G.B. Jr and Frey, W.G. III (1962). Familial aspects of idiopathic hemochromatosis. *J. Am. Med. Assoc.*, **179**, 747–51

269. Balcerzak, S.P. *et al.* (1966). Idiopathic hemochromatosis: a study of three families. *Am. J. Med.*, **40**, 857–73

270. Sinniah, R. (1969). Environmental and genetic factors in idiopathic hemochromatosis. *Arch. Intern. Med.*, **124**, 455–60

271. Schapira, G., *et al.* (1962). Hypersidérémie et surcharge ferrique hépatique chez les descendants d'hémochromatosiques. *Rev. Fr. Clin. Biol.*, **7**, 485–91

272. Mendel, G.A. (1964). Iron metabolism and etiology of iron-storage disease: an interpretive formulation. *J. Am. Med. Assoc.*, **189**, 45–53

273. Powell, L.W. (1965). Iron storage in relatives of patients with hemochromatosis and in relatives of patients with alcoholic cirrhosis and haemosiderosis. *Q. J. Med.*, **34**, 427–42

274. Charlton, R.W., Abrahams, C. and Bothwell, T.H. (1967). Idiopathic hemochromatosis in young subjects: clinical, pathological, and chemical findings in four patients. *Arch. Pathol.*, **83**, 132–40

275. Crosby, W.H. (1977). Hemochromatosis: the unsolved problems. *Seminars in Hematology,* Vol. XIV, No. 2., pp.135–43

276. Crosby, W.H. (1966) Heredity of hemochromatosis. In Ingelfinger, F.J., Relman, A.S. and Finland, M. (eds.) *Controversy in Internal Medicine*, pp.261–70. (Philadelphia: Saunders)

277. Saddi, R. and Feingold, J. Hémochromatose idiopathique: maladie récessive autosomique. *Rev. Fr. Clin.*

278. Scheinberg, I.H. (1973). The genetics of hemochromatosis. *Arch. Intern. Med.*, **132**, 126–8

279. Harris, H. (1970). *The Principles of Human Biochemical Genetics*, pp. 251–3. (New York: American Elsevier Publishing Co.)

280. Williams, R., Scheuer, P.J. and Sherlock, S. (1962). Inheritance of idiopathic haemochromatosis: clinical and liver biopsy study of 16 families. *Q. J. Med.*, 31, 249–65

281. Bothwell, T.H., Charlton, R.W. and Motulsky, A.G. (1983). Idiopathic hemochromatosis. In Stanbury, J.B., Wyngaarden, J.B., Frederickson,

D.S., Goldstein, J.L. and Brown, M.S. (eds.) *The Metabolic Basis of Inherited Disease,* 5th edn., p.1269. (New York: McGraw-Hill Book Co.)

282. Simon, M., Alexaandre, J.L., Rauchet, R., Genetet, B. and Bourel, M. (1980). The genetics of hemochromatosis. *Prog. Med. Genet.*, **4**(new series), 135

283. Schwartz, P. (1970). *Amyloidosis: Cause and Manifestation of Senile Deterioration.* (Springfield, Illinois: Charles C. Thomas)

284. Reimann, H.A., Koucky, R.F. and Eklund, C.M. (1935). Primary amyloidosis limited to tissue of mesodermal origin. *Am. J. Pathol.*, **11**, 977

285. Kyle, R.A. and Bayrd, E.D. (1975). Amyloidosis: review of 236 cases. *Medicine*, **54**, 271–98

286. Wilks, A. (1856). Cases of lardaceous disease and some allied affections: with remarks. *Guy's Hosp. Rep. Ser. 3*, **2**, 103

287. Wild, C. (1886). Beitrag zur Kenntnis der amyloiden und der hyalinen Degeneration des Bindegewebes. *Beitr. Pathol. Anat.*, **1**, 175

288. Ostertag, B. (1932). Demonstration einer eigenartigen familiären 'Paraamyloidose.' *Zentrabl. Path.*, **56**, 253

289. Ostertag, B. (1950). Familiäre Amyloid-Erkrankung. *Ztschr. menschl. Vererb. Konstitutionslehre.*, **30**, 105

290. Maxwell, E.S. and Kimbell, I. (1936). Familial amyloidosis, with case reports. *M. Bull. V.A.*, **12**, 365

291. Andrade, C.A. (1952). Peculiar form of peripheral neuropathy. *Brain*, **75**, 408

292. Da Silva Horta, J. (1956). Pathologische Anatomie der portugiesischen Paramyloidosenfälle mit besonderer Bevorzugung des peripheren Nerven-systems. *Gaz. Méd. Portug.*, **9**, 678

293. Rukavina, J.G., Block, W.D., Jackson, C.E., Falls, H.F., Carey, J.H. and Curtis, A.C. (1956). Primary systemic amyloidosis: a review and an experimental, genetic, and clinical study of 29 cases with particular emphasis on the familial form. *Medicine* (Baltimore), **35**, 239

294. Mahloudji, M., Teasdall, R.D., Adamkiewiez, J.J., Hartmann, W.H., Lambird, P.A. and McKusick, V.A. (1969). The genetic amyloidoses: with particular reference to hereditary neuropathic amyloidosis, type II (Indiana or Rukavina type). *Medicine* (Baltimore), **48**, 1

295. Eisen, H.N. (1946). Primary systemic amyloidosis. *Am. J. Med.*, **1**, 144

296. Lindsay, S. (1948). The heart in primary

systemic amyloid disease. *Med. Cone. Cardiovase. Dis.*, **17**, 6

297. Wessler, S. and Freedberg, A.S. (1948). Cardiac amyloidosis: electrocardiographic and pathologic observations. *Arch. Intern. Med.*, **82**, 63

298. Josselson, A.J. and Pruitt, R.D. (1953). Electrocardiographic findings in cardiac amyloidosis. *Circulation*, **7**, 200

299. Bernreiter, M. (1958). Cardiac amyloidosis. Electrocardiographic findings. *Am. J. Cardiol.*, **1**, 644

300. Fisher, D.L., Campbell, J.A., Baker, L. and Vawter, G. (1950). Hemodynamic studies in a case of primary amyloidosis. *J. Lab. Clin. Med.*, **36**, 821

301. Hetzel, P.S., Wood, E.H. and Burchell, H.B. (1953). Pressure pulses in the right side of the heart in a case of amyloid disease and in a case of idiopathic heart failure simulating constrictive pericarditis. *Proc. Staff Meet. Mayo Clin.*, **28**, 107

302. Gunnar, R.M., Dillon, R.F., Wallyn, R.J. and Elisberg, E.I. (1955). The physiologic and clinical similarity between primary amyloid of the heart and constrictive pericarditis. *Circulation*, **12**, 827

303. Himbert, J. (1959). Deux nouvelles observations anatomocliniques et hémodynamiques d'amylose cardiaque primitive. *Arch. Mal. Coeur*, **2**, 1020

304. Frederiksen, T., Gøtsche, H. and Harboe, N. (1962). Familial primary amyloidosis with severe amyloid heart disease. *Am. J. Med.*, **33**, 328–48

305. Hawley, R.H., Gottdiener, J.S., Gay, J.A. and Engel, W.K. (1983). Families with myotonic dystrophy with and without cardiac involvement. *Arch. Intern. Med.*, **143**, 2134–6

306. Mohr, J. (1954). *A Study of Linkage in Man.* (Copenhagen: Munksgaard)

307. Thomasen, E. (1948). Myotonia. Aahrus. Universitetsforlaget

308. Renwick, J.H., Bundey, S.E., Ferguson-Smith, M.A. and Izatt, M.M. (1971). Confirmation of linkage of the loci for myotonic dystrophy and ABH secretion. *J. Med. Genet.*, **8**, 407–16

309. Harper, P.S., Rivas, M.L., Bias, W.B., Hutchinson, J.R., Dyken, P.R. and McKusick, V.A. (1972). Genetic linkage confirmed between the locus for myotonic dystrophy and the ABH-secretion and the Lutheran blood group loci. *Am. J. Hum. Genet.*, **24**, 310–16

310. Eiberg, H., Mohr, J., Nielsen, L.S. and Simonsen, N. (1983). Genetics and linkage relationships of the C3 polymorphism: discovery of the C3-Se linkage and assignment of LES-C3-DM-SePEPD-Lu synteny to chromosome 19. *Clin. Genet.*, **24**, 159–70

311. Whitehead, A.S., Solomon, F., Chambers, S., Bodmer, W.F., Povey, S. and Fey, G. (1982). Assignment of the structural gene for the third component of human complement to chromosome 19. *Proc. Natl. Acad. Sci. USA*, **79**, 5021–5

312. Swift, M.R. and Finegold, M.J. (1969). Myotonic muscular dystrophy: abnormalities in fibroblast culture. *Science*, **165**, 294–6

313. Schott, J., Jacobi, M. and Wald, M.A. (1955). Electrocardiographic patterns in the differential diagnosis of progressive muscular dystrophy. *Am. J. Med. Sci.*, **229**, 517

314. Gailani, A., Danowski, T.S. and Fisher, D.C. (1958). Muscular dystrophy. *Circulation*, **17**, 583

315. Manning, G.W. and Cropp, C.J. (1958). The electrocardiogram in progressive muscular dystrophy. *Br. Heart J.*, **20**, 416

316. Skiring, A. and McKusick, V.A. (1961). Clinical, genetic and electrocardiographic studies in childhood muscular dystrophy. *Am. J. Med. Sci.*, **242**, 54

317. Gilroy, J., Cahalan, J.L., Berman, K. and Newman, M. (1963). Cardiac and pulmonary complications in Duchenne's progressive muscular dystrophy. *Circulation*, **27**, 484

318. Welsh, J.D., Lynn, T.N. and Naase, G.R. (1963). Cardiac findings in 73 patients with muscular dystrophy. *Arch. Intern. Med.*, **112**, 199

319. Perloff, J.K., DeLeon, A.C. and O'Doherty, D. (1966). The cardiomyopathy of progressive muscular dystrophy. *Circulation*, **33**, 625

320. Perloff, J.K., Roberts, W.C., DeLeon, A.C, Jr and O'Doherty, D. (1967). The distinctive electrocardiogram of Duchenne's progressive muscular dystrophy. *Am. J. Med.*, **42**, 179–88

321. James, T.N. (1962). Observations on the cardiovascular involvment, including the cardiac conduction system, in progressive muscular dystrophy. *Am. Heart J.*, **63**, 48

322. Rossi, L. and James, T.N. (1964). Neurovascular pathology of the heart in progressive muscular dystrophy. *Panminerva Med.*, **6**, 357

323. Friedreich, N. (1863). Über degenerative Atrophie der spinalen Hinterstränge. *Arch. Path. Anat.*, **26**, 391, 433

324. Pitt, G.N. (1886–7). On a case of Friedreich's disease. Its clinical history and postmortem appearances. *Guy's Hosp. Rep.*, **44**, 369

325. Saury, L. (1905). *Le coeur dans la maladie de*

Friedreich. (Lyon: Thèse Méd.)

326. Mollaret, P. (1929). *La maladie de Friedrich*. Thèse de Paris

327. Loiseau, J. (1938). *Les troubles cardiaques dans la maladie de Friedreich*. (Paris: Thèse Méd.)

328. Evans, W. and Wright, G. (1942). The electrocardiogram in Friedreich's disease. *Br. Heart J.*, **4**, 91

329. Hejtmancik, M.R., Bradfield, J.Y. Jr and Miller, G.V. (1949). Myocarditis and Friedreich's ataxia. A report of two cases. *Am. Heart J.*, **38**, 757

330. Manning, G.W. (1950). Cardiac manifestations in Friedreich's ataxia. *Am. Heart J.*, **39**, 799

331. Lorenz, T.H., Kurtz, C.M. and Shapiro, H.H. (1950). Cardiopathy in Friedreich's ataxia (spinal form of hereditary sclerosis). Review of literature and analysis of cases in five siblings. *Arch. Intern. Med.*, **86**, 412

332. Nadas, A.S., Alimurung, M.M. and Sieracki, L.A. (1951). Cardiac manifestations of Friedreich's ataxia. *N. Engl. J. Med.*, **244**, 239

333. Schilero, A.J., Antzis, E. and Dunn, J. (1952). Friedreich's ataxia and its cardiac manifestations. *Am. Heart J.*, **44**, 805

334. Novick, R., Adams, P. Jr and Anderson, R.C. (1955). Cardiac manifestations of Friedreich's ataxia in children. *Lancet*, **75**, 62

335. Russell, D.S. (1946). Myocarditis in Friedreich's ataxia. *J. Path. Bact.*, **58**, 739

336. Ellwood, W.W. (1948). Friedreich's ataxia with unusual heart complications. *California Med.*, **68**, 296

337. Robinson, B.H., Sherwood, W.G., Kahler, S., O'Flynn, M.E. and Nadler, H. (1981). Lipoamide dehydrogenase deficiency. (Letter) *N. Engl. J. Med.*, **304**, 53–4

338. Boyer, S.H., Chisholm, A.W. and McKusick, V.A. (1962). Cardiac aspects in Friedreich's ataxia. *Circulation*, **25**, 493–505

339. Bell, J. and Carmichael, E.A. (1939). On hereditary ataxia and spastic paraplegia. *Treasury of Human Inheritance*, **4**, 41. (London: Cambridge Press)

340. Leers, H. and Scholz, E. (1939). Korrelations pathologische Untersuchungen. 2. Die erbliche Ataxie. *Ztschr. menschl. Vererb.-u. Konstitutionslehre*, **22**, 703

341. Hewer, R.L. (1968). Study of fatal cases of Friedreich's ataxia. *Br. Med. J.*, **3**, 649–52

342. Elias, G. (1972). Muscular subaortic stenosis and Friedreich's ataxia. *Am. Heart J.*, **84**, 843

343. Ackroyd, R.S., Finnegan, J.A. and Green, S.H. (1984). Friedreich's ataxia: a clinical review with neurophysiological and echocardiographic findings. *Arch. Dis. Child.*, **59**, 217–21

344. Winter, R.M., Harding, A.W., Baraitser, M. and Bravery, M.B. (1981). Intrafamilial correlation in Friedreich's ataxia. *Clin. Genet.*, **20**, 419–27

345. Chamberlain, S., Worrall, C.S., South, S., Shaw, J., Farrall, M. and Williamson, R. (1987). Exclusion of the Friedreich ataxia gene from chromosome 19. *Hum. Genet.*, **76**, 186–90

346. Weinberg, T. and Himelfarb, A.J. (1943). Endocardial fibroelastosis (so-called foetal endocarditis): a report of two cases occurring in siblings. *Bull. Johns Hopkins Hospital*, **72**, 299

347. Gowing, N.F.C. (1953). Congenital fibroelastosis of the endocardium. *J. Pathol. Bacteriol.*, **65**, 13

348. Andersen, D.H. and Kelly, J. (1956). Endocardial fibroelastosis. I. Endocardial fibroelastosis associated with congenital malformations of the heart. *Pediatrics*, **18**, 513

349. Dordick, J.R. (1951). Diffuse endocardial fibrosis and cardiac hypertrophy in infancy; report of two cases in consecutive siblings. *Am. J. Clin. Pathol.*, **21**, 743

350. Axtrup, S. (1954). Proceedings of the Pediatric Society of South Sweden, Meeting, Nov. 8, 1953, *Acta Pædiat (Upps.)*, **43**, 501

351. Tulczynska, H. (1957). Elastic fibrosis of endocardium in brother and sister (in Polish). *Pol. Tyg. Lek.*, **12**, 1039

352. Nadas, A. (1957). *Pediatric Cardiology*. (Philadelphia: W. B. Saunders Company)

353. Winter, S.T., Moses, W.S., Cohen, N.J. and Naftalin, J.M. (1960). Primary endocardial fibroelastosis in two sisters. *Am. J. Dis. Child.*, **99**, 529

354. Vestermark, S. (1962). Primary endocardial fibroelastosis in siblings. *Acta Paediatrica*, **51**, 94

355. Forfar, J.O., Miller, R.A., Bain, A.D. and Macleod, W. (1964). Endocardial fibroelastosis. *Br. Med. J.*, **2**, 7

356. Sellers, F.J., Keith, J.D. and Manning, J.A. (1964). The diagnosis of primary endocardial fibroelastosis. *Circulation*, **29**, 49

357. Hunter, A.S. and Keay, A.J. (1973). Primary endocardial fibroelastosis. An inherited condition. *Arch. Dis. Child.*, **48**, 66–9

358. Westwood, M., Harris, R., Burn, J.L. and Barson, A.J. (1975). Heredity in primary endocardial fibroelastosis. *Br. Heart J.*, **37**, 1077–84

359. Olsen, E.G.A. (1975). Pathological recognition

of cardiomyopathy. *Posgrad. Med. J.*, **51**, 277–281

360. Peters, T.J., Wells, G., Oakley, C.M. *et al.* (1977). Enzymatic analysis of endomyocardial biopsy specimens from patients with cardiomyopathies. *Br. Heart J.*, **39**, 1333–9

361. Tripp, M.E., Katcher, M.L., Peters, H.A. *et al.* (1981). Systemic carnitine deficiency presenting as familial endocardial fibroelastosis. A treatable cardiomyopathy. *N. Engl. J. Med.*, **305**, 385–90

362. Engel, A.G. and Angelini, C. (1973). Carnitine deficiency of human skeletal muscle with associated lipid storage myopathy: a new syndrome. *Science*, **179**, 899–902

363. Perheentupa, J., Autio, S., Leisti, S. and Raitta, C. (1970). Mulibrey nanism: dwarfism with muscle, liver, brain and eye involvement. *Acta Paediatr. Scand.*, **59**, 74

364. Perheentupa, J., Autio, S., Leisti, S., Raitta, C. and Tuuteri, L. (1973). Mulibrey nanism, an autosomal recessive syndrome with pericardial constriction. *Lancet*, **2**, 351

365. Tuuteri, L., Perheentupa, J. and Rapola, J. (1974). The cardiopathy of mulibrey nanism, a new inherited syndrome. *Chest*, **65**, 628

366. Voorhees, M.L., Husson, G.S. and Blackman, M.S. (1973). Growth failure with pericardial constriction. *Am. J. Dis. Child.*, **130**, 1146

367. Krause, S., Adler, L.N., Reddy, P.S. and Magovern, G.J. (1971). Intracardiac myxoma in siblings. *Chest*, **60**, 404–6

368. Heydorn, W.H., Gomez, A.C., Kleid, J.J. and Haas, J.J. (1973). Atrial myxoma in siblings. *J. Thorac. Cardiovasc. Surg.*, **65**, 484–6

369. Kleid, J.M., Klugman, J., Haas, J.M. and Battock, D. (1973). Familial atrial myxoma. *Am. J. Cardiol.*, **32**, 361–4

370. Farah, M.G. (1975). Familial atrial myxoma. *Ann. Intern. Med.*, **83**, 358–60

371. Siltanen, P., Tuuteri, L., Norio, R., Tala, P., Ahrenberg, P. and Halonen, P.I. (1976). Atrial myxoma in a family. *Am. J. Cardiol.*, **38**, 252–6

372. Powers, J.C., Falkoff, M., Heinle, R.A., Nanda, N.C., Ong, L.S., Weiner, R.S. and Barold, S.S. (1979). Familial cardiac myxoma; emphasis on unusual clinical manifestations. *J. Thorac. Cardiovasc. Surg.*, **77**, 782–8

373. Tshrakides, V., Burke, B., Mastri, A. *et al.* (1974). Rhabdomyomas of heart. *Am. J. Dis. Child.*, **128**, 639

374. Nevin, N.C. and Pearce, W.G. (1968). Diagnostic and genetical aspects of tuberous sclerosis. *J. Med. Genet.*, **5**, 273

375. McKusick, V.A. (1988). *Mendelian Inheritance in Man*, 8th edn., p. 1095. (Baltimore: Johns Hopkins Univ. Press)

376. Sherlock, E.B. (1911). *The Feeble-minded.* (London: Macmillan & Co.)

377. von Recklinghausen, F. (1862). Monats. *Geburtskunde*, **20**, 1

378. Virchow, R. (1864–65). *Die krankhaften Geschwulste*, **2**, 148

379. Bourneville, D.M. (1880). Sclerose tubereuse des circonvolutions cerebrales, idiotie et epilepsie hemiplegique. *Arch. Neurol.*, **1**, 81

380. Bourneville, D.M. (1880). Contribution a l'etude de l'idiotie; idiotie et epilepsie hemiplegique. *Arch. de Neurol.*, **1**, 81

381. Hartdegen, A. (1881). Ein Fall von multipler Verhaertung des Grosshirns nebst histologisch eigenartigen harten Geschwuelsten der seitenventrikel (Glioma gangliocellulare) bei einem Neugeborenen. *Arch. F. Psychiat.*, **11**, 117

382. De la Cruz, F.F. and La Veck, G. (1962). Tuberous sclerosis: a review and report of eight cases. *Am. J. Ment. Defic.*, **67**, 369–80

383. Bielschowsky, M. and Bielschowsky, G. (1913). Ueber tuberoese Sklerose. *J. F. Psychiat. Neurol.*, **20**, 1

384. Alzheimer. (1907). Die Gruppierung der Epilepsie. *Allg. Sellforsch. Psychiat.*

385. Bouwdijk-Bastiaanse. (1922). Eine familiaere Form tuberoeser Sklerose. *Nederl. Tijdsch. Geneesk.*, **66**, 248

386. Feriz, H. (1930). Ein Beitrag zur Histopathologie der tuberoesen sklerose. *Arch. Path. Anat.*, **278**, 690

387. Berg, H. (1913). Vererbung der tuberosen sklerose durch 2–3 generationen. *Ztschr. Ges. Neurol. & Psychiat.*, **19**, 528

388. Gunther, M. and Penrose, L. (1935). Genetics of epiloia. *J. Genet.*, **31**, 413–30

389. Penrose, L.S. (1954). *The Biology of Mental Defect.* (London: Sidgwick & Jackson Limited)

390. Marshall, D., Saul, G.B. and Sachs, E. Jr (1959). Tuberous sclerosis. A report of 16 cases in two family trees revealing genetic dominance. *N. Engl. J. Med.*, **261**, 22, 1102–5

391. Sybert, V.P. and Hall, J.G. (1979). Inheritance of tuberous sclerosis. (Letter) *Lancet*, **1**, 783

392. Gomez, M.R. (1979). *Tuberous Sclerosis.* (New York: Raven Press)

393. Kandt, R.S., Gebarski, S.S. and Goetting, M.G. (1985). Tuberous sclerosis with cardiogenic cerebral embolism: magnetic resonance imaging. *Neurology*, **35**, 1223–5

394. Journel, H., Roussey, M., Plais, M.H., Milon, J., Almange, C. and Le Marec, B. (1986). Prenatal diagnosis of familial tuberous sclerosis following detection of cardiac rhabdomyoma by ultrasound. *Prenatal Diagnosis*, **6**, 283–9

395. Smith, M., Haines, J., Trofatter, J., Dumars, K., Pandolfo, M. and Conneally, M. (1987). Linkage studies in tuberous sclerosis. (Abstract) *Am. J. Hum. Genet.*, **41**, A186

396. Goldstein, J.L., Schrott, H.G., Hazzard, W.R., Bierman, E.L. and Motulsky, A.G. (1973). Hyperlipidemia in coronary heart disease. II Genetic analysis of lipid levels in 176 families, and delineation of a new inherited disorder, combined hyperlipidemia. *J. Clin. Invest.*, **52**, 1544

397. Duncan, C. and McLeod, G.M. (1970). Angiokeratoma corporis diffusum universale (Fabry's disease). *Aust. Ann. Med.*, **1**, 58

398. Becker, A.E., Schoorl, R., Balk, A.G. and van der Heidl, R.M. (1975). Cardiac manifestations of Fabry's disease. *Am. J. Cardiol.*, **36**, 829

399. Brown, M.S. and Goldstein, J.L. (1986). A receptor-mediated pathway for cholesterol homeostasis. *Science*, **232**, 34

400. Goldstein, J.L. and Brown, M.S. (1983). Familial hypercholesterolemia. In Stanbury, J.B., Wyngaarden, J.B., Frederickson, D.S., Goldstein, J.L. and Brown, M.S. (eds.) *The Metabolic Basis of Inherited Disease*, 5th edn., p. 672. (New York: McGraw Hill Book Co.)

401. Slack, J. (1969). Risks of ischemic heart disease in familial hyperlipoproteinemic states. *Lancet*, **2**, 1380

402. Jensen, J., Blankenhorn, D.H. and Kornerup, V. (1967). Coronary disease in familial hypercholesterolemia. *Circulation*, **36**, 77

403. Goldstein, J.L. (1972). The cardiac manifestations of the homozygous and heterozygous forms of familial type II hyperbetalipoproteinemia. *Birth Defects. Original Article Series*, **8**, 202

404. Sprecker, D.L., Schaefer, E.S., Kent, K.M. *et al.* (1984). Cardiovascular features of homozygous familial hypercholesterolemia. Analysis of 16 patients. *Am. J. Cardiol.*, **54**, 20

405. Fogge, C.H. (1872). General xanthelasma or vitiligoidea. *Trans. Pathol. Soc.*, London, **24**, 242

406. Fox, T.C. (1879). A case of xanthelasma multiplex. *Lancet*, **2**, 688

407. Poensgen, A. (1883). Mittheilung eines seltenen Falles von Xanthelasma multiplex. *Arch. Pathol. Anat. Physiol.*, **91**, 350

408. Lehzen, G. and Knauss, K. (1889). Ueber Xanthoma multiplex planum, tuberosum, mollusciforme. *Arch. Pathol., Anat. Phisiol.*, **116**, 85

409. Muller, C. (1938). Xanthomata, hypercholesterolemia, angina pectoris. *Acta. Med. Scand. (Suppl.)*, **89**, 75

410. Mueller, C. (1939). Angina pectoris in hereditary xanthomatosis. *Arch. Intern. Med.*, **64**, 675

411. Thannhauser, S.J. and Magendantz, H. (1938). The different clinical groups of xanthomatous disease: a clinical physiological study of 22 cases. *Ann. Intern. Med.*, **11**, 1662

412. Thannhauser, S.J. (1950). *Lipoidoses*. (New York: Oxford Univ. Press)

413. Wilkinson, C.F., Hand, E.A. and Fliegelman, M.T. (1948). Essential familial hypercholesterolemia. *Ann. Intern. Med.*, **29**, 671

414. Wilkinson, C.F. (1950). Essential familial hypercholesterolemia: cutaneous, metabolic and hereditary aspects. *Bull. NY Acad. Med.*, **26**, 670

415. Adlersberg, D. (1955). Inborn errors of lipid metabolism. *Arch. Pathol.*, **60**, 481

416. Bloom, D., Kaufman, S.R. and Stevens, R.A. (1942). Hereditary xanthomatosis: familial incidence of xanthoma tuberosum associated with hypercholesterolemia and cardiovascular involvement with report of several cases of sudden death. *Arch. Derm. Syph.*, **45**, 1

417. Epstein, F.H., Block, W.D., Hand, E.A. and Francis, T. Jr (1959). Familial hypercholesterolemia, xanthomatosis and coronary heart disease. *Am. J. Med.*, **26**, 39

418. Khachadurian, A.K. (1964). The inheritance of essential familial hypercholesterolemia. *Am. J. Med.*, **37**, 402

419. Gofman, J.W., DeLalla, O., Glazier, F., Freeman, N.K., Lindgren, F.T., Nicholas, A.V., Strishower, E.H. and Tamplin, A.R. (1954). The serum lipoprotein transport system in health, metabolic disorders, atherosclerosis and coronary artery disease. *Plasma*, **2**, 413

420. Gofman, J.W., Rubin, L., McGinley, J.P. and Jones, H.B. (1954). Hyperlipoproteinemia. *Am. J. Med.*, **17**, 514

421. Frederickson, D.S., Levy, R.I. and Less, R.S. (1967). Fat transport in lipoproteins – an integrated approach to mechanisms and disorders. *N. Engl. J. Med.*, **276**, 32, 94, 148, 215, 273

422. Bailey, J.M. (1973). In Porter, R. and Knight, J. (eds.) *Atherogenesis. Initiating Factors, Ciba Foundation Symposium*, vol. 12, pp. 63–92. (Amsterdam: Elsevier)

423. Rothblat, G.H. (1969). *Adv. Lipid Res.*, **7**, 135

424. Neufeld, E.F. and Fratantoni, J.C. (1970). *Science*, **169**, 141

425. Goldstein, J.L. and Brown, M.S. (1973). *Proc. Natl. Acad. Sci. USA*, **70**, 2804

426. *Ibid.* (1974). **71**, 788

427. Kita, T. *et al.* (1982). *Proc. Natl. Acad. Sci. USA*, **79**, 3623

428. Müller, C. (1938). *Acta Med. Scand. (Suppl.)*, **89**, 75

429. Neufeld, H.N. and Goldbourt, U. (1983). Coronary heart disease: genetic aspects. *Circulation*, **67**, 943

430. Havel, R.J. (ed.) (1982). Symposium on lipid disorders. *Med. Clin. North Am.*, **66**, pp. 317–550

431. Chait, A. and Brunzell, J.D. (1983). Severe hypertriglyceridemia: role of familial and acquired disorders. *Metabolism*, **32**, 209

432. Namboodiri, K.K., Elston, R.C. and Hames, C. (1977). Segregation and linkage analyses of a large pedigree with hypertriglyceridemia. *Am. J. Med. Genet.*, **I**, 157–71

433. Goldstein, J.L., Schrott, H.G., Hazzard, W.R., Bierman, E.L. and Motulsky, A.G. (1973). Hyperlipidemia in coronary heart disease. Genetic analysis of lipid levels in 176 families and delineation of a new inherited disorder, combined hyperlipidemia. *J. Clin. Invest.*, **52**, 1544–68

434. Brunzell, J.D., Hazzard, W.R., Motulsky, A.G. and Bierman, E.L. (1975). Evidence for diabetes mellitus and genetic forms of hypertriglyceridemia as independent entities. *Metabolism*, **24**, 1115–21

435. Fredrickson, D.S. and Levy, R.I. (1972). Familial hyperlipoproteinemias. In Stanbury, J.B., Wyngaarden, J.B. and Fredreickson, D.S. (eds.) *The Metabolic Basis of Inherited Disease*, 3rd edn. (New York: McGraw-Hill Book Co.)

436. Breckenridge, W.C., Little, J.A., Steiner, G., Chow, A. and Poapst, M. (1978). Hypertriglyceridemia associated with deficiency of apolipoprotein C-II. *N. Engl. J. Med.*, **289**, 1265–73

437. Karathanasis, S.K., McPherson, J., Zannis, V.I. and Breslow, J.L. (1983). Linkage of human apolipoproteins A-I and C-III genes. *Nature (London)*, **304**, 371–3

438. Rees, A., Schoulders, C.C., Stocks, J., Galton, D.J. and Baralle, F.E. (1983). DNA polymorphism adjacent to human apoprotein A-I gene: relation to hypertriglyceridaemia. *Lancet*, **1**, 444–6

439. Havel, R.J., Golstein, J.L. and Brown, M.S. (1980). Lipoproteins and lipid transport. In Boudy, P.K. and Rosenberg, L.E. (eds.) *Diseases of Metabolism*, 8th edn., p. 393. (Philadelphia: W.B. Saunders Co.)

440. Brown, M.S., Goldstein, J.L. and Fredrickson, D.S. (1983). Familial type 3 hypercholestorelemia (dysbetalipoproteinemia). In Stanbury, J.B., Wyngaarden, J.B., Fredrickson, D.S., Goldstein, J.L. and Brown, M.S. (eds.) *The Metabolic Basis of Inherited Disease*, 5th edn., p. 655. (New York: McGraw-Hill Book Co.

441. Morganroth, J., Levy, R.I. and Fredrickson, D.S. (1975). The biochemical, clinical and genetic features of type III hyperlipoproteinemia. *Ann. Intern. Med.*, **82**, 158

Section 5

Diagnostic techniques

22   Physical examination

Physical diagnosis is that branch of medical practice whereby the diagnosis of a disease process is made through the use of one or more of our senses: visual, olfactory, gustatory, tactile and auscultatory. These senses are attributes that are universal in mankind, easily refined and improved upon through practice, and readily available at little or no cost.

Utilization of the sense of smell is an uncommon tool in current practice though at one time exaggerated claims were made in its favor such as its ability to diagnose the presence of typhoid fever because of the emission of a characteristic odor on the part of the patient. Still, I can recall from personal experience as a young resident in internal medicine, the 'mousy odor' of cirrhotics and the 'ammoniacal odor' of the uremic patient as well as the sweet 'acetone breath' of diabetic ketosis. The impact, however, of the olfactory sense in cardiology has been virtually non-existent.

The Hindus were the first to utilize taste as a means of determining the sweetness of diabetic urine (Madhumela)[1]. This practice continued during the medieval and renaissance periods of European history. But, again, sense of taste like smell, had no impact in the evaluation of cardiac disease.

Physical diagnosis has developed on the basis of the remaining senses and therefore is commonly described as consisting of four components: inspection, palpation, percussion and auscultation. The art of utilizing these components in the diagnosis and evaluation of heart disease has been an exciting chapter in the history of cardiology.

Physical diagnosis, *per se*, did not spring up overnight but rather evolved over the centuries with its roots as far back as the earliest physicians. In fact, all of the basic techniques of physical diagnosis, including percussion and auscultation, were employed by Hippocrates and his followers.

The development of physical diagnosis in maladies afflicting the cardiovascular system was treated in depth in 1824 by R. J. H. Bertin[2].

For those who cannot read the treatise in the original French, an excellent translation is available by Charles W. Chauncey under the title *Treatise on the Diseases of the Heart and Great Vessels*[3].

Although the other elements of physical diagnosis may have been utilized such as palpation and percussion, visual observation played a leading role among the medicine men of antiquity whether they were part of a primitive tribe bedecked in feathers or a member of a more civilized type of urban population encased in sacerdotal robes.

Mettler[4] recounts the practice in Mesopotamia of exposing the sick in the market place so that the opinions regarding the nature of the malady could be expressed by the casual passer-by. To be sure, this probably was an insignificant method of obtaining medical help and, no doubt, heavily laden with errors. Nevertheless, it points out how important visual inspection was and continued to be for millennia in the evaluation of a subject's state of health.

Vivid descriptions of illness, based mostly on inspection, can be found, as indicated by this Mesopotamian quotation, from Castiglioni's text[5]: 'The sick one coughs frequently, his sputum is thick and sometimes contains blood, his respirations give a sound like a flute, his skin is cold but his feet are hot, he sweats greatly and his heart is much disturbed'.

Detailed clinical pictures containing pertinent visual elements were carried even further by Hippocrates. An example is the following description by Hippocrates as taken from the translation of F. Adams[6]. '... A sharp nose, hollow eyes, collapsed temples, the ears cold, contracted and the lobes turned out; the skin about the forehead being rough, distended and parched; the color of the whole face being green, black, livid or lead-colored'. This is the famous symptom-complex known to generations of physicians as the 'facies Hippocratica' and indicative of impending death.

The Chinese also paid considerable attention to the appearance of the tongue and face[4].

... Each organ is in correspondence with a particular colour which is decided by the prevailing element ... In pathological conditions the prevailing colour indicates the site of the disease. ... the inspection of the colour takes place mostly upon those parts of the head and face which stand in relationship to the organ in question; thus the site for the heart is the tongue. Again, if in disease of the heart, the tongue, which should normally be red, is black (colour of the kidneys), enemies of the heart, have acquired the mastery, whence the prognosis indicates destruction of the heart and a fatal issue[7].

Thirty-seven different types of textures of the tongue were classified by the Chinese physicians of ancient times. It was thought that the specific illness could be identified on the basis of the predominant color. It was also thought that the tongue was 'the window of the heart' and for that reason it was subjected to more careful inspection when a heart disorder was suspected.

The practice of inspecting the tongue for tell-tale signs of disease is still firmly entrenched in medicine.It was particularly popular in the 19th century when physical diagnosis was evolving as an especially important bedside technique. Figure 1 depicts a doctor during this era peering at the tongue of a patient seated before him.

The Hippocratic practice of objective observation was further amplified and refined by the Alexandrians. During Roman times, Aretaeus was particularly prominent as a follower of Hippocrates, placing considerable emphasis on observation and leaving for posterity invariably good descriptions.

... And there is a difference of the discharge, whether it be brought up from an artery or a vein. For if it is black, thick and readily coagulates, if from a vein; it is less dangerous, and is more speedily stopped; but if from an artery, it is of a bright yellow colour and thin, does not readily coagulate, the danger is more imminent, and to stop it is not easy; for the pulsations of the artery provoke the hemorrhage, and the lips of the wound do not coalesce from the frequent movements of the vessel ...[8]

The art of visual observation in cardiac disease continued to flourish in the early and middle part of the 19th century among the Parisian clinicians simultaneously with the advances being made

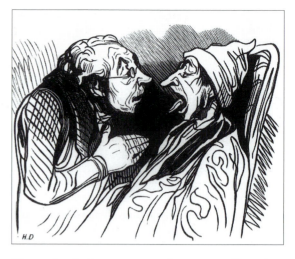

Figure 1 A doctor peers at the tongue of a patient seated before him. *Photo Source National Library of Medicine. Literary Source Dimier, Louis (ed.). Physionomies, Paris, 1930, Planche IV (LC copy). Courtesy of National Library of Medicine*

through palpation, percussion and auscultation. This is aptly illustrated by the following excerpts from Corvisart's section on *The Methods of distinguishing Organic Lesions of the Heart from Hydrothorax*[9,10].

In essential, uncomplicated, confirmed hydrothorax, the appearance is pale, fatigued, emaciated, without being bloated; the eyes are dull, and languid, the lips pale and apparently thinned. In hydrothorax, the involved side of the chest is fuller and more rounded ... Nothing like this is seen in diseases of the heart and great vessels; one sometimes sees an aneurysm which elevates the chest wall, and causes it to protrude in front but the swelling, produced by this disease, happens only at a single point, and never occupies an entire side of the thorax. Moreover, the obvious pulsation of this region in the latter case prevents confusion of the two diseases ... In cardiac diseases the wall of the chest is not edematous unless the disease is very advanced and has proceeded to generalized anasarca ... In cardiac diseases the position is never horizontal; the patients when stretched upon their back elevate their chest and head in such a manner as to be, as it were, sitting up; others entirely resist this position so as to crouch forward. It is unusual to see any of them turned on one or the other side excepting when they are nigh unto death … In cardiac diseases the cadaver is enlarged, bloated, purplish and infiltrated; the cervical veins are often prominent; the abdominal wall is distended by the effusion in the cavity; all the integuments of the body are swollen with infiltration, especially remarkable in the upper and lower extremities; the quantity of water effused into the chest is ordinarily very slight and if there existed a secondary hydrothorax, which rarely occurs, it is always at the same time accompanied by a serous effusion into the abdomen and by generalized anasarca; the lungs are purplish and distended with blood; the heart always presents evidence of a lesion.

Inspection was not necessarily restricted to assessment of the patient. The excreta were also subjected to visual scrutiny. Figure 2 is a mezzotint showing a physician of the 17th century examining the urine flask of a patient, in the presence of other patients. Urine flasks of various sizes are depicted on the counter and shelf behind. This was before microscopic inspection was available.

The employment of palpation in physical diagnosis is a logical corollary to inspection. The limitations imposed upon this method by virtue of the peculiarities of each subject (such as obesity and thickness of chest wall), have, however, relegated its usage to a secondary role in assessing cardiac dysfunction.

The size of the heart has long been considered an important sign of cardiac disease, especially in the latter part of the 19th century when correlation between clinical events and pathologic anatomy became firmly entrenched. During this era, the location of the apical impulse was advanced as a means of determining cardiac size. However, its ability to do so on a consistent basis was found to be hampered not only by the previously mentioned constraints but also by the abnormal conditions affecting the lungs, pleural space or abdominal cavity. It is probably for these reasons that the pulse became a more important parameter of cardiac function as determined by palpation. Because of its ready availability and the ease with which it could be evaluated, the radial pulse at the wrist became the most popular site for evaluation. Other sites were utilized for various reasons and for the delineation of other pathologic states so that a considerable body of knowledge has arisen concerning palpation not only of the radial pulse but

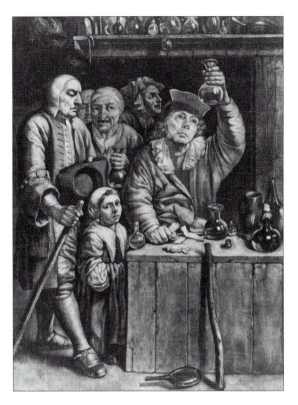

Figure 2 Mezzotint showing physician examining urine flask of patient, in presence of other patients. Urine flasks of various sizes are depicted on counter and shelf behind. *Photo Source National Library of Medicine. Literary Source Whaestem, pinx, Isaac Sarrabat fe. & excud. 1600? Courtesy of National Library of Medicine*

also of epigastric, suprasternal and venous pulsations as well as the pulsations imparted to the palpating hand or fingers by an aneurysm.

For many centuries the tactile examination of the pulse was referred to as 'the messenger that never fails'. The word pulse is derived from the Latin 'pulsare'. It means to throb or beat. It also has connotations such as strike, knock or push. 'Sphygmos' was the Greek name for pulse. They described the changes in rate as being 'sphygmic'. A slow rate was bradysphygmia and a rapid rate would be tachysphygmia. Sphygmology refers to that whole body of knowledge concerned with the pulse. Variation in the strength of the pulse was considered by the Greeks as being analogous to those of a rattle. This is why such variations are called crotic from 'crotolon', a rattle.

The earliest references to the pulse among the ancients are to be found in the Ebers papyrus and the Edwin Smith papyrus. The description in the Ebers papyrus is as follows[11]:

> The beginning of the science of the physician. To know the movements of the heart and to know the heart ... From the heart arise the vessels which go to the whole body ... if the physician lay his finger on the head, on the neck, on the hand, on the epigastrium, on the arm or the leg, everywhere the motion of the heart touches him, coursing through the vessels to all the members ... When the heart is diseased its work is imperfectly performed; the vessels proceeding from the heart become inactive, so that you cannot feel them ... If the heart trembles, has little power and sinks, the disease is advancing.

The Edwin Smith papyrus has the following observations on the pulse and its relationship to the heart beat[12]:

> ... examining is like one counting a certain quantity with a bushel, or counting something with the fingers ... like measuring the ailment of a man in order to know the action of the heart. There are canals in it [the heart] to every member. Now if the priests of Sekhmet or any physician put his hands or his fingers upon the head, upon the two hands, ... upon the two feet, he measures to the heart ... because its pulsation is in every member ... Measure ... his heart in order to recognize the indications which have arisen therein; meaning ... in order to know what is befalling therein.

Figure 3 illustrates the hieroglyphic characters that depict the counting of the pulse. The symbol on the extreme right portrays the counting of seeds or beads being emptied from a container. In actual practice the pulse was counted with the aid of an earthenware vessel that acted as a clock. This vessel had a tiny hole in the bottom which allowed water to escape drop by drop. The pulse rate was determined by correlating the beats with the drops of water. Figure 4 depicts this clock. Although not seen too well, there are markings on the side of the bowl which divide the day into 24 increments. Each increment represents an hour.

The study of the pulse was very important in Chinese medicine dating back as early as 2700 BC, during the reign of Emperor Shen Nung. Evaluation of the pulse continued to be promulgated

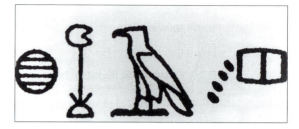

Figure 3 Counting or measurement of the pulse as depicted by hieroglyphic characters in the Smith papyrus. Symbol on the right represents seeds being emptied from the container. *Photo Source University of Central Florida. Literary Source Breasted, J.H. The Edwin Smith Surgical Papyrus. University of Chicago Press. Found in Brewer, L.A. (1983). Sphygmology through the centuries: historical notes. Am. J. Surg., 145, 696–701. With permission*

by Pien Ch'iao during the 6th century BC. Over the centuries, the vast amount of information that accumulated among the Chinese was such that it needed many volumes of tract for its presentation and preservation. There is some confusion as to the actual number of volumes and authorship. One source says it was a 12 volume tract and that the author was Me Ching[13]. Another source names Wang Chu Ho as the author and states that the work consists of 10 volumes[14]. The only certainty appears to be the year of publication which was AD 280, and that it was destined to become a landmark work on the subject.

A great deal of fallacy surrounded the methods for taking the pulse and their interpretation. The Chinese utilized eleven positions for examining the pulse. It was palpated three times using light, medium and strong pressures! An inordinate amount of reliance was placed upon environmental conditions, necromancy and divine influence. Preservation of female modesty was also strictly observed. The female pulse was palpated across a bamboo curtain. Numeration of the pulse was achieved by utilizing the physician's own respirations as a reference point.

The pulse lore of Chinese medicine also had some other interesting aspects. Although it was expected that a capable physician could arrive at the diagnosis from the quality of the pulse, there were times when he could not avail himself of the 'luxury' of personally palpating the pulse. This applied not only to females but, at times, to male patients as well, especially if either one was of a high social status. As I mentioned before, even if the physician were able to personally evaluate the pulse of a female patient, he had to do so not only with the patient sitting behind a bamboo curtain but also with the physician accomplishing the procedure by means of a silk thread. In such cases the silk thread was looped around the wrist of the female patient at the site where the radial pulse would ordinarily be felt. The physician then judged the quality of the pulse by sensing the movement imparted to the thread – sometimes the patient would be in another room, necessitating the usage of a thread several meters in length.

The taboo against any form of physical contact with the female patient brought about the introduction of the so-called diagnostic doll. These were small, naked female figurines made of ivory, jade, porcelain or saponite. The patient would mark the site of the disorder on the figurine. These were usually in the permanent possession of the patient but many a physician carried his own supply as well so that female modesty could never be compromised. There was a fetish at the time, which persisted well into the 19th century, regarding the size of female feet. At an early age, females, especially those of the 'upper crust' would have their feet bound so that they would remain small. The resultant distorted feet were thought to be a mark of beauty and were often referred to as 'lily feet'. Most figurines then had very small feet in accordance with this custom. Authorities on the subject claim that diagnostic dolls with well-formed feet should always be considered as forgeries. It is of interest to note that diagnostic dolls were also used during the Victorian era in England.

India was also preoccupied with the pulse as is evident through its many treatises on the subject and through the Ayurvedic teachings. The Hindus recognized the diagnostic value of the various characteristics of the pulse such as rate, rhythm, and regularity. They advocated palpating the pulse on the right side in men, and on the left side in women! In 1924, Ghose wrote a paper called *A peep into the Ayurvedic system of sphygmology* in which he tells how the Ayurvedics had classified the pulse into 600 types[15]. This would overwhelm, to say the least, any modern practitioner of medicine.

The first Greek to pay much attention to the pulse was Praxagoras of Cos (400 BC)[16]. He described tachycardia and bradycardia. Although Hippocrates is known to have counted the pulse,

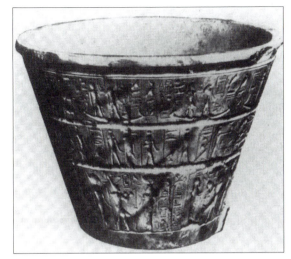

Figure 4 Egyptian Clock. The earthenware vessel has a tiny hole in the bottom through which water escaped drop by drop. The pulse rate was determined by correlating it with the drops of water escaping from the vessel. *Photo Source National Library of Medicine. Literary Source Brewer, L.A. (1983). Sphygmology through the centuries: historical notes. Am. J. Surg. **145**, 696–701. Taken from Encyclopedia of World Art. (New York: McGraw-Hill). With permission*

it was Herophilus who went into detail regarding its frequency, rhythm, size and amplitude[17,18]. Herophilus timed the rate with a waterclock (clepsydra) that he invented[19–22]. Other notables of this era include Aegimius, a contemporary of Praxagoras, whose recorded observations are not to be found, Erasistratus, Aristotle and Rufus of Ephesus. Erasistratus described the transmission of the pulse as 'wave-like'[7]. Aristotle appeared to appreciate a relationship between the pulse and the heart as indicated by the following comments: 'The pulse inheres in the very constitution of the heart and appears from the beginning as is learned both from the dissection of living animals and the formation of the chick in the egg'.[23]

It was left to Rufus of Ephesus, however, to show definitely that the pulse was synonymous with the heartbeat[24]. He also advanced the thesis that the throbbing of the fontanelles in the infant was due to arterial pulsations. Charaka, an ancient Buddhist, also made the same comments[25].

The commentaries of the notable physicians of the first century AD, such as Celsus, Paulus Aeginata and others are neither informative nor enlightening[20,26].

Galen, as usual, was quite prolific. He wrote at least 18 essays on the pulse.

The fundamental principle of Galenic sphygmology is that every organ has its own special pulse and that every disease has its own characteristic pattern of pulse behavior. He amplified and modified the beliefs of Erasistratus and fellow Alexandrian, Herophilus, regarding the mechanisms responsible for the pulse. The pervasive theory during antiquity was that the activity of the arterial pulse was due to the 'pneuma' or air which filled the arteries. It was Erasistratus who advanced the belief that the pneuma in the arteries was derived from respiration. Galen's words were: 'The pulse is that peculiar action initiated of the heart, thence of the arteries, which are moved in diastole and systole; by which a balance of the innate heat is maintained, and animal spirit generated in the brain … The pulsatile faculty of the heart has its source in its own substance …'[20].

Galen described five basic characteristics of the pulse as determined by palpation of the radial artery at the wrist, a site which he favored, claiming it to be the best site for such a maneuver[27]. These characteristics are astoundingly similar to the ones currently evaluated by clinicians throughout the world and which include rate, rhythm, compressibility, and tension of the pulse, condition of the arterial wall, and size and shape of the pulse wave.

The first characteristic, which Galen referred to as speed, would be compared to the current designation of rate. The size of the pulse, a second characteristic, was equivalent to the degree of distention of the artery itself. Since Galen viewed the artery as a solid body, this conception of pulse-size actually embodied the current notions of body and force. The third characteristic was an estimation of the strength of the pulse. In describing this, Galen recognized that physiologically the pulse has both a systolic and diastolic component (the difference between the two constituting our current term of pulse pressure).

The quality of the condition of the artery itself was another characteristic. This would correlate today with the degree of compressibility of the arterial wall and would therefore be an indication of degree of sclerosis or hardness of the arterial wall. The fifth characteristic corresponds to our concept of tension and would be dependent upon the extent to which the artery was filled with blood.

Galen described these basic characteristics of the pulse as types of pulse and, in addition, he described in detail the rhythm, size and shape of the pulse wave, antedating Vierordt's work in the 19th century.

Many varieties of pulse abnormalities were described by Galen and these should be recounted since they so closely resemble the descriptions of the 19th century. Rhythm was denoted by the expressions rhythmic and arrhythmic. The quality of the rhythm was also described. An equal pulse was one in which all the pulsations were alike. On the other hand, unequal pulsations were said to be intermittent if dropped beats or pauses were noted; intercurrent, if extra beats were felt.

Pulsus paradoxicus was recognized by Galen under the term 'myurus recurrens'. Myurus is the Greek word for pulse. The term 'paradoxical pulse' was reintroduced by Adolph Kussmaul in a paper published in 1873[28]. It has since become entrenched as a simple and important sign in the diagnosis of pericardial tamponade and constrictive pericarditis.

It was Vierordt who first described the presence of an 'irregular pulse' despite a regular heartbeat in a patient with purulent pericarditis[29]. Kussmaul acknowledged this and, coupled with his own observations of three patients with constrictive pericarditis, he coined the expression 'paradoxical pulse'. He described the pulse in these patients as becoming fainter and disappearing in regular repetitive intervals during inspiration. Kussmaul called this type of pulse paradoxical, primarily because of the incongruous relationship of an irregular peripheral arterial pulsation in the presence of a regular precordial heartbeat. The repetitive regularity of the progressive faintness of the peripheral pulse and final disappearance was another reason for using the term paradoxical. Unlike Galen, Kussmaul correlated this physical finding with pericardial disease.

Figure 5 is taken from Vierordt's textbook and is a graphic representation of the paradoxical pulse.

It should be noted that current practice utilizes auscultation as a means of eliciting the paradoxical pulse rather than palpation. A drop in systolic blood pressure greater that 10 mmHg at the end of inspiration is the criterion utilized. There is no documentation of who was responsible for the introduction of manometry rather that palpation.

Pulsus alternans of Traube may have also been described initially by Galen if the comparison with Galen's 'goat-leap' is valid. The 'goat-leap' pulse as described by Galen consists of a pulsation followed

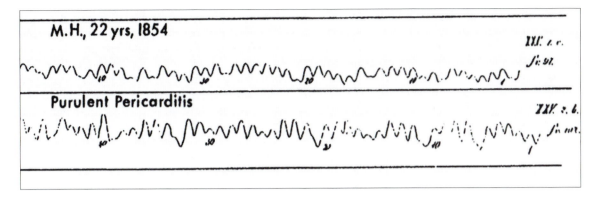

Figure 5 Vierordt's example of paradoxical pulse. *Photo Source University of Central Florida. Literary Source Vierordt, K. (1855). Die Lehre von Arterienpuls in gesunden und kranken zustaenden Braunschiveig. F. Vieqeg, p.226. Public domain*

by another one of greater amplitude and occurring before diastole. Later writers called this type of pulse 'caprizans'. The waning, thready pulse of hemorrhagic shock is probably the equivalent of the one Galen described as a 'failing myurus'. The 'pulsus parvus' that can be seen with aortic stenosis was also described by Galen though not within that context. He called this type of pulse, 'formicans'.

One of the most interesting presentations of pulse lore is to be found in the paper by Schechter, Lillehei, and Soffer which appeared in 1969. It described the reciprocal relationship between the pulse and the brain. This is a relationship that has been well known for centuries but only recently has the biochemical basis for this relationship become unveiled to some extent. I have taken the liberty of paraphrasing freely from this scholarly paper.

Many terms were used in the past to describe the loss of consciousness and the peripheral arteries without realizing the ultimate dependency on cardiac rhythm. Schechter and his associates recount how the carotid arteries were so named. They ascribe the original usage of the label 'carotid' to Rufus of Ephesus, who derived it from the Greek word for torpor or deep sleep, 'karosis'. Carotids mean sleep producers because it was his belief that compression of these arteries produced stupor. This belief persisted even during the Renaissance despite the fact the Curtius in 1551 showed that tying them in animals did not result in such an effect[30]. Even Vesalius was heir to this belief when he named them 'arteriae soporiferae'.

Other descriptive terms for temporary loss of consciousness are to be found in the writings of Celsus and Arataeus of Cappadocia. Celsus used the words 'morbus cardiacus' as a synonym for syncope. 'Leipothymia' was the term used by Arataeus. Thymos means mind and leipen indicates flight, therefore leipothymia means to leave the mind. The word, leipothymia, indicating syncope, was popular until the beginning of the 20th century. It is strange that Celsus should have referred to syncope as morbus cardiacus. He had absolutely no idea that disturbances of cardiac rhythm could have a significant role in the precipitation of fainting episodes.

Again, Schechter and co-authors bring out very clearly the intimate relationship between emotions and the heart. This close kinship was known not only to physicians but apparently to some discerning literary figures as well. Their paper mentions how Robert Burton details the 'pulsus amatorius' in his book *Anatomy of Melancholy*. That great student of human nature, Shakespeare, is also quoted with excerpts from *Coriolanus* and *Hamlet*. The quotation from Hamlet is 'My pulse, as yours, doth temperately keep time, and makes as healthful music. It is not madness that I have uttered: bring me to the test'[31].

Medicine had to wait until the 19th century to correlate the physical findings by palpation with pathologic anatomy. The Parisian clinicians during this era were exemplary of those at the forefront. A quotation from his text as translated by J. Gates concisely summarizes Corvisart's approach[10]. 'The more exactly anatomy is studied by physicians, the sooner they will be able by careful observation to distinguish and establish among diseases, a great number of organic lesions, whose existence has not by a majority of them been even suspected'.

Several important physical findings utilizing palpation were originally described by Corvisart, among them being the diastolic thrill of mitral stenosis. The thrill is a palpable murmur and is akin to the sensation felt by the purring of a cat. The thrill of mitral stenosis is elicited most commonly by palpating the apical impulse. It is intense just before systole.

Systolic thrills are usually felt at the base of the heart just to the right of the upper part of the sternum. They are often transmitted upwards to the neck. Aortic stenosis is the most common cause of a systolic thrill in this area though an aortic aneurysm can also be responsible. It was originally described also by Corvisart[32].

One of the greatest advocates of palpation was Mathew Baillie of Britain. He placed such a great deal of reliance on this element of physical diagnosis that a contemporary of his, Sir Henry Halford, accused Baillie of too much familiarity when using the technique[32].

Hope described in detail the volume and contour of the arterial pulse in the presence of several valvular lesions[33]. The quantitative relationship between the aortic and mitral lesions and pulse volume was clearly elucidated by him. Corrigan's classic account of the celer pulse of aortic insufficiency was anticipated by Hope. Hope was also the first to note the early diastolic pulmonary murmur heard in association with pulmonary hypertension and now called the Graham Steell murmur. At one time this murmur carried the eponym of Hope. James Hope (1801–41) along with Jean Baptiste Bouillaud and C. J. B. Williams were among the most outstanding students and exponents of physical diagnosis immediately following the death of Laénnec. Hope also suffered the same fate as Laénnec, dying prematurely from tuberculosis. What Laénnec did for the clinical diagnosis of pulmonary disease, Hope did for diseases of the heart and aorta. In addition to his observations on the pulse, he provided the experimental evidence that an incompetent valve resulted in regurgitation.

Charles James Blazius Williams' (1805–89) influence in physical diagnosis was felt in both Britain and America. This influence began at the early age of 23, when he published his *Rational Exposition of the Physical Signs of the Diseases of the Lungs and Pleura*. According to Korns, he described pulsus paradoxicus 23 years before Kussmaul[34].

The contributions of Jean Baptiste Bouillaud (1796–1881) were principally in auscultation rather than palpation. These consisted of his discovery of the reduplication of the second sound and his clarification of many of the auscultatory signs of aortic aneurysm. He is also responsible for the best early description of atrial fibrillation as elicited by auscultation[35].

Although it is probably true that the bounding pulse of aortic regurgitation was described by several authors before Corrigan, eponymic recognition should still remain with Corrigan because of his detailed analysis and correlation with the underlying pathophysiologic disorder. Kligfield reports that the classic bounding and collapsing pulse of aortic regurgitation was noted by William Cowper in 1705, Raymond Vieussens in 1715, and James Hope in 1831[36]. He also presents evidence that a Dublin practitioner by the name of Thomas Cuming published a case report describing this peripheral circulatory phenomenon 10 years prior to Corrigan's publication[36].

Dominic Corrigan was a contemporary of such medical giants of Dublin as Graves, Stokes and Adams. He was born in Dublin in 1802 and earned his M.D. degree from Edinburgh in 1825. Although Corrigan made many significant contributions to medicine, his fame rests primarily on a paper he wrote describing the clinical manifestations of aortic insufficiency. The paper was entitled *On Permanent Patency of the Mouth of the Aorta, or Inadequacy of the Aortic Valves*[37]. It was in the detailed analysis of this valvular lesion that Corrigan described the associated peripheral vascular manifestations. He also described in another paper the 'small and contracted' pulse of aortic stenosis in contrast to the collapsing pulse of aortic insufficiency[38].

Corrigan's medical career was punctuated by many honors, among which was his appointment as Honorary Physician-in-Ordinary to Queen Victoria; a unique achievement for an Irish Catholic of that era. He was also created a baronet and represented Dublin in his later years as an elected member of Parliament. His portrait can be seen in Figure 6. A year before his death, the *British Medical Journal* published anonymously a paper written by him that was entitled *Reminiscences of a medical student prior to passing of the Anatomy Act*. This paper recounted his experiences in raids on the graveyard in Bully's acre, Kilmainhaim in order to obtain subjects for the dissecting room[39]. At his death in 1880,

Freeman's Journal of Dublin wrote of him as follows: 'The people of Ireland regarded his career with peculiar interest and his success with gratified pride. This feeling was nowise sectarian. It was rather racial and national. They felt that intellectual triumph was their best and noblest vindication against the contumely which had fallen on them in consequence of the ignorance enforced upon the nation by the Penal Laws'[40].

The collapsing pulse of aortic insufficiency has also been poetically described as a 'vascular dance'[41]. A manifestation of this 'dance' would be the 'abrupt rhythmic extension of one leg when crossed over the other, coincident with systole'. Schwartz recounts how this physical diagnostic sign helped explain the slightly blurred appearance of Abe Lincoln's left foot in a photo of the president while being interviewed by a newspaperman called Brooks[42]. This sign which Schwartz suggests calling the Lincoln-Brooks sign of aortic insufficiency is cited along with the skeletal and visual stigmata that Lincoln had as being sufficient evidence for stating that the awkward looking Lincoln was a victim of Marfan's syndrome[43–45]. Figure 7 depicts the photokymographic evidence. The blurred left boot was attributed to the so-called vascular dance of aortic insufficiency.

The saga of determining the pulse rate is an extremely interesting one and spans a period of time beginning again with the ancients. I have already mentioned how the Chinese used the physician's own respirations as a reference point, since no technical devices were available for the measurement of time during that era. These did not appear until many centuries later.

The Romans used a float-regulated windlass. This was a very inaccurate type of water clock. Refinements and improvements on the water clock did not appear until the Renaissance beginning with Cardinal Krebs of Cues[20,46]. We must turn, however, to Galileo Galilei for inventing the first device that could measure the pulse[47,48]. Galileo, markedly dissatisfied with the inaccuracy of water clocks and the obvious disadvantages of the hourglass, designed a clock with a pendulum. He called it a 'pulsilogium' and it is illustrated in Figure 8. The design was based on the isochronism of pendular objects; a principle he discovered in 1583 by timing the oscillations of a chandelier on the altar of the Cathedral of Pisa against his own pulse[49]. I wonder how many Paternosters Galileo had to say to atone for this distraction while

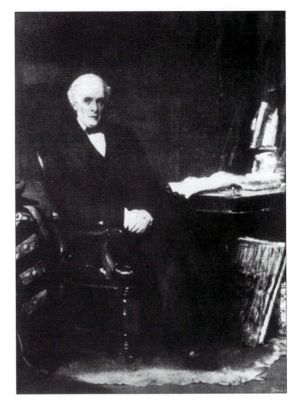

Figure 6 Sir Dominic Corrigan (1802–1880). *Photo Source Royal College of Physicians. Literary Source Photo Archives. Courtesy of the Royal College of Physicians*

attending Mass. The instrument was remarkable for its simplicity. It consisted of a dial with a pointer and a string which acted as a pendulum by virtue of a weight attached to its free end. The string was capable of being wound up on a wheel behind the dial. When the pendulum swung in synchrony with the patient's pulse, the pointer on the dial indicated the rate of that patient's pulse. The amount of concentration so obviously needed in employing this device would indicate that Paternoster or no Paternoster, neither Galileo nor anyone else could afford to be distracted while using it.

Over the next century, pulse clocks of similar design were introduced by Santorio Santorio, Marin Mersenne and Christian Huygen. Santorio's model, introduced in 1625, utilized suspended lead weights that swung in rhythm with the pulse. The frequency of oscillation was registered on a calibrated scale. He also designed a timer that was shaped like a cup and which he named the cotyla after the Greek word for cup, cotylon.

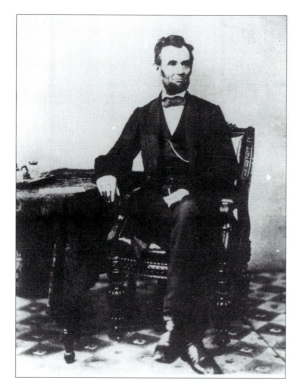

Figure 7 Photokymographic evidence of vascular dance in Abraham Lincoln. Blurred left boot was attributed to the so-called vascular dance of aortic insufficiency. *Photo Source National Library of Medicine. Literary Source Schwartz, H. Abraham Lincoln and aortic insufficiency – the declining of the president (clinical note). Calif. Med., **116**, 82–4, May, 1972. With permission*

In his early history of instrumental precision in medicine, Mitchell quotes Santorio's description of the device he designed[49]. It is as follows:

> For a long time I have been deliberating in what manner the amount of disease could be determined from any region whatever. I have contrived four instruments. The first is my pulsilogium by which with mathematical certainty, and not by conjecture, I can measure the utmost degrees of variation of the pulse both as to frequency and as to slowness, of which instrument I have given some account in lib. 5 of my Meth. With the aforesaid pulsilogium I have found this to be easily done, as is explained in the first figure. It is composed of a little cord made of linen or silk, to which, as may be seen, is fastened a leaden bullet, which being struck,

if the cord be long, the motion of the bullet will be slower and less frequent, if the cord be short, its motion will be quicker and more frequent. When therefore we wish to measure the frequency or slowness of the pulse, we drive the bullet with the fingers, lengthening or shortening the cord until that point be reached where the motion of the bullet exactly coincided with the pulse-beat of the artery; which being found in a certain region to be 70 in degree, shown by a white line on the bullet itself at the point C. This degree being kept in mind again on the same or on the following day, we can make trial with the same instrument whether the pulsation of the same artery be a very little quicker or slower; we say 'a very little', because in the use of this instrument we do not seek those marked differences of rapidity or slowness of pulsation which can be carried in the memory of the physician, but rather those very slight ones of which the differences between one day and another are barely noticeable. For the same purpose is another similar instrument of which a representation may be seen in fol. 78, figure E. But it is to be noted that the impelling of the leaden bullet by a greater or less force does not change the slowness or frequency , because, in striking it, what is lost in space is gained in force. With such an instrument we can measure the pulse in a state of health; then in time of disease we note the departure from the natural state, which is especially necessary in diagnosis, prognosis, and treatment. By this means we can recognize the difference between a slow and a weak pulse, in which thing the physicians are often deceived; the difference being that in fevers the weak pulse does not decrease in frequency, whereas the slow pulse abates, which abatement, so slight is it, cannot be perceived by physicians without an instrument, and in prognosis they are often mightily deceived. We may add that no physician is created with such remarkable skill, that without the aid of the pulsilogium he can retain in his memory the smallest differences of motion and rest of the artery; so that that which other physicians acquire by conjecture concerning the motion of the pulse, we are able to attain unerringly by the infallible skill of the pulsilogium.

Figure 9 is a picture of Santorio's pulsilogium and a partial description of it in Latin from his treatise on the instrument.

By the beginning of the 18th century, watches were coming into vogue. The ordinary watch, however, was unable to measure minutes or seconds. It had only one hand which showed the time in hours. This was remedied by Floyer in 1707 when he introduced his unique watch designed primarily for determining the pulse[20]. Floyer's watch ran for precisely one minute. The inventive genius of Floyer can be better appreciated when it is realized that the pulse could now be counted with great accuracy despite the fact that neither the second hand nor the 24 hour watch were yet in existence.

Sir John Floyer was a Staffordshire physician with an entrepreneurial bent. He attempted to popularize his invention by describing its usefulness and the expectations to be realized from its usage with the publication of a small book entitled *The Physician's Pulse Watch*[50].

> I have for many years try'd pulses by the minute in common watches and pendulum clocks, when I was among my patients; after some time I met with the common sea minute-glass ... and by that I made most of my experiments. But because this was not portable I caused a pulse-watch to be made which ran 60 seconds, and I placed it in a box to be more easily carried, and by this I now feel pulses ... The Art of Feeling the Pulse, which I have proposed for distinction sake, I will call Mechanical; 'tis short, easie, and more certain than the Galenical or Chinese Art, because it requires no more than counting of the Pulse, and observing the time by the Pulse-Watch; this will show the Diseases of the Fluids, that is, of the Blood and Spirits; and the Method to raise or sink the Pulse; and by the same Method the Circulation will be stopt or accelerated; and he who knows and can best regulate the Excesses or Defects in the Pulse and circulation (as I conjecture) in the Learned Ages which are to come, will be esteemed the best Physician.

Floyer's pulse watch is illustrated in Figure 10.

Unfortunately, Floyer's watch added nothing of scientific value to palpating the pulse. All it did was create an inundation of the literature with weird theories and unfounded speculation with respect to the pulse and diet, weather, age, sleep, pregnancy and so on. Mitchell's account of the significance of

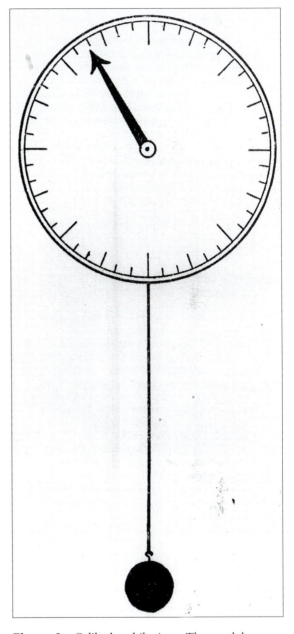

Figure 8 Galileo's pulsilogium. The pendulum was synchronized with the pulse and then the dial pointed to the rate of the pulse. *Photo Source University of Central Florida. Literary Source Hart: Makers of Science. Oxford University Press. With permission*

the pulse during the 18th century, and especially during the aftermath of Floyer's invention provides an interesting insight into the status of the pulse at the time. This is what he says: 'If any man, wishes

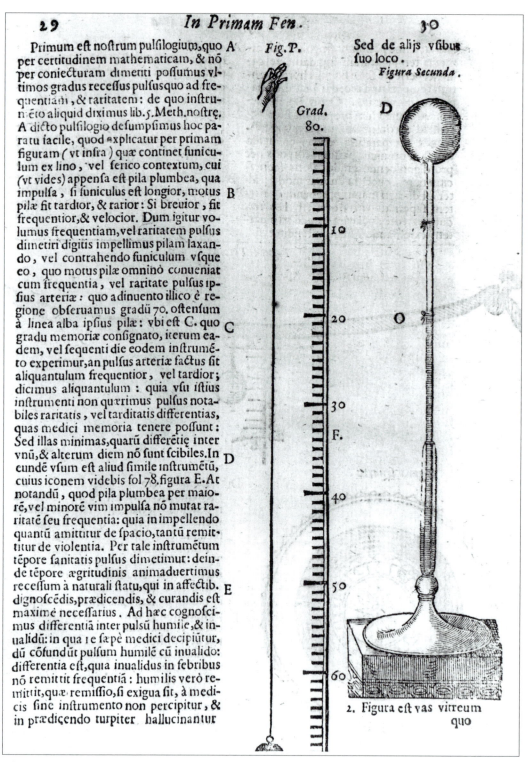

Primum eſt noſtrum pulſilogium, quo
per certitudinem mathematicam, & nõ
per coniecturam dimetiri poſſumus vl-
timos gradus receſſus pulſusquo ad frequentiam, & raritatem: de quo inſtru-
mẽto aliquid diximus lib. 5. Meth. noſtrę.
A dicto pulſilogio deſumpſimus hoc pa-
ratu facile, quod explicatur per primam
figuram (vt infra) quæ continet funiculum ex lino, vel ſerico contextum, cui
(vt vides) appenſa eſt pila plumbea, qua
impulſa, ſi funiculus eſt longior, motus
pilæ fit tardior, & rarior: Si breuior, fit
frequentior, & velocior. Dum igitur vo-
lumus frequentiam, vel raritatem pulſus
dimetiri digitis impellimus pilam laxan-
do, vel contrahendo funiculum vſque
eo, quo motus pilæ omninò conueniat
cum frequentia, vel raritate pulſus ipſius arteriæ: quo adinuento illico è re-
gione obſeruamus gradũ 70. oſtenſum
à linea alba ipſius pilæ: vbi eſt C. quo
gradu memoriæ conſignato, iterum ea-
dem, vel ſequenti die eodem inſtrumẽ-
to experimur, an pulſus arteriæ factus ſit
aliquantulum frequentior, vel tardior;
dicimus aliquantulum: quia vſu iſtius
inſtrumenti non quærimus pulſus nota-
biles raritatis, vel tarditatis differentias,
quas medici memoria tenere poſſunt:
Sed illas minimas, quarũ differetię inter
vnũ, & alterum diem nõ ſunt ſcibiles. In
cundẽ vſum eſt aliud ſimile inſtrumẽtũ,
cuius iconem videbis fol 78. figura E. At
notandũ, quod pila plumbea per maio-
rẽ, vel minorẽ vim impulſa nõ mutat ra-
ritatẽ ſeu frequentia: quia in impellendo
quantũ amittitur de ſpacio, tantũ remit-
titur de violentia. Per tale inſtrumẽtum
tẽpore ſanitatis pulſus dimetimur: dein-
de tẽpore ægritudinis animaduertimus
receſſum à naturali ſtatu, qui in affectib.
dignoſcẽdis, prædicendis, & curandis eſt
maximè neceſſarius. Ad hæc cognoſci-
mus differentiã inter pulſũ humile, & in-
ualidũ: in qua re ſæpè medici decipiũtur,
dũ cõfundũt pulſum humilẽ cũ inualido:
differentia eſt, quia inualidus in febribus
nõ remittit frequentiã: humilis verò remittit, quæ remiſſio, ſi exigua ſit, à medi-
cis ſine inſtrumento non percipitur, &
in prædicendo turpiter hallucinantur

Fig. P.

Sed de alijs vſibus
ſuo loco.

Figura Secunda.

Grad.
80.

2. Figura eſt vas vitreum
quo

Figure 9   Santorio's pulsilogium with partial description. *Photo Source National Library of Medicine.
Literary Source Santorio, S. Opera omnia. Venice, 1660. National Library of Medicine 17th century collection,
v.3, col.30. Courtesy of National Library of Medicine*

to nourish a taste for cynical criticism let him study honestly the books of the 18th century on the pulse. It is observation gone minutely mad: a whole Lilliput of symptoms: an exasperating waste of human intelligence. I know few more dreary deserts in medical literature from the essay on the *Chinese Art of Feeling the Pulse*, with which Floyer loaded his otherwise valuable essay, to Marquet's method of learning to know the pulse by musical notes, an art in which he was not alone. And error died hard. The doctrine of the specific pulse, a pulse for every malady, although rejected by de Haen, is in countless volumes, and survived up to 1827'[49]. The title-page of Floyer's monograph on the physician's pulse watch is reproduced in Figure 11.

It took centuries before Galileo's idea of measuring the pulse would take its proper place in clinical practice. Floyer's watch was a step in the right direction but medicine needed an eminent clinician of Graves' calibre to adopt the measurement of the pulse as an accepted and rigidly utilized element of physical diagnosis. Thus, the picture of the physician counting and assessing the quality of the pulse with watch in hand did not emerge until the 19th century. Graves introduced the practice and put it on a more scientific basis than Floyer. Clendenning's description of how all this came about is worth reading because of the most interesting way in which he narrates the development of this aspect of palpation[51].

Figure 12 is an interesting caricature on the pulse as perceived by Thomas Rowlandson. It is entitled 'Doctor Doubledose killing two birds with one stone'.

Another satire on physicians is depicted in Figure 13 which emphasizes that a doctor can still tote up the bill while palpating the pulse.

Although the art of percussion itself dates back to antiquity as a means of distinguishing between tympanites and ascites in the abdomen, it did not become part of the clinician's diagnostic armamentarium until the publication of Auenbrugger's *Inventum Novum ex Percussione Thoracis Humani* in 1761[52]. Figure 14 is an illustration of the frontispiece.

This small monograph of 95 pages, devoted entirely to immediate percussion, helped initiate the modern period of physical diagnosis. Its arrival was very timely since bedside clinical diagnosis had become exceedingly important in patient evaluation and was in dire need of simple diagnostic modalities.

Boerhaave of Leyden was one of the first of the great clinicians of the era to utilize bedside clinical

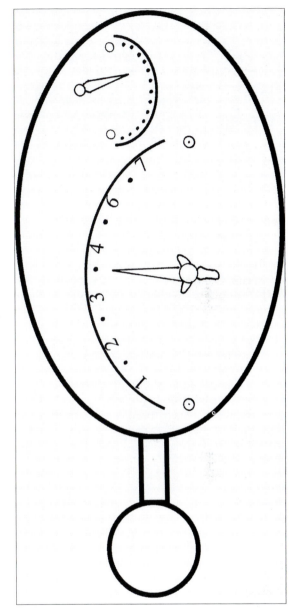

Figure 10 Floyer's pulse watch. *Photo Source University of Central Florida. Literary Source Mitchell, S.W. (1891). The early history of instrumental precision in medicine. The Transactions of the Congress of American Physicians and Surgeons. 2, 159–98. Public domain*

methods in the instruction of the young aspiring physician. His work was carried on by his pupil Gerhard van Swieten in Vienna, to which university the young van Swieten had been invited by the empress, Maria Theresa. Of course, there

THE
Physician's Pulse-Watch;
OR, AN
ESSAY
To Explain the Old Art of FEELING the PULSE, and to Improve it by the help of a PULSE-WATCH.
In Three PARTS.

I. The Old *Galenic* Art of Feeling the Pulse is describ'd, and many of its Errors corrected: The true Use of the Pulses, and their Causes, Differences and Prognostications by them, are fully explain'd, and Directions given for Feeling the Pulse by the Pulse-Watch, or Minute-Glass.

II. A New Mechanical Method is propos'd for preserving Health, and prolonging Life, and for curing Diseases by the help of the Pulse-Watch, which shews the Pulses when they exceed or are deficient from the natural.

III. The *Chinese* Art of Feeling the Pulse is describ'd; and the Imitation of their Practice of Physick, which is grounded on the Observation of the Pulse, is recommended.

To which is added,
An Extract out of *Andrew Cleyer*, concerning the *Chinese* Art of Feeling the Pulse.

By Sir JOHN FLOYER, Knight.

LONDON, Printed for *Sam. Smith* and *Benj. Walford*, at the *Prince's-Arms* in St. *Paul's Church-Yard*, 1707.

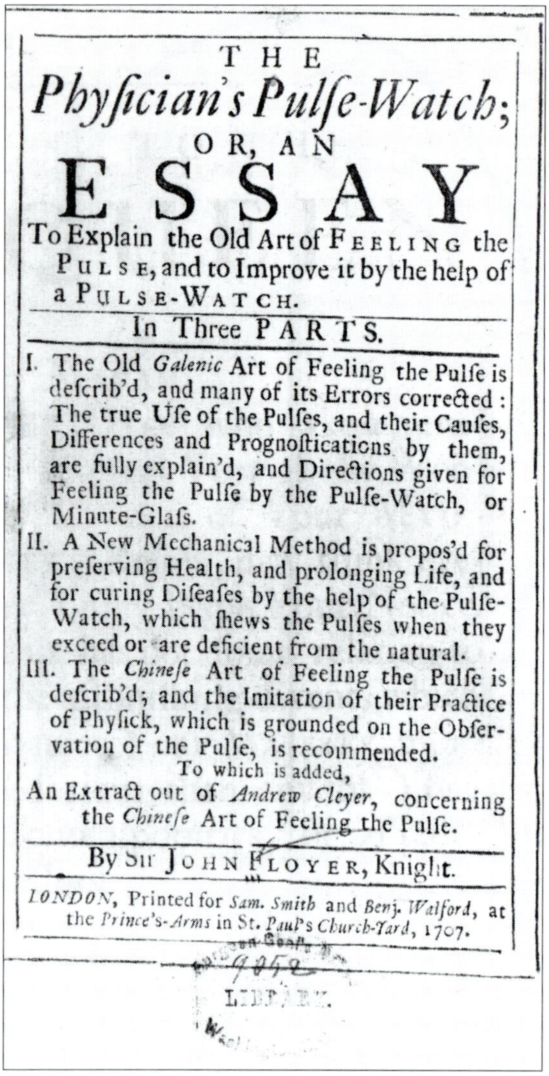

Figure 11 Title-page of Floyer's monograph on the physician's pulse watch. *Photo Source National Library of Medicine. Literary Source Photo Archives. Courtesy of National Library of Medicine*

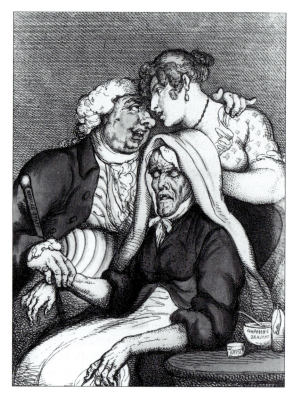

Figure 12 Dr Doubledose killing two birds with one stone. Doctor takes the pulse of an old woman while caressing her daughter. A jar marked 'Opium' and a bottle marked 'Composing Draught' rest on a side table. *Photo Source National Library of Medicine. Literary Source Thomas Tegg (no.47), Nov.20, 1810. Courtesy of National Library of Medicine*

were the usual die-hard bigots who strove to denigrate the potential benefits of any new diagnostic approach. Notable among these was de Haen, also of Vienna, who was adamantly opposed to Auenbrugger's method of clinical diagnosis. Notwithstanding his outstanding reputation as a clinician and teacher, de Haen's vehement opposition was unable to stem the tide, and upon his death, percussion moved toward acceptance as an important diagnostic tool in the school at Vienna under his successor, the brilliant Maximilian Stoll. It was Jean Nicholas Corvisart, however, who was responsible for establishing percussion as an important element of physical diagnosis. Corvisart's interest was aroused when he read a paper on percussion written by Josef Eyeral, a pupil of Stoll. This led Corvisart to Stoll's aphorisms and these, in turn, caused him to study Auenbrugger's original monograph. Corvisart's great prestige, coupled with the publication of his studies on percussion that extended over a period of 20 years, rescued the art of percussion from being merely a diagnostic tool restricted in its usage to Vienna to being an important method of physical diagnosis that was accepted throughout Europe and finally in America. It took 47 years for Auenbrugger's innovative approach to become fixed in clinical practice. And now, Laënnec's 'mediate auscultation,' in

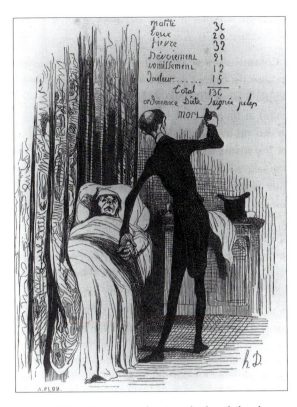

Figure 13   The patient has just died and the doctor totes up the bill. *Photo Source National Library of Medicine. Literary Source Fabre, Antoine Francois Hippolyte: Nemesis médicale illustrée, recueil de satires. Bruxelles, 1841. Woodcut illustrations after drawings by Honore Daumier. Courtesy of National Library of Medicine*

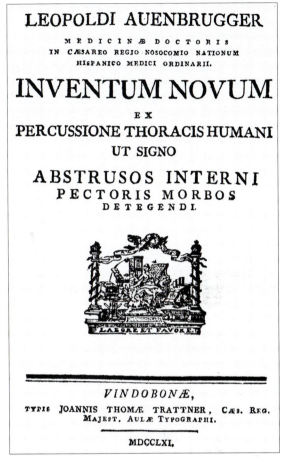

Figure 14   Frontispiece of 'Inventum Novum' by Leopold Auenbrugger. *Photo Source Royal College of Physicians. Literary Source Original. Courtesy of the Royal College of Physicians*

tandem with Corvisart's textbook and fame as a clinician, made Paris the Mecca of physical diagnosis. Parisian medicine rose from the depths brought about by the French revolution to new heights of prominence, attracting student physicians from all parts of Europe and elsewhere.

Corvisart is considered to have been one of the most brilliant physicians of the early 19th century. He was born in the small village of Drecourt which is in the Ardennes region of France. His father wanted him to be a lawyer, but the young Corvisart did not have either the enthusiasm or interest to follow in his father's footsteps, and left law school in favor of the Faculté de Médecine of Paris[53].

He was stocky in stature, vigorous in manner, and rather outspoken. It is said that his disinclination to abide by tradition was responsible for his failure to secure a job after graduation at the newly opened Hôpital des Paroisses. He refused to wear the required powdered wig that went with the position[54]. His reputation as an astute diagnostician and excellent teacher became established while he was professor of medicine at La Charité Hospital, a large teaching center.

As stated before, he was primarily responsible for the popularization of Auenbrugger's technique of percussion, disseminating this important element of physical diagnosis through his teachings and through his translation of Auenbrugger's treatise on percussion. The following quotation indicates how he gave full credit to Auenbrugger in this translation: 'I might easily have elevated myself to the rank of an author, if I had elaborated anew the doctrine of

461

Auenbrugger and published an independent work on percussion. In this way, however, I should have sacrificed the name of Auenbrugger to my own vanity, a thing which I am unwilling to do. It is he, and the beautiful invention which of right belongs to him, that I desire to recall to life'.

On the political scene his position as personal physician to Napoleon is of considerable interest and the source of an anecdote regarding Napoleon and scabies. Corvisart was apparently able to cure Napoleon of a dermal affliction accompanied by marked itching, and which, in turn, Napoleon had managed to transmit to his wife, Josephine. Corvisart was able to clear up the scabetic infection, without knowing that he was dealing with this entity by prescribing a topical mixture containing alcohol, olive oil, and powdered cevadilla[55].

Corvisart's detailed clinical records also contained data correlating the antemortem physical findings of the subject with the morbid anatomical changes seen at autopsy. Although the anatomical basis for such correlation had already been established through Morgagni's work, it needed the arrival of Corvisart to provide the spark plug for the increasing utilization of Morgagni's approach as the basis for interpretation of abnormal physical findings. Corvisart's remarks on certain clinical states are worthy of quotation: 'It is clear that the majority of the individuals reputed to have died of anasarca, leucophlegmasia, and particularly of hydrothorax, and of various species of asthmas and singular dypnoeas, may have perished from diseases of the heart'.

Corvisart utilized all four elements of physical diagnosis in his evaluation of cardiac dysfunction. He was able to delineate the presence of arrhythmias and distinguish between cardiac hypertrophy and cardiac dilatation. He recognized the pathological and clinical picture of vegetative endocarditis, and was aware that aphonia and inequality of the radial pulses could be due to an aneurysm of the arch of the aorta. Among the irregularities of rhythm, he described 'the pulse that was irregular, not coincident with the strokes of the heart'. He was also aware of the palpable thrill of mitral stenosis, and of the pathophysiologic mechanism for right-sided cardiac dilatation[56].

The diastolic thrill that so often accompanies mitral stenosis was described by him as 'a peculiar rushing like water, difficult to be described, sensible to the hand applied over the precordial region, a rushing which proceeds apparently from the embarrassment which the blood undergoes in passing through an opening which is no longer proportioned to the quantity of fluid which it ought to discharge'. Notice how well this description fits in with the deformed narrow orifice of the mitral valve seen at autopsy. This description as well as others culled from this book again attest to his extraordinary ability to diagnose cardiac disorders on the basis of physical findings.

Aneurysm of the heart was the term used for cardiac enlargement. When this enlargement was due to dilatation, he called it passive aneurysm, whereas myocardial thickening (hypertrophy) was labeled active aneurysm. Palpation of both the apical and radial pulse was his method for differentiating between the two types of enlargement. When the radial pulse could not be dampened or obliterated by digital pressure, Corvisart felt that this indicated cardiac enlargement due to hypertrophy. He also noted that the impulse at the cardiac apex was much less forceful in the presence of cardiac dilatation than hypertrophy. One should dwell upon this last statement for a moment and marvel again at how it represents the incredible level of refinement that Corvisart brought to physical diagnosis. Figure 15 depicts Corvisart during his prime, and Figure 16 is the frontispiece of his *Essai sur les Maladies et les Lesions Organiques du Coeur et des Gros Vaisseaux*.

In this discussion, a great deal of space was devoted to Corvisart at the expense of Auenbrugger, and rightfully so. Auenbrugger's role was limited to being the inventor while Corvisart was the propagator. Auenbrugger's fame in clinical medicine rests primarily on his treatise dealing with percussion. The acceptance of the technique needed Corvisart.

Leopold Auenbrugger was born in 1722, the son of an innkeeper. It is widely accepted that he adopted the tapping of the wine barrels in his father's inn to determine how much wine they contained to evaluating pathologic processes capable of causing alterations in sound within the thorax[57].

There are two types of percussion: direct and indirect (also known as mediate). Auenbrugger described and practiced the direct type, striking the subject's chest with glove-encased finger tips and not bothering to remove the patient's shirt. This was not due to elegance or modesty but served rather as a means of preventing the fingers from sliding over the skin of the subject.

Auenbrugger was also an accomplished musician, and perhaps this meant that he had such a good ear for sound that it was not necessary to disrobe the patient. At any rate, in his hands, this impediment to accuracy failed to detract from the overall efficacy of percussion as a diagnostic tool. Corvisart later did do away with the glove and tightly stretched shirt as practiced by Auenbrugger.

Although most of Auenbrugger's observations on percussion concerned themselves primarily with lung disease, he also described in detail the findings in pericardial effusion and in aneurysm of the heart. As would be expected, being analogous to the sounds produced when tapping a wine barrel, pericardial effusion was found to cause the percussion note to be flat.

Aside from this, while observing the various gradations of percussion sounds in different parts of the chest, he noted a dull percussion note (sonus carnis) when tapping over the space occupied by the heart itself. This simple description provided the basis for later observers, especially Corvisart, to detect enlargement of the heart without benefit of such sophisticated techniques as radiology and echocardiography. Of course, the method was crude and markedly subjective, but it marked an important transition point in the physical examination.

It is interesting to note that when Laénnec introduced his mediate auscultation he practiced percussion by striking the chest with his fingers while listening with his stethoscope. True refinement of Auenbrugger's technique, however, did not come about until the introduction of mediate percussion by Piorry in 1828[58]. There were, of course, some serious objections to the usage of immediate or direct percussion. It could be very painful to the patient, and at the same time, unrewarding in terms of localizing a pathologic process. Very few people could master the art of immediate percussion without minimizing or circumventing the above objections. When Piorry introduced his pleximeter, which was initially made of wood, it was to overcome these very disadvantages. Later, he used a small ivory plaque which was applied to the chest with one hand, either alone or attached to a stethoscope, and then struck by a finger of the other hand. This pleximeter is illustrated in Figure 17[59] as published in his atlas of pleximetry in 1851[60].

Further variations of these were introduced by Sansom in 1829[61], and later by Hirschfelder[59] who called his instrument an orthopleximeter.

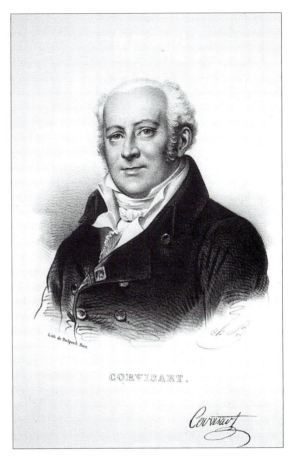

CORVISART.

Figure 15 Portrait of J.N.Corvisart. *Photo Source National Library of Medicine. Literary Source Photo Archives. Courtesy of National Library of Medicine*

For a while, the percussion hammer of Max Anton Wintrich enjoyed some favor. But this, too, along with the numerous and useless modifications of both the original pleximeter and hammer, were tried and found wanting. As early as 1831, James Hope and William Stokes independently found that the usage of the fingers as pleximeter was superior to all other methods, and this method is still in vogue today[62].

Prior to the appearance of his definitive monograph in 1828, Piorry had initially presented a paper on his new method of percussing the thorax at a meeting of the Académie Royale de Médecine. It was held in Paris on February 28, 1826. The paper was published in the *Archives of General Medicine* a few months after[63]. Piorry's presentation precipitated widespread acclaim and soon

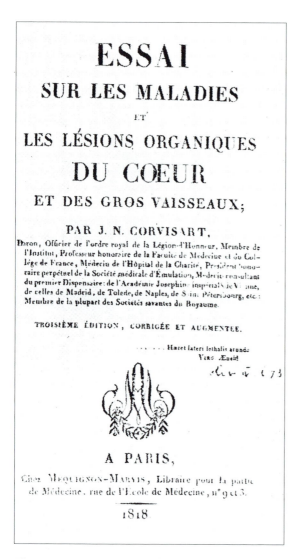

ESSAI

SUR LES MALADIES

ET

LES LÉSIONS ORGANIQUES

DU COEUR

ET DES GROS VAISSEAUX;

PAR J. N. CORVISART,

Baron, Officier de l'ordre royal de la Légion-d'Honneur, Membre de l'Institut, Professeur honoraire de la Faculté de Médecine et du Collége de France, Médecin de l'Hôpital de la Charité, Président honoraire perpétuel de la Société médicale d'Émulation, Médecin consultant du premier Dispensaire de l'Académie Joséphine impériale de Vienne, de celles de Madrid, de Tolède, de Naples, de Saint Pétersbourg, etc.; Membre de la plupart des Sociétés savantes du Royaume.

TROISIÈME ÉDITION, CORRIGÉE ET AUGMENTÉE.

Hæret lateri lethalis arundo
Virg. Æneid.

A PARIS,

Chez MEQUIGNON-MARVIS, Libraire pour la partie de Médecine, rue de l'École de Médecine, n° 9 et 3.

1818.

Figure 16 Frontispiece of Corvisart's monograph. *Photo Source University of Central Florida. Literary Source East, T. The Story of Heart Disease. Plate 6B. Wm. Dawson & Sons, Ltd., 4 Duke Street, London, W.1. Public domain*

transformed him from the relative obscurity of an 'agrégé' to a highly respected clinician. His subsequent monograph in 1828 solidified this perception so that in 1829 he was awarded a prize of 200 francs at a public session of the Academy of Sciences for 'his efforts to perfect the art of medicine'[64].

Piorry practiced the so-called topographical method of percussion and was the first to describe relative and absolute cardiac dullness utilizing this approach. He was also the first to measure the size of the heart on the basis of percussion.

Piorry persistently emphasized the superiority of percussion over auscultation asserting that it reflected more accurately the underlying morbid anatomical change. The patent absurdity of this view is quite obvious to us today since percussion elicits its findings through an entirely different mechanism from that of auscultation; with each modality having its own inherent limitations. It should be pointed out, however, that, to Piorry's credit, he did advocate the use of both methods in actual practice. In his monograph, Piorry states that 'To employ one mode of exploration to the exclusion of others would be proof of poor judgement'[58].

Piorry died in 1879, a widely acclaimed authority on percussion, but also somewhat too pedantic and meticulous in his approach. His meticulous attitude was reflected in his obituary which appeared in *The Lancet* soon after his death. 'There he was in the hospital wards, perched on a high stool, which was taken from bed to bed. He bent over the patient, now knocking the ivory plate gently, now scarcely grazing it with his fingers, with the conviction and love of some great artist, eliciting marvelous notes from a musical instrument'[65].

Another obituary of Piorry appeared 23 years later which anecdotally emphasized his exaggerated claims concerning the accuracy and potentiality of percussion[66]. While on a visit to the Royal Palace at the Tuileries, Piorry insisted upon seeing the king but was put off by the chamberlain with the excuse that the king was not in the reception hall. Not convinced of this, Piorry began percussing the closed door with his pleximeter. As soon as he heard a dull sound, Piorry turned to the chamberlain advising him that this was proof positive that the king was indeed in the chamber. This was showmanship at its best!

In addition to his clinical exploits, Piorry was an ardent linguistic revolutionary. He was opposed especially to the usage of eponyms in medicine. His perception of an adequate nomenclature revolved around terms derived from the Greek. Here too, he tended to exaggerate, creating terms that not only were too pedantic but also were very cumbersome for practical use. He even renamed his 'plessimetre,' introducing instead the word, 'placeplesse.' However, many of the terms he introduced were universally accepted and are still in use today. Examples of these are toxin, toxemia, and septicemia.

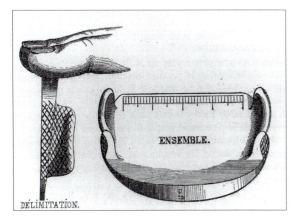

Figure 17 Piorry's pleximeter as published in his atlas of pleximetry in 1851. *Photo Source National Library of Medicine. Literary Source Piorry, P.A. (1851). Traite de Médicine Pranque. Atlas de Plessimetrisme. (Paris: Baillière). Courtesy of National Library of Medicine*

Despite all this, the opening paragraph of the same obituary that reflected his pedantic nature, does acknowledge the great esteem that he deserved: '… One of the most remarkable figures of contemporary medicine in France has just departed this life. He seemed invulnerable, so well did he bear the encroachments of age, and at his advanced time of life he would be seen in the forum of the Paris Academy of Medicine as erect, as firm, and as ardent as ever, fighting his hundredth fight for some favourite theme of medical nomenclature, or some cherished theory in pathology. He has, however, succumbed after a laborious career, full of good work and well deserved honours'[65]. The title page of his classical monograph is displayed in Figure 18.

The technique of percussion along with auscultation became an important part of the physical examination in England and America with the advent of Forbes' book in 1824[67]. Throughout the last half of the 19th century, and well into the first half of the 20th century, numerous contributions on percussion sounds and their meaning were made by a host of clinicians without regard to national boundaries. These included Skoda[68], Ebstein[69], Goldscheider[70], Hirschfelder[59], Camman and Clark[71,72], Brockbank[73], Sibson[74], Rotch[75], Ewart[76], and Bamberger[76]. Some of these men are engraved in posterity by virtue of having their names affixed to certain percussion sounds.

Skoda became the leading non-Parisian advocate of percussion in Europe. The eponym, Skoda's sign,

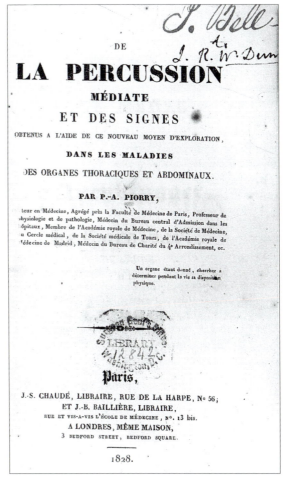

Figure 18 Frontispiece of 'De La Percussion Mediate Et Des Signes' by Piorry. *Photo Source National Library of Medicine. Literary Source Photo Archives. Courtesy of National Library of Medicine*

in massive pleural effusion, is well known to generations of medical students. His treatise on percussion and auscultation was made available to the English speaking world through the translations of Markham, Barth and Roger, and Newbigging[72,77].

Skoda, although influenced no doubt by the Parisian developments, did not abide completely by either their techniques or nomenclature of percussion and auscultation. In an attempt to render these diagnostic aids more scientific rather than artful, he devised a system of description based upon physics and acoustics correlating his clinical conclusions with experiments on cadavers. Skoda was a leading clinician of the new Vienna School of Medicine.

His ability to clarify in more precise terms the various physical signs caused by the anatomic lesion was due, in large part, to a good foundation that he acquired during his preclinical years. Skoda's zeal and faith in the validity of physical diagnosis was so intense that many patients complained about his tiresome repeated examinations. This was finally brought to a head necessitating his transferral by his superiors to a mental ward where, with fewer complaints from these poor unfortunates, he continued his investigations[78].

It is true that Skoda's descriptions and explanatory terms were rudimentary but they represented an important advancement over the flowery and imprecise descriptions of the French. Furthermore, they served as the basis for the addition of further knowledge of physical diagnosis by subsequent clinicians. The Parisian school led by Corvisart and Laénnec, and later by Piorry couched their flowery description in empirical terms. Laénnec's 'cracked pot sound' (bruit de pot fele) is an example of this empirical approach. Later Piorry based the sounds produced on the organ being percussed. In this approach the notes produced over a lung would be described as a 'lung sound,' while those over the liver as an 'hepatic sound,' and so on. Skoda attempted to overcome these imprecise terms by describing four types of percussion notes:

(1) full-empty;

(2) clear-dull;

(3) tympanic-nontympanic; and

(4) high-low[79].

In similar fashion, Skoda's terms for the sounds heard on auscultation were based on pitch and tone. Although most of his work was involved with the lungs, he was one of the first to distinguish between heart sounds and murmurs. He correlated the presence of murmurs with the pathophysiologic changes of individual valves. He also made a special study of pericarditis and the pericardial friction rub; this study was made in collaboration with his long-time friend and colleague, Kollectschka, a pathologist.

Joseph Skoda was born in Pilsen which was then in Bohemia. His father was a locksmith and not situated well financially. Fortunately, a Madame Bischoff, wife of a Viennese manufacturer, overcame this pecuniary status by subsidizing Skoda's attendance at medical school in Vienna. Skoda had two brothers, one of whom also became a physician while the other, Johann, became initially a locksmith like the father. The younger Johann eventually founded a locomotive factory which evolved into the famous Skoda works, noted for armaments and, later, automobiles[80].

Skoda in conjugation with the German pathologist, Karl von Rokitansky, was responsible for the justified fame of Vienna as being at the forefront of medical knowledge during the mid-19th century. Skoda's major work was his *Abhandlung über Perkussion und Auskultation*[81]. It was published in 1839 and went through six editions. It was translated into English by William Orlando Markham, an English cardiologist, who was editor of the British Medical Journal[82]. Figure 19 is the title page from Skoda's text on percussion and auscultation.

At the time Skoda's text was published, he had just lost his position as an assistant physician at the Allgemeine Krankenhaus. Despite his reputation as an excellent clinical teacher his future was still uncertain. To underline the vicissitudes of fortune, Skoda's success was soon secured by virtue of a diagnosis he made on the ailing Duke of Blacas, who was then the French minister to Austria. The source of the Duke's abdominal complaints had eluded a good many of the eminent physicians of the time. Skoda accurately identified it as being due to a leaking abdominal aortic aneurysm and predicted that the patient would die in a very short time. The diagnosis was soon confirmed at autopsy. This greatly enhanced Skoda's reputation as a diagnostician and very soon thereafter he was appointed Primarius for the newly established division of chest diseases at the Allgemeine Krankenhaus. Though still without salary, Skoda was now able to continue his studies without restraint. Six years later he was appointed to the chair of internal medicine in the Vienna medical school, and in contrast to his earlier struggles he began to enjoy financial security. He died in 1881 with his declining years marred by a cardiac disorder. Autopsy revealed aortic stenosis and advanced coronary artery disease[83]. Skilled as a foremost diagnostician, assiduous in his application of scientific principles to medical practice, Skoda had very little respect or faith in the therapeutic modalities of his time. He was probably right for maintaining such a skeptical, and at times, nihilistic attitude, since the fashionable therapeutic measures at that time consisted of bleeding, application of leeches, sweating, and polypharmacy with useless galenicals.

Ebstein's method of percussion depended upon the sense of resistance to the finger rather that alteration in sound[69]. It was known as 'Tastpercussion'. Goldscheider introduced the term 'orthopercussion' in 1905[70]. He used the finger tip method of Plesch. The shaft of his instrument had to be pointed parallel to the border of the heart. Bedford[77] in his classic paper on the history of percussion of the heart noted that the correlation of auscultatory percussion with cadaver experiments was initiated by Camman and Clark. As a result of these experiments, Bedford describes how these men utilized a cedarwood rod, centering one end over the heart, and listening at the upper end while percussing the chest wall from the space overlying the adjacent lung towards the heart itself. The point of transition over which the percussion note changed from resonant to dull indicated the border of the heart thereby providing a quasi-quantitative means of measuring the size of the heart; a rather crude method to be sure, but able to provide some valuable information in this pretechnological era. The extent to which this attempt at quantitation reached an exaggerated level can be gleaned by reference to Figure 20. This figure purports to illustrate how Brockbank differentiated between dilatation and hypertrophy of the heart.

Bedford goes on to recount how Rotch, in 1878, described dullness in the fifth intercostal space as indicating the presence of pericardial effusion. Another sign consistent with pericardial effusion was that described by Ewart.

In the same paper, Bedford also describes some of the issues, myths and vagaries surrounding the use of percussion. Is it better to percuss lightly or heavily? This was and continues to be a bitterly contested point. Should the percussion sounds be expressed in terms of tonality, sonority, intensity and timbre? Austin Flint in America had already added to this plethora of terms in 1852 with his paper describing variations of pitch in percussion, and the interpretation of respiratory sounds as they applied to physical diagnosis[84].

Bedford also related how the myth of Sibson's notch in pericardial effusion was exposed by Blechman in 1922. Blechmann stated that Sibson never described the sign from *in vivo* observations. Sibson's illustrations of pericardial effusion were drawn instead from cadavers after the injection of

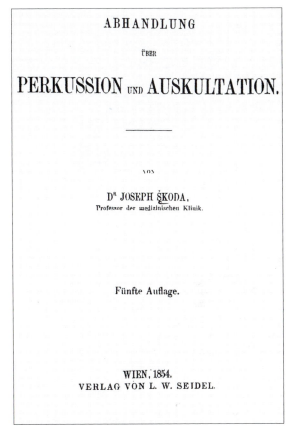

Figure 19 Title page of Skoda's text on percussion and auscultation. *Photo Source Royal Society of Medicine. Literary Source Original. Courtesy of the Royal Society of Medicine*

fluid into the pericardial sac without a comparable clinical model. The alleged pattern of Sibson's notch is depicted in Figure 21.

As a final note, percussion of the heart is rapidly becoming a lost art. There are far better methods today of determining the size of the heart. Echocardiography is an excellent example, among others, of the non-invasive strides that have been made not only in assessing cardiac size but also in delineating between dilatation and hypertrophy; in pinpointing which cardiac chamber is affected; in determining whether the changes are due to pressure overload or volume overload, and in defining other physiologic changes that are important in assessing cardiac status.

However, we should not mourn the passing of a lost art nor denigrate it. Percussion served a useful purpose during an age that relied heavily on one's

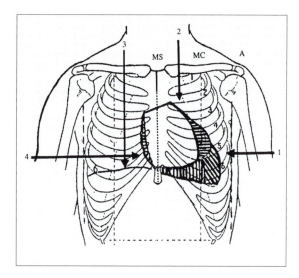

Figure 20 Percussion of the heart after Brockbank. Arrows show order and direction. Dilatation indicated by horizontal shading, hypertrophy by vertical shading and combined hypertrophy and dilatation by diagonal shading. *Photo Source University of Central Florida. Literary Source Brockbank, E.M. (1930). The Diagnosis and Treatment of Heart Disease, 6th ed. (London: H.K.Lewis) With permission*

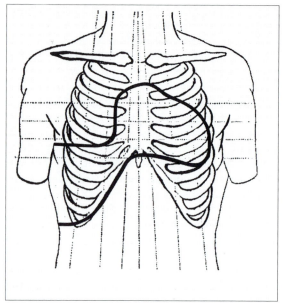

Figure 21 Sibson's notch on left border as a sign of a large pericardial effusion. *Photo Source University of Central Florida. Literary Source Merklen and Heitz, 1914, 5th edition. Masson et Cie. With permission*

senses rather than on electronic equipment. It provided an important link between the ignorance of the past and the explosive knowledge provided by the technological advancements during the last half of the 20th century.

Auscultation was one of the modalities used by Hippocrates in the examination of the patient. He described it in these words: 'You shall know by this that the chest contains water and not pus, if in applying the ear during a certain time on the side, you perceive a noise like that of boiling vinegar'[85]. This mode of examination endured throughout the years during which the Hippocratic precepts held sway. It was carried out by applying the ear directly to the subject's chest or abdomen, and because of the direct application of the ear, it is known as direct auscultation. The friction rub of the pleuritis was clearly described in this manner by Hippocrates. He compared it to the creaking sound of leather. Hippocrates was also the first to describe the succussion splash. This is a noise heard over a body cavity containing air and fluid when the subject is shaken briskly. When this sound is heard in the thorax, it is usually due to pneumohydrothorax. Similar splashing

sounds can also be heard over the abdomen; again, when there is a mixture of air and fluid in the stomach or in a distended bowel. Figure 22 is a half-tone showing Laénnec utilizing direct auscultation on a patient with pulmonary tuberculosis.

Mediate auscultation involves the use of an instrument interposed between the source of origin of the sounds and the observer's ear. It owes its inception to Laénnec, who, in using such a method, created the first stethoscope. Laénnec initially practiced direct or immediate auscultation, a technique he learned from Gaspard-Laurent Bayle.

The possible benefits of auscultation were perceived long before Laénnec by Robert Hooke (1635–1793), secretary of the Royal Society of London. He wrote about his ability to hear very plainly the beating of a man's heart … 'Who knows, I say, but that it may be possible to discover the motions of the internal parts of bodies by the sound they make'[86].

René Theophile-Hyacinthe Laénnec was born in Quimper, West Brittany in 1781[87]. The son of a lawyer, young René was actually raised by his uncles, one of whom, a priest, inculcated in the youth an ardent enthusiasm for the classics. Laénnec's medical training was under the direction of another uncle who eventually became professor of medicine at Nantes. Laénnec then became a pupil of Jean-Nicholas Corvisart des Marets, and later succeeded him as physician to the Charité Hospital in Paris.

Always somewhat frail and burdened by a busy private practice along with his research and teaching activities, Laénnec already began to manifest the sapping effect of pulmonary tuberculosis early in life. However, despite his easy fatigability and inclination to become readily exhausted, he still carried on, in a methodical fashion, his daily activities, dying prematurely at the early age of 45.

Averse to the idea of applying his ear to the chest of an obese woman with symptoms of cardiac dysfunction, Laénnec introduced the art of mediate auscultation by listening to the patient's heart with a quire of paper that he had previously rolled into the form of a cylinder. He applied one end of this roll to the precordial area while listening at the other end. This was the first monaural stethoscope, and with it, a quantum leap was made in the ability to diagnose many disorders of the heart through physical findings. The stethoscope provided the final link, namely, auscultation.

The following translation of Laénnec's description is from John Forbes[88].

The first instrument which I used was a cylinder of paper, formed of three quires, compactly rolled together, and kept in shape by paste. The longitudinal aperture which is always left in the centre of the paper thus rolled, led accidentally in my hands to an important discovery. This aperture is essential to the exploration of the voice. A cylinder without any aperture is the best for the exploration of the heart: the same kind of instrument will indeed suffice for the respiration and rattle; but both of these are more distinctly perceived by means of a cylinder which is perforated throughout, and excavated into somewhat of a funnel shape, at one of its extremities, to the depth of an inch and a half. The most dense bodies do not, as might have been expected from analogy, furnish the best materials for these instruments. Glass and metals, exclusively of their weight and the sensation of cold occasioned by their application in winter, convey the sound less distinctly than bodies of

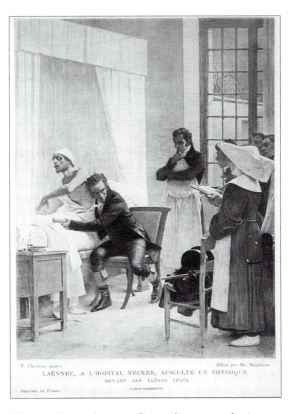

Figure 22 Laénnec utilizing direct auscultation on a patient with pulmonary tuberculosis. *Photo Source National Library of Medicine. Literary Source T. Chartran, peintre. Courtesy of National Library of Medicine*

inferior density. Upon making this observation, which at first surprised me, I wished to give a trial to materials of the least possible density, and, accordingly, caused to be constructed a cylinder of goldbeater's skin, inflated with air, and having the central aperture formed of pasteboard. This instrument I found to be inferior to all the others, as well from its communicating the sounds of the thoracic organs more imperfectly, as from its giving rise to foreign sounds, from the contact of the hand, &c.

Bodies of a moderate density, such as paper, the lighter kinds of wood, or Indian cane, are those which I always found preferable to others. This result is perhaps in opposition to an axiom in physics; it has, nevertheless, appeared to me one which is invariable. In consequence of these various experiments I now employ a cylinder of wood, an inch and a half in diameter, and a foot long, perforated longitudinally by a bore one quarter inch wide, and hollowed out into a funnel-shape, to the depth of an inch and a half at one of its extremities. It is divided into two portions, partly for the convenience of carriage, and partly to permit its being used of half the usual length. The instrument in this form – that is, with the funnel-shaped extremity, – is used in exploring the respiration and rattle; when applied to the exploration of the heart and the voice, it is converted into a simple tube, with thick sides, by inserting into its excavated extremity a stopper or plug traversed by a small aperture, and accurately adjusted to the excavation. This instrument I have denominated the Stethoscope. The dimensions mentioned are not a matter of indifference. A greater diameter renders its exact application to certain parts of the chest, impracticable; greater length renders its retention in exact apposition more difficult, and when shorter, it is not so easy to apply it to the axilla, while it exposes the physician too closely to the patient's breath, and, besides, frequently obliged him to assume an inconvenient posture, a thing above all others to be avoided, if we wish to observe accurately. The only case in which a shorter instrument is useful, is where the patient is seated in bed, or on a chair, the head or back of which is close to him: then it may be more convenient to employ the half length instrument.

Laénnec's original account of what transpired at the bedside of the patient is as follows:

I was consulted in 1816 by a girl who presented the general symptoms of heart disease and in whom palpation and percussion gave little information on account of the patient's obesity. Her age and sex forbade an examination [by direct auscultation]. Then I remembered a well-known acoustic fact, that if the ear be applied to one end of a plank it is easy to hear a pin's scratching at the other end. I conceived the possibility of employing this property of matter in the present case. I took a quire of paper, rolled it very tight, and applied one end of the roll to the precordium; then inclining my ear to the other end, I was surprised and pleased to hear the beating of the heart much more clearly than if I had applied my ear directly to the chest.

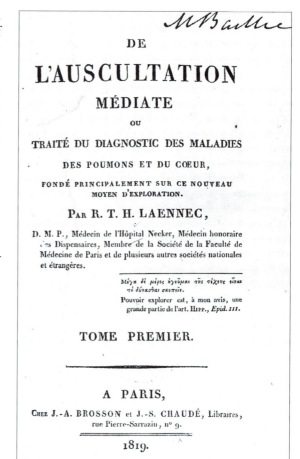

Figure 23 Title page of Laénnec's text on mediate auscultation. The copy belonged to Baillie as indicated by his signature in the upper right hand corner. *Photo Source Royal College of Physicians. Literary Source Original. Courtesy of the Royal College of Physicians*

Figure 23 depicts the title page of his text on mediate auscultation. When Laénnec described the 'well-known acoustic fact' in his original account, he apparently had no inkling that Leonardo da Vinci was also aware of this phenomenon, and perhaps was the first to describe the forerunner of the stethoscope. In his *The Notebooks of Leonardo da Vinci*, MacCurdy quotes Leonardo's notes verbatim[89]: 'If you cause your ship to stop, and place one end of an oar in the water and the other end to your ear, you will hear ships at a great distance from you. You can also do the same by placing the end on the ground and you will then hear anyone passing at a distance from you'.

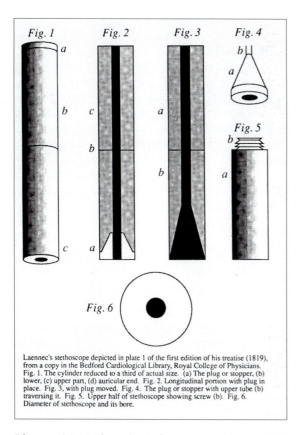

Laennec's stethoscope depicted in plate 1 of the first edition of his treatise (1819), from a copy in the Bedford Cardiological Library, Royal College of Physicians. Fig. 1. The cylinder reduced to a third of actual size. (a) The plug or stopper, (b) lower, (c) upper part, (d) auricular end. Fig. 2. Longitudinal portion with plug in place. Fig. 3, with plug moved. Fig. 4. The plug or stopper with upper tube (b) traversing it. Fig. 5. Upper half of stethoscope showing screw (b). Fig. 6. Diameter of stethoscope and its bore.

Figure 24 Laénnec's stethoscope as depicted in plate 1 of the first edition of his treatise (1819). *Photo Source University of Central Florida. Literary Source Taken from a copy in the Bedford Cardiological Library in the Royal College of Physicians. Courtesy of the Royal College of Physicians*

After numerous designs, Laénnec finally developed the wooden stethoscope that is shown in Figure 24[90]. This model was 18 inches long and 1.5 inches in diameter. It was perforated in the center and fitted with a plug against which the ear was applied. To facilitate portability, it was made in two parts which were screwed together prior to use. The entrepreneurial instinct of Laénnec is evident from the fact that he himself manufactured these instruments in his own home workshop, and gave complementary stethoscopes to every buyer of his book on auscultation. The Royal College of Physicians housed one of these original models. It is the very same one that was presented to C. J. B. Williams by Laénnec[91]. Figure 25 is an illustration of this particular model.

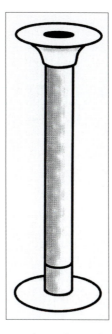

Figure 25 Monaural wooden stethoscope belonging to C.J.B. Williams. Now housed in the Royal College of Physicians. *Photo Source University of Central Florida. Literary Source Williams, C.T. (1907). Laénnec and the evolution of the stethoscope. Br. Med. J., July 6, pp. 6–7. With permission*

The word 'stethoscope' is derived from the Greek, meaning to view the chest. Laénnec's designation of this instrument by the term stethoscope did not come into popular usage until sometime later. It was called by a number of different names such as 'cornet de papier', 'cylindre', 'baton', 'solometer', and 'cornet medical'.

Laénnec experimented with materials of different densities in his earlier models in an attempt to improve the quality of the transmitted sounds. He found that very dense materials such as glass or metal were not good carriers of sounds emanating from the heart or lungs. Prior to settling on the wooden stethoscope, Laénnec experimented with goldbeater's skin inflated with air and with the central aperture formed of pasteboard. This did not satisfy him and after numerous substitutions he finally reached the conclusions that wood and cane, substances of medium density, were the best compromise. He finally settled on boxwood[92]. Some of the earlier stethoscopes were 13 inches in length rather than 18 inches. These were also in the

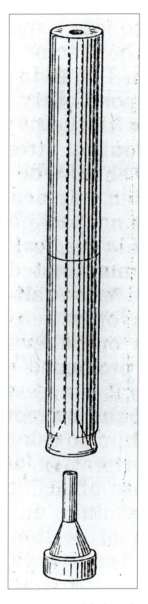

Figure 26 Laénnec's modified stethoscope. *Photo Source National Library of Medicine. Literary Source Williams, C.T. (1907). Laénnec and the evolution of the stethoscope. Br. Med. J., July 6, pp. 6–7. With permission*

form of a cylinder with a diameter of 1½ inches[93]. The entire cylinder was perforated by a longitudinally arranged bore ¾ inch wide, and hollowed out at one end in the shape of a funnel to a depth of 1½ inches[94]. Laénnec was of the opinion that the heart sounds were heard better by inserting at the funnel

shaped opening a stopper or plug. Figure 26 pictures this device.

Initially, there was a great deal of opposition and resistance to the practice of auscultation. There were a number of reasons for this. Many patients were fearful. There was an impression on the part of certain physicians that they might look foolish in the utilization of this technique, or, even worse, that they might be confused with surgeons[95]. There was also the inconvenience of carrying the instrument itself. One way of dealing with this last impediment might have been the one recounted by Hawksley, a reputable medical and surgical instrument maker of London. According to them, most of the stethoscopes manufactured during the first half of the 19th century were made in one piece and of a certain length so that they could be carried by the physician in his high hat which was the fashionable gear for well-dressed gentlemen of that era[96]. By the time Arthur Conan Doyle (1859–1930) wrote his Sherlock Holmes stories, the high hat of the 19th century physician with its discreetly hidden stethoscope, came to be the very symbol of the medical profession, so much so, that Sherlock Holmes in *A Scandal in Bohemia* identifies an individual as a physician by this symbol among other signs. To wit: '... As to your practice, if a gentleman walks into my rooms, smelling of iodoform, with a black mark of nitrate of silver upon his right forefinger, and a bulge on the side of his top-hat to show where he has secreted his stethoscope, I must be dull indeed if I do not pronounce him to be an active member of the medical profession'.

This long stethoscope was eventually modified into three parts by a Dr Judson Doland. By separating the instrument into a stem, bell, and ear piece, Doland was, of course, thinking of the convenience of utilizing the vest pocket as a portable repository[96].

The London Times of December 19, 1824 printed the following paragraph on the recently invented stethoscope. It is of interest not only because of its sociological implications, but also because of the insight it gives concerning the attitude of the lay press towards the new invention.

A wonderful instrument called the Stethoscope, invented a few months ago, for the purpose of ascertaining the different stages of pulmonary affections, is now in complete vogue at Paris. It is merely a hollow wooden tube, about a foot in length (a common flute, with the holes stopped and the top open, would do, perhaps, just as well). One end is applied to the breast of the patient, the other to the ear of the physician, and according to the different sounds, harsh, hollow, soft, loud, etc., he judges of the state of the disease. It is quite a fashion if a person complains of a cough, to have recourse to the miraculous tube, which, however, cannot effect a cure; but should you unfortunately perceive in the countenance of the Doctor, that he fancies certain symptoms exist, it is very likely that a nervous person might become seriously indisposed and convert the supposition into reality.

Despite the opposition, historically predictable as with any form of scientific breakthrough, Laénnec's mediate method of auscultation soon gained widespread popularity and attracted physicians to his clinic from all over Europe so that they could learn about this new method from the master himself. By the 1830s, the stethoscope had become part and parcel of a careful bedside examination. Indeed, by this time, failure to use a stethoscope was considered detrimental to a physician's competency and reputation.

Piorry improved Laénnec's stethoscope by reducing the stem to the thickness of a finger. Several modifications of the pectoral end were then tried to intensify and condense the sounds with minimal discomfort to the patient. In the hands of C. J. B. Williams, this finally evolved into a trumpet-shaped form that seemed to resolve all the problems of the previous designs. Williams made a further improvement by introducing a movable earpiece to facilitate auscultation above the clavicle and the scapula. Figure 27 is a picture of Williams' monaural stethoscope.

In his zeal to make the perfect stethoscope, Williams also experimented with different types of wood. He finally settled on ebonite because of its strength and the ease with which it could be cleaned after each use; a practice he strongly advocated.

The inflexibility of the original stiff wooden tubes caused discomfort to both patient and physician. This led to the introduction of the flexible monaural device. This modification was devised by Nicholas Comens in 1829 and consisted of two rigid tubes joined in such a manner that they could be twisted into various angles[97].

As time went on, it became clear that the solid vibrating wall of wood was not necessary since

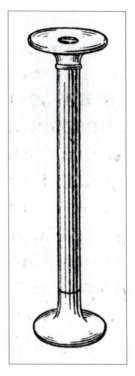

Figure 27 Williams' monaural stethoscope. *Photo Source National Library of Medicine. Literary Source Williams, C.T. (1907). Laénnec and the evolution of the stethoscope. Br. Med. J., July 6, pp.6–7. With permission*

it was the air column that was the conductor of the sound. The flexibility of Comens' modification was enhanced further by the substitution of India rubber tubing. Figure 28 is an illustration of this modification.

Variations and modifications of Laénnec's original model proliferated to such an extent that by 1869 Maw & Son of England was able to offer 24 varieties as indicated in the quarterly price-current (see Figure 29).

The monaural stethoscope, with and without the aforementioned modifications, still survives in certain parts of Europe but its usage appears to be restricted solely to those areas that still employ some form of Piorry's pleximeter[32].

A Dr Arthur Leared claimed to have invented the binaural stethoscope in 1851. However, it is the contention of C. T. Williams (and confirmed by others) that the credit should really belong to his father, C. J. B. Williams[93]. He presents in his paper an illustration of what he claims was the first

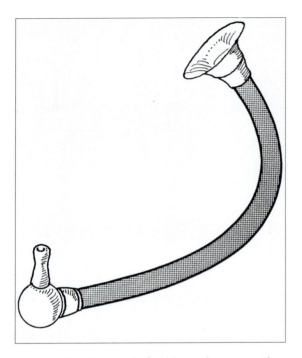

Figure 28 Monaural flexible stethoscope. *Photo Source National Library of Medicine. Literary Source Williams, C.T. (1907). Laénnec and the evolution of the stethoscope. Br. Med. J., July 6, pp. 6–7. With permission*

binaural stethoscope as constructed by his father in 1829, a good 22 years prior to Leared. Figure 30 is taken from Williams' paper illustrating his father's binaural stethoscope.

This stethoscope consisted of a chest piece made of mahogany and shaped like a trumpet. It was connected by means of a screw-like device to two bent lead pipes. The listening end of the pipes must have been very uncomfortable since they lacked earpieces or adaptable fittings of any kind.

In 1850, George Camman substituted rubber tubing for the lead pieces. This was the forerunner of the modern stethoscope. The aural ends of Camman's model fitted nicely into the auditory meatus providing greater comfort and clarity of sound for the physician[98]. Comfort for the physician was enhanced further in time by lengthening the flexible tubes. The optimal length and diameter of the flexible tubing was not established until the mid 20th century. Figure 31 is an illustration of an advertisement by Caswell, Hazard and Company. Three varieties of Camman's 'double stethoscope'

are offered. The prices are rather low from today's inflationary perspective, but hardly so for those times.

It is quite obvious by now that C. J. B. Williams played an important role in the development of the stethoscope, and it would not be remiss at this point to digress a bit with an interesting anecdote concerning him.

C. J. B. Williams was renowned for his clinical abilities, and was held in great esteem by his peers. He cherished this reputation, and, at one time, when his professional ability was challenged, he came to its defense with a vengeance.

Figure 32 is the title page of a pamphlet written by C. J. B. Williams in defense against certain allegations made by the Duchess of Somerset. In essence, she accused Williams of misconduct and incompetence while he was in attendance at her son's illness. Pages 6 and 7 of this pamphlet outline the reasons for the narrative and the following is a direct quotation[99]:

My conscience is clear that throughout this short but anxious and painful charge, I acted in good faith and to the best of my ability and good judgement. And I have no doubt that the verdict of my own profession will be in my favor. It is with feelings of deep satisfaction that I refer to the statement at the end of this preface, which expresses the deliberate opinion of some of the most eminent and enlightened physicians and surgeons in this country.

The retraction and apology of the Duke and Duchess of Somerset in Court (See Appendix) has frankly and freely, and most unreservedly withdrawn all those imputations in the libel which reflect on my professional honor and character. This is so far satisfactory to me, as an act of justice, albeit somewhat tardy. It is still more satisfactory to me to prove that all the charges and imputations were, from the first, absolutely without foundation; but it is far more gratifying to me – I feel it to be a positive honor – that throughout this painful and embarrassing trial, and amid opposing influences of high rank and noble birth, I have received the support and approval of those whom I most esteem and venerate in my own honorable profession, and of my numerous other personal friends.

Charles J. B. Williams
49 Upper Brook Street
March 12, 1870

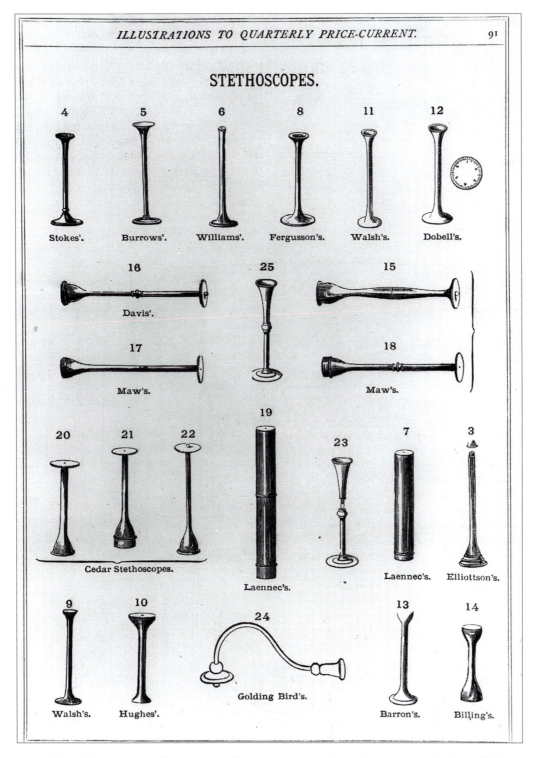

Figure 29 Advertisement of stethoscopes from Maw & Son. *Photo Source National Library of Medicine. Literary Source Maw(S.) & Son. Book of Illustrations to Price-Current. London, p.91, 1869. Courtesy of National Library of Medicine*

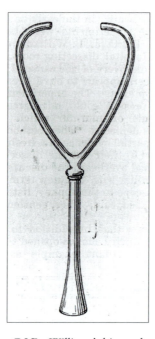

Figure 30 C.J.B. Williams' binaural stethoscope. *Photo Source National Library of Medicine. Literary Source Williams, C.T. (1907). Laénnec and the evolution of the stethoscope. Br. Med. J., July 6, pp.6–7. With permission*

There was no doubt about the overwhelming support accorded Williams by his contemporaries. This is well documented, as he indicated, by the statement at the end of the preface.

An equally interesting aspect of this scenario is the ailment itself that afflicted the patient. This terminal illness of the Earl St Maur was probably due to an aneurysm of the aortic arch, the clinical manifestations of which were caused by pressure against the trachea and its adjacent nerves. The patient was young. He was only 34 when he was seen by the various physicians that the family frantically consulted. One of them, a Dr Fairbanks, described the presence of a depressed sternum. The patient's youth, depressed sternum and the presence of an aortic aneurysm constitute, in the light of present knowledge, enough evidence to advance the hypothesis that the Earl St Maur was probably a victim of Marfan's syndrome.

By the year 1859, even more elaborate variations of the double stethoscope made their appearance. Casper Wistar Pennock introduced a modified version of the flexible stethoscope. It consisted of a coiled wire covered with silk and attached at each end to a metallic cone. Figure 33 depicts in a summary fashion some of the various modifications and improvements beginning with No. 1 which is an example of a monaural stethoscope utilizing pliant tubing.

In 1860, S. Alison invented the so-called differential stethoscope. Kerr's modifications of this is pictured as No. 3 in Figure 33. It consists of two separate chest pieces, each of which directed sound to one ear through its own tubing. Kerr called it a symballophone. The alleged advantage of such an arrangement was that it allowed for simultaneous listening of sounds from different parts of the chest[100]. The symballophone never enjoyed any degree of popularity.

The diaphragm chest piece was developed in 1894, but it was not until 1926 that Howard B. Sprague combined it with the bell[101]. The diaphragm was the invention of R. C. M. Bowles, an engineer from Brookline, Massachusetts.

The physiological and physical laws governing auscultation were outlined by Rappaport and Sprague in 1941[102]. These men also described the effects of tubing bore on stethoscope efficiency in 1951, and a year later they emphasized the relationship between efficiency and the proper fitting of the ear-pieces[103,104].

The popularity of the binaural stethoscope was by no means universal. A short but rather emphatic communication on the preference of the monaural solid stethoscope to the flexible binaural type appeared in *The Lancet* in 1902[105]. The author was H. W. Syers. He attributed the 'decay' of auscultation to the use of the binaural stethoscope. His comments are quite interesting: 'I look upon the use of the binaural stethoscope as being in every way most objectionable … The double stethoscope should be altogether done away with and abolished from the face of the earth – Delenda est Carthago.'

Long before this diatribe appeared, the same type of evaluation regarding the relative merits of the two types of stethoscope are to be found in Sansom's *Physical Diagnosis of the Heart*. It was published in 1881[106].

Even more surprising was the preference for listening with the naked ear by some of the outstanding clinicians of the 19th and even 20th century. Duroziez and Potain described many of their important findings either with the naked ear

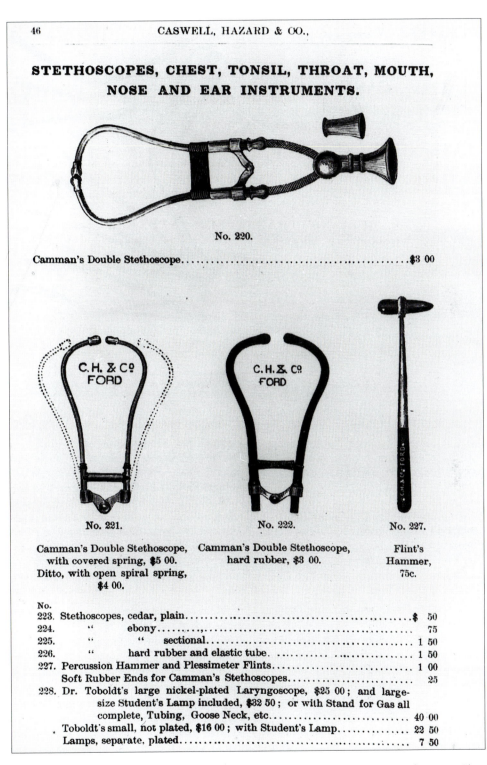

46 CASWELL, HAZARD & CO.,

STETHOSCOPES, CHEST, TONSIL, THROAT, MOUTH, NOSE AND EAR INSTRUMENTS.

No. 220.

Camman's Double Stethoscope..$3 00

No. 221.   No. 222.   No. 227.

Camman's Double Stethoscope,   Camman's Double Stethoscope,   Flint's
with covered spring, $5 00.   hard rubber, $3 00.   Hammer,
Ditto, with open spiral spring,   75c.
     $4 00.

No.
223. Stethoscopes, cedar, plain.............................$ 50
224.   "   ebony.........................   75
225.   "   "   sectional............................. 1 50
226.   "   hard rubber and elastic tube. 1 50
227. Percussion Hammer and Plessimeter Flints.................. 1 00
     Soft Rubber Ends for Camman's Stethoscopes...............   25
228. Dr. Toboldt's large nickel-plated Laryngoscope, $25 00; and large-
     size Student's Lamp included, $32 50; or with Stand for Gas all
     complete, Tubing, Goose Neck, etc..................... 40 00
     Toboldt's small, not plated, $16 00; with Student's Lamp.............. 22 50
     Lamps, separate, plated............................... 7 50

Figure 31   Three models of Camman's double stethoscope and Flint's percussion hammer. *Photo Source National Library of Medicine. Literary Source Caswell & Hazard Co. Illustrated catalogue of Surgical Instruments and Appliances. George C. Frye, p. 46, 1880. Courtesy of National Library of Medicine*

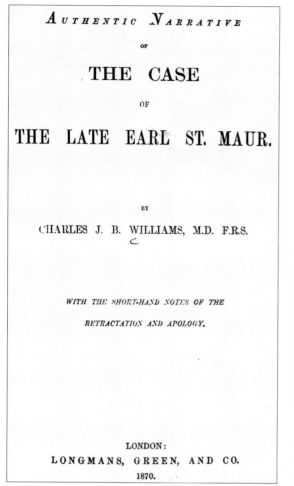

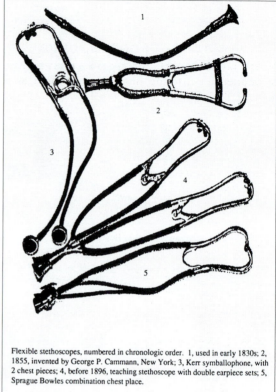

Flexible stethoscopes, numbered in chronologic order. 1, used in early 1830s; 2, 1855, invented by George P. Cammann, New York; 3, Kerr symballophone, with 2 chest pieces; 4, before 1896, teaching stethoscope with double earpiece sets; 5, Sprague Bowles combination chest place.

Figure 32 Title-page of 'The Case of the Late Earl St. Maur' by Charles J.B. Williams. *Photo Source The Royal College of Physicians. Literary Source Original. Courtesy of the Royal College of Physicians*

Figure 33 Modifications and improvements in flexible stethoscopes (numbered in chronological order). *Photo Source University of Central Florida. Literary Source McKusick, V.A., Sharp, W.D. and Warner, A.O. (1957). An exhibition on the history of cardiovascular sound including the evolution of the stethoscope. Bull. Hist. Med., 31, 463–87. With permission from Johns Hopkins University Press, Journals Publishing Division, 701 W. 40th Street, Ste. 275, Baltimore, Md. 21211*

applied to the chest or, only later, by means of the monaural stethoscope.

Lewis A. Conner, a founder of the American Heart Association, always carried a silk handkerchief for use in direct auscultation. He favored this approach for the faint, high-pitched diastolic murmurs of aortic regurgitation[106]. This was as late as 1907.

Although it applies to direct auscultation of the lungs rather than the heart, the illustration in Figure 34 is a perfect example of the satirical perspective the French still had in 1902 regarding this diagnostic modality.

Mediate auscultation with the monaural stethoscope also came in for its share of biting satire as indicated by Figure 35 which is entitled 'Kranker Teufel'.

Other variations of the stethoscope also came and went. An interesting one was the phonendoscope. It was invented by a physicist, Bazzi, in collaboration with a physician, Bianchi[107]. Its inventors claimed that it was able to amplify faint sounds and that it was also capable of precise localization of sounds. This stethoscope contained as part of its components, a stiff diaphragm. It is pure conjecture on my part, but, perhaps, this may have been the inspiration for Bowles' diaphragm. A really versatile one was the instrument that Aydon Smith introduced in 1884[108]. It reminds one of the 'army knives' that the Swiss produce for campers and other outdoorsmen. Smith, in all sincerity, recommended that the instrument be used as a monaural, binaural or a differential stethoscope. In addition he suggested that the tubing could serve as a tourniquet, catheter or gastric lavage tube. He also advised that the chest pieces could serve as a funnel for administering fluids through a tube for enemas or douches. This was a veritable storehouse of accessories.

Following the invention of the microphone, and in the current age of electronic gadgetry, further modifications utilizing this technology have been introduced as a means of amplifying the sounds. These, too, have never achieved any significant degree of popularity since the instruments are not only cumbersome but in exchange for amplification, they transmit the sounds with less clarity. However, electronic innovations have played a very important and beneficial role in the development of apparatus for the teaching of heart sounds and murmurs. A notable example of this is 'Harvey', an electronic mannequin named after a notable and esteemed stethoscopist of this century, Dr Proctor Harvey.

The evolution of the stethoscope has been shown to have been dependent upon contributors from Europe, Britain, and America without regard for international boundaries. What about the role auscultation, *per se*, has played as a clinical diagnostic tool? The answer is self-evident. Auscultation has enabled the physician to capture and appreciate the nuances of heart sounds, murmurs, and disturbances in rhythm to such an extent that this element of physical diagnosis has become firmly entrenched in the clinical evaluation of patients. As in the successive modifications of the stethoscope, the growing knowledge concerning the presence, interpretations and clinical application of auscultatory signs in cardiac dysfunction has also been dependent upon various investigators of different national origins. Little did Laénnec realize the impact that his method of auscultation would have on the clinical practice of cardiology. From its embryonic days in Paris and its growing acceptance by the physicians of continental Europe, it soon crossed the channel into England and then, the Atlantic into America.

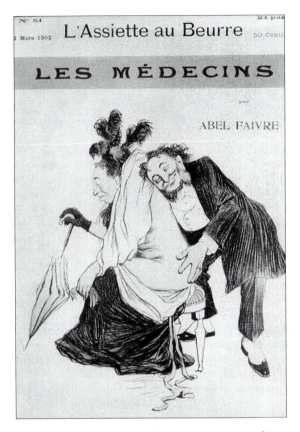

Figure 34 L'Assiette au Beurre. A satire on direct auscultation. *Photo Source National Library of Medicine. Literary Source Faivre Abel: Les Médécins. Courtesy of National Library of Medicine*

It was Sir John Forbes who was mainly responsible for introducing the stethoscope to England. C. J. B. Williams, as noted, was also a leading exponent of mediate auscultation. In 1825, Stokes further enhanced the popularity of this method of auscultation through his book on the use of the stethoscope[109]. In America, the stethoscope was accepted as an important tool of physical diagnosis when Bowditch published *The Young Stethoscopist* in 1846[110]. Along with Bowditch, Austin Flint Sr had a great deal to do with the acceptance of the stethoscope in America. Incidentally, most of the stethoscopes in Flint's time were solid wooden cylinders. These were usually about six or ten inches long. The end to which the ear was applied was concave and rather broad allowing for intimate contact with the listener's ear[111].

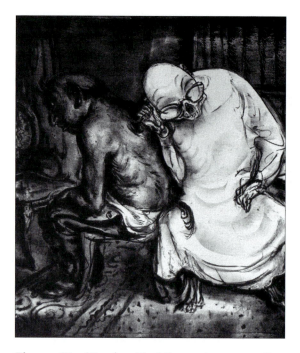

Figure 35 'Kranker Teufel': a satire on mediate auscultation. *Photo Source National Library of Medicine. Literary Source Lithograph by A. Paul Weber. Courtesy of National Library of Medicine*

Another equally important figure in the early development of percussion and auscultation in America was James Jackson Sr at the Massachusetts General Hospital. He was soon joined by many American physicians, a number of whom had gone to Paris to study the new methods of physical diagnosis from the masters themselves. Among them were James Jackson Jr, C.W. Pennock and William Wood Gerhard. Although recognized and esteemed as a teacher, Gerhard never held a professorship. His treatise on diseases of the chest was regarded for many years as an outstanding text ever since its publication in 1848. It was the first American text to incorporate the newer methods of physical diagnosis.

Coming back to Laénnec, the originator of it all, it is ironic that although he invented the stethoscope primarily for the evaluation of cardiac disturbances, his greatest contributions centered about pulmonary rather than cardiac afflictions. In fact, there is a great deal of controversy regarding Laénnec's contributions to cardiology. He has been maligned for his obvious errors in the interpretations, significance and causation of his auscultatory observations on the heart. Some authors have openly ridiculed him while others have been much more indulgent. Yet, it must be remembered that Laénnec (Figure 36) was treading upon virgin ground with an utterly new and untried technique. Prior to Laénnec, there was a 'dearth of recorded interest' in the evaluation of cardiac diseases through physical diagnostic methods[112]. He opened the door to a whole new world of clinical signs fulfilling the antemortem diagnostic potentialities of auscultation.

If one had to select an outstanding attribute of Laénnec, it was his obsessive attention to detail in his clinical observations and the correlation of these observations with the morbid anatomy at necropsy. This was probably the result of the influence of his uncle who had acted for a while as preceptor to the young René. Later, during the first three years as a student at La Charité Hospital where he came under the tutelage of the brilliant Corvisart, Laénnec's devotion to clinical observation was manifested by his compilation of detailed histories of some 400 cases[113]. It was this independent scientific approach that caused Laénnec to be on the cutting edge of medical progress. It is extraordinary, however, that in the face of this attitude, he still felt an obligation to adhere to many of the teachings of Hippocrates. In fact, his doctoral thesis in medicine concerned itself with the doctrines of Hippocrates as applied to clinical practice.

Laénnec's frailty, his untimely death from tuberculosis, and his wonderful discovery were ripe ingredients for romanticizing him. Laénnec is one of the 'witches' in Kipling's *Marklake Witches*. In the story, Laénnec is captured by the British during the Napoleonic Wars and confined to a small English village for the duration. The local medico, called Jerry, is the other 'witch' of the title and the two develop a friendship. Kipling alludes to Laénnec's stethoscope as a 'toy trumpet'. The heroine comes upon the pair one day playing with these 'toy trumpets'. In actuality, the local physician, Jerry, was listening to Laénnec's chest with this so-called trumpet. These are Jerry's words and René's answer:

> Tis wonderfully like hearing a man's soul whispering in his innards; but unless I've a buzzing in my ears, you make about the same kind o' noise as Old Goffer Marklin – but not

quite so loud as young Cooper. It sounds like the breakers in a reef – a long way off. Comprenny?' 'Perfectly'. answered Rene. He knew the significance of these sounds in his chest and in his soul he said, 'I drive on the breakers. But before I strike, I shall save hundreds, thousands, millions perhaps, by my little 'trumpets'[114].

The motion picture industry also remembered Laénnec with the documentary 'Docteur Laénnec' in 1949.

Laénnec's original treatise in 1819, his second edition in 1826, and Forbes' translation in 1834 describe many important discoveries based upon his method[90,91,115,116]. He identified for the first time that each cardiac cycle consisted of two sounds though his explanation for the genesis of the second heart sound was erroneous. As later observations were to confirm, he correctly linked the first sound with the beginning of systole but incorrectly felt that the second sound was due to atrial contraction. It was left to Turner of Edinburgh to point out the error[117].

Laénnec's other important contributions in bedside cardiology include: the 'bruit de soufflet'; the 'bruit de lime'; 'bruit de scie' and 'bruit de rape'; and the sounds audible over the arteries having a characteristic musical or hissing bellows sound. These are purely clinical descriptions of the sounds heard by means of the stethoscope and the analogies relate to the commonalities of Laénnec's time. Thus, 'lime', 'scie', and 'rape' describe the noises produced by filing, sawing and rasping. His explanation for the origin of these sounds as well as other auscultatory findings were often in error but this should not detract from the importance of his basic contribution which was the introduction of the stethoscope.

The cardiology of Laénnec deserves even closer scrutiny since it was he, after all, who opened the flood gates of auscultation. Jacalyn M. Duffin's paper[118] should be read for a scholarly analysis of Laénnec's contributions in this regard. It helps place into proper perspective Laénnec's interpretation of the heart sounds and murmurs – complete with errors, yet notable for the skill with which he navigated through uncharted waters without benefit of physiological understanding. As Duffin states, 'Laénnec's interpretation of the heart sounds and his rejection of the significance of heart murmurs were incorrect, but his observations were sound and some of the sounds he described were

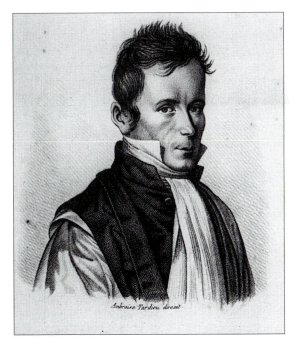

Figure 36 Portrait of Laénnec. *Photo Source National Library of Medicine. Literary Source Photo Archives. Courtesy of National Library of Medicine*

actually useful in predicting the pathological changes that interested him most'[119].

It must also be emphasized that Laénnec made his judgements on the value and significance of stethoscopic signs with no prior guidelines as to their sensitivity and specificity. In fact, these statistical terms did not even exist at the time; nor did the terms 'false negative' and false positive'. He was guided purely by his firm belief in the 'one sign–one lesion' principle. Therefore, he felt that when the sign was present, it had to be indicative of one condition. This was his notion of specificity, and he expressed it by the words, 'constant' or 'pathognomonic'. He also insisted on a certain level of sensitivity, but this was of secondary importance to constant or pathognomonic. He believed so strongly in the 'one sign-one lesion' principle that again he fell into error, when he attempted to classify the qualitative differences in these signs, as they related to the pathologic lesion. Again, Duffin states that Laénnec's qualitative distinctions between murmurs were also 'too subtle to be workable, and since they did not correspond to any reliable clinical or therapeutic distinction, they fell into disuse'[120].

The true nature of the heart sounds and the relationship of murmurs to valvular lesions had to await correlation by future observers with the morbid anatomical changes, newer insights into the hemodynamics governing transvalvular flow, and the introduction of phonocardiography. The graphic representation of the various heart sounds and murmurs enabled succeeding generations of physicians to time precisely their occurrence during the cardiac cycle, and to delineate their relationship to hemodynamic events. Notwithstanding all this, it is still a literary delight to read the various descriptions of the auscultatory events, whether normal or abnormal, by the numerous clinicians who amplified Laénnec's original observations. One of the descriptions that stands out is the famous onomatopoesis of Duroziez for the sounds produced by mitral stenosis. All the components of these sounds (presystolic murmur, accentuated first sound, second sound, opening snap and diastolic rumble) are represented by the expression: *ffout-ta-ta-rou*[121]. My generation was fortunate in having these sounds duplicated orally by Proctor Harvey as he delivered his widely acclaimed lectures on cardiac murmurs.

The stethoscope as a diagnostic tool was also of extreme importance to Stokes. In one of his lectures at Meath Hospital, he strongly defended its usage with the following remarks:

The stethoscope is an instrument not as some represent it, the bagatelle of a day, the brain-born fancy of some speculative enthusiast, the use of which, like the universal medicine of animal magnetism, will soon be forgotten, or remembered only to be ridiculed. It is one of those rich and splendid gifts which science now and then bestows upon her votaries, which while they extend our views and open to us wide and fruitful fields of inquiry, confer in the meantime the richest benefits and blessings on mankind. This instrument was first introduced by one whose works will ever remain as an example of patient investigation, philosophical research, and brilliant discovery, and its use is now supported by the liberal and enlightened and scientific portion of the medical world'.

William Stokes (Figure 37) was part of an extremely capable group of internists that made the Dublin School of Medicine famous. This was during one of Ireland's most trying times; the great potato famine that not only devastated the land but caused the emigration of hordes of Irish to other countries. America was fortunate in receiving a good number of them.

William Stokes was born in Dublin in 1804. His father was a physician, and apparently a very good one, though with a political bent and disturbingly outspoken in this regard. At any rate, notwithstanding his position on the losing side of the political fence, Stokes' father ultimately managed to become Regius Professor of Medicine at Trinity College.

It appears that William was not a very good student during his boyhood. O'Brien tells of how young William had no formal schooling prior to attending medical school in Edinburgh. He had been expelled from school 'after having drawn blood by sending a slate at his Master's head'; and this after only one day of attendance at the local school[122]. He would be categorized in today's pedagogical jargon as a 'late bloomer'. Moreover, he did not seem to be interested in anything, whether it was in sports or school. He would prefer to spend his time with his head 'propped on the neck of a red cow' reading ballads of Sir Walter Scott[123]. Apparently he eventually overcame this deficiency in character and applied himself most diligently to acquiring an education at the hands of his father as well as a tutor. After having been rejected by Trinity College, he was admitted to the Medical School of Edinburgh from which he graduated in 1825. His first claim to fame was a treatise on the use of the stethoscope. This was published immediately after his graduation from medical school.

A year after graduation, Stokes joined the staff at Meath Hospital where he spent the next fifty years. Throughout a good portion of this time he worked very closely with Robert Graves who was initially Stokes' teacher and then close friend and colleague. Stokes published three medical texts after his initial treatise on the use of the stethoscope. The first one appeared in 1837. It was entitled *A Treatise on the Diagnosis and Treatment of Disease of the Chest*. It was hailed as the best treatment of the subject since Laénnec. One of the important topics discussed in this text is the original description of a case of respiratory difficulty, the manifestations of which had been described originally by Cheyne, and are now known to us as 'Cheyne-Stokes respiration'. The case was that of a 60 year old male who had suffered a stroke and was rendered hemiplegic and aphasic. The following quotation is from the text:

> The only peculiarity in the last period of his illness which lasted only eight or nine days, was in the state of the respiration. For several days his breathing was irregular; it would entirely cease for a quarter of a minute, then it would become perceptible, though very low, then by degrees it became heaving and quick, and then it would gradually cease again. This revolution in the state of his breathing occupied about a minute, during which there were about thirty acts of respiration.

The eponym Cheyne-Stokes is applied to this type of respiration because Cheyne's description of the disorder antedates that of Stokes by thirty years[124]. Stokes' contribution lies in his recognition of the fact that this type of disordered breathing could be seen as part of the picture of a weakened and failing heart. Perhaps Hippocrates may have antedated both Cheyne and Stokes if the following quotation is interpreted correctly: 'The respiration throughout like that of a person recollecting himself, was rare and large'[125].

Stokes' second medical text was published 17 years after his first (1854). This one was entitled *Diseases of the Heart and Aorta*. It became quite popular in both Britain and America and was considered a classic for many years[126]. The text dealt extensively with the elements of physical diagnosis emphasizing above all the utility and limitations of the newly introduced auscultation in the diagnosis of heart disease. While stressing the importance of the murmurs delineated by this method, Stokes, nevertheless, realized that though the murmur set the stage, it was clearly the level of cardiac muscular dysfunction that determined the clinical picture. In explaining this, Stokes wrote as follows:

> It is in the vital and anatomical conditions of the muscular fibers that we find the key to cardiac pathology; for, no matter what the affection may be, its symptoms mainly depend on the strength or the weakness, the irritability or the paralysis, the anatomic health or disease of the cardiac muscle. It was long ago observed by Laénnec that valvular diseases had but little influence on health when the muscular condition of the heart remained sound, and every day's experiences confirms this observation.[127]

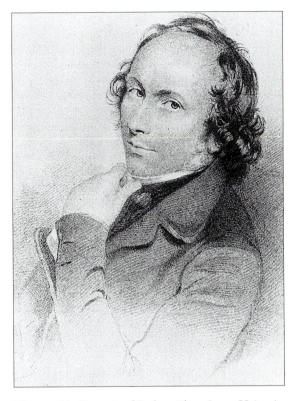

Figure 37 Portrait of Stokes. *Photo Source University of Central Florida. Literary Source Willius, F.A. and Keys, T.E. (1941). Cardiac Classics. (St. Louis, MO: The C.V. Mosby Co.). Courtesy of the Mayo Clinic*

His awareness of this basic dictum that all cardiologists follow today is truly amazing, especially when viewed from the perspective of a technologically oriented approach as in current practice.

As we shall see in the appropriate sections of this book, estimations and assessment of cardiac output, ejection fraction, abnormal wall motion and other parameters of ventricular function are but technological derivations of what Stokes was saying during an era when physical diagnosis constituted the only means of such an evaluation.

Stokes was but one of a group of practical Irish clinicians who, because of their enthusiasm, investigative minds and clear common sense, did a great deal to place Ireland at the forefront of medicine during the first half of the 19th century. This group included Graves, Cheyne and Corrigan, all of whom are eponymously remembered. As Herrick states[128], these men should be commended for their accomplishments though a degree of chauvinism is manifested by Dr Walsh in his *Makers of Modern Medicine* (1907) wherein he claims that 'the Irish school of medicine has in Graves and Stokes and Corrigan a greater group of contemporaries than has been given to any other nation at one time'. The Irish, noted for their gift of hyperbole, should be forgiven for this bit of national pride.

Stokes, in time, became Regius Professor of Medicine at Dublin. He, along with his cohorts, embraced fully the Italian method of bedside clinical diagnosis and instruction utilizing the elements of the Parisian school in physical diagnosis. The group founded medical journals, and wrote books and numerous articles while carrying on an active practice in conjunction with their teaching obligations.

In 1827, Robert Adams published a paper that describes a clinical disorder usually designated as the Stokes–Adams syndrome. According to some, it should rightfully bear the eponym 'Morgagni–Stokes–Adams' since, as noted elsewhere, Morgagni was also aware of some of the components of the syndrome as far back as 1760[129]. Adams described the disorder in a case report of a man seen by him in consultation. The patient manifested not only the same type of respiratory irregularity that characterizes the Cheyne–Stokes respiration, but also a marked slowing of the pulse rate. The hyphenated eponym 'Stokes–Adams' is founded upon Stokes' correlation of the clinical findings with the presence of heart disease. This was based on an analysis of seven cases that Stokes collated from various physicians including two of his own. It was published in 1846, and it antedated by many years the electrocardiographic evidence that the slow pulse was due to a complete heart block with varying degrees of marked bradycardia[130]. Stokes referred to the entire symptom-complex as 'a combination of a singularly slow pulse, tendency to syncope and disease of the aortic valve'. In his description, Stokes mentioned 'semi-beats', heard over the precordium, between the regular contractions, and not accompanied by a pulse. These were probably non-conducted atrial beats though Stokes was not aware that this was the physiologic origin of the 'semi-beats'. Stokes also described in this paper the occurrence in two patients of a peculiar type of pulsation of the veins in the neck which were probably 'cannon waves', and again, was unaware that these pulsations were a reflection of the complete dissociation between atrial and ventricular beats[131]. It should be noted, and again, merely for the sake of completeness, that the syndrome of cardiac syncope, which, in essence, is the major clinical manifestation of complete heart block, had been described by at least six different people prior to Stokes. These were Gerbezius in 1719, Morgagni in 1761, Spens and Duncan in 1793 and Adams and Burnett in 1827 (see Section 4).

The pre-eminence of the French in bedside clinical instruction and its emphasis on physical diagnosis cast its spell not only on the Irish and the English but also, as noted before, on many Americans. Figure 38 is an etching by A. Masson showing a doctor holding forth to a group of students at the bedside in a hospital. This type of teaching persists even today. Figure 39 is a photograph of a class in physical diagnosis in 1903.

Mention has already been made of some of the 'converts' such as Gerhard and Jackson who, in turn, influenced generations of American physicians in training in the art of physical diagnosis. A product of this type of American training was Austin Flint Sr. In truth, he became one of the most outstanding champions of physical diagnosis, enlarging upon and refining many of the diagnostic maneuvers.

Austin Flint Sr was a native of Petersham, Massachusetts, who came from a long line of physicians and who received his education at Amherst and then Harvard. He numbered among his teachers James Jackson Sr, John C. Warren and Jacob Bigelow. A feeling for Flint, the man, can be obtained from Middeton's quotation of a tribute to him by Samuel D. Gross:

Tall, handsome, and of manly form, with a well modulated voice of great compass, he is a lecturer at once clear, distinct and inspiring. During his hour in the classroom no student ever falls asleep. He ranks high as a clinical instructor. As a diagnostician in diseases of the chest he has few equals. Nor is this fact surprising when we bear in mind, the time and the immense labor which, from an early period of his professional life, he has devoted to their investigation. I know of no one who is so well entitled as Austin Flint, Sr. to be regarded as the American Laénnec'[132].

He was indeed a prepossessing figure of a man as this photograph of him in Figure 40 testifies.

Another accolade is the following statement by Korns: 'Flint's remarkable talents, extraordinary versatility, prodigious capacity for work, scientific

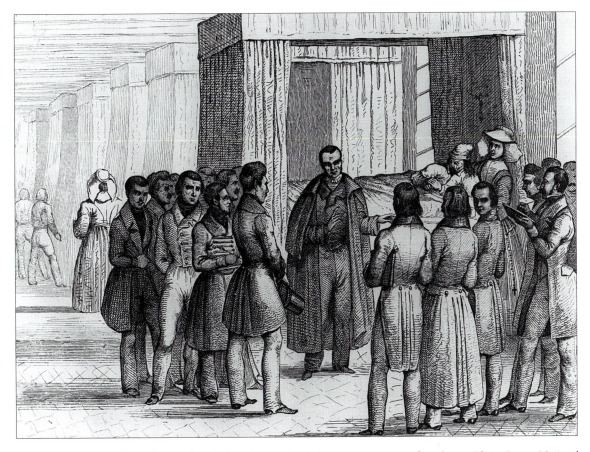

Figure 38 At the bedside in a hospital, a doctor holds forth to a group of students. *Photo Source National Library of Medicine. Literary Source Etching by A. Masson from a painting by Alexandre Lacauchie, working in 1833–1846. Courtesy of National Library of Medicine*

achievements, public spirit, and strength of character made him the greatest figure in American medicine between Benjamin Rush and William Osler'.

Flint's paper on cardiac murmurs is a classic and the bedrock upon which his role in cardiology is assured. This paper appeared originally in 1862. At that time he was Professor of the Principles and Practice of Medicine at Bellevue Hospital Medical College in New York and at the Long Island College Hospital in Brooklyn, NY.

The importance of this paper lies not merely in the classification of the various cardiac murmurs but rather in the presentation of the patho-physiologic scenario that could ensue in the presence of these murmurs. The paper is written in a straightforward and easy manner and on reading it, one can visualize Austin Flint, sitting next to a student and imparting in conversational tones his analysis of the various cardiac murmurs to be encountered.

He classified cardiac murmurs first of all on the basis of their occurrence during the cardiac cycle. He outlined the various factors he utilized in establishing whether or not the murmur was organic or functional in origin. Most of all, he stressed that in the evaluation of the patient, it was not the presence of the murmur that was significant, but rather the effects of the underlying valvular lesion on the myocardium that had to be taken into consideration. In other words, in terms of present day physiological knowledge, the gravity of the lesion should be assessed only by the long term results of either pressure or volume overload. In this, he followed in the footsteps of Stokes.

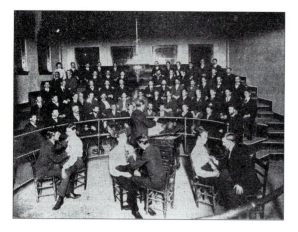

Figure 39 Photograph of a class in physical diagnosis in 1903. *Photo Source National Library of Medicine. Literary Source Photo Archives. Courtesy of National Library of Medicine*

Thus, he writes:

> The murmurs, in themselves, give no information respecting the amount of obstruction from contracted orifices, or of regurgitation from valvular insufficiency ... The truth is, the evils and danger arising from valvular lesions, for the most part, are not dependent directly on these lesions, but on the enlargement of the heart resulting from the lesions ... serious consequences of valvular lesions do not follow until the heart becomes weakened either by dilatation or by degenerative changes in the tissue ... Happily, in most cases, hypertrophy is the first effect of valvular lesions, and, for a time, it keeps pace with the progress of the latter. Dilatation which weakens the hearts action, is an effect consecutive to hypertrophy, and, as a rule, it is not until the dilatation predominates that distressing and dangerous evils are manifested. [133]

This paper also describes for the first time the occurrence and characteristics of a presystolic mitral murmur in the presence of aortic regurgitation, and is now eponymously remembered as the Austin Flint murmur. The following is his account of the murmur; how it can occur in the absence of mitral stenosis and the mechanism for its production.

> ... The murmur is oftener rough than soft. The roughness is often peculiar. It is a blubbering sound, resembling that produced by throwing the lips or the tongue into vibration with the breath of respiration. I suppose that the murmur is caused, in these cases, by the vibration of the mitral currents, and that the vibration of the lips or tongue by the breath of respiration represents the mechanism of the murmur as well as imitates the character of the sound. At one time, I supposed this blubbering murmur denoted a particular lesion, viz., adhesion of the mitral curtains at their sides, forming that species of mitral contraction known as the buttonhole slit; but I have found this variety of murmur to occur without that lesion, and, in fact, as will be seen presently, when no mitral lesion whatever exists ... How is the occurrence of the mitral direct murmur in these cases to be explained? ... Now in cases of considerable aortic insufficiency, the left ventricle is rapidly filled with blood flowing back from the aorta as well as from the auricle, before the auricular contraction takes place. The distension of the ventricle is such that the mitral curtains are brought into coaptation , and when the auricular contraction takes place the mitral direct current passing between the curtains throws them into vibration and gives rise to the characteristic blubbering murmur. The physical condition is in effect analogous to contraction of the mitral orifice from an adhesion of the curtains at their sides, the latter condition, as clinical observation abundantly proves, giving rise to a mitral direct murmur of a similar character ... The practical conclusion to be drawn from the two cases which have been given is, that a mitral direct murmur in a case presenting an aortic regurgitant murmur and cardiac enlargement, is not positive proof of the existence of mitral contraction or of any mitral lesion' [134].

The preceding quotations are a marvel of clarity, incisive logic and deep knowledge of the hemodynamic forces involved in aortic insufficiency; and more than a century before the advent of echocardiography with doppler analysis and color flow imaging demonstrated the very mechanisms he described.

Further developments in cardiac auscultation since Flint's time have concerned themselves primarily with graphic representation of the auscultatory data and technological elucidation of the physiologic and pathophysiologic processes involved in the production of heart sounds, murmurs, and

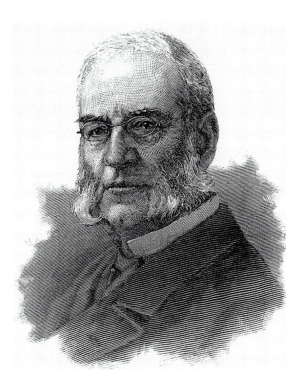

Figure 40 Austin Flint Sr. (Wood engraving after a photograph by Sarony). *Photo Source National Library of Medicine. Literary Source Harper's Weekly **30**, 196, March 27, 1886. Courtesy of National Library of Medicine*

rhythm disturbances. These will be taken up in the section dealing with the newer technological diagnostic techniques.

This portion of the history of auscultation cannot be concluded, however, without presenting a humorous story by C.T. Williams on the usage of the term 'bruit' and the stethoscope song of Oliver Wendell Holmes.

The following paragraph is taken from Williams' article on the evolution of the stethoscope published in 1907[135].

The late Sir Prescott Hewett used to tell a humorous story of the use of the term 'bruit' in the early days of the stethoscope. When the experiments were being carried on by Dr. Hope and Dr. C. J. B. Williams on a donkey in the St. George's Hospital dissecting room, experiments which led to the discovery of the cause of the second sound of the heart, there appears to have been on one occasion a difference of opinion.

The experimenters and several medical men present could not agree as to the audibility of a bruit or murmur which one said was present, while others denied it. They bethought themselves of getting the impartial evidence of a fresh ear to decide the point, and called to their aid the dissecting room porter, who no doubt had overheard the discussion, and was beginning to get familiar with the new terminology. He applied the stethoscope to the donkey, listened attentively, and looking satisfied, said, 'Yes, gentlemen, I hears the brute'.

The doggerel of Oliver Wendell Holmes is considered by some to be a coarse attempt at denigrating the importance of Laénnec's invention. I consider it rather to be a bitterly humorous evaluation of the limitations of any diagnostic tool (which, in this case, happens to be the stethoscope). A ballad of this sort can be written about the usage of any of the sophisticated technological instruments available today at the expense of a logical and common sense approach in the evaluation of cardiac disturbances.

Stethoscope Song
A Professional Ballad

There was a young man in Boston town,
He bought him a stethoscope nice and new,
All mounted and finished and polished down,
With an ivory cap and a stopper too.

It happened a spider within did crawl,
And spins him a web of ample size,
Wherein there chanced one day to fall
A couple of very imprudent flies.

The first was a bottle fly, big and blue,
The second was smaller, and thin and long;
So there was a concert between the two,
Like an octave flute and a tavern gong.

Now being from Paris but recently,
This fine young man would show his skill;
And so they gave him, his hand to try,
A hospital patient extremely ill.

Some said his liver was short of bile,
And some that his heart was oversize,

487

While some kept arguing, all the while,
He was crammed with tubercles up to his eyes.

This fine young man then up stepped he,
And all the doctors made a pause;
Said he, The man must die, you see,
By the fifty-seventh of Louis's laws.

But since the case is a desperate one,
To explore his chest it may be well;
For if he should die and it were not done,
You know the autopsy would not tell.

Then out his stethoscope he took,
And on it placed his curious ear;
Mon Dieu! said he with a knowing look,
Why, here is a sound that's mighty queer!

The bourdonnement is very clear,–
Amphoric buzzing, as I'm alive!
Five doctors took their turn to hear;
Amphoric buzzing, said all five.

There's empyema beyond a doubt;
We'll plunge a trocar in his side.
The diagnosis was made out,-
They tapped the patient; so he died.

Now such as have new-fashioned toys
Began to look extremely glum;
They said that rattles were made for boys,
And vowed that his buzzing was all a hum.

There was an old lady had long been sick,
And what was the matter none did know;
Her pulse was slow, though her tongue was quick;
To her this knowing youth must go.

So there the nice old lady sat,
With phials and boxes all in a row,
She asked the young doctor what he was at,
To thump her and tumble her ruffles so.

Now, when the stethoscope came out,
The flies began to buzz and whiz;
Oh, ho! the matter is clear, no doubt;
An aneurism there plainly is.

The bruit de rape and the bruit de scie
and the bruit de diable are all combined.

How happy Boulliaud would be,
If he a case like this could find!

Then six young damsels, slight and frail,
Received this kind young doctor's care;
They all were getting slim and pale,
And short of breath in mounting stairs.

They all made rhymes with 'sighs' and 'skies,'
And loathed their puddings and buttered rolls,
And dieted, much to their friends' surprise,
On pickles and pencils and chalks and coals.

So fast their little hearts did bound,
The frightened insects buzzed the more;
So over their chests he found
The rale sifflant and the rale sonore.

He shook his head. There's grave disease,–
I greatly fear you all must die;
A slight post-mortem, if you please,
Surviving friends would gratify.

The six young damsels wept aloud,
Which so prevailed on six young men
That each his honest love avowed,
Whereat they all got well again.

This poor young man was all aghast!
The price of stethoscopes came down;
And he was reduced at last
To practice in a country town.

The doctors being very sore,
A stethoscope they did devise
That had a rammer to clear the bore,
With a knot at the end to kill the flies.

Now use your ears, all you that can,
But don't forget to mind your eyes,
Or you may be cheated, like this young man,
By a couple of silly, abnormal flies.

A fitting summary to this entire discussion on physical diagnosis would be Piorry's advice regarding the conduct of the physician in clinical practice. Such conduct would be exemplary of the finest standards of medicine in this era of technological confusion and scientific aloofness. The following quotation is from Handerson's translation of Baas' *History of Medicine*[136].

The art of examining a patient demands long study and extensive knowledge. The examination should generally be short, so as not to weary the patient. To ask a question twice is better than once, and to examine a patient a second time, after an interval of twenty-four hours, is better than a single examination. Emphasis and arrogance should be avoided without becoming commonplace. Questions must be answered, however useless they may be, for in the eyes of the world they have great value, and the physician cannot neglect these little nothings when related to him by the patient. The physician should behave with firmness but with courtesy, unite cold-bloodedness with a certain amount of feeling, and in important matters stand firmly upon what he regards as for the good of the patient. Prejudices which he cannot overcome he must know how to yield to (though always giving them his censure), unless they are accompanied with danger. These precautions the physician should not neglect if he desires to make his fortune in this world, where savoir faire often commands more success than reason and sound understanding.

REFERENCES

1. Mettler, C.C. (1947). *History of Medicine*, 1st edn., p. 287. (Philadelphia: The Blakiston Company)
2. Bertin, R.J.H. in Bouillaud, J.B. (1824). *Traité des Maladies du Coeur et des Gros Vaisseaux*, Paris, 464 pp.
3. Chauncey, C.W. (1833). *Treatise on the Diseases of the Heart and Great Vessels*, 449 pp. (Philadelphia: Carey, Lea and Blanchard)
4. Mettler, C.C. (1947). *Op. cit.*, pp. 281–315
5. Castiglioni, A. (1941). *A History of Medicine*, p. 39. (New York)
6. Adams, F. (1849). *The Genuine Works of Hippocrates*, **1**, 235–6. (London)
7. Neuburger, M. (1910–11). *History of Medicine*, **1**, 67 (London)
8. Adams, F. (1856). *The Extant Works of Aretaeus the Cappadocian*, pp. 264–8. (London)
9. Corvisart, J.N. (1855). *Essai sur les maladies et les lesions organiques du coeur et des gros vaisseaux*, pp. 162–4. (Paris)
10. Corvisart, J.N. (1812). *An Essay on the Organic Diseases and Lesions of the Heart and Great Vessels*, trans. by J. Gates, Philadelphia, Preface VI
11. Ebbell, B. (1937). *The Papyrus Ebers*, (Copenhagen: Levin & Munksgaard)
12. Breasted, J.H. (1930). *The Edwin Smith Surgical Papyrus.* (Chicago: Univ. of Chicago Press)
13. Garrison, F.H. (1929). *History of Medicine*, 4th edn. (Philadelphia: W.B. Saunders)
14. Wong, K.C. and Lien-Teh, W. (1932). *History of Chinese Medicine.* (Tientsin: The Tientsin Press)
15. Ghose, E.N. (1924). A peep into the Ayurvedic System of sphygmology. *J. Ayurveda* (Calcutta), **1**, 43
16. Brewer, L.A. (1983). Sphygmology through the centuries, historical notes. *Am. J. Surg.*, **145**, 696–701
17. Adams, F. (1929). *The Genuine Works of Hippocrates.* (Wm. Woods and Co.)
18. Garrison, F.H. (1929). *History of Medicine*, 4th edn., p. 13. (Philadelphia: W.B. Saunders)
19. Kanada, S. (1891). *Science of Sphygmica* (English transl. by K.R.L. Gupta). (Calcutta: S.C. Addy)
20. Horine, E.F. (1941). An epitome of ancient pulse lore. *Bull. Hist. Med.*, **10**, 209
21. Schöne, H. (1907). *Markellinos' pulslehre, Festschr. z. 49 Versamml. deutscher Philologen u Schulmänner.* (Basel: Birkhauser)
22. Rucco, J. (1827). *Introduction to the Science of the Pulse.* (London: Burgess & Hill)
23. Aristotle. (1931). *The Works* (transl. under the ed. of J.A. Smith & W.D. Ross) (Oxford: Clarendon)
24. Brock, A.J. (1929). *Greek Medicine.* (London: J.M. Dent & Sons)
25. Hoernie, A.F.R. (1907–08). *Arch. Getsch Med. Leipz.*, 29–40
26. Paulus Aeginata. (1844). *Seven Books* (transl. by F. Adams). (London: The Sydenham Society)
27. Sarton, G. (1954). *Galen of Pergamon.* (Lawrence, Kansas: Univ. of Kansas Press)
28. Kussmaul, A. (1873). Über schwielige Mediastino – Pericarditis und den paradoxen Puls. *Berlin Klin Wschr.*, **10**, 433–5
29. Vierordt, K. (1855). Die Lehre vons Arterienpuls in gesunden und kranken zuständen Braunschweig. F. Vieqeg, p. 226 (also Fig. 5–3)
30. Schecter, D.S., Lillehei, W.C. and Soffer, A. (1969). History of sphygmology and heart block. *Dis. of Chest*, vol. 55, Suppl. No. 1, p. 537
31. *Ibid.*, p. 538
32. Williams, C.T. (1907). Laénnec and the evolution of the stethoscope. *Br. Med. J.*, pp. 6–7
33. Hope, J. (1846). *Diseases of the Heart and Great Vessels*, C.W. Pennock (ed.) 2nd American from 3rd London edn., Philadelphia

34. Korns, H.M. (1939). A brief history of physical diagnosis. *Annals of Medical History*, 3rd. sec., **1**, 50–67

35. Korns, H.M. (1939). *Op. cit.*, p. 50–67

36. Kligfield, P. (1979). An annotation on the pulse in aortic regurgitation: Thomas Cuming, 1822. *Am. J. Cardiol.*, **44**, 370–1

37. Corrigan, D.J. (1832). On permanent patency of the mouth of the aorta, or inadequacy of the aortic valves. *Edinburgh Med. Surg. J.*, **37**, 225–45

38. Corrigan (1802–1880) and his description of the pericardial knock. (1980). *Mayo Clin. Proc.*, **55**, 771–3

39. Horgan, J. (1980). Corrigan on cardiac disease. *J. Irish Coll. Physicians and Surgeons*, **10** (1), 27–31

40. Obituary. (1961). Freeman's J. Feb. 2, 1880: Cited by Mulcahy R: Sir Dominic John Corrigan. *Ir. J. Med. Sci.*, series 6, **430**, 454–63

41. Luisada, A. (1950). *Heart*, 2nd edn. (Baltimore: Williams and Wilkins)

42. Schwartz, H. (1972). Abraham Lincoln and aortic insufficiency – the declining health of the president (Clinical Note). *Calif. Med.*, **116**, 82–4

43. Schwartz, H. (1964). Abraham Lincoln and the Marfan Syndrome. *J. Am. Med. Assoc.*, **187**, 473–9

44. Hamilton, C. and Ostendorf, L. (1963). *Lincoln in Photographs*. (Norman, Oklahoma: Univ. of Oklahoma Press)

45. Brooks, N. (1878). Personal Reminiscences of Lincoln. *Scribner's Monthly XV*, 565

46. Viets, H. (1922). De staticis experimentis of Nicolaus Cusanus. *Ann. Med. Hist.*, **4**, 115

47. Hart. *Makers of Science*. (Oxford Press)

48. Laénnec, R.T.H. (1942). Introduction to 'On mediate auscultation.' In Clendenning, L. *Source Book of Medical History*, p. 136. (New York City: Dover Publications)

49. Mitchell, S.W. (1891). The early history of instrumental precision in medicine. *The Transactions of the Congress of American Physicians and Surgeons*, **2**, 159–98

50. Floyer, J. (1707). *The Physician's Pulse-Watch*, (London: S. Smith & B. Walford)

51. Clendenning, L. (1930). The history of certain medical instruments. *Ann. Intern. Med.*, **4**, 176–89

52. Auenbrugger, L. (1761). *Invention Novum ex Percussione Thoracis Humani, ut Signo Abstruso Interni pectoris Morboa Detegendi*, J.T. Trattner, Vienna. Facsimile edition with French, English, and German translations and Neuberger's biography, 1922. (Vienna and Leipzig: S.Safar)

53. Siegrist, H.E. (1933). *The Great Doctors*. (New York: W.W. Norton & Co.)

54. Cantwell, J.D. (1988). Jean-Nicolas Corvisart. *Clin. Cardiol.*, **11**, 801–3

55. Dale, P.M. (1952). *Medical Biographies. The Ailments of Thirty-three Famous Persons.* (Norman, OK: Univ. of Oklahoma Press)

56. Corvisart, J.N. (1962). *An Essay on the Organic Diseases and Lesions of the Heart and Great Vessels*, (translated from the French by J. Gates, with an introduction by D.W. Richards). (New York: Hafner Publishing Co.)

57. Auenbrugger, L. (1974). *Encyclopaedia Britannica, Micropaedia*, 15th edn., p. 664

58. Piorry, P.A. (1828). De la Percussion Mediate et des Signes Obtenus à l'Aide de ce Nouveau Moyen d'Exploration, dans les Maladies des Organes Thoraciques et Abdominaux. (Paris: J.S. Chaudé)

59. Hirschfelder, A.D. (1913). *Diseases of the Heart and Aorta*, 2nd edn. (Philadelphia and London: Lippincott)

60. Piorry, P.A. (1851). Traité de Médecine Pranque. *Atlas de Plessimétrisme*. (Paris: Baillière)

61. Sansom, A.E. (1892). *The Diagnosis of the Diseases of the Heart and Thoracic Aorta*. (London: Griffin)

62. Korns, H.M. (1939). *Op. cit.*, p. 54

63. Piorry, P.A. (1826). Nouvelle méthode de percussion du thorax. *Arch. Gen. Méd.*, **10**, 471–2

64. Risse, G.B. (1971). Pierre A. Piorry (1794–1879), The French 'Master of Percussion'. *Med. Hist. Chest*, **60**, 484–8

65. Obituary of Piorry. (1879). *Lancet*, **1**, 827

66. Obituary (1902). *J. Santé*, **19**, 241–3

67. Forbes, J. (1824). *Original Cases with Dissections and Observations Illustrating the Use of the Stethoscope and Percussion in the Diagnosis of Diseases of the Chest, etc.* (London: T. and G. Underwood)

68. Skoda, J. (1854). *Abhandlung Über Perkussion und Auskultation*, 5th. edn. (Vienna: L. W. Scidel)

69. Ebstein, W. (1876). Zur Lehre von der Herzpercussion. *Berliner Klinische Wochenschrift*, **13**, 501

70. Goldscheider (1905). Ueber Herzperkussion. *Deutsche medizinische Wochenschrift*, **31**, 333, 382

71. Clark, A. (1884). *Lectures on Diseases of the Heart.* (New York and London: Bermingham and Co.)

72. Barth, J.B.P. and Roger, H. (1854). *Traité Pratique d'Auscultation Suivi d'un Précis de Percussion*, 4th. edn. (Paris: Labé)

73. Brockbank, E.M. (1930). *The Diagnosis and Treatment of Heart Disease*, 6th edn. (London: H.K. Lewis)

74. Blechmann, G. (1922). *Les Péricardites Aigües.* (Paris: E. Flammarion)

75. Rotch, T.M. (1878). Absence of resonance in

the fifth right intercostal space diagnostic of pericardial effusion. *Boston Med. Surg. J.*, **99**, 389, 421

76. Ewart, W. (1896). Practical aids in the diagnosis of pericardial effusion, in connection with the question as to surgical treatment. *Br. Med. J.*, **1**, 717

77. Bedford, D.E. (1971). Auenbrugger's contribution to cardiology. *Br. Heart J.*, **33**, 817–21

78. Sakula, S. (1981). Joseph Skoda 1805–81. A Centenary tribute to a pioneer of thoracic medicine. *Thorax*, **36**, 404–11

79. *Ibid.*, p. 406

80. *Ibid.*, p. 404

81. Skoda, J. (1839). *Abhandlung über Perkussion und Auskultation.* (Vienna: Mösle and Braumüller)

82. Skoda, J. (1853). *A Treatise on Auscultation and Percussion*, English translation by W.O. Markham. (London: Highley)

83. Sakula, S. (1981). *Op. cit.*, pp. 404–11

84. Flint, A. (1852). Variation of pitch in percussion and respiratory sounds and their application to physical diagnosis. *Tr. Am. Med. Assoc., Philadelphia V*

85. Hippocrates. *De Morbis*, **2**, 47

86. Hooke, R.A. (1705). A general scheme, or idea of the present state of natural philosophy. In Waller, R. (ed). *The Posthumous Works of Robert Hooke*, p. 39. (London: S. Smith and B. Walford)

87. Laénnec, R.T. (1974). *Encyclopaedia Britannica, Micropaedia*, 15th edn., p. 984

88. Forbes, J. (1827). *A Treatise on the Diseases of the Chest and on Mediate Auscultation*, pp. 5–7. (London)

89. MacCurdy, E. (ed.) (1938). *The Notebooks of Leonardo da Vinci*, vol. 1, p. 277. (New York: Reynal and Hitchcock)

90. Laénnec, R.T.H. (1819). *De l'Auscultation Médiate ou traité du Diagnostic des Maladies des Poumons et du Coeur*, 1st ed., 2 vols. (Paris: Brosson et Chaudé)

91. Bedford, D.E. (1972). Cardiology in the days of Laénnec. *Br. Heart J.*, **34**, 1193–8

92. Chang, L. (1987). Development and use of the stethoscope in diagnosing cardiac disease. *Am. J. Cardiol.*, **60**, 1378–82

93. Williams, C.T. (1907). *Op. cit.*, pp. 6–7

94. *Ibid.*, p. 7

95. Reiser, S.J. (1979). The medical influence of the stethoscope. *Sci. Am.*, **40**, 153

96. Reiser, S.J. (1978). The stethoscope and the detection of pathology by sound. In *Medicine and the Reign of Technology*, pp. 36–7.

(Cambridge: Cambridge Univ. Press)

97. McKusick, V.A., Sharp, W.D. and Warner, A.O. (1957). An exhibition on the history of cardiovascular sound including the evolution of the stethoscope. *Bull. Hist. Med.*, **31**, 463–87

98. Mettler, C.C. (1947). *Op. cit.*, p. 304

99. Williams, C.J.B. (1870). *The Case of the Late Earl St. Maur*, pp. 6–7. (Longmans, Green and Co.)

100. Kerr, W.S., Althausen, T.L., Bassett, A.M. and Goldman, M.J. (1937). The symballophone: a modified stethoscope for the lateralization and comparison of sounds. *Am. Heart J.*, **14**, 594

101. Sprague, H.B. (1926). A new combined stethoscope chest piece. *J. Am. Med. Assoc.*, **86**, 1909

102. Rappaport, M.B. and Sprague, H.B. (1941). Physiologic and physical laws which govern auscultation and their clinical application. The acoustic stethoscope and the electrical amplifying stethoscope and stethograph. *Am. Heart J.*, **21**, 257

103. Rappaport, M.B. and Sprague, H.B. (1951). The effects of tubing bore on stethoscope efficiency. *Am. Heart J.*, **42**, 605

104. Rappaport, M.B. and Sprague, H.B. (1952). The effects of improper fitting of stethoscope to ears on auscultatory efficiency. *Am. Heart J.*, **43**, 713

105. Syers, H.W. (1902). The decay of auscultation and the use of the binaural stethoscope. *Lancet*, **1**, 369

106. Conner, L.A. (1907). Certain acoustic limitations of the stethoscope and their clinical importance. *Trans. A. Am. Physicians*, **22**, 113

107. Bianchi, A. (1898). *The Phonendoscope and its Practical Applications* (translated by A.G. Baker). (Philadelphia)

108. Smith, E.T.A. (1884). A new form of stethoscope. *Br. Med. J.*, **1**, 909

109. Stokes, W. (1825). *An Introduction to the Use of the Stethoscope.* (Edinburgh: Maclachen and Stewart)

110. Bowditch, H.P. (1846). *The Young Stethoscopist or the Student's Aid to Auscultation.* (Reprinted, Hafner Publishing Co. New York, 1964). (Boston)

111. Flint, A. (1856). *A Practical Treatise on the Physical Exploration of the Chest and the Diagnosis of Diseases Affecting the Respiratory Organs*, p. 293. (Philadelphia)

112. McKusick, V.A. (1960). The history of methods for the diagnosis of heart disease. *Bull. Hist. Med.*, **34**, 16

113. Middleton, W.S. (1924). A Biographic History

of Physical Diagnosis. *Ann. Med. Hist.* (Read before the Univ. of Wisconsin Med. Hist. Seminar, Jan. 23)

114. Bragmann, L.J. (1927). Laénnec and Culpepper as depicted by Kipling. *Ann. Med. Hist.*, **9**, 129

115. Laénnec, R.T.H. (1826). *Ibid.*, 2nd edn.

116. Laénnec, R.T.H. (1834). *Ibid.*, English translation with notes and a sketch of the author's life by John Forbes, 4th edn. (London: Longman, Rees, Orme, Brown and others)

117. Turner, J. (1828). Observations on the causes of the sounds produced by the action of the heart. *Edinburgh Medicochirurg. Soc. Trans.*, **3**, 205

118. Duffin, J.M. (1989). The Cardiology of R.T.H. Laénnec. *Med. Hist.*, **33**, 42–71

119. *Ibid.*, p. 67

120. *Ibid.*, p. 70

121. Middleton, W.S. *Op. cit.*, pp 441–2

122. O'Brien, B. (1978). William Stokes (1804–1878). *Irish Med. J.*, **71**, 598

123. *Ibid.*, p. 598

124. Cheyne, J. (1818). A case of apoplexy in which the fleshy part of the heart was converted into fat. *Dublin Hosp. Rep.*, **2**, 216

125. Middleton, W.S. (1924). *Op. cit.*, p. 425

126. Bendiner, E. (1984). The Dublin school: from poverty, a rich legacy. *Hosp. Prac.*, **19**, 221

127. Stokes, W. (1854). *Diseases of the Heart and Aorta*, p. 131

128. Herrick, J.B. (1942). *A Short History of Cardiology*, p. 112. (Baltimore, Md.: Charles C. Thomas)

129. Adams, R. (1827). Cases of diseases of the heart accompanied with pathological observations. *Dublin Hosp. Rep.*, **4**, 353–454

130. Herrick, J.B. (1942). *Op cit.*, p. 119

131. Stokes, W. (1842). *Dublin Q. J.*, Vol **ii**, p. 72

132. Middleton, W.S. (1924). *Op. cit.*, p. 450

133. Flint, A. (1973). On cardiac murmurs. *Am. Med. Sci.*, **265**, 236–55

134. *Ibid.*, pp. 252, 254

135. Williams, C.T. (1907). *Op. cit.*, p. 8

136. Baas, J.H. (1889). *History of Medicine*, trans. from the German by H.E. Handerson, NY

23   Sphygmomanometry

The father of sphygmomanometry is undoubtedly Stephen Hales. It was his marked interest in the hydraulics of animal and plant fluids that caused him to conduct experiments that eventually led to the discovery of the physiologic phenomenon known as blood pressure. Without benefit of graphic recording devices, Hales was also able to measure cardiac output, capacity of the left ventricle and the speed and resistance to the flow of blood, albeit in a very rough manner. Time has shown all of these elements to be instrumental in the regulation of blood pressure[1-3].

Cardiac output was determined in the particular animal being studied by first determining its pulse rate and then by sacrificing the animal for removal of its heart. Wax was then injected into the left ventricle to determine its volume. This figure was multiplied by the pulse rate to obtain the cardiac output. The effect of peripheral resistance on the level of the blood pressure was also roughly assessed by virtue of changes in blood velocity through his perfusion experiments utilizing saline solutions, stimulants and brandy[4]. The changes in blood velocity with these various substances were attributed by him to changes in the diameter of the capillaries, and are known to us today as vasoconstriction and vasodilation; basic mechanisms for alterations in peripheral resistance and hence blood pressure.

Stephen Hales was born on September 17, 1677 in the village of Bekesbourne in Kent. He was the last of six sons. He had a long and fruitful life dying in 1761. Hales matriculated at Corpus Christi College in Cambridge where he studied theology in preparation for his vocation as an Anglican priest. Corpus Christi was then known as Bene't College. Hales became a fellow of the College after receiving a BA. He was later awarded an MA. This seven year span of studies at Cambridge was quite a liberal one with courses in classics, mathematics and science added to the basic theology and philosophy that he needed for his priestly functions[1-3]. It was not unusual during the 18th century for men of the cloth to be interested in natural phenomena since this was the 'Age of Reason based on Faith'[5].

It was while at Cambridge that Hales began his initial experiments on pressure, resistance and flow. He worked at that time with a young and enthusiastic premedical student by the name of William Stukeley[6]. Hales remained one more year, leaving Cambridge to become curate of Teddington in Middlesex, a small rural community just a few miles outside London. In three short years after his arrival at Teddington, Hales was awarded another degree; this one being a Bachelor of Divinity from Oxford. Figure 1 is a portrait of Hales.

Apparently Hales had ample opportunity while curate to pursue his interests in science. Several years after his installation as curate, he began to conduct his studies on the circulation. Twenty-five experiments were conducted in all, utilizing mostly dogs but including also three horses, a sheep, and a doe. These experiments were the result of Hales' intense interest in the quantitative aspects of pressure and flow in living plants and animals emanating from his belief in the order and balance of the universe and his adherence to Newton's teachings in physical science[7].

These observations were published in volume II of the *Statical Essays* in 1733. Although the methodology was rather crude, it was straight-forward to say the least as the following quotation from his essays indicates[8].

In December I caused a mare to be tied down alive on her back; she was fourteen hands high, and about fourteen years of age; had a fistula of her withers, was neither very lean nor yet lusty; having laid open the left crural artery about three inches from her belly, I inserted into it a brass pipe whose bore was one sixth of an inch in diameter ... I fixed a glass tube of nearly the

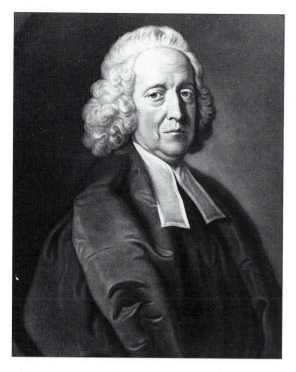

Figure 1 Portrait of Stephen Hales (1677–1761). *Photo Source National Library of Medicine. Literary Source Photo Archives. Courtesy of National Library of Medicine*

same diameter which was nine feet in length: then untying the ligature of the artery, the blood rose in the tube 8 feet 3 inches perpendicular above the level of the left ventricle of the heart; … when it was at its full height it would rise and fall at and after each pulse 2, 3, or 4 inches …'

Figure 2 is an artist's impression of Hales' experiments to determine the blood pressure of a horse. (Note that in the artist's rendering, the cannula is inserted into the carotid artery rather than the crural as described by Hales.) Figure 3 is a page from his *Haemastatics* showing his measurements for correlating blood volume with the blood pressure.

Hales was thus the first to measure arterial pressure. His experiments also led him to determine that since the peak blood pressure occurred with contraction of the heart, it would be a reflection then of cardiac output. He went on to reason further that the lowest level of blood pressure (since it occurred when the heart was relaxed) represented the resistance to flow. This is an absolute documentation of Hales' recognition of the concepts of cardiac output and total peripheral resistance[9].

It is of interest to note that despite the fact that Floyer's physician pulse watch had already been introduced, Hale did not avail himself of the device, preferring instead the pendulum. In the passage wherein he describes blood flow and its measurements, he writes as follows:

Having provided a Pendulum which beat Seconds, and pouring in thro' the Tube known Quantities of warm Water, I found that 342 cubic Inches of Water passed off in 400 Seconds or 6.6 minutes.

Then cutting all the mesenteric Arteries asunder close to the Guts, and taking away the Guts, I found that a like Quantity of Water passed thro' these larger Ramifications of the Arteries in 140 Seconds, or 2.3 Minutes; that is, in one third of the Time.

Then cutting asunder the crural Arteries, which were before tyed, and cutting off the mesenteric and emulgent Arteries close to the Aorta, a like Quantity of Water passed thro' this cut in .38 Minute, that is in 1/21. 4th part of the Time, in which it passed thro' the capillary Arteries of the slit Guts[10].

Perhaps America could claim Hales as one of its own because in 1732 he was elected to the 17 member board of trustees for the colony of Georgia along with James Oglethorpe[11]. There is even a tree native to Georgia that is named in Hales' honor.

Hales never did care much for animal dissection so that after his original 25 experiments, most of his efforts until the age of 83, when he died suddenly, centered about plants.

A century had to pass, however, before increasingly accurate measurements of blood pressure were made. Poiseuille initiated this in 1828 with his usage of the mercury manometer. Poiseuille was both a physician and a physicist. He won the gold medal of the Royal Academy of Medicine for his doctoral dissertation on the measurement of arterial blood pressure by means of a mercury manometer connected to a cannula that was inserted directly into an artery[12]. Potassium carbonate in the cannula acted as an anticoagulant.

Jean Faivre has the distinction of having made the first direct intra-arterial measurements of blood pressure in man. He performed these studies in patients undergoing amputation of a limb and used Poiseuille's hemodynamometer, the mercury-filled U tube. Faivre collaborated frequently with the

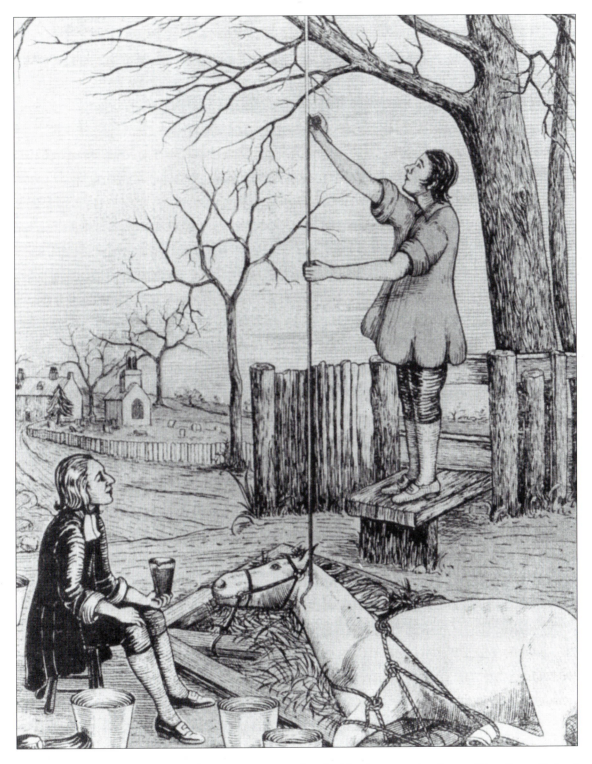

Figure 2 Rev. Stephen Hales and an assistant measuring the blood pressure in a horse. *Photo Source National Library of Medicine. Literary Source Medical Times, 1944. Courtesy of National Library of Medicine*

Hæmaſtatics.

The ſeveral Trials.	The Quantities of Blood let out in Wine Meaſure.		The ſeveral Heights of the Blood after theſe evacuations	
	Quarts	Pints	Feet	Inches
1	0	*5 Ounces	8	3/8
2	1	0	7	8
3	2		7	2
4	3		6	6 1/4
5	4		6	10 1/2
6	5		6	1/4
7	6		5	8 1/2
8	7		4	5
9	8		3	3
10	8	1	3	7 1/4
11	9	0	3	10
12	9	1	3	6 1/4
13	10	0	3	9 1/4
14	10	1	4	3 1/4
15	11	0	3	8
16	11	1	3	10 1/2
17	12	0	3	9
18	12	1	3	7 1/4
19	13	0	3	2
20	13	1	4	1/4
21	14	0	3	9
22	14	1	3	3
23	15	0	3	4 1/4
24	15	1	3	1
25	16	0	2	4

Theſe 5 Ounces loſt in preparing the Artery.

By this time there is a Pint loſt in making the ſeveral Trials, which is not allowed for in this Table.

There was about a Quart loſt in making the ſeveral Trials, ſo there flowed out in all ſeventeen Quarts, and half a Pint after the laſt Trial, when ſhe expired. This whole Quantity of Blood was equal to 1185.3 cubick Inches.

3   5. We

Figure 3 A page from Hale's 'Haemastatics'. *Photo Source National Library of Medicine. Literary Source Original. Courtesy of National Library of Medicine*

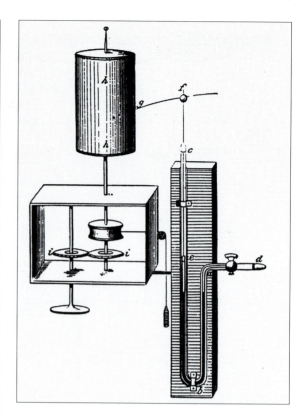

Figure 4 Ludwig's kymograph, described and published in 1847. *Photo Source National Library of Medicine. Literary Source not available. Courtesy of National Library of Medicine*

noted veterinarian physiologist, Chauveau, in other experiments involving cardiac catheterization in horses.

A graphic method for recording the arterial pressure, also through direct cannulation, was then developed by Carl Ludwig. His invention was called the kymograph from the Greek (kyma = wave; grapheion = stylus). Figure 4 illustrates the various components of this recording apparatus and how it registers the movements of the mercury on a revolving smoked drum[13]. Incidentally, this recording device became the model for the sphygmograph, a graphic method developed by Vierordt of Tübingen for monitoring the pulse.

The main drawback in obtaining blood pressure measurements by direct cannulation is, of course, its invasive approach. Clinical application of this important physiologic parameter had to wait until a non-invasive method could be found. The first attempts in this direction were made by Vierordt. He postulated that an indirect non-invasive method of measuring arterial pressure could be obtained by measuring the amount of pressure needed to obliterate the radial arterial pulse. The recording device of Ludwig became the model for Vierordt's sphygmograph. Figure 5 illustrates Vierordt's cumbersome device which proved to be not only difficult to use but also quite inaccurate. Nevertheless, it represented a step in the right direction.

The difficulties inherent in Vierordt's device were ameliorated to some extent five years later when Etienne Jules Marey introduced his

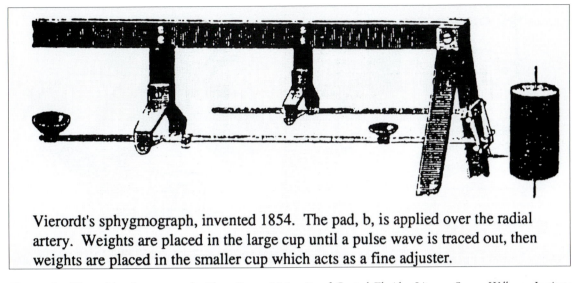

Vierordt's sphygmograph, invented 1854. The pad, b, is applied over the radial artery. Weights are placed in the large cup until a pulse wave is traced out, then weights are placed in the smaller cup which acts as a fine adjuster.

Figure 5 Vierordt's sphygmograph. *Photo Source University of Central Florida. Literary Source Wellcome Institute Library. By courtesy of the Wellcome Trust*

direct sphygmograph. It too, however, was too complicated and unwieldy to be used in the daily management of patients[12].

Widespread non-invasive measurement of arterial pressure had to await the development of newer techniques. Samuel von Basch paved the way by using an inflatable rubber bag with water[12]. The device was still formidable. However, it was, in reality, a simple and more accurate one than those that preceded it. Figure 6 illustrates a device invented by him in 1881 while Figure 7 illustrates a much simpler one developed by him just two years later. Figure 8 depicts von Recklinghausen's sphygmograph in use.

In 1889, Potain substituted air for the water and utilized a rubber bulb for compression of the pulse. The pressure was then recorded by a portable aneroid manometer[12]. Other modifications followed in an effort to obtain more accurate readings. However, it was Potain who noted that spring manometers could not be relied upon for accuracy since the force necessary to move the spring depended not only on the arterial pressure but also on the resistance of the arterial wall itself which imposed a negative interference on the free movement of the spring.

It was in 1896 that Scipione Riva-Rocci reported a non-invasive method of obtaining the arterial blood pressures that ultimately led to the techniques in use today[14]. Figure 9 is an illustration of his model. His technique utilized an inflatable rubber bag encased in a cuff of non-expandable material. The whole circumference of the upper arm was compressed as the rubber bag was inflated with air by means of an attached rubber bulb. The pressure within the cuff was registered by a mercury manometer.

The appearance of definite and pronounced oscillations in the column of mercury would coincide with the reappearance of the radial pulse by palpation as the rubber bag was being deflated. Since, at this time, the cuff pressure was equal to the arterial pulse, the level of the mercury column was taken as the systolic pressure. The diastolic pressure was obtained by recording the level of the mercury column in the manometer at the point of transition from large to small oscillations.

A major defect in Riva-Rocci's model was the narrowness of the cuff, which was only 5 cm wide. This was rectified by Von Recklinghausen in 1901 when he introduced a much wider arm band of 12 cm. Further refinement of Riva-Rocci's basic model occurred in 1897 when Hill and Barnard introduced a portable device utilizing a needle pressure gauge[15]. Clinical measurement of blood pressure remained at this level until N. E. Korotkoff introduced in 1905 his now well-established auscultatory method.

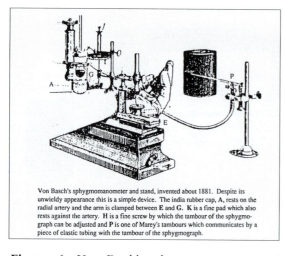

Von Basch's sphygmomanometer and stand, invented about 1881. Despite its unwieldy appearance this is a simple device. The india rubber cap, A, rests on the radial artery and the arm is clamped between E and G. K is a fine pad which also rests against the artery. H is a fine screw by which the tambour of the sphygmograph can be adjusted and P is one of Marey's tambours which communicates by a piece of elastic tubing with the tambour of the sphygmograph.

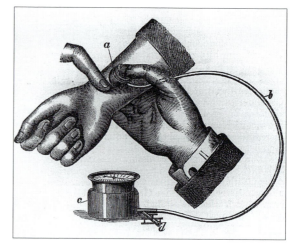

Figure 6 Von Basch's sphygmomanometer and stand, invented about 1881. *Photo source University of Central Florida. Literary Source Wellcome Institute Library. By courtesy of the Wellcome Trustees*

Figure 7 A later sphygmomanometer by Von Basch (1883). *Photo Source National Library of Medicine. Literary Source Basch, S.S.R. von (1883). Ein-Metall-sphygmomanometer. Wien. Med. Woch., 33 (22) 674. Courtesy of National Library of Medicine*

Nicolai Korotkoff was born in 1874 and died at the young age of 46. He received his degree in medicine from Moscow University in 1898 following which he served a residency in surgery at the surgical clinic of Moscow. He then worked for two years at the Military Academy of Medicine as an assistant in the gynecological division. During the Russo-Japanese war of 1904, he became interested in vascular surgery. Upon completion of his war-time tour of duty, Korotkoff returned to St. Petersburg for further study of arterial injuries. It was during this period that he developed the auscultatory method for measuring blood pressure. In 1910, he was awarded a doctorate on the basis of his thesis *Experiments for determining the strength of arterial collaterals.*

Korotkoff was a pioneer in vascular surgery. He was part of that *avant garde* group of surgeons that relied on the stethoscope for differentiating between a solid mass and an arterial aneurysm. In his quest for accuracy he was inclined to use auscultation rather than palpation as a means of determining the presence of complete occlusion of an artery.

The translation of Korotkoff's original report appears in a paper by Lewis on clinical sphygmomanometry and it is as follows [16]:

On the basis of this observation, the speaker came to the conclusion that a perfectly constricted artery under normal conditions, does not emit

any sounds. Taking this fact into consideration, the speaker proposed the sound method for measuring blood pressure on human beings. The sleeve of Riva-Rocci is put on the middle third of the arm; the pressure in this sleeve rises rapidly until the circulation below this sleeve stops completely. At first there are no sounds whatsoever. As the mercury in the manometer drops to a certain height, there appears the first short or faint tones, the appearance of which indicates that part of the pulse wave of the blood stream has passed under the sleeve. Consequently, the reading on the manometer when the first sound appears corresponds to the maximum blood pressure; with the further fall of the mercury in the manometer, there are heard systolic pressure murmurs which become again sounds (secondary). Finally all sounds disappear. The time of disappearance of the sounds indicates the free passage or flow of the blood stream; in other words, at the moment of disappearance or fading out of the sounds, the minimum blood pressure in the artery has surpassed the pressure in the sleeve. Consequently, the reading of the manometer at this time corresponds to the minimum blood pressure. Experiments conducted on animals gave positive results. The first sound tones appear (10–12 mm) sooner than the pulse which (1 ar. radialis) can be felt only after the passage of the major portion of the blood stream.

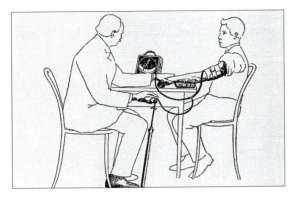

Figure 8 Von Recklinghausen's sphygmograph in use. *Photo Source National Library of Medicine. Literary Source Photo Archives. Courtesy of National Library of Medicine*

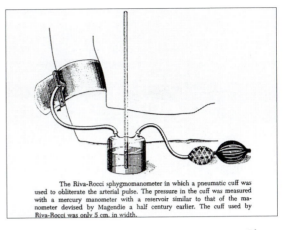

The Riva-Rocci sphygmomanometer in which a pneumatic cuff was used to obliterate the arterial pulse. The pressure in the cuff was measured with a mercury manometer with a reservoir similar to that of the manometer devised by Magendie a half century earlier. The cuff used by Riva-Rocci was only 5 cm. in width.

Figure 9 Riva-Rocci's sphygmomanometer. Photo Source University of Central Florida. *Literary Source Burch, G. and DePasquale, N. (1962) Primer of Clinical Measurements of Blood Pressure. Fig. 14, p.29, (St. Louis MO: C. V. Mosby Co.). With permission*

The discovery was reported to the Imperial Military Medical Academy in St. Petersburg in December 1905; a rather humble and brief presentation for so great a discovery. Indeed, Korotkoff's contribution is one of the most outstanding events in the history of medicine. It put into the hands of clinicians throughout the world an extremely simple diagnostic approach capable at the same time of being very accurate. It literally was the reason for the discovery of a disease that must have been present for millennia and yet exerted its devastating effects on the heart and other target organs in a covert manner. The disease is hypertension, one of the leading causes of death in the world.

The accuracy of the so-called Korotkoff's sounds is quite acceptable for clinical use. Cuff readings are closely related to those obtained by direct cannulation. The crucial element is the size of the cuff as pointed out by von Recklinghausen in 1901. The smaller the cuff in relation to the girth of the arm, the higher the recorded pressure and the greater the error. Another crucial element in obtaining accurate readings is the relationship of the arm and the manometer to the 'heart level'. The arm should be kept level with the fourth intercostal space when the patient is sitting or standing. Figure 10 depicts Korotkoff as a young man. The principle of Korotkoff's method is illustrated in Figure 11.

The development of electronic devices during the past two decades has further refined the means of indirectly measuring blood pressure[17]. Now that the electronic engineers have entered the field who knows what lies ahead with photocells, strain gauges and semi-conductors for measuring blood pressure.

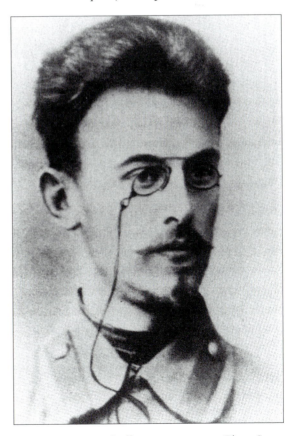

Figure 10 Korotkoff as a young man. *Photo Source National Library of Medicine. Literary Source Comroe, J. Exploring the Heart, 1st edn. (New York: Norton). With permission*

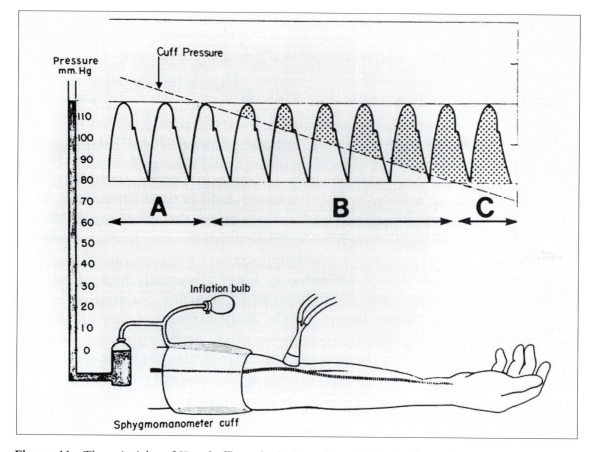

Figure 11 The principles of Korotkoff's method. *Photo Source National Library of Medicine. Literary Source Comroe, J. Exploring the Heart, 1st edn. (New York: Norton). With permission*

REFERENCES

1. Roth, N. (1981). Hales hydraulics: measuring blood pressure, 1706. *Med. Instrumentation*, **15**, 1

2. Burget, G.E. (1925). Stephen Hales (1677–1761). *Ann. Med. Hist.*, **7**, 109

3. Cohen, I.B. (1976). Stephen Hales. *Sci. Am.*, **234**, 98

4. Roth, N. *Op. cit.*, p. 69

5. Whitehead, A.N. (1931). *Science and the Modern World*. (New York: Macmillan)

6. Clark-Kennedy, A.E. (1977). Stephen Hales, D.D., F.R.S. *Br. Med. J.*, **2**, 1656

7. Editorial. (1944). Stephen Hales: father of hemodynamics. *Med. Times*, **72**, 315

8. Hales, S. (1733). *Statical Essays: containing Haemostaticks*. (London: Innys and Manby)

9. *Ibid.*

10. *Ibid.*

11. Wilbur, J.A. (1981). The founding of Georgia and the discovery of blood pressure. *J. Med. Assoc. Ga.*, **70**, 332

12. Booth, J. (1977). A short history of blood pressure measurement. *Proc. R. Soc. Med.*, **70**, 793–9

13. Brunton, L. (1908). *Therapeutics of the Circulation*. (London: John Murray)

14. Riva-Rocci, S. (1986). Un nuovo sfigmomanometro. *Gasetta Medical di Torino*, **47**, vol. 51 & 52

15. Singer, C. and Underwood, E.A. *A Short History of Medicine*, 2nd. edn. (Oxford: Clarendon Press)

16. Lewis, W.H. (1941). Clinical sphygmomanometry. *Bull. NY Acad. Med.*, **17**, 871

17. Longmore, D. (1969). *Machines in Medicine*. (London: Oldus)

24　　Graphic methods

GENERAL SURVEY

In 1885, Marey wrote 'Science meets with two obstacles, the deficiency of our senses to discover facts and the insufficiency of our language to describe them. The object of the graphic methods is to get around these two obstacles; to grasp fine details which would be otherwise unobserved; and to transcribe them with a clarity superior to that of our words'[1].

Graphic methods of diagnosis are, in essence, a means of extending our senses. In cardiology, these methods are based upon the activity of the heart and vessels. The various physiologic parameters whether normal or abnormal can be delineated by means of mechanical, sound or electrical tracings and by the usage of radiation methods. Sphygmography would be a refined extension of palpation, phonocardiography enhances auscultation, while electrocardiography would be a means of evaluating the electrical forces underlying cardiac function. Radiation methods would include all tracings recorded by rays. For example, Roentgen's discovery of the X-ray made possible Stumpf's technique of roentgenkymography[2]. Electrokymography for recording heart motion was introduced by Henny and Boone in 1945[3]. They utilized the roentgenoscope which was made possible through the development of the phototube. Plethysmography uses visible rays through photoelectric recordings. Another example of a radiation method is radiocardiography which was introduced by Prinzmetal in 1949[4]. These are tracings of atomic discharges within the heart.

Graphic registration became an important tool during the 19th century and continued to be an important tool during the first few decades of the 20th century. It helped solidify the rapidly evolving physiologic and pharmacologic knowledge. An example of this was the verification of Harvey's description of the sequence of chamber movements during the cardiac cycle by Etienne Marey and J. B. A. Chauveau[5].

They introduced air-filled ampules into the heart chambers of a horse and then directly recorded the variations in pressure within the atria and ventricles during the cardiac cycle. Figure 1 illustrates the type of tracing they recorded. Notice the correlation of the pressure changes within the right atrium (top), right ventricle (middle) and left ventricle (bottom).

Figure 2 depicts the apparatus they used and the revolving drum holding the paper on which the tracings were made. The apparatus was called the cardiograph and the revolving drum recorder was known as the kymograph.

The invention of the kymograph revolutionized the experimental approach in physiological research[6]. It proved to be an exceedingly important stimulus in the advancement of graphic techniques not only in the laboratory but also in the clinical setting. Karl Ludwig (1816–95) was the first to develop a revolving type of drum recorder. He did this in 1846, calling it a 'kymographion' or 'wave-writer'[7]. Figure 3 is a sketch of the drum having a tracing recorded in synchrony with the motion of a float on a mercury manometer that transmitted changes in blood pressure[7,8]. It was an apparatus that refined intra-arterial blood pressure recordings, helping overcome the intrusive effects of heartbeat and respiration, and the inertia of the mercury column inherent in previous manometers. The smoked paper preserved the minute fluctuations of the stylus in a very sensitive fashion for future analysis and comparative measurements.

Prior to the introduction of the electronic devices, the kymograph was the mainstay of every physiology laboratory and the bane of every medical student. The method, though reliable and effective, was not without its stumbling blocks. I remember too well how many a carefully prepared experiment in physiology and pharmacology

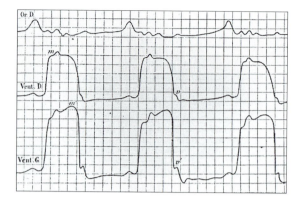

Figure 1 Pressure tracings as obtained by Marey. *Photo Source National Library of Medicine. Literary Source Marey, E. (1878). La Methode Graphique, p.357. Courtesy of National Library of Medicine*

went down the drain, so to speak, because of mechanical difficulties.

The basic principle behind Ludwig's kymograph was modified in a number of ways for the study of various physiological phenomena[8], but it still remained basically a laboratory tool. The major impediment that prevented its routine use in the clinical setting was the necessity for the invasive introduction of a catheter into a blood vessel.

I have already traced the development of blood pressure recording in the section on sphygmomanometry. We have also learned that the pulse was one of the earliest physical signs that came under the scrutiny of palpation. A tracing of the palpatory variations would give us then a more durable graphic representation of the mechanical events.

Karl Vierordt attempted to graphically register the radial pulse with a weighted mechanism that did not penetrate the skin and that directly recorded in the form of a tracing the amplitude and duration of each pulse beat[9]. The apparatus was a step in the right direction but, in actuality, it offered no advantages over the physician's palpating fingers. It was Marey in the 1860s and 1870s who set out to extend and refine Vierordt's sphygmograph. He, too, used a stylus that traced the pulse beat on a smoked surface but he replaced the balance mechanism with a spring. We have already seen how Marey improved the recording of blood pressure with his introduction of pneumatic devices (tambours), that indirectly transmitted pressure changes to the stylus (see Figure 4).

Marey's research efforts in association with Potain led not only to this refinement of the sphygmogram but also to the development of the cardiogram and phlebogram.

The sphygmogram was made even more accurate and more suitable for clinical usage with the advent of the polygraph devised by Mackenzie and later modified in collaboration with Lewis. It was a portable machine which made it extremely handy for the bedside clinician. It had two receiving tambours; one was placed over the radial or brachial artery, and the other over the jugular vein. Figure 5 is an illustration of the polygraph.

A watchmaker by the name of Shaw collaborated with Mackenzie in designing the original machine; the recorder being driven by a windup clock. Mackenzie was the first to study the irregularities of the pulse with this machine.

Mackenzie's polygraph became quite popular, and over the years numerous modifications were introduced so that it became quite versatile in its capabilities. J. Hays became one of the leading exponents on the use of the device within the clinical setting. His text on graphic methods in heart disease appeared in 1909, and in it he relates how he relied quite heavily on Mackenzie's polygraph[10]. By this time, it was so modified that it could record not only the pulses from the radial, carotid, venous or hepatic sites but also the apex beat of the heart and the respiratory curve. Hays also outlined its use in recording various forms of arrhythmia as well as conductivity, excitability, contractility, stimulus production and tonicity.

Hays was so impressed with the clinical usefulness of graphic methods that he stated in his text 'when care is taken to avoid errors due to defective apparatus' the tracing of any movement of the circulation by instrumental methods remains as a true and permanent record of an actual event'[10].

James Mackenzie was born in Scone, Scotland, in 1853, the son of a farmer. Prior to entering the medical school of the University of Edinburgh, he served as a pharmacist's apprentice and then as a pharmacist for a total of six years. His entire training was oriented towards general practice, a love for which stayed with him throughout his entire life. A short study period in Vienna, then the mecca of medicine, did not deter him from his avowed desire to be a general practitioner. Thus, he settled in Burnley, a cotton manufacturing town in Lancashire.

His interest in sphygmology began shortly after he established his practice, and for ten years he spent a good deal of time developing pulse recording

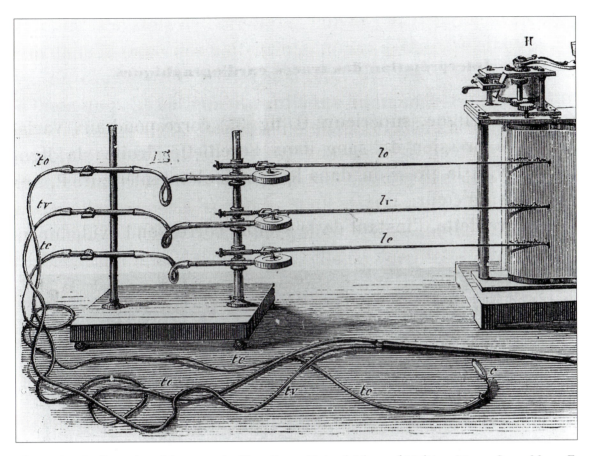

Figure 2 Cardiograph and kymograph. *Photo Source National Library of Medicine. Literary Source Marey, E. (1878). La Methode Graphique, p.358. Courtesy of National Library of Medicine*

instruments. This finally resulted in his invention of the ink polygraph. Despite his desire to be considered a general practitioner, his interest in cardiac abnormalities, concomitant with his investigations with the polygraph, soon brought him renown as an expert in cardiac diseases and as an authority on arrhythmias. His reputation was such that the illustrious Wenckebach, on his visit to England, made it a point to see Mackenzie first before going to London.

Mackenzie was able to make a number of observations on cardiac arrhythmias which were later amplified and confirmed or corrected by electrocardiography. He was correct in his identification of extrasystoles and their points of origin but he erred when he mislabeled atrial fibrillation as nodal rhythm. This is not to his discredit, however, since it was the marked irregularity of rhythm that he was able to record with his polygraph. His conclusion that this irregularity was nodal in origin

was based on the insufficient electrophysiologic knowledge of the time.

The pressures of his growing reputation in cardiac disease finally persuaded him to move to London as a Harley street consultant in cardiology. He was not welcomed with open arms by his highly placed London colleagues, finding it difficult to get adequate hospital appointments. Like many a newcomer, he had ample time to spare so that during his first year he was able to complete his textbook on diseases of the heart[11]. In 1910 he was finally appointed lecturer in cardiac research at the London Hospital, which subsequently led to the chairmanship of the cardiology department. By this time his polygraph had also become widely accepted as a useful tool in the management of cardiac diseases.

Dr Mackenzie became Sir James in 1915 in recognition of his invaluable contributions to

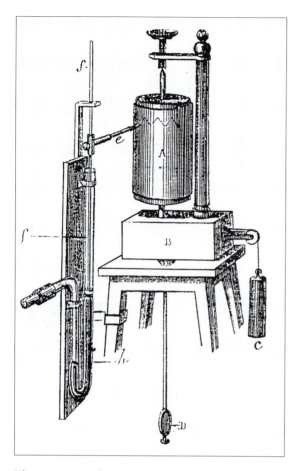

Figure 3 Ludwig's kymographion. *Photo Source University of Central Florida. Literary Source Marey, E. (1868). Du Mouvement, p.132. Public domain*

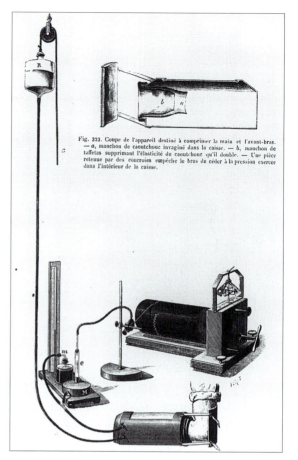

Fig. 323. Coupe de l'appareil destiné à comprimer la main et l'avant-bras. — *a*, manchon de caoutchouc invaginé dans la caisse. — *b*, manchon de taffetas supprimant l'élasticité du caoutchouc qu'il double. — Une pièce retenue par des courroies empêche le bras de céder à la pression exercée dans l'intérieur de la caisse.

Figure 4 Marey's sphygmographic apparatus. *Photo Source National Library of Medicine. Literary Source Marey, E.J. (1878). La methode graphique dans les sciences experimentales, p.614, Paris. Courtesy of National Library of Medicine*

cardiology. At the age of 65, now dissatisfied with life in London, he returned to his homeland, and established in St Andrews the Institute for Clinical Research. In reality, it served as a setting for his first love, general practice. This he attempted to do in partnership with other local practitioners of the same bent. However, his health was now failing and in six years' time he returned to London where he died at the age of 71. Death was attributed to coronary artery disease. He had had a history of angina pectoris during his stay in St Andrews[12,13]. Possibly, part of Mackenzie's dissatisfaction with London may have been due to the straining of a long, friendly, social and professional relationship he had with the rigid and autocratic Lewis. It must have been humiliating to Mackenzie to have had his paper on the vagal component of the action of

digitalis on the heart rejected by the 'high and mighty' Lewis, who was editor of the journal, *Heart*[14]. Ironically, Mackenzie was one of several close colleagues who encouraged Lewis to found the journal, *Heart*, in the first place.

Sir James Mackenzie must be viewed as one of the giants of modern medicine. He practiced during an era that was on the verge of a technological explosion. We are in the throes of this technological revolution today both in and out of the medical arena. The impact of technological advances is such that it warrants a careful evaluation of its effects on the ethical, legal and economic issues surrounding the practice of medicine. Gone are the days of the kindly family doctor, both friend and physician. In his stead there have appeared an array of health providers armed with the newest technological tools but with no apparent concern for the patient as a human being. It is true that these innovations have made the practice of medicine more certain of its diagnoses and more rewarding therapeutically. But in all of this, the art of medicine, that intimate rapport between physician and patient, that feeling of mutual respect, have all but disappeared in the closing years of this century.

Mackenzie must have sensed the present course of events in current medical practice. After an extensive clinical experience with his own polygraph, he was ardent in his exposition of the dangers arising from the misuse of technological developments in medicine, and especially of an uncritical acceptance of and dependance upon them.

In 1919, in a monograph on the future of medicine, Mackenzie wrote:

> Before a new method is introduced into medicine, its limitations must be realized and the nature of the knowledge it reveals must be demonstrated. The first step is to find out the value of the facts which the new method brings to light. No instrument should be allowed to be used in practice until the inventor demonstrates the bearing the facts which it brings to light has upon the diseased condition it reveals, that is to say, he must be prepared to show the effects of the cause of this new sign upon the health of the patient, and show that its recognition gives a guide to treatment. This evidence must not rely on theoretical considerations , but must be based on a report of a sufficient number of individual cases, which have been followed long enough to verify the claims, and in whom the associated phenomena have been studied in accordance with the methods peculiar to clinical medicine … After a new method has been discovered steps must be taken to supersede it. The next thing the discoverer of a mechanical device must do after he has recognized its use in clinical medicine, is, to get rid of it in practice. This seems an absurd recommendation, but it is vital to the progress of clinical medicine. [15]

Of course, the last sentence in this commentary is pure rhetoric. I am sure he expressed this sentiment to emphasize the previous points more forcefully; a device commonly used in debates and known as 'argumentum reductio ad absurdum'.

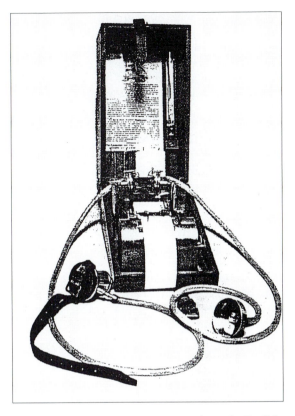

Figure 5 The Mackenzie-Lewis polygraph, English, Cambridge and Paul Instrument Co., ca. 1915. *Photo Source University of Central Florida. Literary Source Bakken Library of Electricity in Life. With permission*

I am quite convinced that Mackenzie was not against technology, *per se*. He was first and foremost a general practitioner who believed that clinical research should be part of the practitioner's daily duties and not restricted to the ivory towers of academia with their 'specialists'. He was also a prudent and cautious man who was weaned during an era when medicine was thought to be predominantly an observational science and where knowledge of the natural history of a disease was all important in appreciating its nuances[16]. Simply stated, diagnostic and therapeutic innovations were not to be used by the practitioner until thoroughly studied and understood. This is why when he finally became a Harley Street consultant he repeatedly criticized the misuse by physicians of his polygraph and later the electrocardiograph. 'I fear the day may come when a 'heart specialist' will no longer be a physician looking at the body as a whole, but one with more and more complicated instruments working in a narrow and restricted area of the body – that was never my idea'[17]. Current cardiologists should have these words firmly implanted in their minds.

PHONOCARDIOGRAPHY

Phonocardiography is a diagnostic technique that graphically records the acoustic phenomena of the cardiac cycle. It has declined in popularity in recent years but for several decades it provided a safe, inexpensive and relatively easy method of obtaining and recording permanently heart sounds and murmurs. Its usage in the clinical setting has always been conducted in conjunction with the palpable signs of cardiac function utilizing the carotid pulse, apex beat and jugular venous tracings. In the clinical laboratory, in combination with echocardiography, it has also proven to be very useful in elucidating the origin of the heart sounds and the physiological basis of cardiac murmurs.

The essential elements of the phonocardiograph include the transducer (microphone), amplifier, equalizer or filter, recording system and the transcription system. The recording device can be either a cathode ray tube or a galvanometer. De Forest in 1906 started the technical development of the modern phonocardiograph with his invention of the amplifying triode. However, amplifier units for audio work did not become commercially available until the 1920s when radio was being developed for common use.

Laénnec's stethoscope began the entire era of cardiac auscultation while phonocardiography and later echocardiography gave the procedure a firm scientific basis. Unfortunately, today's younger generation of physicians, accustomed to the technological superiority of Doppler analysis and color flow imaging, have begun to lose the proficiency in auscultation exhibited by previous clinicians. I am hoping that the pendulum will soon be balanced. To me, it has always been exciting to listen first and then either confirm or negate my auscultatory skills.

In 1895, Huerthle connected a microphone to an inductorium and with this crude apparatus, he was able to record heart sounds for the first time[18]. Einthoven was also working on a similar project at the same time. He used initially a capillary electrometer and then a string galvanometer[18]. Sir Thomas Lewis carried on further investigations within the clinical setting, using also a string galvanometer[19–21]. Frank recorded phonocardiograms directly with his segment capsule[22]. This capsule was later modified by Wiggers[23]. The modified capsule was used extensively by Orias and Braun-Menéndez of Buenos Aires for recording heart sounds and murmurs from the chest wall[24]. Most of this work was done between 1935 and 1939.

The initial efforts of these early investigators were carried on and expanded upon by a host of workers from around the world. In Germany, Schuetz (1929–34) studied the origin of heart sounds and cardiodynamics[25,26]. Studies by Maas and Weber in the 1950s led to improved versions of phonocardiographs which Holldack soon used to advantage in his observations[27,28].

Holldack, of Germany, worked with several colleagues, and also spent some time with Luisada's group in Chicago. In 1956 he co-authored with Wolf an atlas and textbook based primarily on his own investigations. In 1953, he recorded the sounds of stenotic mitral valves after commissurotomy and several years later he published his findings on the pericardial friction rub as recorded with the phonocardiogram[29–31]. Mannheimer introduced the calibrated form of phonocardiography in 1940[32]. His initial study was a clinical-statistical one of normal children and children with congenital heart disease[32,33].

Beginning with the 1940s, the majority of the contributions came from American and English centers. In America, Rappaport and Sprague (1940–42) dealt with linear, stethoscopic, and logarithmic phonocardiography. They helped delineate the physiologic and physical laws governing auscultation and their clinical application, and outlined the utility and limitations of the acoustic stethoscope, the electrical amplifying stethoscope and stethograph[34]. Their observations in the graphic registration of normal heart sounds appeared in 1942. These two workers were indefatigable in improving the modern stethoscope by pointing out the importance of tubing bore and proper fitting of the stethoscope to the ears utilizing phonocardiographic data as the analytical means[35–37]. McKusick's studies, also beginning in the 1950s, were concerned mostly with spectral phonocardiography[38,39]. A number of papers were published by him and his group on the subject.

Musical murmurs were evaluated in a rather extensive manner [40,41].

The literary output of Aldo Luisada in the field, either alone or in collaboration with his assistants or associates, was awesome, to say the least. When Luisada began his studies in the 1940s in Chicago, he used initially a low frequency technique with no accurate timing channel. By 1959 he had built his own experimental phonocardiograph and recorded high-frequency tracings within a clinical setting [18]. Further experimental studies were conducted by him and his group during the 1960s on the hemodynamic correlates of the heart sounds. Rosa from Budapest was now a member of the team concentrating on precordial dynamics. He was truly an international researcher with his papers originating from Germany, Switzerland and America [42–46].

Dimond and his co-workers at La Jolla and Eddleman along with his associates at Birmingham studied ultra-low frequency tracings of the precordium. Dimond and Benchimol correlated the hemodynamic and phonocardiographic findings in atrial septal defect and pulmonary stenosis [47,48]. Eddleman called his method kinetocardiography. He outlined the method of recording precordial movements, described the normal configuration and amplitude of the kinetocardiographic tracings, and studied the distribution of forces over the anterior chest [49–52].

Simultaneous with this intense American activity great strides were being made by Leatham and his cohorts in Great Britain utilizing primarily medium high-frequency tracings. We shall see how important Leatham was when we trace the historical background of phonocardiography in understanding the origin and mechanisms of heart sounds and murmurs.

The first monograph on phonocardiography was written by O. Weiss and G. Joachim in 1911 [53]. Since then many excellent texts appeared. The best known among them are those of Orias and Braun-Menéndez (1939) [24], Luisada (1953) [54], Holldack and Wolf (1956) [30], McKusick (1958) [55], and Ueda, Kaito and Sakamoto (1963) from Japan [56].

It is quite apparent by this time that phonocardiography owed its development to a substantial number of researchers. Although each of the contributors is a giant in his own right, the two superstars are, in my opinion, Luisada and Leatham. Luisada, because of his enormous and beneficial output, and Leatham, because of his incisive observations, merit, at least, a brief biographical sketch.

'Everyone knows Luisada'. This remark was heard quite frequently throughout the greater portion of this century. Luisada's accomplishments are legion. Endowed with boundless energy and self-discipline, Luisada has left an unforgettable imprint on cardiology during more than 50 years of a highly productive professional career. He was a teacher, *par excellence*, and a clinical investigator of equal caliber. His bibliography is awesome, as he was the author or co-author of 5 textbooks, 7 monographs, and some 315 scientific papers. In keeping with the era in which he worked, his scientific output centered about circulatory hemodynamics, electrocardiography and most of all, phonocardiography.

Three of his proteges describe Luisada, the man, as follows [57]:

His personal offices convey his deeper, less apparent attributes. The decor is quite comfortable, orderly and modest. One gets the feeling that here is where the 'action' begins. Orderliness and control seem to be deeply rooted in the character of the 'Chief' as he engages you in conversation. Such conversation is likely to begin with the usual amenities and quickly progresses to a discussion of the latest projects taking place in his research activity. Original ideas flow with unusual rapidity, and one cannot help but be impressed with his dedication and youthful vigor. Interspersed with the conversation and telephone calls will be numerous interruptions by secretaries and technicians, his 'coworkers'. Each incident is handled with aplomb and understanding, and it becomes clear that such organization is at least part of the reason for continued excellence and productivity. There is never any implication of pause (or even slowing down) in accomplishment. The sense of activity is the same now as it was 10 years ago. and it would be difficult to think it has ever been different.

Luisada was born in Florence, Italy in 1901 and died at the respectable age of 86. He obtained his medical degree from the Royal University of Florence. After serving at several universities in Italy including Padua, Naples, Sassari and Ferrara, he transferred his activities to the United States where he remained for the rest of his life. He was initially a professor at Tufts University and later a distinguished professor of physiology and medicine at the Chicago Medical School.

Luisada gained international renown for his prodigious contributions in electromyography, phonocardiography and echocardiography and also for his research on the pulmonary circulation and intracardiac pressures.

At a meeting of the Laénnec Society in 1988, which Luisada helped to found, he was the subject of many commemorative remarks in observance of his death the year before. Those made by Sakamoto are perhaps the most illuminating[58]. Luisada had visited Japan several times where he met with colleagues and former co-workers in cardiovascular sound. Among them were Ueda, Yamakawa and the narrator, Sakamoto. All three men were leaders in the field of phonocardiography. When Luisada first visited Japan in 1960, he acknowledged that the methodology he used in his phonocardiographic studies before 1957 was not reliable, and at the same time, he stressed the necessity of new research techniques to clarify the mechanism of heart sounds. The ultrasonic Doppler technique was still in the developmental stage at the time, and Luisada was quite anxious for a Japanese manufacturer to supply him with a new Doppler machine so that he could investigate heart sounds by this new method. Unfortunately, this was not to be.

Sakamoto, in his recollections, also recounts how Luisada was the guiding spirit behind the formation of the Society of Cardiovascular Sound in Japan, which developed into the Japanese College of Cardiology in 1987. Sakamoto also translated Luisada's last book *The Heart Sound* into Japanese, and, again, in his recollections, he tells how Luisada quoted sentences from Herman Hesse's noble *Siddartha* in the prologue of this book.

> Do you call yourself a seeker, O venerable one, you who are already advanced in years and wear the robe of Gotama's monks?
>
> I am indeed old, said Govinka, 'but I have never ceased seeking. I will never cease seeking. That seems to be my destiny. It seems to me that you also have sought. Will you talk to me a little about it, my friend?

The above quotation illustrates Luisada's spirit as a serious scientist.

A number of references to heart sounds are to be found long before the invention of the stethoscope.

Harvey wrote in his *De Motu Cordis* '… with each movement of the heart, when there is the delivery of a quantity of blood from the veins to the arteries, a pulse takes place and can be heard within the chest'. Although auscultation was practiced as far back as Hippocrates, the auscultatory phenomena that were described referred to sounds originating in the lungs or abdominal cavity but never in the heart. Harvey then appears to be the first to have described sounds emanating from the heart though not without derogatory remarks by some of his contemporaries. The Venetian physician, Aemilius Parisanus was quite sarcastic when he stated 'nor we, poor deafs, nor any other doctor in Venice, can hear them, but happy is he who can hear them in London'[59]. I can inject my own sarcasm by suggesting that Parisanus could not hear heart sounds because of the cacophony produced by erstwhile gondolier tenors as they paddled through the canals.

Fetal heart sounds were also heard not too many years after Harvey's publication. These were described by Massac in 1650, and also greeted with derision and skepticism.

The posthumous works of Robert Hooke, published in 1705, containing his *Cutlerian Lectures and other Discourses* refer also to his ability to hear heart sounds. His description is prescient: 'I have been able to hear very plainly the beating of a Man's Heart … Who knows, I say, but that it may be possible to discover the Motions of the Internal parts of Bodies … by the sound they make, that one may discover the works performed in the several Offices and Shops of a man's Body, and thereby discover what Instrument or Engine is out of order'[60].

Descriptions of heart sounds prior to Laénnec are to be found in the writings of Casper Bartholin, the Elder (1654)[61], Cornelius Stalpert van der Wiel (1687)[62], James Douglas (1715)[63] and William Hunter (1764)[64].

The debate concerning the origin of the heart sounds began with the invention of the stethoscope, and has continued unabated since then. Over the years, however, certain concepts have become more firmly established. It is now generally accepted that valvular closure is an important source of these sounds. What is still debatable is the degree of influence exercised by the muscular portion of the heart.

The ability of the muscular portion of the heart to produce sounds was amply demonstrated by Wiggers and Dean as well as Eckstein[65,66].

They recorded the vibrations produced by the contraction of an isolated perfused strip of myocardium. Wiggers had already shown in 1915 that as the intraventricular pressure suddenly increased with systole, many structures were set into vibration, but he could not identify which structure was involved by the recorded vibrations. He also brought out the asynchronous contraction of the left and right ventricles; an important point in explaining the components of the second heart sound.

Heart sounds can be divided into those that are loud with relatively high frequency, and those that are soft with low frequency. It was William Dock who in 1933 popularized the hypothesis that the major cause of the high frequency sounds was the terminal halt of opening and closing valves[67]. Kountz later tried to emphasize instead the importance of the myocardium in the production of the first sound by eliminating valvular action[68]. He did this by clamping the vena cava or by blocking the atrioventricular orifices. In 1944, he and Wright compared the total vibrations obtained from a normal, rapidly dying, human heart with those obtained in chronic myocardial disease[69]. But Dock had already shown in his original paper in 1933 that upon ligation of the atrioventricular groove or the azygos, there was either complete disappearance or extreme reduction in the loudness of the first heart sound.

It was on the basis of this that Dock concluded that the first heart sound was caused by the 'sudden tension of the previously slack fibers of the atrioventricular valves.' The forces needed to evoke sounds from cardiac activity were elucidated by him even further in a paper that appeared in 1959[70]. I distinctly remember, while serving on the house staff at Kings County Hospital in Brooklyn, New York, how he would occasionally stop during ward rounds to demonstrate with the aid of a handkerchief held between both hands, the creation of a loud snapping noise when he forcefully and rapidly made the limp handkerchief taut.

Orias and Braun-Menéndez were of the opinion that the first sound consisted of vibrations produced by atrial, valvular, muscular, and vascular factors[24]. Rappaport and Sprague joined the South American investigators in agreeing with this concept, thus opposing Dock's purely valvular hypothesis[35]. In 1950, Smith and his co-workers added more experimental evidence to support Dock's view. They used surviving perfused dog hearts to reach the conclusion that the first heart sound is largely due 'to the forceful striking of the valves'[71]. Luisada attempted to pursue the subject further by conducting open-chest experiments in 1952. His group concluded that 'extensive damage of either the atrioventricular valves or the ventricular walls caused extreme reduction in the intensity of the first heart sound'[72].

Throughout this time, investigations in phonocardiography were going on in Great Britain with the same intensity of interest. William Evans was an early pioneer in exploring the potentialities of phonocardiography. He did most of his work at the London Hospital. He must be given recognition primarily for providing the stimulus for further research in the field. One of the major difficulties in recording heart sounds is the broad band of frequencies that they produce and the lack of a 'gold-standard' phonocardiograph that could track the nuances of these vibrations and sift between what is physiologically important and what is not. Evans used an old Cambridge double string galvanometer to record the events. Figure 6 illustrates one of his recordings.

Since no filters were used, marked low frequency oscillations are noted, and, it should be emphasized, these bear no relationship to the auscultatory findings. This deficiency was overcome when Rappaport and Sprague introduced the use of low frequency filtration in 1941. This made possible, for the first time, the graphic registration of sounds that resembled those heard with the stethoscope.

Evans' interest in heart sounds was so all-consuming that Leatham recounts how the London Hospital Gazette published in 1941 a caricature of Evans listening to a patient's heart even though a bombing raid of London was in progress. Figure 7 is a reproduction of this caricature with Evans supposedly asking 'Do I hear more than two sounds?'

This interest was further intensified by Aubrey Leatham when he was appointed as the first Sherbrook Research Fellow at the London Hospital in 1947. Leatham pursued his investigations with such enthusiasm, vigor and productivity, that he soon became an indisputable authority on auscultation and phonocardiography. In the Jubilee editorial of the *British Heart Journal* in 1987, Leatham relates how he first became involved with the phonocardiographic technique[73]. This was in 1946, and at that time, Leatham was serving as a resident medical officer at the National Heart Hospital.

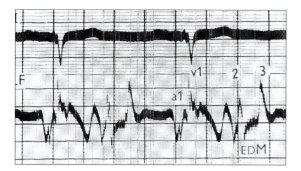

Figure 6 An Evans phonocardiogram (obtained without filters). *Photo Source National Library of Medicine. Literary Source Leatham, A. (1987). Auscultation and phonocardiography : a personal view of the past 40 years. Br. Heart J., **57**, 397–403. With permission*

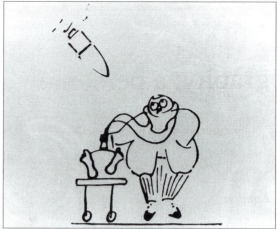

Figure 7 Do I hear more than two sounds? A caricature of William Evans at work. It appeared in the London Hospital Gazette during the heavy bombing of London in the early days of World War II. *Photo Source National Library of Medicine. Literary Source The London Hospital Gazette. With permission*

The following remarks are taken from the editorial wherein in a conversationally personal manner he outlined his approach and contributions in the evolution of auscultation and phonocardiography during his commitment of 40 years.

Auscultation and phonocardiography started for me with the gardener at the country branch of the hospital who while tending his plants was noticeably short of breath. When I examined him I found very abnormal heart sounds which I could not interpret. An earphone harnessed to the hospital string galvanometer electrocardiograph produced puzzling and large low frequency vibrations not at all resembling auscultation. A chest radiograph showed that he had an enormous heart, he died six months later and at necropsy proved to have Lutembacher's syndrome.

Leatham's apparatus, suitably fitted with amplifiers and filters, was able to delineate quite nicely the components of both the first and second heart sounds. He relates, however, how the strings of the galvanometer had a tendency to wrap around each other whenever a large deflection occurred and how only one old technician in Cambridge was able to unwrap these strings. Since the mishap occurred quite often, it necessitated frequent trips from London by Leatham in a 1934 baby Austin in order to set things right again[73].

During this time, we have already seen how Aldo Luisada, the political refugee from fascist Italy, was also exploring the potentialities of phonocardiography in Chicago. During the early 1940s, Luisada was still using a low frequency technique

with no accurate timing channel. It was also at this time that the Mannheimer system was introduced. It utilized multiple channels simultaneously fed by one microphone, with each channel operating in a different frequency range. This system was particularly popular in Sweden and Germany, but no important discoveries were made with it.

A considerable controversy arose between Leatham and Luisada regarding the origin of the first heart sound. Luisada held to the view that mitral activity was entirely responsible for the first sound. Leatham contended that tricuspid closure contributed to the second component of the first sound. On top of all this, a group from Pittsburgh led by Shaver ascribed the first sound to aortic ejection. They called it the root sound.

Echocardiography helped resolve the problem through its ability to time exactly the entire spectrum of valvular movement. This ultrasonic technique demonstrated that the components of the first sound at the apex were initially due to mitral valve closure and then to tricuspid closure. This was in keeping with Wiggers' demonstration of ventricular systolic asynchrony. Leatham's group carried out its early observations on patients with Ebstein's anomaly where the large anterior leaflet could be seen easily[74–77]. As echocardiographic technology improved further confirmation of

Leatham's observations was obtained through the simultaneous efforts of Graham Leech and Earnest Craige[76,77].

Prior to the utilization of ultrasound in his investigations with electrocardiography, Leatham had moved in 1951 to the National Heart Hospital where Paul Wood was the director of the Institute of Cardiology. Again, his early efforts were with 'recycled' instruments. He recounts how the chief technician, John Norman (like a good sergeant in the US Army) managed to find for him a 1918 Cambridge table model string galvanometer on which they mounted a second string and two mirror galvanometers with the aid of the Cambridge Instrument Company[73]. In the same article, Leatham reproduces a tracing taken with this apparatus with the statement 'The quality of the sound recordings made with this apparatus has never been surpassed; it cannot even be equalled with modern apparatus'[73].

The variable intensity of the first sound at the apex and the relationship of this variability to the PR interval occupied the attention of Craige in America and Leatham in England. Craige helped to delineate the relationship between the PR interval and the intensity of the first mitral component with the aid of echocardiography. Subsequent to Craige's work, Leatham's group used high speed echocardiography and demonstrated that the mitral valve was wide open at the initiation of left ventricular contraction when the PR interval was short so that the mitral leaflets closed with a 'bang,' as it were, resulting in a loud first sound. In the presence of a long interval, the mitral leaflets had enough time to be much closer to each other by the time the ventricle contracted. This resulted in a soft first sound[78].

Leatham's group also showed how to distinguish between proximal right bundle branch block and distal or arborization block on the basis of wide splitting of the first sound in the former and no detection of splitting in the latter[79]. This differentiation has an important prognostic significance when the electrocardiogram manifests a right bundle branch block.

Concerning the second heart sound, the major value in understanding the mechanism for its origin, its configuration on the phonocardiogram, and its respiratory variations lies in the examination of children in whom 'innocent' or physiological ejection murmurs are frequently heard. I have already mentioned how Laénnec erroneously attributed the origin of the second sound to atrial contraction. This was a serious error because on the basis of this assumption, he was unable to accurately correlate murmurs and pathological changes.

Hope was the first to accurately time the first and second heart sounds. Utilizing both animal experiments and clinical observations, he reported in 1832 that the second sound was related to closure of the aortic and pulmonic valves[73]. This was a rather astute conclusion, antedating phonocardiographic and electrocardiographic evidence. Rouanet, also in 1832, suggested too that the second sound was caused by the closure of the semilunar valves[80]. However, Wiggers at a much later date believed that the semilunar valves closed without noise, and that the second sound occurred only after these valves had already closed[65].

Leatham's investigations in 1951 and 1954 uncovered the presence of an aortic and pulmonic component in the second sound and traced their production to the closure of their respective valves[81,82]. He recognized that splitting was due to ventricular asynchrony with its consequent effect on the relative closing times of the aortic and pulmonic valves, and he delineated also the role of respiration in the ventricular asynchrony. Leatham furthermore showed that the width of split between the aortic and pulmonic components is almost as accurate as the degree of pressure gradient across the pulmonic valve in assessing the severity of pulmonic stenosis[83].

Leatham credited his technician, Bill Dicks, with alerting the physician researchers to the presence of a fixed split second sound in atrial septal defect[73]. The technician was looking at the moving shadow of the string rather than at the finished graph when he 'triumphantly announced this observation'. Leatham also credited Wolferth and Margolies with the identification of the two components of the second sound (A2 and P2) in bundle branch block by recording simultaneously the carotid pulse with the phonocardiograph.

The true origin of the aortic ejection sound eluded phonocardiographers until the advent of cineaortography and echocardiography. Utilizing cineaortography, Richard Ross and O'Neil Humphries from Johns Hopkins demonstrated that the aortic ejection sound coincided with the final halt of the upward moving aortic cusps during systole[73]. The echocardiogram has been shown to be equally as good in demonstrating this physiologic phenomenon, and without the difficulties inherent in cineaortography. Adequate mobility of the valve was found to be essential for the production of the aortic ejection sound. No sound is produced if the aortic valve is immobilized as could occur with heavy deposition of calcium.

Leatham's initial interest focused on the origin of the heart sounds. It was not until sometime later that he began to investigate the origin and physiologic basis of systolic murmurs, including those heard at the apex. This was an important step because, as he himself stated, most British cardiologists at the time tended to ignore the systolic murmur since it was felt to represent in most cases an innocent aberration but still capable of creating too many 'cardiac invalids' when falsely misinterpreted, a view fostered by Mackenzie, Lewis and other leading cardiologists.

Leatham was the first to describe the systolic murmur of aortic stenosis as an ejection murmur. This was based on his observations with high frequency phonocardiography that the systolic murmur in aortic stenosis ended before the aortic component of the second sound. He also used the phonocardiographic relationship of the apical systolic murmur with respect to A2 to differentiate between mitral regurgitation and a left ventricular outflow tract ejection murmur.

In his Goulstonian lecture which was later published in *The Lancet* in 1958, Leatham made several pertinent remarks regarding heart murmurs[84]. The first is that classification of systolic murmurs into pansystolic regurgitant murmurs and midsystolic ejection murmurs has withstood the test of time and can be easily identified with phonocar-diography. He also alluded to the usefulness of a combined echophonocardiographic evaluation with a synchronous carotid tracing for analyzing an apical systolic murmur to get its relationship to the components of the second heart sound.

The advent of echophonocardiography also brought about an improvement in our understanding of diastolic murmurs. A notable example is the work of Fortuin and Craige in the genesis of mitral diastolic murmurs[85]. They also confirmed Austin Flint's observations on the mechanism of the mitral diastolic murmur in aortic regurgitation; again underscoring the amazing astuteness of our 'bedside cardiologists'[86].

As one would expect, sounds caused by artificial valves are entirely different from those produced by the natural ones. The initial phonocardiographic studies on prosthetic mitral valves were conducted by Starr and his staff in 1962. They evaluated the silicone-covered valves that he and Edwards devised[87]. Shortly thereafter, Segal and his group conducted similar studies in Philadelphia[88]. Both groups demonstrated that the artificial mitral valve causes two high-pitched clicking sounds, one at its closure and one at its opening. In 1963, P. Shah, working as a member of Luisada's group, conducted a physiological study on 5 patients with mitral valve replacement using high speed phonocardiography[89]. Segal also delineated in 1964 the acoustic findings with prosthetic aortic valves[88].

Among the special applications of phonocardiography, mention should be made of the fetal, esophageal, tracheal and epicardial approaches.

Long before the advent of fetal phonocardiography, fetal heart sounds were heard, as I have said, by Massac in 1650, and much later by the surgeon, Francois Mayor of Geneva. Mayor reported this in an address before the Society of Physics and Natural History of Geneva; a few months after Laénnec's preliminary paper on the stethoscope before the Academy of Sciences in Paris in June, 1818. A description of the surgeon's remarks was published in the *Bibliotheque Universelle des Sciences et Arts* which McKusick described as a Readers Digest of the Arts and Sciences[90]. It is as follows: 'M. Mayor believes he has discovered something of importance to the art of obstetrics, namely, a means of determining whether the infant is dead or alive in the mother's womb; if the infant is alive but the pelvis contracted, caesarean operation is performed. M. Mayor has demonstrated that when one places the ear to the abdomen of the woman, the beatings of the heart of the infant are heard'.

The earliest tracings of fetal heart sounds were recorded by Pestalozza in 1891[16]. Utilizing gradually improved phonocardiographic techniques, a number of investigators also recorded fetal heart sounds beginning with Sampson in 1926[91], and followed by Beruti (1927)[92], Hyman (1930)[93], Peralta (1933)[94], Lian and Golblin (1938)[95], Pereira (1939)[96], Cesa and Seganti (1943)[97], Jordan and Randolph (1947)[98] and Fishleder (1960)[16].

Sampson and his group demonstrated that fetal phonocardiography was a relatively simple procedure and far easier to do than fetal electrocardiography. Hyman's study concerned itself primarily with irregularities of the fetal heart between the fifth and eighth months of pregnancy. The observations by Peralta, Lian and Golblin, and Cesa and Seganti did not break new ground, but were rather confirmations of previous studies. Jordan and Randolph pointed out how the technique could give valuable prenatal information on certain severe malformations of the heart. Their paper illustrated how congenital complete heart block could be diagnosed *in utero* with sound tracings and a simultaneous electrocardiogram of the mother. Fishleder and his colleagues in Mexico contributed a great deal towards the subject with the bulk of their observations appearing between the years 1952 and 1963. They delineated the phonocardiographic characteristics of the fetus during the various phases of the cardiac cycle, as well as many cardiac malformations, among them being persistent ductus arteriosus, interatrial septal defects, and aortic and pulmonary stenosis. Bolechowski of Poland also added to the pool of knowledge during this period. His group routinely recorded fetal heart sounds after the 20th week of pregnancy in 164 women[99]. They were able to separate sounds produced by the fetal heart from noises caused by fetal movement, maternal souffles and umbilical cord murmurs.

Luisada's contributions on fetal phonocardiography included the observation that the best tracings were obtainable by using the lower (50 or 100 cps) bands[16].

Taquini of Argentina was the first to utilize the esophageal approach. His initial observations appeared in 1936[100]. A year later he published a much more extensive paper on the subject[101]. Miller and Groedel also took up this approach and published their findings in 1950[102]. The transesophageal approach has certain merits which these workers were quick to point out. Since the heart sounds are registered from inside the chest, their origin is nearer to the transducer, and there is no skeletal impediment in their transmission. Atrial sounds and the murmur of mitral insufficiency are recorded more distinctly with this approach than from the surface of the chest.

Miller and Groedel also recorded sounds from within the trachea. They used this approach in patients who had in place a tracheal cannula. Several authors have recorded tracings directly from the epicardium of the exposed heart or the adventitia of the large vessels. Magri and his colleagues obtained a few tracings in man in 1952[103,16].

Animal experiments of this sort were reported by three different groups working independently of each other. They were Bertrand[104], Zalter[105] and Shah[106] (the latter two working in Luisada's laboratory). The results of all these observations were published in the same year (1963).

The pioneers in intracardiac phonocardiography were Yamakawa and Soulié. Yamakawa's group published its observations initially in 1953, and again, in 1954[107]. Both of these papers appeared in American periodicals. The group's observations were updated in a Japanese periodical in 1960[108].

P. Soulié presented his findings with intracardiac registration at the World Congress of Cardiology that was held in Washington DC in 1954[109]. He and his group subsequently published a number of papers on their continuing observations. A very interesting paper was the one they presented at the Fourth World Congress of Cardiology held in Mexico in 1962[110]. It was a study of the intracardiac sounds picked up in the left heart chambers by means of a micromanometer (pressure-sound transducer).

Numerous studies have been published since the original works of these two pioneering groups. By far the greatest contributions, again, appear to be those by Luisada and his coterie of workers beginning in the 1950s. In 1957, Luisada and Liu described a method of recording intracardiac sound vibrations utilizing the electric signal of a pressure transducer through differentiation and filtration[111]. During the same year, Lewis and his co-workers obtained tracings with a miniature barium titanate tubular element at the tip of an intracardiac catheter[112].

Some of these studies were conducted on animals but the vast majority were carried out on humans during cardiac catheterization. Luisada continued to use his own method for many years investigating various chambers of the heart and aorta[113–115].

Feruglio and his group also conducted extensive studies with this approach. Feruglio's initial paper appeared in the *American Heart Journal* in 1959[116]. Subsequent papers by him or in collaboration with others appeared not only in American but also in Italian and French periodicals[117–123]. His text on intracardiac auscultation and phonocardiography appeared in 1964[121].

Moscovitz and his associates published extensively on their findings with animal experimentation as well as with patients. Most of their work, which appeared between the years 1956 and

513

1959, was concerned with the correlation of mechanical, acoustic, and electric events in the cardiac cycle [124–127]. His atlas of the hemodynamics of the cardiovascular system has excellent phonocardiographic tracings [128].

Luisada's method of obtaining intracardiac tracings was modified by Yarza Iriarte in 1961 [129]. His group used a piezoelectric microphone cemented to the end of a catheter. They studied 20 patients with acquired heart disease and 38 patients with congenital heart disease. In 1965, Luisada modified his method further by applying a flat sonar-type, barium titanate microphone at the end of a catheter [16]. He called the system an FCT phonocardiogram. It proved to be quite adequate for both low and high frequency vibrations. Figure 8 is an illustration of the various devices used for recording intracardiac phonocardiograms [130].

BALLISTOCARDIOGRAPHY

The term 'ballistocardiogram' was coined by Starr in 1939 [131]. It is derived from the Greek: *ballein*, to throw; *kardia*, heart; *gramma*, a drawing. In essence, the ballistocardiogram is a graphic representation of the ballistic impulses experienced by the body to the waves of pressure and blood flow set in motion in the heart and great vessels by systole and diastole of the atria and ventricles. It therefore represents mechanical events, and should give information regarding the efficiency of the heart action as a pump. It was touted as an aid in the diagnosis of coronary artery disease, hypertensive heart disease, congestive heart failure, coarctation of the aorta, and in assessing myocardial function after an acute infarction.

Although Isaac Starr is considered to be the father of ballistocardiography, its roots go back to J. W. Gordon in 1877. He was the first to demonstrate that motion of the body occurs with each heartbeat. This was reported in a paper entitled 'On certain molar movements of the human body produced by the circulation of the blood' [132]. The paper's introduction contains the following remarks: 'A person standing erect in a perfectly easy posture on the bed of an ordinary spring weighing machine, and maintaining, as far as possible, perfect stillness, will be found, if the instrument is delicately adjusted, to impart a rhythmic movement to the index, synchronous with the pulse ... It does not

appear that this phenomenon has heretofore been anticipated by any process of theorizing, or turned to any useful account'.

The banal bathroom scale lends itself very easily to this observation if one stands very still while observing the rhythmic deflection of the pointer in synchrony with the pulse.

In order to record this motion, Gordon initially used a weighing machine with a pointer that graphically reproduced the effects of the bodily movements. He later substituted a light frame table for the weighing machine. The table was suspended from a trestle by four ropes. Figure 9 depicts Gordon's tracings as obtained with the weighing machine (A) and from a table suspended by ropes (B).

Three years later Landois described the vertical ballistocardiogram utilizing Gordon's technique [133]. Henderson in 1905 published a report describing what he called a new method for estimating the volume of blood moved by each heart beat [134]. He designed and utilized a horizontal table suspended by four piano wires and fitted with attachments that prevented lateral movement. This was a design similar to that devised by Gordon. The recorded pattern that resulted from the movements imparted to the suspended table by the subject's heart action was called by Henderson a 'recoil curve of the circulation as a whole'. He considered it to be a quantitative expression of the algebraic sum of all the mass movements of the circulation.

In 1911, as part of a study to determine the effect of altitude on cardiac output, a version of Henderson's table was used by members of the Anglo-American Pike's Peak expedition [135]. Henderson along with the noted physiologist, Haldane, formed part of the group. The study concluded that a low barometric pressure has no effect on the volume of blood ejected during systole.

Heald and Tucker continued to explore the relationship between body movements and mechanical systole [136]. Their apparatus was quite elaborate and used a hot wire microphone for the recording. The tracings obtained with their model were quite good. Both the apparatus and tracings are depicted in their paper entitled *The recoil curves as shown by the hot wire microphone* which appeared in 1922. The complexity of their entire set-up can be easily appreciated by referring to Figure 10. This apparatus not only appeared to provide an effective method for evaluating cardiac function but also demonstrated respiratory variations in the amplitude

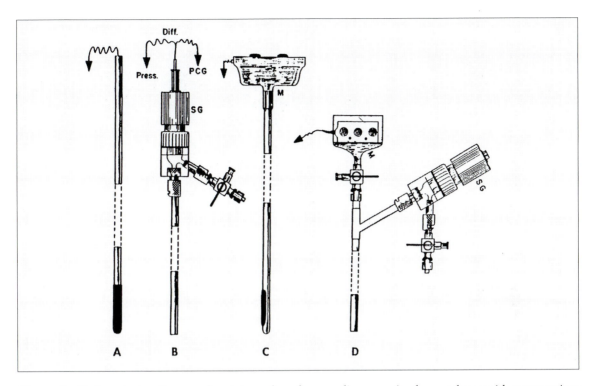

Figure 8   Various devices for recording intracardiac phonocardiograms. A: phonocatheter with sensor unit at the tip (Soulie, Lewis et al.); B: strain gauge with electric differentiation of output (Luisada and Liu); C: catheter closed by a membrane and connected with a regular microphone (M) (Feruglio); D: strain gauge (SG) and microphone mounted on same open catheter (Luisada and Slodki). *Photo Source University of Central Florida. Literary Source Luisada, A.A. (1962). The Heart Beat. Graphic Methods in the Study of the Cardiac Patient. Paul B. Hoeber, Inc., Medical Book Dept. of Harper & Bros., p.142. With permission*

of the recorded complexes. Later studies have shown that these respiratory variations are extremely important in the total interpretation.

In 1928, Angenheister and Lau introduced a seismographic variation of the apparatus[137]. They utilized a firm table with short legs. The impulse created by systole was transmitted to the seismograph via the movement imparted to the table and then recorded by optical means. As a result of this work, Abramson, a Swedish physiologist, became interested in the association between heart beat and bodily movement. With the aid of his brother, an engineer, he devised a chair containing a spring mechanism, the movement of which was magnified by a mirror placed in the center of the spring[138]. The movement was magnified by about 130 000 times and recorded with a camera. Abramson called his records 'kardiodynamograms'. He considered the recordings as representing a change in bodily motion imparted by the beating heart. Abramson

attempted to extrapolate this theoretical conclusion with a formula for determining cardiac output. Unfortunately, the formula was found to be erroneous by none other than Isaac Starr, the so-called father of ballistocardiography.

The arousal of clinical interest in the technique was almost entirely due to Starr's involvement. It was his hope that a truly simple and non-invasive method was at hand for accurately assessing cardiac output and therefore function. As Brown and co-authors recount in their text, *Clinical Ballisto-cardiography*, Starr's objectives throughout his investigations were to 'answer the question whether the heart is strong or weak, and how it is performing the function of pumping the blood'[139-141].

An appreciation of Isaac Starr appeared in the *New England Journal of Medicine* in April, 1979. Eugene Stead wrote it and we are indebted to him for the following remarks: '... How could the physician determine that the muscle of the heart

515

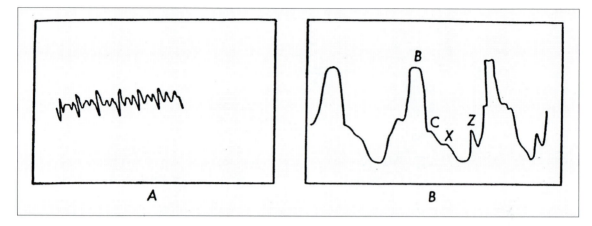

Figure 9 Pictures of Gordon's tracings are shown. A was obtained from his weighing machine and B from a table suspended by ropes. In A the downstroke which is immediately succeeded by a long upstroke is synchronous with the systole; the next downstroke is the second deflection referred to by Gordon. The upstrokes are to be regarded merely as indicating the instrumental tendency to restore equilibrium. In B the letters bear the same significance as in Dr Galabin's figures. *Photo Source University of Central Florida. Literary Source Gordon JW: On certain molar movements of the human body produced by the circulation of the blood., J. Anat. & Physiol., 11:533, 1877. Public domain*

was involved and make the diagnosis in life, in an organ that had been largely in the pathologist's province after death? The ballistocardiograph was the instrument that Starr developed to solve this problem'[142].

However, the ballistograph is not the ideal instrument for determining cardiac output. Hamilton brought this out when he concluded, on the basis of his own investigations, that the method was not capable of yielding dependable information on stroke volume in disease[143]. He felt that the instrument provided patterns of body motion which might be correlated only with clinical entities and prognosis.

Starr's thoughts on cardiac output as a diagnostic denominator of cardiac function were such as to cause him to have no interest in this possible use of the ballistocardiogram. Stead quotes him as saying: 'One must conclude that cardiac output will be worthless for the detection of early cardiac weakness, and I lost interest in it'[142]. The systole of the strong heart has a greater initial velocity than that of the weak heart. Starr knew this and appreciated that the ballistocardiograph provided an excellent method of measuring initial cardiac forces, and thus determining the strength of cardiac muscle.

Stead also recounts how Starr's ballistocardiographic studies documented the same type of

cardiac uncoordination as delineated by invasive tests; how this uncoordination is common in elderly people; how it is associated with coronary artery disease, and how it involves a strong respiratory variation in many patients.

When William Dock transferred his activities to Kings County Hospital in Brooklyn, New York, he too became intensely interested in ballistocardiography. He carried on extensive studies in the field for many years, and contributed invaluable data regarding its utility and limitations within the clinical setting. His book on ballistocardiography written in collaboration with the two Mandlebaums represented a compilation and analysis of all these efforts. It appeared in 1953[143].

I distinctly remember utilizing a model that he devised for the purpose while serving as a young resident at Kings County Hospital. The model cost me only $1.50 to make which was considerably cheaper than the $3200 the commercial entrepreneurs were asking for their instrument at the time. The patient was placed on an X-ray table and the body movements were picked up by this small apparatus placed against the feet. Smoking a cigarette caused evidence of marked cardiac uncoordination in my ballistocardiogram. This was unusual since temporary uncoordination induced by smoking was seen in elderly subjects and not in

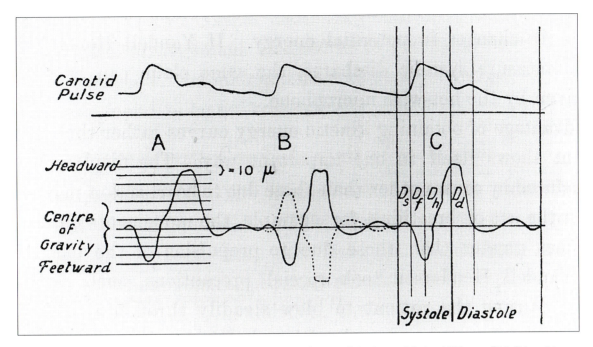

Figure 10 Recoil curves as shown by hot wire microphone. *Photo Source National Library of Medicine. Literary Source Herald, C.B. and Tucker, W.S. (1922). The recoil curves as shown by the hot wire microphone. Proc. R. Soc. (London), Series B, **93**, 281. With permission*

younger people[143]. Unfortunately, I did not take the hint at the time; I waited another 10 years before I gave up the weed.

William Dock played an important role in cardiology for more than a half century. His father, George Dock, was a famous physician in his own right, and one of the first full-time professors of medicine in America. William always spoke of his father with awe and affection. This was apparent especially when he would recount his father's classical description of the clinical manifestations of coronary artery disease.

William Dock received his doctorate in medicine from Rush in 1923. He later studied under Wilson, Merrick, Fred Smith and Sam Levine. He also spent time in Vienna, studying under his father's old friend, K.F. Wenckebach, who was already quite renowned for his electrocardiographic studies. Dock could be quite candid in his comments, and when asked about his opinion of Wenckebach, he answered by saying that Wenckebach was a very poor teacher and guilty of rambling presentations. He went on to say that the students used to recite:

in der Klinik Wenckebach
Nur die erste Banke wacht
(In Wenckebach's clinic
Only the first row stays awake)[144]

Dock had a profound knowledge of the basic sciences, especially pathology. In fact he spent six years at Stanford and Cornell as professor of pathology. He used this solid foundation to advantage in approaching a clinical problem. His original experimental and clinical contributions were quite numerous. Among them were his papers on:

(1) The mechanism of production of heart sounds[145];

(2) Atherosclerosis and hypercholesterolemia[146];

(3) Atherosclerosis in the young[147];

(4) The coronary bed in cardiac hypertrophy[148];

(5) Erosion of the ribs in coarctation of the aorta[149];

(6) The evil sequelae of bed rest[150];

(7) Aging of the myocardium[151]; and

(8)   Cardiac output in arteriovenous fistula [152].

This is certainly a formidable list of contributions, and yet, not surprising, from an individual whom God endowed with a lively and curious mind.

In an interview conducted by Allen B. Weisse, he was asked about ballistocardiography. This was his response:

> We have already talked a bit about my way of fixing things. Ballistocardiography is a sad story. Its potential was never realized. It is one of the best methods of studying patients, not just cardiac patients. It's a wonderful cheap toy. I do it in three planes because doing it in one plane is just like taking only a one lead electrocardiogram. I left my three-plane gadget behind me with more regrets than anything else when I retired. No one else ever had the slightest interest in it [144].

When asked about his long-standing dispute with Aldo Luisada about the genesis of the first heart sound, his candor was even more striking with this response:

> I refuse to dispute with him. Never argue with a man with an obsession and who won't repeat any experiments that are in the literature. In the 1830s, a good Frenchman, Rouanet, pointed out that two leaflets could come together but would not make noise unless you subjected them to tension. I quoted him in my first paper, and this is 140 years old now.
>
> What I like to do is get the answer to things. I've got some new experiments cooking here. I discovered to my horror that people were teaching that when you measure a patient's blood pressure, the Korotkoff sound in the artery is due to blood hitting the blood below the cuff. Well, anybody who has ever squirted a hose under the surface of a pool knows that's nonsense. You don't get that kind of noise that way. I'm working on this now.

[This work was published during Dock's 82nd year in the *New England Journal of Medicine* (1980)].

I knew Dock personally, following him quite religiously on his ward rounds or attending his illuminating clinicopathologic conferences. I found him to be energetic, enthusiastic and a consummate showman. His debating style with his peers made him somewhat controversial, but his attitude towards his staff and students was just the opposite. To us, he was always kind, considerate, ever willing to teach or demonstrate a finding no matter how trivial, and always with an engaging personality. His knowledge of the literature was encyclopaedic, and often, he would sprinkle his discourse with aphorisms and allusions to the humanities. I was always in awe of his demonstrations of almost total recall from the literature on the particular subject being discussed.

Zoneraich in his classical description 'William Dock as I knew him' [153] quotes Dock as being happy to have as his obituary Samuel Johnson's verses on the death of Robert Levet: 'A practicer of physic ... obscurely wise and coarsely kind ... /His vigorous remedy displayed/The power of art without the show ... /His frame was firm-his powers were bright,/though now his eightieth year was nigh./Then with no fiery throbbing pain,/no cold graduation of decay,/Death broke once the vital chain,/and freed his soul the nearest way'.

Interest in ballistocardiography as a non-invasive diagnostic tool has declined considerably since its heyday in the 1950s. This is glaringly revealed by the fact that the highly esteemed current text on heart disease edited by Eugene Braunwald fails to mention it at all.

ELECTROCARDIOGRAPHY AND VECTORCARDIOGRAPHY

Three important factors were necessary before electrocardiography could be accepted as an accurate non-invasive method of detecting and delineating cardiac abnormalities. These included the development of a clinically practical galvanometer, a firm anatomical basis concerning the conduction of electrical impulses throughout the heart and recognition of the electrophysiologic mechanisms controlling and regulating the heartbeat.

The historical background of the electrophysiologic and anatomical aspects has already been presented in Section 3. At this point, I would like to trace first the technical developments that have led to the modern electrocardiographic instrument and then elaborate on some of the more important figures and their contributions in the evolution of the technique as a clinical tool in the diagnosis and management of heart disease.

The first commercial model was sold in 1908. It was manufactured by the Cambridge Scientific Instrument Company of England. The machine was a highly complex piece of equipment made possible by combining brand new and different ideas and utilizing components that did not even exist a couple of decades before its introduction. Its most delicate part was the string galvanometer, the brainchild of William Einthoven. It also used a quartz filament, a component that had first been made only 20 years before Einthoven's galvanometer. The origin, historical development of each component, and their final amalgamation into the electrocardiograph is an interesting chapter in the history of cardiology. It illustrates how medicine, a branch of the biological sciences, took advantage of the concepts of physical science and its instrumentation, incorporating both into its sphere of activities for diagnostic and physiological evaluation.

The string galvanometer had its origin in the oscillograph. It was an instrument originally developed for the power supply industry. The first practical oscillograph was designed by Eugene Blondel (1863–1938) who was professor of electrotechnology at both the École des Ponts et Chaussées and the École des Mines. The design appeared in a paper published in 1893[154]. It had a moving part that would oscillate in accordance with the variations in the current passing through it. The oscillations were recorded by means of a photographic device. It soon became apparent that the oscillograph would help solve the problem of recording any rapidly alternating voltage. William DuBois Duddell, an engineer with the Cambridge Scientific Instrument Company, pursued this thought and designed an instrument capable of doing just that. His design was developed after he had read Blondel's paper. The result was the first satisfactory oscillograph to appear on the market. It was advertised in the company's catalogue just seven years after the publication of Blondel's paper[155].

The crucial issue in electrocardiography was the development of a means of satisfactorily recording the minute and rapidly alternating voltage generated by the heart. Although the oscillograph, which is functionally a galvanometric device, was not ideal or even designed for this purpose, its invention, nevertheless, paved the way for the eventual development of Einthoven's string galvanometer.

Johannes S. G. Schweigger of the University of Halle invented the original galvanometer that served as a model for subsequent ones. The first single string galvanometer was that devised by Clement Ader in 1897[156]. He was a French electrical engineer, highly esteemed for his major contributions to communications, especially in amplification and stereophonic sound. His main interest, however, was in flying. He is now considered a pioneer in aeronautics, credited with being the first to make a powered, manned air flight. This was in 1890, a full 13 years before the much publicized epochal flight of the Wright brothers[157].

Ader's string galvanometer, suspended between the poles of a large magnet, was a fine metal wire, only 0.02 mm in diameter. Ader was well aware that the mass of the coil of wires between the magnets in the previous galvanometers limited the sensitivity and response time of the instruments. It is for this reason that he eliminated the coil and substituted a single wire. The oscillations were transmitted to a quill stuck to the wire. The shadow of the quills' movement as the wire vibrated fell on a sensitized telegraph tape and the recording was made permanent by placing the tape in a bath of fixer. The instrument was devised primarily for transmission of telegraphic data at high speed. To increase its sensitivity, adequate magnification of the movements of the string was necessary. The Cambridge Company accomplished this by resorting to an optical system. This required the use of an apochromatic lens because chromatic aberration was a serious problem. The apochromatic lens was the result of the efforts of Otto Schott, a Westphalian glass manufacturer. He worked under the guidance of Ernst Abbe, a partner of the noted Carl Zeiss firm. The lens became available for commercial use in 1886[158].

Despite all these developments and improvements, the string galvanometer was yet to be tried for electrocardiographic recordings. Early investigators in the field were working with either a Thompson siphon recorder or the Lippmann capillary electrometer. The Thompson siphon recorder was used by Alexander Muirhead of St Bartholomew's Hospital in 1869 or 1870[159]. It had been devised by William Thompson to record signals passing through the newly laid transatlantic cable. Utilizing this device, Muirhead appears to have been the first to successfully record a human electrocardiogram. During the 19th century and prior to him, electric potentials of the heart were obtained from exposed animal hearts[160].

These experiments had their roots in the original observations of Luigi Galvani at the end of the 18th century and those of Carlo Mateucci in 1842. The preferred method for visually demonstrating electrical current associated with muscle activity during the 19th century was the sciatic-nerve gastrocnemius preparation obtained from the frog. It was called a rheocord. Whenever the sciatic nerve was electrically stimulated, the attached muscle would contract. It was a simple experiment and easily reproducible. Electrical activity associated with cardiac muscle was not known until 1856 when it was accidentally discovered by two German scientists, Köllicker and Müller[161]. They prepared a rheocord from one frog and exposed the intact beating heart of the other. While doing so, they unknowingly allowed the sciatic nerve of the rheocord to come into contact with the exposed heart. For some reason or another, they left their work table at this point, and upon resuming their labors on their return, they noticed the gastrocnemius muscle, still attached to its sciatic nerve, contracting in synchrony with the heartbeat[161]. Another example of serendipity in science!

To return to Muirhead, he later became a successful telegraph engineer and contributed nothing further to medical technology.

In 1887, and again in 1888, A. D. Waller published his findings on electric potentials obtained from intact living animals, and then from the limbs and chest of humans[160,162]. He used the Lippmann capillary electrometer to deflect a light beam for the recording of these electrical forces. The Lippmann capillary electrometer was a far better device for measuring the electrical activity of the heart than the siphon recorder.

Gabriel Lippmann described his invention in a paper published in 1873 while he was working in Kirchoffs' physical laboratory in Berlin[163]. It consisted of a thin glass tube partly filled with mercury and overlaid with sulphuric acid. Placing the tube in electrical series with the body's surface would cause the current from that surface to flow through the mercury.

Variations in current flow caused the mercury to expand or contract. This oscillating movement of the column of mercury was magnified with the aid of a microscope, and the image was then projected onto photographic paper. Its response time was slow and therefore could not register high frequency potentials. Despite this and other deficiencies that annoyed Einthoven extremely, Lippmann's electrometer played an important role during the formative years of electrocardiography.

It is unfortunate that the name of Waller is unfamiliar to generations of physicians, including cardiologists. For too long a time his role in the evolution of electrocardiography has been overshadowed by that of Einthoven. Waller was truly a pioneer in electrocardiography, and this role has been championed recently especially by Edwin Besterman and colleagues from the staff of the Waller cardiopulmonary unit at St Mary's Hospital in London[164–167]. Waller's original apparatus and some of the tracings obtained with it are housed in this unit. It is true that Muirhead may have been the first to record a human electrocardiogram but Waller was the first to do so in a combined clinico-physiologic setting, the first to publish a report on his findings, and a pioneer in acquiring an extensive experience with this new diagnostic modality. He called the tracing an 'electrogram'. By 1917, he was able to present before the Physiological Society of London a paper entitled *A preliminary survey of 2000 electrocardiograms*[168]. As can be seen by the title, he was now calling the tracings, 'electrocardiograms'. This paper must have represented 'a change in heart' on his part, because only six years before its presentation, Waller had said 'I do not imagine that electrocardiography is likely to find any very extensive use in the hospital. It can at most be of rare and occasional use to afford a record of some rare anomaly of cardiac action'[169].

Auguste Desire Waller was the scion of an eminent scientist, Augustus Volney Waller, noted for his work on nerve degeneration. Young Waller was born in Paris in 1856, and remained there until his father's death in 1870. He and his mother moved to Scotland where he pursued his medical studies in Aberdeen and Edinburgh. From the very beginning, Waller's primary interest was in physiology, a discipline to which he devoted his entire life, and to which he contributed a great deal. His textbook, *An Introduction to Human Physiology*, published in 1891, was, in actuality, a comprehensive treatise on the subject[170].

Waller's initial work in electrocardiography was conducted at St Mary's Hospital, and it was there that he gave his first public demonstration of his recording device. Waller remained at St Mary's until 1903 when he was appointed professor at the newly established University of London. This was followed in a very short time by his appointment as consulting cardiologist to the National Heart Hospital in London where he continued his clinical investigations in electrocardiography[164].

In his profile of Waller, Besterman relates how Waller's students greeted their instructor after his marriage to one of them[164]. The blackboard bore the inscription 'Waller takes the biscuit'. Apparently not the least offended, and in good humor, Waller added the words 'and the tin as well'. Besterman also quotes a recollection of Robert Marshall which suggests 'a certain unconventionality'. 'Waller presented a very different appearance from that of our physicians, who were always soberly garbed in frock coats or morning coats and silk hats. He was a short, stocky man, very light on his feet. His grey beard and double-breasted blue jacket make him look exactly like a skipper in the merchant navy. Like Sir Winston, he seemed to be habitually smoking cigars, and was invariably followed by his bulldog, Jimmy, who also had a Churchillian quality and had the distinction of having had a question asked about him in the House of Commons.'

> Q. At a conversazione[sic] of the Royal Society at Burlington House on May 12th last, a bulldog was cruelly treated when a leather strap with sharp nails was wound around his neck and his feet were immersed in glass jars containing salts in solution, and the jars in turn were connected with wires to galvanometers. Such a cruel procedure should surely be dealt with under the 'Cruelty to Animals Act' of 1876?
>
> A. The dog in question wore a leather collar ornamented with brass studs, and he was placed to stand in water to which some sodium chloride had been added, or in other words, common salt. If my honourable friend had ever paddled in the sea, he will appreciate fully the sensation obtained thereby from this simple pleasurable experience!

Waller died in 1922 after suffering two strokes. He left behind three sons and a daughter, none of whom married, so that only collateral descendants remain. Figure 11 is a photograph of Waller and his constant companion, Jimmy, 'the dog in question'.

In his initial experiments, Einthoven also used the Lippmann capillary electrometer. In 1895, he published a paper delineating its capabilities in the measurement of minute electric currents[171].

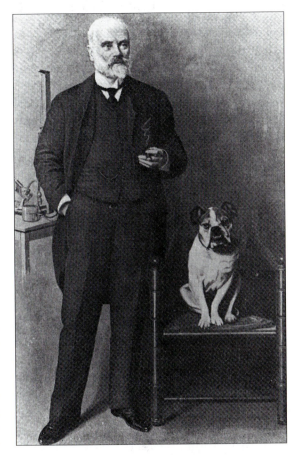

Figure 11 Waller and Jimmy. *Photo Source National Library of Medicine. Literary Source Besterman, E. (1979). Waller – pioneer of electrocardiography. Br. Heart J., 42, 61–4, (Fig. 4). With permission*

When he attended Waller's first demonstration of the device at St Mary's hospital, Einthoven was already familiar with the potentialities of the instrument in electrocardiography and Waller's lecture reinforced this belief to the extent that when Einthoven returned to his laboratory in Holland, he tackled his work with renewed vigor and enthusiasm. As time went on, however, Einthoven became increasingly disenchanted with the capillary electrometer.

One of its major deficiencies was its extreme sensitivity to vibration. Einthoven's laboratory did not help the situation either. It was located on the ground floor of an old wooden-framed building adjacent to a street paved with cobblestones. Every time a team of horses came by, pulling a heavily laden cart, the whole building would shake. It must have been very frustrating, after having spent six hours in setting up at least 3 limb leads on the subject to have to repeat the entire process because of multiple artifacts induced by a jostling column of mercury as the building shook[172]. What a veritable comedy of errors this must have been!

At first, Einthoven tried to improve the situation by removing the floor boards and having a hole dug about 10–15 feet deep and then filling it with large rocks so as to create a stable base for the capillary electrometer[173]. Unfortunately, this too did not solve the problem, causing Einthoven to look for a galvanometer without this frustrating defect. He initially experimented with the d'Arsonval galvanometer. But this too had a major defect. It used a coil between the magnets which limited its sensitivity and response. Apparently, Einthoven then reflected on the thesis that his teacher, Johannes Bosscha wrote in 1854 on *The differential galvanometer*[174]. Bosscha was a professor in Leyden. His thesis, dealing with the forces involved in measuring minute amounts of electricity, pointed out the advantages of a galvanometer in which the moving parts consisted of a single needle hanging from a silk thread. Einthoven was also acquainted with Ader's single string galvanometer, and it is not too inconceivable to conjecture that Ader's device may also have been the fruit of Bosscha's concept. At any rate, fortified with the knowledge derived from both Bosscha and Ader, Einthoven abandoned the coil of the d'Arsonval device and substituted in its stead, a fine wire. It was quite similar to the galvanometer Ader had introduced as a telegraph receiver and Einthoven acknowledged Ader's contribution when he published his landmark paper in 1901[175]. This was the culmination of 11 years of research on the electrophysiology of the heart. Three years after, Einthoven, in another paper, fully delineated the advantages of a string galvanometer over the capillary electrometer[176]. It is interesting to note that many years later, Waller, too, appreciated the technological superiority of Einthoven's invention; so much so that during Waller's tenure as consulting cardiologist to the National Heart Hospital, he used Einthoven's instrument rather than the Lippmann capillary electrometer.

Einthoven's galvanometer was made of a single strand of silver-coated quartz thread suspended between the poles of a horseshoe magnet with a strong magnetic field. The quartz string was only 2.1 μm in diameter; much finer than Ader's string which had a diameter of 0.02 mm. The extreme thinness of the string with its minimal mass assured now a sensitivity and response time capable of recording the rapid deflections of cardiac potentials with a high degree of fidelity. The oscillations of the wire were recorded photographically, after having been magnified with the aid of a microscope. Einthoven used a beam of light aimed through a hole in the poles of the magnet and reflected onto a falling photographic plate by a mirror attached to the string[177].

Ershler relates how the incredible thinness of the string was made possible[172]. 'The tail end of an arrow was attached by an element of quartz to the string of a tightly drawn bow. The quartz was heated, as it melted, the arrow was released and it shot across the room, drawing the quartz into a fine string. At times, the string was picked out of the air where it was held up by air currents in the room'. No doubt this dexterous bit of manipulation was performed by the laboratory assistant, Van de Woerdt, since Einthoven, himself, was rather inept when assembling the 'nuts and bolts' of an apparatus.

Despite the obvious advantages of the string, Einthoven's entire apparatus was still a monstrosity in size and too complicated for routine diagnostic usage. It occupied two rooms and required five people to operate it. A major problem was overheating which he attempted to circumvent with a huge continuous-flow water jacket for cooling the electromagnet. If this were not done, the heat generated caused the string conductance to change rapidly[178]. An arc lamp that needed continuous adjustments was used for projecting the shadow of the string onto the photographic plate. Large trays or bowls of saline were used as electrodes with the subject immersing his hands or feet in them. Figure 12 illustrates the Leyden model. It is a far cry from the minuscule portable instruments of today. Figure 13 shows how cumbersome it was to attach the subject. The buckets are paricularly intriguing.

The enormousness and immobility of the housing for the galvanometer was probably the main reason for Waller's initial feeling that the electrocardiograph would not have much clinical value. They appeared as insurmountable obstacles. It was Einthoven's former teacher, Bosscha, who again came to the rescue and helped change Waller's mind as Einthoven's access to clinical cases began to demonstrate the clinical usefulness of this new diagnostic instrument. Bosscha suggested linking the hospital to Einthoven's laboratory via telephonic transmission. Easy access to hospitalized patients was now realized and laid the foundation for Einthoven's contributions to electrocardiography in the clinical sphere.

Only five years after his landmark paper, Einthoven was able to describe the clinical applications of the electrocardiogram as obtained through telephone lines in a paper entitled 'Le Telecardiogramme'[179]. This, along with Waller's observations, set the stage for the monumental outpouring of studies and great clinical discoveries of the 20th century. In only a few short years, the electrocardiograph was about to take its place, side by side, with Laénnec's stethoscope in the management of heart disease.

The realization of Bosscha's suggestion was accomplished through the efforts of the Holland Society of the Sciences after Einthoven had advised its members of this key to clinical accessibility. Enough money was collected by the society to pay for the underground installation of wires, encased in a special lead cable, that connected Einthoven's electrocardiograph to the hospital, a good 1.5 km away[180]. The local telephone company imposed a nominal annual charge for use of the cable. Its cost was to be shared equally by both Einthoven's laboratory and the department of medicine. The serenity of this arrangement was disrupted soon after Einthoven's paper Le Telecardiogramme appeared. The green eye of envy emerged in the form of Nolen, professor and head of the department of medicine, who, obsessed with the perception that Einthoven was getting all the credit for this innovative technique, refused to pay for his half of the cost. Nolen's refusal to pay created an impasse that was to block further use of the cable system for a good many years. The petty jealousies of academia are quite obvious in this scenario.

Willem Einthoven was born in the Dutch East Indies (Semarang, Java) in 1860 where his father was stationed as a military physician. The family returned to Holland upon the father's death. The similarity of these circumstances surrounding the early years of Einthoven and Waller is quite striking.

Although the name Einthoven is definitely not a Spanish one, biographical sources state that he was descended from Spanish Jews who emigrated to Holland from Spain, probably to escape the inquisition in the late 15th century.

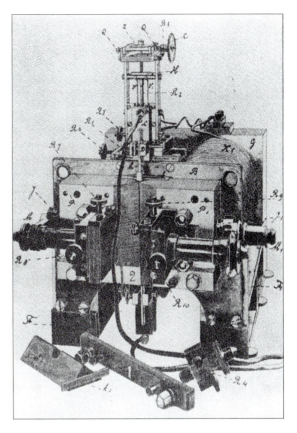

Figure 12 Einthoven's original Leyden model. *Photo Source National Library of Medicine. Literary Source Ciba symposium. Courtesy of Ciba symposium (with permission)*

Einthoven's interest in electrophysiology was stimulated in his medical school days by the illustrious physiologist, Donders, who at the time was studying action currents of the heart. This was part of his broad interest in the whole discipline of physical sciences, a fact that was quite evident then and throughout his entire life. A year after receiving his medical degree from the University of Utrecht, Einthoven, with the support of his teacher, Donders, was appointed professor of physiology and histology at Leyden University. He was only 26 at the time, his reputation already established with the publication of his paper On the Law of Specific Nerve Energies[181]. In the same year he had also published another paper which reflected his basic interest in the physical sciences. It was called On the influence of color differences in the production of stereoscopic effects. Einthoven remained at Leyden throughout his entire professional career, not only working on

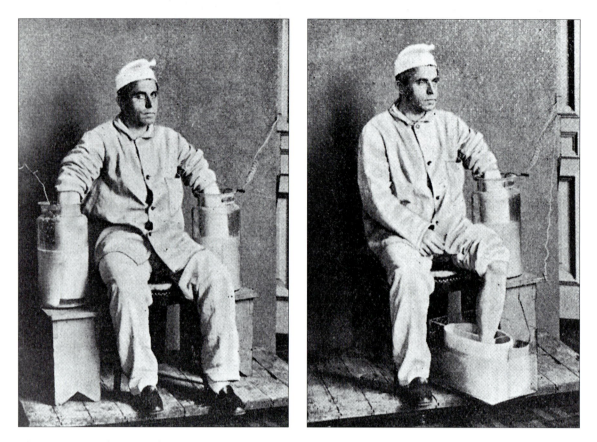

Figure 13 Einthoven's galvanometer attached to a patient. Note the buckets. *Photo Source National Library of Medicine. Literary Source Ciba symposium. Courtesy of Ciba symposium (with permission)*

electrocardiography but also making important contributions to the physiology of the bronchial musculature and the eye.

He must have been a man of incredible integrity and honesty. This is exemplified by his desire to share half of the $40 000 prize money he received as a Nobel laureate in 1924 with his former 'diener' Van der Woerdt. He was quick to admit that his work in electrocardiography, which led to the prize, was made possible only through the collaboration of Van der Woerdt. Learning that his retired laboratory assistant had died, Einthoven sought out the two surviving sisters and prevailed upon them to accept 'justifiably', half of the award money [172,180].

Probably the best portrait of Einthoven in terms of his 'humaneness', is to be found in the obituary written by his colleague, A. V. Hill, upon Einthoven's death in 1927 [182].

Einthoven was a master of physical technique. Despite his medical training, he was essentially a physicist, and the extraordinary value of his contributions to physiology and, therefore, to medicine emphasizes the way an aptitude for physics can aid in the solution of physiological problems. Of the more personal side of Einthoven's life, one might write of the grace, beauty, and simplicity of his character. He spoke with ease three languages as well as his own; he was a regular attendant at international gatherings; he threw all of his weight on the side of good international relations in science. It was a wonderful thing to be his guest and to enjoy the delightful hospitality of his home. He invited me some years ago, while we were attending a German Congress of physiologists at Tübingen, to stay with him at Leiden on my way back to England. We arranged to meet at a station in North Germany and to travel the last part of the journey together. I waited until his train arrived. He came literally running along the platform to meet me, seized my bag out of my hand, carried it to the carriage where he had kept me the best seat, and made me feel whatever the differences of our age and position, I was from that moment his honored guest. In 1924, we sailed together to America and at night under the starlit sky, we walked on the upper deck discussing the random movements of electrons in conducting fibers and other matters equally as strange. These personal details will emphasize what a loss his passing will be, not only to his older colleagues and to his younger friends, but also to all the good fellowship of physiologists throughout the world.

There were other technical difficulties with Einthoven's model. These included the inclusion of a casing that would provide an airtight environment for the string, and protection of the fibers that made up the string. In an attempt to overcome these and other problems of a technical nature, a working arrangement soon developed between Einthoven and the Cambridge Scientific Instrument Company of England.

The Cambridge Scientific Instrument Company was founded in 1881 by Albert George Dew-Smith and Horace Darwin, both members of Trinity College, which for many years was the main center of scientific activity in Cambridge[183]. Horace Darwin was the youngest child of Charles Darwin, the evolutionist. The two men parted in 1891 leaving Darwin in full control of the instrument-making activities of the company, oriented primarily towards physiological research. The company maintained for many years a very close relationship with Trinity College. Many of the instruments that it manufactured were designed by members of the Trinity College Faculty. In 1924, the company changed its name to the 'Cambridge Instrument Company'. The list and variety of its instruments are endless. Its contributions over the years to the various sciences represent a unique model of disdain for financial profit, especially if such profit were to be obtained at the expense of an honest rapport with the scientific community or by compromising intellectual integrity. This represents a most unusual orientation for a commercial enterprise and underscores the respect that scientists have had for this company. Excellence of design and craftsmanship of the highest quality were the hallmarks of Darwin's enterprise.

All the preliminary communications between Einthoven and the company are to be found in the Museum Boerhave at Leyden University. The company was asked to redesign, manufacture and market the instrument. Dudell, the inventor of their oscillograph, played a very important role in the final product. In 1908, the company sold its first version to E. A. Schafer of Edinburgh. This model was to be bought for many years primarily by physiology laboratories. Its size was greatly reduced from Einthoven's model by redesigning the magnet. The field could now be concentrated in the region of the string. Improved optics were also used so that the hole through the magnet could be made smaller. The continuous-flow water jacket was eliminated by substituting a smaller and more manageable water bath.

Further design improvements were necessary to eliminate its bulkiness and improve its portability. The Cambridge Company was firmly committed to the realization of these objectives. It finally brought out a table-model in 1911. It was leased to Sir Thomas Lewis at University Hospital in London[160]. By 1918, the Cambridge Instrument Company had managed to install 35 of its instruments in hospitals in English-speaking countries. A modified version designed by C. B. Williams of Columbia University had already been introduced into the United States. His continued collaboration with the Cambridge Company led to the establishment of the American branch of the company and for many years after, it was the only supplier of these instruments in the United States.

The size remained a problem for many years limiting its use to hospital wards capable of handling long connecting wires and telephone connections between nurse and operator. The breakthrough in size came in 1926 with the introduction by Cambridge of the first truly portable electrocardiograph. It was still a hefty machine at 80 lb, requiring wheeled trolleys, but, indeed, a far cry from Einthoven's behemoth. Reduction in size was accomplished by the use of new magnetic alloys that could produce the same field strength as the much larger electromagnet. Another improvement was the substitution of the falling-plate film with a motor-driven drum wrapped with film. An example of this instrument is illustrated in Figure 14. It is a 1932 advertisement of their Hindle model[184].

The late 1930s saw the introduction of the first electronic or 'valve' instrument. It was advertised

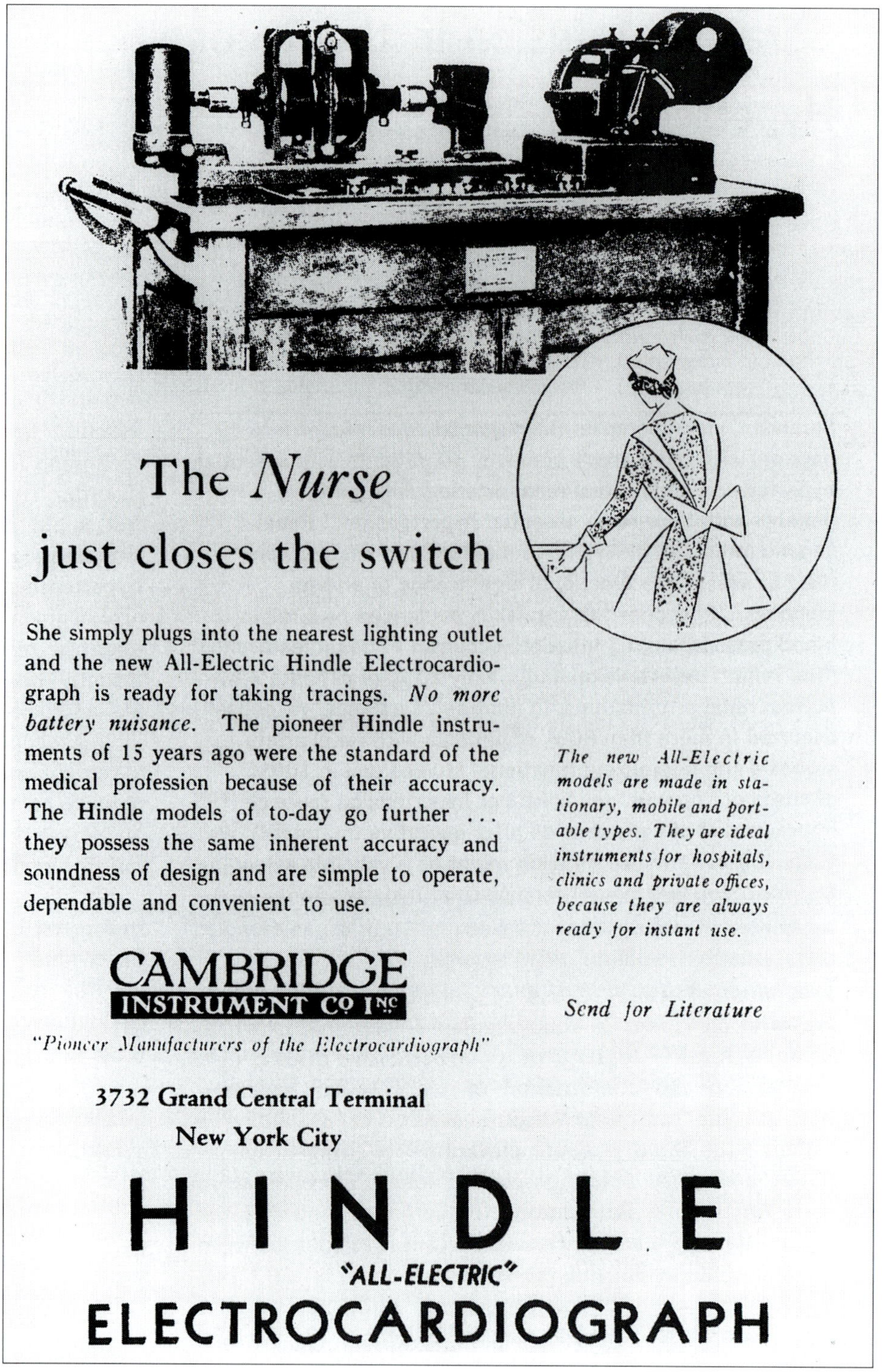

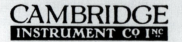

Figure 14 1932 advertisement of Hindle model by Cambridge Instrument Co. *Photo Source National Library of Medicine. Literary Source Burch, G.E. (1977). The Electrocardiograph: a 1932 advertisement. Ann. Int. Med., 87, 35. With permission*

by Cambridge as a portable 'suitcase' model and weighed about 30 lb. It was called a 'suitcase' model because the instrument, along with direct-contact strap-on electrodes, could be stored in one case and easily transported. The electrodes had already been in use since their introduction in 1926. It was a dual-beam galvanometer. A model of this instrument is in the G. E. Burch collection of the Bakken library[178]. This particular model had two light sources, a camera with the film fed by a motor and two string galvanometers. Any electrical outlet would do in America for the source of electrical current.

Immediately after World War II, direct-writing models became available. I was fortunate enough to own one of the earliest Sanborn models. It was my constant companion during my residency, and served me quite well in several of my clinical investigative projects. In fact, I used the machine without need of servicing for the first 25 years of private practice. Many companies have entered the field since then usurping the dominance of both Cambridge and Sanborn. Some of the newer units now weigh even less than 10 lb. They are highly sophisticated electronic instruments, offering acceptable accuracy, ease of operation, rapid results and consistently good performance. Electronic electrocardiographic monitors are now ubiquitous in every coronary care or intensive care unit, as well as in hospital rooms and in surgical suites. NASA developed telemetry methods as part of its space program. In 1959, they were able to record electrocardiograms from Able and Baker, the two squirrel monkeys who were on the first successful round-trip journey between Earth and outer space. If Einthoven could only see us now!

The emergence of electrocardiography as a clinical tool must, definitely, be attributed to Einthoven. Waller's initial contributions were purely physiological in nature, and many years had to elapse before he, too, began to appreciate its potentialities and benefits in the clinical setting.

Waller experimented a great deal with the placement of the leads, and described in detail those arrangements which he found most favorable. He also elaborated on the concepts of the electrical field and the vectors of the electrical forces. Most of these descriptions were derived from studies conducted while he was still using the capillary electrometer. In his paper which appeared very early in these investigations (1889) and entitled *On the electromotive changes connected with the beat of the mammalian heart, and of the human heart in particular*, he erred in his interpretation of the origin of the deflections[185]. He believed the first deflection corresponded to the negativity at the apex of the heart and that the second deflection reflected negativity at the base of the heart. His error lay in the assumption that the electrical forces moved from the apex to the base and not *vice versa*.

Waller utilized the letters A,B,C,D to designate the deflections he obtained with the capillary electrometer. Einthoven substituted instead the letters P,Q,R,S,T. This nomenclature became firmly entrenched immediately and has remained unaltered ever since. Figure 15 illustrates the tracing as obtained with the capillary electrometer and Einthoven's 'corrected curve'. The lowermost record is the photographic one obtained by Einthoven's string galvanometer. The upper and middle records appeared in his paper on the galvanometric registration of the human 'elektro-kardiogramm' published in 1903[186]. The rationale for Einthoven's nomenclature may be gathered from the opening paragraphs of this paper.

Up to the present … Simple inspection of the curve inscribed by means of this instrument results in an entirely fallacious representation of the variations of potential, which, as a matter of fact, actually existed. If one desires accurate value of the latter, the form of the registered curve must be corrected for the size of the capillary tube used, the degree of magnification, and the speed of the photosensitive plate. By this method one arrives at the construction of a new curve, the outline of which actually represents the variations of potential … In explanation of this fact, the following example will be offered.

The upper figure represents the registered curve of Mr. v. d. W. by leads from the right and left hand, while the middle figure represents the corrected curve. The differences are obvious. One immediately likens the deflections C and D in the registered curve to the corresponding deflections R and T in the constructed curve. Only the latter portrays an accurate comparison of the height of the deflections … What holds true for the electrocardiogram, also, in general, holds true for any other curve obtained by the capillary-electrometer, …

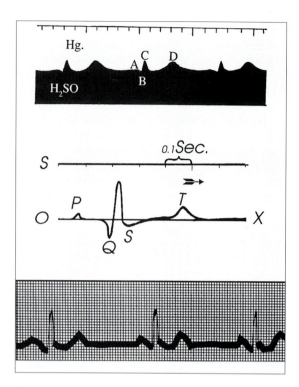

Figure 15 Demonstration of perfect agreement between the record obtained with Einthoven's modified galvanometer and the mathematically corrected curves obtained with the capillary electrometer. *Photo Source University of Central Florida. Literary Source Fleckenstein, K. (1984). The early ECG in medical practice. Medical Instrumentation. vol.18, no.3, May–June. With permission from Association for the Advancement of Medical Instrumentation, 1901 N. Ft. Meyer Drive , Ste 602, Arlington, Virginia, 22209*

The paper was written in German and therefore the German spelling 'elektrokardiogramm' became the source for the universally adopted abbreviation 'EKG'. It was not until World War II that patriotic fervor in America brought about the currently used abbreviation 'ECG'. According to Cooper, Einthoven's usage of the latter part of the alphabet in his lettering was in keeping with the convention used by geometricians at the time: all curved lines were labeled beginning with P while points on straight lines were labeled beginning with Q[187].

As a counterpoint to Einthoven's paper regarding nomenclature it is interesting to read some of the remarks by Waller in the preface to his book on *The Electrical Action of the Human Heart*[188].

The following lectures, delivered in 1913 in the Physiological Laboratory of the University of London, contain a resume of facts and principles relating to the Electrical Action of the Human Heart, which I have studied at some length upon two occasions, during the years 1888–90 by means of Lippmann's capillary electrometer, and during the years 1910–17 by means of Einthoven's string galvanometer … Between these two periods the subject has been greatly elaborated by many Continental and English observers, following in the main the indications and the phraseology of Einthoven, who in 1904 introduced an improved instrument, 'the string galvanometer', in place of the capillary electrometer, by means of which the facts had been first discovered and reviewed by me in 1888–90. Einthoven's instrument has been of great service, and has been widely adopted by clinical observers for purposes of detailed cardiac diagnosis. Its employment has been made extremely easy, and the instrument has become in many hospitals an automatic machine, turning out three kinds of records, I, II and III, each with a series of summits and depression, P, Q, R, S, T, and U, upon which the student is taught to recognize empirically the signs of Right and Left ventricular hypertrophy, and of Heart Block, and of interruption of the Right or Left branch of His's bundle. But this complicated rubric is made to serve as a meaningless trial of memory, while excluding the simple principle of 'strong' and 'weak' leads due to the obliquity of the heart's axis, and the consequent electrical inequality between the right-and left-hand (p.3) leads is altogether ignored … I do not propose to enter upon electrocardiological considerations in terms of the rubric P, Q, R, S, T and U; the terminology, however useful it may have been in Einthoven's hands in 1895 for the analysis of the electrometer record, is misleading and confusing for clinical purposes, and merely serves the evil purpose of imparting a pseudo-scientific air to voluminous publications, amid which facts of real significance are apt to be concealed … As will appear in the course of these lectures, I recognize only three waves in the normal record, viz. one auricular followed by two ventricular, the first and the second ventricular corresponding with the first and second sounds of the heart.

Einthoven's earliest report on the clinical applications of his monstrous machine appeared in his paper *Le Telecardiogramme*. Despite the technical difficulties of transmitting and recording the information, Einthoven was able to describe in his paper, both left and right ventricular hypertrophy, the mitral P wave and complete heart block. Soon after, clinicians in Europe and America began to issue their reports on the clinical use of this new device. It is refreshing to note the complete lack of enmity between Waller and Einthoven during these formative years. Each one openly and repeatedly acknowledged the contributions of the other in the evolution of electrocardiography. In 1922, when Waller published his book on *The Electrical Action of the Human Heart*, he stated in it: 'Einthoven's galvanometer is to the capillary electrometer as a high is to a low power of the microscope. It has opened a new chapter in the clinical study of heart disease, and played a part in medical literature that exhibits no sign of its physiological origin'[188].

The clinical ramifications of the electrocardiograph was also soon apparent. Fetal electrocardiographic monitoring was introduced as early as 1906[189]. In the same paper, Cremer reported his findings on recordings made from the esophagus.

Cremer recorded the fetal electrocardiogram by attaching silver electrodes to the abdominal wall and inserted in the vagina. His report generated no interest at all and no further significant investigations were done until 1936 when Strassman demonstrated the fetal electrocardiogram with standard maternal limb leads[190]. Even this paper failed to attract any clinical interest. In 1957, Southern described the possible relationship between fetal anoxia and changes in the fetal prenatal electrocardiogram[191]. At last, fetal electrocardiography appeared to have some clinical value but the changes were not sufficiently specific for its acceptance yet as a clinical tool.

The relationship between anoxia and electrolyte and lactate levels and acid-base status had become pretty well established during the first half of the 20th century. In 1971, Symonds was the first to document the relationship between electrocardiographic changes and acid-base measurements[192]. The 1970s also saw extensive use of the fetal heart rate as a means of determining fetal distress. This was primarily due to the ease with which a fetal QRS complex could be recorded. Computer analysis techniques were also developed during the same decade, but the use of these methods has been severely restricted because of electrical noise and signal distortion. The recent introduction of real time monitoring may have opened the door to a precise method of constantly evaluating the status of the fetus in relationship to hypoxia.

As noted in the section dealing with disease entities, signs of its future role in the diagnosis and management of coronary artery disease became apparent as early as 1910[193]. At that time, the association between T wave inversion and angina and arteriosclerosis was identified. It took virtually no time at all for the literature to become bombarded with numerous studies concerned with the mechanisms of the heartbeat. The electrocardiograph rapidly supplanted the polygraph in the elucidation and delineation of arrhythmias. Many early workers directed most of their energies towards investigation of cardiac rhythm and its disturbances[194]. Especially prominent among them were Lewis, Rothberger, Wenckebach and Winterberg[195–197]. All of these original workers left behind a host of colleagues and students that continue to expand the horizon in this fascinating aspect of electrocardiography. There has recently been, in fact, an intensification of interest in rhythm disturbances with the highly technological advances of invasive electrophysiologic studies.

In 1913, Einthoven, in collaboration with G. Fahr and A. De Waart, published another landmark paper on the direction and manifest size of the variations of potential in the human heart and on the influence of the position of the heart on the form of the electrocardiogram[198]. This was a theoretical analysis in which the body was considered as a solid conductor and in which the electrical currents generated by the heart could be plotted in terms of magnitude and direction. Waller, too, viewed the body as a solid conductor, well aware of the laws governing the distribution of potential differences within solid conductors. Helmholtz had formulated these laws as early as 1853[199].

Waller visualized the electrical field of the heart as a tetrahedron and obtained 5 cardinal leads from this figure. The details are to be found in his monograph on the electrical action of the human heart published in 1922[200].

Einthoven's paper of 1913 analyzed the direction of the potential difference only in the frontal plane of the body as obtained with three limb leads. The basic assumption was that the electromotive forces of the heart in the frontal plane may be represented by a single vector in the center of an equilateral triangle. Other subsidiary assumptions were implicit in this schema. For more than 30 years after Einthoven's original paper there was considerable debate on the validity of these assumptions. Despite all the controversy, Einthoven's triangle still remains in current usage as a practical basis for determining axis deviation.

Frank N. Wilson and his associates from the University of Michigan were major contributors in the clarification of the involved issues by describing more precisely the laws which govern the distribution of electromotive forces in solid conductors. Wilson's work paved the way for the introduction of the central terminal, V leads, unipolar limb leads and augmented unipolar limb leads [201–204]. This work was carried on between the years 1931 and 1946. In 1942, Emanuel Goldberger described a simple, indifferent electrocardiographic electrode of zero potential, and a technique of obtaining augmented unipolar extremity leads [205]. These are the current AVR, AVL, and AVF leads.

Wilson's concepts became important in analyzing the distribution of action currents and injury currents of cardiac muscle [206]. The practical advantages of these theoretical considerations soon became obvious and remained so despite the discovery later that Wilson's central terminal is not absolutely zero throughout the cardiac cycle.

As time went on the theoretical inadequacies of Einthoven's triangle became even more evident. In 1941, Wolferth and his associates studied the relationship of Lead I, chest leads from C3, C4 and C5 positions, and certain leads from each shoulder region [207]. They reported the bearing their observations had upon the Einthoven triangle hypothesis and upon the formation of Lead I. This rather detailed study went a long way in refueling the debate on the validity of the Einthoven triangle. Further refutation was supplied by the studies of Katz when he described the genesis of the electrocardiogram in 1947 [208], and again by Wilson and his co-workers in 1949 [209].

The non-validity of Einthoven's hypothesis was finally brought to light by a theoretical physicist, H. C. Burger, who was remotely removed from medicine and completely unaware of the controversy surrounding it [210]. His brother sent him a book in 1939 which contained a schematic representation of Einthoven's concept. Figure 16 depicts

the diagram that Burger viewed as an absurdity but which, at the same time, stimulated an interest that held him until he was able to refute Einthoven's concepts [211]. His observations on the electrical conductivity of human tissues and on the voltages obtained from a dipole contained within a glass model of the human body enabled him to do so.

In several years, Burger, now thoroughly enmeshed in the project, was to be regarded as an authority on the theoretical basis of electrocardiography. In 1946, he and his co-worker, van Milaan, introduced lead vectors to replace the geometric lead lines of Einthoven's triangle [211]. A year later, they introduced the concept of 'image surface' [212]. The simple frontal plane of Einthoven's triangle was supplanted by complicated representations of 'lead fields' and their patterns of current flow [213–215]. These concepts represented a definite advancement in the evolution of electrocardiographic theory but they too had their own inadequacies that continue to plague investigators to this day.

Other advances over the years have involved several important aspects of electrophysiologic concepts and include the spread of the wave of excitation (depolarization), the concept of intrinsic deflection, activation of the atria, ventricles and interventricular septum, intraventricular block, pre-excitation syndrome, and repolarization or recovery from excitation. The historical background of all of these items of interest has been presented in the section dealing with electrophysiology.

Another important path of investigation in the evolution of clinical electrocardiography centered about the influence of myocardial injury. There is a direct effect on both activation and recovery. The electrocardiogram has become an invaluable tool in the diagnosis and management of myocardial injury from whatever cause, but especially in coronary artery disease and myocarditis. Wilson and colleagues played a prominent role in delineating the presence of Q or QS waves as a result of transmural myocardial infarction [216]. Alterations in the pattern of activation as another effect of myocardial injury were described by First and his colleagues in 1950 [217].

In 1917, Herrick reported the first case in which the electrocardiogram played a role in the diagnosis of myocardial infarction [218]. Herrick's role in the evolution of our knowledge of coronary artery disease was of the first order of magnitude as we have seen in Section 4. Ten years after Herrick's report, the perception still prevailed, however, that the electrocardiograph was not a useful tool in the diagnosis of acute myocardial infarction. In that year (1927), a paper appeared by Scott and Harvey stating that, for 'obvious reasons', the electrocardiograph was impossible to use in detecting myocardial damage from coronary occlusion[219]. The 'obvious reasons' of Scott and Harvey was the prevailing notion of the time that an acute myocardial infarction was incompatible with life. It was not until George Dock's comments appeared that this erroneous notion was refuted and laid to rest. The early 1940s heralded the recognition of myocardial infarction as we know it today, and the importance of the electrocardiogram in its diagnosis and management became increasingly evident. For many years, it remained the central and most specific diagnostic method for the entity.

The first monograph on clinical electrocardiography was a short pamphlet of 37 pages written by Alexander Samojloff, entitled *Elektrokardiogramme* (Figure 17). It appeared in 1909, and surprisingly was not known to Western physicians even though it was written in German and issued by a reputable German publisher[220,221]. Samojloff was a Russian physiologist who, with his training in electrophysiology, became very much interested in electrocardiography after reading Einthoven's original paper of 1903. He arranged a visit to Einthoven's laboratory at Leyden and familiarized himself with Einthoven's invention. This was the start of a friendship that endured until Einthoven died in 1927. Samojloff was professor of zoology, comparative anatomy and physiology. In 1908, he bought the sixth instrument made by the Cambridge Scientific Company[159].

The first definitive textbook on clinical electrocardiography was that written by Thomas Lewis in 1913. The text was the product of an experience that spanned only four short years but it was written with the conviction that electrocardiography would become essential to the modern diagnosis and treatment of cardiac diseases[222]. The experience was gained from recordings obtained with a machine that was located under a staircase opposite the elevator motor of the hospital[223]. Apparently, Einthoven's original problems with vibration were not encountered by Lewis in this alcove.

Where Samojloff's pamphlet contained only single lead electrocardiograms limited to mitral stenosis and hypertrophy of both ventricles, Lewis' text included descriptions of many arrhythmias.

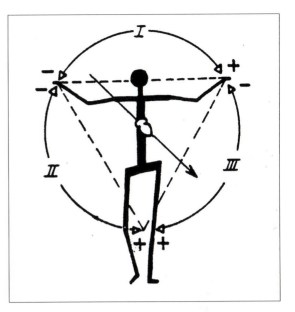

Figure 16 Diagram of Einthoven's equilateral triangle that Burger considered absurd and which stimulated his interest in electrocardiography. *Photo Source University of Central Florida. Literary Source Fishman, A.P. and Richards, D.W. (1982). Circulation of the Blood, Men and Ideas. American Physiological Society, Fig. 20, p.305. With permission*

Lewis was well acquainted with the contributions by Samojloff since his text cites nine works published by the Russian physiologist.

Lewis was only 32 when he published his text. It must have been extremely gratifying to him when he no doubt read the original review which appeared in the *British Medical Journal* of June 20, 1914[224].

The following is the short paragraph that succinctly expresses the reviewer's acclaim for this landmark work.

Dr. Thomas Lewis's book, *Clinical Electrocardiography*, is an excellent summary of the present state of knowledge of the subject. The figures are admirable, and the descriptions of the various curves and what they signify leave little to be desired. He states in his preface that the book is intended as a supplement to his little work *Clinical Disorders of the Heart Beat*, but it is really an independent treatise which can readily be followed by any one acquainted with the other book. In the very brief historical note with which

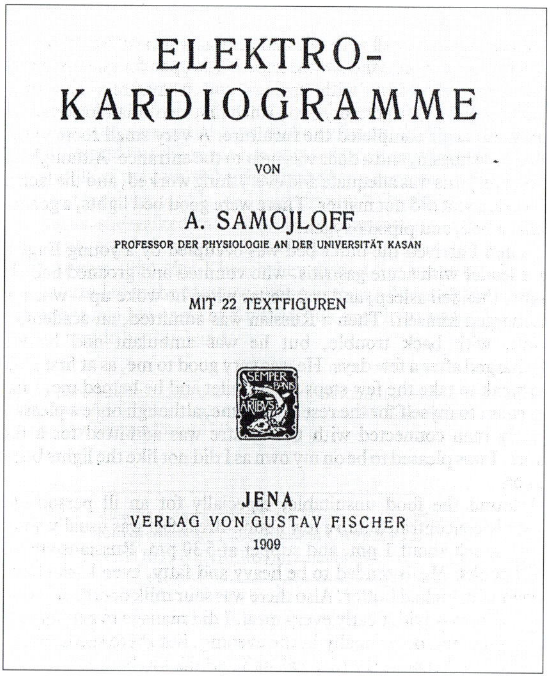

ELEKTRO-KARDIOGRAMME

VON

A. SAMOJLOFF

PROFESSOR DER PHYSIOLOGIE AN DER UNIVERSITÄT KASAN

MIT 22 TEXTFIGUREN

JENA
VERLAG VON GUSTAV FISCHER
1909

Figure 17 Title-page of Samojloff's monograph. *Photo Source National Library of Medicine. Literary Source Krikler, D.M. (1987). The search for Samojloff: a Russian physiologist in times of change. Br. Med. J., 295, 1624–7. With permission*

the first chapter opens, the demonstration in 1856 by Kölicker and Müller of the generation of electric currents in the contracting heart is alluded to, but no mention is made of Waller's work, which was certainly a landmark in the subject. The normal electrocardiogram is first described, and thereafter certain rhythmic but anomalous forms are discussed, including those variations which are thought to indicate right and left ventricular hypertrophy. There then follow descriptions of the electrical signs of heart block, premature contractions, paroxysmal tachycardia auricular flutter and auricular fibrillation. Two chapters are devoted to sinus disturbances and the less marked electrical phenomena of certain valvular lesions. A perusal of the book will convince most readers that the author is justified in his claim that 'there are certain abnormal types of heart action upon which other methods are almost, if not quite, silent; knowledge of these conditions is the almost exclusive possession of electrocardiography.

Sir Thomas Lewis was born in 1881, and led a highly productive life until he died in 1945. He was reared in Cardiff, Wales, and until the age of 16, his entire education was home brewed, almost entirely in the hands of his mother. Like so many boys, he had little interest in books, though his wealthy family boasted a library of several thousand volumes. Most of his time was spent during his early teens, observing the fruits of nature in the surrounding countryside. This indifference to study was probably the reason for his failure to pass the University of London matriculation examination. This failure must have been crucial to him, because he changed his habits, studied intensively, and passed the entrance examination to the University College at Cardiff a year later, at the age of 17. Lewis remained a serious student from then on. While still in medical school, he found the time to write several papers on the lymph glands in mammals and birds that later became standard works of reference.

Lewis pursued his clinical studies at University College Hospital in London, earning his doctorate in medicine in 1902. He was to remain at this hospital for the rest of his life. Private practice was not to his liking, and he soon gave it up in favor of an appointment as clinician and researcher at the University College Hospital.

Lewis met James Mackenzie in 1908 and established a life-long friendship with him. It was Mackenzie who inculcated in Lewis an interest in cardiac arrhythmias. Lewis initially made use of Mackenzie's polygraph but after having been exposed to Einthoven's galvanometer, he had the prescience to realize how the electrocardiograph possessed many advantages over the polygraph.

Although Lewis was engaged in many intellectual activities, he still found time to indulge in his hobby, watching and photographing birds. He founded the journal *Heart* which later was renamed *Clinical Science*, and remained as its editor for 35 years. His editorial standards were so high and rigid that he had no compunction in rejecting manuscripts submitted by many well-known investigators, including among them, James Mackenzie and Frank Wilson.

Lewis should be remembered primarily as a teacher and researcher. He was a prolific writer with a bibliography that lists 12 books and some 240 articles. Until 1924, his main research interests were the spread of electrical excitation and cardiac arrhythmias. He was especially interested in the mechanisms underlying atrial fibrillation and flutter.

Thinking that he had reached the end of the road in his studies with the electrocardiograph, he then turned to the study of skin vessels and their response to injury. The torch for the electrocardiograph was now taken up by his good friend, Frank Wilson, who, in turn, went on to make many significant contributions to the subject.

Lewis suffered a myocardial infarction in 1927, and later became a patient of one of his former students, Paul Dudley White. A fourth myocardial infarction finally took away from this world an indefatigable, precise scientist who left a legacy in electrocardiography that becomes more notable as time goes on[225–229].

In the obituary notices of the Fellows of the Royal Society, the following aphorism is attributed to him: 'Clinical science has the long-established right to wander unimpeded into any branch of medical science in search of information directly relevant to the problems of human disease'[230]. His scientific orientation is aptly described by the following comments in his book on the mechanism and graphic registration of the heartbeat[231,232].

> Inexact method of observation, as I believe, is one flaw in clinical pathology to-day. Prematurity of conclusion is another, and in part follows from the first; but in chief part an unusual craving and veneration for hypothesis, which besets the minds of most medical men, is responsible … The purity of a science is to be judged by the paucity of its recorded hypothesis … Hypothesis is the heart which no man with right purpose wears willingly upon his sleeve.

His photograph in Figure 18 reveals eyes and the facial expression of a man who brooked no nonsense when there was a task to be finished.

A host of investigators have contributed towards the development of electrocardiography, but among them, three men dominated the field during its inception and formative years. I have already presented a short biographical note about Einthoven and Lewis. The third man in this triumvirate was Frank N. Wilson. Once more the absence of national boundaries in scientific inquiry is evident. Einthoven was a native of Holland, Lewis of England, Wilson, of America.

Frank Wilson was an only child. He was born just outside Detroit, Michigan in Livonia township in 1890. His premedical and medical studies took place at the University of Michigan. Upon graduation

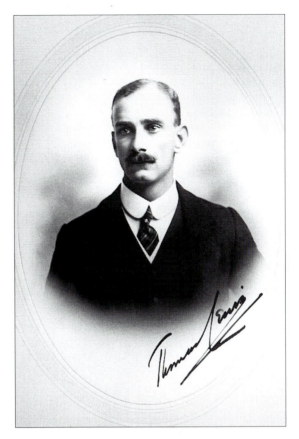

Figure 18 Sir Thomas Lewis. *Photo Source National Library of Medicine. Literary Source Photo Archives. Courtesy of National Library of Medicine*

he was appointed as an assistant in the department of medicine. A year after this appointment, the department purchased one of the early electro-cardiograph machines manufactured by the Cambridge Scientific Instrument Company. There were no more than a dozen of them in the USA at the time (1914). Wilson was put in charge of starting and supervising the electrocardiographic program at the University, and in one year he was able to present his first paper on the subject. It was published in *Heart*, the journal that was founded by Lewis only a few years before.

Wilson met Lewis while stationed at Colchester, England, as an officer in the US Army Medical Corps. Although they were there to help unravel the spectrum of a disease called at that time 'soldier's heart', both men, sharing a common interest in electrocardiography, were also able to pursue a mutually shared interest in bird photography.

A strong friendship developed between the two which lasted throughout their lives. Burchell describes both men as 'kindred souls supported by mutual characteristics, for example, times of detachment and apparent coldness to visitors, a ferocious editing of papers and on occasion an acidulous tongue'[233].

Upon discharge from the military service, Wilson spent three years with George Hermann in St Louis studying the electrocardiographic signs of hypertrophy and bundle branch block. In 1921, he returned to his alma mater in charge of the cardiology service and spent the rest of his career at that institution. Six years later he was relieved of his clinical responsibilities so that he could devote his entire time to electrocardiographic research. By this time he had assembled around him a group of associates from whose collaborative efforts significant contributions in the field were beginning to appear. These men included Barker, Macleod and Johnston.

During an enforced convalescence of two years after a cholecystectomy, Wilson utilized the time to learn the intricacies of physics and mathematics. He was now on a par with both Einthoven and Lewis in being able to wade through the theoretical aspects of electrocardiography. In 1933, he put this knowledge to good use by publishing a highly theoretical monograph on the electrical properties of the heartbeat[206]. It is this monograph that contains his introduction of the dipole theory to explain the electrical basis of the ventricular complex and the injury currents seen in myocardial injury. Wilson readily acknowledged the contributions Lewis made in the development of the analytical principles governing the interpretation of the electrocardiogram. He did this publicly at the International Conference of Physicians in 1947, and again in 1953 when he equated Lewis's theory of limited potential differences in ventricular excitation as being, 'in essence', the dipole hypothesis[234]. Lewis had already expounded on 'limited potential differences' during his American tour in 1922.

The central terminal of Wilson was conceived and developed by him in the early 1930s[235]. During this time he also corrected some of the misconceptions about left and right bundle branch block[236].

His remarkable intellectual abilities, the ease and swiftness with which he could resolve the problem at hand, caused him to earn the sobriquet 'Snake Wilson'[237]. He was also a prolific writer, having authored more that 120 scientific articles.

Wilson died suddenly in 1952, several months after undergoing segmental resection of a tuberculous lesion during which he was revived from an intraoperative episode of cardiac arrest. The last of the triumvirate was now gone but his influence as well as that of the other two will continue to be felt for many years.

The interrelationship that developed between this trio and contemporary electrocardiographic investigators throughout the world is truly amazing. A multitude of physicians were either trained or influenced by them. In the Americas alone the list is quite extensive. Among them may be mentioned such prominent luminaries in their own right as Carl Wiggers, J. B. Williams, George Burch, Demetrio Sodi-Pollares, George Fahr, Paul D. White, Samuel Levine, and Arthur Master. In general, this interrelationship was without rancor, petty jealousies or claims of priority that have so often clouded scientific endeavor through the ages. It was based on mutual respect, admiration for each other and an honest appraisal of the significant contributions made by each individual in the interest of the collective goal. An exception to this tranquility was an engineer, turned physician, who in his memoirs initiated a controversy regarding priority in the conception of the dipole theory. He was W. H. Craib[238,239].

Craib was a Rockefeller research fellow at Johns Hopkins Hospital in 1925 when he first became acquainted with the research activities of Lewis[239]. At this time, according to his memoirs, he, too, developed a theory on the genesis of the electrocardiogram. It was based on a concept of myocardial excitation through 'sequential doublets' (or dipoles), and he claimed it was several years before Wilson's paper on the subject appeared. A bitter controversy ensued as a result of Craib's allegations in his memoirs. He felt that he was not accorded his rightful due, and pointed the finger of this injustice against Wilson, Lewis and Einthoven among others. Wilson's daughter resented what she thought was Craib's slur on her father's honesty[233]. The controversy still continues with some inclined to feel that Craib's claims are invalid while others hold to the view that he should be given credit for priority in the conceptualization of the dipole theory. Three years before Craib's memoirs appeared, McMichael had written that Craib's 'doublet theory became the dipole theory in the hands of F. N. Wilson'[240].

Electrocardiographic monitoring

Monitoring of cardiac events with the electrocardiogram appears to have been ushered in during the early part of this century as an interest in what transpires during anesthesia.

The first electrocardiographic documentation of cardiac arrhythmias occurring during or immediately after ether anesthesia were the reports by Heard and Strauss in 1918[241] and Sam Levine in 1920[242]. Two years later, Levine in collaboration with Lennox and Graves demonstrated the practicality of the electrocardiogram in monitoring patients while under anesthesia[243]. Even though the instrumentation and method of obtaining tracings were markedly primitive in contrast to our current electronic devices, the value of monitoring was demonstrated not only by these workers but also by similar studies over the next two decades[244–246]. The introduction of the direct writing electrocardiograph eliminated the delay associated with processing films but did not alter the impracticality of continuous recording. Ziegler, in 1948, was the first to demonstrate the use of the direct writer during anesthesia[247]. The patients under study had cyanotic congenital heart disease. The first continuous device using a display on a cathode ray screen was introduced by Himmelstein and Scheiner in 1952[248]. It was called a cardiotachoscope. Each beat appeared as a moving line on the calibrated screen. The heart rate was determined by measuring the interval between successive beats. Permanent records could be obtained by attaching a direct writer to the cardiotachoscope.

The introduction of continuous monitoring without the need for paper or photography assured its acceptance as a valid clinical tool during anesthesia. Its use became even more firmly entrenched when subsequent studies brought to light the occurrence of dysrhythmias and myocardial ischemia during anesthesia. Cannard's paper in 1960[249], and that of Russell in 1969[250], were instrumental in alerting the anesthesiologist to the occurrence of the various types of dysrhythmias. The application of the electrocardiogram to detect myocardial ischemia during anesthesia was first proposed by Kaplan and King in 1976[251]. Studies were then conducted by several independent investigators to determine both the incidence and types of arrhythmia as well as myocardial ischemia in the perioperative period[252–254]. These have shown that the most hazardous periods are during induction of anesthesia and immediately after recovery.

The next step in electrocardiographic monitoring was the recording of electrocardiographic data in the ambulant patient. It is my opinion, probably shared by many other cardiologists, that ambulatory electrocardiography represents one of the greatest technological advancements in the history of cardiology. It now carries the eponym 'Holter Monitor' and rightfully so. It's inventor, Norman J. Holter, was trained in physics and chemistry, receiving a master's degree in both. He first became interested in biotelemetry in 1936 while working as an assistant to Lawrence Detrick studying the effect of Vitamin C on frog muscle fatigue. He later joined Joseph A. Gengerelli and in 1939 they began experiments in the stimulation of a frog nerve[255]. It was not until 1961, however, when these two workers, taking advantage of more sophisticated equipment, were able to show that a magnetic field could be detected emanating from an active nerve[256]. Prior to this, telemetry had to rely on relatively primitive equipment. Holter had already established his research foundation in 1947, to carry on his experiments on human electrophysiological phenomena. The Holter Research Foundation, as it was called, was initially subsidized by him personally. He had to wait 5 more years before funds became available from other sources, including grants from the National Institutes of Health. In 1957, Holter reported on a new technique for cardiovascular study, calling it 'radioelectrocardiography'. The device was a far cry from today's miniature models. It weighed a hefty 85 lb. Holter used it strapped to his back. It was based on previous work conducted by him in association with Gengerelli and Glasscock on remote recording of physiological data by radio and its application in medical research[257–261]. The whole system consisted of two units, a transmitter and receiver, and did not allow the subject to wander away from home base.

The next step was obviously to reduce the size and weight of the equipment to a level of portability. This was done by redesigning the device into the form of a briefcase that contained a miniature, self-powered, receiver-recorder unit. A full 24 hours of recording was obtainable through the use of this magnetic tape. Holter abandoned radioelectrocardiography as soon as adequate transistors entered the market. In his own words: 'Having done the briefcase bit, let's invent the telemetry idea. Get rid of the radiobroadcasting and put the whole shebang in one small box and wear it'.

Holter selected Del Mar Avionics to develop his invention and market it. Technological improvements have brought further refinement in fidelity, size and number of channels. There is very little inconvenience today to wearing one strapped around the waist for a 24 hour period.

Paul D. White, as prescient as ever, was the first cardiologist to foresee the impact Holter's invention would have on the practice of cardiology. Roberts and Silver quote White as saying to Holter when the latter as a young man was disheartened about his progress with the device: 'You keep working on this because it's going to result in a great lifesaving device'[262].

Vectorcardiography

A vector is a mathematical representation characterized by sense, magnitude and direction. Vectorcardiography is a form of electrocardiography that utilizes vectorial representation of successive instantaneous mean electric forces from the heart throughout a cardiac cycle. These vectors are displayed in the form of loops.

Einthoven, Fahr and de Waart were the first to utilize the concept of representing the electric forces from the heart by recording vector forces from the surface of the body. They reported their findings in a paper that appeared in 1913[263]. A few years prior to this Waller had already described the electromotive changes connected with the human heartbeat by mapping isopotential lines on the surface of the body using the capillary electrometer[185]. This introduced the concept of the mean electric potential of the heart as a single dipole. In 1916 Lewis described the spread of the excitatory process in the vertebrate heart showing it as a series of vectors constructed from the electrocardiogram. It appeared in the Philosophical Transactions of the Royal Society of London and constituted an important early contribution to vector analysis of the electric activity in the heart[264].

Mann in 1920 was the first to introduce the 'loop' as a means of displaying the series of vectors during depolarization and repolarization[265]. He utilized the body surface recordings of the electric activity as noted in the electrocardiogram, and then manually constructed the loops on the basis of the

vector analysis principles that had been established by Einthoven, Fahr and de Waart. Monocardiogram was his term for the loop[266]. This was a very tedious and time consuming process and fraught with inaccuracy. Fahr was also engaged at the same time with vector analysis of the electrocardiogram[267].

In order to overcome the inherent difficulties in the manually constructed monocardiogram, Mann developed an apparatus that was capable of directly recording the loop. He described this in 1938. However, just before Mann's paper, investigators from Germany and America introduced the cathode ray oscilloscope as an accurate and automatic method of recording the vectorcardiogram. These were Schellong and Hollmann and Hollmann from Germany, and Frank Wilson with his group in the USA[268]. The results of their research activities with the cathode ray oscilloscope, conducted independently of each other and bereft of any communication between the three groups, proved to be of the utmost importance in advancing the use of vectorcardiography. For the first time, accurate vectorcardiograms were obtainable. The cathode ray tube now became an established and reliable component of the recording apparatus. The paper by Schellong in 1936 was a landmark report on spatial vectorcardiography[269]. Wilson and his group had already introduced the central terminal for more reliable electrocardiographic recordings, and they used this terminal along with the standard limb electrodes to obtain their vectorcardiographic recordings. This was initially reported in 1937[270]. and a year later Wilson and Johnston elaborated in greater detail on this method in a paper which appeared in the American Heart Journal[271]. This paper also illustrated in a diagrammatic fashion the relationship between the vectorcardiogram and the 3-standard lead electrocardiogram.

Hollmann and Hollmann introduced the concept of the 'scroll', which Burch explains is a 'continuous recording of the vectorcardiogram in an attempt to record the time course of the cardiac rhythm and time intervals as well as the vectorcardiogram of successive and entire heartbeats[272].

In 1950, Burch and co-workers reported in the Transactions of the Association of American Physicians their method for recording stereoscopic views directly from two cathode ray tubes using a simple electrode arrangement[273]. The use of this method enabled the group to construct accurate wire models of the loops for detailed study at leisure.

Both the loop models and equipment are in the Smithsonian Institution[274].

The term vectorcardiogram was suggested by Wilson and Johnston in 1938, and it has supplemented Mann's monocardiogram. The clinical application was investigated by a number of workers including the already mentioned individuals chiefly responsible for the technical development of the recording devices. By 1938 several centers throughout the world were actively engaged in studying its clinical utility and limitations. Both manual construction methods and automatic electronic cathode ray oscilloscopic techniques were utilized.

In 1939, Schellong presented in a classic paper, the vectorcardiographic changes in various abnormalities of the heart[275]. One of the chief arguments with regard to its clinical application was the type of reference system that would best serve the recording of the vectorcardiogram and the resultant spatial form. A number of investigators attempted to resolve this problem, and the debate among them continued for almost two decades between the late 1930s and well into the 1950s.

Arrighi (1939), an Argentinian, preferred a sagittal view obtainable with his so-called triangle method[276]. Two workers from Switzerland adopted the 'double cube' (rectangular) method of electrode placement[277,278]. It gained considerable popularity which was, however, short-lived. It is no longer used today.

Important contributions concerning reference frames and standardizing factors came from H. C. Burger and van Milaan in their series of papers dealing with heart-vector and leads[279–281]. Wilson, Johnston and Kossman advocated as their reference frame the tetrahedron[282]. Burch and his group contributed by delineating the correction factors for lead placement and by helping to standardize reference frames[283]. Most centers are now using the Frank system which was introduced in 1956[284]. Burch was at a loss to explain its wide acceptance[285]. To quote him:

At present the Frank system is used in most areas of the world[43,44,45]. Introduced in 1954 (sic), it is based upon one torso plastic model and theoretical mathematic considerations. The reasons for its acceptance are not very clear. The reproducibility of electrode placement from time to time is quite variable and poor and is impossible in routine recordings. The system

is difficult to use correctly in all patients, it is time-consuming to apply, and it is especially difficult to apply the electrodes properly on fat women with large breasts and almost impossible on newborn infants.

George Burch, among his many other achievements, was highly instrumental in the clinical investigation of vectorcardiography as a diagnostic tool. Over the years he and his associate, De Pasquale, published a number of papers describing the normal patterns and those seen with such abnormalities as diffuse myocardial damage, myocardial infarction, ventricular aneurysms, and bundle branch disturbances, among others.

Despite all these careful studies by Burch and others, vectorcardiography failed to receive an enthusiastic welcome by clinical cardiologists. First of all, it had to show some aspect of cardiac electrical activity that was not already evident from the scaler electrocardiogram. The procedure itself was too time-consuming, necessitating many steps. In addition, the electronic equipment was rather elaborate. Instruments for Cardiac Research, an American company, attempted to overcome some of the impediments with its introduction of a direct-writing, high-fidelity machine. Although the method of recording vectorcardiograms was simplified somewhat, this diagnostic modality still failed to gain universal acceptance. Although of value in research and education, vector analysis failed to prove itself as a valid diagnostic clinical tool. Among its many shortcomings, in addition to the ones previously mentioned, is its inability to record heartbeats continuously. Only a random cardiac cycle can be studied at one sitting. It cannot measure time intervals and a standard and accurate reference frame for electrode placement has yet to be accepted. This last item is important for obtaining reliable, reproducible recordings.

BODY TEMPERATURE MEASUREMENTS

At first glance it seems rather incongruous to include in a history of cardiology the evolution of the thermometer. However, the ubiquitous vital signs sheet in any hospital chart with numerical values for body temperatures, respiration, pulse, and blood pressure should convince anyone that this graphic representation must be of some value in the management of all patients regardless of the underlying malady. Febrile states could be of the utmost importance in cardiac disorders. The transitory rise in temperature is a common finding in acute myocardial infarction, but more importantly, the level of body temperature is a useful diagnostic and monitoring modality in infectious and malignant states affecting the heart.

The knowledge that elevation of body temperature is an important sign of disease was well known to the physicians of antiquity. Their methods of determining this, however, were crude. Reliance was placed on the patient's statements of unusual warmth or on the sensation of unusual warmth being imparted to the physician's palpating hand. Many of us should remember how mothers often assessed their child's body temperature by applying their lips to the child's forehead.

The first device for measuring ambient temperature was the brainchild of Galileo. Bolton in his book on the evolution of the thermometer quotes a contemporary of Galileo in his description of the experiments that Galileo conducted with his invention[286].

The year was 1603, and the description is found in a letter written by a priest, Benedetto Castelli. 'Galileo took a glass vessel about the size of a hen's egg, fitted to a tube the width of a straw and about two spans long; he heated the glass bulb in his hands and turned the glass upside down so that the tube dipped in water held in another vessel; as soon as the bulb cooled down the water rose in the tube to the height of a span above the level in the vessel. This instrument he used to investigate degrees of heat and cold'.

Santorio Santorio, a physician of the early 17th century, was the first to assess body temperature with a thermometric device[287]. He built several models, all grossly inaccurate. Figure 19 depicts three such devices.

Heat was transferred to the instrument by blowing upon it or holding it in the hand or mouth. The device was calibrated with horizontal markings. The lower end was immersed in water. It relied on Boyle's law (still unformulated at the time) that gases expanded when heated. Thus, as the air in the instrument expanded when heated by blowing upon it or holding the device in the hand or mouth, it would force the water downwards.

The lack of precision and inaccuracies of these instruments precluded their general acceptance.

Atmospheric pressure was known to alter considerably the response of air to temperature changes. Ferdinand II attempted to overcome this variable factor by enclosing the fluid within a hermetically sealed glass tube. It did help resolve this particular aspect of the problems but the remaining issues centered about the best type of fluid and the standards to be used for calibrating the measuring scale. Among the various types of fluid tested, quicksilver appeared to be the most reliable and is still in use today. The freezing or boiling points of water emerged as the most convenient reference frames but they remained as a hotly contested issue with no resolution in sight until Gabriel Fahrenheit, a Dutch instrument maker, became interested in the problem. He used mercury as the fluid, and utilizing improved techniques of construction he designed a thermometer with three points on the scale that corresponded respectively with zero, 32 degrees and 96 degrees. The last was the external temperature of the human body as recorded by his instrument. These reference points added appreciably to the practical view of the thermometer in a clinical setting.

Despite the improvements, only a handful of physicians remained enthusiastic about this thermometric modality either in the laboratory or at the bedside. Boerhave's pupil, Anton de Haen, showed more interest in it than his mentor. De Haen used it as a clinical guide in the patients' response to therapy[288]. James Currie used changes in temperature as a prognosticator[289]. During the remainder of the 18th century, a debate flourished with regard to the relative clinical merits of the pulse and body temperature. Moreover, the thermometer still remained unreliable casting doubt on its value at the bedside. The palpating hand was still considered far superior.

It was not until the fourth decade of the 19th century when Gabriel Andral lectured on temperature changes that a turn-around in interest occurred[290]. This was followed by a poorly documented paper by Henri Roger[291].

Two prominent German physicians helped to establish the use of the thermometer as a valuable clinical tool. Traube and von Bärensprung proposed that it be used as a means of diagnosis, prognosis and therapy[292]. One of them (von Bärensprung) fell into the same trap that ensnared the followers of Floyer with his pulse watch. Von Bärensprung reduced the temperature readings to an absurdity by carrying out the measurements to two decimal places, and

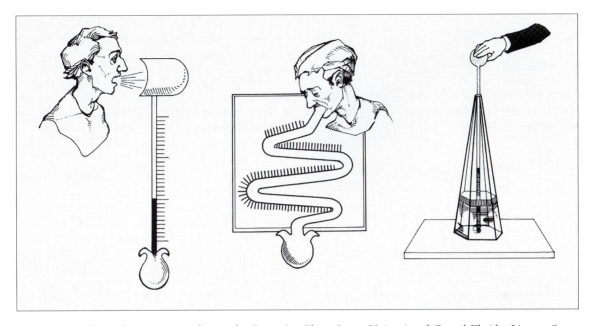

Figure 19 Three thermometric devices by Santorio. *Photo Source University of Central Florida. Literary Source Mitchell, S.W. (1891). The Transactions of the Congress of American Physicians and Surgeons, 2, 159–98. Public domain*

advising that at least 30 minutes be spent in obtaining measurements. Traube's main contribution lay in his ability to stimulate an intense interest in his colleagues in thermometry as a clinical tool. Among them was Carl Wunderlich who was destined to become the leading authority on thermometry. His first paper was published in 1857. His treatise *On the Temperature in Diseases* appeared 11 years later[293]. It was a landmark monograph which served to present for the first time detailed data documenting the utility of temperature recordings in clinical practice. It was based on a large number of objective observations. Although Wunderlich was certainly biased in stating that thermometry was the best of all diagnostic modalities available at the time, he fortunately shied away from von Barensprung's absurdities. He also stressed the point that the physician could delegate the task of actual measurement to any dependable individual, even a lay person. This was, indeed, a radical departure from the past. Taking one's temperature appears to be a banality, but, in truth, it was part of the entrepreneurial armamentarium of the attending physician and was used as a tool to cajole, reassure, or intimidate the patient. Wunderlich also brought out in his treatise two important facts regarding body temperature. The first was the observation that

a healthy body has a fairly constant temperature, and the second was that alterations of temperature occurred in disease with certain diseases manifesting their own characteristic pattern. He initiated the graphic representation of pulse, temperature, and respiration which has become the standard component of all hospital charts.

In America, Austin Flint's prestige helped stimulate an interest in the clinical usage of the thermometer though not without some resistance by some of his peers. Some of the alleged negative factors both in America and abroad were: a perception that excessive data were being accumulated that would only confuse the physician; blind reliance on the measurements and not on the patient; using reduction of temperature as the sole criterion of success with the therapeutic approach in force; and objections on the part of the patients to frequent temperature readings. Figure 20 is a lithograph by Faivre lampooning thermometry. It shows a doctor attempting to take a man's temperature with a barometer.

The persistent inaccuracies and variability in measurements among the various commercially available models continued to remain a legitimate source of dissatisfaction. This was finally resolved by subjecting all the manufactured thermometers to a certification

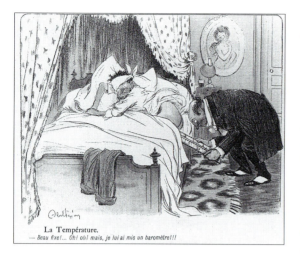

Figure 20 La Température. Doctor attempts to take a man's temperature with a barometer. *Photo Source National Library of Medicine. Literary Source L'Assiette au Beurre, no. 51, Les Medicins. Courtesy of National Library of Medicine*

process; a procedure initiated and carried out by the astronomical laboratory of Yale University[294].

SPHYGMOLOGIC METHODS

Apexcardiography

Apexcardiography is the graphic registration of precordial movements. There are certain significant limitations in the method and for that reason it has never gained wide acceptance in clinical practice. In actuality, the technique is an extension of palpation, and therefore its roots lie in the evolution of sphygmology in general.

James Hope's text (1842) contains excellent descriptions of precordial movements in the presence of aortic aneurysm as well as in a number of cardiac abnormalities[295]. We have already seen how Marey led the movement in sphygmography[5]. He was followed by Potain who was well aware of the value of simultaneous recordings involving the pulse[296]. Many of his tracings are examples of apex movements in combination with venous and arterial curves.

Over the years, many of the limitations have been addressed and solved but the popularity of the technique, despite its simplicity, continues to be overshadowed by the more sophisticated current non-invasive methods. Numerous studies have

yielded a better understanding of the characteristics of the transducer-recording system that assures reproducible and accurate results. This has been an international effort with the participants being Craige and Roberts of America, Willems of Belgium, and the Japanese group led by Mashimo. The studies conducted by Willems in dogs using catheter-tipped manometers in the left ventricle established the temporal relationship between the intraventricular pressures and the left ventricular apexcardiogram. Willems also established the relationship between the right apexcardiogram and right ventricular dynamics, recording the tracings during right heart catheterization. The origins of the left ventricular apex movements were delineated by Dellyannis and co-workers in 1964 by means of angiocardiographic studies[297]. Differentiation between normal and hyperdynamic movements required quantitative measurements. The methods for accomplishing this were provided by Craige's and Willems' groups[298–300].

In 1966, Fishleder of Mexico and later Willems, suggested the use of the term 'mechanocardiography'[301,302]. In their opinion this would have eliminated the perception that the recordings are restricted to observations of the cardiac apex only while at the same time emphasizing the preferred usage of multi-channel recordings with varying combinations of carotid and venous pulsations, precordial movements, phonocardiograms, and more recently, echocardiograms.

Systolic time intervals

Systolic time intervals, as a parameter of left ventricular function, also owes its introduction to Marey's sphygmograph. It was his instrument that provided Garrod, a contemporary, with the means to explore the significance of the duration of ventricular systole[303]. In 1874, Garrod described the inverse relationship between heart rate and the duration of left ventricular ejection. Two years after Garrod's presentation of his sphygmographic tracings before the Royal Society of London further studies were reported by Thurston[304]. Both this paper and the one that appeared by Chapman and Lond[305] in 1894 attempted to bring to light the relationship of the duration of systole to cycle length, and to apply this measurement in analyzing cardiac performance. Bowen in 1904 described the effects of exercise on the systolic ejection period utilizing sphygmographic recordings of the carotid pulse to measure the duration of ejection[306].

The classical studies of Wiggers on the consecutive phases of the cardiac cycle appeared in 1921. There were two papers in the same issue of the *American Journal of Physiology*[307,308]. The first one dealt with the duration of the consecutive phases of the cardiac cycle and the criteria for their precise determination. The laws governing the relative duration of ventricular systole and diastole were outlined in the second paper.

Katz and Feil were the first to apply modern electronic recording techniques for determining the phases of systole in the presence of left ventricular disease. Their recordings registered simultaneously, the central arterial pulse, electrocardiogram and heart sounds. Three papers were published by this team between 1923 and 1927[309-311]. The first explored the dynamics of left ventricular function in the presence of atrial fibrillation, the second in hypertensive patients, and the third was a beautifully designed study evaluating the dynamics of ventricular contraction in a heart-lung preparation.

In 1926, Lombard and Cope demonstrated the influence of posture and the subject's sex on the systolic ejection phase[312]. Blumberger's contribution appeared in 1942 and was based on extensive studies in a wide variety of cardiac disorders[313]. He demonstrated their potential clinical usefulness especially in valvular heart disease and in disorders of left ventricular contraction. In America, Arnold Weissler was a leading investigator of systolic time intervals and established himself as an authority on the subject through his numerous studies. His paper on *Systolic Time Intervals in Man* which appeared in 1968 documented that a defect in the mechanical performance of the heart was responsible for the abnormal systolic time intervals[314].

REFERENCES

1. Marey, E.J. (1885). *La Méthode Graphique dans les Sciences Expérimentales et Principalement en Physiologie et en Médecine*, (edn. 2). (Paris: Masson)
2. Stumpff, P. (1931). Archiv und Atlas der normalen und pathologischen Anatomie in typischen Roentgenbildern: Das roentgeno-graphische Bewegungsbild und seine Anwendung (Flacchenkymographie und Kymoskopie). *Fortschr. Geb. Roentgenstr.: Erganz.*, **41** (Leipzig: Thieme)
3. Henny, G.C. and Boone, B.R. (1945). Electrokymograph for recording heart motion utilizing the roentgenoscope. *Am. J. Roentgenol.*, **54**, 217
4. Prinzmetal, M. *et al.* (1949). Radiocardiography and its clinical applications. *J. Am. Med. Assoc.*, **139**, 617
5. Marey, E.J. (1878). *La Méthode Graphique dans les Sciences Expérimentales et Particuliérement en Physiologie et en Médecine*, pp. 357–66. (Paris: G. Masson)
6. Cranefield, P.F. (ed.) (1982). Foreward to Estelle Du Bois-Reymond and Paul Diepgen, *Two Great Scientists of the Nineteenth Century: Correspondence of Emil Du Bois-Reymond and Carl Ludwig*, Sabine Lichtner-Ayèd trans., p. viii. (Baltimore: The Johns Hopkins University Press)
7. Ludwig, C. (1967). *Beiträge zur Kenntniss des Einflusses der Respirations bewegungen auf den Blutlauf im Aortensysteme*, Müller's Archiv (1847), pp. 242–302; see also Heinz Schröer: Carl Ludwig: *Begründer der messenden Experimentalphysiologie*, pp. 104–14. (Stuttgart: Wissenschaftliche Verlagsgesellschaft M.B.H.)
8. Marey, E.J. (1868). *Du mouvement dan les fonctions de la vie: lecons faites au Collège de France*, pp. 130–68. (Paris: Baillière)
9. Keele, K.D. (1963). *The Evolution of Clinical Methods in Medicine*, pp. 77–8. (Springfield, Ill.: Charles C. Thomas)
10. Hays, J. (1909). *Graphic Methods in Heart Disease.* (London: Henry Frowde and Oxford Univ. Press)
11. Mackenzie, J. (1908). *Diseases of the Heart.* (London: Henry Frowde)
12. Krikler, D.M. (1988). Profiles in cardiology. Sir James Mackenzie. *Clin. Cardiol.*, **11**, 193–4
13. Seipp, C. (1986). Sir James Mackenzie and the spectre of medical technology. *Family Med.*, **18**, 163–5
14. McMichael, J. (1981). Sir James Mackenzie and atrial fibrillation. A new perspective. *J. R. Coll. Gen. Pract.*, **31**, 402
15. MacKenzie, J. (1919). *The Future of Medicine*, pp. 194–6. (London: Henry Frowde and Hodder and Stoughton)
16. McWhinney, I.R. (1977). The naturalist tradition in general practice. *J. Fam. Pract.*, **5**, 375–8
17. Mair, A. (1973). *Sir James Mackenzie, M.D. 1853–1925: General Practitioner.* (Edinburgh:

Churchill Livingstone)

18. Luisada, A. (1965). *From Auscultation to Phono-cardiography*, p. 4. (St. Louis: C.V. Mosby Co.)

19. Lewis, T. (1913). Illustrations of heart sound records. *Q. J. Med.*, **6**, 441

20. Lewis, T. (1915). *Lectures on the Heart.* (New York: Paul B. Hoeber, Inc., Medical Book Department of Harper & Row, Publishers)

21. Lewis, T. (1925). *The Mechanism and Graphic Registration of the Heart Beat.* (London: Shaw & Sons)

22. Frank, O. (1904). Die unmittelbare Registrierung der Herztoene. *München med. Wchnschr.*, **51**, 953

23. Wiggers, C.J. and Dean, A. Jr (1917). The principles and practice of registering heart sounds by direct methods. *Am. J. Med. Sci.*, **153**, 666

24. Orias, O. and Braun-Menéndez, E. (1939). *The Heart Sounds in Normal and Pathological Conditions.* (London: Oxford University Press)

25. Schuetz, E. (1958). *Physiologie des Herzens.* (Berlin: Springer-Verlag)

26. Schuetz, E., Dieter, E. and Rosa, L. (1959). Das tieffrequente Herzschallbild. Zur Frage der Vortöne und zur Messung der Anspannungszeit des Herzens. *Pflueger's Arch. Ges. Physiol.*, **268**, 229

27. Maas, H. and Weber, A. (1952). Herzschallregistrierung mittels differenzieren-der Filter: Eine Studie zur Herzschallnormung. *Cardiologia* (Basel), **21**, 773

28. Holldack, K. (1952). Die Phonokardiographie, ihre Bedeutung für die sinnesphysiologischen Grundlagen der Herzauskultation und ihre diagnostische Verwendung. Ergebn. *Inn. Med. Kinderh.*, **3**, 407

29. Holldack, K. and Bayer, O. (1953). Phonokardiographische Untersuchungen bei Mitralstenosen nach Kommissurotomie. *Ztschr. Kreislaufforsch.*, **42**, 721

30. Holldack, K. and Wolf, D. (1956). *Atlas und kurzgefasstes Lehrbuch der Phonokardiographie und verwandter Untersuchungsmethoden.* (Stuttgart: Georg Thieme Verlag)

31. Holldack, K., Heller, A. and Groth, W. (1959). The pericardial friction rub in the phonocardiogram. *Am. J. Cardiol.*, **4**, 351

32. Mannheimer, E. (1940). Calibrated phonocardiography and electrocardiography. A clinical-statistical study of normal children and children with congenital heart disease. *Acta Paediatr.*, **28** (suppl. 2), 1–287

33. Mannheimer, E. (1951). Calibrated phono-cardiography. A new technique for clinical use. *Am. Heart J.*, **21**, 151

34. Rappaport, M.B. and Sprague, H.B. (1941). Physiologic and physical laws that govern ausculation and their clinical application. The acoustic stethoscope and the electrical amplifying stethoscope and stethograph. *Am. Heart J.*, **21**, 257

35. Rappaport, M.B. and Sprague, H.B. (1942). The graphic registration of the normal heart sounds. *Am. Heart J.*, **23**, 591

36. Rappaport, M.B. and Sprague, H.B. (1951). The effects of tubing bore on stethoscope efficiency. *Am. Heart J.*, **42**, 605

37. Rappaport, M.B. and Sprague, H.B. (1952). The effects of improper fitting of stethoscope to ears on auscultatory efficiency. *Am. Heart J.*, **43**, 713

38. McKusick, V.A., Talbot, S.A. and Webb, G.N. (1954). Spectral phonocardiography; problems and prospects in the application of the Bell sound spectrograph to phonocardiography. *Bull. Johns Hopkins Hosp.*, **94**, 187

39. McKusick, V.A., Murray, G.E., Peeler, R.G. and Webb, G.N. (1955). Musical murmurs. *Bull. Johns Hopkins Hosp.*, **97**, 136

40. McKusick, V.A. (1964). Musical murmurs: spectral phonocardiographic studies. In Segal, B.L. (ed.) *The Theory and Practice of Auscultation*, p. 93. (Philadelphia: F.A. Davis Co.)

41. McKusick, V.A., Webb, G.N., Humphries, J.O. and Reid, J.A. (1955). On cardiovascular sound. Further observations by means of spectral phonocardiography. *Circulation*, **11**, 849

42. Rosa, L.M. (1940). Diagnostische Untersuchungen mit Kathodenstrahlen. *Ztschr. Ges. Exp. Med.*, **107**, 441

43. Rosa, L.M. (1948). Cardiokinetics. A study on circulatory pulsatoric oscillations, *Cardiologia* (Basel), **13**, 33

44. Rosa, L.M. (1958). *Einführung in die ballistische Kardiographie.* (Münster: Regensberg)

45. Rosa, L.M. (1959). The "displacement" vibrocardiogram of the precordium in the low frequency range. *Am. J. Cardiol.*, **4**, 191

46. Rosa, L.M. (1962). The accelerogram of the precordium. In Luisada, A.A. (ed.) *Cardiology*, vol. II, part 3, suppl. 1, p. 70H. (New York: Blakiston Division, McGraw-Hill Book Co., Inc.)

47. Dimond, E.G. and Benchimol, A. (1959). Phonocardiography in atrial septal defect: correlation between hemodynamics and phonocardiographic findings *Am. Heart J.*, **58**, 343

48. Dimond, E.G. and Benchimol, A. (1960). Phonocardiography in pulmonary stenosis: special correlation between hemodynamics and phonocardiographic findings. *Ann. Int. Med.*, **52**, 145

49. Eddleman, E.E. Jr (1962). The kinetocardiogram: ultra-low frequency precordial movements. In Luisada, A.A. (ed.) *Cardiology*, vol. II, part 3, (suppl. 1), p. 63. (New York, Blakiston Division, McGraw-Hill Book Co., Inc.)

50. Eddleman, E.E. Jr and Willis, K. (1953). The kinetocardiogram. III. The distribution of forces over the anterior chest. *Circulation*, **8**, 569

51. Eddleman, E.E. Jr, Willis, K., Reeves, T.J. and Harrison, T.R. (1953). The kinetocardiogram. I. Method of recording precordial movements. *Circulation*, **8**, 269

52. Eddleman, E.E. Jr, Willis, K., Christianson, L., Pierce, J.R. and Walker, R.P. (1953). The kinetocardiogram. II. The normal configuration and amplitude. *Circulation*, **8**, 370

53. Weiss, O. and Joachim, G. (1911). Registrierung von Hertzönen und Herzgeräuschen mittels des Phonoskips und ihre Beziehungen zum Elektrokardiogramm. *Ztschr. Klin. Med.*, **73**, 240

54. Luisada, A.A. (1953). *The Heart Beat.* (New York: Paul B. Hoeber, Inc., Medical Book Department of Harper & Row, Publishers, Inc.)

55. McKusick, V.A. (1958). *Cardiovascular Sound in Health and Disease.* (Baltimore: Williams & Wilkins Co.)

56. Ueda, H., Kaito, G. and Sakamoto, T. (1963). *Clinical Phonocardiography* (Japanese). (Tokyo: Nanzand)

57. Kaplan, M.A., Sarnoff, S.J. and Liu, C.K. (1985). Aldo A. Luisada, M.D. FACC: Physician, Scientist, Teacher. *Am. J. Cardiol.*

58. Laénnec Society remembers Aldo Augusto Luisada. (1989). Aldo Luisada and the origin of the Laénnec Society: commemorative remarks. *Can. J. Cardiol.*, **5** (3), 139–42

59. Parisanus Aemilius (1870). De cordis et sanguinis motione ad Harvaeum et contra eum. 1633 In Daremburg, C.V. *Historie des Sciences Médicales*, vol. 2, p. 614. (Paris: J.B. Baillière)

60. Hooke, R. (1705). *The Posthumous Works of Robert Hooke, containing his Cullerian Lectures and Other Discourses Read at the Meeting of the Illustrious Royal Society, etc.*, Published by Sam. Smith and Benj. Walford (Printers to the Royal Society) at the Princes Arms in St. Paul's Churchyard. (The method of improving natural philosophy), p. 39

61. McKusick, V.A. (1958). *Cardiovascular Sound in Health and Disease.* (Baltimore: Williams and Wilkins Co.)

62. Stalpert van der Wiel, C. *Observationum Rariorum Medic. Anatomic. Chirurgicarum*, Cent. l, obs. 36. Quoted by Morgagni, loc. cit., p. 394

63. Douglas, J. (1715). An extraordinary dilatation or enlargement of the left ventricle of the heart. *Trans. R. Soc. London*, p. 181 (no. 345)

64. Hunter, W. (1764). *Medical Observations and Researches*, vol. II, p. 403

65. Wiggers, C.J. (1949). *Physiology in Health and Disease*, edn. 5. (Philadelphia: Lea & Febiger)

66. Eckstein, R.W. (1937). Sounds due to muscular contraction and their importance in auscultatory qualities of the first heart sound. *Am. J. Physiol.*, **118**, 359

67. Dock, W. (1933). Mode of production of the first heart sound. *Arch. Intern. Med.*, **51**, 737

68. Kountz, W.B., Gilson, A.S. and Smith, J.R. (1940). The use of the cathode ray for recording heart sounds and vibrations. I. Studies on the normal heart. *Am. Heart J.*, **20**, 667

69. Kountz, W.B. and Wright, S.T. (1944). Comparison of total vibrations obtained from a normal, rapidly dying, human heart with those obtained in chronic myocardial disease. *Am. Heart J.*, **27**, 396

70. Dock, W. (1959). The forces needed to evoke sounds from cardiac tissues, and the attenuation of heart sounds. *Circulation*, **19**, 3766

71. Smith, H.L., Essex, H.E. and Baldes, E.J. (1950). Study of movements of heart valves and of heart sounds. *Ann. Intern. Med.*, **33**, 1357

72. Luisada, A.A., Alimurung, M.M. and Lewis, L. (1952). Mechanisms of production of the first heart sound. *Am. J. Physiol.*, **168**, 226

73. Leatham, A. (1987). Auscultation and phonocardiography: a personal view of the past 40 years. *Br. Heart J.*, **57**, 397–403

74. Luisada, A. (1975). 'Tricuspid' component of the first heart sound. In Monograph no. 46 of *Am. Heart Assoc.*

75. Crews, T., Pridie, R., Benham, R. and Leatham, A. (1972). Auscultatory and phonocardiographic findings in Ebstein's anomaly: correlation of first heart sound with ultrasonic recordings of tricuspid valve movement. *Br. Heart J.*, **34**, 681

76. Leatham, A. and Leech, G. (1975). Observations on the relationship between heart sounds and valve movements by simultaneous echo and phonocardiography. *Br. Heart J.*, (abstr.), **37**, 557

77. Waider, W. and Craige, E. (1975). First heart sound and ejection sounds: echocardiographic and phonocardiographic correlation with valvular events. *Am. J. Cardiol.*, **35**, 3

78. Leech, G., Brooks, N., Green-Wilkinson, A. and Leatham, A. (1980). Mechanism of influence of PR interval on loudness of first heart sound. *Br. Heart J.*, **43**, 138

79. Brooks, N., Leech, G. and Leatham, A. (1979). Complete right bundle branch block. Echophonocardiographic study of first heart sound and right ventricular contraction times. *Br. Heart J.*, **41**, 637

80. Rouanet, J. (1832). *Analyse des bruits du coeur*, thesis no. 252. (Paris)

81. Leatham, A. and Towers, M. (1951). Splitting of the second heart sound in health. *Br. Heart J.*, **13**, 575

82. Leatham, A. (1954). Splitting of the first and second heart sounds. *Lancet*, **2**, 607

83. Leatham, A. and Weitzman, D. (1957). Auscultatory and phonocardiographic signs of pulmonary stenosis. *Br. Heart J.*, **19**, 303

84. Leatham, A. (1958). Auscultation of the heart: Goulstonian lecture. *Lancet*, **1**, 757

85. Fortuin, N.J. and Craige, E. (1973). Echocardiographic studies of genesis of mitral diastolic murmurs. *Br. Heart J.*, **35**, 75

86. Fortuin, N.J. and Craige, E. (1972). On the mechanism of the Austin Flint murmur. *Circulation*, **45**, 558

87. Starr, A., Edwards, M.L. and Griswold, H. (1962). Mitral replacement: late results with a ball-valve prosthesis. *Prog. Cardiovasc. Dis.*, **5**, 298

88. Segal, J.P. (1964). Acoustic findings following aortic valve surgery. In Segal, B.L. (ed.) *The Theory and Practice of Auscultation*, p. 515. (Philadelphia: F.A. Davis Co.)

89. Shah, P.M., MacCanon, D.M. and Luisada, A.A. (1963). Spread of the 'mitral' sound over the chest. A study of five subjects with the Starr-Edwards valve. *Circulation*, **28**, 1102

90. Mayor, F.L. (1818). Bruits du coeur du foetus. *Bibliotheque universelle des sciences et arts*, **9**, 248

91. Sampson, J.J., McCalla, R.L. and Kerr, W.J. (1926). Phonocardiography of the human fetus. *Am. Heart J.*, **1**, 717

92. Beruti, J.A. (1927). Fernauskultation und Registrierung der fötalen Herztöne. *Arch. Gynäk.*, **132**, 52

93. Hyman, A.S. (1930). Irregularities of the fetal heart. A phonocardiographic study of the fetal heart sounds from the fifth to eight months of pregnancy. *Am. J. Obstet. Gynecol.*, **20**, 332

94. Peralta Ramos, A. (1933). Algunos progresos en el diagnóstico de la vida intrauterina (fonocardiografia, aminografia). *Prensa Med. Argent.*, **19**, 2181

95. Lian, C. and Golblin, V. (1938). Les bruits du coeur foetal in utero (étude phonocardiographique). *Arch. Mal. Coeur*, **31**, 173

96. Pereira, J.C. (1939). *Estudio fonocardiografico y hemodinamico de embarazadas y fetos en los últimos meses del embarazo normal.* (Buenos Aires: Thesis)

97. Cesa, I. and Seganti, A. (1943). Ricerche di eletrocardiografia fetale. *Cuore Circolaz.*, **27**, 184

98. Jordan, F.C. and Randolph, H. (1947). Congenital complete heart block diagnosed in utero with sound tracings and simultaneous electrocardiograph of the mother. *Am. Heart J.*, **33**, 109

99. Bolechowski, F., Kledecki, Z., Pietrzyk, B., Christman, R. and Fiwek, T. (1961). Fonokardiogramy pladowe, *Kardiol. Pol.*, **4**, 47

100. Taquini, A.C. (1936). *Exploración del corazón por via esofágica.* (Buenos Aires: El Ateneo)

101. Taquini, A.C. (1937). Los ruidos cardíacos normales por via esofágica. *Rev. Soc. Argent. Biol.*, **13**, 24

102. Miller, M. and Groedel, F.M. (1950). Esophageal phonocardiography. *Exp. Med. Surg.*, **8**, 34

103. Luisada, A.A. and Magri, G. (1952). The low frequency tracings of the precordium and epigastrium in normal subjects and cardiac patients. *Am. Heart J.*, **44**, 545

104. Bertrand, C.A., Milne, I.G. and Hornick, R. (1956). A study of heart sounds and murmurs by direct heart recordings. *Circulation*, **13**, 49

105. Zalter, R., Hardy, H.C. and Luisada, A.A. (1963). Acoustic transmission characteristics of the thorax. *J. Appl. Physiol.*, **18**, 428

106. Shah, P.M., Mori, M., MacCanon, D.M. and Luisada, A.A. (1963). Hemodynamic correlates of the various components of the first heart sound. *Circulation Res.*, **12**, 386

107. Yamakawa, K., Shinonoya, Y., Kitamura, K., Nagai, T., Yamamoto, T. and Ohta, S. (1954). Intracardiac phonocardiography. *Tohoku J. Exp. Med.*, **58**, 311, 1953; *Am. Heart J.*, **47**, 424

108. Yamakawa, K. (1960). Intracardiac phonocardiography: recent observations. *Jap. Circ. J.*, **24**, 932

109. Soulié, P. (1954). Intracardiac phonocardiography. Presented at *World Congress of Cardiology*, Washington, DC

110. Soulié, P., Joly, F., Carlotti, J., Forman, J., Azerad, N. and Osty, J. (1962). Study of the intracardiac sounds picked up in the left heart chambers by means of a micromanometer. *Fourth World Congress of Cardiology,* Mexico, p. 332 (Abst.)

111. Luisada, A.A. and Liu, C.K. (1957). Simple methods for recording intracardiac electrocardiograms and phonocardiograms during left or right heart catheterization. *Am. Heart J.,* **54**, 531

112. Lewis, D.H., Deitz, G.W., Wallace, J.D. and Brown, J.R. Jr (1958). Present status of intracardiac phonocardiography. *Circulation,* **18**, 991

113. Luisada, A.A. and Liu, C.K. (1958). Intracardiac phonocardiography in mitral and aortic valve lesions. *Circulation,* **18**, 989

114. Luisada, A.A. and Liu, C.K. (1958). *Intracardiac Phenomena in Right and Left Heart Catheterization.* (New York: Grune & Stratton, Inc.)

115. Luisada, A.A., MacCanon, D.M. and Slodki, S.J. Intracardiac phonocardiography. Description of a new simplified system, in press

116. Feruglio, G.A. (1959). Intracardiac phonocardiography: a valuable diagnostic technique in congenital and acquired heart disease. *Am. Heart J.,* **58**, 827

117. Feruglio, G.A. (1960). Utilité del fonocardiogramma intracardiaco nella diagnosi differenziale delle sindromi che si accompagnano ad un soffio continuo. *Boll. Soc. Ital. Cardiol.,* **5**, 541

118. Feruglio, G.A. (1962). Aortic diastolic musical murmurs: a conventional and intracardiac phonocardiographic study. *Malattie Cardiovas.,* **3**, 181

119. Feruglio, G.A. (1962). An intracardiac sound generator for the study of the transmission of heart murmurs in man. *Am. Heart J.,* **63**, 231

120. Feruglio, G.A. (1963). A new method for producing, calibrating, and recording intracardiac sounds in man. *Am. Heart J.,* **65**, 377

121. Feruglio, G.A. (1964). *Intracardiac Auscultation and Phonocardiography.* (Torino: Edizioni Minerva Medica)

122. Feruglio, G.A. and Gunton, R.W. (1960). Intracardiac phonocardiography in ventricular septal defect. *Circulation,* **21**, 49

123. Feruglio, G.A., Dalla Volta, S., Lewis, D.H. and Wallace, J.D. (1959). La phonocardiographic intra-cardiaque chez l'homme. *Arch. Mal. Coeur,* **52**, 1156

124. Moscovitz, H.L. and Wilder, R.J. (1956). Pressure events of the cardiac cycle in the dog. Normal right and left heart. *Circ. Res.,* **4**, 574

125. Moscovitz, H.L., Donoso, E., Gelb, I.J. and Welkowitz, W. (1957). Intracardiac phonocardiography: correlative study of mechanical, acoustic and electric events in experimental valve lesions. *Circulation,* **16**, 918 (Abstr.)

126. Moscovitz, H.L., Donoso, E., Gelb, I.J. and Welkowitz, W. (1958). Intracardiac phonocardiography. Correlation of mechanical, acoustic and electric events of the cardiac cycle. *Circulation,* **18**, 983

127. Moscovitz, H.L., Donoso, E., Gelb, I.J. and Henry, E. (1959). Fourth heart sound; studies with intracardiac phonocardiography. *Circulation,* **20**, 742 (Abstr.)

128. Moscovitz, H.L., Donoso, E., Gelb, I.J. and Wilder, R.J. (1963). *An Atlas of Hemodynamics of the Cardiovascular System.* (New York: Grune & Stratton, Inc)

129. Yarza Iriarte, J.M., Iriarte Ezcurdra, M., Rodriguez de Azua, C., Calderón Sanz, A. and Laso Nuñez, J.L. (1961). Valor diagnóstico de la fonocardiografia intracardiaca. *Rev. Española Cardiol.,* **14**, 194

130. Luisada, A.A. (1962). *The Heart Beat. Graphic Methods in the Study of the Cardiac Patient,* p. 142. (Paul B Hoeber, Inc. Medical Book Dept. of Harper and Brothers)

131. Starr, I., Rawson, A.J., Schroeder, H.A. and Joseph, N.R. (1939). Studies on the estimation of cardiac output in man and of abnormalities in cardiac function from the heart's recoil and the blood's impact. The ballistocardiogram. *Am. J. Physiol.,* **127**, 1

132. Gordon, J.W. (1877). On certain molar movements of the human body produced by the circulation of the blood. *J. Anat. Physiol.,* **11**, 533

133. Landois, L. (1880). *Lehrbuch der Physiologie des Menschen, Vienna* (quoted by Lamport, H. (1941). *Science,* **93**, 305)

134. Henderson, Y. (1905). The mass-movements of the circulation as shown by a recoil curve. *Am. J. Physiol.,* **14**, 287

135. Douglas, C.G., Haldane, J.S., Henderson, Y. and Schneider, E.C. (1913). VI. Physiological observations made on Pike's Peak, Colorado, with special reference to adaptation to low barometric pressures, *Trans. R. Soc. (London),* Series B, **203**, 185

136. Heald, C.B. and Tucker, W.S. (1922). The recoil curves as shown by the hot wire microphone. *Proc. R. Soc. (London),* Series B, **93**, 281

137. Angenheister, G. and Lau, E. (1928). Seismographische Aufnahmen der Herztatigkeit. *Naturwissenschaften,* **16**, 513

138. Abramson, E. (1933). Die Rückstosskurve des Herzens (Kardiodynamogramm) *Skand. Arch. Physiol.*, **66**, 191

139. Starr, I., Rawson, A.J., Schroeder, H.A. and Joseph, N.R. (1939). Studies on the estimation of cardiac output in man, and of abnormalities in cardiac function, from the heart's recoil and the blood's impacts; the ballistocardiogram. *Am. J. Physiol.*, **127**, 1

140. Starr, I. (1946–7). *The Ballistocardiograph: an Instrument for Clinical Research and for Routine Clinical Diagnosis*, Harvey Lect., Series 42, p. 194. (Lancaster, Pa.: The Science Press)

141. Brown, H.R., de Halla, V., Epstein, M.A. and Hoffman, M.J. (1952). *Clinical Ballistocardiography*, p. 16. (New York: The Macmillan Co.)

142. Stead, E.A. (1979). An appreciation of Isaac Starr. *N. Engl. J. Med.*, **300**, 930–1

143. Dock, W., Mandelbaum, H., Mandlebaum, R.A. (1953). *Ballistocardiography*. (St. Louis: C.V. Mosby Co.)

144. Weisse, A.B. (1987). Conversations in medicine. Wilbam Dock, M.D. *Hospital Practice*, Aug.15

145. Dock, W. (1933). Mode of production of the first heart sound. *Arch. Intern. Med.*, **51**, 737–46

146. Dock, W. (1952). Hypercholesteremia: its clinical significance and management. *Med. Clin. N. Am.*, **36**, 865–74

147. French, A.J. and Dock, W. (1944). Fatal coronary arteriosclerosis in young soldiers. *J. Am. Med. Assoc.*, **124**, 1233–7

148. Dock, W. (1941). The capacity of the coronary bed in cardiac hypertrophy. *J. Exp. Med.*, **74**, 177–86

149. Railsbach, D.C. and Dock, W. (1929). Erosion of the ribs due to stenosis of the isthmus (coarctation) of the aorta. *Radiology*, **12**, 58–61

150. Dock, W. (1944). The evil sequelae of complete bed rest. *J. Am. Med. Assoc.*, **125**, 1983–5

151. Dock, W. (1945). Presbycardia, or aging of the myocardium. *NY State J. Med.*, **45**, 983–6

152. Harrison, R.T., Dock, W. and Holman, E. (1924). Experimental studies in arterio-venous fistulae: cardiac output. *Heart*, **11**, 337–41

153. Zoneraich, S. (1986). William Dock as I knew him. *Am. J. Cardiol.*, **57**, 467–70

154. Blondel, A.E. (1893). Oscillographes; nouveaux appareils pour l'etude des oscillations electriques lentes. *C.r. hebd. Séanc Acad. Sci. Paris*, **116**, 502–6

155. Barron, S.L. (1950). *The Development of the Duddell Oscillograph*, p. 4. (London: Cambridge Instrum. Co.)

156. Ader, C. (1897). Sur un nouvel appareil enregisteur pour cables sous-marins. *C.r. hebd Séanc Acad. Sci. Paris*, **124**, 1440–2

157. Zahm, A.F. (1945). *Early Powerplane Fathers*. (Indiana: Univ. Press, Notre Dame)

158. Bradburg, S. (1967). *The Evolution of the Microscope*, pp. 153–6. (Oxford: Pergamon Press)

159. Burnett, J. (1985). The origins of the electrocardiogram as a clinical instrument. *Med. Hist., Suppl.*, **5**, p. 60

160. Burch, G.E. and De Pasquale, N.P. (1964). *A History of Electrocardiography*. (Chicago: Year Book Medical Publishers Inc.)

161. Köllicker, A. and Muller, H. (1856). Nachiveis der negativen Schwankung des Muskelstromes am naturlich sich contrahirenden. *Muskel. Verh. Phys. Med. Ges.*, **6**, 528–33

162. Waller, A.D. (1887). A demonstration on man of electromotive changes accompanying the heart beat. *J. Physiol.*, **8**, 229

163. Lippman, G. (1873). Beziehungen zwischen den capillaren und elektrischen Erscheinungen. *Ann. Phys. Chem.*, **149**, 546–51

164. Besterman, E. (1979). Waller – pioneer of electrocardiography. *Br. Heart J.*, **42**, 61–4

165. Besterman, E. (1982). Waller before Einthoven in the clinical development of noninvasive ECG. *Am. Heart J.*, **103**, 572

166. Waller, A.D. (1950). Discovery of the electrocardiogram (Lett.). *Br. Med. J.*, **1**, 1008

167. Cope, Z. (1973). Augustus Desire Waller (1856–1922). *Med. Hist.*, **17**, 380

168. Waller, A.D. (1917). A preliminary survey of 2000 electrocardiograms. *J. Physiol.*, **51**, 18 (*Proc. Physiol. Soc.*, July 28)

169. Barker, L.F. (1910). Electrocardiography and phonocardiography: a collective review. *Bull. Johns Hopkins Hosp.*, **21**, 358–9

170. Waller, A.D. (1891). *An Introduction to Human Physiology*. (London: Longmans, Green & Co.)

171. Einthoven, W. (1895). Ueber den Einfluss des Leitungswiderstandes auf die Geschwindigkeit der Quecksilberbewegung in Lippmann's Capillarelectrometer. *Pflugers Arch.*, **60**, 91–100

172. Ershler, I. (1988). Willem Einthoven – the man. The string galvanometer electrocardiograph. *Arch. Intern. Med.*, **148**, 453–5

173. Fahr, G.E. (1962). Einthoven: Ik Wilde Weten. *George E. Fahr Festschrift*, pp. 15–25. (Minneapolis: Lancet Publications)

174. Bosscha, J. (1854). *De galvanometro differential*. (Lyons: Batavia Academy)

175. Einthoven, W. (1901). Un nouveau

galvanométre. *Arch. Néerland. Sci. exactes naturelles, Serie 2*, **6**, 625–33

176. Einthoven, W. (1904). Enregisteur galvanométrique de l'électrócardiogramme humain et controle des resulats obtenus par l'emploi de l'électrométre capillaire en physiologie. *Arch. Néerland. Sci. exactes naturelles, Serie 2*, **9**, 202–9

177. Einthoven, W. (1903). Ein neues Galvanometer. *Ann. Phys. S4*, **12**, 1059–71

178. Fleckenstein, K. (1984). The early ECG in medical practice. *Med. Instrum.*, **18**, (3)

179. Einthoven, W. (1906). Le telecardiogramme. *Arch. Int. Physiol.*, **4**, 132–64

180. George, E. (1962). *Fahr Festschrift*. (Minneapolis: Lancet Publications)

181. Willius, F.A. and Keys, T.E. (1941). *Cardiac Classics*, pp. 719–21. (St. Louis: C.V. Mosby Co.)

182. Hill, A.V. (1927). An obituary of Einthoven. *Nature (London)*, **120**, 591

183. Burnett, J. (1985). *Op. cit.*, p. 67

184. Burch, G.E. (1977). The Electrocardiograph: a 1932 advertisement. *Ann. Int. Med.*, **87**, 35

185. Waller, A.D. (1889). On the electromotive changes connected with the beat of the mammalian heart, and of the human heart in particular. *Phil. Trans. B.*, **180**, 169

186. Einthoven, W. (1903). Die galvanometrische Registrirung des menschlichen Elecktrokardiogramms, zugleich eine Beurtheilung der Anivendung des Capillar-Elecktrometers in der Physiologie. *Pflügers Arch. Ges. Physiol.*, **99**, 472

187. Cooper, J.K. (1986). Occasional notes. Electrocardiography 100 years ago. Origins, pioneers and contributors. *N. Engl. J. Med.*, **315**, 461–3

188. Waller, A.D. (1922). *The Electrical Action of the Human Heart*. (London: Univ. of London Press)

189. Cremer, M. (1906). Über die direkte Ableitung der Aktionsstiome des menschlicken Herzens vom Oesophagus und über das Elektrokardiogramm des Fötus. *München Med. Wochenschr.*, **53**, 811–13

190. Strassman, E.O. (1936). The fetal electrocardiogram in late pregnancy. *Proc. Staff Meet. Mayo Clinic*, **II**, 778

191. Southern, E.M. (1957). Fetal anoxia and its possible relation to changes in the prenatal fetal electrocardiogram. *Am. J. Obstet. Gynecol.*, **73**, 233

192. Symonds, E.M. (1971). Configuration of the fetal eletrocardiogram in relation to fetal acid-base balance and plasma electrolytes. *J. Obstet. Gynaecol. Br. Commonw.*, **78**, 957

193. James, W.B. and Williams, H.B. (1910). The electrocardiogram in clinical medicine. I. The string galvanometer and the electrocardiogram in health. *Am. J. Med. Sci.*, **140**, 408–21

194. Peck, A., Langendorf, R. and Katz, L.N. (1957). Advances in the electrocardiographic diagnosis of cardiac arrhythmias. *Med. Clin. N. Am.*, p. 269

195. Lewis, T. (1925). *The Mechanism and Graphic Registration of the Heart Beat*, 3rd edn. (London: Shaw)

196. Rothberger, C.J. (1926). Allgemeine Physiologie des Herzens. In *Handbuch der normalen und pathologischen Physiologie*, **7**, 523. (Berlin: Springer)

197. Wenckebach, K.F. and Winterberg, H. (1927). *Die unregalmässige Herztätigkeit*. (Leipzig: Engelmann)

198. Einthoven, W., Fahr, G. and De Waart, A. (1913). Über die Richtung und die manifeste Grösse der Potentialschwankungen im menschlichen Herzen und über den Einfluss der Herzlage auf di Form des Elektrokardiogramms. *Pflügers Arch. Ges. Physiol.*, **150**, 275

199. Helmholtz, H. (1853). Über einige Gesetze der Verteilung elektrischer Ströme in körperlichen Leitern, mit Anivendung auf die tierschelektrischen Versuche. *Poggendorff's Ann.*

200. Waller, A.D. (1922). *Op. cit.*

201. Wilson, F.N., Macleod, A.G. and Barker, P.S. (1931). The potential variations produced by the heart at the apices of Einthoven's triangle. *Am. Heart. J.*, **7**, 207

202. Wilson, F.N., Macleod, A.G. and Barker, P.S. (1931). The interpretation of the initial deflection of the ventricular complex of the electrocardiogram. *Am. Heart J.*, **6**, 637

203. Wilson, F.N., Johnston, F.D. and Hill, I.G.W. (1934). The interpretation of the galvanometric curves obtained when one electrode is distant from the heart and the other near or in contact with the ventricular surface. Part II. Observations on the mammalian heart. *Am. Heart J.*, **10**, 176

204. Wilson, F.N., Johnston, F.D., Rosenbaum, F.F. and Barker, P.S. (1946). On Einthoven's triangle. The theory of unipolar electrocardiographic leads, and the interpretation of the precordial electrocardiogram. *Am. Heart J.*, **32**, 277

205. Goldberger, E. (1942). A simple, indifferent, electrocardiographic electrode of zero potential and a technique of obtaining augmented, unipolar, extremity leads. *Am. Heart J.*, **23**, 483

206. Wilson, F.N., Macleod, A.G. and Barker, P.S. (1933). The distribution of the currents of action and of injury displayed by heart muscle and other excitable tissues. *Scientific Series*, vol. **18**, 58. (Ann Harbor, Mi.: Univ. of Michigan Press)

207. Wolferth, C.C., Livezey, M.M. and Wood, F.C. (1941). The relationship of Lead I, chest leads from C3, C4 and C5 positions, and certain leads made from each shoulder region. The bearing of these observations upon the Einthoven equilateral triangle hypothesis and upon the formation of Lead I. *Am. Heart J.*, **21**, 215

208. Katz, L.N. (1947). The genesis of the electrocardiogram. *Physiol. Rev.*, **27**, 398

209. Wilson, F.N., Bryant, J.M. and Johnston, F.D. (1949). On the possibility of constructing an Einthoven triangle for a given subject. *Am. Heart J.*, **37**, 493

210. Katz, L.N. and Hellerstein, H.K. (1982). Electrocardiography. In: Fishman, A.P. and Richards, D.W. (eds.) *Circulation of the Blood. Men and Ideas*, p. 303. (Betheseda, Md: Am. Physiol. Soc.)

211. Burger, H.C. and van Milaan, J.B. (1946). Heart-vector and leads. *Br. Heart J.*, **8**, 157

212. Burger, H.C. and van Milaan, J.B. (1947). Heart-vector and leads. Part II. *Br. Heart J.*, **9**, 154

213. Brody, D.A. (1954). The meaning of lead vectors and the Burger triangle. *Am. Heart J.*, **48**, 730

214. Frank, E. (1954). The image surface of a homogeneous torso. *Am. Heart J.*, **47**, 757

215. McFee, R., Stow, R.M. and Johnston, F.D. (1952). Graphic representation of electrocardiographic leads by means of fluid mappers. *Circulation*, **6**, 21

216. Wilson, F.N., Macleod, A.G., Barker, P.S., Johnston, F.D. and Klostermeyer, L.L. (1954). The Electrocardiogram in myocardial infarction with particular reference to the initial deflections of the ventricular complex. In Johnston, F.D. and Lepeschkin, E. (eds.) *Selected Papers, F.N. Wilson.* (Ann Arbor: Edwards)

217. First, S.R., Bayley, R.H. and Bedford, D.R. (1950). Peri-infarction block; electrocardiographic abnormality occasionally resembling bundle branch block and local ventricular block of other types. *Circulation*, **2**, 31

218. Herrick, J.B. (1944). An intimate account of my early experience with coronary thrombosis. *Am. Heart J.*, **27**, 1–18

219. Scott, J.W. and Harvey, J. (1927). Myocardial damage in coronary occlusion. *South. Med. J.*, **20**, 510–15

220. Samojloff, A. (1909). *Elektrokardiogramme.* (Jena: Verlag von Gustav Fischer)

221. Krikler, D.M. (1987). The search for Samojloff: a Russian physiologist in times of change. *Br. Med. J.*, **295**, 1624–7

222. Lewis (1913). *Clinical Electrocardiography*, p. 11. (New York: Shaw and Sons)

223. Shapiro, E. The first textbook of electrocardiography. Thomas Lewis: *Clinical Electrocardiography*

224. Anonymous (1914). Book Review. *Br. Med. J.*, **1**, 1357

225. Hollman, A. (1973). Lewis, Thomas. In *Dictionary of Scientific Biography*, vol. 8, pp. 294–6. (New York: Charles Scribner's Sons)

226. White, P.D. (1945). In memoriam: Thomas Lewis 1881–1945. *Am. Heart J.*, **29**, 419–20

227. GWP (1948). In memoriam: Thomas Lewis. *Clin. Sci.*, **6**, 2–11

228. Obituary (1945). Sir Thomas Lewis. *Br. Med. J.*, **1**, 461–3

229. Drury, A.N., Grant, R.T. and Parkinson, J. (1946). Thomas Lewis. *Br. Heart J.*, **8**, 1–5

230. Drury, A.N. and Grant, R.T. (1948). Thomas Lewis: 1881–1945. In *Obituary Notices of Fellows of the Royal Society: 1945–1948*, vol. 5, pp. 178–202. (London: Morrison & Gibb)

231. Lewis, T. (1920). *The Mechanism and Graphic Registration of the Heart Beat*, second edition, p. vii. (London: Shaw & Sons)

232. Callahan, J.A., Key, J.D. and Keys, T.E. (1981). Sir Thomas Lewis. The centennial of a medical human dynamo. *Mayo Clin. Proc.*, **56**, 749–52

233. Burchell, H. (1981). Sir. Thomas Lewis: his impact on American cardiology. *Br. Heart J.*, **46**, 1–4

234. Wilson, F.N. (1953). Foreward to McFee, R. and Johnston, F.D. Electrocardiographic leads. *Circulation*, **8**, 554–68

235. Wilson, F.N., Johnston, F.D., Macleod, A.G. and Barker, P.S. (1934). Electrocardiograms that represent the potential variations of a single electrode. *Am. Heart J.*, **9**, 447

236. Wilson, F.N., Macleod, A.G. and Barker, P.S. (1932). The order of ventricular excitation in bundle branch block. *Am. Heart J.*, **7**, 305

237. Kahn, J.K. and Howell, J.D. (1987). Profiles in cardiology. Frank Norman Wilson. *Clin. Cardiol.*, **10**, 616–18

238. Pruitt, R.D. (1976). Doublets, dipoles and the negativity hypothesis: an historical note on

W.H. Craib and his relationship with F.N. Wilson and Thomas Lewis. *Johns Hopkins Med. J.*, **138**, 279–88

239. Craib, W.H. (1979). For the amusement of cardiologists. *Perspect. Biol. Med.*, **22**, 205–31

240. McMichael, J.A. (1976). *A Transition in Cardiology: the MacKenzie-Lewis Era.* (London: R. Coll. Physicians, London)

241. Heard, J.D. and Strauss, A.E. (1918). A report on the electrocardiographic study of two cases of nodal rhythm exhibiting R-P intervals. *Am. J. Med. Soc.*, **75**, 238–51

242. Levine, S.A. (1920). Acute cardiac upsets occurring during or following surgical operations. *J. Am. Med. Assoc.*, **75**, 795–9

243. Lennox, W.G., Graves, R.C. and Levine, S.A. (1922). An electrocardiographic study of fifty patients during operation. *Arch. Intern. Med.*, **30**, 57–72

244. Maher, C.L., Crittenden, P.J. and Shapiro, P.T. (1934). Electrocardiographic study of viscerocardiac reflexes during major operations. *Am. Heart J.*, **9**, 664–76

245. Kurtz, C.M., Bennet, J.H. and Shapiro, H.H. (1936). Electrocardiographic studies during surgical anesthesia. *J. Am. Med. Assoc.*, **106**, 434–41

246. Feil, H. and Rossman, P.L. (1939). Electrocardiographic observations in cardiac surgery. *Ann. Intern. Med.*, **13**, 402–14

247. Ziegler, R.F. (1948). Cardiac mechanism during anesthesia and operation in patients with congenital heart disease and cyanosis. *Bull. Johns Hopkins Hosp.*, **83**, 237–71

248. Himmelstein, A. and Scheiner, M. (1952). The cardiotachoscope. *Anesthesiology*, **13**, 62–4

249. Cannard, T.H., Dripps, R.D., Helwig, J. Jr and Zinsser, H.F. (1960). The electrocardiogram during anesthesia and surgery. *Anesthesiology*, **21**, 194–202

250. Russell, P.H. and Coakley, C.S. (1969). Electrocardiographic observation in the operating room. *Anesth. Analg.*, **48**, 474–88

251. Kaplan, J.A. and King, S.B. (1976). The precordial electrocardiographic lead V5 in patients who have coronary artery disease. *Anesthesiology*, **45**, 570–4

252. Kaplan, J.A. (1979). Electrocardiographic monitoring. In *Cardiac Anesthesia*, pp.149–51. (New York: Grune and Stratton)

253. Coriat, P., Harari, A., Doloz, M. and Viars, P. (1982). Clinical prediction of intraoperative myocardial ischemia in patients with coronary artery disease undergoing non-cardiac surgery. *Acta. Anaesth. Scand.*, **26**, 287–90

254. Roy, L.W., Edelist, G. and Gilbert, B. (1982). Myocardial ischemia during non-cardiac surgical procedures in patients with coronary artery disease. *Anesthesiology*, **51**, 393–7

255. Gengerelli, J.A. and Holter, N.J. (1941). Experiments on stimulation of nerves by alternating electrical fields. *Proc. Soc. Exp. Biol. Med.*, **46**, 532–4

256. Gengerelli, J.A., Holter, N.J. and Glasscock, W.R. (1961). Magnetic fields accompanying transmission of nerve impulses in the frog's sciatic nerve. *J. Psychology*, **52**, 317–26

257. Holter, N.J. and Gengerelli, J.A. (1949). Remote recording of physiological data by radio. *Rocky Mountain Med. J.*, **46**, 747–51

258. Glasscock, W.R. and Holter, N.J. (1952). Radioelectroencephalograph for medical research. *Electronics*, **25**, 126–35

259. Holter, N.J. (1957). Radioelectrocardiography: a new technique for cardiovascular studies. *Ann. NY Acad. Sci.*, **65**, 913–23

260. Holter, N.J. (1961). New method for heart studies. *Science*, **134**, 1214–20

261. Macinnis, H.F. (1954). The clinical application of radioelectrocardiography. *Can. Med. Assoc. J.*, **70**, 574–6

262. Roberts, W.C. and Silver, M.A. (1983). Norman Jefferis Holter and ambulatory ECG monitoring. *Am. J. Cardiol.*, **52**, 903–6

263. Einthoven, W., Fahr, G. and de Waart, A. (1913). Über die Richtung und die manifest Grösse der Potentialschwankungen im menschlichen Herzen und über den Einfluss der Herzlage auf di Form des Elektrokardiogramms. *Pflügers. Arch. Ges Physiol.*, **150**, 275–315

264. Lewis, T. (1916). The spread of the excitatory process in the vertebrate heart. *Phil. Trans. R. Soc. Lond.*, **207**, 221–310

265. Mann, H. (1920). A method of analyzing the electrocardiogram. *Arch. Intern. Med.*, **25**, 283–94

266. Mann, H. (1938). The monocardiograph. *Am. Heart J.*, **15**, 681–99

267. Fahr, G. (1920). An analysis of the spread of the excitation wave in the human ventricle. *Arch. Intern. Med.*, **25**, 146–73

268. Burch, G.E. (1985). The history of vectorcardiography. *Medical History*, suppl. no. 5, pp. 113–4

269. Schellong, F. (1936). Elektrographische Diagnostik der Herzmuskeler-krenkungen, Verhandl. *Dt. Gesell. Inn. Med.*, **48**, 288–310

270. Wilson, F.N., Johnston, F.D. and Barker, P.S. (1937). The use of the cathode-ray oscillograph in the study of the monocardiogram. *J. Clin. Invest.*, **16**, 664–5

271. Wilson, F.N. and Johnston, F.D. (1938). The vectorcardiogram. *Am. Heart J.*, **16**, 14–28

272. Burch, G.E. (1985). *Op. cit.*, p. 118

273. Burch, G.E., Cronvich, J.A., Abildskov, J.A. and Jackson, C.E. (1950). A derivation for stereoscopic vectorcardiograms and analysis of vectorcardiograms by high-speed motion pictures. *Trans. Assoc. Am. Physicians*, **63**, 268–71

274. Burch, G.E. (1985). *Op. cit.*, p. 119

275. Schellong, F. (1939). Grundzüge einer klinischen Vektordiagraphie des Herzens. *Ergebn. Inn. Med. Kinderheilk.*, **56**, j1657–743

276. Arrighi, F.P. (1939). El eje eléctrico del corazón en el espacio con el estudio, y empleo de las derivaciones sagitales. Eje eléctrico y electrocardiogramma en el plano sagital. *La Prensa Argent*, **26**, 253–82

277. Sulzer, R. and Duchosal, P.W. (1942). Principes de cardiovectographie. I. La planographie. *Cardiologia*, **6**, 236–50

278. Sulzer, R. and Duchosal, P.W. (1945). Principes de cardiovectographie. II. La stéréographie. *ibid.*, **9**, 106–20

279. Burger, H.C. and van Milaan, J.B. (1946). Heart-vector and leads. *Br. Heart J.*, **26**, 769–831

280. Burger, H.C. and van Milaan, J.B. (1947). Heart-vector and leads. Part II. *ibid.*, **9**, 154–60

281. Burger, H.C. and van Milaan, J.B. (1948). Heart-vector and leads. Part III: Geometrical representation. *ibid.*, **10**, 229–33

282. Wilson, F.N., Johnston, F.D. and Kossman, C.E. (1947). The substitution of a tetrahedron for the Einthoven triangle. *Am. Heart J.*, **33**, 594–603

283. Burch, G.E., Abildskov, J.A. and Cronvich, J.A. (1953). *Spatial Vectorcardiography*, pp. 67–72. (Philadelphia: Lea and Febiger)

284. Frank, E. (1956). An accurate clinically practical system for spatial vectorcardiography. *Circulation*, **13**, 737–94

285. Burch, G. (1985). *Op. cit.*, p. 126

286. Bolton, H.C. (1900). *Evolution of the Thermometer*, 1592–1743, p. 18. (Easton, Pa.: Chemical Publishing Co.)

287. Mitchell, W.S. (1892). *Early History of Instrumental Precision in Medicine*, p. 13. (New Haven: Tuttle, Morehouse and Taylor)

288. Wunderlich, C.A. (1871). *On the Temperature in Diseases: A Manual of Medical Thermometry*, pp. 21–3, trans. W. Bathurst Woodman. (London: New Sydenham Society)

289. Currie, J. (1797). *Medical Reports on the Effects of Water, Cold and Warm, as a Remedy in Fever and Febrile Diseases.* (Liverpool: Cadell & Davies)

290. Wunderlich, C.A. (1871). *Op. cit.*, p. 31

291. *Ibid.*, p. 32

292. *Ibid.*, pp. 37–8

293. *Ibid.*

294. Reiser, S.J. (1978). *Medicine and the Reign of Technology*, p. 121. (Cambridge: Cambridge Univ. Press)

295. Hope, J. (1842). *A Treatise on the Diseases of the Heart and Great Vessels*, p. 427. (Philadelphia: Lea and Blanchard)

296. Potain, C. (1875). Du rhythme cardiaque appelé bruit de galop. *Bull. Hôp. (Paris) Ser. 2*, **12**, 137

297. Dellyannis, A.A., Gillam, P.M.S., Mounsey, J.P.D. and Steiner, R.E. (1964). The cardiac impulse and the motion of the heart. *Br. Heart J.*, **26**, 396–411

298. Sutton, G.C. and Craige, E. (1967). Quantitation of precordial movement. I. Normal subjects. *Circulation*, **35**, 476–82

299. Williams, J.L., Kesteloot, H. and De Ocest, H. (1972). Influence of acute hemodynamic changes on the apex cardiogram in dogs. *Am. J. Cardiol.*, **29**, 504–13

300. Sutton, G.C., Prewitt, T.A. and Craige, E. (1970). Relationship between quantitated precordial movement and left ventricular function. *Circulation*, **41**, 179–90

301. Groot, H., Willems, J. and van Vollenhoven, E. (1960). On the physical principles and methodology of fonomecanocardiography. *Acta Cardiol.*, **24**, 147–60

302. Fishleder, B.L. (1966). Exploracion cardiovascular y fonomecanocardiographia. *Med. Mex*, p. 1

303. Garrod, A.H. (1874–75). On some points connected with circulation of the blood arrived at from a study of the sphygmograph. *Proc. R. Soc. London*, **23**, 140

304. Thurston, E. (1876). The length of the systole of the heart, as estimated from sphygmographic tracings. *J. Anat. Physiol.*, **10**, 494–501

305. Chapman, P.M. and Lond, M.D. (1894). Abstract of the Goulstonian Lectures on the physics of the circulation. *Br. Med. J.*, **1**, 511–15

306. Bowen, W.P. (1904). Changes in heart rate, blood pressure and duration of systole resulting from bicycling. *Am. J. Physiol.*, **11**, 59–77

307. Wiggers, C.J. (1921). Studies on the consecutive phases of the cardiac cycle. I.

The duration of the consecutive phases of the cardiac cycle and the criteria for their precise determination. *Am. J. Physiol.*, **56**, 415–38

308. Wiggers, C.J. (1921). Studies on the consecutive phases of the cardiac cycle. II. The laws governing the relative duration of ventricular systole and diastole. *Am. J. Physiol.*, **56**, 439–59

309. Katz, L.N. and Feil, H.S. (1923). Clinical observations on the dynamics of ventricular systole. I. Auricular fibrillation. *Arch. Intern. Med.*, **32**, 672–92

310. Feil, H.S. and Katz, L.N. (1924). Clinical observation on the dynamics of ventricular systole. II. Hypertension. *Arch. Intern. Med.*, **33**, 321–9

311. Katz, L.N. (1927). Observations on the dynamics of ventricular contraction in the heart-lung preparation. *Am. J. Physiol.*, **80**, 470–84

312. Lombard, W.P. and Cope, O.M. (1926). Duration of the systole of the left ventricle of man. *Am. J. Physiol.*, **77**, 263

313. Blumberger, K. (1942). VI. Die untersuchung der dynamik des herzens beim menschen. Ergeb. *Inn. Med. Kinderheiks.*, **62**, 424–531

314. Weissler, A.M., Harris, W.S. and Schoenfeld, C.D. (1968). Systolic time intervals in heart failure in man. *Circulation*, **37**, 149–59

25   Radiologic methods

CHEST ROENTGENOGRAPHY

The roots of radiology are to be found in the experiments that were being conducted in the late 19th century concerning cathode rays and their properties. These rays were produced by discharging electric currents through air in a partially evacuated tube made of glass and containing a positive and negative electrode. The tube was named Crookes, after its inventor. In the early part of 1894, Wilhelm Roentgen also became interested in these rays. The prevailing thought at the time was that cathode rays could not penetrate through glass. Apparently, Roentgen was not convinced that this was so, and this doubt was the stimulus that caused him to embark on a series of experiments which, with the help of serendipity, led to the discovery of the X-rays.

The belief that cathode rays were unable to pass through glass was considered a handicap by the physicists engaged in this field of research. In order to overcome this limitation, Philipp Lenard, a German physicist, redesigned Crookes' tube. Hertz had already demonstrated that cathode rays could pass through aluminum and Lenard took advantage of this fact by creating an 'aluminum window' in the Crookes tube through which the cathode rays could pass. It was already known that a paper saturated with barium platinocyanide would become fluorescent when cathode rays came into contact with it. Lenard observed that fluorescence occurred only when he used the Crookes tube modified with his aluminum window. This, in his mind, confirmed the perception that glass was an impenetrable barrier against the passage of cathode rays.

Despite these observations there was a lingering doubt on the part of Roentgen concerning the validity of Lenard's conclusion. Roentgen set out to duplicate Lenard's experiments but for some unknown reason he gave up the project after only a few months. A hiatus of several months ensued

during which Roentgen's doubts about the impenetrability of glass to cathode rays must have continued to fester within him so that once again he took up experiments to explore the problem further.

Roentgen now entertained the hypothesis that the ability of cathode rays to induce luminescence on a fluorescent screen could be blocked by light generated within the Crookes tube itself as the electric current was being discharged. In order to prove this he covered an unmodified Crookes tube with black cardboard, darkened the room and discharged the tube while watching carefully to be sure that no light was coming through. To his astonishment, the fluorescent screen containing the barium platinocyanide suddenly began to emit a faint glow. The screen had been placed on a bench about a meter away from the tube. Roentgen discharged the tube again and again, placing the screen at increasingly greater distances from the tube, with the same result each time.

Six weeks of intense concentration with a countless number of observations and experiments followed this serendipitous discovery. He knew the phenomenon could not be attributed to the cathode rays, because it was very well documented that these rays could not travel through air for more than several centimeters. Since he did not know the nature of the factors responsible for the fluorescence, he decided to call them X-rays.

Prior to publishing this discovery, Roentgen was well aware of the reverberations his announcement would create and therefore took every precaution to be sure that his observations and conclusions were accurate, valid and reproducible. In the process, he delineated some important characteristics of the newly discovered rays. He found that they travelled in straight lines; that they could not be refracted or reflected; that a magnet could not alter their course; and that they could travel through air for a distance of two meters. He was also able to ascertain their penetrance capability, finding that, in general, the lower the density of the object, the greater the penetrance of the X-ray through it. Lead constituted an impenetrable barrier. Bone, being denser than the surrounding tissue, was relatively impenetrable and could not only be visualized on the fluorescent screen but also be registered permanently on photographic plates. His wife was caught up in his enthusiasm and allowed him to obtain a bony portrait of her hand. The original photograph is housed in the Frances A. Countway Library of Medicine in Boston. It is the first X-ray film of a human being. Figure 1 is a reproduction of this radiograph.

On December 28, 1895, only six days after the photograph was taken, Roentgen submitted his paper for publication in the Proceedings of the Physio-Medical Society of Würzburg. Köllicker, a member of the society, was so impressed with Roentgen's work that upon his motion the society passed a resolution to abandon the term 'X-rays' in favor of 'Roentgen rays'. The eponym has persisted when alluding to the general field of radiology (roentgenology) despite the xenophobia of World War II, but the rays themselves are more commonly referred to as X-rays. They are no longer an unknown quantity since they were subsequently found to be part of the electromagnetic spectrum with a very short wave length in the region of 0.01 to 50 angstrom units.

Whether it was entrepreneurship or simply excess enthusiasm on his part, Roentgen lost no time in disseminating the fruits of his work as rapidly and as widely as possible. Only three days after his paper appeared in the Proceedings, on the first day of the new year, he mailed reprints of his paper along with X-ray prints to a number of well-known physicists. Roentgen realized his objectives immediately because in several days Emil Warburg displayed some of the photos at a meeting of the Berlin Physical Society. Never in the history of medicine had a report of a scientific discovery been disseminated so swiftly and so widely. In another two days following the Berlin meeting the newspapers broke the story around the world[1].

Crookes' tube had been in use in laboratories for more than 30 years. Roentgen's announcement came as a shock to the entire scientific world. In addition, the lay press continued to fan such an intense interest in it that at every turn one was reminded of Roentgen's outstanding discovery. As with the popularization of any item, many excesses were committed in the name of X-ray. Charlatans soon enjoyed a lucrative response from those willing to be duped. Fiction soon overcame fact as the public's fascination with the X-ray remained unsatisfied.

In medical circles, the X-ray soon came to symbolize the most advanced scientific approach to medicine. At last a diagnostic modality was available that overcame many of the limitations of physical diagnosis.

Wilhelm Konrad Roentgen was the only son of a cloth manufacturer. He was born in Lennep, Germany in 1845, and died in Munich in 1923. Although he led a highly productive intellectual life, there was no discernable indication of this potentiality during his youth. There are some cloudy elements in his early education. He was never a regular student at the University of Utrecht, remaining there for only nine months while pursuing courses in philosophy. Apparently his failure to be enrolled as a fully matriculating student was based on the incompleteness of his pre-university schooling. He had been expelled from the Utrecht Technical School for refusing to identify the classmate who had drawn an unpleasing caricature of one of the masters. Despite this obstacle Roentgen did manage to pass the examinations for entrance into the mechanical engineering program at the Polytechnic School in Zurich. Now, perfectly disciplined, he not only received a diploma in mechanical engineering but a doctorate in philosophy as well a year later.

Roentgen's academic career began immediately after receiving his doctorate. He remained at his alma mater as assistant to August Kundt who was then professor of physics. A bond was established between teacher and pupil that was to remain unbroken for many years and highlighted by many collaborative efforts. When Kundt transferred his activities to the University of Würzburg, Roentgen accompanied his mentor. Again following Kundt, Roentgen went to Strasbourg, beginning as a tutor at the Physical Institute. In several years his reputation and research productivity were such that he was offered the chair of physics at the University of Giessen. He remained at Giessen for 9 years without a break in his numerous research activities. In 1888 he left Giessen to become professor of physics and director of the Physical Institute at the Royal University of Würzburg. In 1894 he was appointed rector of the university.

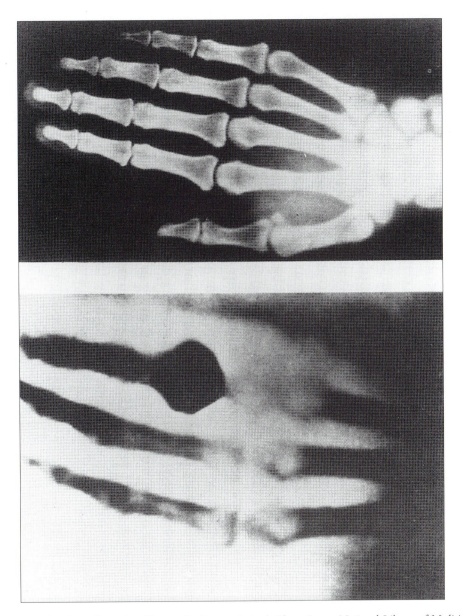

Figure 1 Reproduction of the first X-ray of a human being. *Photo Source National Library of Medicine. Literary Source Reiser, S.J. (1978). Medicine and the Reign of Technology, p.121, Cambridge University Press. Permission from the Countway Library of Medicine or from Cambridge University Press, Edinburgh Bldg., Shaftesbury Road, Cambridge CB2 2RU, England*

His administrative duties did not deter him from continuing his research efforts which were to lead him a year later to the discovery of X-rays and the establishment of his international fame.

The succeeding years saw him the recipient of many honors among which was the Nobel prize in 1901. Throughout all this Roentgen remained a simple, truth-loving man who preferred his laboratory to the limelight. When controversy arose as to whether he or his assistant was the true discoverer of X-rays, he withdrew more and more from the public view. The privations of World War I and the loss of his wife in 1919 added to his distress in the remaining years of his life.

In all, Roentgen authored or co-authored 58 papers. Before his discovery of X-rays his research interests focused on the rates of the specific heat of gases, the conductivity of heat in crystals, and the rotation of the plane of polarization of light in gases. He also concerned himself with the magnetic effects produced in a dielectric, such as a glass plate, when it was moved between two electrically charged condenser plates. This resulted in a contribution equally as important as the X-ray because his conclusion and documentation led to some of the theories of electricity[2].

A keen scientist, a humanist, a tireless worker who retained his modesty despite his fame – these are the attributes that made up the man, Roentgen; a fitting obituary for an adopted son of medicine.

Only one short month after the X-ray machine was introduced, the technique of fluoroscopy came on the scene. The fluoroscope is a relatively simple apparatus. It consists of an X-ray generating component and a screen covered with a fluorescing chemical. Almost a year after Roentgen's paper appeared, Williams was able to report on the value of fluoroscopy in the X-ray examination of the heart. His *Notes on x-rays in medicine* appeared in the Transaction of the Association of American Physicians[3]. Williams' first medical case was a man with an enlarged heart. Muir recounts how Williams was able to image the heart despite the fact that the man was wearing two shirts and a waistcoat[4].

Although radiology, in general, continued to flourish for many years, its application to cardiac diseases was not received with any degree of enthusiasm. Williams' paper, in particular, failed to generate any interest at all. The noted Sir James Mackenzie did not help matters either when he wrote as late as 1920: 'Indeed I am doubtful if an x-ray examination of the heart has ever thrown the slightest light on any cardiac condition'[5].

However, despite the authoritarian negativism on the part of Mackenzie, younger members of the profession diligently continued their observations on the radiologic examination of the heart, and by 1933, three important papers appeared in the same issue of the *British Medical Journal*. These were written by three different men: John Parkinson, Chricton Bramwell and Peter Kerly[6–8]. These papers were the catalysts that caused radiology of the heart to become an established procedure. Roesler's textbook on *Clinical Roentgenology of the Cardiovascular System* appeared in 1937[9]. It was very

well received and created a further stimulus for the routine use of X-rays in cardiologic evaluation. In an attempt to standardize the methodology for measuring heart size, the teleroentgenogram was introduced. This provided a standard reference point for the later utilization of the cardiothoracic ratio in assessing the presence of cardiomegaly.

Despite its marked limitations, and since nothing better was available, fluoroscopy became an essential part of the cardiac evaluation. The ingestion of barium sulphate to visualize the esophagus was practiced with regularity as an aid in delineating indirectly the borders of the cardiac chambers. The popularity of the fluoroscope remained unaltered until the 1960s when newer technological advancements rendered its use obsolete. Today, the fluoroscopic screen serves as a guiding and monitoring device for the various invasive and interventional modalities.

Kymography also appeared, stayed awhile and then faded into oblivion. It was devised to analyze the motion of the heart during contraction and relaxation. X-rays were passed through the chest to a film which moved at a uniform rate behind a grid of lead strips.

CARDIAC CATHETERIZATION AND ANGIOGRAPHY

The introduction of cardiac catheterization has been undoubtedly a far greater boon to cardiology than any other technological innovation. It has not only played an important role in experimental and clinical physiology, but also refined the diagnostic accuracy of cardiac disturbances, whether congenital or acquired, to a level hitherto unattainable. At the same time, it has provided a safe method for the utilization of highly innovative and specific therapeutic approaches that, at times, are astoundingly varied in their application. It has truly become, in the hands of young aggressive cardiologists, the cutting edge of exploration in diagnosis and therapy.

Andre Cournand, a leading pioneer in the field, divided the evolution of cardiac catheterization into three periods[10]. The first was the experimental period, the second started with the young urologist who first demonstrated the feasibility of cardiac catheterization in humans, and the third witnessed the elaboration, extension and universal acceptance of the technique in all phases of cardiac management.

The first two periods lay the groundwork for its development while the last period, still evolving, has borne and continues to bear the many fruits of its application.

The initial period began in 1844 with Claude Bernard. He was the first to perform the procedure, and he is responsible for naming it cardiac catheterization. Bernard was, first and foremost, a physiologist, who had the foresight and conviction that medical advances could be made only from sound physiologic studies coupled with clinical observations. In accordance with this view, he set out to resolve, if possible, a controversy that had been debated ever since Lavoisier first suggested that animal heat is produced as a result of respiratory gas exchange during the blood's passage through the lungs[5]. Although this was not accepted as the gospel truth by various physiologists, interest in the subject waxed and waned over the years. The controversy was rekindled many years later (1837) when Gustav Magnus asserted that combustion takes place in the tissues rather than in the lungs[11]. Bernard addressed the problem initially while working as an assistant in Magendie's laboratory. According to Bechat, it appeared that Magendie had already perceived cardiac catheterization many years earlier as a potentially valuable means of physiological research. It was he who suggested this approach to Bernard as indicated by Bechat in the footnotes to the 4th edition of his *Recherches Physiologiques sur la Vie et la Mort* originally published in 1822[12]. Bernard had reasoned that if pulmonary combustion did occur then the blood returning from the lungs would be warmer than the blood entering the pulmonary artery. Acting on his mentor's suggested approach, Bernard recorded the temperature of the blood in the left ventricle by passing a long mercury thermometer through the exposed carotid artery of a horse. The temperature of the blood in the right ventricle was determined by passing the thermometer through the jugular vein. He did find a difference in the temperature of the blood between the two ventricles. Since the temperature of the blood in the right ventricle was slightly higher than that in the left, he concluded that pulmonary combustion was not possible. Bernard repeated these experiments many times over the next 30 years using also sheep and dogs as subjects. His observations were consistently the same as those of the original experiment in 1844. He refined his technique somewhat in his later experiments by using a very sensitive thermoelectric probe capable of differentiating temperatures by as little as 0.01 degrees Celsius.

In an article that appeared in the *American Journal of Cardiology* in 1959, Buzzi recounts how Bernard gave a rather detailed description of the technique in his textbook *Lecons de Physiologie Operatoire*, published posthumously in 1879[13,14].

In addition to addressing the combustion problem, Bernard utilized his technique to measure intracardiac pressures. We have already seen how Hales demonstrated in the preceding century the feasibility of intra-arterial pressures through cannulation. Bernard went one step further by entering the cardiac chambers through the appropriate vascular channels. His purpose for doing so was to determine the influence of the nervous system on blood pressure. His initial experiment was confined to the right ventricle with the dog as a subject. When the animal was sacrificed, it was seen that the glass tube Bernard used had perforated the wall of the ventricle. Despite this untoward complication seen with his first experiment, Bernard continued with his studies and over a number of years he was able to measure intracardiac blood pressures under a variety of physiological states.

Another controversy also existed during this period of experimentation. It was concerned with the nature and timing of the cardiac apex beat. Was the apical beat due to ventricular contraction, and when it was felt on palpation, did this indicate the beginning of ventricular systole? Harvey thought so and Laénnec as well. This view was also shared by Chauveau and Faivre. The following quotation is from a book they published in 1865 wherein they described their investigations of the cardiac movements and heart sounds[15]: 'The apical thrust corresponds to the instantaneous change of the ventricular form and consistency of the beginning of systole transmitted to the anterior thoracic wall but felt only where there is no bony structure'. Incidentally, these two workers were also the first to record pulmonary artery pressure experimentally, using a needle to obtain the measurement, rather than advancing the probe beyond the right ventricle. Chauveau was professor of veterinary medicine in Lyons, but at heart and in his work, he was an experimental physiologist.

Chauveau's interest in the nature and timing of the cardiac apex beat caused him to join forces with Marey in an attempt to resolve the controversy.

Marey's work and experience with the sphygmograph was an all important factor in the way the two men approached the problem. It was based on the generally accepted view at the time that intraventricular pressure rose with systole. The sphygmograph lent itself easily to measuring the pressure changes within the ventricle. The crucial point was the correlation of intraventricular pressure rise with the onset of the apex beat. The initial transmitting device they designed failed to give accurate and reproducible results[16]. They then resorted to a system based on one developed by Pierre Buisson[17]. The experiments were conducted on a horse and provided what they thought was irrefutable evidence in support of the hypothesis that the apical beat is caused by ventricular systole. These observations were published in the *Gazette Medicale de Paris* in 1861. The objections raised regarding the validity of their conclusions prompted them to publish another paper several months later in an effort to silence the critics. The conclusions of Chauveau and Marey were upheld by a committee of the Academy of Sciences specifically convened to resolve the issue[18].

Chauveau and Marey continued with their investigations and by 1863 they were able to publish the first systematic description and interpretation of intracardiac pressure recordings[19]. This report was identified by Cournand as a milestone in cardiac physiology. Equally important as a landmark publication was Marey's book which also appeared in 1863, and which reiterated in detail the instrumentation and the many physiological firsts as observed and recorded by this physician and his veterinarian colleague[20]. Among these are:

(1) the first recorded simultaneous measurement of pressures in the left ventricle and in the central aorta;

(2) the identification of the isometric phase of left ventricular systole;

(3) a description of a double-lumen catheter, and a special catheter for introduction into the carotid artery for recording left ventricular pressure.

The remainder of the 19th century saw further elaboration of the groundwork laid by Chauveau and Marey. National boundaries were again transcended by such workers as Fick, Porter, Rolleston, Roy and Adams.

Fick's recording system differed from that of the sphygmograph in that the pressure recordings were inscribed on Ludwig's kymograph. In 1873, Fick published his findings on the form and level of blood pressure variations from both sides of the heart[21]. Despite Fick's contention that his technique and instrumentation was more accurate than that of Chauveau and Marey, it soon became apparent that such was not the case. The issue of accuracy now embroiled the scientific community and was fought over the succeeding years with the introduction of individually championed manometric systems. Friction was thought to be the most important adverse factor affecting accuracy. Porter favored a single- or a double-lumen rigid catheter made of silver-plated brass[22]. Rolleston concentrated on minimizing the role of friction along the tube and connectors[23]. Roy and Adams substituted a short cannula for the catheter[24]. It was introduced through the apex of the heart and connected via its distal end to a piston manometer filled with oil. It was finally left to Otto Frank to settle the issue. Beginning in 1913, he issued a series of papers in which he outlined the theoretical and mathematical basis for the accurate and reproducible recording of intracardiac events[25-27].

The following is an English translation of that part of the page relating to Fick's contribution (Figure 2)[28] as taken from *Circulation of the Blood, Men and Ideas*[29].

Herr Fick had a contribution on the measurement of the amount of blood ejected by the ventricle of the heart with each systole, a quantity the knowledge of which is certainly of great importance. Varying opinions have been expressed in this. While Thomas Young estimated the quantity at about 45 cc, most estimates in modern textbooks, supported by the views of Volksmann and Vierordt, run much higher, up to 180 cc. It is surprising that no one has arrived at the following procedure by which this important value is available by direct determination, at least in animals. One measures how much oxygen an animal absorbs from the air in a given time, and how much CO_2 it gives off. One takes during this time a sample of arterial and a sample of venous blood; in both samples oxygen content and CO_2 content are measured. The difference of oxygen content gives the amount of oxygen each cubic centimeter of blood takes up in its passage through the lungs; and as one knows how much total oxygen has been taken up in given time, one can calculate how many cubic centimeters of blood have passed through the lungs in this time, or if one divides by the number of heartbeats during this time, how many cubic centimeters of blood are ejected with each beat. The corresponding calculation with CO_2 quantities gives a determination of the same value, which provides a control for the other calculation.

Fick, convinced of the soundness of his concept, never bothered to subject it to experimental proof. Sixteen years had to elapse before this was provided by Grehant and Quinquaud in their experiments concerning the measurement of blood flow in 6 dogs[30]. Further experimental proof was supplied by the lengthy and detailed studies of Zuntz with the help of Hagemann. He was the first to combine blood flow measurement with direct recording of blood pressure in the pulmonary artery, aorta or both for the determination of cardiac work, and the first to combine these hemodynamic measurements with studies of respiratory gas transport. These findings were initially published by him in 1893[31]. Zuntz and Hagemann continued to work together for some time after Zuntz's initial paper. Their combined efforts culminated in the publication of a remarkable monograph in 1898, acclaimed for its detailed presentation of observations and analyses, its scientific integrity and the high quality of the work performed[32].

There was a long hiatus of almost a quarter of a century between the experiments in the physiology laboratory and the first controlled catheterization of the right atrium in man which initiated Cournand's so-called second period. This period is generally conceded to have begun with Werner Forssmann's self-experiment in 1929.

There is no doubt that Forssmann was the catalyst for stimulating interest in the clinical application of cardiac catheterization, but he was not the first to have tried the procedure in a human. According to A. J. Benatt, whose historical note on cardiac catheterization appeared in *The Lancet* in 1949, Fritz Bleichröder may have been the first to have had a catheter passed into his heart[33]. In 1912, Bleichröder, in collaboration with Unger and Lob, published three articles on intra-arterial therapy which described the passage of ureteric catheters through veins and arteries in

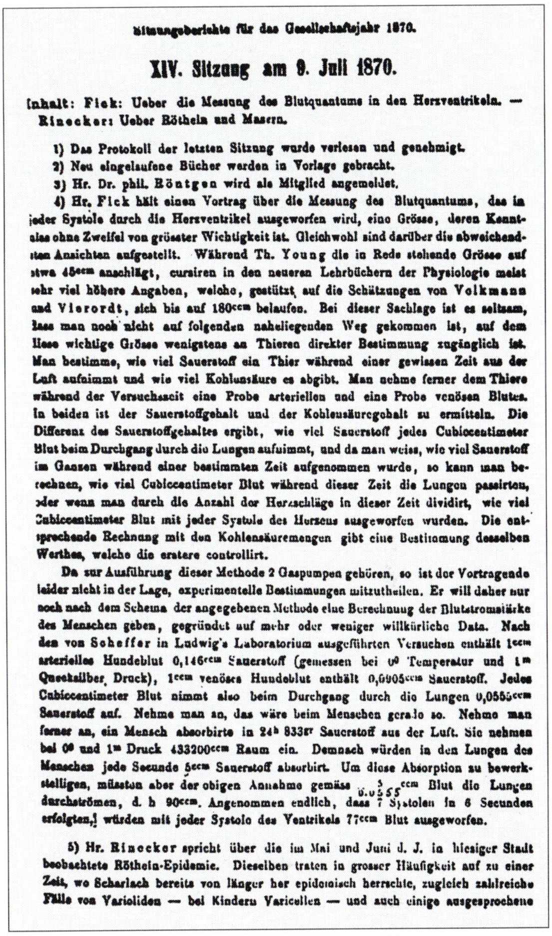
Sitzungsberichte für das Gesellschaftsjahr 1870.

XIV. Sitzung am 9. Juli 1870.

Inhalt: Fick: Ueber die Messung des Blutquantums in den Herzventrikeln. — Rinecker: Ueber Rötheln und Masern.

1) Das Protokoll der letzten Sitzung wurde verlesen und genehmigt.

2) Neu eingelaufene Bücher werden in Vorlage gebracht.

3) Hr. Dr. phil. Röntgen wird als Mitglied angemeldet.

4) Hr. Fick hält einen Vortrag über die Messung des Blutquantums, das in jeder Systole durch die Herzventrikel ausgeworfen wird, eine Grösse, deren Kenntniss ohne Zweifel von grösster Wichtigkeit ist. Gleichwohl sind darüber die abweichendsten Ansichten aufgestellt. Während Th. Young die in Rede stehende Grösse auf etwa 45ccm anschlägt, cursiren in den neueren Lehrbüchern der Physiologie meist sehr viel höhere Angaben, welche, gestützt auf die Schätzungen von Volkmann und Vierordt, sich bis auf 180ccm belaufen. Bei dieser Sachlage ist es seltsam, dass man noch nicht auf folgenden naheliegenden Weg gekommen ist, auf dem diese wichtige Grösse wenigstens an Thieren direkter Bestimmung zugänglich ist. Man bestimme, wie viel Sauerstoff ein Thier während einer gewissen Zeit aus der Luft aufnimmt und wie viel Kohlensäure es abgibt. Man nehme ferner dem Thiere während der Versuchszeit eine Probe arteriellen und eine Probe venösen Blutes. In beiden ist der Sauerstoffgehalt und der Kohlensäuregehalt zu ermitteln. Die Differenz des Sauerstoffgehaltes ergibt, wie viel Sauerstoff jedes Cubiccentimeter Blut beim Durchgang durch die Lungen aufnimmt, und da man weiss, wie viel Sauerstoff im Ganzen während einer bestimmten Zeit aufgenommen wurde, so kann man berechnen, wie viel Cubiccentimeter Blut während dieser Zeit die Lungen passirten, oder wenn man durch die Anzahl der Herzschläge in dieser Zeit dividirt, wie viel Cubiccentimeter Blut mit jeder Systole des Herzens ausgeworfen wurden. Die entsprechende Rechnung mit den Kohlensäuremengen gibt eine Bestimmung desselben Werthes, welche die erstere controllirt.

Da zur Ausführung dieser Methode 2 Gaspumpen gehören, so ist der Vortragende leider nicht in der Lage, experimentelle Bestimmungen mitzutheilen. Er will daher nur noch nach dem Schema der angegebenen Methode eine Berechnung der Blutstromstärke des Menschen geben, gegründet auf mehr oder weniger willkürliche Data. Nach den von Scheffer in Ludwig's Laboratorium ausgeführten Versuchen enthält 1ccm arterielles Hundeblut 0,146ccm Sauerstoff (gemessen bei 0° Temperatur und 1m Quecksilber Druck), 1ccm venöses Hundeblut enthält 0,0905ccm Sauerstoff. Jedes Cubiccentimeter Blut nimmt also beim Durchgang durch die Lungen 0,0555ccm Sauerstoff auf. Nehme man an, das wäre beim Menschen gerade so. Nehme man ferner an, ein Mensch absorbirte in 24h 833gr Sauerstoff aus der Luft. Sie nehmen bei 0° und 1m Druck 433200ccm Raum ein. Demnach würden in den Lungen des Menschen jede Secunde 5ccm Sauerstoff absorbirt. Um diese Absorption zu bewerkstelligen, müssten aber der obigen Annahme gemäss $\frac{5}{0.0555}$ccm Blut die Lungen durchströmen, d. h 90ccm. Angenommen endlich, dass 7 Systolen in 6 Secunden erfolgten, würden mit jeder Systole des Ventrikels 77ccm Blut ausgeworfen.

5) Hr. Rinecker spricht über die im Mai und Juni d. J. in hiesiger Stadt beobachtete Rötheln-Epidemie. Dieselben traten in grosser Häufigkeit auf zu einer Zeit, wo Scharlach bereits von länger her epidemisch herrschte, zugleich zahlreiche Fälle von Varioliden — bei Kindern Varicellen — und auch einige ausgesprochene

Figure 2 First page of 'Proceedings' describing the Fick principle. *Photo Source University of Central Florida. Literary Source Original. Public domain*

humans for the purpose of delivering medication to target organs. Forssmann, himself, related in 1929, how one of the authors, Unger, recounted these experiments to him, emphasizing the unpublished perception that Bleichröder's right atrium had been invaded during one of these experiments as far back as 1905, seven years before their papers on intra-arterial therapy appeared[34].

Be that as it may, and as is usual with so many innovative procedures, it is at times very difficult to pinpoint the individual or individuals who were responsible for the initial introduction of a particular procedure. Such is the case even here. Though Fritz Bleichröder may have had a catheter passed into his heart in 1905, antedating Forssmann by 24 years, it appears that even he may not have been the first to undergo this procedure, self-imposed or otherwise. N. Howard-Jones describes a report on the passage of an elastic catheter into the left side of the heart by Johann Friedrich Dieffenbach, a prominent Prussian surgeon[35]. Dieffenbach published the report in 1832 and reprinted the paper two years later in his monograph on physiological–surgical observations in cholera[36,37]. Utilizing the brachial artery, the surgeon introduced the catheter into a patient dying of cholera under the mistaken notion that these patents needed to be bled in order to effect a cure. Dieffenbach's description of the procedure is as follows[37]:

> In an almost dying [cholera] patient suffering from great anxiety and breathlessness I opened, with the agreement of Herr Medical Counsellor Casper, the brachial artery in its upper third. As not a drop of blood flowed, I introduced, as I had planned, an elastic catheter into the vessel approximately as far as the heart. Nevertheless no blood appeared through the catheter. The heartbeat became clearer and more rapid, and I now withdrew the catheter. It was completely empty and no drop of blood had entered it, as must have happened if fluid blood had been present in the heart … It is greatly to be regretted that this operation of interest for all physiology was performed on a man who was so near to death and who shortly afterwards was seized by convulsions and rendered his soul.

Of course, there is no proof that the heart was actually entered. The same reservations apply regarding Unger's communication to Forssmann as indicated by these lines in Forssmann's paper: 'He has even, in the case of Dr. Bleichroder, as he concluded from the length of the catheter and the stabbing pain, reached the right heart'[34]. Forssmann, then, must be given credit for priority in the deliberate insertion of a catheter into a human heart under roentgenological control, and with this control constituting proof of entry.

Werner Forssmann was a surgical resident at the Eberswalde Clinic in Germany when he became interested in the procedure. His objective was to develop a technique for the rapid administration of drugs directly into the heart. Although he did not spell it out in so many words, Forssmann probably also saw the potentialities of the technique in the clinical evaluation of the heart. In his initial experiment, he introduced a ureteral catheter through an arm vein of a cadaver and noted how easily it could be guided into the right atrium[38]. Pleased with the facility with which he entered the right atrium in the cadaver, Forssmann utilized the technique for the first time, *in vivo*, in a patient with purulent peritonitis administering a solution of glucose, epinephrine and strophanthin. Despite what could be considered a heroic measure for the time, but lacking, unfortunately, the ingredients of the antibiotic age, the patient died. At autopsy, the tip of the catheter was seen to be near the opening of the inferior vena cava.

Encouraged by this initial attempt, and imbued with the brashness of youth, he persuaded his colleagues to try the procedure on him. They were unsuccessful in their attempt, and refused to try again, fearful of the possible consequences. Undaunted, Forssmann took the matter into his own hands by exposing one of his own left arm veins, and under fluoroscopic control, aided by a mirror held by a nurse, he introduced a ureteral catheter and advanced it to the right atrium. Anxious to obtain a permanent record of his entry into the chamber, he went to the x-ray department, a few steps away, and recorded the event with a chest film.

The transition from physiological experimentation to clinical application was assured when his report appeared in 1929[34]. Forssmann's interest was now thoroughly aroused. In the succeeding two years he explored the radiologic examination of the heart in dogs utilizing the radiopaque medium available at the time to outline the atrial chamber[39]. The results were somewhat disappointing through no fault of his since contrast media at the time were still inadequate in terms of both efficacy and toxicity.

Because there was a general attitude of hostility, and especially, unsubstantiated fears regarding the dangers of the technique, Forssmann's work was taken up by only a few investigators. Two researchers, however, whose interest was stimulated by Forssmann's report in 1929, did publish papers of excellent quality. They appeared only one year later. One was by O. Klein of Prague[40]. He reported 11 successful placements of a catheter into the right side of the heart in 18 attempts. In three of these cases, Klein was able to establish for the first time an arterio-venous oxygen differential[40]. This work indicates that Klein should be given credit for being the first to measure cardiac output, using Fick's principle. Klein then visited Boston in an attempt to convince the local clinicians of the feasibility of the technique for gathering blood samples from different areas of the heart. Unfortunately, the Bostonian establishment turned a deaf ear to his proposals, and medicine had to wait another 12 years for Cournand and Richards to alert the profession to the enormous potentialities of cardiac catheterization. The team of Jimenez Diaz and Sanchez Cuenca published two papers, also in 1930. The first paper described their successful attempt to introduce a ureteral catheter through a cannula in the arm vein of a patient near death[41]. Their second paper which appeared several months later was laden with suggestions concerning the therapeutic and diagnostic potentialities of Forssmann's procedure[42]. In 1932, a trio of part-time clinicians from the medical clinic of the University of Buenos Aires (Padilla, Cossio, and Berconsky), published four articles in succession describing the technique[43], radiologic identification of the superior vena cava[44], determination of cardiac output using Fick's principle[45], and possible clinical applications of cardiac catheterization[46]. The foresight of Klein and these South American investigators was amazing but unfortunately, neither they nor others conducted further studies regarding the utility of cardiac catheterization for some time.

Aside from the rapidly developing studies in pulmonary angiography, the state of interest in cardiac catheterization as a clinical tool remained almost non-existent with only undirected and sporadic reports until 1936. That year marked the beginning of Cournand's so-called third period; an era that saw the establishment of cardiac catheterization as a highly accurate and useful diagnostic tool in cardiology. The two leaders in the field were Andre Cournand and Dickinson Richards. The breadth of their work and the brilliance of its execution allowed these two men eventually to share with Werner Forssmann the Nobel Prize for Medicine and Physiology in 1956[47].

Cournand (Figure 3) described the prelude to the period as beginning in 1932 when he was chief resident of the Columbia University Chest Service, Bellevue Hospital in New York City. He, in collaboration with Richards, set out to investigate the hypothesis formulated by Lawrence Henderson that 'the lungs, heart and circulation form a single system for the exchange of respiratory gases between the atmosphere and the tissues of the organism'[48]. After four years of effort failed to provide them with adequate data to validate

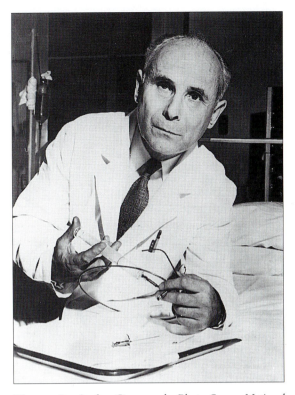

Figure 3   Andre Cournand. *Photo Source National Library of Medicine. Literary Source Photo Archives. Courtesy of National Library of Medicine*

Henderson's hypothesis, Cournand and Richards resorted to the technique of right heart catheterization in the hope that this approach might be the avenue through which they could obtain the mixed venous blood necessary for the determination of respiratory gas concentrations. The following is Cournand's description of what transpired[49]:

In 1936 we considered whether the technique of right heart catheterization might provide help in obtaining the mixed venous blood needed for determination of respiratory gas concentrations, in accordance with our general plan. I arranged, therefore, to visit with Dr. Ameuille, one of my former teachers, who had completed pulmonary angiography in 100 patients in his hospital in Paris. The protocols of these cases convinced me of the safety of the technique. Dick Richards and I, in collaboration with Robert Darling, then familiarized ourselves with the method, first in canine experiments and eventually in a chimpanzee. Meanwhile, George Wright, a former student of Carl Wiggers and then a resident of the Chest Service at Bellevue Hospital, offered to advance ureteral catheters, under fluoroscopic control, into the right atrium of human cadavers, in order to measure the distance between the catheter tip and a landmark on the anterior chest wall on lateral chest X-rays; this datum would be needed to establish a reference point for measuring intracardiac pressures.

In 1940, their attention was directed towards a study involving an accurate calibration of the ill-fated ballistocardiograph. The hypertensive clinic at Bellevue Hospital was interested in utilizing ballistocardiography as a means of determining cardiac output, but needed assurance of its accuracy. Homer Smith, who was then professor of physiology at New York University, suggested that this could be done by correlating the values obtained with the ballistocardiograph with the simultaneous determination of cardiac output utilizing Fick's formula. Cournand addressed the problem in collaboration with Ranges, and one year later they published their first report in a paper entitled *Catheterization of the right auricle in man*[50]. The value of the paper lay not in its elucidation of the inaccuracy of the ballistocardiograph but rather in its indication of the importance of cardiac catheterization as an accurate clinical tool. It emphasized its acceptability by the patients, the reproducibility of the results, and the relative ease with which the procedure could be performed. This classical paper codified the technique of catheterization, and outlined a precise method for the determination of cardiac output and intra-cavitary and pulmonary artery pressures. The authors provided irrefutable evidence supporting the validity of the Fick principle under basal conditions and after physical effort as well, provided certain criteria were met.

In a memorial to Cournand who died in his 93rd year, J. Lequime, a former student and later professor of cardiology at the University of Brussels, summarized Cournand's view of the primacy of the clinical aspect in all of his research efforts in Cournand's own words[51]:

To be fruitful in useful results, the application of new methods requires not only a profound knowledge of the techniques used but also that of the patient under examination: the value of precise physiological measurement is all the greater when the clinical study is more elaborated; before presenting his conclusions, the investigator must always ensure that he has explored in all its clinical aspects the problem which he proposes to resolve.

Between 1941 and 1945 Cournand and Richards, working with other associates, were able to improve on the technical aspects of cardiac catheterization. These included the design of a more readily manipulable catheter, a better type of cannula that facilitated insertion into the brachial or femoral artery, pressure recordings with the Hamilton manometer, and many other improvements in instrumentation[52]. In 1942, Cournand's group reported their observations with the catheter advanced into the right ventricle. Two years later, the catheter was advanced even further into the pulmonary artery.

An important technical advancement introduced by Cournand and his co-workers was the development of a double-lumen catheter. Pressure recordings could now be obtained simultaneously with the procurement of blood samples. The number and type of their clinical studies began to cover a wide range of problems. Many of their trainees and collaborators went on to different centers in the United States and elsewhere, extending cardiac catheterization into new fields, and adding their own original contributions to a rapidly growing field. For example, the first two reports on the usage of cardiac catheterization in the diagnosis of interatrial and interventricular septal defects were published by Warren's group in Atlanta[53], and Eleanor Baldwin with Robert Noble at Columbia University[54].

John McMichael and Sharpey-Schafer, influenced by Cournand's group, introduced cardiac catheterization into England. Despite strong opposition, these two men forged forward in the application of this new technique and made significant contributions in the hemodynamics of shock, heart failure, and the vasovagal syndrome. They were the first to study the effects of intravenous digoxin. This report appeared a year before the end of World War II[55].

Just after the end of the war, McMichael diligently searched out Forssmann as part of his attempt to restore Forssmann to his rightful place in the evolution of cardiac catheterization. McMichael bridled at the fact that orthodox medicine had banished Forssmann from the academic world.

When Forssmann, elated by his early success, approached Ernst Sauerbruch with the good news, the reaction on the part of Sauerbruch was the all too typical one of entrenched authoritarianism. Sauerbruch, at that time an internationally esteemed authority in thoracic surgery, dismissed Forssmann with the statement that he ran a clinic, not a circus[56].

The Parisian efforts were led by Jean Lenegre and Pierre Maurice. At the time of their work, Paris was occupied by Hitler's military machine. The restrictions and trials of a military occupation obviously did not interfere with their studies nor with their publication in 1944 of the first endocardial electrocardiogram, the first X-ray film illustrating the tip of the catheter in the pulmonary artery, and their report on right ventricular pressure measurements using a saline manometer[57,58].

In 1947, Dexter and his associates published three papers describing their findings in patients with congenital heart disease, who were studied by means of a modified version of Cournand's technique[59–61]. They found that venous catheterization was a highly useful tool for investigating cardiac malformations provided that allowances were made for the effect of shunts or any other disturbing effect on blood flow and oxygen content. Venous catheterization continued to provide significant contributions in the study of congenital lesions during the remainder of the 1940s, though, of course, not the last word as subsequent studies have shown.

The need for access to the left ventricle became quite evident quite early. The first to report left heart catheterization in man was Zimmerman and his group in 1950[62]. They used a 6F catheter devised by Cournand. It was introduced into the ulnar artery and advanced in a retrograde fashion into the left ventricle. During the same year the team of Limon-Lason and Bouchard also reported their attempts at retrograde left heart catheterization[63]. Two years later, J. Facquet and others introduced an approach via a transbronchial left atrial puncture[64]. A year later, Björk utilized a transthoracic left atrial puncture[65]. This was a rather complicated affair. A right thorasectomy had to be done first as a precautionary measure. Björk then inserted the needle into the left atrium through the 7th or 8th intercostal space under fluoroscopic control. The bore of the needle was large enough to allow passage of a plastic catheter through it. Despite fluoroscopic control, the catheter would at times pass through the azygos vein. This caused a hematoma which was usually insignificant. A more worrisome complication was the inadvertent passage of the catheter through the esophagus before entering the left heart.

In 1959, a trans-septal approach was introduced. A plastic 70 cm long plastic sheathed needle was passed through the saphenous vein into the right atrium, and then advanced into the left atrium by puncturing the interatrial septum. All of these various methods of entering the left heart made the retrograde arterial approach, the obvious method of choice. Entry into the artery was facilitated when Seldinger introduced his percutaneous technique, circumventing the necessity for exposing the artery by dissection. Strangely though the percutaneous approach did not gain wide acceptance until it was advocated by Ricketts and Abrams in 1962[66].

This approach was solidified even further in 1967, when Melvin P. Judkins described his results with a catheter of his own design, gaining entry through the femoral artery[67]. Judkins' percutaneous femoral arterial approach is the one used most extensively today. The transeptal approach is also still in use today, both for therapeutic intervention and diagnosis. A whole new world was opened with the relatively safe and easy retrograde arterial approach. It permitted localization of the level of left ventricular outflow tract obstruction, assessment of aortic and mitral lesions and, most importantly, selective coronary arteriography. In 1966, Shirey reported on the ability to assess mitral stenosis utilizing his uniquely designed catheter[68].

William Willis, professor of medicine at Loma Linda University, knew Dr Judkins quite well. This is what he told me about him:

> Dr. Judkins first became interested in catheters as a family practitioner when he was assigned to a military post that was short of urologists. Dr. Judkins became fascinated with catheters and their shapes, so that after leaving the military he went into the field of vascular radiology. He spent a year in Sweden with one of the leading vascular radiologists and subsequently developed the Judkins technique of coronary arteriography. The two things I find most memorable about Dr. Judkins were: First, he was a technical perfectionist. The catheters which he designed by forming and shaping wires over heating pipes have hardly changed over the last twenty years.

With regard to the left coronary catheter, one of Dr. Judkins' favorite phrases was 'this catheter will seek the left coronary lumen unless thwarted by the operator'. The second thing which is prominent in my memory of Dr. Judkins is that he very strongly was the patient's advocate. He felt that the safety and completeness of coronary arteriography were of utmost importance. If a study was technically incomplete or of poor diagnostic quality, he felt that this was almost of equal magnitude as a complication. Dr. Judkins truly was a giant in the field of diagnostic coronary angiography.

Very few academic and community hospitals were involved in cardiac catheterization during the 1940s, but by the time the mid-20th century arrived, the picture had begun to change considerably. Rather than having a purely experimental orientation, the newly established centers emphasized clinical research and application. The spectrum of cardiac diseases subjected to cardiac catheterization began to broaden, ranging from congenital heart disease to cor pulmonale. For the most part only right heart or limited arterial catheterization were performed. Angiography was still in its infancy.

In the early days, total darkness of the room was the order of the day. Red goggles were utilized for 20–30 minutes prior to turning off the lights so that the eyes would become adapted to the dark. Operator, assistants and observers were properly attired and gathered around a relatively primitive fluoroscopic screen. Gentility and caution were the guidelines. Radiation exposure was carefully monitored in the interests of all concerned. Zimmerman quotes the rule 'three seconds on, five seconds off'[69]. Resuscitative measures were rather crude. Current antiarrhythmic pharmacologic agents were lacking. There were no DC defibrillators or automatic cycling respirators.

Image intensifiers were introduced in the 1950s but their usage did not become widespread until well into the late 1960s. This was a welcome technical advancement. A dimly lit ambience made the performance of the procedure much easier. Further technical advances included the registration of intracardiac phonocardiographs and electrocardiograms, development of better manometers for intracardiac pressure recordings, superior cinegraphic equipment, and less toxic angiographic contrast media. Dilution techniques

were made practical and were being used with more frequency. The 1950s and 1960s also saw closer collaboration between the cardiac catheterization laboratory and the surgical theater.

All in all, it had become an exciting era during which a vast amount of clinical experience was being accumulated from centers rapidly sprouting throughout the world. Aided by remarkable technological advances in all the aspects of instrumentation and equipment, and propelled by a cadre of well-trained and innovative young cardiologists, a new type of cardiologic practice was unfolding. This was interventional cardiology, and as we shall see later, brought with it astounding advances in diagnosis and therapy.

Although today's highly sophisticated cardiac catheterization laboratory is a far cry from the primitive ones of yesteryear, history has taught us, time and again, that improvements are always possible. In the past, advances in medicine occurred at a snail's pace. The frontiers today are expanding at an exponential rate. It is interesting to speculate on what an historian of cardiology fifty years hence will have to say.

In time, cardiac catheterization expanded its role from assessment of purely physiological parameters to the anatomical and functional delineation of the valvular structures and coronary arteries. Although the transition evolved in concert with the development of less toxic and more effective contrast agents, and with the exploration of the feasibility and safety of coronary arteriography *per se*, many factors had to be resolved before the coronary arteries could be safely visualized in humans. The initial factor was the necessity for a more detailed knowledge of the anatomy of the coronary arteries.

Accurate descriptions of the epicardial coronary arteries were provided by Leonardo da Vinci and later by Vesalius. The smaller intramural branches were more difficult to visualize and required postmortem injection techniques for proper study. One of the first to employ an injection technique was Richard Lower. In his treatise (1669), he wrote that 'the coronary arteries come together again, and here and there communicate by anastomosis. As a result, fluid injected into one of them spreads at one and the same time through both. There is everywhere an equally great need of vital heat and nourishment, so deficiency of these is very fully guarded against by anastomosis'[70].

Although only indirectly, the matter remained at this level until the advent of roentgenography. This new technique served as a stimulus initially for the visualization of the arterial system in general, and it was the evolution and refinement of these early studies, superimposed on the newly developed technique of cardiac catheterization that eventually led to coronary arteriography.

In January of 1896, only 10 weeks after Roentgen's report on the discovery of X-rays, the Viennese team of Hascheck and Lindenthal published a paper demonstrating the arterial supply of the hand by injecting a radiopaque substance into the brachial artery of a cadaver[71]. The contrast medium was a thick emulsion of chalk and required an exposure time of 57 minutes to adequately visualize the arterial tree with Roentgen's X-rays. Figure 4 is a reproduction of their arteriogram. It shows clearly the opacified digital arteries. A copper ring around the index finger is also discernible[72].

There were also other Europeans, as well as Americans who were now focusing their efforts on the exploration of the vascular system with contrast media. Several months after the report by Hascheck and Lindenthal, Destot and Bérard in France described their observations following the injection of a mixture of powdered bronze, alcohol and xylol into the arterial tree of the kidney, spleen and thyroid[73]. During the same time, McIntyre of Glascow experimented with the usage of barium sulphate as a contrast medium[74]. The next few years saw a number of reports published concerning the usage of different agents for injection. These experiments were all conducted as before on cadavers and utilized suspensions of lead salts, bismuth salts, or metallic mercury. In 1899, Musgrove, an American, published a radiograph with contrast visualization of a full-term stillborn infant[75].

Simultaneously with these studies, the unresolved issue of the functional significance of coronary anastomosis continued to attract interest among other investigators. Among them was Robert Baumgarten of Harvard University. He carried out his experiments with radiopaque agents on cats and dogs, and in 1899, he published an extensive review on the subject[76]. In 1907, the first roentgenographic atlas of the human coronary arteries was published by Friedrich Jamin and Hermann Merkel[77]. The atlas contained stereoscopic roentgenograms of 29 cadaver hearts in which the coronary arteries were injected with a suspension of red lead in gelatin.

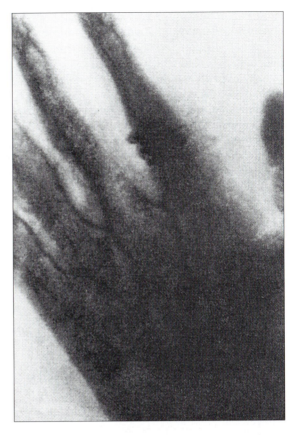

Figure 4 Reproduction of the arteriogram obtained by Hascheck and Lindenthal. The opacified digital areries and a copper wire wound around the index finger are clearly visible. *Photo Source National Library of Medicine. Literary Source Killen, D.A.(1973). Angiographic contrast media. Surgery, 73, 336–46, Fig. 1. Taken from Wien. Klin. Wochenschr., 9, 63, 1896. With permission*

Some of their X-ray pictures demonstrated anastomotic channels or even coronary occlusions.

The year 1910 witnessed the first use of liquid contrast media *in vivo*. It was the work of Franck and Alwens[78]. They injected soluble mixtures of heavy metals (e.g. Bismuth in oil) directly into the heart or into the large veins of dogs and rabbits. Under fluoroscopy, they were able to follow the radiopaque material as it passed through the right heart into the lung field. Schepelmann also investigated the use of oil suspensions and solutions of heavy metal salts for contrast angiography. His subjects were rabbits and frogs[79].

These pioneering investigators all came to the same conclusion. A trial with living humans was unthinkable until contrast media could be found that did not cause the potentially lethal systemic toxicity of heavy metal salts or the embolism of the oily suspensions.

Iodinated poppy seed oil (lipiodol) was an agent that initially seemed to meet the above requirements. It was introduced as a contrast agent in 1921 by Sicard and Forestier[80]. The radiopaque properties of lipiodol were well know since it was a popular remedy in France ever since its introduction in 1901. After initial experimentation with animals, the two French physicians injected small amounts of the agent into the antecubital vein of humans and followed its course through the right heart, pulmonary artery and into the pulmonary capillary bed under fluoroscopic visualization. The only ill effect was coughing, apparently not too troublesome.

In 1923, Berberich and Hirsch published reproductions of human angiograms obtained during life[81]. Their work represented the first clinically successful realization of angiography. They tried a variety of agents but found that strontium bromide was the most promising whether it was used intra-arterially or intravenously. During the same year both Osborne's group at the Mayo clinic and Dunner from Germany used sodium iodide as the contrast medium[81,82]. Some experience had already been gained with the introduction of sodium iodide in 1918 as a contrast agent for urography. Incidentally, the development of contrast agents for urography played a great role in finding a suitable agent for arteriography.

An attempt was made by Sicard and his associates in 1924 to visualize the femoral artery using lipiodol[83]. This proved to be impractical and was therefore abandoned. In the same year, Barney Brooks, a vascular surgeon, also described the clinical application of sodium iodide, adding his experience to that of Dunner and the Osborne team[84]. He was able to show that despite the marked systemic toxicity of sodium iodide, contrast angiography with this agent could prove to be an invaluable aid in delineating occlusive as well as other pathologic changes in the arterial tree. The exact site and extent of the occlusion in the arteries was an exact analogue of what we know occurs in the coronary arteries. It would have taken but a single step to use this agent for the visualization of the coronary arteries. The fly in the ointment was that at that time nobody had the faintest notion of how to go about it.

Significant contributions came in the early 1930s from the pioneering efforts of Egas Moniz and his associates[85]. They explored initially the potentialities of cerebral angiography but soon extended their studies to the cardiovascular system. In 1931, Carvalho and Moniz were the first to perform, *in vivo*, pulmonary arteriography by injecting sodium iodide directly into the right side of the heart utilizing the recently introduced catheter technique of Werner Forssmann.

Despite its marked systemic toxicity, sodium iodide was the agent of choice for several years. The toxic manifestations were headache, thirst, feeling of heat, nausea, vomiting and fever. Even death could result. The amount of sodium iodide had to be carefully determined to minimize these reactions. It was soon obvious that the adoption of angiography as a standard clinical procedure required the formulation of a relatively safe agent. The evolution and development of such an agent was a tedious process involving the cooperation of industry and the trial of many agents.

Again, the needs of cardiology were not the driving force in the search for a non-toxic radiopaque substance. The stimulus was provided by the need for such a substance that was capable of renal clearance at a rate rapid enough to permit realization of an excretory nephropyelogram. A major step forward came with the introduction of an organic iodide compound. The iodine toxicity was minimized or eliminated by incorporating the iodine into an organic radical. Numerous variations of these compounds were introduced over the succeeding years, and a few of them were found to be safe enough to subject them to clinical trials.

In 1931, Pearse and Warren used a 40% solution of Abrodil marketed under the trade name, Skiodan, for peripheral angiography with no markedly significant untoward reactions[86]. It soon began to replace sodium iodide as the contrast agent of choice but not for long. The arrival of Uroselectan B and Perabrodil soon replaced it. The utilization of these latter two compounds as angiographic media was not made possible until it was learned that they needed to be given in a highly concentrated solution. Uroselectan B (Neo-Ioprax) was marketed as a 75% solution for this purpose. In the late 1930s, Castellanos and associates[87], and

Robb and Steinberg[88,89]. conducted their angiographic studies with a 70% solution of Perabrodil (Diodrast). These agents continued to enjoy their popularity through the 1940s.

Despite the general acceptance of the organic iodide compounds, an effort was made to substitute an entirely different type of contrast agent. It was a particulate suspension of thorium dioxide known commercially as Thorotrast. It was originally introduced by Radt in 1929 for the liver and spleen[90,91]. This was made possible because of its affinity for the reticuloendothelial cells. It was this very property that caused concern among physicians because it was never eliminated, predisposing to the possibility of long term hazards resulting from its permanent residence in the reticuloendothelial cells. In fact, three years after its introduction the Council on Pharmacy and Chemistry of the American Medical Association voted that the compound not be accepted for intravenous administration[92].

Vernon Wallingford made the next major breakthrough in the development of angiographic contrast media. He investigated many of the triiodobenzoic acid derivatives. He was able to synthesize first the acetrizoates and later the diatrizoates and iothalamates[93]. These all have in common a benzene ring nucleus. All of the modern angiographic contrast media contain the triiodinated benzene ring as their basic structure. Urokon (sodium acetrizoate) was the first agent that he developed. It proved to be a very suitable contrast agent for intravenous pyelography. Nesbit and Lapides were the first to report this application in 1949 and 1950[94,95]. It had a very low toxicity with a high degree of contrast. When made up as a 70% solution, it became, during the 1950s, the contrast medium of choice for angiocardiography, aortography and venography. In the 1960s this agent was supplanted to a great extent by its congeners, the triiodinated benzoic acid derivatives. These proved to be far less toxic than those compounds containing the acetrizoate molecule.

Another contrast agent that did not gain much clinical acceptance in angiocardiography was carbon dioxide. It was introduced in 1955 by Stauffer and colleagues[96]. Since this produces a negative shadow in contrast to the relatively opaque surrounding tissues, Durant and Stauffer in 1957 combined carbon dioxide with a positive contrast agent[97]. This too did not generate much enthusiasm clinically.

Current radiopaque compounds are relatively free of significant toxic reactions due to the triiodinated benzene ring. Even large quantities can be injected without ill effect. It is true that anaphylactic reactions can still occur, but this too can be prevented with the prior administration of steroid derivatives and antihistamines.

Now that we have seen in some detail the historical development of the modern angiographic contrast agent, let us retrace our steps again and focus our attention on the evolution of clinical angiocardiography and its sequel, coronary arteriography.

As far back as 1931, Castellanos of Cuba applied the technique of injecting sodium iodide followed immediately by a chest X-ray in the diagnosis of congenital heart disease. The toxic reactions associated with sodium iodide caused him to discontinue his *in vivo* investigations. He continued to investigate the diagnostic potentialities of contrast visualization in cadavers. He resumed his studies in living humans when Diodrast, with much less toxicity, appeared. In 1932, Peter Rousthöi of Sweden demonstrated the coronary circulation in rabbits by injecting thorium dioxide into the proximal aorta[98]. He also showed that the catheter could be advanced in a retrograde fashion from the aorta into the left ventricle without damaging the aortic valve. This immediately assured the obsolescence of the complicated procedures previously described for gaining access to the left ventricle. In 1937, Castellanos and his group published the results of their studies on a number of congenital cardiac abnormalities utilizing Diodrast. This initial report was followed by a succession of papers between September of 1937 and July of 1938, elaborating on the technique and diagnostic criteria of many forms of congenital heart disease. Despite an automatic injection device which they designed, and which carefully regulated the amount of contrast being injected, their studies were hampered by two limitations. The first was inadequate opacification of the left heart chambers. This restricted their diagnostic ability to only those anomalies wherein the right chambers were involved. The second limitation was a temporary one. In their early investigations, their results were inconsistent in children over the age of 6. As the group gained more experience, however, the age window was extended to 14[99].

During this time, Robb and Steinberg were also involved in contrast studies. By January of 1939, they were able to report on their observations in 127 patients who were subjected to a total of 238 injections[89]. They used ether and cyanide circulation times as a guide to the timing of successive X-ray exposures. This approach resulted in films showing sequential opacification of the right and left heart. Thus, although Castellanos and his group attempted four chamber opacification, it was Robb and Steinberg who obtained consistently good results in all four chambers as well as the great vessels. Sussman's group, also from New York, designed a practical device for multiple exposures during angiocardiography. With the aid of this device, they were able to illustrate and report in 1941, the first angiocardiographic diagnosis of a case of Tetralogy of Fallot in the American literature. During the same year Fariñas, an associate of Castellanos, described a new technique for the arteriographic examination of the abdominal aorta and its branches[100]. Access to the aorta was gained by blunt dissection of the femoral artery followed by puncture of the artery with a trocar through which a catheter was passed. Two years before, Castellanos and Pereiras had already demonstrated the feasibility of retrograde brachial aortography. Fariñas' method opened the path for Seldinger's technique of percutaneous transfemoral catheterization which he introduced in 1953.

In 1945, Nathan Grossman demonstrated the feasibility of instilling substances directly into the coronary circulation without opening the chest[101]. He did this by inserting a ureteral catheter into the exposed right common carotid artery. The catheter tip was advanced to the ascending aorta just above the aortic valve. The contrast medium was injected into this area with no attempt made to enter the openings of either of the main coronary arteries. These experiments were carried out in dogs. The reader will recall Rousthöi's attempts with thorium dioxide in his animal experiments[98].

Radner of Lund, Sweden was the first to outline the coronary arteries in a human during life[102]. He entered the ascending aorta through a sternal puncture. This not only gave rise to significant complications but also failed to provide adequate visualization of the coronary arteries. Radner's work was followed by Meneses Hoyos and Gomez del Campo in 1948[103] and also by Jönnson during the same year[104].

The efforts of these early investigators represent the first period in the evolution of coronary arteriography. The results were abysmally poor,

inconsistent and fraught with danger; all preclusive for general clinical acceptance.

During the 1940s, a polyethylene catheter was introduced for clinical use in cardiac catheterization. Helmsworth and his colleagues at Cincinnati studied six patients with this new catheter inserted into the brachial artery and passed retrograde to the ascending aorta[105]. The results were presented by Helmsworth at the 50th Annual Meeting of the American Roentgen Ray Society. Although acknowledged to describe an interesting means of exploring the anatomy of the coronary arteries *in vivo*, the paper was greeted with marked reservations because of the perception that the procedure could prove to be quite hazardous. Harold Kolte, in his discussion of the paper, made the following remarks:

> Coronary angiography presents an intriguing problem. One cannot deny the importance of a method whereby narrowing or obstruction of the coronary arteries can be demonstrated. However, the technical difficulties of adequate filling and proper exposure may be hard to overcome. The danger of introducing a foreign, oxygen-free medium into a coronary circulation already seriously compromised by arteriosclerosis is probably great, and anginal pain, dangerous arrhythmias or sudden death are to be feared[105].

This perception was not unique to Kolte. His remarks were reflective of the general attitude prevailing at the time concerning contrast visualization of the coronary arteries.

The first monograph on non-selective coronary arteriography in the living was written in 1952 by DiGuglielmo and Guttadauro[106]. It was based on observations noted in 235 patients while they were working in Gunnar Jönnson's radiology department in Stockholm. The monograph was well illustrated with most of the X-ray films taken as the contrast medium was injected into the proximal ascending aorta via a catheter advanced in a retrograde fashion from the radial artery.

Following these early studies a second period ensued punctuated by experimental animal studies, and a search for a relatively innocuous method that selectively and satisfactorily visualized the coronary arteries[107–114]. However, deliberate selective visualization had to await the arrival of Sones in 1959. Prior to the introduction of Sones' technique, several avenues of approach were tried utilizing:

(1)   random 'brute force',

(2)   phasic injection,

(3)   reduction of cardiac output,

(4)   occlusion aortography, and

(5)   differential opacification of the aortic system.

Each one will be taken up in turn.

The earliest and most simple approach, as we have seen, was the random 'brute force' method. It consisted of flooding the aortic root with about 50 ml of contrast material in one or two seconds. The results were often inconsistent and lacking in detail. It did result in one important observation; better studies were produced when the injection took place during diastole. This led to the adoption of a phasic method of injection. Under electronic control, automatic high-pressure injections were made into the proximal aorta timed to begin with closure of the aortic valves and lasting throughout diastole.

In 1958, and again a year later, Arnulf explored the application of acetylcholine arrest as a method of reducing cardiac output in human coronary arteriography[115,116]. The contrast agent was injected into the ascending aorta as soon as asystole occurred. The patient was under general anesthesia throughout the entire procedure. He had to use atropine only once to restart the heart. Several American investigators pursued Arnulf's approach of deliberate temporary cardiac arrest. Among them were Lehman[117], Dotter and Frische[118], Gensini[119], Bilgutay and Lillehei[120]. Technical disadvantages, the large doses of acetylcholine, and the need for general anesthesia, were all considerably negative factors inherent in this approach. Arnulf's original technique imposed the additional danger and inefficiency of gaining entry into the aorta via a needle puncture. Although this last factor was circumvented later by substituting a percutaneous transfemoral approach, the procedure, in general, still left much to be desired.

Another method of reducing cardiac output was the intrabronchial pressure elevation technique. It was tried initially in animals by Boerema and Blickman in 1955[121]. Its application in clinical arteriography was reported by Dotter in 1960[122]. The technique was then investigated by Nordenstrom and Gensini[123–125]. The physiological principle underlying the procedure was a decrease in cardiac output caused by obstruction of the inflow of blood into the heart as the intrabronchial

pressure increased. Although it was based on a simple concept, its implementation had too many drawbacks because of the technical complexities and potential hazards.

Two years before Dotter reported his experience with the intrabronchial pressure elevation technique, he had also experimented with the occlusion aortographic approach. He occluded the aorta just above the openings of the two main coronary arteries with a double-lumen balloon catheter that he and Lukas had devised[126]. The balloon was inflated with carbon dioxide, sealing that part of the aorta just beneath it. Contrast agent was then injected into this temporary pocket and the agent would then drain off naturally into the openings of the coronary arteries. Occlusion aortography was also tried by Cannon and his co-workers at UCLA. They used a balloon-tipped, single end-hole catheter[127]. Gensini, too, tried this method, but rapidly abandoned it because its drawbacks were too many and too significant[128]. General anesthesia was necessary, and often, the aorta proved to be too large to be effectively sealed with the available balloon.

A different principle was adopted by Bellman and his associates in 1960[129]. This was a semi-selective method. They gained entry into the aorta of dogs through an exposed carotid or femoral artery. The exploring end of the catheter was preformed in the shape of a loop, and contained multiple radial holes arranged in a spiral manner. The tip of the catheter was straightened out over a spring guide while being advanced towards its target site. Once there, the guide spring was removed, and the tip allowed to resume its preformed loop. The jet of injected contrast agent issued from the holes towards the periphery of the bloodstream at the base of the aorta. This resulted in selective opacification of the coronary arteries. The group also reported their clinical experience with the loop-end catheter in the same issue of the *New England Journal of Medicine*[130]. In humans, the percutaneous transfemoral approach was used. Gensini recounts in his text that 'this ingenious technique never became popular because of the lack of a commercially available, professionally made loop-end catheter, which would have obviated the clumsiness and lack of standardization of homemade equipment'[131].

During all this time, technical advances in film taking were being made; all crucial for the successful implementation of Sones' technique for the visualization of the coronary arteries. These advances included the development of a rapid film changer by Gedlund, biplane film changers by Axen and Lind, the application of cineangiocardiography, and image intensification. Chamberlin was the first to suggest image intensification in 1942. Coltman developed it further and published his results in 1948. The following year Sturm and Morgan published their observations and helped pave the way for the general acceptance of image intensification in the late 1960s. The evaluation of ventricular volume utilizing biplane cinefluorography was described by Chapman in 1958. Biplane image amplified cineangiocardiography was also introduced in 1958 by Abrams.

Although selective visualization of the main branches of the aorta was suggested and practiced by Odman of Jönsson's group as far back as 1956, he made no mention when he reported this of attempting to catheterize the coronary arteries[132]. In fact, the general feeling was that the procedure should not be attempted because of the perceived possible adverse effects. During the late 1950s – the very place where selective coronary arteriography was to be developed – all investigators, including Sones, did their very best to avoid inserting the catheter into the coronary ostia. They attempted to augment opacification by placing the tip of the catheter as near as possible to the ostia, but never dared enter. It was during these investigations that Sones discovered while performing aortographic examinations in patients with rheumatic valvular disease, that some injections would preferentially fill one coronary artery without apparent ill-effect. This was a form of semi-selective coronary arteriography, and he pursued the usage of this methodology in further studies on dogs and then humans. He utilized a Gidlund pressure syringe so that he could inject the contrast agent into the aortic root under increased pressure. At times, he purposely directed the contrast into one of the sinuses of Valsalva. His initial experiences with this method were presented at the 32nd Scientific Session of the American Heart Association in Philadelphia in 1959.

Although Sones' paper at this meeting was concerned only with this form of semi-selective coronary arteriography, he had already begun his investigations on true selective coronary arteriography a year before. In fact, several months before the Philadelphia meeting, Sones had begun to work with a new catheter specially designed and made for him by the US Catheter and Instrument Company. The catheter had a preformed tapered tip that permitted easy entry into the coronary ostia without completely obstructing the artery.

This background on Sones' investigation along with his observations on 'deliberate selective opacification of individual coronary arteries in more than 1020 patients' is to be found in his paper entitled *Cine Coronary Arteriography*. It was published in July, 1962 by the American Heart Association in their monthly *Modern Concepts of Cardiovascular Disease*[133]. The opening paragraph of this landmark paper is worth reproducing since it underscored the need for the new technique, and established the basis for our current intervention procedures[133].

> During the past four years, the technique of cine coronary arteriography has been developed in an effort to provide a more objective and precise standard of diagnosis for human coronary artery disease. Heretofore, the diagnosis of coronary atherosclerosis has been primarily dependent on the physician's interpretation of the efforts of distressed patients to describe chest pain, and upon recognition of transient or chronic electrocardiographic changes which usually indicate the presence of myocardial ischemia or necrosis. Although conscientious, knowledgeable, history taking and electrocardiographic study require no apologist for their contributions to understanding, their limitations have been responsible, even in the hands of experts, for the production of iatrogenic disability on the one hand, and unjustified reassurance on the other, in a significant number of patients. A safe and dependable method for demonstrating the physical characteristics of the human coronary artery tree, which could be applied in any phase of the natural history of coronary artery disease, was needed to supplement available diagnostic methods.

The impact of Sones' paper was explosive to say the least. It demonstrated conclusively how ill-founded the previous perception was regarding the dangers of coronary arteriography, while acting as a stimulus for the rapid growth of the technique during the 1960s. The development of the tools permitting modern cardiac surgery such as the cardiopulmonary bypass machine, the improvements in anesthesia, and the evolution of myocardial revascularization established in conjunction with Sones' technique a heretofore unknown symbiosis between cardiologist and surgeon.

Sones' basic technique still survives practically unchanged in concept. The ensuing years have seen only modification of the catheter tip configuration to facilitate entrance into the coronary arteries. The percutaneous approach, especially the transfemoral one introduced by Judkins in 1967, and utilizing his pre-shaped catheters is currently the favored approach[134].

REFERENCES

1. Glasser, O. (1934). *Wilhelm Conrad Röntgen and the Early History of the Roentgen Rays.* (Springfield: Thomas)

2. Turner, G. L'E. (1975). Wilhelm Conrad Röntgen (Roentgen). In Gillepsie, Charles C. (ed.) *Dictionary of Scientific Biography*, pp. 529–531, vol. II. (New York: Charles Scribner's Sons)

3. Williams, F.H. (1896). Notes on X-rays in medicine. *Trans. Assoc. Am. Physicians*, **XI**, 375–82

4. Muir, A.I. (1987). Cardiac imaging 50 years on. Jubilee Editorial. *Br. Heart J.*, **58**, 1–5

5. Mackenzie, J. (1920). Chronic diseases of the heart. In Christian, H.A. and Mackenzie, J. (eds.) *The Oxford Medicine*, pp. 387–492. (Oxford: Oxford University Press)

6. Parkinson, J. (1933). Radiology of heart disease. *Br. Med. J.*, **2**, 591–4

7. Bramwell, C. (1933). Radiology in heart disease. *Br. Med. J.*, **2**, 597–9

8. Kerley, P. (1933). Radiology in heart disease. *Br. Med. J.*, **2**, 594–7

9. Roesler, H. (1937). *Clinical Roentgenology of the Cardiovascular Diseases.* (Springfield, Ill.: Charles C. Thomas)

10. Cournand, A. (1975). Cardiac catheterization. *Acta. Med. Scand. Suppl.*, **579**

11. *Ibid.*

12. Bechat, X. (1822). *Recherches Physiologiques sur la Vie et la mort. L'Imprimerie de L.T. Celot*, Paris, 4th. edn.

13. Buzzi, A. (1959). Claude Bernard on cardiac catheterization. *Am. J. Cardiol.*, **4**, 405

14. Bernard, C. (1879). *Lecons Physiologie Opératoire.* (Paris: J.B. Baillière et Fils)

15. Chauveau, A. and Faivre, B. (1856). *Nouvelles Recherches Experimentales sur les Mouvements et les Bruits Normaux du coeur Envisagés du Point de Vue de la Physiologie Medicale.* (Paris: J.B. Baillière et Fils)

16. Chauveau, A. and Marey, E.J. (1861). Détermination graphique du rapports du choc du coeur avec les mouvements des oreillettes et des ventricles: expérience faite à l'aide à un appareils enregistreur (sphygmographe). *Compt. rend. des Séances de l'Academie des Sciences LIII*, p. 622

17. Buisson, P.C. (1862). Quelques recherches sur la circulation du sang a l'aide d'appareils enregistreurs. *Faculté de Médecine de Paris*

18. Cournand, A. (1975). *Op. cit.*, p. 13

19. Chauveau, A. and Marey, E.J. (1863). Appareils et Expériences Cardiographiques: Demonstration nouvelle du mécanisme des mouvements du coeur par l'emploi des instruments enregistreurs à indications continues. *Mémoires de l'Academie de Médecine*, **26**, 268

20. Marey, E.J. (1863). *Physiologie Médicale de la Circulation du Sang.* (Paris: Delahaye)

21. Fick, A. (1873). Ueber die Schwankungen des Blutdruckes in verschiedenen Abschnitten des Gefass-Systems (Zum Theil nach Versuchen von D. Naceff aus Belgrad in Rumänien). *Vorhandl. der Wurzburg Physiol. Med. Gesellsch.*, N.B. IV, p. 223

22. Porter, W.T. (1892). Researches in the filling of the heart. *J. Physiol.*, **13**, 513

23. Rolleston, H.D. (1887). Observations on the endocardial pressure curve. *J. Physiol.*, **8**, 235

24. Roy, C.S. and Adams, J.G. (1890). Heart beat and pulse wave. *Practitioner*, **44**, 88, and **44**, 161

25. Frank, O. (1903). Kritik der elastischen Manometer. *Z. Biol.*, **44**, 445

26. Frank, O. (1905). Die puls in den arterien. *Z. Biol.*, **46**, 441

27. Wiggers, C.J. (1928). *The Pressure Pulse in the Cardiovascular System.* (New York: Longmans)

28. Fick, A. (1870). Über die Messung des Blutquantums in den Herzventrikeln. *Würzburg Physickalische-medizinische Gesellschaft*

29. Fishman, A.P. and Richards, D.W. (1964). *Circulation of the Blood – Men and Ideas*, pp. 96–7. (New York: Oxford Univ. Press)

30. Grehant, N. and Quinguaud, C.E. (1886). Recherches expérimentales sur la mesure du volume du sang qui traverse le poumon en un temps donné. *Compt. Rend. des Séances hebdo-madaires de la Société de Biologie*, tome 5, série 8, p. 159

31. Zuntz, N. (1893). Eine neue Method zur

Messung der circulierende Blutmenge und das Arbeit des Herzens. *Ebenda*, **IV**, 1

32. Zuntz, N. and Hagemann, O. (1898). Untersuchungen über den Stoffwechsel des Pferdes bei Ruhe und Arbeit. Landwirtschaftliche Jahrbücher, Zeitschrift für wissenschaftliche Landwirtschaft und Archiv der Königlich Preussischen Landes Ökonomie Collegiums. XXVII Band, Ergänzungsband III, pp. 1–438. (Berlin: Paul Parey Publisher)

33. Benatt, A.J. (1949). Cardiac catheterization. A historical note. *Lancet*, **2**, 746

34. Forssmann, W. (1929). Die Sondierung des Rechten Herzens. *Klin. Wochnschr.*, **8**, 2085

35. Howard-Jones, N. *Cardiac catheterization. A historical note*

36. Dieffenbach, J.F. (1832). Physiologisch chirurgische Beobachtungen bei Cholera-Kranken. *Cholera-Archiv.*, **1**, 86–105

37. Dieffenbach, J.F. (1834). Physiologisch-chirurgische Beobachtungen bei Cholera-Kranken. *Güstrow*, 2nd edn., p.IV

38. Benatt, A.J. (1949). *Op. cit.*, p. 746

39. Forssmann, W. (1931). Über Kontrastdarstellung der Höhlen des lebenden rechten Herzens und der Lungenschlagader. *Münch. Med. Wchnschr.*, **78**, 489

40. Klein, O. (1930). Zur Bestimmung des zirkulatorischen minutens Volumen nach dem Fickschen Prinzip (Gewinnung des gemischten venösen Blutes mittels Herzsondierung). *Münch. Med. Wchnschr.*, **77**, 1311

41. Jimenez Diaz, C. and Sanchez Cuenca, B. (1930). El Sondaage del Corazón Derechio. *Archivas de Cardiologfica y Hematologia*, vol. **11**

42. Jimenez Diaz, C. and Sanchez Cuenca (1930). Studios de Insuficiencia Circulatore. *Archivas de Cardiologia Y Hematologia*, vol. **11**

43. Padilla, O., Cossio, A. and Berconsky, I. (1932). Sondeo del Corazón; tecnica. *Semana Medica*, **21**, 79

44. Padilla, O., Cossio, A. and Berconsky, I. (1932). Sondeo del Corazón: la vena cava superior y el bordo derectio de la sombra de proyeccion de las grandes vasas de la base. *Semana Medica*, **2**, 391

45. Padilla, O., Cossio, A. and Berconsky, I. (1932). Sondeo del Corazón: determinación del Volumen Minuto Circulatorio. *Semana Medica*, **2**, 445

46. Padilla, O., Cossio, A. and Berconsky, I. (1932). Sondeo del Corazón: diversas tipos de circulacion periferica. *Semana Medica*, **2**, 645

47. Sourkes, T.L. (1966). *Nobel Prize Winners in Medicine and Physiology 1901–1965*. (New York: Abelard Schuman)

48. Cournand, A. (1975). *Op. cit.*, p. 24

49. *Ibid.*, p. 24

50. Cournand, A. and Ranges, H.A. (1941). Catheterization of the right auricle in man. *Proc. Soc. Exp. Biol. Med.*, **46**, 462

51. Lequime, J. (1988). Andre Cournand (1895–1988). His role in the development of modern cardiology. *Acta Cardiol.*, vol. **XLIII** (4), pp. 437–42

52. Cournand, A. (1975). *Op. cit.*, pp. 25–6

53. Brannon, E.S., Weens, H.S. and Warren, J.V. (1945). Atrial septal defect. Study of hemodynamics by the technique of right heart catheterization. *Am. J. Med. Sci.*, **210**, 480

54. Baldwin, E. de F., Moore, L.V. and Noble, R.P. (1946). The demonstration of ventricular septal defect by means of right heart catheterization. *Am. Heart J.*, **32**, 152

55. McMichael, J. and Sharpey-Schafer, E.P. (1944). The action of intravenous digoxin in man. *Q. J. Med.*, **13**, 1123

56. Carlson, P.A. (1980). Three contributors to cardiac catheterization. *J. Thorac. Cardiovasc. Surg.*, **79**, 782–8

57. Lenegre, J. and Maurice, P. (1944). Premiers recherchs sur la pression ventriculaire droite. *Bull. Mém. Soc. Méd. d'Hop. Paris*, **80**, 239

58. Lenegre, J. and Maurice, P. (1945). La derivation derecte intracavitaire des courants electriques de l'oreillette et du ventricule droit. *Paris Méd.*, **35**, 23

59. Dexter, L. *et al.* (1947). Studies of congenital heart disease. I. Technique of venous catheterization as a diagnostic procedure. *J. Clin. Invest.*, **26**, 547–53

60. *Ibid.*, II. (1947). The pressure and oxygen content of blood in the right auricle, right ventricle, and pulmonary artery in control patients, with observations on the oxygen saturation and source of pulmonary 'capillary' blood. *J. Clin. Invest.*, **26**, 554–60

61. *Ibid.*, III. (1947). Venous catheterization as a diagnostic aid in patent ductus arteriosus, tetralogy of Fallot, ventricular septal defect, and auricular septal defect. *J. Clin. Invest.*, **26**, 561–76

62. Zimmerman, H.A., Scott, R.W. and Becker, N.D. (1950). Catheterization of the left side of the heart in man. *Circulation*, **1**, 357–9

63. Limon-Lason, R. and Bouchard, A. (1950). El

cateterismo intracardico: cateterizacion de las cavidades iz quierdas en el hombre. Registro simultaneo de presion y electrocardiograma intracavetarios. *Arch. Inst. Cardiol. Mexico*, **21**, 271–85

64. Bing, R.J. (1952). Catheterization of the heart. *Adv. Intern. Med.*, **5**, 59–141

65. Bjork, V.O., Malmstrom, G. and Uggla, L.G. (1953). Left auricular pressure measurements in man. *Ann. Surg.*, **138**, 718–25

66. Ricketts, J.H. and Abrams, H.L. (1962). Percutaneous selective coronary arteriography. *J. Am. Med. Assoc.*, **181**, 620–4

67. Judkins, M.P. (1967). Selective coronary arteriography: a percutaneous transfemoral technique. *Radiology*, **89**, 815–24

68. Shirey, E.K. (1966). Retrograde transaortic and mitral valve catheterization for physiological and morphological evaluation of the left side of the heart. *Circulation*, **34** (Suppl.) III-216–III-217

69. Zimmerman, H. (1975). Then and Now. *Catheterization Cardiovasc. Diagn.*, **1**, 3–5

70. Lower, R. (1932). *Tractatus de Corde item de Motu & Colore Sanguinis*, Franklin, K.J., translator. (Oxford: Oxford University Press)

71. Haschek, E. and Lindenthal, O.T. (1896). Ein Beitrag zur praktischen verwerthung der Photographie nach Röntgen. *Wiener Klin. Wochenschr.*, **9**, 63

72. Killen, D.A. (1973). Angiographic contrast media: a historical résumé. *Surgery*, **73**, 336–46

73. Destot, Bérard (1896). Les rayons X appliqués à la découverte des circulations artérielles viscérales. *Lyon Med.*, **83**, 445

74. Stirling, W.B. (1957). *Aortography*. (Edinburgh, London: E. & S. Livingston, Ltd)

75. Musgrove. C.I. (1899). A radiograph of an injected full-term foetus. *J. Anat. Physiol.*, **33**, 672

76. Baumgarten, W. (1899). Infarction in the heart. *Am. J. Physiol.*, **2**, 243

77. Jamin, F. and Merkel, H. (1907). *Die Koronarterien des menschlichen Herzens unter normalen und pathologischen Verhältnissen*. (Jena: Gustave Fischer)

78. Franck and Alwens (1910). Kreislaufstudien im Röntgenschirm. *Munch. Med. Wochenschr.*, **57**, 950

79. Schepelmann (1910). Ueber Blutgefässchatten im Röntgenbilde munchen. *Med. Wochenschr.*, **57**, 1614 (cited by Edwards)

80. Sicard, J.A. and Forestier, J. (1921). Méthode radiographique d'exploration de la cavité épidurale par la lipiodol. *Rev. Neurol.*, **28**, 1264

81. Berberich, J. and Hirsch, S. (1923). Die röntgenographische Darstellung der Arterien und Venen am lebenden Menschen. *Klin. Wochenschr.*, **2**, 2226

82. Osborne, E.D., Sutherland, C.G., Scholl, A.J. Jr and Rowntree, L.G. (1923). Roentgenography of urinary tract during excretion of sodium iodide. *J. Am. Med. Assoc.*, **80**, 368

83. Sicard, J.A. and DeGennes, Coste (1924). Radiodiagnostic lipiodole de la thrombose arterielle. *Bull. Mem. Soc. Méd. Hôp. Paris Ser. 3*, **31**, 1483

84. Brooks, B. (1924). Intra-arterial injection of sodium iodide. *J. Am. Med. Assoc.*, **82**, 1016

85. Moniz, E., Pinto, A. and Lima, A. (1932). Die Vorzügedes Thorotrast bei arterieller Enzephalographie. *Röntgenpraxis*, **4**, 90

86. Pearse, H.E. and Warren, S.L. (1931). The röntgenographic visualization of the arteries in peripheral vascular disease. *Ann. Surg.*, **94**, 1094

87. Castellanos, A., Pereiras, R. and Garcia, A. (1937). La angio-cardiografia radio-opaca. *Arch. Soc. Estud. Clin. Habaña*, **31**, 523

88. Robb, G.P. and Steinberg, I. (1938). A practical method of visualization of the chambers of the heart, the pulmonary circulation, and the great vessels in man. *J. Clin. Invest.*, **17**, 507

89. Robb, G.P. and Steinberg, I. (1939). Visualization of the chambers of the heart, the pulmonary circulation, and the great blood vessels in man. *Am. J. Roentgenol.*, **41**, 1

90. Radt, P. (1929). Eine Methode der röntgenologischen Kontrastdarstellung von Milz und Leber. *Klin. Wochenschr.*, **8**, 2128

91. Radt, P. (1930). Eine neue Methode sur Röntgenologischen Sichtharmachung von Leber und Milz durch Injektion eines Kontrastmittels. *Med. Klin.*, **26**, 1888

92. Leech, P.N. (1932). Thorotrast (report of the Council on Pharmacy and Chemistry), *J. Am. Med. Assoc.*, **99**, 2183

93. Wallingford, V.H. (1943). The development of organic iodine compounds as X-ray contrast media. *Am. Pharm. Assoc. J.*, **42**, 721

94. Nesbit, R.M. and Lapides, J. (1949). Urokon, a new excretory pyelographic medium. *Mich. Univ. Hosp. Bull.*, **15**, 43

95. Nesbit, R.M. and Lapides, J. (1950). Observations on Urokon, a new excretory pyelographic medium. *Mich. Univ. Med. Bull.*, **16**, 37

96. Stauffer, H.M., Oppenheimer, M.J., Durant, T.M. and Lynch, P.R. (1955). Experimental

demonstration of cardiac structure and function by gas-contrast roentgen cinematograph. *Clin. Res. Proc.*, **3**, 107

97. Durant, T.M., Stauffer, H.M., Oppenheimes, M.J. and Paul, R.E. Jr (1957). The safety of intravascular carbon dioxide and its use for roentgenologic visualization of intracardiac structures. *Ann. Intern. Med.*, **47**, 191

98. Rousthöi, P. (1933). Über angiokardiographie vorläufige mitteilung. *Acta Radiol.*, **14**, 419

99. Abrams, H.L. (1964). Angiocardiography and thoracic aortography. In Brewer, A.J. (ed.) *Classic Descriptions in Diagnostic Roentgenology*, vol. 1, p. 492. (Springfield: Charles C. Thomas)

100. Fariñas, P.L. (1941). A new technique for the arteriographic examination of the abdominal aorta and its branches. *Am. J. Roentgenol.*, **46**, 641

101. Grossman, N. (1945). Visualization of the coronary arteries in dogs. *Am. J. Roentgenol.*, **54**, 57

102. Radner, S. (1945). Attempt at roentgenologic visualization of coronary blood vessels in man. *Acta Radiol.*, **26**, 497–502

103. Meneses Hoyos, J. and Gomez del Campo, C. (1948). Angiography of thoracic aorta and coronary vessels with direct injection of opaque solution in aorta. *Radiology*, **50**, 211–3

104. Jönsson, G. (1948). Visualization of coronary arteries: preliminary report. *Acta Radiol.*, **29**, 536–40

105. Helmsworth, J.A., McGuire, J. and Felson, B. (1950). Arteriography of the aorta and its branches by means of the polyethylene catheter. *Am. J. Roentgenol.*, **64**, 196

106. DiGuglielmo, L. and Guttadauro, M. (1952). A roentgenologic study of the coronary arteries in the living. *Acta Radiol. Suppl.*, **97**, 1–82

107. Pearl, F., Friedman, M., Gray, N. and Friedman, B. (1950). Coronary arteriography in intact dog. *Circulation*, **1**, 1188–92

108. Helmsworth, J.A., McGuire, J. and Felson, B. (1950). Arteriography of aorta and its branches by means of polyethylene catheter. *Am. J. Roentgenol.*, **64**, 196–213

109. Cannon, J.A., Clifford, C.A., Diesh, G. and Barker, W.F. (1956). Accurate diagnostic coronary arteriography in the dog. *Surg. Forum*, **6**, 197–9

110. Hughes, C.R., Sartorius, H. and Kolff, W.J. (1956). Angiography of coronary arteries in the live dog. *Cleveland Clin. Q.*, **23**, 251–5

111. Miller, E.W., Hughes, C.R. and Kolff, W.J. (1957). Angiography of the coronary arteries in the live dog. II Detecting abnormalities. *Cleveland Clin. Q.*, **24**, 41–50

112. Miller, E.W., Kolff, W.J. and Hughes, C.R. (1957). Angiography of the coronary arteries in dogs. III Lung perfusion with a heart-lung machine in combination with cardiac arrest in coronary artery surgery. *Cleveland. Clin. Q.*, **24**, 123–7

113. Anlyan, W.G., Baylin, G.J., Fabrikant, J.I. and Trumbo, R.B. (1959). Studies in coronary angiography. *Surgery*, **45**, 8–18

114. Nelson, S.W., Molnar, W., Christoforidis, A. and Britt, C. (1960). Coronary arteriography: development of a method in animals with particular attention to physiologic effects. *Radiology*, **75**, 34–49

115. Arnulf, G. (1958). L'artériographie méthodique des artères cornoaries grâce l'utilisation de l'acétylcholine. Données expérimentales et clinique. *Bull. Acad. Natl. Med.*, **142,** 661–7

116. Arnulf, G. and Buffard, P. (1959). Artériographie des coronaries grâce à l'acétylcholine. *Ann. Radiol.*, **2**, 685–701

117. Lehman, J.S., Boyer, R.A. and Winter, R.A. (1959). Coronary arteries. *Am. J. Roentgenol.*, **81**, 749–63

118. Dotter, C.T. and Frische, L.H. (1958). Visualization of the coronary circulation by occlusion aortography: a practical method. *Radiology*, **71**, 50

119. Gensini, G.G., Di Giorgi and Black, A. (1961). New approaches to coronary arteriography. *Angiology*, **12**, 223–38

120. Bilgutay, A.M. and Lillehei, C. (1962). New method for coronary arteriography: acetycholine asystole with controlled return of heart rate using a cardiac pacemaker. *J. Am. Med. Assoc.*, **180**, 1095–9

121. Boerema, I. and Blickman, J.R. (1955). Reduced intrathoracic circulation as an aid in angiocardiography: an experimental study. *J. Thorac. Surg.*, **80**, 129–42

122. Dotter, C.T., Veatch, W., Wishart, W. and Dotter, P. (1960). The effects of specific gravity upon the distribution of cardiovascular contrast agents. *Circulation*, **22**, 1144–8

123. Nordenstrom, B., Overtors, C.O. and Tornell, G. (1962). Coronary angiography of 100 cases of ischemic heart disease. *Radiology*, **78**, 714–24

124. Nordenstrom, B. (1960). Contrast examination of the cardiovascular system during increased intrabronchial pressure. *Acta. Radiol. Sto. Suppl.*, **200**, 1–110

125. Gensini, G.G. and Ecker, A. (1960). Percutaneous aortocerebral angiography. A diagnostic and physiologic method. *Radiology*, **75**, 885–93

126. Dotter, C.T. and Lukas, D.S. (1950). Cor pulmonale: an experimental study utilizing a special cardiac catheter. *Proc. Am. Fed. Clin. Res.*, **6**, 48

127. Cannon, J.A., Clifford, C.A., Diesh, G. and Barker, W. (1955). Accurate diagnostic coronary arteriography in the dog. *Surg. Forum*, **6**, 197

128. Gensini, G.G. (1975). *Coronary Arteriography*, p. 6. (Mt. Kisco, NY: Futura Publishing Co.)

129. Bellman, S., Frank, H.A., Lambert, P.B., Littman, D. and Williams, J.A. (1960). Coronary arteriography. I. Differential opacification of the aortic stream by catheters of special design: experimental development. *N. Engl. J. Med.*, **262**, 325–8

130. Williams, J.A., Littmann, D., Hall, J.H., Bellman, S., Lambert, P.B. and Frank, H.A. (1960). Coronary arteriography. II. Clinical experiences with loop-end catheter. *N. Engl. J. Med.*, **262**, 328–32

131. Gensini, G.G. (1975). *Op. cit.*, p. 7

132. Odman, P. (1956). Percutaneous selective angiography of the main branches of the aorta. *Acta Radiol.*, **45**, 1

133. Sones, F.M. Jr and Shirey, E.K. (1962). Cine coronary arteriography. *Mod. Concepts Cardiovasc. Dis.*, **31**, 735–8

134. Judkins, M.P. (1967). Selective coronary artiography. I. A percutaneous transfemoral technique. *Radiology*, **89**, 815–24

26   Echocardiography

Ultrasonic ocean floor detectors were developed during World War II and were quite useful for tracking the ubiquitous German submarine. The concept proved to be quite appealing to Dr Inge Edler in its potential application towards the visualization of cardiac structures. He was already aware of its usage in attempting to locate brain tumors. In pursuing this goal, he called upon Dr Helmuth Hertz, the physicist, to help conduct the initial investigations. The project was begun with a sonar device borrowed from a local shipyard and with Dr Hertz recording the echoes from his own heart. These early observations aroused their interest to the extent that Edler and Hertz jointly designed a modified version of the borrowed device and then successfully prevailed upon a medical electronics firm to construct a prototype. It was called an 'ultrasonic reflectoscope', and for several years, it served as the means for the extensive exploration of cardiac echoes and their genesis[1–3].

Their initial report appeared in 1954 and addressed itself towards the continuous recording of the movements of the heart walls[1]. Two years later, Edler and Hertz described the ultrasound cardiogram in mitral valvular diseases[3]. They thought they were recording echoes from the left atrial wall and that the various patterns from these recordings were sufficiently distinct and different to allow them to diagnose the presence of mitral stenosis. Further studies revealed that the echoes were really arising from the anterior leaflet of the mitral valve. Edler, on his own and then in conjunction with colleagues, pursued further anatomical and physiological studies which were instrumental in identifying the origin of the various echo patterns. In 1961, they reported an experimental study that led specifically to the proper labeling of aortic and mitral valve movements[4,5].

It was but a few short years between this latest study by Edler and his initial paper in 1954, but, by this time, the new technique had captured the interest of several investigators throughout Europe.

From among these converts, the most extensive studies were those originating from Effert's laboratory in Germany. He and his group published their original paper in 1957[6] stressing the diagnostic value of 'ultrasonic cardiography'. Another paper on the diagnostic value of ultrasound in cardiac diseases was published by him and another group of associates in 1964[7]. Effert's team visited the USA in the early 1960s. It was during a visit to Dr Claude Joyner's laboratory that they easily convinced him of the clinical potentialities of ultrasound and of its non-hazardous nature. Joyner was a radiologist, and he was soon joined in this interest by Gramiak, another radiologist. Both men foresaw the development of the technique within the boundaries of radiology. For years, there was an acrimonious debate as to who should be responsible for the clinical application of echocardiography, the radiologist or the cardiologist. It was finally resolved in favor of the cardiologist.

Echocardiography was looked upon, initially, mainly as a means of assessing mitral stenosis or diagnosing the rare case of atrial myxoma. The pioneering efforts of the early European investigators helped to remove this perception somewhat but in America, realization of its usefulness in many cardiac disorders was attributable primarily to the well-designed studies of Harvey Feigenbaum. He attracted many young cardiologists to his basement laboratory at the Krannert Institute in Indiana. Many of these young men, armed with their newly acquired knowledge, set up their own investigative centers and their own training programs. It is a tribute to Feigenbaum's integrity, enthusiasm for teaching and altruism, that this was made possible. Feigenbaum has been called the father of American echocardiography and rightfully so.

He wrote the first American text on the subject. It was a small book but a treasure house of information based mostly on his personal observations. Sonya Chang was his technologist during these formative years, and the quality of her work still remains unsurpassed. She, too, subsequently wrote a text on echocardiography. It was written for her fellow technologists. All of the echoes at the time were obtained in the so-called M-mode. These patterns bore no relationship to the true anatomical make-up of any of the cardiac structures, making it all the more remarkable for these early investigators to correlate the patterns with physiological and pathophysiological events.

The 1970s saw a phenomenal explosion of interest and studies in both the clinical and technical aspects of echocardiography. The American College of Cardiology now began to assign at its annual convention entire sections devoted to the presentation of papers dealing with the subject. The authors of the vast majority of these papers were Feigenbaum's former trainees who were now becoming leaders in their own right. Commercial instrument makers, initially small and dedicated, now began to play a greater role in refining the technical capabilities of their equipment. Many of these companies leased individual booths at the conventions exhibiting their latest products, and enticing the professional to buy a machine for the office. Echocardiography was now becoming a standard component of cardiac evaluation. Unfortunately, my generation of cardiologists began to see the increasing popularity of the technique occurring at the expense of the skills in physical diagnosis. This trend appears to have abated somewhat in that physical diagnosis has re-established itself as an important complementary element in the overall evaluation, working hand in hand with the capability and accuracy of current instrumentation.

The two main drawbacks of M-mode echocardiography, namely, the so-called 'ice pick' view, and the inability to visualize the true anatomy, were overcome by the introduction of what is now termed '2-D echocardiography'.

A spatially oriented M-mode examination can be obtained by tracking electronically the spatial orientation of the transducer. This type of approach was first used in Japan[8]. Another approach for the creation of a cross-sectional image is the one that tracks the ultrasonic beam to create a spatially oriented B-mode. This rapid B-mode scan is also known as a 'real-time' scan[9]. Today, the real-time B-mode scan is commonly called 'cross-sectional' or 'two dimensional' echocardiography. A good deal of confusion in terminology existed before the

adoption of this term by the American Society of Echocardiography. One of the first investigators labeled it 'ultrasonic cinematography'[10]. Terms favored by subsequent investigators included 'cine ultrasound cardiography' by Gramiak[11], 'ultrasonic tomography' suggested by Kratochwil and his associates[12], a tongue twister, 'ultrasonocardiotomography' adopted by Ebina[13], 'cardiac ultrasonography', offered by King[14], and lastly, 'ultrasonic cardiokymography' advanced by Nagayama's group[15]. Fortunately, the standard terminology today is the previously mentioned 'cross-sectional' or '2-dimensional'.

Two types of real-time, two-dimensional scanners were developed: mechanical and electronic. The mechanical scanners used an electric motor to move the ultrasonic beam within a given angle[11–13]. Another mechanical system using a mirror was developed independently by A. Asberg in 1967 and later by C. Hertz and K. Lundstrom[14,16]. Both approaches failed to achieve any commercial success, and are no longer available.

Two variations of electronic real-time scanners were introduced in an effort to improve upon the mechanical device. The first practical one to become commercially available was the multi-element linear array transducer. The ultrasonic beam could be moved in a linear fashion by firing the elements in a sequential manner. Three groups, working independently of each other, reported their experience with this transducer between the years 1971 and 1977. The principals involved included a group from the Netherlands headed by Bom[17,18], Yoshikawa and his associates from Japan[19], and the Scandinavian team of Pedersen and Northeved[20]. The early enthusiasm for two-dimensional echocardiography was due primarily to the highly satisfactory images obtained with this device. The original scanner has undergone many refinements. Despite these improvements, its principal disadvantage, the necessity for a large acoustic window, continues to plague the industry. Since the probe is quite large so that it must overlie the ribs, it cannot be angled easily in the plane of the scan axis.

The other real-time scanner utilizes the phased array principle. It was introduced and developed primarily by von Ramm, Thurstone and Kisslo[21–24]. The scanner also uses a multi-element transducer which, however, creates a single electronic beam. It was soon determined that a computer or microprocessor could control the sequential firing of each element, and thus it was possible to control the direction of the ultrasonic beam. This device has become the most popular of the real-time scanners. Comparatively speaking, it has more advantages than disadvantages with respect to the mechanical scanner. Its most important advantage is its ability to get a wide-angle scan through a small acoustic window. The phased array technology, because of the random access available through electronic steering, also paved the way for the simultaneous recording of Doppler and two-dimensional echocardiography.

Doppler echocardiography has become an important component of the complete echocardiographic evaluation. It is based on the Doppler effect which was first described by Christian Johann Doppler in 1842. He demonstrated that the frequency of sound reflected from an object is altered if that object is moving. An example would be a person hearing a higher-pitched note if the sound source is moving toward him and a lower-pitched note if it is moving away from him. The Doppler effect is, in essence then, this change or shift in frequency in relation to the direction of movement of its source. Blood cell movements also produce a Doppler shift of ultrasound frequencies. The extent and direction of shift of the ultrasound frequency are related to the velocity and direction of blood flow.

As the technique was being developed, cardiologists rapidly became aware of its potentialities as a method for evaluating the manner in which blood moves through the cardiovascular system. Both laminar and turbulent flow patterns can be detected. Turbulent flow occurs when blood is flowing across an obstruction or a narrowed area.

Laminar flow lends itself quite readily to Doppler assessment of blood velocity[25]. This ability was very instrumental in fueling the interest for investigating further the precise role of Doppler echocardiography in the estimation of pressure changes across an orifice[26–28]. This led several investigators to introduce a modified Bernoulli formula as a means of relating velocity distal to a narrowed orifice to the pressure gradient across that orifice[27–30].

One of the major limitations of Doppler echocardiography was the lack of an adequate graphic display. This had to be overcome before the technique could realize its full potential as a non-invasive diagnostic tool. Two groups of investigators led respectively by De Maria with Mason[31] and

Burckhardt[32], helped to resolve the problem by introducing the fast Fourier transform approach for displaying the Doppler signal. This results in a spectral display that has now become the dominant type of Doppler recording.

Another important development was the combination of Doppler and two-dimensional echocardiography for color flow mapping. A good deal of the original investigations came from the Japanese groups led by Omoto and Miyatake[33–36]. Ever since its introduction, it has enjoyed an ever increasing popularity for the demonstration of blood flow patterns through the cardiac chambers, in the blood vessels, both venous and arterial, and across intracardiac and extracardiac shunts.

Computers have also played an important role in the evolution of echocardiography. First of all, the development of more powerful microprocessors capable of digitally manipulating the new scan converters, has considerably enhanced the quality of the image. Computers were introduced that enabled the echocardiographer to obtain a continuous cine loop presentation of a single cardiac cycle which has proven invaluable in detecting abnormalities of myocardial wall motion. Still other computer derived benefits include

(1) the ability to display simultaneously multiple views of the heart so that side by side comparisons of sequential studies can be made;

(2) the ability to store images on relatively inexpensive floppy disks with no loss of resolution as one would expect from videotapes; and

(3) the ability to manipulate the image so as to enhance definition of desired structures such as endocardial or epicardial borders.

Although echocardiography was introduced and popularized as an accurate non-invasive procedure without hazard, recent developments have seen increasing usage in an invasive setting. Small transducers have been placed at the tip of cardiac catheters so that intracardiac recordings are now possible. This approach was reported by Glassman and Conti's group[37,38]. Schluter and Hisanaga were the first to describe transesophageal echocardiography. This provides images of the heart not distorted by ribs or lungs. They obtained their images by placing a two-dimensional transducer on a fiberoptic endoscope[39–42]. It is rapidly becoming an increasingly popular approach as the indications for its use continue to expand. Transesophageal echocardiography was also suggested by Topol, Dubroff and Ren as a means of monitoring patients during surgery, especially cardiac surgery, and in the immediate post-operative period[43–45].

REFERENCES

1. Edler, I. and Hertz, C.H. (1954). The use of ultrasonic reflectoscope for the continuous recording of the movements of heart walls. *Kungl. Fysiogr. Sällsk. i Lund Förhandl.*, **24**, 5

2. Edler, I. (1955). The diagnostic use of ultrasound in heart disease. *Acta Med. Scand. Suppl.*, **308**, 32

3. Edler, I. and Hertz, C.H. (1956). Ultrasound cardiogram in mitral valvular diseases. *Acta Chir. Scand.*, **111**, 230

4. Edler, I. (1961). The use of ultrasound as a diagnostic aid and its effects on biological tissues. Continuous recording of the movement of various heart structures using an ultrasound echo method. *Acta Med. Scand. Suppl.*, **370**, 7

5. Edler, I., Gustafson, A., Karlefors, T. *et al.* (1961). Mitral and aortic valve movements recorded by an ultrasonic echo method: an experimental study. *Acta Med. Scand. Suppl.*, **370**, 68

6. Effert, S., Erkerus, H.. and Grosse-Brockhoff, F. (1957). Ueber die Anwendung des Ultrashall echoverfahrens in der Herzdiagnostick. *Dtsch. Med. Wochenschr.*, **82**, 1253

7. Effert, S., Bleifeld, W., Deapmann, F.J. *et al.* (1964). Diagnostic value of ultrasonic cardiography. *Br. J. Radiol.*, **37**, 920

8. Matsumoto, M., Matsuo, H., Ohara, T. and Abe, H. (1977). Use of kymo-two-dimensional echocardiography for the diagnosis of aortic root dissection and mycotic aneurysm of the aortic root. *Ultrasound Med. Biol.*, **3**, 153

9. Eggleston, R.C. *et al.* (1975). Visualization of cardiac dynamics with real-time B-mode ultrasonic scanner. In White, D. (ed.) *Ultrasound in Medicine*. (New York: Plenum Press)

10. Asberg, A. (1967). Ultrasonic cinematography of the living heart. *Ultrasonics*, **6**, 113

11. Griffith, J.M. and Henry, W.L. (1974). A sector scanner for real time two-dimensional echocardiography. *Circulation*, **49**, 1147

12. Eggleton, R.C. *et al.* (1975). Visualization of cardiac dynamics with real-time B-mode ultrasonic scanner. In White, D. (ed.) *Ultrasound in Medicine*. (New York: Plenum Press)

13. Ebina, T. *et al.* (1967). The ultrasonotomography of the heart and great vessels in living human subjects by means of the ultrasonic reflection technique. *Jpn. Heart J.*, **8**, 331

14. Asberg, A. (1967). *Op. cit.*, ref. 10

15. Nagayama, T., Nakamura, S., Hayakawa, K. and Komo, Y. (1962). Ultrasonic cardiokymogram. *Acta. Med. U. Kagoshima*, **4**, 229

16. Hertz, C.H. and Lundstrom, K. (1972). A fast ultrasonic scanning system for heart investigation. *3rd. International Conference on Medical Physics*. (Sweden: Gotenburg)

17. Bom, N., Lancee, C.T., Honkoop, J. and Hugenholtz, P.C. (1971). Ultrasonic viewer for cross-sectional analyses of moving cardiac structures. *Biomed. Eng.*, **6**, 500

18. Bom, N., Lancee, C.T., Van Zwieten, G., Kloster, F.E. and, Roelandt, J. (1973). Multiscan echocardiography. I. Technical description. *Circulation*, **48**, 1066

19. Yoshikawa, J. *et al.* (1977). Electroscan echocardiography: application to the cardiac diagnosis. *J. Cardiogr.*, **7**, 33

20. Pedersen, J.F. and Northeved, A. (1977). An ultrasonic multitransducer scanner for real-time heart imaging. *J. Clin. Ultrasound*, **5**, 11

21. Morgan, C.L., Trought, W.S., Clark, W.M., Von Ramm, O.T. and Thurstone, F.L. (1978). Principles and applications of a dynamically focused phased array real time ultrasound system. *J. Clin. Ultrasound*, **6**, 385

22. Von Ramm, O.T. and Thurstone, F.L. (1975). Thaumascan: design considerations and performance characteristics. In White, D (ed.) *Ultrasound in Medicine*. (New York: Plenum Press)

23. Kisslo, J.A., Von Ramm, O.T. and Thurstone, F.L. (1977). Dynamic cardiac imaging using a focused, phased array ultrasound system. *Am. J. Med.*, **63**, 61

24. Von Ramm, O.T. and Thurstone, F.L. (1976). Cardiac imaging using a phased array ultrasound system. *Circulation*, **53**, 258

25. Hatle, L. and Angelsen, B. (1984). *Ultrasound in Cardiology: Physical Principles and Clinical Applications*, 2nd edn. (Philadelphia: Lea and Febiger)

26. Baker, D.W., Rubinstein, S.A. and Lorch, G. (1977). Pulsed Doppler echocardiography: principles and applications. *Am. J. Med.*, **63**, 69

27. Hatle, L., Brubakk, A., Tromsdal, A. and

Angelsen, B. (1978). Noninvasive assessment of pressure drop in mitral stenosis by Doppler ultrasound. *Br. Heart J.*, **40**, 131

28. Hatle, L., Angelsen, B. and Tromsdal, A. (1979). Noninvasive assessment of aortic stenosis by Doppler ultrasound. *Br. Heart J.*, **43**, 284

29. Stam, R.B. and Martin, R.P. (1983). Quantification of pressure gradients across stenotic valves by Doppler ultrasound. *J. Am. Coll. Cardiol.*, **2**, 707

30. Berger, M., Berdoff, R.L., Gallerstein, P.E. and Goldberg, E. (1984). Evaluation of aortic stenosis by continuous wave Doppler ultrasound. *J. Am. Coll. Cardiol.*, **3**, 150

31. Bommer, W.J., Miller, L.R., Mason, D.T. and DeMaria, A.N. (1978). Enhancement of pulsed Doppler echocardiography in the evaluation of aortic valve disease by the development of computerized spectral frequency analysis. *Circulation* (Suppl. II) Abstr., **58**, 187

32. Burckhardt, C.B. (1981). Comparison between spectrum and time interval histogram of ultrasound Doppler signals. *Ultrasound Med. Biol.*, **7**, 79

33. Omoto, R. (1984). *Color Atlas of Real-Time Two-Dimensional Doppler Echocardiography.* (Tokyo: Shindan-To-Chiryo Co. Ltd)

34. Miyatake, K., Okamoto, M., Kinoshita, N., Izumi, S., Owa, M., Takao, S., Sakakibara, H. and Nimura, Y. (1984). Clinical applications of a new type of real-time two-dimensional Doppler flow imaging system. *Am. J. Cardiol.*, **54**, 857

35. Omoto, R., Yokote, Y., Takamoto, S., Kyo, S., Wuda, K., Asano, H., Namekawa, K., Kasai, C., Kondo, Y. and Koyano, A. (1984). The development of real-time two-dimensional Doppler echocardiography and its clinical significance in acquired valvular regurgitation. *Jpn. Heart J.*, **25**, 325

36. Brandestini, M.A., Eyer, M.K. and Stevenson, J.G. (1979). M/Q-mode echocardiography. The synthesis of conventional echo with digital multigate Doppler. In Lancee, C.T. (ed.) *Echocardiography.* (The Hague: Martinus Nijhoff)

37. Glossman, F. and Krouzon, I. (1981). Transvenous intracardiac echocardiography. *Am. J. Cardiol.*, **47**, 1255

38. Conetta, D.A., Christie, L.G. Jr, Pepine, C.J., Nichols, W.W. and Conti, C.R. (1979). Intracardiac M-mode echocardiography for continuous left ventricular monitoring: method and potential application. *Cathet. Cardiovasc. Diagn.*, **5**, 135

39. Hisanaga, K., Hisanaga, A., Hibi, N., Nishimura, K. and Kambe, T. (1980). High-speed rotating scanner for transesophageal cross-sectional echocardiography. *Am. J. Cardiol.*, **46**, 837

40. Hisanaga, K., Hisanaga, A., Nagata, K. and Ichie, Y. (1980). Transesophageal echocardiography. *Am. Heart J.*, **100**, 605

41. Schluter, M. *et al.* (1982). Transesophageal cross-sectional echocardiography with phased array transducer system. Technique and initial clinical results. *Br. Heart J.*, **48**, 67

42. Schluter, M. et al. (1982). Assessment of transesophageal pulsed Doppler echocardiography in the detection of mitral regurgitation. *Circulation*, **66**, 784

43. Topol, E.J. *et al.* (1984). Immediate improvement of dysfunctional myocardial segments after coronary revascularization: detection by intraoperative transesophageal echocardiography. *J. Am. Coll. Cardiol.*, **4**, 1123

44. Dubroff, J.M., Clark, M.B., Wong, C.Y.H., Spotnitz, A.J., Collins, R.H. and Spotnitz, H.M. (1983). Left ventricular ejection fraction during cardiac surgery: a two-dimensional echocardiographic study. *Circulation*, **68**, 95

45. Ren, J.F. et al. (1985). Effect of coronary bypass surgery and valve replacement on left ventricular function: assessment by intraoperative two-dimensional echocardio-graphy. *Am. Heart J.*, **109**, 281

27   Nuclear imaging techniques

The beginnings of nuclear cardiology are to be found in the studies on the velocity of blood flow conducted by H. L. Blumgart and S. Weiss in 1927[1]. They measured the circulation time by injecting into an arm vein a dose of radium C salt and determined its arrival in the opposite arm by recording the radioactivity at this location with a Wilson cloud chamber. This method of tracing the transmigration of a radioactive substance was based upon experiments conducted by G. Hevesey in 1923 on the absorption and translocation of lead in plants[2]. No further exploration of this method was noted until 1948 when Myron Prinzmetal announced his technique of 'radiocardiography' for determining circulation time and for recording the passage of radioactivity through the heart and lungs[3]. In essence, Prinzmetal's work was a repetition of the experiments carried out by Blumgart and Weiss. He used radioactive sodium chloride. Although the method had its limitations, Prinzmetal suggested it could be used as a means of evaluating left ventricular function and in the detection of shunts. Radioactive sodium chloride emits gamma rays at high energies, and cannot be used as a specific marker for blood. In measuring radioactivity, Prinzmetal was restricted to the Geiger-Muller tube which is primarily a beta particle counter and not very sensitive to high-energy gamma rays. However, there was nothing else available at the time.

When Prinzmetal announced his discovery of the radiocardiogram, it did not generate much enthusiasm among the cardiologists of the time. I was serving my residency in medicine then, and I remember that when I read his paper, it appeared to me as merely a sophisticated method of determining circulation times. At that time we were using decholate or paraldehyde intravenously as vehicles for this parameter. Little did I or anyone else realize the prescient nature of Prinzmetal's report.

Several technical and pharmaceutical developments had to emerge before evaluation of the heart with radioactive substances could be utilized as a reliable non-invasive technique. As it turned out, these evolving techniques gave the cardiologist the means to assess non-invasively various aspects of cardiac function hitherto unobtainable in the clinical setting. Indeed, radionuclide imaging has secured for itself a prominent role in cardiology, especially in the diagnosis and management of coronary artery disease and the cardiomyopathies.

A year after Prinzmetal's report, Kety and his colleagues described a method of determining rate of blood flow by measuring the rate of clearance of radioactive sodium chloride from a subcutaneous or intramuscular injection site[4]. Further exploration of radiocardiography was reported by Veall and associates in 1954[5], MacIntyre and his group in 1958[6], Donato in 1962[7], and van Dyke in 1972[8]. Both Veall and MacIntyre demonstrated how the cardiac output could be derived from the left ventricular portion of the radiocardiographic portion of the radiocardiographic curve while Donato and van Dyke added their refinements to the technique.

In the same year that saw Prinzmetal's report, Robert Hofstadter of Princeton University announced his synthesis of thallium-activated sodium iodide scintillation crystals[9]. This was the first of the technical developments so necessary in the evolution of nuclear medicine. These scintillation crystals were very sensitive to gamma rays and because of this, the capability of recording numerically the radioactive counts per second increased tremendously. This resulted in much better resolution. There still remained, however, an inherent inaccuracy in counting at a distance from the source because the instruments available at the time were not able to separate primary from scattered gamma rays. This is known as external counting and needed Bell's gamma X-ray spectrometer for correction of the problem. Bell introduced his device in 1951, but he did not report on its application in medicine until 1955[10].

Another step forward in external counting was Cassen's gamma ray scanner[11]. He invented it in 1949, and in the subsequent decade it became the most widely used instrument in nuclear diagnostic procedures. It was found to be quite satisfactory except for assessment of cardiac function; being too slow for this purpose.

Nuclear imaging of the heart was actually made feasible with the advent of Hal Anger's scintillation camera. He exhibited his machine for the first time at a meeting of the Society of Nuclear Medicine at Estes Park in 1958[12]. It was able to operate at a very high speed so that the scanner could now accumulate counts within the time constraints of a cardiac cycle.

So much for the rapidity of the scanner. What was needed now was a good blood tag before radiocardiography could be utilized as an accurate clinical tool. This was answered to a certain degree with the availability of a newly developed tracer called ^{131}I-labeled human serum albumin (IHSA). The tracer was made possible through the foresight of Hymer Friedell, chairman of the Department of Radiology at Western Reserve University. Utilizing his experience during the war as part of the Manhattan Project team, and capitalizing on his many contacts made during his tenure there, Friedell reoriented the direction of his department upon his return to the university so that in several years it became the mecca of nuclear research in medicine. His department now included physicists and chemists to help the research oriented medical staff in exploring untapped sources and modes of radiation.

Friedell tried to measure cardiac output by imaging the cardiac chambers with a blood–volume technique. This necessitated the use of a tracer that would stay in the bloodstream long enough for the purpose. Radioactive sodium chloride was tried but found wanting because it left the bloodstream at too rapid a rate. Fortunately, an associate, John Storaasli, extrapolated his wartime experience on capillary permeability after traumatic shock wherein the loss of blood was traced with radioactively iodinated bovine serum albumin. He substituted human albumin for the bovine variety and found that it was a good blood tag making it an effective agent for blood–volume studies[13]. Abbott Laboratories immediately made the human albumin tracer commercially available acting on the advice of one

of their chemists, Donalee Tabern, who had heard of Storaasli's work through an Abbott pharmaceutical representative. American industrial entrepreneurship was quite manifest with Abbott's entry into the nuclear pharmaceutical field. For many years, the Atomic Energy Commission was the sole source of practically all isotopes. This monopoly was broken when Abbott led the way for other pharmaceutical houses to make isotopes commercially available. IHSA was a good source of income for Abbott since it dominated nuclear medicine for at least twenty years.

Storaasli's original investigations underwent further elaboration by other members of Friedell's department. A year after the publication of Storaasli's paper, MacIntyre, a physicist in the department described, in collaboration with other members, a method of determining cardiac output in dogs using IHSA and a continuous recording system that he devised[14]. Because exsanguination was involved, the clinical potentialities of MacIntyre's technique was not recognized until later in the year when his paper was being discussed by a radiologist, Robert Robbins, at the convention of the Radiological Society of North America in Chicago[15]. Robbins pointed out that exsanguination was not necessary since the procedure could be done with external counting alone. He also pointed out, at the same time, that the procedure lent itself quite nicely to the detection and evaluation of intracardiac shunts.

However, another seven years had to elapse before blood pool imaging with IHSA was more fully explored. In 1958, Friedell's group, this time led by Rejali, described for the first time, the use of IHSA in the diagnosis of a clinical entity[16]. Their images were used initially to detect pericardial effusion. It was based on the reasoning that if IHSA were injected into a vein, and allowed to come into equilibrium in the body vascular space, then an image of that space could be obtained. They used a rectilinear scanner. This was a reasonably good technique for the non-invasive detection of pericardial effusion, but its use for this purpose was short-lived, supplanted by the superior advantages of echocardiography.

In several short years, it was soon determined that blood pool imaging was not only useful in the detection of pericardial effusion, but also of value in identifying cardiac chamber enlargement and intracardiac tumors; in differentiating between solid tumors and aneurysms within the thorax and abdomen; and in outlining the anatomical configuration of mediastinal arteries and large veins. Friedell's department was again active in this regard but other groups headed by Bonte, Sklaroff and Wagner, working independently of each other, also added their contributions to the field[17–22].

The first attempts to measure coronary blood flow were also made with IHSA. In 1952, Peter Waser and Werner Hunzinger intubated the coronary arteries and injected them with IHSA, which is non-diffusible, and then again with a diffusible agent, rubidium-84 followed by a radioactive gas, krypton-85. All three agents gave consistent results[23]. However, these studies were handicapped because Anger's fast gamma camera had not yet been invented.

Initially no distinction was made between coronary blood flow and myocardial dispersion. The difference became meaningful only when more was learned about 'buildup' and 'washout' of the tracers. Burch's group at Tulane used rubidium-86 as an index of coronary flow in 1953[24]. Then in 1957, Love and Burch reported their study in dogs concerning methods for estimating the rate of myocardial uptake of ^{86}Rb, and suggested that they were suitable also in man, and that ^{86}Rb could be used as a myocardial scanning agent[25]. Just a year later, Donato's group at Pisa presented their observations on the evaluation of myocardial blood flow with ^{86}Rb at a meeting in Geneva[26]. Further work on myocardial flow was carried out at Johns Hopkins under the direction of Richard Ross. In 1964, he injected xenon-133 into the coronary arteries to prove that blood flow measured in this way included not only coronary flow but also a large component of myocardial blood flow[27].

Development of tracers for imaging the heart was uppermost in the minds of many investigators in the field. We have already seen how a number of isotopes were tried. In addition to blood pool imaging, the quest was on to find an agent that would be specific for normal and abnormal myocardium. Metabolic activity as an indication of the status of an intact heart was one method of approach[28]. Richard Bing in 1961 used radioiodinated fatty acids in addressing this aspect[29]. Evans and his group also showed in 1965 that radioiodinated long chain fatty acids could be used as a tracer for perfusing the myocardium[30]. It was not entirely satisfactory, however, for single photon imaging.

Much of the important research in the development of 'tracer families' was in the hands of Carr, Beierwaltes and their associates. They were the first to successfully detect experimentally produced myocardial infarcts by scanning. This was in 1962. They used [203]Hg-chloromerodrin, an agent which was thought to label necrotic tissue[31]. Unfortunately, it was not found to be satisfactory when used clinically. In 1967, Malek tagged radioactive mercury with fluorescein but this too proved wanting[32]. A much better infarct-avid tracer was developed in 1973 by Holman and his group[33]. It was ^{99}Tc-tetracycline. Soon after, Bonte and his colleagues described their results in experimentally produced infarcts in animals with ^{99m}Tc-stannous pyrophosphate[34]. Further clinical studies by the same group found this phosphate isotope to be highly satisfactory in labeling necrotic myocardium, in detecting extensions of infarct, in picking up ventricular aneurysms, and in the evaluation of myocardial damage following coronary artery bypass surgery[35–37].

Throughout this time several other centers were involved in exploring the potentialities of nuclear cardiology. In 1966, Quinn of Northwestern University was the first to demonstrate the ability of a tracer agent to visualize the coronary bed[38]. He injected radioiodine-albumin into the coronary arteries of dogs and demonstrated the distribution of each vessel's arteriolar bed. He never did carry out this experiment in humans telling Marshall Brucer in 1970 that he was 'afraid to try coronary dispersion scans in humans'[39]. Brucer then recounts how Masahito Endo, a cardiovascular surgical resident in Tokyo's Women's Medical College had no such reservations. After trying the procedure on eight dogs and being satisfied that there were no untoward effects, Endo catheterized the coronary arteries in four patients and then injected them with radioiodine-albumin. He was able to visualize in 30 minutes the coronary arteriolar bed. He found that the area of myocardial ischemia was clearly outlined on both dog and human scans[40]. Although the technique had no advantages over radiopaque angiography, it was an important step in that it proved nuclear capillary dispersion was not only feasible but apparently innocuous.

Richard Gorlin also demonstrated the ability to visualize regional myocardial blood flow with a nuclear approach[28]. He used krypton-85 injected directly into the myocardium. In 1971, Hurley and his associates described their findings with a newly developed radiopharmaceutical agent, potassium chloride-43[41]. Two years later Strauss and his co-workers demonstrated its utility in detecting areas of transient ischemia during exercise testing[42]. Incidentally, these were the first cardiac scans in an exercise stress test.

In 1972, Harper and associates demonstrated the clinical feasibility of myocardial imaging with ammonia-13, a positron-emitting tracer[43]. In 1975, Ter-Pogossian and his co-workers also used a positron-emitter, imaging the myocardium with the radionuclide carbon-11 incorporated into carbon monoxide or palmitate[44].

The currently popular myocardial perfusion tracer is thallium-201. It was introduced by Lebowitz and associates in 1973. The work was done at the Brookhaven National Laboratory. The initial report describes how three days after the injection of thallium-201 very high concentrations of the tracer were found in muscle, including the myocardium[45]. It is able to demonstrate areas of transient ischemia following exercise, and also fixed non-perfused areas as a result of infarction.

Blood-pool imaging techniques and agents also had their cadre of investigators elaborating on the initial studies with iodinated human serum albumin. The introduction of Anger's large-crystal scintillation camera and the development of technetium-99m-labeled tracers brought about considerable improvement in blood pool imaging[46]. It came to be known as radionuclide angiocardiography. Richards and Harper's group spearheaded the use of technetium-99m as the preferred agent[47–51]. It was now the 1960s, and for the first time it was possible to view the passage of a tracer bolus through the central venous and arterial circulation in a series of camera images[52]. The new camera produced images as a dynamic series of events rather than as a static image created by a summation of events collected by a rectilinear scanner over a long period of time.

Storage and processing of images was another factor that had to be addressed as nuclear cardiology evolved. MacIntyre and later Bonte were instrumental in using magnetic tape and specialized electronic circuitry for the storage and processing of the data[53,54]. Within a span of five short years, Brown improved the processing significantly even though the images were derived from a rectilinear scanner[55]. A video system for recording dynamic studies with the Anger scintillation camera was described by Ashburn's group in 1968[56]. During the same year Wellman's group described their findings using a similar system[57]. They suggested the term 'quantitative cinescintivideography' – a new concept in dynamic function studies.

By this time gating mechanisms were already in place. The procedure had been introduced by Eugene Braunwald in 1962 during his tenure at the National Institutes of Health. An electrical signal from the heart itself, utilizing the electrocardiogram, allowed the scanner to image during an 'open period'. By so doing, images could now be taken at the end of systole and diastole.

1971 became the banner year for nuclear cardiology. Working now with rather sophisticated systems, a number of important confirmatory contributions were made during this year. This was due to the independent efforts of teams led by Kriss[58], Ashburn and Mullins[59] and Strauss and Zaret[60]. It was now possible to measure volume changes in the various chambers of the heart. Braunwald had already indicated how ejection fractions could be derived from the volume measurements with his gating approach. These men solidified these approaches and thereby offered cardiologists an easy means of obtaining these parameters for assessing cardiac function. Zaret and Strauss also described in the same year a method for detecting regional myocardial wall motion, again with the aid of Braunwald's gating mechanism[61]. Now cardiac function could be assessed in both global and segmental terms without the need for cardiac catheterization. Incidentally, these workers, rather than Braunwald, were responsible for coining the term 'gating'.

Three-dimensional image reconstruction was another important advancement in radiocardiography. The concept of computer assisted reconstruction was originally introduced by Kuhl and Edwards in 1964[62]. They used a single-photon tomographic technique. In 1973, Hounsfield introduced computerized axial tomography. It was described in the *British Journal of Radiology*[63]. In Brucer's words: 'CAT scanners revolutionized diagnostic imaging'[63].

The technique though immediately popular required very expensive equipment and availability of a cyclotron; much beyond the financial resources of most hospitals, and most definitely beyond the resources of physicians in private practice.

Moreover before the technique could be used for cardiac evaluation, it needed an acceptable single-photon emitting radionuclide. Technetium-99m and thallium-201 were already available and had proven to be quite satisfactory single-photon emitting agents. David Kuhl supplied the solution in 1975. He had been working with the concept for some time, having adapted Hounsfield's CAT technology to his cross-sectional nuclear scans, which finally culminated in his invention of SPECT, an acronym for single-photon emitting computerized tomography[64]. Although his studies were focused on local cerebral volumes as determined with three-dimensional reconstruction of radionuclide scan data, the *modus operandi* that he described in combination with thallium-201 proved to be the key to the modern era of nuclear cardiology. SPECT became firmly established as an acceptable tool in assessing myocardial perfusion, and thus, indirectly, the pathophysiologic consequences of coronary artery disease. Electronic entrepreneurship soon made available to cardiologists equipment that could be bought at a reasonable cost. Nuclear imaging could now be performed on an out-patient basis. Many cardiologists learned the technique and after being duly licensed set up nuclear scanning centers in their offices.

Technetium-99m fits the bill quite nicely for evaluating abnormalities of wall motion, leakage of the valves and cardiac function in general but it could not be used for myocardial perfusion. Thallium-201, on the other hand, proved to be quite useful for myocardial perfusion. As clinical experience began to accumulate with these new approaches, and, again, typical of any new development in medicine, cardiologists began to look for further improvements and refinements. In particular, there was a desire to assess simultaneously wall motion and myocardial perfusion. The ability to do so would not only increase the specificity of radiocardiography but would also prove to be a useful strategy in the early diagnosis of myocardial infarction or in stress studies for evaluation of a myocardium in jeopardy. This was facilitated by Du Pont when they developed a tracer capable of achieving these objectives. Its commercial name is Cardiolite; another example of the ever increasing collaboration between industry and medicine as the 20th century unfolded.

At this point, the prescient nature of Prinzmetal's original report on radiocardiography is quite obvious. Radiocardiography has come a long way from those early and, in retrospect, rather crude beginnings. But the technique is still evolving, and even more exciting improvements and discoveries are waiting to see the light of day.

REFERENCES

1. Blumgart, H.L. and Weiss, S. (1927). Studies on the velocity of blood flow. *J. Clin. Invest.*, **4**, 15
2. Hevesy, G. (1923). The absorption and translocation of lead by plants: a contribution to the application of the method of radioactive indicators in the investigation in the change of substance in plants. *Biochem. J.*, **17**, 439
3. Prinzmetal, M., Corday, E., Bergman, H.C. *et al.* (1948). Radiocardiography: a new method for studying the blood flow through the chambers of the heart in human beings. *Science*, **108**, 340
4. Kety, S.S. (1949). Measurement of regional circulation by the local clearance of radioactive sodium. *Am. Heart J.*, **38**, 321
5. Veall, N., Pearson, J.D., Henley, E. *et al.* (1954). A method for determination of cardiac output. Radioisotopes Conference, Oxford – *Medical and Physiological Applications*, p. 183. (London: Butterworth)
6. MacIntyre, W.J., Pritchard, W.H. and Moir, T.W. (1958). The determination of cardiac output by the dilution method without arterial sampling. I: Analytic concepts. *Circulation*, **18**, 1139
7. Donato, L., Giuntini, C., Lewis, M.L. *et al.* (1962). Quantitative radiocardiography. I: Theoretical considerations. *Circulation*, **26**, 174
8. Van Dyke, D., Anger, H.A., Sullivan, R.W. *et al.* (1972). Cardiac evaluation from radioisotope dynamics. *J. Nucl. Med.*, **13**, 585
9. Hofstadter, R. (1949). Detection of X-rays with thallium activated sodium iodide crystals. *Phys. Rev.*, **75**, 791–810
10. Francis, J.E., Bell, P.R. and Harris, C.C. (1955). Medical scintillation spectrometry. *Nucleonics*, **13**, 82–8
11. Cassen, B., Curtis, L. and Reed, C.W. (1951). A sensitive directional gamma ray detector. *Nucleonics*, **9**, 46–8
12. Anger, H. (1958). *Exhibit at Estes Park Meeting of the Society of Nuclear Medicine*
13. Storaasli, J.P., Krieger, H., Friedell, H.L. *et al.* (1950). Use of radioactive iodinated plasma protein in the study of blood volume. *Surg. Gyn.*

Obstet., **91**, 458–64

14. MacIntyre, W.J., Pritchard, W.H., Eckstein, R.W. *et al.* (1951). Determination of cardiac output by continuous recording system using iodinated ^{131}I human serum albumin: animal studies. *Circulation*, **4**, 552–6

15. Robbins, R. (1952). Discussion of paper by MacIntyre W.J. *et al.*: Determination of cardiac output. *Radiology*, **59**, 849–56

16. Rejali, A.M., MacIntyre, W.J. and Friedell, H.L. (1958). Radioisotope method of visualization of blood pools. *Am J. Roentgenol.*, **79**, 129

17. Bonte, F.J., Krohmer, J.S., Tseng, C.H. *et al.* (1961). Scintillation scanning in differential diagnosis: thoracoabdominal midline masses. *J. Am. Med. Assoc.*, **175**, 221

18. Bonte, F.J., Andrews, G.J., Elmendorf, E.A. *et al.* (1962). Radioisotope scanning in the detection of pericardial effusion. *South. Med. J.*, **55**, 577

19. Bonte, F.J., Christensen, E.E. and Curry, T.S. (1969). Tc-99m pertechnetate angiocardiography in the diagnosis of superior mediastinal masses and pericardial effusions. *Am. J. Roentgenol.*, **107**, 404

20. MacIntyre, W.J., Crespo, G.G. and Christi, J.H. (1963). The use of radioiodinated (I-131) iodipamide for cardiovascular scanning. *Am. J. Roentgenol.*, **89**, 315

21. Sklaroff, D.M., Charkes, N.D. and Morse, D. (1964). Measurement of pericardial fluid: correlation with I-131 cholografin IHSA heart scan. *J. Nucl. Med.*, **5**, 101

22. Wagner, H.N. Jr, McAfee, J.G. and Mozley, J.M. (1961). Diagnosis of pericardial effusion by radioisotope scanning. *Arch. Intern. Med.*, **108**, 679

23. Brucer, M. (1991). Radiocardiography evolves into different directions. *J. Myocardial Ischemia*, **3**, 64–82

24. Love, W.D. and Burch, G.E. (1953). Comparison of K-42, Rb-86, Cs-134. *Lab. Clin. Med.*, **41**, 351–62

25. Love, W.D. and Burch, G.E. (1957). A study in dogs of methods suitable for estimating rate of myocardial uptake of Rb-86 in man. *J. Clin. Invest.*, **36**, 468–84

26. Monasterio, G. and Donato, L. (1958). Investigation of central hemodynamics. *Proceedings of the 2nd Atoms for Peace Conference*, Geneva, Switzerland, United Nations, pp. 83–93

27. Brucer, M. (1991). *Op. cit.*, p. 71

28. Sullivan, J.M., Gorlin, R., Taylor, W.J. *et al.* (1967). Regional myocardial blood flow. *J. Clin. Invest.*, **46**, 1402–12

29. Bing, R.J. (1961). Metabolic activity of the intact heart. *Am. J. Med.*, **30**, 679–91

30. Evans, J.R., Gunton, R.W., Baker, R.G. *et al.* (1965). Use of radioiodinated fatty acid for photoscans of the heart. *Circ. Res.*, **16**, 1

31. Carr, E.A., Beierwaltes, W.H., Pateno, M.E. *et al.* (1962). The detection of experimental myocardial infarcts by photoscanning. *Am. Heart J.*, **64**, 650

32. Malek, P., Vavrejn, B., Ratusky, J. *et al.* (1967). Detection of myocardial infarction by in vivo scanning. *Cardiologia*, **51**, 22

33. Holman, B.L., Dewanjee, M.K., Idoine, J. *et al.* (1973). Detection and localization of experimental myocardial infarction ^{99m}Tc-tetracycline. *J. Nucl. Med.*, **14**, 595

34. Bonte, F.J., Parkey, R.W., Graham, K.D. *et al.* (1974). A new method for radionuclide imaging of myocardial infarcts. *Radiology*, **110**, 473

35. Parkey, R.W., Bonte, F.J., Meyer, S.L. *et al.* (1974). A new method for radionuclide imaging of acute myocardial infarction in humans. *Circulation*, **50**, 540

36. Willerson, J.T., Parkey, R.W., Bonte, F.J. *et al.* (1975). Technetium stannous pyrophosphate myocardial scintigrams in patients with chest pain of varying etiology. *Circulation*, **51**, 1046

37. Buja, L.M., Parkey, R.W., Stokely, E.M. *et al.* (1976). Pathophysiology of technetium-99m stannous pyrophosphate and thallium-201 scintigraphy of acute anterior myocardial infarcts in dogs. *J. Clin. Invest.*, **57**, 1508

38. Quinn, J.L., Serratto, M., Kedzie, P. *et al.* (1966). Coronary artery bed photoscanning using [131]IMAA. *J. Nucl. Med.*, **7**, 107–13

39. Brucer, M. (1991). *Op. cit.*, p. 76

40. Endo, M., Yamacaki, T., Konno, S. *et al.* (1970). Direct diagnosis of human myocardial ischemia using ^{131}I-MAA via elective coronary catheters. *Am. Heart J.*, **80**, 498–506

41. Hurley, P.J., Cooper, M., Reba, R.C. *et al.* (1971). [43]KCl: a new radiopharmaceutical for imaging the heart. *J. Nucl. Med.*, **12**, 516

42. Strauss, H.W., Zaret, B.L., Martin, N.D. *et al.* (1973). Non-invasive evaluation of regional myocardial perfussion with potassium-43. Technique in patients with exercise induced transient myocardial ischemia. *Radiology*, **108**, 85

43. Harper, P.V., Lathrop, K.A., Krizek, H. *et al.* (1972). Clinical feasibility of myocardial

imaging with $^{13}NH_3$. *J. Nucl. Med.*, **13**, 278

44. Ter-Pogossian, M.M., Phelps, M.E., Hoffman, E.J. *et al.* (1975). Positron-emission transaxial tomograph for nuclear imaging (PETT). *Radiology*, **114**, 89

45. Lebowitz, E., Bradley, P.R., Green, M.W. *et al.* (1973). Thallium-201 for medical use (abstract). *J. Nucl. Med.*, **14**, 421

46. Anger, H.O. (1958). Scintillation camera. *Rev. Sci. Instrum.*, **29**, 27

47. Richards, P. (1960). A survey of the production at Brookhaven National Laboratory of radioisotopes for medical research. In *Trans. 5th. Nuclear Congress*, New York, IEEE, pp. 225–44

48. Harper, P.V., Lathrop, K.A., Jimenez, F. *et al.* (1965). Technetium-99m as a scanning agent. *Radiology*, **85**, 101

49. Bonte, F.J., Christensen, E.E., Curry, T.S. III (1969). *Op. cit.*, ref. 19

50. Gottschalk, A. (1966). Radioisotope scintiphotography with technetium-99m and gamma scintillation camera. *Am. J. Roentgenol.*, **97**, 860

51. Kriss, J.P., Yeh, S.H., Farrer, P.A. *et al.* (1966). Radioisotope angiocardiography. *J. Nucl. Med.*, **7**, 367

52. Rosenthall, L. (1966). Radionuclide venography using technetium-99m pertech-netate and gamma-ray scintillation camera. *Am. J. Roentgenol.*, **97**, 874

53. MacIntyre, W.J., Friedell, H.L., Crespo, G.G. *et al.* (1959). Accentuation scintillation scanning. *Radiology*, **73**, 329

54. Bonte, F.J., Krohmer, J.S. and Romans, W.E. (1963). Magnetic tape recording of scintillation scan data. *Int. J. Appl. Radiat. Isot.*, **14**, 273

55. Brown, D.W. (1964). Digital computer analysis display of the radioisotope scan. *J. Nucl. Med.*, **5**, 802

56. Ashburn, W.L., Harbert, J.C., Whitehouse, W.C. *et al.* (1968). A video system for recording dynamic radioisotope studies with the Anger scintillation camera. *J. Nucl. Med.*, **9**, 554

57. Wellman, H.N., Hunkar, D., Kerelakes, J. *et al.* (1968). A new concept in dynamic function studies: quantitative cinescintivideography. *J. Nucl. Med.*, **9**, 420

58. Kriss, J.P., Enright, L.P., Hayden, W.G. *et al.* (1971). Radioisotopic angiocardiography. *Circulation*, **43**, 792

59. Mullins, C.B., Mason, D.T., Ashburn, W.L. *et al.* (1969). Determination of ventricular volume by radioisotope angiography. *Am. J. Cardiol.*, **24**, 72

60. Strauss, H.W., Zaret, B.L., Hurley, P.J. *et al.* (1971). A non-invasive scintiphotographic method for measuring left ventricular ejection fraction in man without cardiac catheterization. *Am. J. Cardiol.*, **28**, 575

61. Zaret, B.L., Strauss, H.W., Hurley, P.J. *et al.* (1971). A non-invasive scintiphotographic method for detecting regional ventricular dysfunction in man. *N. Engl. J. Med.*, **284**, 1165

62. Kuhl, D.E. and Edwards, R.Q. (1964). Cylindrical and section radioisotope scanning of the liver and brain. *Radiology*, **83**, 926

63. Brucer, M. (1991). *Op. cit.*, p. 82

64. Kuhl, D.E., Reivich, M., Alavi, A. *et al.* (1975). Local cerebral volume determined by three dimensional reconstruction of radionuclide scan data. *Circ. Res.*, **36**, 610–9

28   Magnetic resonance imaging

Nuclear magnetic resonance (NMR) is a phenomenon exhibited by certain atomic nuclei that have magnetic properties due to their charge and spin. When an object containing these nuclei is placed within a magnet, the nuclei reorient and align within the magnetic field. The cardiovascular system has several types of elements that contain these sensitive nuclei. These are the protons of hydrogen, phosphorous, sodium, fluorine and the nuclides of carbon and carbon-13. These protons as well as others scattered throughout the body are detectable with the greatest sensitivity by current resonance imaging techniques.

Knowledge of the physical principles underlying nuclear magnetic resonance can be traced to the efforts on the part of physicists at the turn of this century to explain the structure of the atom and the interactions between its nucleus and surrounding electrons. Spectroscopy was already highly developed by this time, and its inability to explain why the wavelength of visible light split into two wavelengths when a substance was placed in a magnetic field probably opened the door to further investigation of magnetic phenomena. It was Pauli who first recognized in 1924 that the splitting of the wavelength was caused by magnetic interactions between the nucleus and electrons and that these interactions could be altered by an external magnetic field. An important corollary to this was the implication that nuclei have magnetic properties[1].

Attention was now focused on delineating the magnetic properties of nuclei. Hydrogen was used initially since it was the simplest element, containing only one proton and no neutrons in its nucleus. Stern was one of the original workers in the field[2]. He and his colleagues described in 1933 the magnetic properties of both hydrogen and its isotope, deuterium. Deuterium has a proton and a single neutron in its nucleus[3,4]. The neutron has no net electrical charge but to their surprise, they found that the neutron of deuterium also had magnetic properties.

Rabi, a former student of Stern, achieved a major breakthrough in understanding the magnetic properties of nuclei. His paper on a molecular beam resonance method for measuring nuclear magnetic movements was published in 1939[5,6]. He was also able to describe with his apparatus the behavior of a molecule in a radiofrequency-alternating magnetic field of prescribed frequency. This is the very principle upon which nuclear magnetic resonance is based, namely, the ability of nuclei to reorient and align within a magnetic field. Rabi received the Nobel Prize in 1944 for his fundamental achievements on the subject.

Bloch and Purcell, working independently of each other, conducted similar experiments in 1945, using methods that overcame the limitations of Rabi's apparatus and achieving the astounding accuracy of measuring the magnetic properties of the proton to within one part per million[7,8]. It was through their efforts that the foundation was laid for the subsequent application of nuclear magnetic resonance in clinical medicine. Both men were awarded the Nobel Prize for their work in 1952.

Analysis of the amplitude and frequency distributions of the emitted signal yields information about the chemical composition of the sample containing the nuclei. It was for this reason that the chemists were the first to take advantage of Bloch's and Purcell's methods since the analysis supplied by these methods constitutes the principle of nuclear magnetic resonance spectroscopy. The chemists led the way, followed by the biochemists, physiologists and finally physicians.

Bloch's group, continuing to make further progress in magnet technology, published in 1951 observations that stimulated others in pursuing the finding that simple frequency shifts in organic chemical groups could be used to delineate the chemical structure of organic compounds with nuclear magnetic resonance techniques. Another advance was the introduction of pulsed nuclear

591

magnetic resonance. It was proposed by Hahn in 1950[9]. By this method, the sample is exposed to a pulse of radiofrequency energy utilizing a wide range of frequencies. Further advances in solid state electronics and computer technology were needed, however, before it could be used on a routine basis. Among these advances was the important one of Fourier transformation capability. A Fourier transformation is a mathematical technique to separate a signal into distinct frequencies. Fourier transformation techniques were first proposed by Kumar and his colleagues in 1975[10]. Once this was made possible, and in conjunction with the advances in signal summation and the development of high-strength superconducting magnets, NMR was poised for application in clinical medicine.

This occurred in 1971 with Damadian's investigation of the relaxation behavior of water in bacterial cells as a function of the intracellular concentration of sodium and potassium. Damadian's research was conducted at Downstate University in Brooklyn, New York. His later efforts were concerned primarily with the identification of cancerous tissue[11]. After numerous animal experiments he applied his method to humans suggesting it as a means of identifying malignant cells[12]. He also invented an NMR device for the sole purpose of detecting and localizing cancer in the body. Although his method did not bear fruit in clinical oncology, Damadian deserves credit for arousing among clinicians a widespread interest in the biological potentialities of NMR.

In another branch of SUNY at Stony Brook, only a few short hours away from Brooklyn by automobile, Lauterbur was busy establishing the principles of NMR tomographic imaging[13]. His images were rather crude but they marked the beginning of all NMR imaging techniques in use today. He coined the term 'zeugmatography' from the Greek zeugma, 'that which joins together'. He arrived at this term presumably because his method was based on computer reconstruction of an image from numerous projections, that is, computer tomography. The term never did gain any measure of popularity.

Further research was carried on in Great Britain with two centers dominating the field for a number of years. These were at Aberdeen, Scotland and Nottingham, England.

The first image of a biological specimen was that of a mouse. It was obtained by Mallard and his co-workers at the University of Aberdeen in Scotland. They were encouraged by this 'first' to turn their attention to human observations, publishing their findings in 1979[14]. Their early images in humans, however, were not quite satisfactory. Meanwhile, the Nottingham group was also involved with human imaging. Led by P. Mansfield and A. Mandsley, they tried to enhance the images with a line scan method that they devised[15]. Despite this new approach, their results were also unsatisfactory as exemplified by their images of a human abdomen in which resolution was so poor that the viscera and blood vessels were only dimly visualized[16].

Undaunted by the poor quality of their earlier images, the Aberdeen group, still under the aegis of J. Mallard, continued to seek a method for improving the images. Utilizing Nottingham's line scan approach, they introduced a minor change by applying radiofrequency pulses of constant duration but different amplitudes rather than pulses of constant amplitude but different durations (as suggested in the original Fourier transformation paper). The Aberdeen group called their system the 'spin-warp' method. The images produced were of such good quality that clinical trials were begun immediately. Their observations were published in 1980[17]. Edlestein's group also used this method. They described their findings as applied to human whole-body imaging the same year the Aberdeen group described theirs[18].

The Nottingham group now adopted planar scanning. They were able to get good quality images with this mode of image construction in conjunction with the described modification of the line scan technique. Their initial observations were published in 1977[19]. In 1980, the same group described the first successful imaging of the brain[20].

Other techniques of imaging involving a pulsed sequence approach were developed. One of them described by Buonanno in 1977 was called the steady-state free precession method (SSFP)[21]. Although the images had a high resolution and excellent contrast, the method was handicapped by a high sensitivity to motion which precluded its use for clinical imaging. Pulse sequences that gained acceptance by clinicians included saturation recovery, inversion recovery, and spin–echo.

Spin echo is the most commonly used pulse sequence as of this writing. It produces the standard images for anatomic display. They are sometimes called 'black-blood images' since the rapidly moving blood produces little or no signal and therefore appears black! Another kind of pulse-sequence is the gradient-echo technique. It is more useful for the study of cardiac function and blood flow. The sequences are called 'white blood' images. As of now, (March 1991), echo-planar imaging is undergoing clinical trials. It may ultimately replace spin-echo and gradient-echo as the technique of choice in most cardiac studies.

In imaging the heart, physiological synchronization with the heart beat is necessary for optimal results. This is known as gating. Mansfield introduced the echo planar gating technique in 1981[22]. In 1984, Lanzer accomplished gating by using the arterial wave form or the electrocardiogram[23]. It has been found that more precise timing has been obtained when using electrocardiographic gating.

In the late 1980s, a movement was started to take the N out of NMR. This was predicated on the fear among laymen regarding the word 'nuclear'. The movement succeeded so that the technique currently carries the label 'MRI' (magnetic resonance imaging). The technology has finally developed to the stage where consistently high quality images are obtained. MRI is a very exciting approach simply because it has the potential to provide high resolution, high-contrast, tomographic 2-dimensional or 3-dimensional images without radiation or contrast medium. Not enough experience has accumulated as yet to state with any degree of certainty the amount of impact this modality will have on the practice of cardiology. The most important foreseeable applications in clinical cardiology are as follows:

(1) non-invasive angiography,

(2) high-resolution regional myocardial perfusion analysis,

(3) characterization of myocardial pathology,

(4) evaluation of hypertrophy, chamber size, contractibility and congenital malpositions, and

(5) myocardial metabolism.

Two groups demonstrated the feasibility of detecting and quantifying obstruction in the coronary vessels[24,25]. These were led by Kaufman and Crooks, both of whom published their findings in 1982. The importance of their observations is unquestionable. Imagine having a non-invasive modality that can consistently provide accurate visualization of the coronary arteries. Rubinstein and his associates demonstrated in 1987 the possibility of using MRI to evaluate the patency of aortacoronary bypass grafts[26]. Higgins described in 1985 the detection of acute myocardial infarction in humans using spin-echo derived images[27]. A year later, Johnston's group described similar findings using the same technique[28]. Dinsmore also showed that infarcts can be accurately localized[29] while Johns was able to calculate infarct volume[30].

Investigations regarding the other foreseeable applications are currently going on at a furious pace, but it is too early at this time to present in its proper perspective the evolution of these efforts. I will leave that to a future historian.

REFERENCES

1. Morgan, C.J. and Hendee, W.R. (1988). Mr: *Introduction to Magnetic Resonance Imaging*, p. 1. (Denver, Colorado: Multi-Media Publishing Co.)

2. *Ibid.*, p. 1

3. Friesch, R. and Stern, O. (1933). Uber die magnetische ablenkung von wasserstoff: Molekulen und das magnetische moment das protons I. *Z. Physik*, **85**, 4–16

4. Esterman, I. and Stern, O. (1933). Ueber die magnetische ablenkung von wasserstoff: molekulen und das magnetische moment das protons II. *Z. Physik*, **85**, 17–24

5. Rabi, II *et al.* (1939). Molecular beam resonance method for measuring nuclear magnetic moments. *Phys. Rev.*, **55**, 526–35

6. Kellog, J.M.B., Rabi, I.I. and Ramsey, N.F. (1940). An electrical quadrapole moment of the deutron. The radiofrequency spectra of HD and D2 molecules in a magnetic field. *Phys. Rev.*, **57**, 677, 695

7. Bloch, F. (1964). The principle of nuclear induction. In *Nobel Lectures in Physics: 1946–1962*. (New York: Elsevier Publishing Company)

8. Purcell, E.M. (1964). Research in nuclear magnetism. In *Nobel Lectures in Physics: 1946–1962*. (New York: Elsevier Publishing Company)

9. Hahn, E.L. (1950). Spin echoes. *Phys. Rev.*, **80**, 580–94

10. Kumar, A., Welti, I. and Ernst, R.R. (1975). NMR Fourier zeugmatography. *J. Mag. Reson.*, **18**, 69–83

11. Damadian, R. (1971). Tumor detection by nuclear magnetic resonance. *Science*, **171**, 1151

12. Damadian, R. *et al.* (1973). Nuclear magnetic resonance as a new tool in cancer research: human tumors by NMR. *Ann. NY Acad. Sci.*, **222**, 1048–76

13. Lauterbur, P.C. (1973). Image formation by induced local interactions: examples employing nuclear magnetic resonance. *Nature (London)*, **242**, 190–1

14. Mallard, J. *et al.* (1979). Imaging by nuclear magnetic resonance and its bio-medical implications. *J. Biomed. Eng.*, **1**, 153–60

15. Mansfield, P. and Mandsley, A.A. (1977). Medical imaging by NMR. *Br. J. Radiol.*, **50**, 188–94

16. Mansfield, P., *et al.* (1978). Short Communications: human whole body line-scan imaging by NMR. *Br. J. Radiol.*, **51**, 921–2

17. Mallard, J. *et al.* (1980). In vivo NMR imaging in medicine. The Aberdeen approach, both physical and biological. *Phil. Trans. R. Soc. Land.*, **289**, 519–33

18. Edelstein, W.A. *et al.* (1980). Spin warp NMR imaging and applications to human whole-body imaging. *Phys. Med. Biol.*, **25**, 751–6

19. Hinshaw, W.S., Bottomley, P.A. and Holland, G.N. (1977). Radiographic thin-section image of the human wrist by nuclear magnetic resonance. *Nature (London)*, **270**, 722–3

20. Holland, G.N., Moore, W.S. and Hawkes, R.C. (1980). Nuclear magnetic resonance tomography of the brain. *J. Comput. Assist. Tomogr.*, **4**, 1–3

21. Buonanno, F.S. *et al.* (1982). Proton NMR imaging of normal and abnormal brain. Experimental and clinical observations. In Witcofski, R.L., Karstaedt, N. and Partain, C.L. (eds.) *Proceedings of the International Symposium in NMR Imaging*, pp. 147–57. (Winston-Salem, N.C.: Bowman Gray School of Medicine Press)

22. Ordidge, R.J., Mansfield, P. and Coupland, R.E. (1981). Rapid biomedical imaging by NMR. *Br. J. Radiol.*, **54**, 850–5

23. Lanzer, P. *et al.* (1984). Cardiac imaging using gated magnetic resonance. *Radiology*, **150**, 121–7

24. Kaufman, L. *et al.* (1982). Evaluation of NMR imaging for detection and quantification of obstructions in vessels. *Invest. Radiol.*, **17**, 554

25. Crooks, L.E. *et al.* (1982). Visualization of cerebral and vascular abnormalities by NMR imaging. The effects of imaging parameters on contrast. *Radiology*, **144**, 843

26. Rubinstein, R.I., Askenase, A.D., Thickman, D. *et al.* (1987). Magnetic resonance imaging to evaluate patency of aortocoronary bypass grafts. *Circulation*, **76**, 786–91

27. McNamara, M.T., Higgins, C.B., Schechtmann, N. *et al.* (1985). Detection and characterization of acute myocardial infarctions in man with the use of gated magnetic resonance imaging. *Circulation*, **71**, 717

28. Johnston, D.L., Thompson, R.C., Liu, P. *et al.* (1986). Magnetic resonance imaging during acute myocardial infarction. *Am. J. Cardiol.*, **57**, 1059–65

29. Dinsmore, R.E., Johns, J.A., Yasuda, T. *et al.* (1985). Characterization of myocardial signal intensity by magnetic resonance imaging in proven normal and infarcted myocardial segments. *Radiology*, **157**, 147

30. Johns, J., Leavitt, M.B., Newell, J.B. et al. (1990). Quantitation of acute myocardial infarct size by nuclear magnetic resonance imaging. *J. Am. Coll. Cardiol.*, **15**, 143–9

Section 6

Therapeutic modalities

29   Surgical modalities

BACKGROUND SURVEY

The foundations of modern cardiovascular surgery are firmly imbedded in the basic disciplines governing all of cardiovascular practice. These disciplines are, of course, anatomy, physiology, pathophysiology and pharmacology. The fabulous advances in these basic sciences allowed for the development of the proper anatomical and physiological approaches that were needed to bring the surgical techniques to their present level of competency. As evolutionary advances were made in these basic disciplines, a number of practical factors were resolved, all intertwined with each other, and which, once solved, allowed cardiac sugery to achieve the pre-eminent position it enjoys today.

Among these factors were the development of suitable thoracic anesthetic techniques that would allow the surgeon to work safely and in a more leisurely manner in the open chest; innovative techniques and instruments for suturing blood vessels; eliminating the major causes of transfusion reactions; development of blood storage techniques; adequate pre-operative diagnostic techniques; and the introduction of hypothermia, cross-circulation and the heart-lung machine. The last three modalities acted as a catalyst for the rapid development of surgical procedures that were no longer extirpative but rather physiologically oriented[1]. This unique and logical approach was most instrumental in the successful management of many forms of both congenital and acquired heart disease – so much so that by 1970, virtually every complicated congenital abnormality was amenable to surgical correction. This included even the Tetralogy of Fallot, transposition of the great vessels and complicated ventricular septal defect as well as all valvular lesions and coronary artery disease.

One of the most important advances in the repair of complicated congenital lesions in infants weighing less than 10 lb was the reintroduction of deep hypothermia and potassium citrate cardiac arrest by Merendino and his group[2]. The use of these two techniques, previously tried and discarded as being worthless, were instead demonstrated by this group as an essential element in the surgical repair of these lesions. The utilization of deep hypothermia and complete potassium citrate cardiac arrest provided the surgeon with the opportunity to operate on an open dry heart in complete circulatory arrest.

When Dwight Harken delivered the first Laurence Brewster Ellis lecture at Boston City Hospital on November 5, 1965, he cited the beginning of the modern era of cardiac surgery as occurring at the end of the 19th century[3]. Moreover, he described four major epochs in the evolution of this surgery from that point in time. The first was surgery directed towards the great vessels, the pericardium, and stab wounds of the heart. This was the period of extracardiac surgery. However, its beginnings can be traced beyond Harken's starting point of the end of the 19th century. Stab wounds of the heart were seen on the battlefield long before and needed to be treated with urgency and without benefit of anesthesia.

The second era consisted of initially blind attempts at removal of foreign bodies from within the heart and later surgery of the heart valves and septal defects. Dwight Harken played a leading role in the development of surgical techniques during this era and provided the experience necessary for the pioneering efforts in the repair of septal defects and valvular lesions.

Open heart surgery was the third era of evolution. It needed the introduction of hypothermia and cardiopulmonary bypass for implementation. Its success has been barely short of incredible.

The last and most current era is that of replacement. Many obstacles still remain. Immunologic processes are the major stumbling blocks in transplantation procedures and these problems remain far from solution. Further advances are also needed in the replacement of valves whether of natural or mechanical origin.

Although it is generally conceded that William Harvey's *De Motu Cordis* provided the physiological foundation for cardiac surgery, the probability exists that Leonardo da Vinci, once again, may have priority in still another aspect of cardiovascular knowledge by providing the earliest observations on the heart functioning as a pump. This conclusion is based on an experiment he conducted with a pig's heart 136 years before Harvey's classical monograph. As usual, Leonardo's work went unnoticed because of his propensity to hide his recorded observations leaving to Harvey the presentation and dissemination of the modern concepts of circulation. This Harvey did, basing the concepts on deductive reasoning as derived from an experimental approach to the problem. Leonardo's notes when finally discovered and deciphered, also had the same approach.

Figure 1 depicts a cork borer which Leonardo da Vinci stuck into a pig's heart allowing him to observe the rhythmic contraction of the heart[3]. This led da Vinci to conceptualize the heart as a pump. This concept was fortified by his demonstration that the valves were constructed for movement of blood through the chambers in only one direction. The unidirectional movement of blood was demonstrated by him by putting small fragments of leaves in water, allowing them to circulate through the heart, and then through a glass cylinder tied in the position of the aorta. According to Harken, this was the first pulse duplicator[3].

Leonardo's experiment is a classical example of the scientific method in testing a hypothesis. He erred in that he failed to realize that the pumping action was related to the circulation of the blood. He reasoned that since, with fever, the heart rate increased, the pumping activity was instrumental in circulating heat rather than blood.

Priority aside, since in and of itself, it has no true importance unless it is the key for further advancements in scientific knowledge, Harvey's contributions, openly disseminated, must take precedence over the secretive observations of Leonardo da Vinci. Harvey's ideas, rather than da Vinci's unknown observations, were primarily responsible for providing the physiological basis for today's precise cardiac surgical techniques. In Chauncey Leake's words, Harvey established the central principle of modern physiology and indeed

of medicine, but he also demonstrated the most effective method of procedure in the natural sciences:

(1) Careful and accurate observation and description of a phenomenon;

(2) A tentative explanation of how the phenomenon occurs;

(3) A controlled testing of the hypothesis; and

(4) Conclusions based on the results of the experiments.

In addition, he introduced the method of quantitative reasoning which enforced the validity of the conclusions[4].

The application of Harvey's concepts in clinical practice needed of course the corollary knowledge provided by the previously mentioned disciplines of anatomy, pathology and pharmacology. As we have seen in the previous chapters, advances in these fields took years before they yielded the fruits of modern surgery.

In concert with the above disciplines cardiac surgery is also highly indebted to a number of other investigators in such diverse fields as mathematics, chemistry, physics and immunology. Examples of this indebtedness abound without end in the scientific literature. To begin with, only a few years after Harvey's publication, a group of Oxford physiologists described a series of experiments which were crucial to our understanding of respiratory physiology. These included such names as Boyle, Hooke, Mayow and Lower[5]. These men proved without a doubt Harvey's contention that an exchange of substances between blood and air was part and parcel of the circulatory process, a fact fundamental to the success of open-heart surgery, and which culminated in the construction of the first artificial heart-lung machine by von Frey and Gruber in 1885[6]. Other examples include the work of Magnus on the absorptive capacity of the blood for oxygen, Bert's investigations in Claude Bernard's laboratory on the effects of different partial pressures of oxygen on respiration, Haldane's many contributions to respiratory physiology, and the application of the second law of thermodynamics to all physical and chemical phenomena by Willard Gibbs[6].

Several technological advances were also important in the evolution of cardiac surgery. These include Roentgen's discovery of the X-ray, the development of the electrocardiogram, and the various modalities of cardiac resuscitation.

Against this background the story of cardiac surgery can now begin. In a purely arbitrary fashion, I have decided to develop this by adopting Harken's four major epochs as the basic scaffold upon which the historical development can be appended, complete with the numerous tangential contributions of the various scientific and practical factors previously mentioned in the opening paragraphs of this survey.

EXTRACARDIAC SURGERY

This is Dwight Harken's first major epoch. As stated before, its roots lie in antiquity with the surgical attempts directed throughout its evolution towards the repair of the great vessels, the pericardium and stab wounds of the heart.

Vascular surgery as a self-contained cohesive specialty did not emerge until the end of the 19th century. Prior to this its history can be characterized as consisting of sporadic efforts by daring individuals, limited in scope, and with a disappointingly high rate of failure. The simple act of suturing and ligation alone was fraught with difficulties, and proved to be an almost insurmountable barrier for centuries. Most of the vascular surgery during the greater part of this epoch was, with virtually no exception, limited to traumatic lesions of the peripheral arteries. Ligation was the chief method of repairing these injured vessels, representing in actuality just a method of preventing death from exsanguination but not protecting at all the viability of the part dependent upon the involved artery. It was probably introduced by the Alexandrian school. During the Hellenistic period Galen's contemporary, Antyllus, may have been the first to apply this technique in the treatment of aneurysms[7]. Antyllus recommended that peripheral aneurysms be treated by proximal and distal ligation of the affected artery, and that the contents of the aneurysmal sac be evacuated by puncturing a hole through the wall. This was, in essence, an aneurysmotomy[8]. Galen once used ligation as the basis for disproving the notion that the arteries carried air. He did this by opening in a live animal the arterial segment between two tightly placed ligatures. Ligatures were also known to Celsus, but there is nothing in his

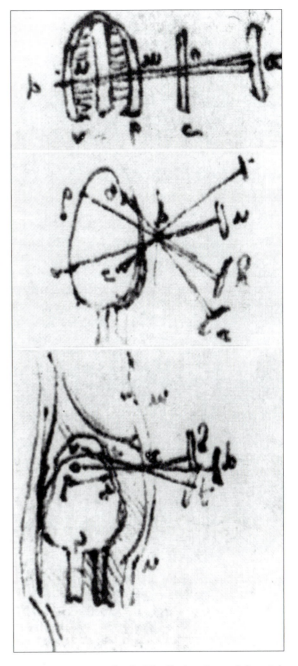

Figure 1 Leonardo da Vinci's drawings of the pig's heart experiments. *Photo Source National Library of Medicine. Literary Source Quad. d'Anatomia, published by O. C. L. Vangensten, A. Fohnan, and H. Hopstock. Christiana, 1911–1916, vol.II. Public domain*

writings to suggest that he used ligation as a regular procedure.

Guy de Chauliac reintroduced the term ligature during the medieval ages, though not in the same sense as in the modern definition of the word. In his treatise *Chirurgia Magna*, which appeared in 1363, during the height of the plague, he described the application of an encircling bandage to draw the margins of a wound together as a means of controlling hemorrhage, an approach that was soon abandoned in favor of boiling oil or actual cautery. This barbaric method remained in vogue until the 16th century, when the Frenchman, Ambroise Paré advocated on an empirical basis, the return to ligation rather than cautery.

During the early part of the 18th century, blood-letting was still a popular mode of treatment. This foolish practice gave Hallowell in 1759 the opportunity to operate on a brachial artery aneurysm which was an all too frequent complication of the procedure. He closed the small opening in the brachial artery by placing a pin through its margin and twisting a thread about it until the opening was entirely closed. Arterial continuity was still maintained even though in a very short period of time both the thread and the pin were sloughed off as part of the so-called post-operative period of 'laudable pus'[8]. The procedure came to be known as the Lambert-Hallowell operation since it was Lambert who had referred the patient to Hallowell.

There is some controversy as to whether Lambert was a physician or surgeon. Although it represents historical trivia, this vignette is of some interest. Matas referred to Lambert as a surgeon while Creech described him as a physician. Creech goes on to recount how Lambert is identified as a barber-surgeon in Hume's *The Infirmary Newcastle on Tyne 1751–1951*. Furthermore, he goes on to say that research by the staff of the National Library of Medicine 'disclosed that for three generations the Lamberts of Newcastle-on-Tyne had been physicians, but that a Lambert in the fourth generation was a surgeon, and it was he who was responsible for the first successful suture of an arterial wound'[9]. In a publication by Lambert entitled *Medical Observations and Inquiries* published in 1762, Lambert described a conversation he had with Hunter on the merits of the procedure, stating that he was not entirely convinced of its suitability but expressing the hope that this method of arterial suturing would be found successful[10].

The Lambert-Hallowell technique induced Asman to try it on experimentally produced lacerations of small arteries in animals[11]. His efforts were unsuccessful, and when he published his observations in 1773, the negative results caused the rapid abandonment of this approach as a clinical procedure. The main fault of the Lambert-Hallowell operation was that the suture invariably obliterated the lumen of the artery. Another 127 years had to elapse before a second attempt of a lateral suture of an artery was reported. It was described by Postempski in a presentation before the Italian Surgical Society in 1886[12]. In 1897, John B. Murphy, an American, performed the first clinical end to end suture of an artery[13]. His technique consisted of first invaginating the severed ends of the artery, then inserting the proximal end into the lumen of the distal end, and finally holding all of this together with sutures. A year before this, Mathieu Jaboulay, instead, everted the margins, and then anastomosed the severed ends with interrupted silk sutures[14]. In 1897, the same year that saw the introduction of Murphy's technique, the German, Erwin Payr, developed a device for folding the proximal end of an artery back over an absorbable magnesium ring which allowed him to insert that end into the cut end of the recipient artery[15]. This device is known as a Payr ring. It too failed to gain any semblance of acceptance, because of the fibrosis it induced. According to Höpfner, M. Nitze of Berlin demonstrated at the Moscow International Congress an ivory ring prosthesis over which the vessel ends could be folded. The ring was removed after suturing[16].

Experiments in arterial suturing continued without success for at least another decade with reports from the hands of Jassinowsky[17], Burci[18], Silberberg[19], Dörfler[20], and Napalkow[21]. Claims were made in favor of approximating just the outer layers while most insisted on using all the layers in the suture. In 1895, Heidenhain had already described the continuous over-and-over suture approximating intima-to-intima[22].

All of these approaches were doomed to failure simply because the major complications of disruption, infection, and local thrombosis were not controlled. The world had to wait for Alexis Carrel before a truly successful procedure was available.

Before outlining Carrel's extraordinary and yet simple achievement, we must backtrack a little and recount the evolution of vein to vein and vein to artery anastomosis. Successful suturing of these vessels constitutes an important element not only in the development of the entire field of vascular surgery but also in the evolution of organ transplantation and current myocardial revascularization procedures.

The first description of a veno-venous anastomosis is ascribed to a Russian, Nicolai Vladimirovich Eck (1849–1908). In 1877, he described a side-to-side anastomosis of the portal vein to the vena cava in a series of animal experiments[23]. He was only 30 years old at the time, an assistant in Professor J. R. Tarchanov's laboratory in St Petersburg. The project was initiated after Eck had read an abstract describing a new function of the liver by B. F. Lautenbach, a young doctor from Philadelphia. Lautenbach described the almost invariable occurrence of death in dogs, cats and rabbits following ligation of their portal vein. He erroneously concluded that the animals died because their livers were unable to detoxify the poisons normally brought to them via a patent portal vein[24]. This was interpreted as a newly discovered function of the liver. Eck set out to test his hypothesis and found that the portal vein in dogs can be ligated without dire consequences provided the blood flow through it was shunted upstream from the ligature[24,25].

Modifications of Eck's method were introduced by Stolnikow in 1882[26], Hahn in 1893[24], Fischler and Schröder in 1909[27], Jerusalem in 1910[28], and Lobb in 1956[29]. The first ligation of the portal vein in a human was reported by George Brewer of New York City in 1908. The vein was already partially occluded from external compression due to an enlarging Echinococcus cyst. The final coup was brought on by an inadvertent laceration of the vein while Brewer was attempting to remove the cyst[30].

Portal-caval shunts involving varying anastomotic approaches were already being carried out in a number of centers, one of which was Palermo, under the direction of I. Tansini[31,32]. The first successful side-to-side portal-caval anastomosis in a human was reported from the Krankenhaus Hasenheide zu Berlin by Paul Rosenstein in 1912[33].

Throughout all this, suture repair of veins suffered from the same complications that plagued arterial repair. H. Braun in 1882 advised the use of disinfected fine silk or catgut and reported the successful repair of an accidental laceration of the femoral vein during an operation for removal of a metastatic carcinomatous lesion[34]. During the same year Gluck also described the successful repair of accidental tears of the jugular veins[35]. Max Schede's report in 1892 is of interest in that his patient revealed at postmortem (18 days after repair of an accidental laceration of the inferior vena cava during surgery for renal carcinoma) a vein that was healed with an intact intima and no evidence of clotting. Clermont became interested in venous repair after he successfully sutured a lacerated internal jugular vein while removing tuberculous lymph nodes. This experience in 1899 caused him to survey the literature and conduct a series of animal experiments, the results of which he reported in 1901[36]. He concluded that infection was the primary factor in causing thrombosis and obviously advised strict asepsis for its prevention.

The first recorded renal graft was reported in 1902 by Emerich Ullmann, a Privatdozent at the University of Vienna. Using dogs, he was able to anastomose the renal artery to the carotid artery and the renal vein to the external jugular vein using a magnesium ring as an aid in suturing[37]. Hermann Kümmell of Hamburg-Eppendorf reported two cases of end-to-end anastomosis in 1900. Both patients underwent surgery for removal of metastatic cancerous lesions to the groin. In the second case, the femoral vein was so heavily infiltrated and encased in the malignant growth that a 2 cm portion of the vein had to be removed. He was able to successfully suture together each end of the severed vein[38]. This was the first reported successful end-to-end anastomosis of a severed vein.

Alexis Carrel was responsible for introducing a leak proof technique for anastomosing blood vessels without constricting the lumen or causing thrombosis. His initial work was conducted on human cadavers and then dogs in Soulier's laboratory in Lyons, France. Anastomosing blood vessels was a critical element in the successful transplantation of organs, and it was for this reason that Carrel turned his attention towards the resolution of this problem and why I feel it necessary to outline in some detail the historical development of both arterio-venous and veno-venous anastomosis. Carrel, in collaboration with Morel and Berard, demonstrated repeatedly the feasibility of grafting veins to arteries, and arteries to arteries[39–41]. Utilizing his innovative anastomotic approach, Carrel in conjunction with Morel, was able to successfully transplant the kidney of a dog from its normal location to the neck by suturing the renal artery and vein to the dog's common carotid artery and external jugular vein respectively[39]. Their approach was radically different from that of

Ullmann who, it should be recalled, used a magnesium ring to aid him in his suturing.

Carrel's background is of some interest. Unsuccessful at passing the clinical examinations for a surgical position on the faculty at Lyons, and also under attack by both clergy and his colleagues for his description of a miraculous recovery of a supplicant at Lourdes that was cloaked in a satirical combination of gullibility and skepticism, Carrel thought that discretion was the better part of valor. He left France to pursue his career in a more favorable environment, French Canada. In the latter part of 1904, only a few months after his arrival, he presented a paper on vascular anastomosis to the Second Medical Congress of the French Language of North America[42]. Karl Beck, a Chicago surgeon, was present at the meeting. He was so impressed with Carrel that he urged the young Frenchman to migrate once again; this time to the United States. In no time at all, Carrel took Beck's urging to heart and left Canada. Within 2 months he settled in Chicago. He was appointed to the physiology department of the University of Chicago and immediately began a fruitful working relationship in the Hull physiological laboratory with Charles Claude Guthrie, a young physiologist. In 21 months, they co-authored 28 papers[43]. Their work included refinement and perfection of vascular anastomotic techniques, the usage of vein grafts in the arterial system, development of tissue preservation techniques, and organ as well as limb transplantation[44–46].

Carrel and Guthrie were successful in transplanting both fresh vascular grafts and those that were stored at near freezing temperature. The latter demonstrated that the latent life of nearly frozen blood vessel grafts was quite considerable, and should be considered as an important physiological discovery in vascular surgery.

It is primarily because of these early endeavors that Steven Friedman likened Carrel to Jules Verne. Both men possessed 'extraordinary imagination and foresight'[43]. Friedman's analogy seems appropriate because the world was to see the implications of Carrel's contributions in the form of saphenous vein bypasses beginning in 1948[47], the routine transplantation of organs beginning with the first successful human renal transplant in 1955[48], followed by Barnard's first human heart transplant in 1967[49], and the successful reimplantation of severed limbs beginning in 1962[50].

Carrel, eager for better financial support, left Chicago in 1906 to accept an appointment at the well endowed Rockefeller Institute. Guthrie also left at this time to accept a position as professor of physiology and pharmacology at Washington University in St Louis.

Carrel's endeavors at the Rockefeller Institute continued to gain for him world-wide respect and admiration. During this time he became involved with the preservation of vascular homografts to replace segments of abdominal aortas, using the cat as his laboratory model[51], development of improved methods for the preservation of arterial segments prior to transplantation[45], experimental surgery of the thoracic aorta involving vena cava grafts and utilizing paraffin tubes as shunts to prevent spinal cord ischemia[52], experimental operations on the orifices of the heart[53], and numerous contributions in the field of tissue culture[54,55].

His relationship with Charles Lindbergh began sometime after World War I. Lindbergh had already became famous as the first aviator to make a solo non-stop flight from New York to France. Carrel at this time was devoting his attention to the development of a perfusion pump for the preservation of organs. Working together, he and Lindbergh constructed a pyrex pump in 1935 which sustained a cat's thyroid gland for 18 days[56]. This paved the way for the preservation of other organs.

Carrel received many honors during his tenure at the Rockefeller Institute including the Nobel Prize in 1912 for his work in vascular surgery and organ transplantation[57]. But all this came to naught with his forced retirement from the Institute in 1935 at the age of 65. He denounced the Institute and science in general and returned to his native France where he continued to enjoy the esteem of his compatriots until 1943 when he was accused of being a Nazi collaborator; a charge that was never proven. This was the beginning of his decline, and amidst accusations, he died one year later as a result of a second heart attack; an unfortunate end to a brilliant career, and for a man who played a pivotal role in laying the groundwork for the remarkable accomplishments of modern day surgery. His photograph is shown in Figure 2 as he appeared in 1914, quite vigorous looking at the age of 41.

An epilogue to Carrel's unmistakable contributions in the evolution of cardiovascular surgery, is the amazing fact that despite his prodigious literary output and the personal intercommunications he maintained with the leading surgeons of his time, many years had to elapse before his work was duplicated in the clinical arena. According to Brewer, Dr Hufnagel of Georgetown was 'perhaps, the only vascular surgeon in the 1950s who knew about his work, collecting Carrel's papers in the library of the Georgetown University Medical Center'[58,59].

While all these advances were being made in experimental surgery, a young man in Louisiana began a notable career in clinical surgery that spanned a half century. This young surgeon was Rudolph Matas, regarded today as the clinical pioneer of modern vascular surgery[60]. His achievements were spectacular when one considers that his early endeavors were conducted in the absence of an effective method to prevent blood clotting, inability to control infection, and inability to replace arteries with a reliable substitute.

Perhaps, the most important contribution of Matas was his technical development of surgical procedures that ensured effective occlusion of peripheral arterial aneurysms without hemorrhage or recurrence[61]. In his own recollections, he performed 620 vascular operations between 1888 and 1940. Only 101 cases represented attempts at restoration of the arteries. The overwhelming number of procedures were arterial ligations[61]. It is noteworthy that Matas was among the leading American surgeons who did not capitalize on Carrel's experimental advances.

Another great contribution by Matas was the chapter he wrote on vascular surgery which barely made it in time for inclusion in volume V of Keen's compendium on surgery in 1909[9]. This work, although reduced markedly in length under editorial pressure, can, nevertheless, be considered a classic because of the scope of its presentation, and the historical basis of its treatment of the subject matter. In the section dealing with surgery of the arteries, he pointed out that many of the early symptoms of arterial disease of the lower extremities were due to an occlusive process rather than rheumatism, flat feet, hysteria or fallen arches (the prevailing notions of the time).

He also described in detail the various types of arterial wounds, the process of healing after arterial injury, and the various methods of treating such wounds. He usually elected to ligate them but considered suturing as the ideal method. A great deal of his management of wounded arteries is,

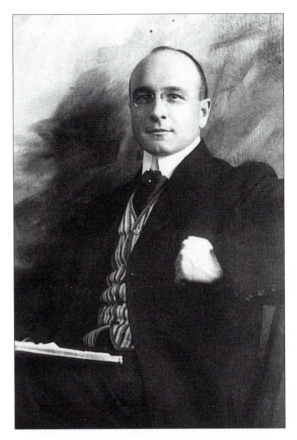

Figure 2 Alexis Carrel. *Photo Source National Library of Medicine. Literary Source Photo Archives. Courtesy of National Library of Medicine*

indeed, devoted to ligation, emphasizing the rules and exceptions in implementing the procedure[9].

Matas brings out in his recollections, how, time and again, he considered his approach to peripheral arterial aneurysms as the epitome of his contributions. He conceived the technique very early in his career constantly refining it over the years. It was the dangers and inherent defects of the previous methods of ligation that led Matas to develop his technique of endoaneurysmorrhaphy. It was conceived on May 30, 1888, while he was operating on a patient with a traumatic brachial aneurysm which proximal and distal ligation of the artery failed to cure. In his initial description, he wrote

This consisted of repair of a large aneurism of the brachial artery in the middle third of the arm resulting from a gunshot wound approximately two months earlier. After opening the sac and removing the clots three orifices were detected at the bottom of the sac and stitched with fine silk, and thus were sealed completely ... This operation was devised as an expedient ... The exigencies of the case made it necessary that hemostasis should be obtained and the occlusion by suture appeared to be so easy and plain that it seemed to be that any surgeon similarly situated would have instinctively adopted this simple way of getting out of the difficulty.[62]

Figure 3 is a reproduction of the title of the original article by Matas[62]. Figure 4 depicts schematically the collateral circulation in the patient who underwent the surgical repair.

In time, there were three variations of his technique. The initial approach was described by him as 'obliterative endoaneurysmorrhaphy'. He called a later variation 'restorative endoaneurys-morrhaphy', while his operation for fusiform aneurysms was described as 'reconstructive endoan-eurysmorrhaphy'. This last approach consisted of reconstructing the wall of the vessel from within using a rubber tube as a stint[9]. A good part of his chapter in Keen's surgery is devoted to this subject, and remarkable for its detail. The appel-lation, 'father of modern vascular surgery' was bestowed upon him primarily for his technique of endoaneurysmorrhaphy.

Although primarily a surgical treatise, the chapter also describes the various modalities he advocated in the management of thoracic and abdominal aneurysms. All of these measures were designed to promote clotting within the aneurysm. An especially interesting one was the usage of gelatin by subcutaneous injection to increase the coagulability of blood. Matas recognized it for what it was, a worthless procedure.

Unfortunately, the advances made by Matas were due mainly to his highly developed clinical skills, and were markedly limited in scope. The maturation of vascular surgery could not depend upon this. It needed several essential elements that were only beginning to evolve during the first half of the 20th century. It is true that the experimental techniques of Carrel and Guthrie went a long way in resolving some highly critical problems, but they were still far from meeting all the requirements[63]. The continuing growth of vascular surgery needed the development of contrast angiography, the introduction of heparin as a safe anti-coagulant, and the availability of synthetic materials for replacement of arterial segments[64].

The maturation process began with Cid dos Santos in 1947[65]. He was the son of Raimundo dos Santos, who, as already noted, was responsible for the development of translumbar aortography[66], an important advance in the visualization of the arterial circulation of the lower extremities. Cid dos Santos should be credited as being the first to remove an obstructive atherosclerotic complex. His target was the femoral artery and this trail-blazing procedure was reported by him in 1947[65]. Four years later, Wylie described his experimental and clinical experience with the use of fascia lata applied as a graft about major arteries after thromboendarterectomy and aneurysmorrhaphy[67]. He used the technique in the sacro-iliac area.

Heparin has proven to be an important adjunct in vascular surgery but it was never intended as a substitute for improper technique. This was amply demonstrated by the results of Carrel and Guthrie, the portacaval transpositions and shunts that have been described and the grafts soon to be described – all of which owe their success to rigid observation of sound technical measures without benefit of heparin[68–77]. Donald Murray appears to be the first to have used heparin in vascular surgery. In 1932, while experimenting with venous autografts in dogs at the University of Toronto, he showed that thrombosis could be prevented by administering heparin. He then described its clinical efficacy in a series of articles[78–82]. In 1950, the San Francisco team of Freeman, Wylie and Gilfillan introduced the clinical usage of regional heparinization[83].

Bridging of large vascular defects was another major step in the maturation process. It is quite likely that the same Englishman, Hallowell, who first used a thread and pin in the repair of the brachial artery[8], was also the first to use an arterial patch prosthesis. This was in 1759, at which time Paré's ligation for repair of an arterial injury was still in vogue. Hallowell's prosthesis was a sliver of wood which he inserted at the margins of the arterial laceration. He then everted the edges around the wood and brought the lacerated edges together by winding a thread around the wooden sliver. It was a brilliant concept in its attempt to preserve the integrity of the blood vessel. Unfortunately, neither infection nor thrombosis could be controlled, preventing its widespread usage.

Subsequent early efforts focused on the usage of other inert materials such as ivory (Nitze)[84], glass (Abbe)[85], paraffined silver (Tuffier)[86] and even paraffined or gold–plated aluminum which Carrel tried for permanent intubation of the thoracic aorta[87]. They were disappointingly inadequate; again, because of the high incidence of clotting but also because of the frequency of disruption at the site of the anastomoses. This led several investigators to the use of homologous or heterologous vessel transplantation either from preserved or fresh specimens. As usual, international boundaries were again crossed with the pioneers in this approach coming from Spain, Germany and America.

A number of steps were involved beginning with replacement of a segment of artery with venous autografts in animals. These experiments were conducted by Jose Goyanes of Spain and the team of Carrel and Guthrie, working independently of each other. In 1905 Carrel and Guthrie performed the first successful biterminal transplantation of a vein in dogs[44], and later pointed out the clinical possibilities with free venous autografts. The next year, Goyanes reported his results with similar experiments[88]. In some of his experiments he tried to replace the infrarenal aorta with the vena cava. His results, complicated by a high incidence of thrombosis, were rather on the negative side in comparison to those of Carrel and Guthrie, who, buoyed by their results, went so far as to say that the ideal method for repairing an aneurysm was 'to extirpate the sac and to restore immediately the continuity of the artery – interposing a venous segment between the cut ends of the artery[44]. Erich Lexer of the University clinic at Königsberg in what was then Russia seized upon this 'ideal method' and tried it for the first time in man. The patient was a 69 year old man who had a large aneurysm of the axillary artery. This was excised and arterial continuity was re-established by anastomosing an 8 cm autograft of his saphenous vein to the cut ends of the artery. He followed carefully the Carrel method of anastomosis using fine silk and embracing all layers of the arterial wall including the intima[89]. J. Hogarth Pringle of Glasgow also used this approach in 1913 and 3 years later Bertram M. Bernheim of Johns Hopkins tried a similar approach[90–92]. Both were successful; presumably, because they rigidly followed Carrel's technique. In 1944, William G. Austen and co-workers from Boston advised certain critical steps

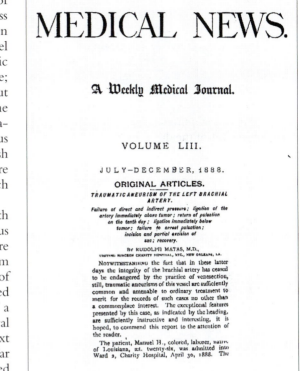

Figure 3 Reproduction of the first page of Matas' original article on endoaneurysmorrhaphy. The name of the periodical was superimposed to indicate when and where it appeared. *Photo Source University of Central Florida. Literary Source Matas, R. Traumatic aneurism of the left brachial artery. Medical News, vol LIII, July–Dec., 1888. Public domain*

when preparing the vein as a free graft in order to minimize injury to the vein[93]. They suggested that a satisfactory immersion medium was a balanced saline solution at 4°C, and a pH of 7, and that the vein should not be stretched too much when irrigated before implantation.

Prior to the advent of heparin, René Leriche of Paris advised that free venous autografts should not exceed 6 cm in length because of the danger of thrombosis. Heparin eliminated this restriction on length so that many years after this advice his assistant, J. Kunlin, was able to report the successful use of saphenous vein autografts as femoro-popliteal shunts that were 14 to 47 cm long. However, the nuances of heparin dosage needed to be defined before the long shunt became firmly established[93–96].

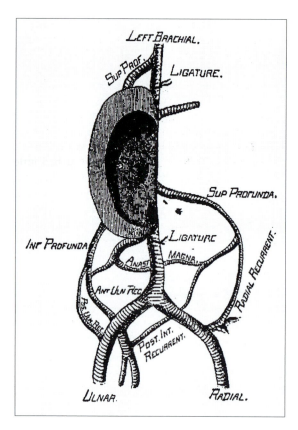

Figure 4 Schematic depiction of the collateral circulation in Matas' patient who underwent the endoaneurysmorrhaphy. *Photo Source University of Central Florida. Literary Source Matas, R. Traumatic aneurism of the left brachial artery. Medical News, vol LIII, July–Dec., 1988. Public domain*

Venous autografts in man were first used in the lower extremities. The experimental approach for their use as aortocoronary shunts was, however, reported by Carrel as early as 1910[97]. Even though he could not anastomose the coronary end of the graft because of the continuous motion of the heart, his prescience regarding the validity of the procedure can be appreciated by his remarks in the paper that described these attempts: 'In certain cases of angina pectoris, when the mouth of the coronary arteries is calcified, it would be useful to establish a complementary circulation for the lower part of the arteries'[97]. This was long before the advent of the heart-lung machine that allowed surgeons to operate on a motionless and bloodless heart. Claude Beck's approach in 1951 did not have as sound a basis. He utilized a vein graft from the aorta to the coronary sinus[98]. Later clinical attempts with this procedure by Beck in the Cleveland clinic and by Mercier Fauteux of Boston were disastrous to say the least. This illustrates once more how a sound physiologic basis was imperative in this as well as in all the other evolutionary aspects of cardiology. Aortocoronary shunting demands precise knowledge of the site of the obstruction in order to bypass it effectively. This was to come later as we have already seen when selective coronary arteriography finally became established.

When Carrel was experimenting with venous autografts, he also considered the possibility of substituting homografts when veins for autografts were not available. He reported this in 1906 at which time he homografted the canine external jugular vein into the common carotid artery[99]. The homograft was relatively fresh having been in cold saline for only a day. In 1907, Levin and Larkin demonstrated that devitalized homografts would function but only for brief periods[100]. The end-results of arterial restoration with devitalized tissue were also described by Guthrie in 1919. In 1908, he had tried to transplant a vein preserved by fixation in a formalin–saline solution. The recipient dog died 11 years after the procedure and the graft, although still functioning, had undergone a fusiform dilatation and consisted of partially calcified fibrous tissue with an endothelial lining[101–103]. Yamanouchi had already described in 1911, the gradual dilatation of canine venous homografts with eventual replacement of the graft by the host's connective tissue. He found no essential difference between formalin-fixed homografts and heterografts[104].

The efforts at prosthetic grafting up to this point should serve to underscore the enormousness of the problem and the difficulties that had to be overcome. Many more difficulties still remained. The high incidence of circulatory injuries during World War II served to emphasize the urgency of resolution. Matas had shown the way on a clinical level. It now remained for others to take up the gauntlet.

Robert Gross of Harvard was particularly active in the field and by the 1940s he was able to demonstrate that preserved arterial homografts could be used in the major arteries such as the aorta[105]. Dubost reported the use of an arterial homograft in the repair of an abdominal aortic aneurysm in 1951[106]. Almost a year later, Oudot resected an occluded aortic bifurcation and replaced it with an allograft[107]. Homografts, however, suffered from several intrinsic disadvantages. These were their limited supply with the concomitant difficulty of preserving them for future use, and most importantly, their propensity to degenerate over time. Obviously another approach was needed. Fortunately, the combined efforts of innovative vascular surgeons and chemists in the textile industries led to the resolution of this most distressing problem.

Although the inert materials of Nitze, Abbe and others had already been discarded, the concept of grafting with inert material was still alive. As late as 1947, Hufnagel, a protege of Gross, anastomosed a multiple point, pressure retaining, serrated ring at the junctional site of his highly polished Lucite tube and the host thoracic artery[108]. It enjoyed a modicum of success but it was still not able to meet the necessary clinical criteria. It was at this time that Arthur Voorhees of Columbia University entered the scene. In his own words:

It was in this atmosphere of excitement over the theoretical possibilities of reconstructive arterial surgery that, while serving in a fellowship at Columbia in 1947, I stumbled on the notion of using a permeable fabric tube as an arterial graft. This followed a serendipitous observation in an experimental animal that endocardium would grow around a silk suture traversing the ventricular cavity of the left heart. My observation gave rise to the speculation that a cloth would provide a latticework of strands on which the body might build its own graft by laying down cells in the interstices of the cloth. This speculation was born in ignorance of Guthrie's conclusions 30 years previously, and that an implant need serve only as a scaffolding for ingrowth of tissue derived from the host.

Proceeding on this assumption, our research group selected the most biologically inert fabric available, with appropriate dernier, and started stitching up grafts and implanting them in laboratory dogs. To our surprise and satisfaction the theory worked. To dignify our discovery we coined the word arteriogenesis and embarked on a systematic study. Our first tubes, stitched from parachute scraps on a home sewing machine, were, by present standards, less than elegant. They did support, however, the concept of a semipermeable cloth tube converting itself into a blood-tight arterial conduit.

Thanks to invaluable advice from Jim Blunt, MD, concerning the biological characteristics of different plastic fabrics, the caring genius of Daisy Mapes, RN, whose innate nursing skills kept the experimental animals alive, and the unflagging scientific and physical support of Dr. Blakemore, the project took on substance. The Union Carbide Company provided us with their only bolt of Vinyon cloth that was perfect for our needs. Too inert to take a dye, it had little commercial value, but, it had all the physical characteristics we were looking for. It served us well throughout our experimental period. Later, in about 1953, Dacron, well-established in the garment industry, had become easier for medical fabricators to obtain. Fortunately it proved to be an equally successful graft material. [109]

After extensive experimentation, Voorhees and his team started to replace aortic segments in the human in 1953[110].

Sheldon M. Levin recounts an interesting anecdote concerning the first time Vinyon was used in a patient's aorta. This occurred while he was serving a surgical fellowship on Dr A. H. Blakemore's service at Columbia-Presbyterian. At that time, Voorhees was the senior resident in the program, and Levin had already been led through the intricacies of the Vinyon project that Voorhees had been conducting for some time. This is Levin's account[111]:

Late in 1952, I began my research period, and I, too, joined the Vinyon project. Voorhees led me through several procedures placing Vinyon tubes in the abdominal aorta of dogs. He was an excellent instructor and demonstrated there was a great difference in sewing arteries together compared with sewing ends of bowel together. I was soon left on my own to carry out the same operation again and again. I was able to compare simple, everting, simple running, and running everting suturing techniques.

The stage was set. It was customary while in the research program to be on call one night in three. Late one night in February 1953, I was paged to see a new patient in the emergency room. The patient had severe back pain, a pulsating abdominal mass, and hypotension. The diagnosis was clearly a ruptured abdominal aortic aneurysm. I called my senior resident, Dr. Voorhees. He called his attending, Dr. Blakemore, and shortly we were all in the operating room. An urgent request for a graft was phoned to the aorta bank. While we were waiting, Dr. Blakemore quickly opened the abdomen and placed the proximal clamp. The float nurse then entered the operating room and grimly announced, 'The aorta bank is empty. there isn't an aortic graft in New York City!' there was shocked silence. Finally Dr. Blakemore drawled, 'Well, I guess we'll just have to make one'. Voorhees and I broke scrub, ran down a flight of stairs to the dog laboratory, sewed two sheets of Vinyon into a bifurcation shape on a sewing machine, cut off the excess, ran back to the operating room, gave it to the nurse to autoclave, and scrubbed in again. Dr. Blakemore sewed in the bifurcation graft and took off the clamps. It worked! It was the first time a synthetic graft was placed in a patient's aorta.

Extensive clinical experience since then has shown that synthetic materials such as Dacron or Teflon seem to work well in the large arteries but not in the smaller ones. Autogenous vein replacement is still the method of choice for the peripheral arteries. Unfortunately, synthetic substitutes are prone to clotting if they are less than 9 mm in diameter and longer than 30 cm [112].

The maturation process of vascular surgery did not end with the introduction of the Vinyon cloth. This was an important step, but other aggressive surgical measures were necessary. Lesions of the aorta, in particular, were still in dire need of innovative corrective techniques. In addition, the newly discovered role of carotid lesions in the causation of strokes presented another challenge to the surgical innovators. The Vinyon cloth gave us a glimpse of what was possible, and further efforts translated the possibilities into actual fact.

The current state of the art can be best appreciated by continuing with the further evolution of vascular surgery, looking first at the tremendous strides made in the surgical management of aortic lesions. In terms of surgery, three major types of aortic lesions have been involved historically. These are acute traumatic aortic transection, acute aortic dissection and chronic thoracic and thoracoabdominal aneurysms.

The first report of successful repair of traumatic transection of the thoracic aorta is ascribed to Dshanelidze [113]. This was in 1923. In 1957,

Gerbode and his group resected the transected portion and then repaired the aorta with a graft under cardiopulmonary bypass [114]. A year later Klassen and his group also reported a successful repair of an acute traumatic aortic transection [115]. This group acquired an extensive experience so that by 1977, its members were able to describe their results in an article with the leading author being J. S. Vasko [116].

The early operations for acute aortic dissection attempted to create either a reentry passage or restoration of circulation directly to the major branches sheared off by the dissection. These procedures were reported initially by Gurin and co-workers in 1935, and later by Shaw in 1955 [117,118]. The failure rate with these approaches was quite high, and for this reason Paullin and James suggested in 1948 that the area of dissection undergo wrapping [119]. Johns on the other hand reported the successful repair of a dissecting aneurysm that involved the abdominal aorta by merely suturing the ruptured area [120].

The modern treatment of aortic dissection was initiated by Michael DeBakey in 1954. His colleagues at the time were Denton Cooley and O. Creech. All three Americans were to become world-renowned in cardiovascular surgery. DeBakey's first case was reported in 1955 [121]. The descending thoracic aorta was involved in the dissection. He resected the aneurysmal dilatation of the false channel and then oversewed the distal entry into the false channel. The procedure was completed with an end-to-end anastomosis.

Spencer and Blake were the first to describe the successful repair of chronic ascending aortic dissection in 1962 [122]. Their procedure is still used today and includes suspending the aortic valve commissure. Aortic valve replacement was carried out in a patient with persistent aortic insufficiency, 15 years after undergoing what was reported as a successful repair of an acute aortic dissection with aortic incompetence. Both procedures were carried out by G. C. Morris; the initial surgery being performed in 1963 and the valve replacement in 1977 [123,124]. The patient was still alive 8 years after the valve replacement.

DeBakey with his colleagues and former pupils accumulated quite an extensive experience in the surgical management of aortic dissection of the ascending aorta which formed the basis for an excellent summary of the subject published in 1964 [125].

Incidentally, the authors of this paper included Henly, Cooley, Morris, Crawford, and Beall, all of whom became highly esteemed cardiovascular surgeons in their own right.

In the evolution of surgical measures used in the repair of aneurysms involving the peripheral arteries, I have already described how important the endoaneurysmorrhaphy of Matas was in this regard. Matas was fully familiar with the manner in which Antyllus treated traumatic aneurysms of the peripheral arteries nearly 1800 years before. Although spears and not gunshots were the culprits in the time of Antyllus, the resultant aneurysms had the same structural composition. In particular, Matas was impressed with the following advice by Antyllus[126]: 'Those who tie the artery, as I advise, at each extremity, but amputate the intervening dilated part, perform a dangerous operation … open the tumor at its top, and, after evacuating the contents, remove the superfluous skin, leaving the part tied by threads. In this way the operation is effected without hemorrhage'. When Antyllus spoke of 'the part tied by threads', he was referring to ligation of all the feeding vessels supplying the aneurysm. Matas modified the procedure, and, as we already know, called it endoaneurysmorrhaphy.

As modern aneurysm surgery of the aorta began to develop, Antyllus' advice and Matas' modification were totally ignored. I have already described how Dubost and his colleagues in Paris were the first to successfully resect an abdominal aortic aneurysm and restored continuity of the aorta with a preserved homograft. This was in 1951[106]. The Mayo group became interested in the problem also in 1951, and by 1953, this group led by J. W. Kirklin reported their results with aneurysm reinforcement, aortoplasty and complete wrapping with fascia lata[127]. Their surgery was also limited to aneurysms involving the abdominal aorta. DeBakey and Cooley were also resecting aneurysms of the abdominal aorta and bridging the gap with a homograft. Their classical paper on the subject appeared in 1953[128]. The procedure was lengthy and tedious with the resection itself fraught with danger. Frustration with this approach prompted DeBakey and his group to resurrect Matas' concept and to suggest that it be utilized in the repair of all aortic aneurysms[129]. The inclusion technique of sewing the graft in place from within the aneurysm was put to actual use by Javid and colleagues in 1962[130], Creech in 1966[131], and by the Mayo group[129].

Working within the aneurysm required availability of homografts. This led to the establishment of arterial homograft banks not only at the Mayo clinic but also in the other centers engaged in this work[132].

Homograft replacement was now used after resection of both thoracic as well as abdominal aortic aneurysms. Numerous reports on the technique began to emanate from several centers. In Boston, Gross and his colleagues were impressive with their success in the clinical use of homografts for treating complex coarctations, including those with aneurysms[133]. Aneurysms of the ascending thoracic aorta were also being resected and replaced with homografts even before the advent of the heart-lung machine. Cooley and DeBakey (1952)[134], Bahnson (1953)[135], and the Mayo group (1953)[136] also participated in the development and refinement of this approach. Cardiopulmonary bypass was first used by Cooley and DeBakey in 1956[137]. They resected a fusiform aneurysm of the entire ascending aorta; a remarkable achievement.

The introduction of the Vinyon cloth by Voorhees inaugurated the synthetic phase of graft replacement. At about the same time, Hufnagel successfully placed an Orlon graft in a patient at Georgetown University Hospital[138]. During a symposium on vascular grafting held by the National Research Council in 1954, Blakemore and Voorhees presented a report on their extensive experimental and clinical work with the Vinyon graft[139]. The leading vascular surgeons of the time, all working on synthetic grafts, shared the symposium. Among them were Hufnagel, Gross, Shumacher, and DeBakey. There was a unanimous opinion among them to continue exploring the clinical use of synthetic grafts. Knitted and woven fabrics have been widely used since then. Dacron was reported by Deterling and Bhonslay as being the most suitable for blood vessel replacement, and still appears to be the favored fabric[140].

This improvement went a long way in overcoming the limitations of homografts. It was followed by another series of improvements, all of which became incorporated into the surgical techniques employed today. Among these are the usage of profound hypothermia and total circulatory arrest in conjunction with cardiopulmonary bypass[141,142]; as well as certain technical improvements such as the single anastomosis in transverse arch surgery by Bloodwell, Hallman, and Cooley in 1968[143]. In 1981, Crawford and Saleh applied the inclusion technique in transverse arch aneurysms[144]. They worked entirely within the aneurysm and wrapped the graft with aneurysm wall.

It is obvious by this time that many men participated in the evolution of modern vascular surgery. At the time of this writing, DeBakey should be considered as the 'elder' of the group. It is for this reason that a few words will be devoted to him. This is not to say that he deserves more recognition than the others. He did, however, act as a catalyst in the field.

The list of cardiovascular surgeons that he trained or influenced attests to his dedication and skills as a teacher. He was also an inventor as well and an innovator in the surgical theater. A pump that he devised while still a medical student was integrated years later as an essential component of the heart–lung machine.

He and his group were the first to perform successful resection and graft replacement of aortic arch aneurysms. He and his associates were also the first to perform aortocoronary artery bypass with autogenous saphenous vein graft, and in 1968 he led a team of surgeons in a multiple transplantation procedure. This was an historic event in that the heart, kidneys, and one lung of a donor were each transplanted to four different recipients.

DeBakey played a prominent role in the establishment and development of the National Library of Medicine. His literary output has been prodigious, as he authored more than 1000 medical articles, chapters and books. These have been reflective of his broad and varied interests, covering surgery, medicine, research, and medical education as well as sociological topics. In 1976, his students founded The Michael E. DeBakey International Cardiovascular Society in recognition of his dedication to the training of young physicians. Great as his accomplishments have been in the field of vascular surgery, his greatest legacy lies in the number of surgeons he trained and who in turn carried on his innovative enthusiasm in centers throughout the world.

Carotid artery surgery

Initial attempts at carotid artery surgery were ligation procedures for the repair of traumatic wounds. Although, as we now know, the history of arterial ligation dates back to antiquity, there is no record of carotid artery ligation being tried until the last decade of the 18th century.

Jesse Thompson credits John Abernathy of England as being the first to deliberately ligate the carotid artery. His patient was bleeding from a torn left carotid artery after being gorged by the horn of a cow[145]. Attempts at controlling the hemorrhage failed him, and for this reason Abernathy resorted to ligation. The patient died 30 hours later. Abernathy (1764–1831) was one of the more famous of John Hunter's pupils[146].

David Fleming was probably the first to successfully ligate the cervical portion of the carotid artery. His patient also had a traumatic lesion. Fleming was a young British naval surgeon at the time with very little clinical experience. The patient was a servant on HMS Tournant who had cut his throat in a suicidal attempt. He appeared to have responded well to compression until 8 days after the incident when, during a coughing spell, the injured and now friable carotid artery burst with an uncontrollable and life-threatening loss of blood. Young Fleming's ingenuity saved the day. With no experience to guide him, but apparently with a sound knowledge of the direction of blood flow, this intrepid surgeon cut down on the carotid artery below the wound and tied a ligature around it. The ship's log indicates that the patient made an uneventful recovery[147].

Numerous reports since then concerning carotid ligation appeared in the literature. By 1868, Pilz had been able to collect 600 recorded cases of carotid ligation for control of hemorrhage or repair of a cervical aneurysm[148]. The mortality up to that time was unacceptably high with a death rate of 43%.

Sir Astley Cooper was the first to ligate the carotid artery for a cervical aneurysm. He performed the procedure twice; the first time in 1805 with an unsuccessful outcome and the second in 1808. Cooper reported that the second patient lived for another 13 years[149]. Valentine Mott of Long Island, New York, compiled a record of 51 common carotid artery ligations and 2 internal carotid ligations. Mott was a pioneer in vascular surgery during the first half of the 19th century. He performed his first carotid ligation in 1829. He also performed a simultaneous ligation of both left and right carotid arteries in 1833. William MacGill of Maryland is credited though of being the first American surgeon to ligate both common carotid arteries. This was in 1823[150].

During the first half of the 19th century, carotid artery ligation was also performed for the treatment of epilepsy, psychoses, and trigeminal neuralgia[151]. Benjamin Travers of London also attempted the procedure and with success in 1809 in a patient who had a pulsating exophthalmos due to carotid-cavernous fistula[152].

In 1911, Matas made an interesting statement concerning carotid artery ligation. He stated that 'the possible occurrence of cerebral disturbance has invested a simple technical procedure with a gravity associated with but few operations'[153]. There was no doubt about the cerebral complications that could arise following ligation but the procedure is still being used for various neurovascular lesions. Harvey Cushing had no compunction about ligating the internal carotid. In 1932 he said, 'I have ligated the internal carotid many times without apparent symptoms. I don't now recall any accidents, but there may have been some. I have been careful to restrict these ligations to young or middle-aged persons without vascular disease'[154]. But hemiplegia or other neurologic defects have occurred. In 1965, Gibbs introduced a rather clever device to ward off these possible complications when ligation of the internal or common carotid appears to be the only therapeutic option. His device twists the subject artery. The torsion is capable of completely shutting off the blood supply. However, if any adverse reaction occurs, restoration of circulation can be rapidly restored by releasing the torsion[155].

The changing concepts in etiology and management of ischemic stroke syndromes since the 1950s brought with them an increased interest in surgery of the carotid arteries.

In Section 1, I described how the word carotid was derived from the Greek, meaning to stupefy or place one into a deep sleep. The 31st metope from the Parthenon shows a centaur applying left carotid compression to the neck of a Lapith warrior. Figure 5[156] illustrates the maneuver, a technique apparently not only well known to the Greeks but also to the modern youths of all nations exposed to American movies and television. I am referring to the 'Vulcan grip', popularized in the science-fiction series called 'Star Trek'. The maneuver is performed repeatedly by the Vulcans, 'aliens' from outer space, in neutralizing their opponents. It is also alleged that modern day wrestlers are also acquainted with the neutralizing effects of carotid artery compression. They call it the 'sleeper'.

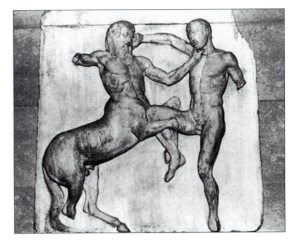

Figure 5 31st metope from the Parthenon showing a centaur applying left carotid pressure to the neck of a Lapith warrior. *Photo Source National Library of Medicine. Literary Source Thompson, J.E. (1986). History of carotid surgery. Surgical clinics of North America, vol. 66, no. 2, pp. 225–31. With permission*

Despite the fact that several observers such as Gull in 1855, Savory in 1856[157], Broadbent in 1875[158], and Penzoldt in 1881[159], had all described cases of stroke due to blockage of the main extracranial arteries supplying the brain, the widely held opinion was that apoplexy was almost invariably due to cerebral hemorrhage or blockage of the intracranial segments.

The first one to describe an ulcerating plaque in the carotid artery was Chiari[160]. This was in 1905. His paper points out quite clearly that such ulceration could be the seat of stroke-causing emboli. Ramsey Hunt of New York City was the first to use the term 'cerebral intermittent claudication' in 1914[161]. He was referring to cerebral ischemic syndromes brought about by recurrent obstructions of the innominate and carotid arteries.

When Egas Moniz of Portugal introduced cerebral arteriography in 1927, the clinical stage was set for the increasing recognition of extracranial occlusive disease. However, many years had to elapse before clinicians took full advantage of this technique in searching for the precipitating cause of a stroke. By 1951, Johnson and Walker had been able to collect from the literature only 101 cases wherein carotid artery thrombosis was diagnosed with arteriography[162]. It was that same year though in which Fisher described the pathophysiology of cerebrovascular insufficiency syndrome due to atherosclerosis of the carotid arteries[163]. He suggested bypassing the blockage by anastomosing the external carotid artery or one of its branches with the internal carotid artery above the stenotic area. Fisher's suggestion was taken up immediately by Carrea, Molins and Murphy of Buenos Aires. They restored blood flow in their patient with an end-to-end anastomosis of the external carotid to the internal carotid. Their case was not reported until four years later[164]. Some claim that this operation initiated the modern era of carotid surgery. Perhaps this is true for the anastomotic approach they took. Endarterectomy is another approach, and currently seems to be the favored one when feasible.

Although their work was confined to the aortoiliac tree, E. J. Wylie and his colleagues also described in 1951 their success with thromboend-arterectomy in the removal of atherosclerotic plaques from this area[165]. Their paper was based upon both experimental and clinical experience. After removing the atherosclerotic plaques they did an aneurysmorrhaphy and finished the procedure by applying the fascia lata as a graft around the aortoiliac segments. The first reported attempt at thrombo-endarterectomy of the cervical internal carotid artery was described by Strully, Hurwitt and Blankenberg just two years after Wylie's report[166]. They were unable, however, to obtain retrograde flow and suggested that endarterectomy would be of value only when the vessels distal to the block were patent.

The first successful carotid endarterectomy was performed by DeBakey in a patient who had a major stroke due to total occlusion of the left carotid artery. Good retrograde flow from the internal carotid artery was obtained, and an immediate postoperative arteriogram confirmed that there was complete patency of the entire internal carotid tree. DeBakey reported this experience in 1975 although he performed the operation on August 7, 1953[167]. The patient survived for 19 years with no recurrences.

DeBakey's effort and success should not be minimized but, in terms of impact on the surgical community, it had little or no effect since it was reported so many years later. A truly historic first in this regard was the feat accomplished at St. Mary's Hospital in London in 1954. It provided the spark for further surgical interventions of lesions involving the carotid arteries. The patient had been suffering from repeated episodes of transient ischemia due to stenosis of the left carotid bifurcation. Utilizing hypothermia during carotid clamping, the team of Eastcott, Pickering and Rob then resected the bifurcated area and restored blood flow with an end-to-end anastomosis between the common carotid and distal internal carotid arteries. Their paper was published in late 1954, six months after they had performed the procedure[168].

During the ensuing 3 decades, concomitant with the development of non-invasive diagnostic techniques, carotid surgery became firmly established. Endarterectomy continues to be the favored approach though resection and grafting as well as bypass procedures are utilized when circumstances mandate these alternative techniques.

The importance of transient ischemic episodes due to occlusive disease of the cervical carotid arteries cannot be overemphasized. The lives of many people and the political fate of nations have been at stake and either sacrificed or altered when their leaders have unknowingly or knowingly suffered from the consequences of these lesions. In 1972, W. J. Friedlander published, in *Stroke*, a paper about 3 old men: Woodrow Wilson, Paul von Hindenburg and Nikolai Lenin[169]. He presented a neurologist's view on how their cerebral arteriosclerosis altered world politics. To this list we must add the episodes of cerebrovascular insufficiency manifested by Franklin Delano Roosevelt. Although it is purely speculative, one cannot help but wonder how his illness affected the outcome of the Yalta conference in 1945.

Pulmonary embolectomy

Pulmonary embolectomy is another evolutionary aspect of vascular surgery that deserves consideration – since it too forms part of the techniques developed during the era of extracardiac surgery.

Removal of emboli from the pulmonary artery was first described and practiced by Friedrich Trendelenburg of Germany. The intervention was based on experience acquired initially from calves and then from cadavers. In clinical trials, Trendelenburg and his associates, despite 12 attempts in selected cases, were never able to achieve success. All of their patients died. The same held true for other surgeons with their patients dying either on the table or several days later from blood loss, infection or pneumothorax[170–175].

Despite the drastic mortality rate, Trendelenburg's technique continued to attract the attention of other European surgeons. The procedure was a simple one, and could be performed within a matter of seconds. But many years had to pass before the first truly successful pulmonary embolectomy could be done. It occurred in the hands of M. Kirschner, also from Germany. He used both the technique and instruments developed by Trendelenburg and announced his results at a meeting with the now elderly Trendelenburg in attendance. This was in 1924 and was immediately reported in the USA by the Berlin correspondent of the *Journal of the American Medical Association*[176–178].

Following Sauerbruch's address, Professor Kirschner of Königsberg presented the first case of pulmonary embolism in which a cure was effected by the Trendelenburg operation. The patient was a woman, aged 38, in whom the embolism developed the third day after operation for femoral hernia, just as she sat up for an examination of the lungs. Fifteen minutes after the onset of the embolism, the operation on the apparently moribund patient was begun. For forty-five seconds, the large vessels were closed off, during which brief space, after exposure and opening of the pericardium, the pulmonary artery was opened and blood clots extending a distance of 17 cm were removed. The cured patient was presented to the assembly, and the chairman was fully justified in congratulating the operator and the aged originator of the operation, Professor Trendelenburg, who was in attendance. [178]

A slightly better mortality rate was realized when A. W. Meyer modified the Trendelenburg technique and redesigned the original instruments. These modifications were also adopted by Craford of Stockholm and Nystrom of Upsala[179–181].

The optimism created by the successful attempts of these surgeons was implanted in two outstanding surgeons in Boston, Elliott Cutler and Edward Churchill. However, despite their skills, and those of their assistants, the mortality rate remained, in their hands, an unacceptable 100%. This was a very distressing state of affairs, for which reason the Boston group almost completely abandoned the procedure. The 100% mortality rate was finally reversed in 1958 when Richard Steenburg and his associates performed at Peter Bent Brigham Hospital a successful modified Trendelenburg operation on a 65 year old woman[182].

By this time, however, new advances had been made in blood transfusions, endotracheal anesthesia, antibiotic therapy, and most importantly, in the management of potentially lethal cardiac arrhythmias. Also, the lessons learned from other cardiac surgical procedures were, no doubt, important in the further reduction of the mortality rate.

This survey concludes the historical development of vascular surgery. It is by no means complete, but sufficient in depth to underscore the importance of proper surgical techniques not only in the restoration of circulatory integrity but also in the successful evolution of cardiac surgery *per se*.

The reader will recall that the historical background of vascular surgery was but one component of what Harken dubbed as the epoch of extracardiac surgery. The term extracardiac connotes no entry into the chambers of the heart. It is for this reason that stab wounds of the heart and pericardial lesions are included in this epoch. But heart wounds are not always induced with bladelike instruments. Cardiac disruption due to blunt injuries must also be considered. Foreign bodies in the heart can also be categorized as traumatic in origin. Since many of these foreign bodies can be found in the chambers of the heart, the historical development of the management of these lesions was rightfully placed by Harken as having occurred predominantly during the era that he labeled blind intracardiac surgery. I shall do the same.

Stab wounds of the heart

Throughout the centuries, a fatalistic attitude existed regarding all wounds of the heart. As was to be expected, wounds of the heart were rather common, but considered by all the authorities during antiquity as being incapable of correction. Aristotle was one of the first to express this nihilistic view[183]. 'The heart alone of all the viscera cannot withstand injury. This is to be expected because when the main source of strength [the heart] is destroyed there is no aid that can be brought to the other organs which depend upon it'[183].

It was not until the 17th and 18th centuries that a reappraisal and more optimistic view appeared. This came about because of the increasingly frequent observations at postmortem of healed lesions that were obviously traumatic in origin[184–187]. The most complete postmortem study that proved that recovery from heart wounds was possible did not appear, however, until the latter part of the 19th century. This was the classical monograph of George Fischer which was published in 1868[188]. His paper was based on a statistical analysis of 452 cases which revealed a recovery rate of 10%. Though rather small, the 10% recovery rate documented in a statistically significant manner that not all heart wounds spelled certain death. Many years had elapsed between the statement of Aristotle and the fecundity of such statistical analysis.

Whether or not Fischer's paper had a catalytic effect is difficult to say, but shortly thereafter, several investigators began to explore the possibility of surgical intervention in the management of heart wounds. Animal experiments were conducted first. In 1882, Block reported the successful repair of heart wounds by suture in rabbits[189]. In 1894, Del Vecchio presented a paper at the 11th International Medical Congress in Rome confirming Block's work[190]. Del Vecchio created heart wounds in dogs, and then repaired them by suture.

These experimental observations, however, did not create any intense interest in the clinical arena. In fact such noted surgeons of the time as Billroth, Paget and Riedinger were quite vocal in their resistance to any attempt of this sort in humans[191,192].

The chief allegation concerning Billroth is that he took advantage of his reputation as the dominant European surgeon of the time, and that, unfortunately, he was markedly counterproductive by his adamant and vociferous remarks concerning the very thought of operating on the heart. Just one year after Block's report, Billroth was supposed to have stated rather bluntly that 'any man who would attempt to operate on the heart should lose the respect of his colleagues'[193].

There are several discrepancies concerning both Billroth and his oft-quoted statement. Absolon rises to his defense with the following remarks: 'The reason for putting into Billroth's mouth provocative statements and twisting the truth can be explained by personal interests of the propagators and by a malicious pleasure of proving a great and famous man wrong. Once made, such statements are easily repeated and make a good highlight for an after-dinner speech. Thus Billroth was accused of anti-Semitism even though his daughter married a Jew, and he was accused of being the forefather of cardiac

surgery even though he never performed a cardiac operation. Other Billroth pronouncements in the well-documented book of medical quotations by Maurice B. Strauss certainly do not include the aforementioned figments of vivid imaginations!' Absolon goes on to say that paragraph no. 118 in Billroth's *Die Verletzungen und Krankheiten der Brust* contains the famous and often misquoted pronouncement of Billroth on cardiac surgery:

> Paracentesis of the hydropic pericardium is an operation which in my view reaches what some surgeons call prostitution of the surgical art, others surgical frivolity. Just to avoid the reproach of being incomplete, we do mention these operations of more interest to the anatomist than the physicians. Future generations may judge differently; internal medicine is becoming more and more surgical and physicians practicing mostly internal medicine are planning the most audacious operations. These suggestions fortunately were not realized.

Absolon concludes his defense by remarking that

> Theodor Billroth, ever so careful, did not even adopt the above statements of 'prostitution of the surgical art' and 'surgical frivolity' to himself but rather to other surgeons … Indeed, later, Billroth himself performed a trocar pericardiocentesis.[194]

Absolon's views are supported by D. C. McGoon who in the John H. Gibbon lecture delivered to the American College of Surgery in 1982 vowed 'I shall never quote this rather inadequately documented statement again!'[195]

There seems to be no doubt, however, about the stance adopted by Riedinger and Paget. In 1888, Riedinger wrote 'The suggestion to suture a wound of the heart, although made in all seriousness, scarcely deserves mention'[196]. Sir Stephen Paget added his own authoritarian opinion 8 years later when he proclaimed 'ex cathedra' that 'the heart alone of all viscera has reached the limits set by nature on all surgery. No new method and no new techniques will overcome the natural obstacles surrounding a wound of the heart. It is true that heart suture has been vaguely proposed as a possible procedure, and that it has been done on animals, but I cannot find that it has ever been attempted in practice'[197].

Fortunately for humanity, the spirit of scientific discipline in medicine was very much alive at this

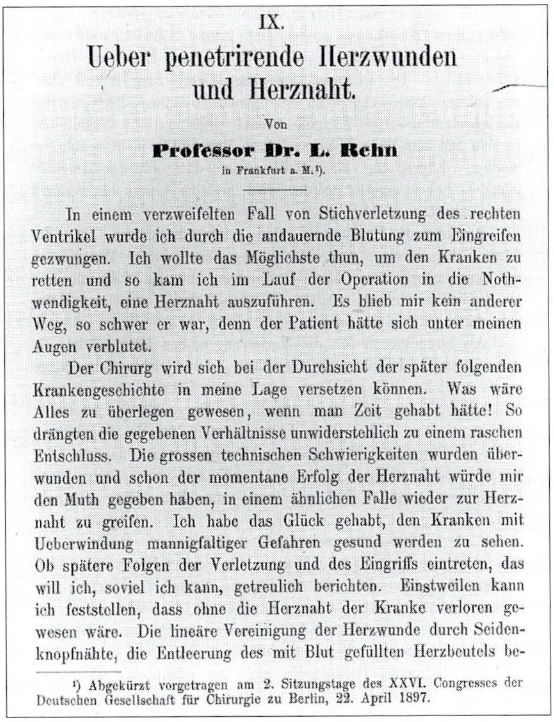

IX.

Ueber penetrirende Herzwunden und Herznaht.

Von

Professor Dr. L. Rehn

in Frankfurt a. M.[1].

In einem verzweifelten Fall von Stichverletzung des rechten Ventrikel wurde ich durch die andauernde Blutung zum Eingreifen gezwungen. Ich wollte das Möglichste thun, um den Kranken zu retten und so kam ich im Lauf der Operation in die Nothwendigkeit, eine Herznaht auszuführen. Es blieb mir kein anderer Weg, so schwer er war, denn der Patient hätte sich unter meinen Augen verblutet.

Der Chirurg wird sich bei der Durchsicht der später folgenden Krankengeschichte in meine Lage versetzen können. Was wäre Alles zu überlegen gewesen, wenn man Zeit gehabt hätte! So drängten die gegebenen Verhältnisse unwiderstehlich zu einem raschen Entschluss. Die grossen technischen Schwierigkeiten wurden überwunden und schon der momentane Erfolg der Herznaht würde mir den Muth gegeben haben, in einem ähnlichen Falle wieder zur Herznaht zu greifen. Ich habe das Glück gehabt, den Kranken mit Ueberwindung mannigfaltiger Gefahren gesund werden zu sehen. Ob spätere Folgen der Verletzung und des Eingriffs eintreten, das will ich, soviel ich kann, getreulich berichten. Einstweilen kann ich feststellen, dass ohne die Herznaht der Kranke verloren gewesen wäre. Die lineäre Vereinigung der Herzwunde durch Seidenknopfnähte, die Entleerung des mit Blut gefüllten Herzbeutels be-

[1] Abgekürzt vorgetragen am 2. Sitzungstage des XXVI. Congresses der Deutschen Gesellschaft für Chirurgie zu Berlin, 22. April 1897.

Figure 6 Title page of Rehn's report describing the first successful cardiorrhaphy. *Photo Source National Library of Medicine. Literary Source Rehn, L. (1897) Ueber penetrirende Herwunden und Herznaht. Arch. Klin. Chir., 55, 315. Courtesy of National Library of Medicine*

point in our civilization, and could not accept a return to Galenic pontification. That very same year saw Paget's myopic opinion refuted with Rehn's successful attempt at suturing a stab wound of the heart in a human[198].

Rehn's surgical skills were largely self-taught. Apparently this was no handicap since in the course of only 4 years, he rose from the level of general practitioner who had opened his own small private surgical clinic to become, at first, surgical director of the Frankfurt State Hospital, and later, professor of surgery at the newly founded University of Frankfurt[199].

Figure 6 depicts the title page of his eye-opening report that ends on the pleasing note regarding not only the possibility but also the feasibility of cardiorrhaphy. The irony of it all is that it was presented to the establishment by someone who had never been a product of their hierarchy.

The opening remarks describe rather graphically the urgency of the situation that led him to suture a

gaping wound of the right ventricle that was about 1.5 cm long. 'In the desperate case of a stab wound of the right ventricle, I was forced to operate … There was no other option open to me, with the patient lying before me, bleeding to death. After a perusal of the following case history, the surgeon will be able to place himself in my position. Though one would have liked to have had time to carefully consider the problem, it demanded an immediate solution'[198].

He was able to say before this august gathering of the German Society of Surgery that 'I am in the fortunate position to be able to tell you that the patient returned to good health. He occupies himself with light work, as I have not yet permitted him physical exertion … The patient has every prospect of remaining well'. His concluding remarks were an attempt to lay to rest any misgivings concerning his conduct: 'Gentlemen! The feasibility of cardiorrhaphy no longer remains in doubt. I need not fear any objections as to its propriety; the operation not only was lifesaving, but prevented the subsequent development of constrictive pericarditis. I trust that this case will not remain a curiosity, but rather, that the field of cardiac surgery will be further investigated. Let me speak once more my conviction that by means of the cardiorrhaphy, many lives can be saved that were previously counted as lost'.

Rehn was not the only one that helped demolish the entrenched beliefs of the ancients. Two other reports also appeared at about the same time. They were by Farina of Rome[200], and Cappelen of Norway[201]. Farina's report appeared a few months before that of Cappelen. It was a rather brief communication, more in the form of a petulant note rather than a purely scientific discussion. Cappelen's report described the presence of a large quantity of blood in both the pleural and pericardial sacs, the ligation of a coronary artery from whence the massive bleeding was coming, and the suturing of a superficial wound of the ventricular myocardium[201]. Among the three reports only Rehn's patient survived, and it is because of this that he is considered to have been the first to have successfully sutured a heart wound in a human, and which no doubt provided the impetus for attempts of the same nature by others.

Ten years after his initial attempt, Rehn had accumulated a surgical experience of 124 cases with a mortality rate of 60%. This was quite a significant achievement for the time[202]. Many obstacles had to be overcome, and much more extensive experience was needed before the mortality rate could be reduced to a currently acceptable level. Of course, as with all other endeavors in medicine, the further evolution of surgical repair of traumatic lesions of the heart required a multidisciplinary effort. Modalities had to be developed for the prevention and treatment of infection, a predominant postoperative cause of death. The surgically induced pneumothorax had to be prevented. Anesthesia itself had to emerge from its primitive beginnings.

Despite all this and before the advent of such sophistication, aggressive surgeons continued to report their experience with individual cases. An example of this was the case report of a 'country doctor' in Alabama, Dr Luther Hill, who described the successful repair of a wound that had penetrated the ventricular chambers. A more primitive setting for the intervention is hard to imagine. The surgical theater was a run-down shack. The kitchen table served as the operating table and lighting was provided by means of two kerosene lamps. Apparently a feat of this sort was not unique. He went on to report in 1902 a 'Case of successful suturing of the heart' with a 'table of 37 other cases of suturing by different operators with various terminations'[203]. Hill's report is generally accepted as being the first published report by an American who was able to duplicate Rehn's successful experience.

Another example is of some interest in that the surgery was performed by a negro surgeon in 1893; a period of time in the United States of America that rarely saw a black professional. He was Daniel H. Williams, a surgeon from Chicago who described a patient still alive 3 years after he sutured a stab wound of the pericardium[204].

In 1926, Claude Beck published an outstanding paper on wounds of the heart[205]. It contained the first English description of the technical steps in heart wound repair. The paper is considered a classic in that it not only presented Beck's own experimental observations on the best technique for approaching various injuries, but also because it reviewed the historical background of heart wound surgery up to that time. The icing on the cake was his presentation of a clear translation of Sauerbruch's earlier technical observations. Beck's research on the subject and his paper generated a wide interest in America, encouraging many surgeons to try their hand in such wounds. Among them were Daniel Elkin and R. Arnold Griswold. In 1936, Elkin presented the results of his series of 13 patients at the annual meeting of the American Association for Thoracic Surgery[206]. The work was conducted at Emory University. Meanwhile, Griswold had already repaired the heart wounds of 12 patients, having acquired interest in this type of surgery while working with Beck at the Cleveland clinic. Griswold continued to maintain an active interest in heart wound repair long after he left Cleveland to join the faculty at the University of Louisville in Kentucky. He transmitted this interest to many of his residents, who in turn became the source of many investigations and papers on the subject[207–217].

Griswold established in 1936 the tenets of a plan for the management of acute cardiac injuries that, for the most part, are still followed today. He was honored for this with the presentation of a paper before the 53rd Annual Assembly of the Southeastern Surgical Congress in 1985. This paper described the first 70 years of experience managing cardiac disruption due to penetrating and blunt injuries at the University of Louisville.

Griswold's final publication on heart wounds represented 20 years of personal experience[214]. It was written in opposition to the views held by Elkin and Campbell[217], and before them by Ravitch and Blalock[218], that pericardiocentesis was the treatment of choice for traumatically induced hemopericardium, and that open operation was advisable only if the bleeding could not be controlled. The need to know what was going on within the heart itself as well as in the adjacent structures, mandated, in Griswold's opinion, the opening of the chest.

The presentation honoring Griswold summarized very nicely in the following paragraph the evolution of cardiac wound surgery up until the 1980s:

Subsequent publications have focused further attention on defining criteria for exploration after chest trauma and describing operative technique. Important contributions have included early documentation of the high percentage of patients with clotted blood in the pericardium, the criteria necessary not to explore a transmediastinal penetrating injury, the usefulness of vascular clamps to control atrial wounds, the large percentage (at least one third) of patients with cardiac disruption who have atypical presentations complicating initial evaluation, and the benefit of subxyphoid or transdiaphragmatic pericardiotomy in thoracoabdominal trauma[216,219–223].

Pericardial surgery

The remaining component of the extracardiac era is the evolution of the surgical management of pericardial lesions.

The earliest interventions aimed at the pericardium were most certainly concerned with the removal of fluid from the sac, and in particular, with the removal of blood caused by injury. Kotte and McGuire traced the first pericardiocentesis to Romero in 1819[224]. This is disputed by W. Edmund Farrar Jr[225]. According to him, the first pericardial puncture was described at least 600 years before Romero. He cites as evidence a passage in *Parzival*, the epic poem written by Wolfram von Eschenbach around 1200. The passage is as follows, and I am quite sure that the reader will be as ready as I am to support Farrar's view – provided the poem was actually written around 1200.

> Then my lord Gawan dismounted. There lay a man pierced through, with his blood rushing inward. He asked the hero's lady whether the knight were still alive or in the throes of death.
>
> 'Sir', she replied, 'he is still alive, but I think it will not be for long. God has sent you here for my comfort. Now advise me as your good faith bids you. You have witnessed more dreadful things than I. Let your comfort be shown to me so I may see your help'.
>
> 'That I shall do, Lady', said he. 'I could keep this knight from dying and I feel sure I could save him if I had a reed. You would soon see and hear him in health, because he is not mortally wounded. The blood is only pressing on his heart'.
>
> He grasped a branch of the linden tree, slipped the bark off like a tube and inserted it into the body through the wound. Then he bade the woman suck on it until the blood flowed toward her.
>
> The hero's strength revived so that he could speak and talk again. When he saw Gawan bending over him he thanked him profusely and said it was to his honor to have saved him from his faint.[226]

What is more interesting is the question: How did Wolfram von Eschenbach come to know about pericardial puncture? Farrar states that his research indicated that the author of the poem was a knight and poet. As far as he could discover, the author had no formal training in medicine or surgery. Jousting was a favorite sport of medieval court society. Farrar rightfully mentions this. It is my guess that many a hemopericardium occurred as a result of these jousts and that one or a number of medical professionals of the time probably practiced aspiration of the pericardium without recording the procedure for posterity. If he were not trained in medicine or surgery, von Eschenbach described the procedure so well probably because he personally observed it performed many a time. Attention must also be drawn to the fact that the author must have had some knowledge of the physiological consequences of blood in the pericardial sac. This is evident by Lord Gawan's remark that 'the blood is only pressing on his heart'.

Saul Jarcho, an eminent medical historian, described in 1973 the role played by Thomas Jowett in the evolution of pericardial paracentesis[227]. Jarcho was told by J. N. Allen, Deputy City Librarian of Nottingham, England that Jowett was born at Colwick near Nottingham in 1801, and that he practiced surgery in Nottingham. Jowett's report was written in the form of a letter and carried the title *Case of Dropsy of the Pericardium, in which the Operation of Tapping was performed*[228]. The report was based on some experience he appeared to have developed regarding the nature of pericarditis and its complications based on clinical and post-mortem observations. It appeared in the *Medico-Chirurgical Review* in 1827, some 8 years after Romero's description.

On reading the report as published in Jarcho's paper, I found the following remarks to be the most pertinent[227].

> Last June, a case of acute pericarditis came under my care, in which the accumulation of fluid interrupted the heart's action so materially, that I expected the issue to prove fatal, unless it were evacuated by the operation. I at that time inserted the following observations in my note book.
>
> June 14th, 8 AM I attribute the interruption of the heart's action to the fluid filling the pericardium; and from a careful examination by the stethoscope, percussion, &c. I think the

pericardium might be cautiously punctured with a trocar between the 6th and 7th left cartilages, without wounding the heart, and the fluid be abstracted. At the same time, I consider that, in the present stage of our knowledge, the operation would only be justifiable under desperate circumstances, and, when it is clear that death must ensue without it, and I have mentioned it to the friends as a chance of life, when no other chance remained. Should the case become desperate, I think I should do it, if he consented.

In the performance of the operation, I think two things are essentially necessary to be guarded against. (1st) Not to wound the heart, and (2nd) not to admit air into the pericardium.

The opportunity to actually perform the procedure presented itself several months later when a 14 year old girl with pericarditis came under his care, and who, in his opinion would benefit from aspirating the pericardim. He performed the puncture with a trocar but was able to get only 2 or 3 drops of fluid. A second attempt higher up yielded no fluid. The patient died 10 days later. Jowett was given permission to conduct a postmortem examination. It was obvious why he did not obtain any fluid; there was none. The pericardium was almost totally adherent to the heart and surrounding structures with the sac containing 'firmish recent lymph'.

Jowett's concluding remarks are as follows:

To this long account I may add, that I have since tried the experiment of puncturing the free portion of the pericardium on the dead body, and I have found, that the point of the trocar readily penetrates the sac; but as soon as the edge of the cannula (which of course is always rather larger than the instrument it contains) comes in contact with it, it pushes the pericardium before it, and does not enter it, unless it be introduced to a considerable depth. This explains the supposed failure of the operation in the first instance.

I conclude by observing, that the following propositions appear to me fair practical deductions from the case: 1st, That the operation of tapping the pericardium may be performed without injuring the heart, or endangering the life of the patient. 2nd, that the operation affords a probable chance of saving life, when all other means have failed. 3rd, That it is proper and justifiable under

urgent circumstances. Believe me, Dear Sir,
Your most obliged servant,
Thomas Jowett.

This entire communication represents Jowett's sole contribution to pericardiocentesis. Actually, he played a very small role in the development of the procedure. The report is of historical interest, however, in that it pointed out the feasibility of aspirating the pericardium, and the benefits to be derived if done properly. What is more astounding is the revelation that the diagnosis of pericardial effusion was entertained and indeed possible utilizing only the basic elements of physical diagnosis.

As diagnostic techniques became more accurate, pericardiocentesis became more frequent. This has been especially so with the introduction of echo-cardiography in the 20th century. The non-invasive nature of echocardiography along with its safety and ability to provide an immediate diagnosis, have been instrumental in establishing pericardial aspiration as a useful and often life-saving procedure.

Constrictive pericarditis has also lent itself quite readily to surgical intervention. Weill was the first to suggest a surgical approach in 1895[229]. Delorme performed decortication and removal of segments of pericardium on cadavers, and reported this experience in 1898[230]. Carl Beck also suggested this type of approach in the opening years of the 20th century[231]. In 1902 Brauer, a German physician, suggested that surgeons perform what he termed 'cardiolysis'. This involved removal of ribs and cartilage overlying the pericardial scar with no attempt being made to remove the adhesions[232]. Although this procedure was tried by Peterson and Simon during the ensuing decade[233], it was obviously not a truly physiological remedy whereas the decortication approach advocated by Weill, Delorme and Carl Beck was.

Several scattered reports appeared which confirmed the results of these early pioneers, but it was not until Ludwig Rehn entered the scene that pericardial resection was established as the procedure of choice[234]. His paper appeared in 1920, and was based on his experience with 4 patients. Victor Schmieden, a German physician, was so markedly impressed with the physiological rationale offered by Rehn that he became quite aggressive in applying pericardial resection for the relief of constrictive pericarditis. He also called the procedure cardiolysis, and acquired more experience with the procedure than all the other surgeons of the time. His results were published in 1926, and established him as an international authority in the field[235].

The first successful pericardial resection in the USA was performed by Edward Churchill in Boston in 1929[236]. The case was referred to him by Paul D. White, who, as noted in Section 2, was responsible for reactivation of interest in constrictive pericarditis. Claude Beck along with Griswold and Moore helped refine the techniques of pericardiectomy[237,238].

Before proceeding to the epoch of blind intracardiac surgery, I would like to present at this time the historical background of both thoracic anesthesia and blood transfusions. Both of these techniques have proven invaluable. Without them, intrathoracic surgery of any kind could not advance. Later, we shall see how hypothermia, circulatory arrest, and cardiopulmonary bypass contributed towards the feats of open heart surgery.

Thoracic anesthesia

Methods for keeping subjects alive during surgical procedures involving the thorax can be found even during the 16th century. When Vesalius practiced dissection he kept his animals alive during his experiments on the lungs by blowing air through the lumen of a reed or cane placed in the trachea[239].

After anesthesia was discovered, a very significant step forward was made by John Snow of London in 1858. He is credited with being the first full time anesthesiologist – a precedent which, unfortunately, was not routinely adopted by hospitals until the 20th century. He demonstrated the feasibility of maintaining both respiration and anesthesia by means of a tube with one end attached to a bag filled with chloroform vapor and the other end inserted into the trachea through a tracheotomy[240]. Rabbits were used as subjects. Trendelenburg applied this technique to a human subject in 1869 as a means of preventing aspiration of blood into the lungs while operating on the upper air passages[241]. His endotracheal tube had an inflatable cuff which sealed off the lower part of the trachea from blood coming from above while allowing air to pass through the tube. Various modifications of endotracheal intubation then appeared during the remaining years of the 19th century. These were introduced by William Macewan in 1880[242], Karel Maydl in 1893[243], and Victor Eisenmenger, also in 1893[244].

Prevention of pneumothorax with its attendant shock and asphyxia had to be overcome if thoracic surgery were to advance. Initial attempts utilized intralaryngeal or endotracheal intubation as a means of maintaining artificial respiration. Tuffier and Hallion introduced an insufflation technique in 1896[245]. They described the successful resection of part of a lung with artificial respiration maintained via a tube inserted through the larynx into the trachea. The distal end of the tube had a fitting in the shape of a T allowing for the administration of chloroform at one end and air through a bellows at the other end. A similar type of technique was also described by Doyen in 1897[246].

Rudolph Matas whom we have already met was also a leading pioneer in thoracic surgery. In his quest for developing a safe approach, he too turned his attention to solving the problem of surgically induced pneumothorax. He resorted to a modification of the Fell–O'Dwyer apparatus. The original apparatus was designed by Fell of Buffalo, New York. It consisted of a simple foot bellows connected to an endotracheal tube or a face mask[247]. O'Dwyer's modification consisted of fitting the endotracheal end of the tube with variously sized conical tips for easier insertion into the larynx. The device was originally introduced as a means of relieving respiratory distress in diphtheritic obstructive lesions or opium poisoning[248]. The Fell–O'Dwyer apparatus is illustrated in Figure 7. F. W. Parham, a colleague of Matas, used it for the first time during the removal of a sarcoma of the chest wall[249,250].

Although Matas was rapidly establishing himself as a leader in the surgical management of aneurysms, this reputation did not prevent his modified Fell–O'Dwyer apparatus from being discarded in favor of other approaches that were evolving. The variety and complexity of the newer modalities were marvels of ingenuity, very interesting, and often quite cumbersome. Quenu's approach, described in 1896, was based on the concept that surgical pneumothorax could be avoided by keeping the lungs inflated during surgery with ambient air at greater than atmospheric pressure. This required the use of a positive pressure chamber in the form of a diver's helmet that had an air-tight seal at the neck when placed over the patient's head. A compressed-air pump supplied the air

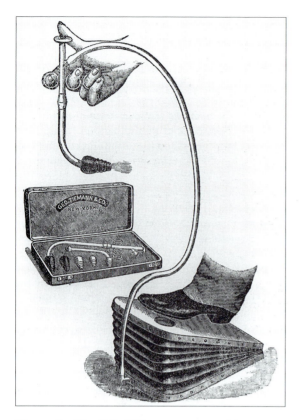

Figure 7 The Fell–O'Dwyer apparatus. *Photo Source National Library of Medicine. Literary Source Matas, R. (1899). On the management of acute traumatic pneumothorax. Ann. Surg., **29**, 428. Courtesy of National Library of Medicine*

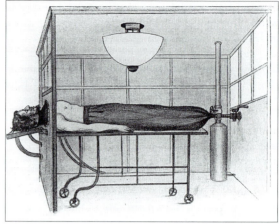

Figure 8 A depiction of an early version of Sauerbruch's negative-pressue chamber. *Photo Source National Library of Medicine. Literary Source Johnson, S.L. The History of Cardiac Surgery, 1896–1955. Johns Hopkins University Press, Journals Publishing Division, 701 W. 40th Street, Ste. 275, Baltimore MD, 21211. With permission*

which flowed through a simple sponge saturated with chloroform[251].

In 1903, Ferdinand Sauerbruch proposed the placement of the patient's thorax within an air-tight negative pressure chamber. The subject's head remained outside the chamber with an air-tight seal at the neck. After being satisfied with the experimental results on dogs, this approach was tried for the first time on a human with Sauerbruch at the controls and his mentor, von Mikulicz as the surgeon, performing the operation while within a specially constructed 500 cubic feet chamber of glass and iron[252,253]. Figure 8 depicts an early version of Sauerbruch's negative pressure chamber.

This had all the trappings of modern technology and created quite a sensation throughout Europe. It was introduced to the USA by Willie Meyer of the Rockefeller Institute. He had personally observed its use by its inventor in 1904, and became so impressed with its possibilities that over the next five years he continued to pursue the applicability of both negative and positive pressure chambers in thoracic surgical procedures. Meyer's efforts culminated in his design of a universal pressure chamber. This consisted of a small positive pressure chamber for the anesthetist and the patient's head, and a rather large negative pressure chamber that accommodated the entire surgical team as well as the rest of the patient's body. In essence, it was a self-contained surgical theater constructed exclusively for thoracic surgery. Lenox Hill Hospital in New York was the first to have such a chamber built for the purpose. This was in 1911 with Meyer in charge of all the details[254]. Figure 9 is an illustration of Meyer's chamber.

Meyer and Sauerbruch were not alone in implementing this approach. Modifications and refinements from other investigators were soon forthcoming. Brauer's positive pressure device enclosed the patient's head in an air-tight chamber with only a 5 cubic feet capacity[255]. Masktype pressure devices were introduced by Brat and Schmieden[256]. This eliminated the necessity of a special chamber for the patient's head. Positive pressure within the lungs was maintained by a spring valve. Tiegel's refinement was essentially the same except that he regulated the pressure with a water column[257].

These were all steps in efforts to avoid the special and cumbersome chambers of Sauerbruch and Meyer. But they all had inherent disadvantages and before the chambers could be discarded, further advances had to be made in endotracheal anesthesia. The door was opened, so to speak, in 1907 with the discovery of the insufflation principle of endotracheal anesthesia by Barthelémy and Dufour[258]. The same discovery was made independently by Meltzer and Auer at the Rockefeller Institute in 1909[259]. These two physiologists devised an apparatus for administering endotracheal anesthesia that completely eliminated the inhalation principle in the normal inflow and outflow of air. It maintained the lungs at constant expansion by air flow under external pressure. Insufflation endotracheal anesthesia in thoracic surgery gained an enthusiastic adherent in the person of Charles Elsberg, a New York surgeon. It was mainly through his efforts that the procedure became firmly established[260].

The development of direct laryngoscopy provided another step for the routine use of the insufflation technique. Although introduced by Alfred Kirstein as early as 1895, it was not widely adopted until Chevalier Jackson's modification appeared in 1913[261,262]. Concomitant with the introduction and refinement of direct laryngoscopic methods, the era of insufflation anesthesia also saw further improvements in endotracheal intubation with its advantages in maintaining an open airway and removal of secretions. Modifications in the technique of endotracheal intubation allowed for a return in due time to the inhalation principle. World War I provided a major opportunity for implementing it. Magill and Rowbotham were the pioneers. They acquired an extensive experience while attached to the British Army Plastic Unit, and reported the details of this experience in the *Proceedings of the Royal Society of Medicine*[263]. They administered the anesthetic agent via a single large-bore endotracheal tube that was attached to a semi-closed anesthesia machine. The work of these two men caused a radical change in thoracic anesthesia methodology that prevailed until the 1930s. Inhalational endotracheal intubation gradually replaced not only the insufflation technique but also the cumbersome differential pressure machines introduced by Sauerbruch. It is of interest to note, though, that even in the face of these advances

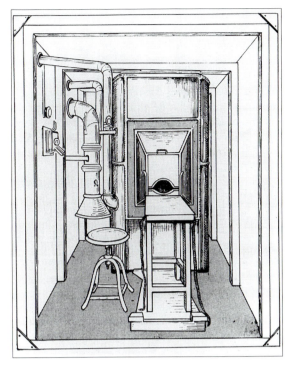

Figure 9 Meyer's universal pressure chamber. *Photo Source National Library of Medicine. Literary Source Johnson, S.L. The History of Cardiac Surgery, 1896–1955. Johns Hopkins University Press, Journals Publishing Division, 701 W. 40th Street, Ste. 275, Baltimore, MD, 21211. With permission*

pockets of Sauerbruch adherents still used his machine as late as the beginning of World War II[264].

Further advances were now made along several interrelated pathways. Attention was focused on modifications of the semi-closed anesthesia machine of Magill and Rowbotham, development of controlled respiration techniques, and pharmacologic research in the creation of newer anesthetic agents. Most important was the tremendous impact made by the introduction of methods for monitoring and management not only of respiration, but also of cardiovascular activity.

The advances began with the introduction of closed-system anesthesia machines utilizing absorbing agents for carbon dioxide. The first such machine used sodium or potassium hydroxide solutions for absorption of the expired carbon dioxide. It was designed by Dennis Jackson, a pharmacologist, who first described its use in experimental animals in 1915[265]. Clinical application was not realized, however, until 1924, when Waters introduced a machine based on a to-and-fro principle utilizing soda lime as the carbon dioxide absorbent[266]. This machine enjoyed a high degree of acceptance on the part of anesthesiologists, undergoing several modifications with continued usage[267]. The possibility of transmitting infectious agents to the patient while anesthetized with Waters' machine was reduced when Sword and his associates strategically relocated the soda lime cannister and breathing bag[268].

The first paper devoted to cardiac anesthesia was from Merel Harmel and Austin Lamont, both from Johns Hopkins University. It was published in 1946 under the title *Anesthesia in the surgical treatment of congenital pulmonary stenosis*[269]. As the epoch of blind intracardiac surgery evolved, Keown then reported on the anesthetic management of closed mitral commissurotomy[270].

As time went on, and just prior to the era of open heart surgery, it was becoming quite obvious that anesthesiologists were needed who were quite knowledgeable in the anesthetic nuances of cardiac surgery. More and more anesthesiologists took up the challenge and began to restrict their activities to cardiac surgery. A subspecialization was in the making, but it was not until 1967 that Harry Wollman and Alan Ominsky 'proclaimed' themselves cardiac anesthetists[271]. Monitoring devices at the time of their statement were still rather rudimentary but a movement was already in place to remedy this with electronic equipment capable of keeping tabs on various hemodynamic parameters. I remember distinctly how I monitored for the first time a cardiac oscilloscope connected to my patient who was prone to paroxysms of ventricular tachycardia, and who was undergoing a spinal fusion at the time. The situation was unique for me but cardiologists in the operating room were becoming 'standard equipment' in both cardiac and non-cardiac surgery. Cardiologists in attendance at these exercises persisted only until we learned that anesthesiologists were becoming quite skilled in the diagnosis and management of cardiac arrhythmias during surgical procedures.

The beginnings of surgical approaches in revascularizing the myocardium proved to be an important impetus in formulating and structuring a comprehensive plan for the management of all cardiac surgical cases. The underlying concept was teamwork between the anesthesiologist, the surgeon, blood gas technicians, and the rest of the panoply that emerged with each notable advance. Various types of monitoring devices were introduced and needed a collator to render them effective. Pulmonary care services and post-operative intensive care units came into being. The anesthesiologist was given due recognition that he was an integral part of the intensive care unit, and that the immediate postoperative care was within his purview.

Succeeding innovations, even though minor in themselves, served to promote even more, the maturation of cardiac surgery. These included the introduction of lung ventilators, the replacement of Cournand needles with Rochester needles, reinstatement of narcotic anesthesia, usage of intra-jugular lines, and a host of newer pharmacologic agents with inotropic, vasodilating and anti-arrhythmic properties. When the Swan–Gans catheter was introduced, hemodynamic monitoring was raised to a highly refined level.

The reader is by now certainly aware that refinements in thoracic and cardiac anesthesia were major factors in securing the high level of efficacy enjoyed by cardiac surgery. However, the reader should also be aware that despite the perceived sophisticated level of today we cannot rest on our laurels. There are still many improvements in the offing, and what may seem so wonderful today may prove to be quite primitive in the next century.

Blood transfusions

Along with anesthesia, the ability to transfuse blood safely constituted another critically important element in the evolution of cardiac surgery. Many factors had to be resolved before it became the simple and relatively safe therapeutic modality that it is today. Paramount among these factors were the much feared transfusion reaction; the transition from a direct to an indirect mode of transfusion; prevention of blood clotting; development of methods for the collection and preservation of blood; and last, but certainly not least, the matter of transmissable diseases. Resolution of all these problems was a long and arduous affair requiring the skills of various disciplines.

References to blood transfusions can be found in the writings of antiquity. Animal blood was used with often fatal reactions. The first clear description of the use of human blood appeared in 1615. Andreas Libavius was the author of this report[272].

It did not have any impact since animal blood, with its attendant and often fatal complications, continued to remain the main source for transfusion.

The earliest attempts at a disciplined approach did not appear until 1824 with the publication of a paper by James Blundell, a London obstetrician[273]. This paper described 3 methods of blood transfusion as utilized in 5 women and using only human blood. This was his first attempt, and despite the fact that he used only human blood all of the women died. Ignorant of the nuances of blood transfusion, he was unable to unravel the reasons for their death. He did manage to successfully transfuse human blood in subsequent attempts reporting this 4 years after his initial paper[274]. Again, this was but a chance affair since he was still unaware of the underlying pathophysiology.

The mechanism underlying the fatal reactions with animal blood was finally brought to light in 1875. This was the result of investigations by two men working independently of each other. They were Emil Ponfick and Leonard Landois[275,276]. Their work put an end to the usage of animal blood but failed to shed any light on the fatal mechanisms involved when using human blood as the donor source.

Karl Landsteiner finally clarified the mechanism while working as an assistant in the Institute of Pathological Anatomy at the University of Vienna. In his paper, published in 1901, he was able to show that clumping of the donor's red blood cells was responsible for the clinical manifestations of the transfusion reaction[277]. Furthermore, this initial paper, based on a study of 22 subjects, revealed that the clumping was due to the presence of iso-agglutinins in the recipient's serum. He described 3 different types of iso-agglutinins. These formed the basis for his blood group classification known to us initially as A, B, and C.

This was a remarkable achievement, but unfortunately, its potentiality was not widely appreciated until several years later when Hektoen, an American, emphasized the clinical importance of agglutination in causing transfusion reactions[278]. By this time another blood type had been added to Landsteiner's original three. It was labeled O when discovered by Alfred von Decastello and Adriano Sturli in 1902[279].

Further work on iso-agglutination was carried on by other American investigators. Hoekten's work had led John Funke at Jefferson Medical College

Hospital to utilize the iso-agglutination phenomenon as the basis for cross-agglutination tests while John Gibbon, a Philadelphia surgeon, lent his prestige to Funke's suggestion that these tests be done prior to the transfusion as a method of assuring compatibility[278,280]. Reuben Ottenberg also described in 1911 the value of these tests in reducing the incidence of transfusion reactions[281]. Statistical evidence finally led to the establishment of 'typing and cross-matching' as a requisite and mandatory procedure for all future blood transfusions.

Landsteiner was awarded the Nobel Prize in 1930 for providing the immunologic basis for transfusion reactions, and for providing the groundwork that was so essential for the development of proper testing procedures prior to transfusion. Before Landsteiner's contributions several tests had been devised to minimize the possibility of transfusion reactions. A 'biologic test' was one of the most popular. This was really a trial and error method of determining incompatibility. A small amount of the donor's blood was injected into the recipient's bloodstream. If no manifestations of a transfusion reaction occurred, the assumption was that the donor's blood did not have the potential to bring about the recipient's death. This was hardly a scientific approach and underscores once more that knowledge of pathophysiologic mechanisms is the key to clinical success.

Initially, blood transfusions were carried out by tapping the donor and allowing the blood to pass directly into the recipient's bloodstream. This direct technique was plagued by the frequent clotting of the blood during the procedure. An important advance in the technique was made with the introduction of Crile's arterio-venous approach in 1907[282,283]. Crile utilized Carrel's method of anastomosing the blood vessels end-to-end. Blood clotting did not occur presumably because the donor's blood always remained in contact with the inner lining of the donor's peripheral artery and that of the anastomosed vein of the recipient. Usually the donor's radial artery was used along with any suitable arm vein of the recipient. It was a rather cumbersome and time-consuming technique. Despite its obvious disadvantages, Crile's method proved to be quite practical, and for that era, an acceptable method for transfusing blood. He later modified the anastomosis by using a ring-like device with a handle attached to it. This enabled him to slip the isolated radial artery over the recipient's arm

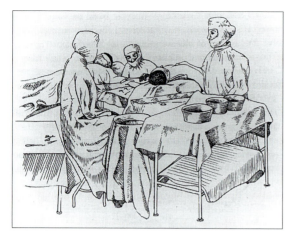

Figure 10 The Crile method of direct arterio-venous blood transfusion, with the donor on the right and the recipient on the left. *Photo Source National Library of Medicine. Literary Source Johnson, S.L. The history of Cardiac Surgery, 1896–1955. Johns Hopkins University Press, Jounals Publishing Division, 701 W. 40th Street, Ste.275, Baltimore, MD, 21211. With permission*

vein, thus providing a continuous surface without the need of sutures[283]. Figure 10 illustrates Crile's method of direct arteriovenous blood transfusion.

The many disadvantages of direct transfusion, however, stimulated the search for methods that would ensure the success of delivering stored blood. This became known as indirect transfusion. It is the prevailing method of our time. The first step in this direction was the use of citrate to prevent the blood from clotting. This discovery alone had the potentiality to assign Crile's arterio-venous approach to the dustbin of historical memorabilia.

As early as 1774, William Hewson had described the use of 'neutral salts' as a means of preventing clotting[284]. This finding was an isolated report, and in reality, it had no impact on the development of means to prevent this phenomenon. A unique approach was the use of defibrinated blood. It was first described by Prévost and Dumas in 1821, and remained for several decades a widely used method[285]. The defibrinated blood was prepared by churning until enough fibrin was deposited on the churning instrument. In 1890, Arthus and Pagés were the first to report that the essential ingredient in initiating the clotting mechanism was calcium[286]. They found that when citrate was added to the donor's blood, it prevented clotting by combining with the donor's calcium ions. This technique remained a laboratory modality for many years before it was adopted by the clinicians. Actually the clinical usage of citrate became established only when efforts were exerted for the implementation of the indirect mode of transfusion, which of course necessitated finding some means for preserving donor's blood.

A major consideration before citrated blood could be used in man was the question of its toxic potentiality, if any. A. Hustin of Belgium provided the answer when he reported in 1914 that in animals the small amount of citrate needed to prevent clotting was non-toxic, and that, in addition, it did not lower the blood calcium level[287,288]. Later in the year, he reported his success with indirect blood transfusion in man using citrated blood[289]. Two other reports appeared within a year of Hustin's paper describing a similar pattern of success in indirect blood transfusion. These were by L'Agote of Buenos Aires and Lewisohn of New York[290,291]. In all of these early attempts, the donor's blood was given to the recipient as soon as possible. Methods for long term preservation were not available as yet. Within these constraints, indirect blood transfusion with citrated blood proved to be of exceptional value during World War I. Many lives were saved while research efforts continued in search of a safe method for preserving the donor's blood as long as possible[292].

Weil was the first to demonstrate that blood containing isotonic sodium citrate had a safe lifespan of only 3.5 days[293]. This was expanded up to several weeks by the addition of dextrose. Peyton Rous and J. R. Turner of the Rockefeller Institute were responsible for this discovery[294,295]. The first large-scale application of preserved blood using the method of Rous and Turner occurred in the latter part of World War I[296,297]. Oswald Robertson reported this in 1918[296]. He used blood from group O donors preserved with isotonic citrate-dextrose solution and stored under refrigeration.

When World War I ended no further advances in blood preservation were made until the Russians became interested in the problem. The leading figure in the search was a celebrated Russian surgeon, Sergei Yudin. His initial attempts centered on the use of cadaver blood with the first successful transfusion of such blood performed in March, 1930[298–300]. Yudin was quick to point out the many advantages of cadaver blood. It could be stored easily and its safety against transmissable diseases could be established by autopsy as well as by using the Wasserman serologic test for syphilis. By 1932, Yudin was able to report on his experience with stored cadaver blood in 100 cases[301]. He presented his findings at a meeting of the Société National de Chirurgie in Paris.

Russian investigators continued to dominate the field of blood transfusion throughout the 1930s. Blood transfusion centers were set up in several of the Russian cities. Extensive experience was also gained with the usage of stored blood from living human donors. By 1936, Bagdassarov of Moscow was able to describe his experience with over 6000 transfusions of stored human blood[302].

The Spanish Civil War provided another opportunity to demonstrate the value and safety of stored human blood. In 1936, F. Duran Jorda established a blood transfusion service for the Spanish Republican Army. This was a massive effort operating within the city of Barcelona[303]. At the same time another transfusion center was established in Madrid. It was organized by the Sanidad Militar of the Spanish Republic. These two centers were actually blood banks containing a pool of blood from thousands of donors, and stored under rigidly controlled conditions regarding preservation and safety from transmissable diseases, especially syphilis[304]. Unfortunately, transmissable diseases are still a problem. The current epidemic of AIDS is a poignant example with many hemophiliacs and others infected with the human immunodeficiency virus by direct contamination with blood transfusion. Even if AIDS and hepatitis could be purged from the blood supply, threats still remain. Two reasons account for this. These are the so-called open window and lack of routine screening for certain infectious disturbances. To minimize the risks, the trend now is to store one's own blood prior to elective surgery. This safeguard, however, is not available during emergency surgery or for hemophiliacs. Still another threat is that of receiving incompatible blood from a bedside mix-up or through mislabeling. The Spanish concept of blood banks was rapidly adopted in England and the USA. During the 1930s blood banks were established in Cook County Hospital in Chicago, the Philadelphia General Hospital and the Kings County Hospital in Brooklyn (where I did my residency in Internal Medicine)[305]. The term 'blood bank' was coined by Bernard Fantus when he set up the first preservation depot at Cook County Hospital[306,307].

In England, blood banks were being established not only for civilian use but also in preparation for the anticipated casualties from the imminent outbreak of World War II. In fact, World War II provided the next opportunity for perfecting blood preservation techniques. In 1938, Cotter and MacNeal demonstrated that the *in vitro* destruction of red blood cells in a trisodium–citrate–glucose solution could be reduced by adjusting the pH to near neutrality with citric acid[308]. In 1944, Loutit and colleagues stationed at the Southwest London Blood Supply Depot, found that Cotter and MacNeal's method also increased the survival time of the donor's red blood cells[309]. The resultant mixture was called the ADC solution. This method of preservation was soon adopted throughout the world.

BLIND INTRACARDIAC SURGERY

The historical highlights of that epoch of cardiac surgery characterized by Harken as the era of blind intracardiac surgery can now be related. Indeed, it began with Harken himself leading the way with his successful removal of foreign bodies followed by surgery of the heart valves and certain congenital defects.

Prior to Harken the removal of foreign bodies from the heart was also, like so many other developments in cardiology, a sporadic event, performed under trying conditions and limited to personal involvement with single cases. We are indebted to Ryerson Decker for his summation of 109 of these cases compiled from the literature[310]. An amazing collection of items were identified at surgery or postmortem. Among them were such items as needles, nails, toothpicks and wooden splinters. Even dental plates and an aluminum pipe stem were found. Even more amazing was Decker's notation that quite a few of these people went about their daily activities without undue effect. He even described one man as still being able to indulge in his hobby – mountain climbing. It is perhaps the lack of untoward effects in some of these individuals that led Decker to title his paper 'Foreign bodies in the heart and pericardium – should they be removed?'

It was not until the latter part of World War II that an opportunity arose for the development of an extensive experience in the removal of foreign bodies from the heart under relatively controlled conditions. The major factors ensuring an ultimately successful outcome were already in place as described in the preceding section dealing with anesthesia, blood transfusion, infections, and the like. All that was needed now was an aggressive and well-trained thoracic surgeon. This appeared in the person of Dwight Harken. He seized the opportunity while serving in the medical corps of the United States Army. He was able to perform 134 operations in which foreign bodies, mostly shell fragments, were removed from the heart chambers, walls or adnexae and great vessels[311]. It was this military experience that aroused in Harken an intense interest in cardiac surgery, and which, soon after the war, became the focus of his career. In time, this interest was to establish him as one of the leading lights of cardiac surgery.

At the start of World War II, Dwight Harken was RSO to Tudor Edwards at the Brompton Hospital in London. When the United States entered the war, Harken returned to the United States only to return again to Britain in 1944. While serving in London, Harken was fortunately under the command of Elliott Cutler who had been professor of surgery at Harvard, and who, though a general surgeon, could be considered as one of the pioneers of thoracic surgery. In view of the anticipated heavy workload from the soon to be launched allied invasion, a course was planned to train medical officers in the new techniques of cardiac surgery that were emerging and Harken was designated to supervise them. Several centers were also set up in England for the treatment of thoracic wounds. Dwight Harken was made director of the 15th Thoracic Center in Cirencester. This was an opportunity that Harken pursued with all the vigor that he possessed. He immediately surrounded himself with a highly competent staff of surgeons, anesthesiologists and nurses. As the casualties from D-day began arriving in ever increasing numbers, Harken and his team worked ceaselessly around the clock. This intensive effort continued in an intermittent fashion as the allied forces advanced towards Germany. After receiving approval from his military superiors, Harken began his aggressive approach in the removal of missiles embedded within the heart or its chambers[312-316]. This important chapter in the history of cardiac surgery is vividly recounted by Johnson as follows:

Harken used the latest surgical techniques to remove the missiles. Prior to operation, the position of the missile was pinpointed by fluoroscopy. At operation, the patient was induced by intravenous pentothal sodium anesthesia; intubated with a large bore endotracheal tube; and maintained with nitrous oxide, ether, oxygen, and assisted respiration. To remove the missile, the heart was often split wide open, with tremendous blood loss. Rapid, massive, blood transfusions were needed to keep the patient alive. Whole blood was often administered, under pressure, at rates up to one and one-half liters per minute. Penicillin, which was just beginning to make an impact on thoracic surgery, was often given in 10 000 unit injections, either intra-muscularly or into the pleural or pericardial sac.[317]

Johnson also narrates an innovative approach in the removal of missiles as communicated personally to him by Harken himself[318]. This is worthy of quotation if for no other reason than as an indication of Harken's willingness to leave no stone unturned in refining his technique.

One of the stories Harken remembers from his year in Cirencester was the 'giant magnet episode'. Several visitors, who had watched the operations suggested that he try magnetic force to remove the missiles. It was an intriguing idea, so a giant electromagnet was ordered. When it arrived, it was mounted above the operating table, suspended by a large crane. Finally, the day arrived to try out the new device. The patient who had been selected was brought to the operating room, the thorax was opened and the heart exposed. The giant magnet was then lowered and the pole-piece positioned just above the heart. The electric switch was thrown to energize the magnet. Instantly, all the nearby instruments jumped to the pole-piece of the magnet, and there was a tremendous commotion in the operating room. Someone had forgotten to use demagnetized instruments. When the commotion subsided, they looked for the missile, but alas, it was still in place within the heart. They used the magnet on several other patients, but it never was successful.

Harken operated on a total of 135 patients, 17 of whom had shell fragments removed from the chambers themselves. All of the patients survived –

a remarkable achievement, and representative of the first consistently successful elective intra-cardiac surgery.

As the war ended, Harken now turned his attention once more to valvular lesions. Just before the war, Harken had already been engaged in animal experimentation regarding mitral valve surgery at the Boston City Hospital. Upon returning to civilian life, Harken took up where he left off and continued his work not only at Boston City but also at the Peter Bent Brigham Hospital.

Harken, however, was not the first to become interested in the surgical repair of valvular lesions. The earliest rumblings on the subject appeared in a paper written by D. W. Samways. It was published in *The Lancet* in 1898 under the title *Cardiac peristalsis: Its nature and effects*[319]. In his summation he concluded with the following remarks: 'I anticipate that with the progress of cardiac surgery some of the severest cases of mitral stenosis will be relieved by slightly notching the mitral orifice and trusting to the auricle to continue its defense'. Figure 11 is a photograph of the title and concluding statement of Samways' paper[320].

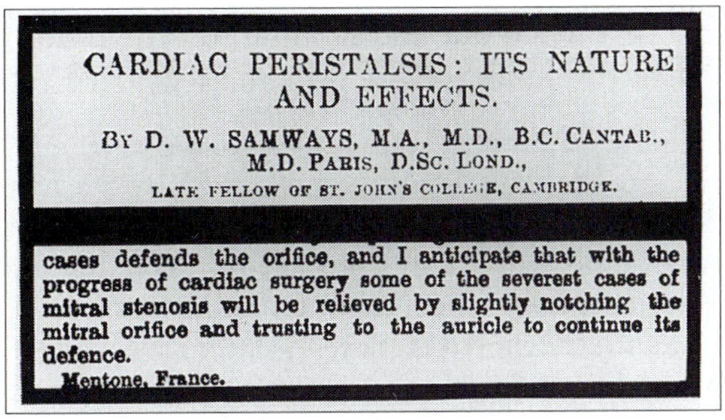

The prescient nature of these remarks must have fallen on deaf ears for he was completely ignored. Sir Lauder Brunton too, was not only completely ignored but also castigated for his views when he suggested four years later that surgery was indeed feasible for the relief of mitral stenosis[321]. His suggestion was part of a preliminary note wherein he propounded the concept that the stenotic mitral slit could be opened by elongating its 'natural opening' and without necessarily creating a leak. This was a notion that was not fully appreciated until the 1940s though in 1927, Bourne stated 'it would seem that an extension of the natural slit at its extremities is preferable to one made laterally into the cusp itself'[322]. This was to remain an essential objective of mitral commissurotomy.

Brunton's suggestion was based on experience acquired on diseased valves of cadavers and on the normal mitral valve of dead cats using a transventricular tenotomy knife[322]. At first he questioned whether the valve should be elongated or cut at right angles, but as we saw, he opted for elongating the 'natural opening'.

Brunton's note also appeared in *The Lancet*. A week later, the editors of this prestigious journal left no doubt as to their opposition to Brunton's views[323]. In an editorial response, they challenged

Figure 11 Title and concluding statement of Samways' paper in 'The Lancet' in 1898. *Photo Source National Library of Medicine. Literary Source Shumaker, H.B. (1968). Authority, research and publication. Reflections based upon some historical aspects of vascular surgery. Ann. Surg., **168**, 169–82. With permission*

his proposal citing the difficulties of the operation and the uncertainty of success. The editorial concluded with this biting sentence: 'But we can only repeat that the mere suggestion of surgical operation for the relief of mitral stenosis casts a grave responsibility upon Sir Lauder Brunton, and a responsibility that he does not lessen by now leaving it to other workers to prove or to disprove its value'. At least the editors had the courtesy to allow Sir Lauder to respond to their editorial criticism. This he did in the following words[324]:

I cannot hope from my own experiments alone to prove the advisability of an operation against which, as stated in your leader, so many a priori arguments can be brought, and therefore hope that others will take up the subject as well as myself. I am quite aware of the responsibility that rests upon me for my suggestion, but I must state that while my experiments on the valves were made only on dead animals my knowledge of the manipulation of the living heart and of the effect upon it of wounds and punctures is based upon very numerous experiments made at intervals during the last 35 years.

Though short-lived, a flurry of interest was created by Brunton's comments and the editorial response. The same issue of *The Lancet* that contained Brunton's response also contained letters from W. Arbuthnot Lane, D. W. Samways, and Theodore Fisher. Samways merely wanted to establish priority in suggesting surgery[325]. Fisher, siding with the editors, felt that the operation would be associated with a high incidence of failure because of irreversible fibrotic changes in the myocardium[326]. Irreversibility of myocardial function in long-standing mitral stenosis was a point well-taken and an important factor in determining the expectant degree of improvement following surgery. W. Arbuthnot Lane was initially in favor of the operation having conceptualized his own approach. Though he believed that the operation was feasible he never attempted it on the advice of his colleague, Lauriston Shaw. He stated that

> it may interest your readers to know that this suggestion was made by me to my colleague, Dr. Lauriston Shaw, some years ago. I then went into the matter fully, both as to the surgical measures to be adopted and the physical conditions of the valve which seemed most suitable for such interference, and was quite prepared to act as soon as Dr. Shaw succeeded in finding a case likely to derive benefit. It was entirely due to his wise caution that the operation has not yet been performed by me. The method by which I proposed to divide the contracted valve through the ventricle was practically identical with that described by Sir Lauder Brunton. Personally I believe that the operation is feasible and under certain circumstances, justifiable.[327]

Shaw corroborated Lane's remarks in another letter that appeared a week later in *The Lancet*[328].

> Lest, however, it should appear from Mr. Lane's letter that I am still hoping to succeed 'in finding a case likely to receive benefit' therefrom, I shall be obliged if you will allow me to state that the a priori arguments against the probability of any patient deriving benefit from this operation seemed to me so conclusive that I deliberately decided against regarding it as a justifiable therapeutic measure. These arguments are so clearly summarized in your leading article of February 15 (p. 461) that your readers will, I think, agree with me that Sir Lauder Brunton's chief task is not to show his surgical colleagues that it is possible to enlarge the stenosed mitral orifice, but to persuade his medical colleagues that such a proceeding is useful. It is possible to do many things that are useless and some things that are harmful.

The debate was not confined to the British Isles. In the same year that saw the publication of Brunton's article, a source of support came from the European continent. It was a paper written by Tollemer wherein he expressed the hope that Brunton's suggestion might indeed be possible[329]. Clinically, though, Brunton's concept was effectively laid to rest until 1913 when Doyen resurrected it in his tenotome correction of a stenotic lesion in the pulmonic area[330]. At this time, he too suggested that the tenotome might be useful in mitral stenosis. However, in the laboratory several investigators were still pursuing the possibility that mitral stenosis was amenable to surgical repair. Strangely enough, one of the earliest experimental investigators was Harvey Cushing, the famous neurosurgeon from Boston[331]. Although his work was restricted to some unsuccessful attempts to create mitral stenosis in dogs, he did provide encouragement to Elliott Cutler, at that time a young and aspiring surgeon. Cutler was to carry out the first clinical trial of mitral valvulotomy while working in Cushing's department some 15 years later. Cushing assigned the fourth experimentation on the problem to B. M. Bernheim. In 1909, Bernheim published his results in a paper which described the technical difficulties involved in the creation of mitral stenosis in dogs but consoled the readers by the relative simplicity of its surgical repair, concluding that the results boded well for its clinical application in humans[332].

E. Jeger in Germany toyed with the possibility of alleviating the symptoms in mitral stenosis by bypassing the valve altogether through a shunt between the pulmonary vein and the left ventricle[333]. This notion failed to arouse any interest and was soon forgotten. In fact, he also never contributed anything further on the matter.

World War I interrupted all further investigation in the field until 1922 when Allen and Graham published their initial work on the problem[334]. These two men devised an instrument for visualizing the interior of the heart. They called it a cardioscope. By trial and error they found that the best way to insert it was through the left atrial appendage. After inducing mitral stenosis, the mitral valve was then easily resected with a small knife attached to the cardioscope. Thirty dogs in all were subjected to this procedure and despite the creation of mitral insufficiency, they appeared to tolerate the procedure well. The leakage did not bother these investigators because they shared the belief prevalent at the time that mitral regurgitation was less damaging than mitral stenosis, since the pulmonary hypertension in mitral insufficiency was thought to be intermittent rather than constant as in mitral stenosis[335].

It was a long time before Allen and Graham were able to try their 'cardioscope cum knife' on a human. It came when a country doctor referred a rather sick patient to them. Meade describes this in his *History of Thoracic Surgery*. '… Finally, a country doctor referred a patient to them who was very sick as a result of mitral stenosis. They planned to carry out the operation in two stages. At the first, they only made the chest-wall incision. At the second operation, they had only opened the pleura when the patient's condition became so critical that the operation had to be stopped. At the third operation, they had gotten to the point of introducing the cardioscope when she suddenly died'[336].

Alexis Carrel had also shown an interest in the surgical management of valvular lesions. In 1914, he described how in his experimental attempts, he exposed the aortic valve in an animal after 'clamping en masse the pedicles of the heart'[337]. Exposure was limited to 2–3 minutes; hardly enough time for a serious attempt at reconstruction. Nevertheless, the experiment was another step in reinforcing the possibility of a surgical repair if the technical problems could be resolved.

When Doyen in 1913 passed a small knife through the right ventricle to correct a stenotic lesion in the pulmonic area, it represented the first clinical attempt of its kind[330]. Unfortunately , since the stenosis was infundibular rather than valvular, the relief was incomplete. At autopsy, the patient was also seen to have been suffering from an interventricular septal defect. That same year, Tuffier attempted to dilate a stenosed aortic valve by invaginating the wall of the aorta with his finger[338]. He also was not favored with a completely successful result, but in his case, it was the concept that was ill-conceived, and not the location of the stenosis.

Several years later (1923), Samuel Levine, the eminent Bostonian cardiologist, collaborated with Elliott Cutler in a palliative procedure for mitral stenosis by producing mitral insufficiency. Cutler and Levine called the procedure a valvulotomy. It was the culmination of two years of experimentation in the laboratory. Their subject was a desperately ill 12 year old girl who was confined to her bed for six months prior to the operation. The girl underwent surgery on May 20, 1923 and the first successful report of cardiotomy and valvulotomy appeared in the June 28, 1923 issue of the *Boston Medical and Surgical Journal*[339].

Although Cutler and Levine were acquainted with Allen and Graham's cardiotome with the self-contained knife, they preferred to resect the mitral valve with their own device. In commenting on this they wrote: 'Our experimental work with the cardioscope left us with the impression that the greater intricacy of the operation and the greater amount of time consumed with this method was such that it seemed wiser to use the simpler and more speedy route through the ventricular wall with the valvulotome in the first human case'.

The essentials of this historical surgical procedure are described very vividly with the following words:

> … the valvulotome, an instrument somewhat similar to a tenotome or a slightly curved tonsil knife … was taken in the right hand and plunged into the left ventricle … The knife was pushed upwards about 2½ inches, until it encountered what seemed to us must be the mitral orifice. It was then turned mesially, and a cut made in what we thought was the aortic leaflet, the resistance encountered being very considerable. The knife was quickly turned and a cut made in the opposite side of the opening. The knife was then withdrawn and the mattress sutures already in place were tied over the point at which the knife had been inserted … The experience with this case … is of importance in that it does show that surgical intervention in cases of mitral stenosis bears no special risk, and should give us further courage and support in our desire to attempt to alleviate a chronic condition, for which there is now not only no treatment, but one which carries a terrible prognosis …

The title page of Cutler and Levine's report is reproduced in Figure 12.

Cutler presented the valvulotome that he used in the procedure to his protege, Harken, who, in turn, used it many times in resecting stenotic lesions of the pulmonary valve[340].

In 1925, Henry Souttar of London used for the first time a transatrial approach to fracture the stenotic mitral valve with his finger[341]. The patient, a 19 year old girl, survived, and thus his attempt represents the first successful digital commissurotomy for the relief of mitral stenosis. Brunton's vision had come true. An important feature of the operation was the use of

The Boston Medical and Surgical Journal

TABLE OF CONTENTS

June 28, 1923

Original Articles.

CARDIOTOMY AND VALVULOTOMY FOR MITRAL STENOSIS. EXPERIMENTAL OBSERVATIONS AND CLINICAL NOTES CONCERNING AN OPERATED CASE WITH RECOVERY.

BY ELLIOTT C. CUTLER, M.D., BOSTON,

AND

S. A. LEVINE, M.D., BOSTON.

[From the Surgical Clinic of the Peter Bent Brigham Hospital and the Laboratory of Surgical Research of the Harvard Medical School.]

DURING the recent decennial celebration of the former and present members of the nursing and professional staff of the Peter Bent Brigham Hospital, we presented (May 24, 1923) a case of mitral stenosis upon which we had operated four days previously in an attempt to alleviate the condition by diminishing the degree of stenosis of the valve.

It so happened that Professor Wenckebach of Vienna was visiting our clinic just at this time. The great enthusiasm and approval of the method of attack of the problem that he manifested, and the considerable discussion and general interest that the presentation of the case aroused, made it appear advisable to us to detail as exact a preliminary report as is possible at the present time. So far as we can determine, this is the only case on record of such a surgical attack upon a mitral stenosis being completed. Doyen[1] previously attempted a similar case, but his patient did not survive the operation.

Ever since Sir Lauder Brunton[2] in 1902 suggested the possibility of the surgical treatment of valvular disease of the heart, investigators have studied the experimental creation of valvular lesions. Papers by McCallum,[3] Cushing and Branch,[4] Bernheim,[5] Schepelmann,[6] and Carrel and Tuffier[7] from 1906 to 1914 describe fully the experimental methods in use. All of these methods were only successful in creating defective valves resulting in regurgitation. The most successful methods consisted in inserting a knife-hook (valvulotome) into the apex or down the aorta and cutting or tearing out valve cusps. Carrel and Tuffier added a new method of creating an insufficiency by the use of an endothelial transplant over the region of valves, the ring at the base of the valve then being cut, thus permitting a bulging at that point. In 1922 Allen and Graham[8] reported investigations of a similar nature with the addition that they used a cardioscope in which a small knife was carried, and by inserting the instrument *via* the left auricular appendage

Figure 12 First page of Cutler and Levine's report of the first succesful operation for mitral stenosis. *Photo Source National Library of Medicine. Literary Source Cutler, E.C. and Levine, S.A. (1923). Cardiotomy and valvulotomy for mitral stenosis. Boston Med. Surg. J.,* **188**, *1023. With permission*

endotracheal anesthesia which allowed excellent transpleural exposure of the atrial appendage. The clarity and logic of his approach and surgical skill are manifestly evident with his description of the procedure. After clamping the base of the atrial appendage he incised it and then inserted his finger.

The whole of the inside of the left auricle could now be explored with facility ... The finger was kept in the auricle for perhaps two minutes and during that time, so long as it remained in the auricle, it appeared to produce no effect upon the heart beat or the pulse. The moment, however, that it passed into the orifice of the mitral valve the blood pressure fell to zero, although even then no change in the cardiac rhythm could be detected. The blood stream was simply cut off by the finger which presumably just fitted the stenosed orifice. As, however, the stenosis was of such moderate degree, and was accompanied by so little thickening of the valves, it was decided not to carry out the valve section which had been arranged, but to limit intervention to such dilatation as could be carried out by the finger. It was felt that an actual section of the valve might only make matters worse by increasing the degree of regurgitation, while the breaking down of adhesions by the finger might improve the condition as regards both regurgitation and stenosis. It appears to me that the method of digital exploration through the auricular appendage cannot be surpassed for simplicity and directness. Not only is the mitral orifice directly to hand, but the aortic valve itself is almost certainly within reach, through the mitral orifice. Owing to the simplicity of the structures, and, oddly enough, to their constant and regular movement, the information given by the finger is exceedingly clear, and personally I felt an appreciation of the mechanical reality of stenosis and regurgitation which I never before possessed ... I could not help being impressed by the mechanical nature of these lesions and by the practicability of their surgical relief.[341]

The title page of Sir Henry Souttar's landmark report is illustrated in Figure 13.

The operation was Souttar's first and only attempt. He was never sent another case. Harken learned of Souttar's case only after he, himself, had performed several hundred operations for mitral stenosis. Sir Henry Souttar (he had been knighted

for his exploit) was now 93 years old when Harken wrote to him to find out why he never again performed the procedure. Souttar's answer was reproduced by Harken in his Lawrence Brewster Ellis lecture delivered at Boston City Hospital; the first of an annual series[342]. The letter is illustrated in Figure 14.

Perhaps, Souttar's failure to get other referrals may have been for the best. As he said, he was ahead of his time and without the sophisticated advances of thoracic anesthesia, blood transfusions and antibiotics, the procedure might have been doomed to failure with its attendant ill-repute.

Cutler and Levine, later with Beck's collaboration, subjected five more patients to their partial valvulectomy between 1924 and 1928. Their valvulotome was designed so that it would resect only a portion of the valve leaflet. Figure 15 is a photograph of the tenotomes and valvulotome used by Cutler for the treatment of mitral stenosis[343].

In 1925, Pribram of Germany also performed a partial valvulectomy using a valvulotome similar to that of Cutler and Levine[344]. When Cutler and Beck published their paper in 1929 describing the status of surgical valvular procedures up to that time they were rather discouraged by their failures[343]. 'It may seem that the information obtained from the 12 cases of chronic valvular disease in which operation was performed is so meager that further attempts are not justified. However, ... we feel that further attempts are necessary ... Unfortunately, our own attempts along this line have been as unsuccessful as the attempts of other and more experienced investigators'[343].

In retrospect, these workers were trading a tight valve for a leaking one. It is no wonder that only two of their twelve patients survived. They did not take into account that volume overload from a leaking valve could be just as disastrous as a pressure overload from a tight valve. This criticism on my part is easy to make from the advantage of current knowledge, and may not be a fair one. However, it does serve to emphasize how important physiology was in the conceptualization of cardiac surgical procedures.

Smithy was another worker actively involved in mitral valve surgery. He modeled his approach after that of Cutler and Beck, and for this purpose, he too designed a cardiovalvulotome which could be inserted through the ventricular wall and passed up to the mitral orifice where it could be manipulated so that a portion of one of the valve leaflets

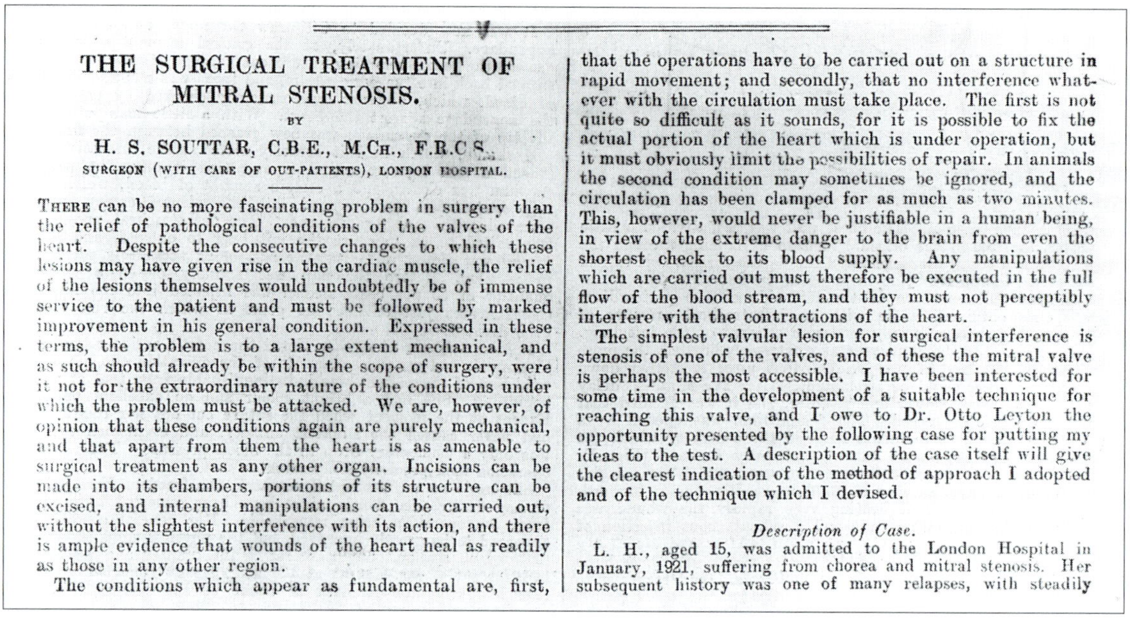

THE SURGICAL TREATMENT OF MITRAL STENOSIS.

BY

H. S. SOUTTAR, C.B.E., M.CH., F.R.C.S.,

SURGEON (WITH CARE OF OUT-PATIENTS), LONDON HOSPITAL.

THERE can be no more fascinating problem in surgery than the relief of pathological conditions of the valves of the heart. Despite the consecutive changes to which these lesions may have given rise in the cardiac muscle, the relief of the lesions themselves would undoubtedly be of immense service to the patient and must be followed by marked improvement in his general condition. Expressed in these terms, the problem is to a large extent mechanical, and as such should already be within the scope of surgery, were it not for the extraordinary nature of the conditions under which the problem must be attacked. We are, however, of opinion that these conditions again are purely mechanical, and that apart from them the heart is as amenable to surgical treatment as any other organ. Incisions can be made into its chambers, portions of its structure can be excised, and internal manipulations can be carried out, without the slightest interference with its action, and there is ample evidence that wounds of the heart heal as readily as those in any other region.

The conditions which appear as fundamental are, first, that the operations have to be carried out on a structure in rapid movement; and secondly, that no interference whatever with the circulation must take place. The first is not quite so difficult as it sounds, for it is possible to fix the actual portion of the heart which is under operation, but it must obviously limit the possibilities of repair. In animals the second condition may sometimes be ignored, and the circulation has been clamped for as much as two minutes. This, however, would never be justifiable in a human being, in view of the extreme danger to the brain from even the shortest check to its blood supply. Any manipulations which are carried out must therefore be executed in the full flow of the blood stream, and they must not perceptibly interfere with the contractions of the heart.

The simplest valvular lesion for surgical interference is stenosis of one of the valves, and of these the mitral valve is perhaps the most accessible. I have been interested for some time in the development of a suitable technique for reaching this valve, and I owe to Dr. Otto Leyton the opportunity presented by the following case for putting my ideas to the test. A description of the case itself will give the clearest indication of the method of approach I adopted and of the technique which I devised.

Description of Case.

L. H., aged 15, was admitted to the London Hospital in January, 1921, suffering from chorea and mitral stenosis. Her subsequent history was one of many relapses, with steadily

Figure 13 First page of Sir Henry Souttar's historic report of his succesful operation for mitral stenosis. *Photo Source National Library of Medicine. Literary Source Souttar, H.S. (1925). The surgical treatment of mitral stenosis. Br. Med. J.,* ***2****, 603. With permission*

was resected. Seven patients underwent this procedure. Two died, four improved, and one remained unchanged. It seems to me that Smithy fell into the same trap as Cutler, Levine and Beck regarding the pathophysiologic mechanisms following a surgically induced acute mitral insufficiency. Smithy's work was published posthumously in 1950[345,346]. It was concerned with experimental methods and early results. Smithy did not live to see its clinical application in the hands of Bailey in 1950[347].

At least two decades were to pass after the discouraging report of Cutler and Beck before a resurgence of interest in valvular surgery was seen. Many prominent physicians were still opposed to surgical intervention *per se*. Mackenzie and Orr wrote in 1923: 'In these cases there are other factors present in addition to the mitral stenosis. The muscle substance is not infrequently damaged and then heart failure is readily induced'[348]. Up to the time of his death, Sir Thomas Lewis was still opposed to surgical treatment. This is what he had to say about it in his textbook: 'I think it will continue to fail, not only because the interference is too drastic, but because the attempt is based upon what, usually at all events, is an erroneous idea, namely that the valve is the chief source of trouble'[349]. Shades of Galen – authoritarianism was still alive in the 20th century!

The late 1940s saw the emergence of several imaginative and capable men who were to lead the way for a renewed direct attack on the mitral valve as well as on the other valves. At the same time, others appeared on the scene with indirect methods for relieving the obstructive mechanisms of mitral stenosis. The leading exponents of the direct attack were Murray, Bailey, Harken and Brock. Men from other nations also contributed their share as we shall see. Smithy's contribution probably would have been greater if it were not curtailed by his untimely death. Ironically, Smithy died of aortic stenosis the same year he tried his transventricular approach for that very lesion. He was only 34 years old.

Murray's interest in valvular surgery began soon after the Boston group's efforts were publicized. By 1938 he had developed an experimental technique in animals similar to that of Cutler[350]. His differed in the steps he took to avoid the precipitation of acute mitral insufficiency. Murray also inserted the valvulotome through the ventricular wall. The regurgitation was controlled with the aid of a vein graft lined with palmaris longus tendon. Parts of the posterior mitral leaflet were excised with the valvulotome, and then the vein graft was passed blindly through the cavity of the left ventricle and positioned just below the valve so that the mitral orifice would be occluded during systole. Murray began using this technique in humans in 1945 and by 1950 he had performed the operation on 10 patients with two fatalities[351,352]. Murray's role was not as intensive or prolonged as the others' but equally important because he too was expanding the frontiers of cardiac surgery.

Bailey's interest in the problems was also pursued initially in the laboratory[353]. His experiments led him to realize several important factors. The most important among them was that mitral insufficiency was poorly tolerated. He soon learned that the left atrial approach was the most satisfactory and that the heart tolerated quite well an exploring or manipulating finger in the atrium. In addition, he learned that the valve must be palpated before using the valvulotome.

Bailey's first clinical attempt occurred in 1945. Unfortunately, the left atrium was torn during surgery, and the patient succumbed from uncontrollable hemorrhage. In his second attempt a year later, the patient became markedly hypotensive before he could position the valvulotome. He immediately removed the instrument and just as quickly inserted his finger. This is what he said about those trying moments.

> I … palpated the valve and pushed my finger through the diminished slit. Although the leaflets were calcified, both commissures split well and I immediately appreciated three things. One was that there was now an opening many times larger than that which had existed previously. Second, the diastolic thrill … disappeared. At the same time I was unable to recognize any regurgitant jet of blood from the valve … I was therefore convinced that I had both relieved the stenosis and failed to produce any regurgitation.[354]

Thirty hours later this patient was also dead. At autopsy, the torn commissural edges were found to be reagglutinated. Despite the fact that the patient died, this second attempt was a crucial one for Bailey in that it firmly established in his mind that commissurotomy was a physiologically sound procedure while at the same time it abolished once and for all the commonly accepted belief that mitral

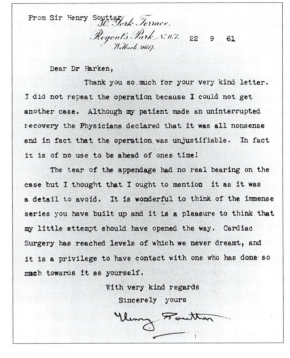

Figure 14 Letter from Sir Henry Souttar to Dr Dwight Harken, written in Sir Henry's 93rd year. *Photo Source National Library of Medicine. Literary Source Harken, D.W. (1967). Heart surgery – legend and a long look. Am. J. Cardiol., 19, 393–401. With permission*

insufficiency must necessarily accompany relief of stenosis. The 'notching' of Samways was indeed possible.

Bailey's two failures put him temporarily in the same predicament that Souttar experienced in England with his one and only venture. No referrals were forthcoming to the 'butcher' of Hahnemann Hospital. Bailey had to wait until 1948 for the tide to turn in his favor. On June 10th of that year he achieved his first successful valvulotomy. The operation was performed in Philadelphia's Episcopal Hospital. Bailey did not even have surgical privileges there.

That morning, Bailey and his associates had experienced their third depressing failure. The future professor of medicine at Temple University, Thomas Durant, had come to watch Bailey operate at the Philadelphia General Hospital. Bailey's home base, the Hahnemann Hospital, had refused to allow him to perform the procedure anymore after his two previous failures. When this third patient died during surgery a necropsy was

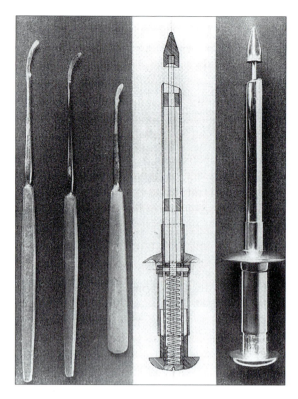

Figure 15 Tenotomes and valvulotome used by Cutler for the surgical relief of mitral stenosis. *Photo Source National Library of Medicine. Literary Source Cutler, E.C. and Beck, C.S. (1929). The present status of the surgical procedures in chronic valvular disease of the heart: final report of all surgical cases. Arch. Surg.,18, 403–16 (Jan., Pt. 2). With permission*

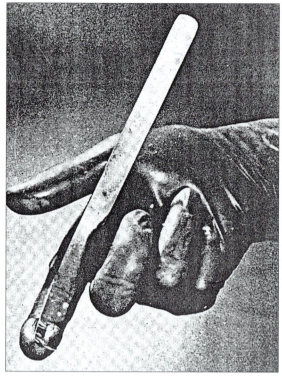

Figure 16 Mitral valve knife that Bailey developed and used in his first clinical attempt at commissurotomy. *Photo Source University of Central Florida. Literary Source Bailey, C.P., et al. (1950). J. Thorac. Surg., 19, 16-45. With permission*

immediately performed. As Bailey turned to Durant in an attempt to explain to him the elements of the procedure, Bailey demonstrated with his finger how he could separate his tightly pursed and fixed lips. Upon seeing this, Durant said: 'Charlie, you mean you are trying to open the commissures?' Bailey responded: 'That's right – and that's what we'll call the procedure – commissurotomy!'[355]

The second operation of the day was the one that propelled Bailey finally into a favorable limelight. Sometime later, he recounted the events of the day. Apparently the second operation had already been scheduled with the patient waiting for his arrival. These are his words: 'We gathered up the frustrated team, including Durant, and promptly drove to Episcopal Hospital to commence the other operation before the morning's bad news could be effective in possibly having the Episcopal

Hospital administration forbid us from doing the procedure'[355].

Using the transatrial approach, he described the crucial moment as follows: 'The hooked knife was inserted through the valve orifice and engaged on the lateral commissure under direct digital guidance. The knife was then drawn backward an inch, widely cutting the commissure. The finger was now inserted through the cut valve and some fine remaining fibrous strands were broken up. The valve was now widely patent'.

The modern era of mitral valve surgery had now begun. The extirpative approach was now replaced with a physiological one. Figure 16 shows the mitral valve knife developed by Bailey and used in his first clinical attempt.

By 1950, Bailey had reported 10 transatrial mitral dilatations or commissurotomies with a mortality rate of 50%[356]. In 1956, Bailey published the results of his experience during the eight years since that first successful attempt[357]. The 'butcher' of Hahnemann had now become the redeemer; the dreamer had become the achiever. During a short span of eight years, he and his group performed more than a thousand of these procedures. Improvement was noted in 89.9% with an operative mortality of 7.9% and a late mortality of 5.6%[357].

A close friend of mine underwent the procedure at the hands of Bailey in 1958. She came under my care in 1984, and although she has chronic atrial fibrillation (adequately controlled with digoxin) she is still active and just celebrated her 65th birthday. Just before she underwent the surgery she asked Dr Bailey if he would be kind enough to explain the procedure to her. He did so through the medium of an artist on his staff. Figure 17 is a photograph of the artist's rendition of the transatrial approach as given to her by the artist.

Boston and London also participated in the birth of the physiologic approach for the correction of mitral stenosis. Harken and Ellis were the collaborators in Boston while Sir Russell Brock (later Lord Brock) was the protagonist in Great Britain.

In the laboratory, Harken found that the anterior leaflet of the mitral valve should not be incised or partially excised; to do so caused a lethal regurgitation. Damage to the posterior leaflet was better tolerated.

Aware now of the danger of creating a marked leakage, Harken and his group formulated the concept of 'selective insufficiency'. This implied that some degree of leakage had to occur. On the basis of this concept they performed wedge-shaped resections of the fused commissure bridges with the valvulotome. This is why they labeled their procedure valvuloplasty rather than commissurotomy. Harken also favored the transatrial approach that Bailey espoused.

Harken's first clinical opportunity to implement these views came in March, 1947. After he had removed two small pieces of tissue from the posterior leaflet, the patient developed uncontrollable tachycardia and died in acute pulmonary edema[358]. This sad experience caused him to realize that a rapid heart action in the presence of mitral stenosis or insufficiency must be avoided since its occurrence within this setting would surely precipitate pulmonary edema.

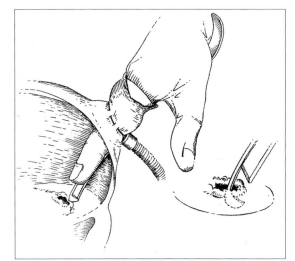

Figure 17 Mitral valve approach from left atrial appendage as described to my patient. *Photo Source Charles P. Bailey Thoracic Clinic. Literary Source None. Courtesy of my patient*

No doubt this experience also caused him and Ellis to suggest cardiac denervation as an alternative approach in the management of mitral stenosis[359]. By so doing, they hoped to abolish episodes of rapid heart action with its attendant pulmonary edema. They presented a single patient on whom this procedure was performed shortly before their first successful valuloplasty[359].

It was only six days after Bailey's proud achievement that Harken experienced the first of his. He described it as follows[357]: 'Through ... the left auricular appendage ... the cardiovalvulotome was introduced with the cutting edge directed at the lateral commissure, the valvulotome hook engaged, and the instrument closed. The cutting sensation and sound were elicited, but the segment was not recovered. The maneuver was repeated with the instrument directed at the medial commissure. Finally, a segment of the stenotic funnel was removed in a third maneuver directed at the posterior aspect of the lateral commissure'. After 12 years of experience in 1571 patients, Ellis and Harken reported the short and long term results of their 'closed valvuloplasty' in the *New England Journal of Medicine* (1964)[360].

In retrospect, Bailey had achieved his initial successes with finger fracture while Harken relied more on the valvulotome. As time went on Bailey came to use the knife more extensively while

Harken favored splitting the valve with his finger, abandoning the use of the valvulotome[361-363]. When Harken reported in 1950 his experience with his first five valvuloplasties he was quick to say: 'The correction of mitral stenosis is no longer directed at the production of insufficiency but at reducing the stenotic block with the greatest possible restoration of valvular function. While much previous work has been based on the concept of exchanging regurgitation for stenosis, it does not follow that this is either desirable or necessary'[361]. It is quite obvious that by now he had abandoned completely his concept of 'selective insufficiency'.

In September of 1948, just three months after Bailey and Harken, the eminent British surgeon, Russell Brock, joined their ranks with his first successful intervention. He called it mitral valvotomy. He did not report this, however, until 1950 when he described his success in six cases[364]. This is what he wrote:

> We also have designed a flat knife, thin and adapted to the curve of the index finger, that can be introduced into the atrium with the finger. We have found it necessary to use this in two cases only; in all others it was possible to split the valve along the line of the commissure by using the finger.
>
> It is not entirely accurate to describe this manoeuvre as 'dilatation' of the valve, which implies that the orifice is merely stretched. The valve is split, and in most cases the split is begun and continued with considerable accuracy … One must have a suitable knife or guillotine that can be passed in with the finger to divide the thickened margin of the stenosed orifice quickly and efficiently if the least difficulty is experienced in splitting with the finger.[364]

Lord Brock had already enjoyed considerable success with direct intracardiac division of stenotic pulmonary valves[365]. His fellow countryman, T. Holmes Sellors, had also described in 1948 (just 2 weeks after Brock's report) a case of pulmonary stenosis in which the pulmonary valve was successfully divided[366]. Brock's success with this lesion was achieved through a right ventricular approach. He had previously failed on three different occasions when he attempted the pulmonary valvotomy through the pulmonary artery. According to Harken, it was O'Shaughnessy who first suggested surgery for the correction of pulmonary stenosis[367]. We shall meet this gifted young man again in the narrative devoted to myocardial revascularization. O'Shaughnessy was to present this suggestion as part of a Hunterian lecture. He never did – he was killed during the Dunkirk evacuation in 1940. The unpublished text has a sketch of the surgical procedure depicting the incision of the stenotic valve with a valvulotome inserted through the right ventricle. Sellors applied O'Shaughnessy's technique in the case he reported. The patient was a 20 year old whose pulmonic stenosis was part of a Fallot's tetralogy.

Returning again to mitral stenosis, indirect methods were also tried as an alternative to the direct attack on the mitral valve. I have already mentioned cardiac denervation which was tried by Harken and Ellis but never pursued beyond their one and only attempt. An intriguing approach was the one suggested by Sweet and Bland in 1949. They were aware, as other clinicians were, that patients with Lutembacher's syndrome did not suffer with episodes of pulmonary edema as did those with mitral stenosis alone. They reasoned that the atrial septal defect in Lutembacher's syndrome acted as a 'safety valve' allowing blood to go from the right atrium to the left atrium when acute pulmonary hypertension appeared. On the basis of this reasoning they attempted to simulate the conditions of Lutembacher's syndrome by anastomosing the pulmonary vein to the azygos vein, creating in effect a constant right to left shunt. Six patients were subjected to this procedure. Improvement was obtained in only three patients and only for a short while, presumably because the anastomosis was occluded by thrombus[368,369].

Harken and Ellis also became intrigued with this approach, but went one step further in actually producing a Lutembacher's syndrome by creating an atrial septal defect[359]. The two patients who underwent this procedure also showed only temporary improvement. No further work along these lines was ever done by anyone.

In retrospect, the reasoning of these investigators was flawed in terms of pathophysiology. Pulmonary hypertension in mitral stenosis results from three factors operating in sequence. Initially, the stenosis creates a pressure overload on the left atrium which in time causes an increase in left atrial pressure and which ultimately is transmitted in a backward manner to the pulmonary capillary bed. This in turn provokes constriction of the pulmonary arterioles and perpetuates a reactive pulmonary hypertension. In time, the persistent hypertension brings about obliterative changes in the vascular bed.

When atrial septal defect is present as an isolated lesion, there is a left to right shunt with volume overload on the right side of the heart. Mitral stenosis tends to augment the left to right shunt because of the increased left intra-atrial pressure. Thus, the creation of an atrial septal opening in an individual with mitral stenosis would have a decompression effect on the left atrium because of the augmented left to right shunt. Symptomatically the patient appears to be improved because the decompressant effect attenuates the orthopnea, paroxysmal dyspnea, hemoptysis and pulmonary edema. But there is a reduction in systemic cardiac output so that fatigue now replaces the pulmonary signs and symptoms. The final answer is that the patient is really no better because of the newly created atrial septal defect. On the other hand, the anastomosis created by Bland and Sweet was actually a bypass procedure. It helped control the level of pressure in the pulmonary vasculature by circumventing the obstruction imposed by the narrowed mitral valve, and in this sense may have brought about temporary relief until occluded by the thrombus.

It is for these reasons then that a direct surgical repair of the mitral stenosis appeared to be the most logical approach and continued to enjoy widespread acceptance. The succeeding years saw improvements in surgical technique aimed at producing as large an opening as possible with minimal regurgitation so as to bring the diseased valve to as nearly a normal functional status as possible. This was more easily said than done. Serious mitral leakage was still encountered. Other distressing problems also arose such as serious arrhythmias, torn atria, atrial thrombosis and systemic embolism.

In 1953, Charles Dubost of Paris began using a transatrial dilator. By 1962 he was able to report a remarkably low mortality rate of only 2% in a series of 1000 cases[370,371]. Despite this, it did not prove to be popular. Only two other Europeans were initially impressed with Dubost's dilator technique. These were Edwards of England[372] and Logan of Edinburgh. Logan, however, used the trans-ventricular route[373,374]. He utilized Brock's aortic dilator for the widening of the mitral valve orifice. It was inserted through a small incision near the apex of the left ventricle. It was later modified by Tubbs. Brock's dilator could expand to only 3.3 cm.

Tubbs modified it with an instrument capable of being expanded to 4.5 cm and controlled in a more accurate fashion by means of a screw. Logan also adopted Tubbs' modification, and between the two of them they managed to subsequently impress most of the surgeons in Great Britain. Tubbs' experience in a series of 124 patients was described by him in 1962[375].

Derom's attempt at refining the methods for relieving the stenosis consisted of performing a posteromedial commissurotomy by means of a special pair of scissors of his own design[376]. No one else seemed to be interested in pursuing this. In 1958, Bailey tried complete hinging of the aortic leaflet as an aid in reaching the primary objective of minimal or no regurgitation[377]. He called the procedure 'neostrophingic mobilization'. This, too, did not gain any foothold among his colleagues. Better methods had to wait for the era of open heart surgery.

The notable success achieved with the blind techniques of mitral valve surgery was not shared by the other valves. Stenosis of the aortic valve, in particular, proved to be an insurmountable problem. Blind manipulation under digital guidance was definitely not the answer. Experimental valvotomy of the aortic valve had already been tried by Becker in 1872[378] and subsequently by Klebs[379]. As early as 1912, Jeger tried to make an aortic valve prosthesis by suturing a graft of the jugular vein between the innominate artery and the left ventricle[380]. Brock attempted to relieve aortic stenosis with a mechanical dilator which, as we have seen, had a greater degree of application in mitral stenosis. Bailey also tried an expanding dilator positioning the device through a transventricular approach. Harken used an oper-ating tunnel stitched to an aortotomy incision in the ascending aorta. In the 1950s, Glenn and his group at Yale reported a technique using the finger or instrument inserted through a fabric diverticulum sutured into the aortic valve. The diverticular approach was adopted also for mitral and pulmonary valve operations[381].

In contrast to the aggressive approaches for mitral stenosis, the development of surgical techniques for the correction of mitral insufficiency really did not evolve satisfactorily until the advent of open-heart surgery. Initially, there was very little interest because of the mistaken belief that a leaking mitral valve was not a serious lesion and was well tolerated by the heart. In due time, it became apparent that mitral regurgitation had a multifactorial etiology, some conditions not lending themselves at all to correction with a blind technique. A case in point would be mitral regurgitation due to ruptured papillary muscle or chordae tendinae.

Except for Carrel's efforts in 1910, no serious experimental studies were reported until 1930 when Carrel published his paper on experimental surgery of the thoracic aorta and heart. He wrote that he had tried to develop an operation for mitral insufficiency which could be performed without opening the heart. 'It consists of producing a slight stenosis of the upper part of the left ventricle. It can be obtained by a partial cuneiform resection of the wall of the ventricle just below the coronary artery. A dog which has undergone this partial ventriculectomy two months ago is still in good health'[382].

In 1930, Wilson was producing mitral obstruction in animals as a basis for developing surgical techniques to reverse the stenosis. He used the animal's own pericardium to do this[383]. Usage of autogenous tissue was then adopted a few years later by several investigators as a means of reducing the size of the orifice. Murray, Wilkinson and MacKenzie used an everted autogenous vein as a subvalvular sling. During systole, it would balloon upwards to effectively occlude the mitral orifice[384]. Templeton and Gibbon tried pericardium in making the sling[385]. Pedunculated atrial flaps were also tried by Botwin in 1954[386].

Another approach utilized plastic materials. These were aimed at supporting or enhancing the closure of the posterior leaflet. Plexiglas, Lucite and Ivalon were used in these experiments[387–391]. Prosthetic valves that were inserted blindly in the region of the mitral orifice were still another approach[392–394]. The uniform failure of these attempts led other investigators to experiment with a technique known as circumferential suturing. It had been used initially as an experimental means of producing mitral stenosis, and was accomplished by placing a ligature around the left atrioventricular groove which would narrow the mitral orifice as it was tightened. Ellison and his group were the first to adopt this as a means of correcting mitral insufficiency due to a dilated mitral ring[395]. Reports describing the results with this experimental technique came from McAllister and Fitzpatrick in 1954[396,397], Davila and his associates also in 1954 and then a year later[398,399], and Borrie of New Zealand in the same years[400,401].

A few surgeons were confident enough to apply some of these experimental techniques in actual clinical practice. When the Canadian surgeon, Murray, excised a portion of the stenotic mitral valve, he attempted to correct the resultant leakage with a transventricular (blind) placement of autogenous tissues[352]. Bailey used pericardium rolled up in the form of a pedicle. This proved to be unsatisfactory because of subsequent shrinkage and fibrosis[385,402]. Johnson tried intact cardiac tissues to reinforce the posterior leaflet[403].

Harken devised a spindle-shaped prosthesis made of Lucite. It was fixed just beneath the valve. He reported this in 1954 with only three deaths in a series of 17 patients[404,405]. Davila, Glover and their associates spearheaded the clinical application of circumferential suturing in mitral insufficiency due to dilated mitral ring. After acquiring an extensive experience in experimental animals they subjected 58 patients to the procedure. The surgical mortality was quite high in those who had intractable heart failure but far less (17%) in those who were not that ill[405–408].

As time went on it became quite obvious that blind techniques, no matter how ingenious, were not the answer. A bloodless field with open heart surgery was the only satisfactory approach, and this needed the introduction of hypothermic cross-circulation and the heart-lung machine. The final evolution of these three factors ushered in Harken's third epoch – the era of open heart surgery.

OPEN HEART SURGERY

Investigators have been interested in hibernation with its marked decrease in body temperature for at least the past two centuries. But these early researchers were not thinking in terms of human application.

In 1797, two books were published by a Dr James Currie of Liverpool, wherein he described his cold water baths as a remedy for fever, convulsions, and insanity. This seems to be the first time that general hypothermia was used in a clinical setting. Unfortunately his imagination knew no bounds and did not correlate well with the clinical facts. He used a deep bath of sea water at 7°C with no deaths. He forgot to mention that his thermometer was of doubtful accuracy[409].

Temple Fay, a Philadelphia surgeon, appears to be the first to have created a clinical interest in hypothermia. He attempted to ameliorate or control cancer and certain other disorders of the brain by bringing the body temperature down to 31°C and maintaining these patients in this moderately hypothermic state for several days. Although he treated over 100 patients in this manner, his methods did not gain general acceptance[410–413].

Several fundamental questions had to be answered regarding hypothermia and its relationship to metabolism before the lowering of body temperature could have any significant application in cardiac surgery. These appeared to be answered through a series of experiments conducted at the Banting Institute in Toronto under the direction of W. G. Bigelow.

W. G. Bigelow was a surgeon at the University of Toronto who first became interested in generalized hypothermia for direct vision intracardiac surgery in the late 1940s[414–418]. A simple but important fundamental discovery was reported by him and his associates during the initial phases of their experiments. They found that if they eliminated the shivering and heightened muscle tone caused by the cold with careful anesthesia, then the body's oxygen requirements fell in almost a linear fashion as the body temperature dropped. It was this simple observation that provided the foundation for the application of hypothermia in humans.

They continued working and after three years of experimentation, they had pretty well established the basic physiological responses to hypothermia. It was now time to test the open heart theory. This was in 1949, and the subject was a dog whose body temperature had been lowered to 20°C. The circulation was interrupted by placing clamps on the superior and inferior vena cavae. The heart was beating very slowly and as soon as it appeared to be empty of blood it was opened. The circulation was stopped in this manner for 15 minutes. The dog survived the procedure fully validating the thesis that hypothermia could be a viable tool in open heart surgery and with a bloodless field. The experiment was tried again and again in a series of 39 animals in all. It proved to be a high risk procedure with only a 51% survival rate. Nevertheless, when the observations were reported at a meeting of the American Surgical Association in Colorado Springs in 1950, it created quite a stir, acting as a stimulus for further research in hypothermia throughout the world.

Another five years were needed for this team to iron out some of the pitfalls of the technique and to increase its safety so that it could be tried in human open heart surgery. Time restrictions limited their choice of candidates to children with simple atrial defects or pulmonary stenosis. These lesions could be surgically corrected within the 8–10 minute window that prevailed with the body temperature at 28–30°C and the circulation stopped with the heart open. Since they were working in an adult hospital, pediatric referrals were not available. This was an impediment they could not surmount, and despite their breakthrough experimentation, they were deprived of being the first to apply the open heart hypothermia technique in a human. John Lewis of Minneapolis 'beat them to the draw'. He was the first to report the successful closure of an atrial septal defect. This was in 1953[419]. The only consolation was the knowledge that Lewis had acquired considerable experimental experience before his first human attempt by utilizing the technique that Bigelow and his group had developed. John Lewis and his collaborator, Mansur Taufic, did their work at the University of Minnesota Medical School. They were initially encouraged to begin their dog experiments by Richard Varco. Throughout these trials, Varco was always ready to offer his advice and repeated encouragement. When the first human attempt presented itself, Varco assisted Lewis during the surgery. The patient was a five year old girl with a large atrial septal defect. The defect was closed under direct vision. The operating field was dry having been rendered so by occluding the vena cavae for the 5½ minutes needed for repair of the defect. There were no complications and the patient made an uneventful recovery[419].

Henry Swan and his associates also expressed their enthusiasm for hypothermia. They reported on their experience in 1953 and again in 1954[420,421]. Swan's ice bath for the induction of hypothermia was generally recognized as being the most acceptable. Four of their patients had atrial septal defect and nine had pulmonary stenosis. The heart was completely excluded from the circulation with bone dry chambers by first clamping the vena cavae, and then the aortic root and pulmonary artery. Swan's group tried to resolve the problem of ventricular fibrillation by hyperventilation, and if not successful, they were usually able to convert to regular sinus rhythm by an intracoronary injection of potassium chloride. They prevented air embolism on reclosure by filling the chest cavity with saline. The year 1952 also saw two other favorable reports on hypothermia, these by Charles Bailey[422,423].

In addition to Swan's ice water bath, other techniques were being tested. During the same period of time, Boerema and Delorme used bloodstream cooling in their experimental animals by means of an external cooling coil connected to a vein and an artery with the animal's heart serving as a pump[424,425].

Sellors working at the Middlesex Hospital in London was one of the first to adopt Swan's technique. In 1960, he reported a series of over 200 cases of closure of atrial septal defect[426].

Sir Russell Brock working at Guy's Hospital encountered too many difficulties with Swan's ice bath technique. He found it rather cumbersome and messy, with a slow rewarming process adding to his woes. It was for this reason that he adopted initially the method suggested by Boerema and Delorme. Brock also encountered too many difficulties with this method and soon abandoned it for one designed by him and D. N. Ross. Heparin had become available by this time and therefore clotting was not a problem. The method devised by Brock and Ross consisted of cooling the venous blood by means of an external circuit consisting of a blood cooling coil and a hand operated rotary pump connected via input and output cannulas to the vena cava[427–429]. They used this method in more than 20 patients.

Meanwhile, Bigelow's efforts and continued research at the Banting Institute spawned an imposing list of trainees that were attracted to the laboratory from all over the world, and who, in time, added their own contributions.

Professor Donald Ross of London dubbed the decade between the mid 1950s and the mid 1960s, 'The first ice age'. He was referring to the inundation of the surgical literature during this time span with reports resulting from the intense activity in researching the utility of hypothermia. It seemed to do for the simple defects but surgical correction of the more complicated lesions required the heart-lung machine with hypothermia offering added protection to the vital organs. Some surgeons were now beginning to practice the so-called 'ice-chip arrest' technique. This was done by packing the heart in ice while the patient was under cardiopulmonary bypass, and which effectively stopped the heart from beating. It was later abandoned.

In London, open heart surgery using 'deep general hypothermia' became quite popular. Japanese surgeons in Sendai, Japan used surface cooling and deep hypothermia in infants[430]. A team from Kyoto, Japan combined deep ether anesthesia with deep hypothermia and partial pulmonary bypass[431].

Denton Cooley now began to report his success with the technique of 'anoxic arrest'. Normal body temperature with cardiac bypass constituted the elements of this approach. This proved to be so popular that by the late 1960s, hypothermia was relegated to a secondary and infrequently used role. However, death from subendocardial necrosis and late muscle scarring brought about a revival of hypothermia in the 1970s. Cold cardioplegia was now introduced. It simplified open heart surgery and reduced the risk. The technique is used universally today, and for this reason Bigelow refers to current times as 'the second ice age'.

The heart–lung machine

When John Gibbon successfully closed an atrial septal defect in a 19 year old girl on May 6, 1953 using his heart–lung machine, the viability of open-heart surgery as a feasible therapeutic modality was assured. Hypothermia with inflow occlusion was certainly a catalyst in starting the era, but time constraints imposed by this method precluded its use in the more complicated cardiac abnormalities such as valve replacement or myocardial revascularization, to mention but two.

'Gibbon's idea and its elaboration take their place among the boldest and most successful feats of man's mind – with invention of the phonetic alphabet, the telephone or a Mozartian symphony. Not a Deus ex machina but a machina a Deo'[432]. These are the words of Eloesser in his *Milestones in Chest Surgery* – rather strong words, but justifiable to a certain degree. Gibbon, of course, deserves a great deal of credit. He was imaginative, daring, innovative, and above all, tenacious in pursuit of a dream. But he was not alone. Many investigators besides him were involved in developing a suitable heart–lung machine, and many workers preceded him in sorting out the many problems in blood oxygenation, and in the creation of adequate cardiorespiratory support systems.

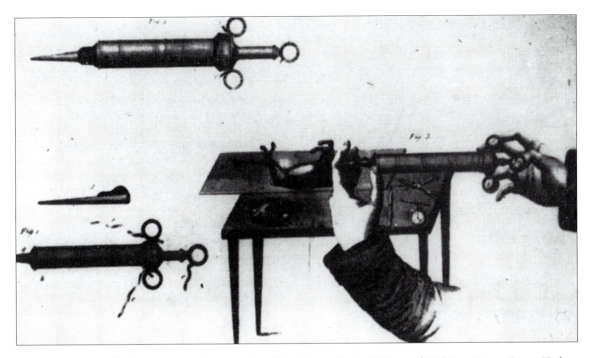

Figure 18 La Gallois' experimental preparation. *Photo Source National Library of Medicine. Literary Source Harken, D.W. (1967). Heart surgery – legend and a long look. Am.J. Cardiol.,* **19**, *393–401. Taken from La Gallois, C.J. (1813). Experiments on the principle of life. (Translated by N.C. & J.G. Nancrede) (Philadelphia: M.Thomas). With permission*

In actuality, the roots of cardiopulmonary bypass systems are to be found in the physiological experiments of the 19th century, but the concept was first promulgated by Cesar Julian La Gallois in 1812[433]. He wrote: 'But if the place of the heart could be supplied by injecting, and if with a regular continuance of this injection there could be furnished a quantity of arterial blood, whether naturally or artificially formed, supposing such a function possible, then life might be indefinitely maintained in any portion'. La Gallois' experimental preparation is illustrated in Figure 18.

La Gallois kept his decapitated rabbits alive for a while with his injection method. Blood clotting prevented the prolonged use of this technique. It was not until 1821 when Prévost and Dumas showed that clotting could be prevented by defibrinating the blood that the possibility arose of confirming La Gallois' attempts[434]. This did not occur, however, until 1849 when Loebell was able to perform isolated perfusion of the kidney with defibrinated blood[435].

Blood was first artificially oxygenated in 1869 when Ludwig and Schmidt simply shook the blood in a balloon containing air during extracorporeal circulation[436]. The blood was kept flowing by displacing it with mercury; an idea that was introduced by Bidder seven years earlier when he was perfusing isolated kidneys with defibrinated blood[437]. In 1882, von Schröder appears to have devised the first truly artificial lung[438]. His method of oxygenation consisted of introducing air directly into a venous reservoir. The oxygenated blood was now forced to enter an 'arterial reservoir' as it was being displaced by the increasing air pressure within the venous reservoir. Hydrostatic pressure served to propel the blood from the arterial reservoir into a perfusing line connected to the isolated organ.

Bubble oxygenation, as this was called, continued to remain the primary focus of interest among other physiologists of the late 19th and early 20th centuries. Among these were Jacobi[439], Brodie[440], and Hooker[441]. Jacobi used a hand bulb for the pumping mechanism. Clark and his group introduced further improvements in bubble oxygenation technique by dispersing oxygen through a sintered glass filter[442].

The first film oxygenator was developed by von Frey and Gruber in 1885[443]. The machine they devised was a rather crude affair with the pumping mechanism consisting of a 10 ml syringe with two unidirectional valves, driven by an electric motor. The blood was pumped to a slanting rotating cylinder with gas exchange occurring as the blood flowed in a thin film over the inner surface of this cylinder.

Refinements in film oxygenation appeared soon after the initial attempt by von Frey and Gruber. Some of them were rather clever. The film oxygenator developed by Richards and Drinker in 1915 consisted of a silk screen suspended from a glass ring[444]. Hooker's device was the forerunner of the modern disk oxygenator. It was a hard rubber disk that was made to rotate in an inverted bell jar filled with air[441]. The blood was oxygenated as it was filmed over this rotating disk. Bayliss refined this in 1928 by using a column of cones that rotated on a vertical axis within a series of stationary plates[445]. Another refinement was the modification of Hooker's disk apparatus by using three oxygenators arranged concentrically. This was the brainchild of Daly and Thorpe and was designed primarily for perfusing a mammalian heart preparation over a prolonged period of time[446].

Björk described the modern rotating disk oxygenator in his classic paper on brain perfusion[447]. He was working in Craford's laboratory at Sabatsberg Hospital at the time. Craford provided Björk with the inspiration by showing that the flow of blood to all the other organs could remain suspended for up to 25 minutes without organic damage provided flow to the brain was adequate. In 1956, Cross and co-workers modified the rotating disk oxygenator by substituting stainless steel, Teflon-coated disks and a pyrex silicone-coated chamber[448].

The film oxygenator devised by Jongbloed consisted of multiple rotating spiral coils arranged in a parallel fashion. It was able to support the circulation and respiration of dogs for up to four hours. He described it in 1949[449,450]. The blood was driven by a modified Dale–Schuster pump. The original Dale–Schuster pump was described by them in 1928[451]. It was a piston pump with a very interesting mechanism. It had a crankshaft driven by a pulley which moved a vertical pumping rod connected to a diaphragm. The diaphragm moved water into and out of a vertical finger stall which expanded to force blood from a glass dome cylinder and then contracted to allow filling.

Carrel and Lindbergh's perfusion pump differed in that it propelled fluid from a reservoir to the isolated organ by means of pulsatile gas pressure. The pump was made of pyrex glass. It was described in 1935[452]. When Gibbon originally maintained the circulation during experimental occlusion of the pulmonary artery, he too used a pump oxygenator[453].

Dogliotti and Costantini were the first to use a pump oxygenator in a human[454]. This was in 1951. They used it to partly bypass the right side of the heart while removing a mediastinal tumor. Their oxygenator was similar to that devised by Clark a year earlier.

Bypassing the right side of the heart was not a new approach. It was pioneered by Sewell and Glenn of Yale University[455]. Their system shunted the venous blood past the right side of the heart directly into the pulmonary artery. William Glenn recounts how their system cost less than $25 (USA). It was 'a simple, air-powered pressure vacuum pump ... constructed from ordinary laboratory parts and a small motor obtained from an Erector set' (a popular toy of the time in the USA)[456]. He and Sewell were able to keep the right atrium and right ventricle wide open for up to two hours. Sewell was a third year medical student when he designed the pump used in their earliest experiments. Figure 19 illustrates the pump. It is now on permanent display at the Smithsonian Institution.

A year after the publication of Sewell and Glenn's report, Clowes described his method for bypassing the left side of the heart[457]. He used a modified Dale–Schuster pump which propelled defoamed oxygenated blood from a reservoir connected to the left atrium. Dodrill and his co-workers also used a modified Dale–Schuster pump when they completely bypassed the right side of the heart in the repair of a stenotic pulmonary valve[458]. This was the first successful open-heart operation in man aided by a mechanical pump.

While all this was going on, a rather ingenious method at oxygenation was being explored by a distinguished group at the University of Minnesota. It was a young group of bright, enthusiastic and motivated surgical residents with an equally young attending staff working under the chairmanship of Owen H. Wangensteen. Lillehei describes him as a 'truly visionary surgeon who created a favorable environment uncluttered by the cobwebs of tradition'[459]. 'Do the experiment! And do think!' was Wangensteen's dictum to his staff[459]. The young group included Lillehei, Dennis, Cohen, Warden and De Wall.

The ingenious method that was being explored was based on the concept of biologic oxygenation. Blum and Megibow in 1950 developed this idea in which the dog's heart was excluded from the circulation by a process they termed 'parabiosis'[460]. It was actually Morley Cohen who first proposed using a human donor as the biologic oxygenator. Cohen and Warden, while still in surgical training, repeatedly conducted the procedure, correcting errors and refining the technique in animals until by 1954 they felt able to recommend it as a clinical tool[461,462].

The first attempt with cross circulation (as this method was also called) was on an infant in intractable heart failure due to a large ventricular septal defect. The boy's father was the donor. The patient survived the surgery but died eleven days later from pneumonia. The second patient also had a ventricular septal defect and again the father was the donor. This patient survived despite total inflow occlusion to his heart for 26½ minutes[463]. Six more young patients with ventricular septal defect were subjected to this procedure with only one more death. The team was now bold enough to attempt a correction of Tetralogy of Fallot. Again they were successful, marking this as the first surgical correction of both the ventricular septal defect and the pulmonic stenosis utilizing the cross circulation technique as the oxygenating mechanism[464].

The details of the technique are fascinating. Both donor and patient were anesthetized and heparinized. The patient's aorta was cannulated and then connected via a tube to a cannula inserted into the donor's superficial femoral artery. This served as the arterial line. The venous line was set up in the same fashion with the patient's superior and inferior vena cavae connected to the donor's superficial femoral vein. A sigmamotor pump was used for both lines and its speed set so that blood flow was less than 50% of normal cardiac output. A properly placed clamp on the patient's vena cavae effectively prevented any blood from entering the heart, thus creating the dry field necessary for the surgery.

By early 1955, the team had enjoyed considerable success in a total number of 45 patients, reporting this in *Surgery* and in the *International Symposium of Cardiovascular Surgery*[465,466]. There was no donor mortality.

The 'azygos flow concept' was the moving force behind the introduction of cross circulation as a

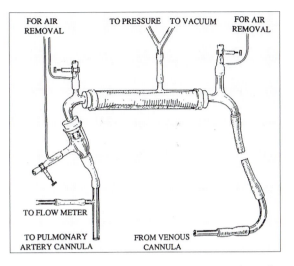

Figure 19 Ventricle type pump designed in the Yale Surgical Laboratory by William H. Sewell, Jr in 1948–49 when he was a third year medical student and used in our earliest experiments on cardiac surgery. Both this pump and the one designed by Lindbergh are on permanent display at the Smithsonian Institution. *Photo Source University of Central Florida. Literary Source Sewell, W.H. Jr. and Glenn, W.W.L. (1950). Experimental cardiac surgery: I. Observation on the action of a pump designed to shunt the venous blood past the right heart directly into the pulmonary artery. Surgery, 28, 474–94. With permission*

clinically useful modality. The team's initial experiments were intended merely as an interim method of gaining open heart experience without the need of the cumbersome, complex and highly expensive pump oxygenators available at the time. They soon realized that application of the 'azygos flow concept' with its attendant reduction in cardiac output not only did not harm the dogs but also resulted in a higher survival rate.

Lillehei's recollections and thoughts on the matter are quite revealing:

It is my opinion that the single most important discovery that made clinical open heart surgery successful was the realization of the vast discrepancy between the total body flow rate that was thought necessary, and what was actually necessary. During some early experiments in which the cavae were temporarily occluded to test tolerance limits of the brain and heart to ischemia, we discovered that if the azygos vein was not clamped (but all other inflow to the heart was), the resulting very small cardiac output was sufficient to sustain the vital organs safely in every animal for a minimum of 30 mins at normothermia. To even mention, at that time, that such a low flow might be adequate for perfusions was heresy; and thus, we were pleased to learn of a similar observation in 1952 in England by Andreason and Watson. Both of these studies agreed that only about 10% of the basal cardiac output was needed to sustain animals unimpaired physiologically for a reasonable period of time (30 mins) at normothermia. The universally accepted minimum for cardiopulmonary bypass (at normothermia) was considered by the authorities of that time to be 100 ml/kg body wt/min. I immediately appreciated this discovery at that time for what it was, namely, the sword that would eventually sever the Gordian Knot of complexity that had garotted perfusion technology. I was convinced that some way could be found to successfully perfuse only 20 to 25 ml/kg/min which we set as a flow rate with a comfortable safety margin. This 'low flow' quantity was only 10 to 20% of what others deemed necessary. Consequently, armed with this information in 1952, I believed that successful open heart surgery was not only possible, but inevitable'[459].

On the clinical application of cross circulation Lillehei went on to say:

Clinical cross circulation for intracardiac surgery was an immense departure from established surgical practice. The thought of taking a normal human to the operating room to serve as a donor circulation (with potential risks however small), even temporarily, was considered by critics at that time to be unacceptable, even 'immoral' as one prominent surgeon was heard to say. Some others, skilled in the art of criticism, were quick to point out that this proposed operation was the first in all of surgical history to have the potential (even the probability in their judgment) for a 200% mortality. This breakthrough with extracorporeal circulation by the cross circulation method rapidly moved the technique of total heart–lung bypass for intracardiac surgery from the experimental laboratory into the arena of clinical surgery. Further, the unprecedented success of the cross circulation technique in patients with complex defects, and often in intractable heart failure, played a crucial role in rapidly dispelling (virtually overnight) the widespread pessimism that had prevailed at that time amongst cardiologists and surgeons concerning the feasibility of open heart surgery in man. The conclusion that the sick human heart represented an insurmountable barrier was clearly untenable, and attention was directed once again to the previously unrecognized deficiencies of the existing pump oxygenators and in particular to perfusion physiology. Cross circulation was the major force that got open heart surgery moving. Knowing, now, what we did not know in 1954, it seems very probable that the only method for extracorporeal circulation that could possibly have succeeded in the face of such primitive knowledge and in the many high risk infants with complex anatomic lesions was cross circulation. The homeostatic mechanisms of the donor automatically corrected the many aberrations that had not even been discovered yet. Doubtless, pump oxygenator perfusions would have continued to have had an unacceptable clinical mortality for a long time.[459]

Southworth and Peirce were also involved in cross circulation experiments. They reported on its potential role in intracardiac surgery in 1952[467].

The group at Minnesota developed another approach to open heart surgery. They called it the reservoir technique and used it primarily for infants. It had one major impediment. The surgery had to be done within a short and fixed period of time[468].

W. T. Mustard and his colleagues used a monkey or dog lung as the biologic oxygenator. The blood was propelled with a Cowan perfusion pump[469–473]. This type of biologic oxygenation was also tried by still another team at the University of Minnesota. The team included Gilbert Campbell, Norman Crisp and E. B. Brown. They described their experimental and clinical experience utilizing dog lungs in 1956 with results that left much to be desired[474].

All these alternative approaches for establishing and confirming the feasibility of open heart surgery were being intensively pursued because of the pervasive opinion in the surgical community that total cardiopulmonary bypass with a heart–lung machine acting as the oxygenator was impractical.

Gibbon's initial success in 1953 notwithstanding, the pessimism concerning the future of the heart–lung machine continued throughout the first half of the 1950s. It was even augmented by Gibbon himself when he too became discouraged after his temporary inability to repeat his initial atrial septal success with the more complex ventricular defects. The initial dampening effect was created by Clarence Dennis, also a part of the enterprising Minnesota group. He was the first to use a heart–lung machine in a human. This was in 1951, two years before Gibbon's successful attempt in 1953[475]. Dennis' system consisted of a Gibbon screen, Björk disk oxygenators and a Dale–Schuster pump. Dennis was unsuccessful in his first as well as in his second attempt; both carried out within a month of each other. These were perceived as disastrous consequences. Dennis and most of his team soon moved to Brooklyn, New York. I remember so distinctly that when he began to work at Kings County Hospital it was in the midst of an atmosphere of skepticism and distrust with overtones of disdain.

Despite all this gloom, efforts at perfecting the heart–lung machine continued unabated. Both European and American investigators were participating in breaking down the barriers. These included not only Gibbon, but also the Lillehei group, Björk of Stockholm, Melrose in London, and Kirklin's group from the Mayo clinic with their enviable interdisciplinary and financial resources.

Lillehei's group felt that the problem lay not in the concept *per se*, but rather with the technical complexities involved and that if the entire assembly could be reduced to a simple design, then many of the complications could be avoided with a marked reduction in mortality. Björk's apparatus consisted of stainless steel disks rotating in a bath of blood. The machine designed by Melrose was a refinement of Björk's device. Efficiency was increased by rotating an inclined drum through which blood flowed slowly by gravity across a series of shallow trough-like disks so that the blood was passed from one disk to the next, and was thus able to take up a greater proportion of oxygen[476,477]. Melrose conducted his animal experiments at the Royal Veterinary College. By 1953, he and his team felt that they were ready for their first human subject. Rose Pilgrim, who had severe aortic and mitral valve disease, underwent a double closed valvotomy with the bypass machine acting purely in a supportive capacity[478].

Kirklin and his group at the Mayo clinic modified the machine that Gibbon developed in collaboration with the International Business Machine Corporation; more about this collaboration later. Although Kirklin's group had a 50% mortality in their series of 38 patients, their observations rather than their results gave heart to enthusiasts of the heart–lung machine.

In 1950 Leland Clark, Frank Gollan and Vishiva Gupta devised a bubble oxygenator consisting of a bubbler, defoamer, and a blood settling chamber. It was initially made of glass and later of pyrex. The crucial element in the design was the silicone resin that was used to coat the inner surface of all the glass parts. This was very effective in removing the gas bubbles thereby eliminating a potential source for gas embolism. James Helmsworth was the first to use this assembly in a human[479–482].

Most importantly, the defoaming element helped revitalize research efforts in bubble oxygenation. Despite their success with cross circulation, the Lillehei group realized the limitations of biologic oxygenation. Because of this, parallel efforts were instituted, while their cross circulation trials were going on to develop a simple, practical, reliable and inexpensive bubble oxygenator. DeWall was tapped as the lead man in this project. DeWall's first two models, though apparently successful, needed further refinement. He then, in collaboration with Vincent Gott, developed an experimental model which utilized a disposable plastic bag bubble oxygenator. This was used in conjunction with a vertical blood–oxygen mixing tube, a debubbling tube to remove the large bubbles and a central blood reservoir. A sigmamotor pump was used to deliver low flow rates[483–486]. Researchers from Tulane and Copenhagen also designed similar oxygenators[487,488]. In time, the sigmamotor pump was replaced by the DeBakey pump. DeBakey described his roller pump in 1934. It was initially designed for use in direct blood transfusions[489]. The pump consisted of a circular base plate and a compressible tube. No internal valves were needed to ensure flow in only one direction. The amount of blood pumped could be regulated by the size of the tubing and the speed of the pump. Moreover, the flow was non-pulsatile.

According to Denton Cooley, the roller pump was actually invented by Porter and Bradley and they obtained a patent on it in 1855. He claimed that John Gibbon was in error when he called it the 'DeBakey pump'[490]. He did not document this statement.

During the 1950s, there was general acceptance of the belief that the blood circulating through the heart–lung machine should not come in contact with ambient air. This eventually led to the development of membrane oxygenators. It was a simple refinement but an important one. The membrane was a thin plastic sheet that separated the blood from air but still allowed the diffusion of gases. Kolff had originally used this device in his artificial kidney. In 1956 he collaborated with Clowes in designing 'membrane lungs' for the heart–lung machine similar in principle to the membranes used in his artificial kidney[491–493]. Its complexity in design and operation hindered its general acceptance for a period of time, but its physiological soundness could not be avoided. Peirce[494], Bramson[495] and Lande[496] were also active in introducing membrane oxygenation. Incidentally, Lee and associates were the first to elucidate the adverse effects of a direct blood-gas interface on proteins[497,498].

The currently used perfusion equipment is much simpler and more reliable than those of the past. The present equipment can effectively oxygenate at much higher perfusion rates. Gollan and Neptune introduced the concept of hemodilution so that whole body perfusion could be achieved even more safely[499,500].

The last decade of the 20th century has benefited a great deal from the efforts of so many people. Extracorporeal circulation has allowed cardiac surgeons to perform feats that border on the miraculous. This would seem a good point to end this historical survey of the heart–lung machine but I cannot do so without considering again John Gibbon's role in its development. Was he really the catalyst that ushered in the modern era of open heart surgery? So many personalities were involved that one would hesitate to say so. But he does deserve a special niche in the entire scenario. He did provide the one critical experiment in 1937 when he demonstrated that the cardiorespiratory function of cats could be maintained by a heart–lung machine during the clamping of the pulmonary artery for prolonged periods. He was also a dreamer who by sheer tenacity lived to see his dreams come true.

The idea occurred to Gibbon because of an experience he had while a surgical fellow at Harvard under the tutelage of Edward Churchill. It took many long years before the idea was brought to fruition, and was a perfect example of how,

many times, tenacity and careful experimentation are absolutely essential ingredients in the practical application of a concept. This was the one great defect in Leonardo da Vinci. He was primarily a conceptualist, and once he realized the validity of the concept he lost all interest and failed to pursue it to its ultimate conclusion.

In an article published just 18 days prior to his death, John Gibbon gave a brief account of how 'an idea was born and then developed into a reality'[501]. Some of his comments are as follows:

In February, 1931, a female patient whose gall-bladder had been removed fifteen days previously developed a severe pain in the chest in the substernal region … A correct diagnosis of massive pulmonary embolus was made and Dr. Churchill had the patient moved to the operating room where she could be continuously observed and operated on immediately should her condition become critical. At that time no successful pulmonary embolectomy had been performed in the United States and only a very few in Europe. Because the procedure was so hazardous, Dr. Churchill decided not to operate unless it was apparent that death was imminent without operative intervention. My job in the operating room was to take and record the patient's pulse and respiratory rates and blood pressure every 15 minutes. From 3:00 PM one day to 8:00 AM the next day the operating team and I were by the side of the patient. Finally at 8:00 AM respirations ceased and blood pressure could not be obtained. Within 6 minutes 30 seconds Dr. Churchill had opened the chest, incised the pulmonary artery, extracted a large pulmonary embolus, and closed the incised wound in the pulmonary artery with a lateral clamp. Despite the rapidity of the procedure, the patient could not be revived. During that long night's vigil, watching the patient struggle for life, the thought naturally occurred to me that the patient's life might be saved if some of the blue blood in her veins could be continuously withdrawn into an extracorporeal blood circuit, exposed to an atmosphere of oxygen, and then returned to the patient by way of a systemic artery in a central direction. Thus, some of the patient's cardiorespiratory functions might be temporarily performed by the extracorporeal blood circuit while the massive embolus was surgically removed.

Shortly after this episode I married Dr. Churchill's first technician, Mary Hopkinson and returned to Philadelphia. During the next three years I practiced surgery in the mornings and pursued research projects in the afternoons. During these three years I had constantly in the back of my mind the idea of attempting to construct an extracorporeal blood circuit that would perform a part of the cardiorespiratory functions in animals and, hopefully, later in man. I thought then, and it turned out later to be true, that the most difficult part of the extracorporeal circuit would be the construction of the artificial lung. I therefore read everything I could find on the subject. Imagine for a moment the way research was carried on in a research laboratory in the 1930s. The Federal Government was not then pouring out hundreds of millions of dollars to doctors to perform research. Harvard provided my fellowship and the Massachusetts General Hospital provided the laboratory. I bought an air pump in a second hand shop down in East Boston for a few dollars, and used it to activate finger cot blood pumps. Valves were made from solid rubber corks with the small end cut transversely three quarters through to form a flap about 2 mm thick. With this flap held up, a cork borer was passed longitudinally through the center of the rubber stopper, thus creating a channel for the stream of blood. These simple valves worked well. Plastic materials were not available, so our circuit was largely rubber and glass. Heparin had just become available, but its antagonist, protamine, was not. However, with the dosage of heparin we used, the coagulation time returned to normal in a few hours. We were able to maintain life with the pulmonary artery completely occluded in twenty-one experiments using our extracorporeal circuit. During World War II the work was interrupted for five years. After my discharge from the Army, I accepted the position of professor of surgery and head of surgical research at the Jefferson Medical College of Philadelphia. Here we tackled again our everpresent problem of adequate oxygenation of a large volume of blood. We needed some good engineering advice. The dean of our medical school was aware of this and put me in touch with a freshman in the medical school who had been an aviator in World War II and who also had

invented a machine which transcribed musical notes to paper when a piano keyboard was played by a composer. This device was patented under the aegis of the International Business Machines Corporation. The student thought it quite likely that IBM might give me engineering help. Therefore, during the Christmas vacation of 1946 I went to the IBM building in New York to see the director of research of the corporation, armed with reprints of the articles I had written on the subject. After the director of research had glanced through the articles, he said that he thought that Mr. Thomas J. Watson, Sr., chairman of the board of the corporation, might be interested. We went to the top floor of the building to Mr. Watson's office and I waited in the waiting room while the director of research took my reprints to Mr. Watson. A few minutes later Mr. Watson appeared, greeted me cordially, and asked how he could help. Having arrived at an understanding that neither I nor IBM was to make any money out of our cooperative effort, I said that I needed engineering help. This he said he would provide and we arranged a meeting in my office with five of his engineers early in January 1947. From then on we had a very productive and rewarding association with Mr. Watson and the IBM Corporation.

With the help of these engineers, Gibbon succeeded in greatly improving the performance of the heart–lung machine.

After this demonstration of the greatly improved performance of our new heart-lung machine, we proceeded to carry out further experiments in which we opened the right atrium and ventricle, creating and closing atrial and ventricular septal defects, using the machine. These experiments were performed with a steadily decreasing mortality and morbidity. Finally I thought we had reached the point where it would be safe to employ the apparatus to correct an intracardiac defect under direct vision in a human patient. Our first patient was a year old infant who weighed only 11 pounds. The child had been in cardiac failure since birth. Because of her small size and edematous limbs, attempts at cardiac catheterization failed. Consulting cardiologists were all agreed that the child had a large atrial septal defect. With this diagnosis in mind, we operated on the infant through the right chest.

With the child connected to the heart-lung apparatus, the right atrium was opened, but no defect in the septum could be found. The child was in a precarious condition from the start of the operation and she died on the operating table. At autopsy she was found to have a huge patent ductus arteriosus. A more adequate exposure with a more thorough exploration of the heart might have allowed us to close the ductus and save the child's life. The next patient we operated on using the heart-lung machine was an eighteen year old girl who had been admitted to a hospital three times in the preceding six months because of heart failure. She had been catheterized and had been shown to have a large atrial septal defect with a left-to-right shunt of 9 liters per minute. The situation was carefully explained to the patient and to her mother. They agreed to the operation with the heart-lung machine and on May 6, 1953 I operated on her at the Jefferson Medical College Hospital using the heart-lung machine. All the patient's cardio-pulmonary functions were maintained by the apparatus for 26 minutes, while the large atrial septal defect was closed with a running silk suture. The patient's convalescence was uneventful, the murmur disappeared after the operation, and cardiac catheterization in July 1953 showed that the defect was completely closed without any evidence of a right-to-left shunt. The patient has remained alive and well up to the present time. This operation was the first successful open heart operation in the world using a heart-lung machine.

The above is a brief account of how an idea was born and then developed into a reality and finally was employed successfully in an operation on the heart of a human patient twenty-two years later, an event that I hardly dreamed of in 1931.

Valvular surgery under direct vision

The reliability and efficacy of the heart–lung machine with the ability to perform complex surgical procedures under direct vision and without haste now set the stage for the explosive growth of physiological cardiac surgery. Valve repair and replacement lent itself quite readily to this approach. Repair of congenital lesions was, of course, also a logical objective but this will be dealt with in the section devoted to this category of cardiac lesions. As we have already seen, open heart surgery was first employed primarily for management of the congenital lesions, especially the septal defects and pulmonary stenosis. It was the experience gained with these lessons that made it possible for surgeons to attempt intervention in the complicated acquired valvulopathies.

Repair of mitral insufficiency under direct vision became a primary objective as soon as it became evident that total cardiopulmonary bypass was a truly workable modality. The blind procedures that had been tried were severely hampered by lack of a dry field and adequate vision with a resultant high failure rate in terms of both adequate repair and mortality.

The earliest techniques in open heart valve surgery were reconstructive procedures since prosthetic valves whether mechanical or tissue had yet to be introduced.

Priority for the first successful surgery in acquired mitral insufficiency probably goes to C. Walton Lillehei and his group. It was carried out at the University of Minnesota on August 29, 1956. The lesion was a pure mitral insufficiency and it was corrected by suture plication of the valve commissures under direct vision[502,503]. Two months later, Merendino at the University of Washington successfully performed the same type of procedure in an individual with a similar lesion[504]. Subsequent attempts by both these men and their associates were initially concerned with reconstruction of regurgitant lesions but in a very short time stenotic lesions were also subject to repair under direct vision. Also as time went on, repair by direct suture was carried out for regurgitant lesions caused not only by rheumatic fever but also by tears and perforations precipitated by infective endocarditis or caused by surgeons during a previous blind commissurotomy.

Many surgeons from around the world became involved with direct vision repair. Among the pioneers were Nichols of Philadelphia[505], Belcher[506] and Barrat-Boyes[507] from England and Barnard[508] from South Africa to mention but a few.

Increasing the surface of the mitral leaflet was another method of restoring competency to the valve. Spencer and the groups headed by King and Johnson experimented with patches of Teflon and Nylon while Sauvage and associates attacked autogenous pericardial tissue[509–512]. On a clinical level

Nichol's group used a compressed polyvinyl sponge. This was fashioned into an elliptical shape and inserted between the mitral annulus and the leaflet[505]. Four patients were subjected to this procedure with no deaths reported. Merendino and his co-workers used Teflon and Nylon in two patients[513] while Sauvage[512] and Frater[514] used autogenous pericardium with somewhat better results. However, it soon became evident that this type of approach rarely functioned and it was rapidly abandoned.

Cumulative surgical experience and increasing diagnostic accuracy brought the striking revelation that rupture of the chordae tendinae was a common cause of mitral regurgitation[515]. This led to the introduction of a number of techniques for the repair of the chordae. These included plication of the ruptured leaflet and creation of artificial chordae. Leaflet plication in conjunction with annuloplasty of the posteromedial variety was introduced in 1960 by the Mayo group under the direction of Dwight McGoon[516]. Silk was used by Kay and Egerton[517,518] Dacron and Teflon were used by Sanders[519], and Morris[520,521].

Reducing the gap between the mitral leaflets in the closed position was another approach. Narrowing the circumference of the mitral annulus presented itself as a seemingly good method to do so. This was not a new idea since it was already tried as a blind technique with variable results. Lillehei and his group were the first to narrow the mitral annulus under direct vision. They called their technique bicommissural since it consisted of placing heavy silk sutures in the mitral annulus in the region of both commissures[502,503]. Despite the fact that the approach appeared to have a sound physiological basis, both short and long term results were variable and mostly unfavorable. This led to numerous modifications. In the hands of Merendino[513], Kay[522,523], and Wooler[524], a posteromedial annuloplasty resulted in the greatest number of long term improvements. Carpentier introduced a prosthetic ring annuloplasty in 1971. He also introduced a variant technique in leaflet resection and chordoplasty[525]. Both of Carpentier's techniques gained acceptance throughout the world. By 1980 at least 2000 patients had been subjected to his procedures. In the late 1970s, Duran developed a flexible ring in place of Carpentier's rigid one. The rigid ring had the potential disadvantage of not allowing the annulus to change shape during the cardiac cycle.

During this reconstructive phase of repair under direct vision, many failures were encountered; enough to make early investigators aware of the necessity of another approach, namely, valve replacement. Early efforts were aimed at partial replacement with an immobile prosthesis. This was later followed by the insertion of a mobile prosthesis as a partial replacement, and finally total replacement with a prosthetic device.

Little was known about the problems to be encountered nor the necessity for intensive efforts and numerous revisions and modifications. Clinical results often went contrary to the expectations of the laboratory. Many patients died during the process; sometimes due to the brashness of the surgeon; many times due to an inadequate experimental base; but often because of the inability to test a new hypothesis in the available animals.

The present level of competency in valvular surgery came about only after a long and arduous process. It is a tribute to the concept of the interdisciplinary approach in research that saw its greatest implementation during the latter half of the 20th century. Physiologists, engineers, biochemists, surgeons, scientists in so many other disciplines, and businessmen forged a cooperative linkage that culminated in the present level of sophistication in all of cardiology with valvular surgery being one of its stellar elements.

Initially plastic elements were used in partial replacement. Gott and his co-workers at Minnesota were the first to successfully use a cylinder of compressed Ivalon which they sutured to the undersurface of the leading edge of the posterior mitral leaflet[526]. Barnard and Schrire used the same technique but their Ivalon prosthesis was shaped in the form of a dumb-bell[508]. The appearance of a high rate of complications was responsible for abandoning the technique altogether.

One of the main difficulties with a rigid prosthesis was that often the mitral orifice was narrowed too much so that in effect the surgeons were trading insufficiency for stenosis. Obviously this was not a desirable exchange. Thus other approaches were tried. Knitted Teflon leaflets with chordae extensions were tried experimentally by King[509]. In addition, Barnard[527] and McKenzie[528] used leaflets made of Silastic while Schimert and his group used Silastic covered Teflon leaflets with attached chordae tendinae[529]. In 1963, Frater and his associates replaced a dog's posterior mitral leaflet with autogenous pericardial tissue, properly sized and shaped[530].

Total prosthetic replacement had a very difficult beginning. The experimental approaches were beset with so many problems, both technical and biological, that clinical implementation seemed quite remote and unlikely. Nevertheless, these dog experiments did contribute towards the ultimate design of a clinically useful valve.

A host of shapes was tried, some based on anatomical forms and others based on sound physiological principles. Initially mechanical valves were tried and then as their covert difficulties became known, attempts were made with tissue valves. The different functional designs included the monocusp flap valves, multi-cusp valves, valves with attached artificial chordae tendinae, ball valves, and disk- and lens-shaped valves. Many different types of material were used in fabricating these valves. Mylar, knitted Teflon fabric, Silastic, polyurethane, Dacron and Lucite were all tried. Each had its proponents. All were introduced to overcome the many difficulties and complications that were surfacing as clinical experience accumulated. Thrombosis, durability, difficulty in fixation and encroachment on chamber space were among the problems that arose. Some of the valves were designed primarily for insertion into the mitral area while others were used for either mitral or aortic valve replacement.

Among the first prosthetic valves to be used in humans were flap valves consisting of either single or multiple leaflets. Ellis was the first to try a flap valve in 1960[531,532]. His had only one cusp which was made of laminated Mylar and covered with knitted Teflon. It was used primarily for mitral valve replacement. Late dysfunction with its attendant complications were deficiencies that could not be overcome[533]. Young was more successful with a Silastic bicuspid hinged valve[534]. This was also used only for mitral disease. In 1960, N. S. Braunwald tried to replace the mitral valve with a flexible polyurethane prosthesis with attached synthetic chordae tendinae made of Teflon tape[535].

The greatest advance in mechanical valves was the ball-valve prosthesis introduced by Albert Starr from the University of Oregon Medical School. The valve was designed in collaboration with Lowell Edwards, who was a retired electrical engineer when he began to work with Starr. At first, their goal was to build an artificial heart but it was too ambitious for the time so they revised their objectives in favor of a prosthetic heart valve. The original model was intended for mitral valve replacement[536–538]. An aortic model with three struts was developed later, and after certain modifications, it was introduced commercially in 1968 as model 1260[539]. Prior to these modifications, Cartwright used Starr's original model of 1960 for multiple valve replacements[540]. Starr was not the first, however, to use a mechanical valve. Hufnagel, as far back as 1951 showed that man-made materials could be well-tolerated in the blood stream. He used a caged-ball valve in the descending aorta for the relief of aortic insufficiency[541].

The Starr–Edwards valve had three components: a rigid cage of Vitallium, a Silastic ball, and a suturing ring covered with Teflon[536]. Starr's original report was described at the Conference on Prosthetic Valves for Cardiac Surgery in Chicago in 1960. Most of the report was devoted to the experimental results in dogs who had their mitral valves replaced with the prosthesis. Up to that time, he had tried it in only one clinical case. The patient died during surgery because of an air embolus. At autopsy, there was no evidence of endothelial damage or compromising infringement of space in the left ventricular chamber. This led him to state that 'this type of valve holds much promise'[542].

The original model with certain modifications was accepted and used by several of the leading cardiac surgeons of the time. However, the model was associated during the early years of its implementation in both mitral and aortic valve surgery with a rather high operative mortality rate, varying between 10–20% depending on the surgeon. It was also subject to the dangers of late complications such as infection, leakage, anemia and thromboembolism[543–550]. Harken modified the valve by substituting a hollow silicone ball and a Dacron skirt[551]. He used it for both aortic and mitral valve replacement[552]. Smeloff and his colleagues' modification utilized a double-caged ball valve[553]. Magovern and Cromie designed a version that was fixed with pins instead of sutures[554–556].

The Capetown university group headed by Christian Barnard designed a lens-shaped valve[557]. Their original model was a lenticular, silastic prosthesis suspended by a spindle from a Teflon-coated stainless steel ring and attached to the mitral annulus by means of a polyvinyl sponge ring.

During this time, aortic valve surgery was also moving forward. Prosthetic aortic valves came into use in the mid 1950s following Hufnagel's demonstration in 1951 that partial control of aortic insufficiency was possible by placing a caged plastic ball device in the descending aorta[558]. The advent of cardiopulmonary bypass made possible the replacement of the aortic valve in the subcoronary position, and it was in 1961 that Starr first suggested that his prosthetic mitral valve be modified for insertion in this position. Just one year prior to this, Harken had already demonstrated the feasibility of inserting the caged ball valves at the subcoronary position[552]. He used it successfully twice in 1960 with patients surviving for more than a decade. Incidentally, like Starr, Harken also had a capable design engineer with him. He was W. Clifford Birtwell.

The caged ball valve of Hufnagel was not a new idea. A US patent was given to J. B. Williams of New York in 1858 for a bottle stopper that had the same design. Even Williams didn't claim that the ball valve was original with him. In a letter to the editor of the *American Journal of Cardiology*, Williams is quoted as saying: 'I would state that I am aware a ball valve is not new and I lay no claim to it in its general application; but what I do claim as a new article of manufacture is – a bottle stopper'[559]. Figure 20 is a drawing from Williams' US Patent No. 19323 (February 9, 1858).

Starr's original aortic model had two major drawbacks. Blood tended to clot at the apex of the struts, and where the struts joined the stainless steel orifice. The silastic balls had a tendency to absorb lipid from the blood so that in due time they would swell, crack or both[560]. In the process, the ball would become so deformed that, at times, it could not effectively occlude the orifice in the closed position, or swell so much that it would jam in the open position. Starr tried to overcome the problem of ball variance and thromboembolism by replacing the silastic ball with a hollow metal ball composed of Stellite with the rest of the valve enclosed in woven Dacron. The ball variance problem was solved but thromboembolism was still an important complication despite the laying down of smooth endothelial tissue over the rest of the valve exposed to the bloodstream. Ironically, the fibrous tissue under the endothelial layer created another set of problems. The struts became thicker as the fibrous tissue grew around them. This made it increasingly difficult for the silastic ball to move freely and in some cases the ball actually remained frozen in place. Fibrous tissue

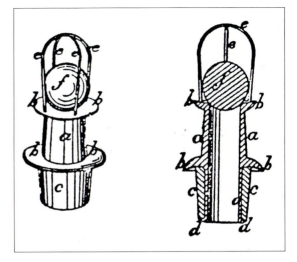

Figure 20 Drawing from Williams' US Patent No. 19323 (February 9, 1858). *Photo Source University of Central Florida. Literary Source Schwartz, D.C. and Kaplan, S. (1966). The caged ball valve circa 1858. Am. J. Cardiol., **18**, 942. With permission*

also grew across the orifice creating severe aortic stenosis. Starr and Edwards now widened the struts so as to provide more leeway for the moving ball. In addition, they inserted metallic projections around the valve's orifice where the ball would be seated. Every time the valve closed, the ball would act as a chopping device effectively trimming back the fibrous growth. These were rather ingenious modifications but two more problems had to be resolved. These were hemolysis and obstruction of the space between the perimeter of the ball in the open position and the aortic wall. Hemolysis was found to be due to wear and tear on the cloth which in due time exposed the sharp spicules of Dacron. As the red blood cells flowed by, many of them were sheared by these sharp projections. This was solved by incorporating a track on the inner aspects of the struts thereby protecting the Dacron from the ball. No amount of modification, however, could eliminate the so-called tertiary orifice obstruction.

The spherical occluder is still popular although attempts had been made to reduce the overall height of the valve by putting a disk occluder in a flattened cage. Unsuccessful models designed in this manner were introduced by Magovern and the team of Smeloff and Cutter. The Magovern model had the propensity to be dislocated from its anchorage at the annulus, especially when the annulus was calcified. The tilting or hinged leaflet valves had all the earmarks of being superior to the Starr–Edwards valve, even with its numerous modifications. They had a smaller profile height and promised not to produce as much occluder-induced turbulence in the flow through and distal to the valve. The Kay–Shiley version was subject to early wear. This was eliminated by Björk and Shiley in 1961 with their free-floating disk. A similar design was introduced a year later by Lillehei and Kaster. It too was based on the concept of a free floating disk which, in the open position, tilted to an angle. The degree of tilt was restricted by how the disk retaining struts were designed. Initially, the Björk–Shiley valve used a Delrin occluder. Later pyrolitic carbon was substituted for the Delrin. Both the Björk–Shiley and the Lillehei–Kaster valves were still subject to sticking and thrombosis.

St Jude Medical Inc. introduced a bileaflet pyrolitic carbon valve; the two pyrolitic occluders being hinged and shaped in a semi-circular fashion. The main advantage of this design was that in the open position, the valve provided minimal disturbance to flow. Emery's clinical evaluation published in 1979 augured well for the success of this valve, and currently, it is still enjoying a high degree of popularity[561].

The risk of thrombosis with mechanical valves carries with it the mandate that the patient be on continuous anticoagulant therapy. Another disadvantage is the less than optimum hemodynamic function, no matter how the mechanical valve is designed. In an attempt to overcome these major disadvantages, subsequent efforts were directed towards finding the ideal tissue valve. There were several stages in the evolution of these bioprostheses.

Aortic valves removed from cadavers were the first to be tried. Ross initiated this approach in 1962[562]. Even though, in 1980, Wain reported satisfactory long-term results with these valves, the potential for long-term damage is still present since these cadaveric allografts are dead and thus unable to combat any damage with regenerating cells[563]. Ross was well aware of this, and as far back as 1967 he used the patient's own pulmonary valve as a means of preventing this outcome. This seemed to be a logical step for two other reasons besides the above. First of all, the pulmonary valve has the same number of cusps as the aortic valve and therefore could be considered as an ideal replacement in terms of function. Moreover, patients could get on quite well despite the loss of their pulmonary valve. Ross tried this technique in 176 patients, and even 13 years later he was able to report that there was no apparent degeneration in these transplanted valves[564]. This was acceptable insofar as aortic valve replacement was concerned but unfortunately, the patient's pulmonary valve could not be used to replace the mitral or tricuspid valves. On went the search for alternative tissue valve substitutes.

Ross remained interested in the subject, intent on finding an alternative to transplanting the pulmonary valve. In 1969, he reported his experience with frame mounted autologous fascia lata. Senning also used autologous fascia lata but his were free standing rather than frame mounted[565]. Whether fascia lata were free or mounted, long-term results were unsatisfactory and in less than a decade their use was abandoned[566]. The fascia lata were simply not strong enough to withstand the cyclic stressing of the heart over a long period of time.

Kaiser and his co-workers were the first to use a pig's aortic valve. It was fixed with glutaraldehyde. He reported his experience with it in conjunction with Hancock in 1969[567]. The glutaraldehyde fixation was an important step in that it reduced the antigenicity of the foreign tissue as well as the occurrence of autolysis while at the same time it rendered the tissue quite flexible with markedly enhanced strength characteristics. In the original design, the porcine valve was mounted on a rigid supporting frame. It was later modified by replacing the rigid frame with one that had a rigid base but flexible posts. This was the design that was produced commercially and known as the Hancock porcine xenograft. The bioprosthesis designed by Carpentier and Edwards used a totally flexible support frame. It was introduced by the Edwards laboratory in 1976[568]. Both bioprostheses are still highly popular at this writing.

Still another approach was the use of glutaraldehyde treated pericardial tissue. This was developed by Ionescu and co-workers, described by them in 1971, and marketed finally as the Ionescu–Shiley pericardial xenograft in 1976[569]. This valve has a tricuspid configuration. It too became quite popular especially because the valves could be made in various sizes. A bicuspid form was introduced by Black and his associates in 1982[570]. It was designed especially for replacement of the mitral valve. According to the inventors, it reproduces more closely the physiological behavior of the normal mitral valve.

A world congress on heart valve replacement was held in January, 1989 in San Diego, California. There was, of course, the usual hyperbole of the various companies regarding the valves each was marketing, but this was tolerable since without their entrepreneurial interest, advances in design and efficiency would have been surely slower in forthcoming. Besides a presentation of the current state of the art in valve surgery, and an analysis of the statistical results of the various types of prostheses, pioneers in the field reminisced about their role in the evolution of valvular surgery. Rather pertinent and interesting remarks were made by Swanson and Starr, Carpentier, Siposs, and Smeloff.

Swanson and Starr categorically stated that the modern version of the Starr–Edwards valve 'remains, even today, the mechanical valve of choice'. No mechanical failures have been reported with it, and the incidence of thrombosis is less than in others[539].

Carpentier's remarks were as follows:

The first successful xenograft implantation in humans was carried out in September 1965 by Jean-Paul Binet, Jean Langlois, and myself … Contrary to experimental findings and despite early good clinical results, the xenograft valves preserved in a mercurial solution tended to deteriorate after 6 months … It became obvious that to prolong the durability of these valves it would be necessary to prevent cellular penetration … Among the many substances tested, glutaraldehyde, a product widely used in electron microscopy, appeared to be the most effective for decreasing the antigenicity and increasing the stability of the tissue as shown by subcutaneous implantation of treated tissue in the rat and by numerous physical or immunological tests … Calcification of the tissue remains a stumbling block in younger patients. The current efforts of my wife, Sophie, who has helped me since 1974, and myself are directed toward the development of chemical methods of calcium mitigation so that, one day, children will have the benefit of a durable, non- thrombogenic valvular prosthesis.[571]

Smeloff waxed enthusiastic about the valve that he and Cutter designed. He described how he and his group focused on three aspects of research: anatomical, engineering and laboratory studies, and how the results of these studies were responsible for the final design of their mechanical valve. The Smeloff–Cutter valve still used the silastic ball. By careful curing of the ball it was possible to 'turn all its elastomers to elastic and therefore eliminated the problem of deformation and splitting'[572]. At the congress, Smeloff claimed that no structural failures of the valve had been reported in 22 years of use, and that the incidence of thromboembolic events for fully anticoagulated patients had been 0.7% for the aortic prosthesis and 1.7% for the mitral one[572].

George Siposs recounted how:

twenty-five years ago I began a career that was the culmination of my childhood dreams: to be an engineer working with surgeons. As a heart-valve design engineer at Edwards Laboratories I was working on my first heart-valve patent within 4 months. While others tried to duplicate the natural shape of human heart valves, Lowell Edwards opted for function, with the elegant simplicity of the caged-ball valve. My job was to design a series of valve sizes and sewing rings. Dr. Albert Starr, my mentor, explained that heart valves cannot be equally proportioned as a ratio of diameter to length, much as a man's pants are not proportionally larger as the waist size increases. We had to tread softly and test carefully because we were in uncharted territory. I obtained calf hearts from the slaughterhouse so that I could learn cardiac morphology. I witnessed, photographed, and filmed many open heart operations, and I attended postmortem examinations. One of my most unforgettable experiences was listening with a stethoscope to the chest of a patient who had one of my valves implanted that morning. Day by day the impossible became reality. It was exhilarating because the lead time from concept to product was so short. The FDA was not yet on the horizon. Early in 1964 I developed a fast-implanting valve based on Dr. Arthur Beall's concept that had spring-loaded pins incorporated in the suture ring and held back by a ripcord suture. When the key suture was cut, the 16 pins sank into the aortic tissue to anchor the valve in place. A photographer was supposed to take pictures during the first animal implantation, but he was so awestruck at the sight of an open heart that he forgot to load his camera. When Dr. Beall signaled him to shoot, the cameraman's mouth dropped open.

653

Heart valves have come a long way, but I am proud to say that the Starr-Edwards valve's longevity is still the gold standard against which all others are measured.[573]

Despite these glowing remarks and those of others at the World Congress, it behooves us to recall the words of Paton and Vogel regarding the 'perfect valve' that the pioneers and others visualized but has yet to be realized. We may never have definitive results. At best, we may be able to say to patients. 'Here and now, with this valve, at your age and with your ventricular function, you have certain percent chance of living 5 years, a different chance of living 10 years, and your chances of living without any complications are such and such. With your new valve you may have problems but we hope that the problems you have will be less serious than the problems you have had'[574].

Surgery in congenital cardiac lesions

The advent of cardiovascular surgery in children is generally accepted as being due to the courage, enthusiasm and highly disciplined approach of Robert Gross of Harvard. Gross was the first to ligate a patent ductus arteriosus successfully. This daring and successful attempt caught the imagination of thoracic surgeons throughout the world. The story behind his landmark procedure is fascinating because it reflects the aspirations and foibles of surgeons as human beings.

The need for such surgery was first suggested to Gross by the cardiologist, Hubbard. After several proddings from Hubbard, the young surgeon decided to take up the challenge, and in his characteristically thorough fashion, he spent time both in the laboratory and at the autopsy table perfecting a suitable technique. When Gross told Hubbard that he was finally ready to comply, the proposal was submitted to Dr Blackfan, who was chief of pediatrics but not a cardiologist. Feeling unqualified to render a decision, Blackfan suggested that they consult Paul D. White. After examining the child, whose parents were the only ones to consent to the surgery among the several solicited, White said 'a brave procedure, and obviously one that has been carefully considered. In my opinion, it should proceed as planned'. In the meanwhile, Gross was already aware of his chief's reluctance to

proceed with this untried operation. Wary of a probable refusal, Gross decided to operate while his chief was vacationing. He could thus easily circumvent the chain of command. There is an undocumented story that soon after the operation was a *fait accompli* and with the chief still on vacation, Gross in a casual encounter with him at the local cricket club was asked as to the status of affairs at the hospital. Gross carefully answered that 'nothing unusual' was happening – a remarkable bit of understatement, considering the waves of excitement that he generated throughout the world.

It is strange though that not too many years later when his fame was established, Gross also succumbed to the eventual authoritarianism of so many pioneers and flatly refused to help Helen Taussig when she proposed to him that he perform an aortic-pulmonary shunt to relieve the cyanosis in Tetralogy of Fallot.

The thought of ligating a patent ductus arteriosus did not originate with Hubbard. Munro appears to have been the first to propose the procedure. The idea came to him in 1907 while performing an autopsy on a child in whom the only cardiac abnormality he could find was a patent ductus[575]. At that time ether anesthesia was available and Munro thought the duct could be ligated through a sternal-splitting incision. Figure 21 depicts the title and opening paragraph of his presentation before the American Surgical Society in 1907[576].

According to Russell Brock, Evarts Graham also entertained the idea in the early 1920s but was rebuffed by the professor of pediatrics at the St Louis Children's Hospital. Instead of referring a child to Graham, this stalwart pediatrician sent instead a man 53 years of age. Brock stated 'I have no doubt that he thought this was a clever act, powerful enough to stop once and for all this imaginative but troublesome surgeon. It was, of course, a cruel and stupid thing to do and, as Graham said, delayed the advent of cardiovascular surgery in children for some 15 years'[575].

Various techniques were tried over the three decades since Munro's original suggestion; but no real progress was made until Gross and Hubbard reported their landmark success in 1939[577]. Just two years before, Graybiel, Strieder and Boyer had been unsuccessful when they ligated a patent ductus in a 22 year old woman with bacterial endarteritis of the duct[578]. She died a few days later.

Eleven months after Gross' first case, Jones of Stanford University presented his results in seven cases at a meeting of the American Association for Thoracic Surgery[579]. When Lewis Bullock referred the first patient to Jones, the patient's parents refused to have their son undergo the operation when in response to their question, they were told that the operation had never been done before. Within several weeks, Gross' article was published, and now the patient's parents agreed to have their son subjected to the procedure based upon the successful outcome reported by Gross[580].

On December 5, 1939, despite the failure reported by Graybiel and his associates a year earlier, Oswald Tubbs of St Bartholomew's Hospital in London, successfully ligated an infected patent ductus[581]. This cured the infection. Four years later, Tubbs described in his Hunterian lecture his results with nine infected ducts[582]. Six patients survived in this series. It must be emphasized that Tubbs' patients had the benefit of adjunctive chemotherapy.

The ensuing decade saw the introduction of numerous closed procedures for other congenital abnormalities. Surgery of the great vessels lent themselves quite readily to intervention without benefit of cardiopulmonary bypass. Thus in 1945, two teams independently described their techniques in correction of coarctation of the aorta. These were Gross and Hufnagel who described their experimental studies concerning its surgical correction[380] and Crafoord and Nylin from Sweden[583]. Crafoord performed his procedure on October 19, 1944. He demonstrated his technique in January 1946 at Westminster Hospital having been invited to do so by Price Thomas, a close friend of Crafoord. The patient made such a wonderful recovery that he was able to play football and even won a medal for boxing[584].

The year 1945 also saw the introduction by Blalock and Taussig of the first shunt procedure for the relief of cyanosis[585]. It was truly a physiological approach, and although purely palliative, it was a remarkable breakthrough until corrective procedures could be implemented with the advent of open heart surgery. Taussig had correctly realized that cyanosis in congenital lesions of the heart was dependent on pulmonary blood flow; the less flow, the deeper the cyanosis.

The technique for connecting a systemic artery to the pulmonary artery had been highly refined by this time; starting with Carrel's initial contributions in

I. LIGATION OF THE DUCTUS ARTERIOSUS.

BY JOHN C. MUNRO, M.C.,
OF BOSTON, MASS

THAT I may be allowed to bring this suggestion for a new operation before your Society, I ask on the basis that it has not been hastily conceived. On the contrary, long ago I demonstrated its technical possibility on the cadaver of newborn children, and felt that it was justifiable on the living. At various times I have tried to inspire the pediatric specialist with my views, but in vain. Now, in view of the recent advances in cardiac surgery, for much of which we are indebted to the surgeons of this city, I will venture to place my ideas before you, asking that you do not dismiss them hastily.

Figure 21 Title and opening paragraph of Munro's paper on ligation of the ductus arteriosus. *Photo Source National Library of Medicine. Literary Source Ann. Surg., 46, 335, 1907. Courtesy of National Library of Medicine*

vascular anastomosis. In 1939, Levy and Blalock had already published the results of their experiments in dogs in which a systemic artery was anastomosed in the left main pulmonary artery[586]. The subclavian artery was chosen originally because of the need to preserve blood flow through one lung while the anastomosis was being performed. Remember, there was no heart–lung machine at the time.

Their first patient was 15 months old, and managed to survive with a marked reduction in the degree of cyanosis. Blalock used the innominate artery in the next two patients because of the technical difficulties in dealing with the tiny left subclavian artery. Figure 22 is a diagram of the first Blalock-Taussig anastomosis.

Twenty years later when Taussig gave the T. Duckett Jones Memorial Lecture at the scientific session of the American Heart Association she reminisced about her rebuff at the hands of Robert Gross, and portrayed quite vividly the salient features of the third operation and the surgical skills of Dr Blalock. These are her words:

Again I am grateful to Harvard and to Dr. Robert Gross that while in his first flush of success of closure of a patent ductus, when in answer to my inquiry, he told me he had built many a ductus but was not in the least interested in my suggestion of creating a ductus for a cyanotic child. So I returned to Baltimore to bide my time until Dr. Alfred Blalock became surgeon-in-chief. He was known for his work on thymoma and on shock and he was considered a vascular surgeon as he had operated

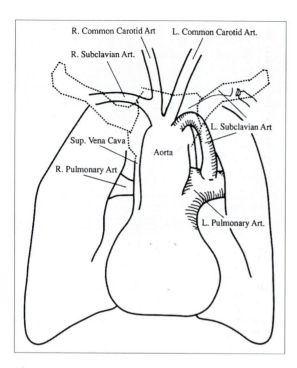

Figure 22 Diagram of the first Blalock-Taussig anastomosis. *Photo Source University of Central Florida. Literary Source Blalock, A. and Taussig, H.B. (1945). The surgical treatment of malformations of the heart in which there is pulmonary stenosis or pulmonary atresia. J. Am. Med. Assoc., **128**, 189. With permission*

successfully on three children with patency of the ductus arteriosus! The fact that the first three operations were successful attests to the brilliancy of Dr. Blalock's surgical skill. It was, however, only at the end of the third operation that we saw the value of the operation. That operation was on an utterly miserable, small, 6-year-old boy who had a red-blood-cell count of 10 million and was no longer able to walk. When Dr. Blalock first removed the clamps, the blood welled up in the child's chest. Dr. Blalock quickly controlled the hemorrhage and poured in plasma. Suddenly Dr. Merrill Harmel cried, 'He's a lovely color now' and I walked around to the head of the table and saw his lovely normal pink lips! The child woke up in the operating room and asked, 'Is the operation over?' When Dr. Blalock said 'Yes', the child said 'May I get up now?' From that moment on he was a happy and active child. [587]

After Blalock and Taussig's paper appeared, there was a veritable odyssey to Baltimore. Within two years, 500 patients underwent the procedure [588]. Of course, the operation was not the definitive answer, either in terms of palliation or correction. Over a 5 year follow-up many of the shunts closed or became smaller requiring a second operation. Moreover, neurologic defects occurred in at least 25% of the patients when the innominate artery was used [588]. In a short time other palliative procedures appeared beginning with those used by Willis Potts, and soon thereafter by William Glenn and later by David Waterston and Denton Cooley.

Potts appreciated immediately the physiological soundness of the Blalock–Taussig shunt. He was the first to adopt the procedure in his own practice, but as his experience developed, he began to realize that in the smaller infants, where it was most needed, the tiny subclavian artery might impede blood flow into the pulmonary artery or that clotting could occur at the anastomotic site. His search for an alternative method of producing an effective systemic-pulmonary anastomosis excluding the varying availability of the brachiocephalic arteries resulted finally in his version of the shunt. This was an anastomosis of the left main pulmonary artery and the descending thoracic aorta. The major hazard in such a procedure was the ischemic damage to the spinal cord with resultant paraplegia during total occlusion of the descending aorta while performing the anastomosis. In collaboration with Sidney Smith, a young research fellow on his staff, and Bruno Richter, a talented craftsman, Potts succeeded in devising an instrument to overcome this potential hazard. It came to be known as the Potts–Smith aortic exclusion clamp. It was made from a modified lid retractor and so designed that the medial lip of the descending aorta could be excluded while the rest of the aorta within the loops of the clamp remained open so that flow to the spinal cord would not be compromised. Potts' procedure became quite popular because it was easy to perform, and did not result in the neurologic defects seen in those patients that underwent anastomosis with the innominate artery [589,590].

William Glenn bypassed the right side of the heart completely. He created a shunt between the superior vena cava and the right pulmonary artery. The success of this shunt depended upon a pulmonary artery of large diameter and a low pulmonary vascular resistance [591]. He tried this approach in a

7 year old boy with transposition of the great arteries and left outflow tract obstruction. The Glenn operation had limited application, however.

Waterston and Cooley developed almost identical techniques in anastomosing the ascending aorta to the right pulmonary artery. Although Waterston had presented his technique in Czechoslovakia in 1960, it was unknown to Cooley since the western world was not privy to Waterston's presentation behind the Iron Curtain[592,593]. The technique became quite popular as a palliative procedure in Tetralogy of Fallot, especially in small infants and neonates in whom the subclavian artery, again, would be too small for a successful shunt.

Some of the uncertainties surrounding the original Blalock–Taussig operation were overcome to a certain extent with the development of microvascular techniques. Still later, synthetic arterial grafts were introduced as the connecting conduit for the shunt but these were plagued with a high rate of thrombosis[594].

In the wake of these palliative shunt procedures, Lord Brock introduced his technique for correction of the pulmonic stenosis in Tetralogy of Fallot with instruments of his own design. These were valvulotomes in different sizes, pinch forceps and expanding dilators. In June of 1948, Brock performed his first closed pulmonary valvotomy[595]. Two weeks later, Sellors' report appeared in *The Lancet*[596]. In it, he described three succesful pulmonary valvotomies performed through the right ventricle. The first one was done on February 16, 1948. The combined procedure of pulmonary valvotomy and pulmonary resection became known as the 'Brock procedure'. It was quite popular in Great Britain, less so in the USA. Total one-stage correction of Fallot's Tetralogy replaced Brock's operation when open heart surgery became possible with the heart–lung machine. Today, corrective intracardiac repair is the method of choice but indications for the palliative shunt still exist as Kirklin pointed out in 1979[597]. De Laval's modification of the shunt is probably the most widely used palliative procedure when a two-stage repair is contemplated[598]. It uses a Grotex conduit from the side of the intact subclavian artery to the side of the pulmonary artery.

Perhaps the apogee of blind intracardiac surgery was reached when attempts were made during this era to correct atrial septal defects. Some methods were ingenious, others were bizarre and all were not truly physiological as we shall see.

The first closed attempts to repair atrial septal defects occurred in the 1940s. Some were experimental while others were tried on humans. Roy Cohn's method, used only in dogs, and described in 1947, invaginated the right atrial wall so that it could be sutured to the periphery of the defect. Mattress sutures were used. The patch was then cut free and the hole closed by tightening the previously placed mattress sutures[599]. A year later, Gordon Murray of Toronto described his method[600]. After experimenting with the technique in animals, he tried it on a 12 year old girl but failed to close the defect completely, resulting in her death a little more than a year later. It was a simple procedure but subject to the uncertainty of closing the defect completely. Sutures were passed through the atrial septum from front to back and when in place, were simply tightened so that the walls of the defect would be drawn together[600,601].

Forest Dodrill designed a double ring clamp. His attempts were confined to dogs only. The clamp was used to press the lateral atrial wall against the septum and held there while it was sutured against the rim of the defect[602]. Still another approach was that devised by Marion and Termet in 1950[603]. Only one human was subjected to it, and happily, it proved successful. It was also an invagination technique. This time the right atrial appendage was invaginated completely through the defect until the invaginated tip could be sutured against the lateral wall of the left atrium. This to me had neither rhyme nor reason because of the obvious encroachment on atrial hemodynamics. Nevertheless, it illustrates the somewhat bizarre means utilized during the blind intracardiac epoch.

A slightly better approach was the one reported by Swan and his group from the University of Colorado, also in 1950[604]. They attached a suture to a curved probe which was then maneuvered blindly from the right atrial appendage through the defect to the left atrial appendage. Once the suture was in place, the probe was withdrawn, and a plastic button on the outside of each appendage was then threaded to each end of the suture. As the suture ends were pulled, the atrial appendages were invaginated until the defect was closed. Again, this technique did not take into account the resultant hemodynamic distortions.

Several other leading cardiac surgeons also became involved with the problem. These were Hufnagel, Merendino, Bailey and Gross. Merendino attempted to close the defects with a pericardial bag filled with autogenous fat[605]. Hufnagel of Georgetown inserted the two halves of a plastic button into the defect by means of a special instrument he designed[606].

Marvels of blind intracardiac surgery were realized in 1952 with the accomplishments of Bailey and those of Gross[607,608]. Bailey devised the atrio-septopexy procedure while Gross introduced his remarkable well technique.

Bailey's concept of atrio-septopexy came to him from his observations at the autopsy of a patient who had a Lutembacher syndrome. The atrial septal defect was closed in this operation by suturing the peripheral portions of the right atrial wall to the edges of the defect. The sutures were placed under digital guidance alone. This was truly an extraordinary feat and reflective of his keenly honed surgical skills. He used the technique in 21 patients describing his results in a series of articles. His first attempt was in 1952 in a 38 year old female, and, encouraged by his success, he proceeded to do his best with the remaining 20 patients.

The approach pursued by Gross took advantage of the relatively low intra-atrial pressure. He sutured an open-ended, funnel-shaped atrial well to an excluded part of the right atrial wall. As soon as the excluding clamp was removed, blood rose in the well up to a level where its pressure was equal to that of the atrium. The surgeon now inserted his finger in the well of blood, located the defect by palpation and then closed the defect by suturing to the edges of the defect a plastic patch – a truly novel and physiologically sound approach, but demonstrating again the need for a highly skilled surgeon. Simpler methods had to be found because skilled surgeons of Gross' calibre were hard to come by. Despite his skill the first three patients died because the plastic double disk button he used as the patch worked its way loose. Gross then substituted a Nylon patch with considerably more success[609–611].

In 1966 Rashkind introduced balloon atrial septostomy as a palliative approach in complete transposition of the great arteries[612]. McNamara stated that this was one of the most important therapeutic procedures developed during the 20th century[613]. The Rashkind procedure not only provided a non-surgical means of creating an atrial septal defect in this anomaly but also made cardiologists more conscious of the circulatory changes in other anomalies in which there is either volume or pressure overload on the right or left atrium[613].

The procedure enabled infants so afflicted to reach an age and size so that definitive repairs could be made. Although not as widely used today, balloon septostomy played an important role in this regard.

As experience accumulated with the simpler lesions, when open heart surgery appeared on the scene, cardiac surgeons were now prepared to tackle the more complex ones. In addition, the age for surgical intervention was being steadily lowered.

One of the first surgeons to operate on children under the age of 5 was McMillan. In 1965, he reported his results in 14 children under that age who were subjected to total correction of the Tetralogy of Fallot[614]. He had only three deaths. Bypass and deep hypothermia were used. Ten years later surgeons were operating on infants during the first year of life.

Liverpool Hospital became one of the leading cardiac surgical centers in Great Britain. It reached that position of eminence under the leadership of Edwards and continued to remain esteemed under Hamilton, his successor. Waterston, Aberdeen and Stark developed their interest in repair of transposition of the great vessels at the Great Ormond Street Paediatric Hospital. Backed by an excellent staff, their open heart operations in the repair of this important malformation also gained for them a well-deserved world-wide reputation[584].

Other English leaders emerged such as Anderson and Allwork, Magdi Yacoub at Harefield Hospital, and Chris Lincoln at the Brompton Hospital. Anderson and Allwork contributed significant anatomical and embryological data. The others devised and introduced improved methods of perfusing the neonate, intensive care and surgical advances in the form of internal and external conduits with or without valves. Double outlet ventricles and persistent truncus arteriosus were now amenable to repair[584].

Myocardial revascularization

Evolution of the various surgical modalities for revascularizing the myocardium occurred in several stages. The first stage was actually devoted to symptomatic relief from the distress of angina rather than physiological alleviation of the cause of the pain. The remaining stages were truly physiological approaches that continued to be refined over the years with the aid of new surgical techniques and such parasurgical advances as cardiopulmonary bypass and cine coronary arteriography.

The first known proposal for surgery in coronary artery disease was the sympathectomy suggested by Francois-Franck in 1899 for the relief of pain in angina pectoris[615]. Twenty years elapsed before the suggestion was actually tried. In 1916, Jonnesco of Bucharest performed a bilateral extirpation of the cervical sympathetic chain and removal of the first dorsal ganglia bilaterally[616]. This historic event caught the attention of many surgeons so that in the short span of just 10 years, cardiac denervation with numerous variations became quite the thing to do for relief of angina. The claims and counter-claims of the procedure became so numerous and confusing that Elliott Cutler in 1927 complained of 'the tangled mess of operative procedures' which could not be subjected to a proper analysis regarding the efficacy of any one of the surgical interventions. Soon thereafter, the procedure fell into disrepute because it was definitely associated with a high mortality and with no relief from pain in at least 15 to 25% of the patients. Cardiac denervation was indeed bereft of any physiological soundness. Resection of the sensory sympathetics eliminated the pain but did not alter in any way the ischemia that was responsible for the pain. Thus, patients and physicians were lulled into a false sense of security as well as being deprived of an important signal.

Claude Beck of the Cleveland Clinic was well aware of the inadequacies of cardiac denervation, and concentrated instead on developing a method for either increasing or redistributing the blood supply to the myocardium. The idea of utilizing the pericardium came to him during the course of his numerous pericardial decortication procedures. Every time a band of pericardial adhesions was cut, brisk bleeding ensued from both ends of the transected adhesions. The adhesions were obviously well-supplied with blood and since many of the adhesions were embedded in the overlying epicardium, it seemed quite logical to conclude that the vascular supply of the adhesions was also nourishing the involved epicardium. It seemed like an excellent way of revascularizing the myocardium. Confirmation of the potentiality of this approach was already available in experimental circles through the work of Hudson, Moritz, Wearn and Orgain[617,618]. By simply injecting a suspension of carbon particles, they were able to demonstrate the

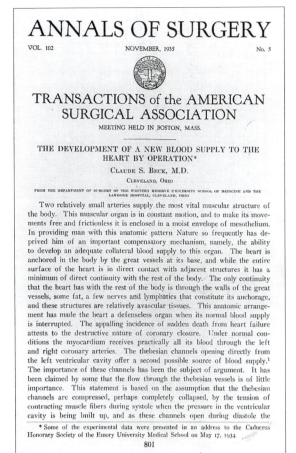

Figure 23 Reproduction of title and first page of Beck's paper on the development of a new blood supply to the heart by operation. *Photo Source National Library of Medicine. Literary Source Beck, C.S. (1935). The development of a new blood supply to the heart by operation. Ann. Surg., 102, 801. With permission*

existence of arterial anastomosis within the heart and surrounding tissues, and augmentation of such collateral channels through pericardial adhesions.

Beck tested his hypothesis in the animal laboratory by artificially creating an inflammation of the epicardium so that a network of vascular channels would be laid down as a byproduct of the inflammatory process. In 1935, Beck published his classic paper on 'The development of a new blood supply to the heart by operation'[619]. In it, he described his methodology in minute detail – how he opened the pericardium, removed the visceral layer, mechanically abraded the epicardium, then added bone dust to further irritate the epicardium, and finally grafted into place over the exposed epicardium a flap of the pectoralis muscle. Figure 23 is a reproduction of the title page from Beck's paper.

At about the same time, a young British surgeon, Laurence O'Shaughnessy was also impressed with the possibility of revascularizing the myocardium[620]. A good deal of animal experimentation was conducted by both O'Shaughnessy and Beck before they attempted the procedure on humans. O'Shaughnessy's untimely death at Dunkirk was a great loss for humanity[621].

The papers by Beck and O'Shaughnessy captured the imagination of many surgeons with each one advocating his own modification. A multitude of mechanical and chemical irritants were used. Among them were sand, asbestos, and Ivalon sponge as mechanical irritants. The chemical agents included irritant pastes, caulk, magnesium silicate and phenol. Some surgeons tried to create a new blood supply by suturing to the epicardial surface segments of small intestine, omentum, lungs, spleen or skin. O'Shaughnessy's experiments led him to conclude that the most promising approach was the use of omental pedicle grafts. It was brought up through an incision in the diaphragm. However, clinically he had only an occasional success in the face of a high mortality[622]. He termed his operation cardio-omentopexy. In order to stimulate more adhesions between the heart and omentum, O'Shaughnessy later used as an adjunct the insertion of aleuronat paste. Key introduced the use of the small intestine. Moran was responsible for introducing a tubed pedicle graft of skin while Lezius described the use of lung tissue calling it cardiopneumonopexy.

Beck's first patient was a 48 year old coal miner who was totally disabled because of severe coronary artery disease with intractable angina. The operation was performed on February 13, 1935. After roughening the epicardial surface, Beck grafted to this surface a pedicle of the left pectoral muscle. The patient recovered without complications and several months later, presumably after enough collateral circulation had been established, the patient was free of angina and able to work as a gardener. Beck, encouraged by this initial result, performed this procedure with various modifications on 15 other patients over the next two years. His results on this small series were reported in 1937[624]. The following year

O'Shaughnessy reported the results with his approach in 20 patients. All of his work was carried out at the Lambeth Cardiovascular Clinic in London before the outbreak of World War II with further work curtailed by his military service and unfortunate death[623].

Retrograde flow from the heart chambers via the Thebesian veins was another idea advanced for revascularizing the myocardium. It was based on Wearn's description in 1933 of the nature of the vascular communications between the coronary arteries and the chambers of the heart[625]. Two years later Gross and Blum described the results of some experiments in dogs[626], that had interesting implications. They showed that when the coronary sinus was occluded, not only was the blood supply to the myocardium increased, but at the same time there was exerted on the myocardium a protective effect against infarction when the feeding coronary arterial branch was ligated[626]. When Beck learned of this, he added subtotal ligation to his procedure. This was tried out at first in the laboratory and as soon as he was satisfied with the validity of the concept he implemented it on a clinical level. The modified approach became known as the Beck I operation[627,628].

Claude Beck's pioneering efforts in myocardial revascularization spanned more than three decades. He recapped the progress that had been made in this field in a paper he wrote in 1958[629]. The mortality in his hands as well as in those of O'Shaughnessy was very high. In addition, not all of their patients remained free of angina. Despite this, both men deserve a niche in the annals of cardiology since their innovative and aggressive efforts established the feasibility and potential benefits of myocardial revascularization.

Two Canadians were responsible for two other approaches in the continuing search for a satisfactory operation. One was the utilization of the internal mammary artery as a new source of blood supply. The other was a direct attack on the diseased coronary arteries via an endarterectomy.

Tunneling the internal mammary through the myocardium was introduced by Vineberg in 1946[630], but many years before him, it was tried experimentally and discarded by Gordon Murray[631]. The popularity of Vineberg's operation, as it came to be known, was stupendous. He, himself, reported in 1975 that more than 5000 such operations were performed between 1950 and 1970[632].

Notwithstanding its popularity, and the fact that angina was relieved in the majority of the patients, there was still considerable controversy regarding the alleged physiological improvement in blood supply. Using krypton-85 as a marker, Gorlin was able to demonstrate that the pattern of perfusion in the myocardium was the same whether the blood was supplied through the mammary implant or via normal coronary arteries. Furthermore, he pointed out that his studies with the Brigham implant series indicated that in the areas of successful mammary implantation, anaerobic metabolism did not occur. This was advanced by Gorlin as evidence that there was no ischemia in these areas since a non-ischemic myocardium has no need for anaerobic metabolism[633].

Sones subjected Vineberg's patient to cine coronary arteriography 8 years after implantation of his left internal mammary artery. Harken called this an historic event because it not only proved sustained patency of the donor vessel but also showed retrograde filling of the left anterior descending artery which was considered to be evidence of collateral circulation. Subsequent studies by Sones and later Gorlin indicated that patency persisted in more than 80% of the patients[634].

It would appear that such documentation had sufficient weight to validate the physiological soundness of the Vineberg operation. In retrospect, it obviously did not. There was still too much doubt concerning the adequacy of blood volume provided by the internal mammary implantation, and further events finally caused the abandonment of the procedure. I, myself, was appalled at the brutality of the operation. How the heart could withstand all the pummeling and manhandling was completely beyond my comprehension. But, contrary to the prevailing opinion of our medical forebears, the heart has an amazing capacity to withstand even the most monstrous of surgical assaults.

After Vineberg introduced his procedure in 1946 there were essentially no modifications until those of Smith and his associates in 1957[635]. This group used both Nylon tubes and free grafts of saphenous vein anastomosed end-to-side to the descending thoracic aorta. These were to act as conduits. Multiple holes were made in the distal portions before the conduits were placed in a myocardial tunnel. In that same year, Sabiston and co-workers utilized the carotid artery rather than the internal mammary artery[636]. This was purely an experimental study. His group

did document the development of anastomotic channels between the arterial graft and the coronary arteries, but these were rather small.

Throughout all this, Russia too had its innovator. He was Vasilii I. Kolesov, an outstanding cardiac surgeon from Leningrad (now St. Petersburg again with the recent demise of Soviet communism). Some authors credit him with being primarily responsible for laying the foundation of coronary vascularization with the internal mammary artery[637].

Kolesov performed his first sutured internal mammary artery-coronary artery anastomosis on February 25, 1964[638-644]. He used the mammary artery in the form of a pedicle, and for this reason it was referred to as Kolesov's pedicle. While performing the procedure on the second patient in his series, he detected beadlike nodules, and a dimpling of the epicardium over the diseased coronary arteries. This finding also acquired an eponym – Kolesov's groove[645]. It was thought to be indicative of underperfusion of the area as a result of the atherosclerotic lesion. Kolesov relied heavily on this sign during surgery as a means of localizing the diseased segments of the coronary artery. This was especially so during those earlier years when he did not have available the benefits and accuracy of pre-operative coronary arteriography[643,644].

Just 3 years after his first attempt, Kolesov introduced mechanical suturing of the mammary artery to the recipient coronary artery. He used a circular apparatus with bushings that allowed end-to-end anastomosis of vessels from 1.3 to 4.0 mm in diameter with an average time of 5 to 7 minutes. The device underwent several refinements in design over the next 20 years, but Kolesov was never completely satisfied with the final product though still believing in the concept.

As his experience with internal mammary artery grafting increased, Kolesov extended the indications for its use towards the treatment of acute myocardial infarction and unstable angina[644,646,647]. By 1976, Kolesov and his associates had performed coronary revascularization with internal mammary artery grafting in 132 patients. The majority of the operations were performed with the heart–lung machine in a standby position. The machine was used only in those who needed a hand suture anastomosis or who were hemodynamically unstable.

Olearchyk published a detailed overview of coronary revascularization in 1988, at which time he placed in perspective Kolesov's contributions on the subject[648]. In another paper, Olearchyk recounts how Kolesov's work was neither recognized nor appreciated in his own country for some time. This is what he had to say: 'However, the work of Kolesov was not recognized or appreciated even in his own country. Ironically, when Kolesov presented his results with IMA grafting during the plenum of the All-Union Cardiological Society in June of 1967 in Leningrad, the importance of his report was not understood or appreciated. That plenum accepted a resolution that the surgical treatment of coronary artery disease was impossible and without prospects for the future'[649].

Donald Effler, himself, acknowledged Kolesov's role as a pioneer in coronary revascularization. In a letter to the editor, Effler commented on how he was instrumental in 1967 in having Kolesov's paper on *Mammary artery-coronary artery anastomosis as method of treatment for angina pectoris* accepted by Brian Blades for publication in the *Journal of Thoracic and Cardiovascular Surgery*. Effler's comments are rather pertinent: At that time coronary arteriography (Sones' technique) was not available to Professor Kolesov; case selection had to be done on the basis of the electrocardiogram, conventional cardiologic evaluation, and direct inspection of the heart and vessels during the operation. Evaluation of the surviving patient relied entirely on basic vital signs and symptomatic changes. In a sense, Professor Kolesov was ahead of this time and could not prove to the critical observer that (1) the operation was indicated and (2) the surviving patient could attribute the alleged benefits to a patent anastomosis and direct revascularization. It seemed at the time that Professor Kolesov faced the same situation that had been presented to Claude Beck, Arthur Vineberg, and others who had made aggressive approaches to revascularization surgery by one method or another.[650] Gordon Murray was the other Canadian who was actively involved in searching for improved methods of myocardial revascularization. It seems that he may very well have been the first to operate directly on the coronary arteries. His attempts, begun in 1950, were restricted to experimental trials in the laboratory and consisted of resecting segments of the coronary arteries and bridging the gaps with vein grafts[651]. His paper, published in 1954, was essentially negative as to the feasibility of this approach. It should be noted, however, that cardiopulmonary bypass was not available as yet. In 1956, Bailey also tried his hand at endarterectomy without benefit of the heart–lung machine[652]. Longmire tried endarterectomy in 9 patients with only 5 survivors, but presumably the remainder improved[653]. He devised tiny curettes and performed the procedure with the aid of a binocular magnifying loop. Coagulation was said to be prevented by the instillation of heparin powder into the vessel. Other investigators used pericardial or venous patches over the site of the endarterectomy. These approaches did not gain any wide acceptance because of the associated high mortality. They were to be resurrected again with the advent of cardiopulmonary bypass, especially in the hands of Dudley Johnson of Milwaukee.

In 1939, Fieschi introduced the concept of internal mammary ligation[654]. It lay dormant until 1956 when DeMarchi and Battezzati revitalized it with their paper published in *Minerva Medica*[654]. They were in agreement with Fieschi in that by ligating both internal mammary arteries, blood was diverted to the pericardiophrenic branches. This was supposed to increase the circulation to the myocardium. Glover introduced the procedure to the USA just a year later, and for a while, it was accepted enthusiastically and with no regard to controlled evaluation[655]. Unfortunately, over the next decade thousands of patients were subjected to this procedure before its usefulness was disproved by controlled sham studies[656].

In the same paper wherein Murray commented so discouragingly on the usage of venous grafts as bridging conduits, he described on a more optimistic note another approach. He noted that the dog could be protected against a myocardial infarction when the left anterior descending artery was ligated if he had previously anastomosed an axillary artery to it just distal to the site of ligation[651]. This experimental fact alone demonstrated clearly the feasibility of a bypass procedure. Another important experimental attempt in the same direction was that described by Sauvage in 1963. He was able to successfully insert in dogs a jugular vein bypass between the aorta and coronary artery[657]. The feasibility of utilizing a saphenous vein bypass in a clinical situation was further demonstrated serendipitously by Edward Garrett[658]. He used it as a means of successfully weaning a patient from the heart–lung machine. He was in training at the time on DeBakey's service in Houston, Texas.

The time was ripe now for a truly physiological approach in the surgical management of coronary artery disease – the bypass procedure. Success in this approach was assured because of the availability of three important ingredients; two technical and one diagnostic. The technical factors had been provided through the efforts of all those engaged in the development of the heart-lung machine and Carrel's unique method of vessel anastomosis. The diagnostic ingredient was supplied by Mason Sones' breakthrough in coronary arteriography.

When Carrel refined the anastomosis of vessels in 1902 with his triangulation technique he made possible the technical skills required to graft arteries to veins. Figure 24 is a diagram showing how Carrel bridged the gap between the severed ends of an artery with a segment of a vein[659].

By substituting a segment of vein for a defect in an artery, Carrel showed that with his meticulous technique the vein was a suitable nonclotting conduit of the blood. The vein gradually thickened to withstand the greater arterial pressure. The coronary arteriographic technique developed by Sones made for precison in anatomical location of the obstructive lesions, the severity and extent of these lesions and the number of coronary arterial branches involved. What more could a surgeon ask for? He was given pre-operatively a detailed map of what to expect. Effler was quick to emphasize the importance of Sones' technique: 'It pried the lid open of a veritable treasure chest and brought forth the present era of revascularization surgery'[660]. The Cleveland Clinic was fortunate in having Sones at the time. He not only lent his technical ability: he was one of the prime movers in the development of bypass surgery at the clinic, offering encouragement as well during the formative years of the program.

Sabiston in 1962 was the first to use the autogenous saphenous vein as a coronary artery bypass graft[661]. He did this without cardiopulmonary bypass. The patient had a stroke shortly after surgery and died. The autopsy finding was significant in that it revealed a thrombus at the proximal end of the anastomosis. The stroke was no doubt due to an embolus from this clot.

At this time Effler and Groves were doing endarterectomies and patch grafting. By 1967, Effler had performed 71 endarterectomies[662,663]. These patients were selected from a total of 6000 patients that had undergone coronary arteriogra-

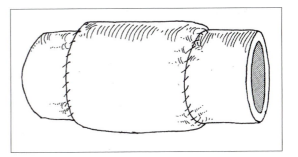

Figure 24 Diagram illustrating the bridging of a gap between the severed ends of an artery with a segment of vein. *Photo Source University of Central Florida*

phy in close collaboration with Sones. Consonant with Effler's example, the Houston group was also doing endarterectomies during the early 1960s. They had planned to do one on a 42 year old man in 1964[664]; the same year that Effler had presented his results on 4 patients before the American Association for Thoracic Surgery. The group consisted of Garrett, Dennis and DeBakey. At surgery, they found the culprit lesion was so badly diseased that an endarterectomy was impossible. At that moment, a segment of saphenous vein was used as a bypass conduit between the aorta and left anterior descending artery, just distal to the diseased portion. The patient survived and 7 years later the graft was found to be still patent at coronary angiography while the previously diseased portion of the left anterior descending artery was now completely occluded.

It was May, 1967 when René Favaloro performed his first coronary artery operation. He used a saphenous vein autograft to replace a stenotically excised segment of the right coronary artery[665]. It was in the latter part of the year that he began to use the saphenous vein as a bypassing channel. In his subsequent early attempts he limited the bypassing to the right coronary artery.

In a special article written for the *International Journal of Cardiology* many years later he reminisced about his initiation and subsequent experience in coronary revascularization. The following are a few excerpts from this fascinating historical survey[666].

I was lucky enough to arrive at the Cleveland Clinic in February, 1962 shortly after two significant landmarks had occurred. On 5 January, Effler and associates were able to repair a severe obstruction at the left main trunk coronary level by the patch graft technique following Senning's idea and, on 12 January, Sones demonstrated, by direct injection of the left mammary artery in a patient operated by Vineberg in 1946, that myocardial perfusion deficit can benefit from collateral circulation originating in a systemic artery implanted in a small tunnel parallel to the anterior descending coronary artery. This was further corroborated in March 1962 in another patient operated on previously by Bigelow. Since the beginning, I was attracted by a unique collection of hundreds of beautiful cine coronary angiograms properly kept in the basement where Sones and associates performed daily studies with advanced equipment only available at the Cleveland Clinic. B10 – the name of Sones' Department at that time – was the place where I spent my free time, once my duties at the Department of Thoracic and Cardiovascular Surgery were over. Living in a small and old apartment only across the street allowed me to be there in a silent and peaceful atmosphere for many hours, while most members of the staff were on their way back home through difficult roads covered with snow during the bitter winter time of the Ohio Great Lakes' area. In May, 1967 I performed the first operation on a 51-year-old lady. With a segment of saphenous vein the proximal and totally occluded right coronary artery was connected to its distal segment. A repeat cine coronary angiogram demonstrated an excellent reconstruction a few days later. I will always remember the time when they called me from the Cardiac Laboratory, and I saw an extremely happy Sones showing all his joy, talking and laughing while the film was running in the Tage-Arno. He left for Europe a few days later carrying a 16-mm movie with the pre- and postoperative study of the first interposed saphenous vein graft. Very early in our experience, we realized the limitation of the technique mainly when dealing with very proximal obstructions. As a consequence, bypasses from the anterolateral wall of the aorta were performed using the same approach frequently utilized in renal artery reconstruction at our institution. Our presentation read at the Fifth Annual Meeting of the American Association for Thoracic Surgery in April 1970 discussed the application of the

bypass technique to the left coronary artery and its divisions. It was gratifying to see how coronary bypass surgery was spreading. Eleven colleagues from different centers participated in the discussion of our presentation. This paper would be incomplete without two final remarks. First, I want to express my everlasting gratitude to Donald B. Effler who always gave me freedom to work. Second, this modern era of revascularization surgery has been made possible only through the introduction of cine coronary angiography by Mason Sones in 1958 which allowed us to:

(1) understand the proper anatomy of the coronary artery tree of ischemic heart disease and its implications with the state of the heart muscle;

(2) clarify the natural history of coronary arteriosclerosis and the correlation with the clinical spectrum;

(3) select the candidates for the revascularization procedure and contribute to organize and simplify the operation;

(4) give us objective postoperative evaluation of the different operative techniques employed. All of us should be grateful and recognize him as the true father of coronary bypass surgery. I will always thank God for having given me the opportunity to share with Mason Sones many years of common work, understanding and deep friendship.

The pioneering efforts of Favaloro were adopted immediately by Dudley Johnson, and in a short time, his fame and experience were as solidly established as those of Favaloro. In fact, it was he who extended the procedure to the left coronary system and blazed the trail for multiple bypasses[667].

There was now a return to the usage of the internal mammary artery but in a different fashion. In February, 1968, Bailey demonstrated that an excellent result was obtained when he did a right internal mammary–distal right coronary artery bypass with cross-clamping of the coronary artery during the anastomosis[668]. During the same month, Green and his team at New York University were successful in anastomosing the left internal mammary artery to the left anterior descending artery. This was the first time this was successfully performed in the USA[669]. The heart–lung machine was used. Nine patients underwent the procedure in their initial series. Three patients died, all within 30 days, and at postmortem, the cause of death was attributed to myocardial infarction. The significant anatomical detail that emerged from the necropsy was that in each case the infarction occurred in those segments of the myocardium that were not perfused by the mammary graft bypass. This detail caused Green to modify his approach by adding multiple saphenous vein grafts[670]. His three year experience with this modification was quite encouraging.

Other surgeons soon realized the advantages of double internal mammary artery grafting with or without simultaneous saphenous vein bypass in contrast to saphenous bypass alone[671–673]. In several years it became the procedure of choice. Today, coronary artery bypass graft surgery is probably the most common operation performed. Indeed, there are now emerging attempts at restricting its use on the part of third-party payers because of their perception that the surgery is being overly performed without regard to sound medical indications.

CARDIAC TRANSPLANT AND ARTIFICIAL HEART

The idea of replacing an irreversibly damaged heart is intriguing both in concept and in its implementation. It is the one last hope for those poor unfortunates in the terminal phase of their cardiac disability. Contrary to popular belief, the concept of maintaining life through artificial means was not the brain-child of the 20th century. Although it is purely speculative on my part, I would not be at all surprised if some future historian found a reference to it in one of the yet undiscovered comments by that quintessential conceptualist of all time, Leonardo da Vinci. In a non-speculative vein, the concept of an artificial heart forms the basis of a short story written in 1882 by Ronald Ross[674]. He was a young British medical officer at the time who wrote this weird tale while serving in India. The novelette is entitled *The Vivisector Vivisected*. Ross was no scatterbrained conjurer of fairy tales. He won the Nobel Prize many years later for discovering the mosquitoes that transmitted malaria. He apparently had an active interest in the classics and spent a considerable amount of time writing poems, plays and novels[675]. The story is about a man who after bleeding to death was revived by an artificial heart. Despite the wierdness, an excerpt from this imaginative tale underscores the foresight of Ronald Ross.

At last on the morning of October 5, 1840, a patient was brought into the Infirmary with a cut wound on the head from which he had bled profusely. [H]e had been cut with a knife in a street row. He was a tall, vigorous man, with an immense amount of red hair and beard and with a vicious leering kind of expression. When I saw him he was fast sinking; for the evident drunken habits of the patient did not predispose him to recovery. I only saw him and attended him (except the nurses); and I had him removed to a private ward when he died at 2:00 PM. I having previously acquainted Maculligan of the case, waited below while the gentleman was preparing the apparatus. I sent the nurses out of the ward after the patient's death. I wrapt him in a blanket and drawing his hands over my shoulders carried him out. A violent storm, which had just broken gave me greater security. I locked the door of the private ward and struggled as I best could with my burden up the narrow stairs of the turret. When I arrived in the laboratory, the apparatus was ready, and the pumps were standing in their baths of hot-water (which was procured from the stove boiler). The donkey had been killed and his fresh blood was in the cavities of our machine. Maculligan was flushed with excitement; 'Now' he exclaimed, 'We shall get at least some knowledge; either a useful negative result, or a world-reforming fact.'

I placed the body on the bed; on his left side was the pump which I was to work and which sent the blood all over his body; on his right side Maculligan supplied his lungs. In a minute I had fastened the limbs, and made bare the chest of the man. Maculligan seized the knife, and at one swoop cut down to the heart. I held apart the severed parts. Almost immediately it seemed he had inserted the tubes into the arteries and veins, and a few seconds sufficed to sew up the chest again, joining the cartilages as well as the skin, and covering all the incision with a quickly congealing gum to exclude the air, and permit breathing. The whole was done by ten minutes after death. The corpse was pale, slightly cold, the eyelids half open, and the eyes turned upwards beneath them. Blankets were thrown upon it to retain the heat.

The storm outside had increased in fury: the rain drenched the window-panes, and the violence of the wind was such that the whole tower seemed to rock sensibly. Most unearthly noises, too, were caused by it; and the darkness was so great that we could barely see to do our experiment. I could observe Maculligan trembling with excitement. I myself though generally stolid was much moved. 'Are you ready', said he, taking hold of his pump and speaking hoarsely, 'Then away', and down went the pistons simultaneously. We told twelve strokes – no blood had oozed from the cut in the chest – all was satisfactory. Another twelve – a slight flushing [of] the cheeks. Maculligan stopped, and we both took off our coats, the wind howling with tenfold fury. We resumed – suddenly the eyes closed. We went on for fully a quarter of an hour. 'He is breathing!' cried my companion. Most certainly there was some slight action of the diaphragm. Maculligan suddenly motioned me to stop, and going up to the patient listened to hear the breathing. While he looked into the man's face the eyes suddenly opened, following my friend, who sprang back to his pump, trembling violently. We went on silently; the man, all the while, watching Maculligan whose hair seemed stiff, and whose face was so changed that I should hardly have known him. I myself was so astounded, that I could not conceive the occurrence as real. We had never expected that there would be any recovery beyond a comatose condition. Suddenly the man, who appeared as if recovering from chloroform, said aloud, 'Lave it, will you'.

'Lave what?' asked Maculligan hoarsely.

'Lave pulling that out of the ground, for sure it goes bang through the wurrld, and is clamped on the other side. Its o' no use'.

'Bedad!' he continued 'but ye're the rummiest egg-flip iver I came across'.

'Egg-flip! eh? boy?', cried Maculligan, laughing excitedly; 'You're another'.

'What!' said the man, smiling with one side of his mouth, 'you air a wag, you air a kind o' wag as tells loodicrus tales to tay-totallers at taymatins, you air'.

The original manuscript is conserved in the Library of the Royal College of Physicians and Surgeons of Glasgow. It is written in brown ink on folded sheets of rice paper[676].

The actual transition from fancy to fact did not take place until 1958. At that time Akutsu and Kolff reported their results with replacement of the heart in an animal with a mechanical device[677]. The feasibility of the method was amply demonstrated even though the animal survived for only 90 minutes. Many others since then focused their efforts on the use of an artificial heart. Among them were Kusserow, Hastings, Cooley and De Bakey, and De Vries[678–681]. They had to contend with many technical problems such as thrombosis, size of the prosthesis, and methods of powering the device.

The first left ventricular assist device to be used in a human was implanted at Baylor College of Medicine in 1963. It was called a left ventricular bypass pump. This pump was donated to the Smithsonian Institution and is now on permanent display there[682]. In April, 1969 Cooley and his group achieved another 'first' when they implanted an artificial heart in a 47 year old man[681]. The insertion of the device was intended as a stop-gap procedure until a human heart could be found for transplantation. The patient survived for 65 hours. Cooley was severely criticized for attempting to do this without previous adequate trials in experimental animals[683]. Cooley waited 12 years before he tried again. This time he was able to maintain the patient on artificial support for 54 hours before subjecting him to an orthotopic transplantation with a human heart. Although the patient died 8 days later, the point was made that an artificial heart could prove to be useful as part of a 2-stage procedure in cardiac transplantation[684].

The first attempt at permanent replacement of the heart with a mechanical prosthesis was the widely publicized one by De Vries and his group in 1982. The patient, Barney Clark, was a retired dentist. The media were enthralled with this 'space-age' approach and described in detail on a daily basis the entire clinical scenario from installation to early demise. Undaunted, De Vries installed shortly after, the mechanical prosthesis designed by Jarvik in another cardiac cripple by the name of Schroeder. This too received in-depth attention from the lay press. The patient managed to survive for several weeks after the installation, tethered constantly to a monstrously sized power unit. He too succumbed to the diverse complications associated with the prosthesis. Humana, an HMO type of medical provider underwrote the entire project. It was another grandstand spectacle under the guise of altruism but, in reality, a means of advertising Humana as a 'caring' purveyor of medical needs.

Concomitant with the preceding steps in total replacement, research continued in the hope of finding mechanical measures to support a failing heart. The surgical team at Kings County Hospital in Brooklyn, NY was probably the first to be clinically successful in supporting a failing heart with mechanical measures[685]. This was in 1957. The patient was still alive and actively running his store 12 years later.

Clauss and his associates in 1961 introduced the concept of counterpulsation[686]. They were part of Harken's group. The technique removed the blood from the arterial circulation during ventricular systole and returned it during diastole. Moulopoulos, Topaz and Kolff introduced the intra-aortic balloon pump as another method of counterpulsation[687]. It proved to be quite effective in the management of cardiogenic shock as demonstrated initially by Schilt and Kantrowitz[688].

Currently, all of these mechanical devices, whether oriented towards supporting a failing heart or as a total replacement (permanently or otherwise) have yet to reach a level of refinement that would be universally acceptable. The technical problems and associated complications still defy solution. Cardiac transplantation, on the other hand, evolved in a more satisfactory manner despite what seemed to be the almost insurmountable problem of rejection.

The first surgeons of the 20th century to conduct experiments in heart transplantation were Carrel and Guthrie. They began their investigations in 1905 with Carrel reporting further observations in 1907[689,690]. A rat was used in the initial experiments, and in the later ones, the donor heart was grafted to the neck vessels of the recipient dog. Similar experiments were carried out by Mann and Yaterin 1933[691]. In the 1940s, Demikhov succeeded in developing a technique whereby he could carry out cardiopulmonary transplantation without the use of artificial means of recipient support during the procedure. Demikhov's interest in transplantation embraced many types of organs but his most notable efforts centered on the heart and heart–lung transplants[692–698]. After experimenting with many different methods of providing a dog with an accessory heart, he attempted to carry out orthotopic transplantation of the heart[699]. He was successful only twice in 22 attempts with the transplanted heart functioning for only several hours.

While Demikhov was carrying on with his work, other men were studying the effects of transplantation. Almost to a man, they were using the neck as the transplant site. Sinitsyn, a co-national of Demikhov, concerned himself with homotransplantation of the frog's heart. He was interested in obtaining physiologic data from this procedure[700–702].

In the late 1950s, several centers were actively involved in orthotopic transplantation of the heart. The pioneers in the field were Goldberg, Berman and Akman[703], Webb, Howard and Neely, and Cass and Brock[704]. None of them was successful in terms of prolonged survival.

In 1964 Hardy carried out the first cardiac transplant in a human with a xenograft. The donor heart was from a chimpanzee[705]. Although it ended in failure, it did not prevent others from using the same approach. As a matter of fact, in the late 1980s, the Loma Linda University group transplanted a baboon's heart in an infant, also without success.

Throughout this multiple experimental activity, the rejection phenomenon remained paramount as the major impediment to success. The attempts at resolution of this problem were intensified as a result of the increasing desire on the part of clinicians to transplant kidneys in end-stage kidney disease. The answer, however, came from a totally unrelated source, and from a man who had absolutely no interest initially in the failures of either renal or heart transplants. He was P. B. Medawar. We are indebted to him for providing the key to successful transplantation. He was the first to develop the immunological concepts as applied to transplantation.

Medawar's first paper published in 1944 described his classic experiments with skin transplants in rabbits; a project begun at the behest of the British government[706]. During World War II, the British authorities established a research program aimed at finding new methods of skin coverage for children extensively burned by the bombings of the Battle of Britain in 1939. Medawar spearheaded these efforts. He determined that the skin transplant from another rabbit developed a cellular infiltrate which in 7–10 days destroyed the transplant. He coined the word 'rejection' for this process. In this and a subsequent paper published in 1961, Medawar formulated a number of fundamental concepts that explained further the entire process of rejection[707].

Armed with this knowledge, investigators now set to work to find immunosuppressive modalities.

However, it was not until 1962 that any headway was made, though very modestly. Just two years before, Lower and Shumway made the first significant breakthrough in the technical aspects of cardiac transplantation. They reported the first successful canine orthotopic cardiac transplants[708]. The three important elements of their technique were cardiopulmonary bypass, mid-atrial excision and grafting of the heart with topical hypothermic myocardial preservation. The technique was so well thought out that it served as a model for further investigative procedures. But further advances could not be made until they could overcome the rejection process.

The corticosteroids had been available to clinicians since the 1940s but their immuno-suppressive capability had yet to be exploited. When Murray and Merrill reported their successful 'kidney transplantation in modified recipients' they used steroids as the modifying agent. The success rate of renal transplantation was increased with this therapeutic approach, but it was a moderate one and accompanied by its own bag of complications. Imuran was known to possess immunosuppressive properties but it was still an investigational drug at the time.

This is the way matters stood when in December 1967 Christian Barnard (who had been a trainee with Shumway at the University of Minnesota) upstaged Shumway and other investigators with the first clinical human heart transplant[709]. The world was electrified. At last, total replacement was a reality. Contrary to the general enthusiasm generated by Barnard's announcement, I reacted with dismay and disdain for what I perceived as a grandstand display without regard for scientific discipline and human life. The patient died from acute rejection only 18 days after surgery. This, in itself, should have caused Barnard to take inventory of the facts. Instead, carried away by the wave of enthusiasm that swept the world (mainly due to the sensationalism of the press) Barnard tried again with the patient dying about 18 months later from severe atheroma of the coronary vessels in the newly transplanted heart. This was another complication that had not been anticipated.

Centers around the world blindly followed suit with predictably tragic results; ethically as well as scientifically. In Britain, only the National Heart Hospital followed Barnard's trail. The surgical team was led by Donald Ross and Donald Longmore.

Three patients underwent transplantation by Ross. All died with the longest survivor lasting 43 days.

As disillusionment set in, a more sober orientation took place and cardiac transplantation was no longer the bright hope that it had seemed to be. Meanwhile in the solitude of his laboratory at Stanford, Shumway continued to plod away with carefully thought out experimentation and trials. Gradually, the results improved in terms of rejection, complications and survival. The introduction of cyclosporine in 1980 as an immunosuppressive agent set the stage for renewed interest in cardiac transplantation. Gradually, the Stanford group began to acquire an extensive clinical experience and slowly but surely cardiac transplantation began to re-emerge as a viable procedure. Many factors were brought into play to account for its acceptance today as a standard therapeutic modality. They include not only Shumway's highly disciplined approach that combined technical refinements with a rational and intensive immunosuppressive protocol but also the development of distant heart procurement programs and the new knowledge brought to light as a result of Medawar's concepts of acquired immune tolerance. The current immunosuppressive protocol at Stanford University consists of cyclosporine, azathioprine, equine anti-thymocyte globulin and steroids. Shumway's group also introduced endomyocardial biopsy as the only sure method for diagnosing rejection in the cyclosporine group.

The ethics behind cardiac transplantation was also a factor that had to be dealt with in a forthright manner. The Nuremberg trials with its lurid tales of human experimentation was still fresh in the minds of the public when cardiac transplantation first exploded on the world. Obviously, advances in medicine could never have occurred without imaginative and innovative approaches. But was there really a need for such drastic surgery? In 1865, Claude Bernard wrote: 'It is our duty and our right to perform an experiment on man whenever it can save his life, cure him or give him some personal benefit[710]. Perhaps in his defense, this is what may have motivated Barnard in his first attempt. He did state in his reflections that he had spent considerable time before the operation in studying in depth the various aspects of rejection and felt confident that the immunosuppressive agents available at that time were adequate defensive measures[711]. I will not belabor the point. The record speaks for itself.

At any rate, the particular issues regarding the ethical aspects of human experimentation were addressed by the Helsinki declaration of the World Medical Association in 1965. The statements have a unique relevance with respect to cardiac transplantation or the usage of the artificial heart. They are:

(1) In the treatment of the sick person, the doctor must be free to use a new diagnostic and therapeutic measure, if in his or her judgement, it offers hope of saving life, reestablishing health or alleviating suffering;

(2) the potential benefits, hazards and discomfort of a new method should be weighed against the advantages of the best current diagnostic and therapeutic methods.[712]

De Vries and his group won the praise of all when they adhered to these statements prior to selecting patients for their untried artificial heart. In fact, their initial application was filed almost 2½ years before they performed the implantation in December, 1982[713]. The delay was caused by the need to examine the many ethical issues raised by the contemplated procedure to ensure that the patient was adequately informed and that all rights of the patient were protected.

More than nine decades have elapsed since Carrel's early attempts. Current survival is in excess of 80% with the majority of these survivors enjoying a life of good quality. All of the breakthroughs described in the evolution of cardiac transplantation form a part of Harken's fourth epoch; that of valvular or complete heart replacement. We have already seen the remarkable progress made with valve replacement but what the future will bring in total replacement is difficult to ascertain at this writing. Many technical and biological problems still exist, but are they insurmountable? Will the final answer be a mechanical or a biological heart, either human or animal? By this time the reader should have realized that with the evolution of cardiology as a scientific discipline, as each question was answered a new one was created.

INTERVENTIONAL TECHNIQUES

For more than three decades, cardiac catheterization served only as a diagnostic modality. A change in this orientation occurred in the early 1980s when it became obvious to some of the more imaginative cardiologists that cardiac catheterization had the potential of serving in a therapeutic role as well. We were merely reverting to Forsmann's original motive for suggesting cardiac catheterization as a clinical tool. A new word was coined to identify this approach. It was 'interventional' and signified any treatment that was based on cardiac catheterization. In due course this new breed of cardiologist became quite facile in delivering mechanical, pharmacological, thermal, microsurgical, or light energy modalities in the treatment of cardiovascular disease. Lysis of blood clots, dilatation of stenotic blood vessels or cardiac valves became part of the therapeutic armamentarium. As invasive electrophysiologic studies evolved, arrhythmias, in turn, came under attack through electro-invasive means.

Dotter and Judkins were the first to realize that the lumen of a peripheral blood vessel could be enlarged by first passing a guidewire and then a catheter or rigid dilator through the stenotic area. They described this new technique in 1964 for relieving stenosis of the ileofemoral arteries[714–716]. It was adopted by the European community in a limited manner, and for at least a decade after its introduction, the Dotter technique, as it became known, did not gain general acceptance primarily because of the local complications that were so frequently associated with its use. The main difficulty was the trauma caused by introducing rather large caliber rigid dilators[717].

The breakthrough came in 1974 when Gruentzig and Kumpe substituted a balloon-tipped catheter for the rigid dilator[718]. Initially, the Gruentzig technique was applied to obstructive lesions involving the peripheral arteries. It was called percutaneous transluminal angioplasty[718]. Very shortly thereafter, renal artery stenosis became another indication for its use[719]. It was not until 1977 that attempts were made to widen the stenotic areas of the epicardial coronary arteries[720]. In no time at all, percutaneous transluminal coronary angioplasty became established as a valid method for treating coronary arterial obstruction. Gruentzig had devised his own special type of catheter to do this. It had two lumens. One was devoted to monitoring or to the injection of radiopaque material for visualization of the coronary tree. The other lumen served as a means of inflating or deflating the balloon. A small flexible guidewire attached to the tip of the catheter served as the steering mechanism. The concept was brilliant in its simplicity. The catheter could be guided to the stenotic area with the balloon in a deflated state and when in place inflated to a predetermined size. Gruentzig's modification gained for him a well-deserved niche among the 'giants' of cardiology.

Andreas Gruentzig was characterized by J. Willis Hurst as a free-spirited genius. His untimely death in a plane crash in 1985 robbed the world of a man whose full potentiality was as yet untapped. His wife died with him when the plane he was piloting crashed while returning to Emory University Hospital during a bad storm.

Hurst described him as a 'multifaceted personality, tall and lean, confident but not arrogant, tough and yet thoughtful of others, elegant, charismatic and fearless'[721]. A memorial fund was created in his honor to finance the Andreas Grüntzig Cardiovascular Center at Emory University. It was hoped that this center would continue to find 'new directions in cardiovascular disease', a phrase that Gruentzig used to describe research.

The Gruentzig technique took the cardiological community by storm. In a few short years, a variety of technical improvements coupled with an increasing number of experienced operators assured the establishment of this procedure as a valid therapeutic measure. Indications for its use were expanded to include not only relief of ischemia from stenosed coronary arteries[722,723], but also for the management of unstable angina[724–726], acute myocardial infarction[727–729], recurrent angina after bypass surgery due to obstruction of a bypass graft[730–732], those in whom bypass surgery poses too great a risk, and also in stenosis of the peripheral vessels. The last represented a return to Dotter's original indication with the rigid dilator.

Beginning in 1982, pediatric cardiologists began using balloon dilatation to split the commissures for relief of pulmonary valve stenosis[733–735]. This eventually replaced open surgical repair of this lesion because of its relative freedom from complications and high success rate. Aortic stenosis was also helped with this technique[735,736]. In 1985, Lock and his group described its use in mitral stenosis approaching the valve from the right atrium through a transseptal puncture[737]. The results were so encouraging that soon after, several centers tried their hand at it with rather promising results though

with severe restrictions as to patient selection[738–741]. The procedure was aptly called balloon valvuloplasty, and, as of this writing, appeared to be gaining even wider acceptance[742–744].

Rashkind was instrumental in utilizing the balloon catheter for the creation of a functional atrial septal defect in such conditions as transposition of the great arteries, atresia of the pulmonic, mitral and tricuspid valves and in single ventricles[745]. Park and co-workers modified Rashkind's technique by attaching a surgical blade to the catheter[746]. They created the atrial septal defect by first passing the catheter from the right atrium to the left atrium via a transseptal puncture, and then incising the septum during withdrawal. Laser ablation for creating an atrial septal defect was reported by Bommer and colleagues in 1983[747]. On the opposite side of the coin, an innovative interventional technique for closing an atrial septal defect or a patent ductus arteriosus was the one introduced by Rashkind in 1983. It involved the use of a 'double-disk' prosthesis[745]. Lock and his colleagues described the transcatheter 'umbrella closure' in congenital defects in 1987[748].

Balloon angioplasty paved the way for the introduction of other techniques in the management of obstructive lesions whether in the coronary or peripheral vessels. Although heralded as an approach with great promise, their potentialities have not been fully realized as yet; and further investigation is necessary before their true level of efficacy can be appraised[749–754]. One approach was atherectomy. An example of this was the 'cut and retrieve' system devised by Simpson[755,756]. Miniature drills and rotating wires are other examples of these cutting techniques that are still under investigation. Permanent vascular stents were introduced in 1987 as a means of preventing recurrent stenosis after balloon angioplasty[757]. Their final place in this ever expanding interventional armamentarium has not been stabilized as yet.

One of the most exciting advances during the 20th century was the introduction of thrombolysis as a means of reperfusing the heart in the face of an acute thrombotic occlusion of a major coronary artery. The history of thrombolysis itself dates back to 1933. After a short burst of enthusiasm, it was consigned to obscurity, all but forgotten, only to be revived again in 1958[758]. Despite the revival there was relatively little progress or acceptance of this modality in the immediate management of acute myocardial infarction until angiography provided visual proof that a clot indeed was a major cause of the infarction, and that lysis of this clot could be effected with beneficial results to the myocardium.

The story of thrombolysis begins in 1933 when Tillett and Garner discovered that Lancefield Group A beta-hemolytic streptococci isolated from patients produced a fibrinolytic substance[759]. They called it streptococcal fibrinolysin. Milstone pointed out 8 years later that streptococci-mediated fibrinolysis needed a lysing factor found in plasma, and which, for lack of a better name, he dubbed 'plasma lysing factor'[760]. The entire mechanism of streptococcal fibrinolysis was worked out in 1945 by L. Royal Christensen, a microbiologist[761,762]. He showed that this type of fibrinolysis was the result of a proteolytic enzyme system that consisted of a cascade of events stemming from a proteolytic precursor which he called plasminogen, and which was activated by the streptococcal fibrinolysin which he called streptokinase. Both names are still in current usage. Thus, under the influence of streptokinase (the activator) plasminogen is converted to plasmin which is capable of lysing protein, fibrin and its precursor, fibrinogen. The cascade is prevented from running amuck by the presence of inhibitors in plasma.

It was not until 1947, however, that Tillett was given a crudely purified preparation of streptokinase by Christensen for both animal and human trials[763]. Since he was not a clinician, he asked Sol Sherry to direct the clinical studies. A team of 5 men now constituted the research group with Tillett supervising the animal studies. Even at that time the ultimate purpose of the trials was to determine its efficacy in the treatment of acute coronary thrombosis.

By 1952, Johnson and Tillett were able to lyse experimental thrombi in rabbit ear veins with intravenously administered streptokinase[764]. A year later Daniel Kline succeeded in obtaining purified human plasmin[765].

According to Sherry, the late 1950s was the most productive period in the development of thrombolytic therapy[766]. Anthony Fletcher and his wife joined Sherry during this exciting period to help delineate the best clinical approach with this modality. They soon determined that plasminogen activators were superior to plasmin in initiating and perpetuating the fibrinolytic process[766–769].

Tillett's crudely purified streptokinase was replaced by a more highly purified preparation developed by Lederle Laboratories. The first experimental study with this purified batch was reported by Sherry and Fletcher in 1958[770]. There was no angiographic control in this pilot study but the results were very encouraging in terms of in-hospital mortality. Sherry recounted how his center now became the mecca for thrombosis, attracting eager fellows from far and wide[758]. Many of these fellows in due time set up their own investigative centers and training programs as well. In 1964, one of them, Fedor Bachmann, while still working in Sherry's laboratory, was responsible for the first major purification of a tissue plasminogen activator from pig heart[758]. Abbott Laboratories and Sterling-Winthrop also joined Sherry's group in a cooperative effort regarding the role of urokinase[771]. Macfarlane and Pilling had isolated urokinase from human urine[772]. Later studies demonstrated that it was also a plasminogen activator. It took a long time to produce sufficient quantities of urokinase for clinical trials. Sophisticated methods of refinement were needed before large-scale production could be effected.

Many clinical trials of both urokinase and streptokinase were conducted between 1963 and 1979 throughout Europe and America. Many of the results were inconclusive because of faulty study designs. More importantly, failure to create acceptance of this mode of treatment in acute myocardial infarction was due mainly to a mistaken notion prevalent during this span of time. Many cardiologists had forgotten the findings of the pathologists during the 1930s with respect to the relationship between coronary thrombosis and myocardial infarction.

The role of thrombosis in acute myocardial infarction became firmly established only when angiographic evidence began to appear in the 1980s. Contrast visualization of the coronary arteries was not even considered safe in acute myocardial infarction until DeWood showed otherwise in 1980[773]. His breakthrough encouraged others to perform such studies during the acute phase of myocardial infarction. These, when performed during the first several hours of an acute transmural infarction, repeatedly revealed that in the vast majority of cases thrombotic occlusion was the final common pathway for the event with the atherosclerotic process being the predisposing ingredient[774–778]. Other investigators also demonstrated that when the infarction did not involve the entire wall, there was a wide variability in the frequency of thrombosis as determined by angiographic means[779–781].

DeWood's demonstration of the safety of angiography during the early phase of myocardial infarction plus the validation with this technique that a thrombotic process was responsible for the sequence of events became the prime movers in the reactivation of interest in thrombolytic therapy. The modern era of thrombolytic therapy thus began with him.

Rentrop and his group demonstrated that infusion of streptokinase directly at the site of the coronary thrombus resulted in recanalization in most cases[782]. He was not, however, the first to use the intracoronary route. It had already been tried by Boucek and Murphy in 1960, but they had no angiographic proof of the results whereas Rentrop did. A team from Israel headed by E.L. Chazov also administered fibrinolysin in acute myocardial infarction via the intracoronary route. This was in 1979. Two years later Gans and his associates described their experience with intracoronary thrombolysis in evolving myocardial infarction[783]. That same year Markis and Braunwald delineated the degree of myocardial salvage with the same technique[784]. Schroeder, in 1983, reintroduced the intravenous route utilizing a high dose of streptokinase over a short period of time[785].

Systemic lytic reactions were of some concern as more experience with this renascent modality accumulated. This reaction assumed a considerable degree of importance since logistics and lack of adequate numbers of trained personnel mandated an intravenous route of administration rather than one requiring cardiac catheterization. A quest was on for the development of clot-specific antithrombolytic agents with little or no systemic lytic action. Close cooperation between clinicians, geneticists and the pharmaceutical industry forged the way with rt-PA (tissue plasminogen activator) as an example of this collaborative effort[779]. The end is by no means in sight. The search for the ideal thrombolytic agent is still in progress[786,787].

REFERENCES

1. Johnson, S.L. (1970). *The History of Cardiac Surgery, 1896–1955*, p. X. (introduction by Vincent L. Gott). (Baltimore: Johns Hopkins Press)

2. Merendino, A. (1970). In Johnson, S.L. *Op. cit.*, p. XI. (introduction by Vincent L. Gott)

3. Harken, D.W. (1967). Heart surgery – legend and a long look. *Am. J. Cardiol.*, **19**, 393–401

4. Leake, C.D. (1962). The historical development of cardiovascular physiology. In Hamilton, W.F. and Dow, P. (eds.) *Handbook of Physiology, Circulation*, sect. 2, vol. I. (Washington: Am. Physiol. Soc.)

5. Gollan, F. (1959). *Physiology of Cardiac Surgery*, p. v. (Springfield, Ill.: Charles C Thomas)

6. Galletti, P.M. and Brecher, G.A. (1962). *Heart-Lung Bypass*. (New York: Grune and Stratton)

7. Voorhees, A.B. (1985). The development of arterial prostheses. *Arch. Surg.*, **120**, 289–95

8. Shumacher, H.B. Jr and Muhn, H.Y. (1969). Arterial suture techniques and grafts: past, present and future. *Surgery*, **66**, 419–33

9. Creech, O. (1967). Rudolph Matas and Keen's surgery. *Am. J. Surg.*, **113**, 791–801

10. Lambert (1909). Medical observations and inquiries, vol. II, 1762. Cited by Smith, E.A. *Suture of Arteries: An Experimental Research*. (London: Oxford University Press)

11. Asman, C. (1773). *De aneurysmate*. Gronique, Dissertatio inaugr.

12. Postempski, P. (1886). La sutura dei vasi sanguini. Recerche sperimentali. *Arch. ed atti d. Soc. Ital. Chir.*, **3**, 391

13. Murphy, J.B. (1897). Resection of arteries and veins injured in continuity: end-to-end suture: experimental and clinical research. *M. Rec. Ann.*, **51**, 73

14. Jaboulay, M. and Briau, E. (1896). Recherches experimentales sur la suture et la greffe arterielle. *Lyon Med.*, **81**, 97

15. Payr, E. (1900). Beitrage zur Technik der Blutgefasse und Nervennacht hebst Mitthellungen uber die Vervendung elnes resorbirbaren Metalles in der Chirurgie. *Arch. Klin. Chir.*, **62**, 67–93

16. Höpfner, E. (1903). Ueber Gefässnaht, Gefässtransplantationen und Replantation von Ampurititen Extremitàten. *Arch. Klin. Chir.*, **70**, 417–71

17. Jassinowsky, A. (1889). Die arteriennaht. Eine experimentellchirurgische Studie. Dorpat, Inaug. Diss.

18. Burci, E. (1891). Ricerche sperimentali sul processo di reparazione delle ferite longitudinali delle arterie. *Atti della soc. Toscana di Sc. Nat.*, **11**, 36

19. Silberberg, O. (1899). Über die Naht der

Blutgefasse, Klinische und experimentelle Untersuchungen. Breslau, Inaug. Diss.

20. Dörfler, J. (1889). Über arteriennaht. *Beltr. Klin. Chir.*, **25**, 781

21. Napalkow (1900). Naht von Herz und Blutgefassen, Moskow, Inaug. Diss. Abstracted in *Ztschr. Chir.*, **27**, 596

22. Heidenhain, L. (1893). Über Naht von Arterienwunden. *Centralbl. Chir.*, **49**, 1113

23. Eck, N. (1877). Ligature of the portal vein. *Voen Med. Zh.*, **1**, 120

24. Hahn, O., Massen, M., Nencki and Pawlow, J. (1893). Die Eck'sche Fistel zwischen der unteren Hohlvene und der Pfortader und ihre Folgen für den Organismus. *Arch. Exp. Pathol. Pharm.*, **32**, 161–210

25. Child, C.G. (1953). Eck's fistula. *Surg., Gyn., Obst.*, Has transl. of Eck's paper from Russian by I.N. Kovarsky, **96**, 375–6

26. Stolnikow (1882). Die Stelle vv. hepaticarum im Leber – und gesammten Kreislaufe. *Pflüg. Arch. Ges. Physiol.*, **28**, 255–86

27. Fischler, F. and Schröder, R. (1909). Eine einfachere Ausführung der Eck'schen Fistel. *Arch. Exp. Path. Pharm.*, **61**, 428–33

28. Jerusalem, E. (1910). Eine Vereinfachung in der Operationtechnik der Eckschen Fistel. *Zentralblatt Physiol.*, **24**, 837–40

29. Lobb, A.W., Wagner, C.W. and Crystal, D.K. (1956). The history of vascular repair. *West. J. Surg., Obst., Gyn.*, **64**, 574–7

30. Brewer, G.E. (1908). Hydatid cyst of the liver with ligation of the portal vein. *Ann. Surg.*, **47**, 619–22

31. Tansini, I. (1902). Ableitung des portalen Blutes durch die direkta Verbindung der V. portae mit der V. cava. Neues operatives Verfahren. *Centralblatt Chir.*, no. **36**, 937–9

32. Vidal (1903). Traitement chirurgical des ascites. *La Presse médicale*, no.**85**, 747

33. Rosenstein, P. (1912). Ueber die Behandlung des Lebercirrhose durch Anlegung einer Eck'schen Fistel. *Arch. Klin. Chir.*, **98**, 1082–92

34. Braun, H. (1882). Ueber den seitlichen Verschluss von Venenwunden. *Arch. Klin. Chir.*, **28**, 654–72

35. Schede, M. (1892). Einige Bemerkungen über die Naht Venenwunden, nebst Mittheilung eines Falles von geheilten Naht der Vena cava inferior. *Arch. Klin. Chir.*, **43**, 338–70

36. Clermont, G. (1901). Suture latérale et circulaire des veines. *La Presse médicale*, pt. l, 229–33

37. Ullmann, E. (1902). Experimentelle Nieren-transplantation. *Wiener Klin. Wochenschr.*, **15**, 281–2

38. Kümmell, H. (1900). Ueber cirkuläre Gefässnaht beim Menschen. *Beitr. Klin. Chir.*, **26**, 128–32

39. Carrel (1958). La Technique Operatoire des Anastomoses Vascularies et la Transportation des Viscères, Lyon Médical (1902). (Translation, Carrel: The operative technique of vascular anastomoses and the transplantation of organs, from Alfred Hurwitz and George A. Degenshein, *Milestones in Modern Surgery*, pp. 374–9.) (New York: Paul B. Hober, Inc.)

40. Carrel (1904). Les Anastomoses Vasculaires, Leur Technique Opératoire et Leurs Indications. *Congrés des Médicines de Langue Francaise de l'Amerique du Nord*

41. Carrel and Morel (1902). Anastomoses Bont – Bont de la Jugulaire et de la Conotide Interne. *Lyon Médical*, **99**, 114

42. Carrel A. (1904). Les anastomoses vasculares et leum technique operatoire. *Union Med. Can.*, **33**, 521–7

43. Friedman, S.G. (1988). Alexis Carrel: Jules Verne of cardiovascular surgery. *Am. J. Surg.*, **155**, 420–4

44. Carrel, A. and Guthrie, C.C. (1906). Uniterminal and biterminal venous transplantations. *Surg. Gynecol. Obstet.*, **2**, 266–86

45. Carrel, A. (1912). The preservation of tissues and its applications in surgery. *J. Am. Med. Assoc.*, **59**, 523–7

46. Carrel, A. and Guthrie, C.C. (1905). The transplantation of veins and organs. *Am. Med.*, **10**, 1101–2

47. Kunlin, J. (1949). Le traitement de l'arterite obliterante par la greffe veineuss. *Arch. Mal. Coeur*, **42**, 371–2

48. Murray, J.E., Merril, J.P. and Harrison, J.H. (1955). Renal homotransplantation in identical twins. *Surg. Forum*, **6**, 432–6

49. Barnard, C.N. (1968). What we have learned about heart transplantations. *J. Thorac. Cardiovasc. Surg.*, **56**, 457–68

50. Malt, R.A. and McKhann, C.F. (1964). Replantation of severed arms. *J. Am. Med. Assoc.*, **189**, 716–22

51. Carrel, A. (1910). Graft of the vena cava on the abdominal aorta. *Ann. Surg.*, **52**, 462–70

52. Carrel, A. (1910). On the experimental surgery of the thoracic aorta and the heart. *Ann. Surg.*, **52**, 83–95

53. Carrel, A. (1914). Experimental operations on the orifices of the heart. *Ann. Surg.*, **60**, 1–6

54. Carrel, A. and Burrows, M.T. (1910). Human sarcoma cultivated outside of the body. *J. Am. Med. Assoc.*, **55**, 1732–8

55. Carrel, A. (1914). Present condition of a strain of connective tissue twenty-eight months old. *J. Exp. Med.*, **20**, 1–2

56. Carrel, A. and Lindbergh, C.A. (1938). *The Culture of Organs*. (New York: Hoeber)

57. Alexis Carrel (1913). Nobel lecture: suture of blood-vessels and transplantation of organs, from *Les Prix Nobel en 1912*, pp. 1–25. (Stockholm: Imprimerie Royale, P.A. Norstedt & Söner)

58. Brewer, L.A. (1987). Alexis Carrel: a cardiovascular prophet crying in the wilderness of early twentieth century surgery. *J. Thorac. Cardiovasc. Surg.*, **94**, 724–6

59. Carrel, A. (1973). Papers of the Centennial conference at Georgetown University, June 28, 1973. Chambers, R.W. and Durkin, J.T. (eds.) (Washington DC: Georgetown Unitersity)

60. Cohn, I. (1960). *Rudolph Matas, Biography of the Great Pioneer in Surgery*. (New York: Doubleday)

61. Matas, R. (1940). Personal experiences in vascular surgery. *Ann. Surg.*, **112**, 802

62. Matas, R. (1888). Traumatic aneurism of the left brachial artery. *NY Med. News*, **53**, 412

63. Guthrie, C.C. (1959). In Harbinson, S.P. and Fisher, B (eds.) *Blood Vessel Surgery and Its Applications* (Reprint), p. 360. (Pittsburgh: University of Pittsburgh Press)

64. Murray, D.W.G. and Best, C.H. (1938). The use of heparin in thrombosis. *Ann. Surg.*, **108**, 163

65. Dos Santos, J.C. (1947). Sur la désobstruction des thromboses arterielles anciennes. *Mem. Acad. Chir.*, **73**, 409

66. Dos Santos, R., Lamas, A. and Pereira, C.J.J. (1929). L'arteriographie des membres de l'aorte et ses branches abdominales. *Bull. Soc. Nat. Chir.*, **55**, 587

67. Wylie, E.J. *et al.* (1951). Experimental and clinical experiences with the use of fascia lata applied as a graft about major arteries after thromboendarteriectomy and aneurysm-orrhaphy. *Surg. Gynecol. Obstet.*, **93**, 257

68. Child, C.G., Barr, D., Holswade, G.R. and Harrison, C.S. (1953). Liver regeneration following portacaval transposition in dogs. *Ann. Surg.*, **138**, 600–8

69. Ono, H., Kojima, Y., Brown, H. and McDermott, W.V. (1968). A technique for porta-renal transposition in dogs. *Surgery*, **63**, 653–7

70. Julian, O.C. and Dye, W.A. (1951). Venous shunts in portal hypertension. *Arch. Surg.*, **63**, 373–8

71. Reynolds, J.T. and Southwick, H.W. (1951). Portal hypertension. Use of venous grafts when side-to-side anastomosis is impossible. *Arch. Surg.*, **62**, 789–800

72. Johnson, J., Kirby, C.K., Allam, K.W. and Hagan, W. (1951). The growth of vena cava and aorta grafts: an experimental study. *Surgery*, **29**, 726–30

73. Rousselot, L.M. (1952). Autogenous vein grafts in splenorenal anastomosis. A description of technique and its clinical application in seven patients. *Surgery*, **31**, 403–10

74. Sauvage, L.R. and Harkins, H.N. (1952). Growth of vascular anastomoses: an experimental study of the influence of suture type and suture method with a note on certain mechanical factors involved. *Bull. Johns Hopkins Hosp.*, **91**, 276–97

75. Sauvage, L.R. and Wesolowski, S.A. (1954). The influence of suture method upon the incidence of thrombosis in artery-artery, vein-vein, and artery-vein-artery anastomosis. *Surgery*, **36**, 227–32

76. Sauvage, L.R. and Wesolowski, S.A. (1955). Anastomoses and grafts in the venous system with special reference to growth changes. *Surgery*, **37**, 714–9

77. Maluf, N.S.R. (1956). Effect of complete portalisation of the renal effluent blood upon arterial pressure. *Am. J. Physiol.*, **187**, 466–8

78. Murray, D.W.G., *et al.* (1937). Heparin and thrombosis after injury. *Surgery*, **2**, 163–87

79. Murray, D.W.G., Jacques, L.B., Perrett, T.S. and Best, C.H. (1936). Heparin and vascular occlusion. *Can. Med. Assoc. J.*, **35**, 621–2

80. Murray, D.W.G. and Best, C.H. (1938). The use of heparin in thrombosis. *Ann. Surg.*, **108**, 163–77

81. Murray, D.W.G. (1940). Heparin in thrombosis and embolism. *Br. J. Surg.*, **27**, 567–98

82. Murray, D.W.G. (1940). Heparin in surgical treatment of blood vessels. *Arch. Surg.*, **40**, 307–25

83. Freeman, N.E., Wylie, E.J. and Gilfillan, R.S. (1950). Regional heparinisation in vascular surgery. *Surg. Gynecol. Obst.*, **90**, 406–12

84. Nitze, F. (1897). Kleinere Mitthellungen Kongress in Moskau. *Centralbl. Chir.*, **24**, 1042

85. Abbe, R. (1894). The surgery of the hand. *NY Med. J.*, **59**, 33–40

86. Tuffier, T. (1902). Intervention chirugicale directe pour un aneurysme de la crosse de l'aorte, ligature du sac. *Bull. Soc. Chir.*, **28**, 326–44

87. Carrel, A. (1912). Results of permanent intubation of the thoracic aorta. *Surg. Gynecol. Obstet.*, **15**, 245

88. Goyanes, J. (1906). Neuvos trabajos de chirurgia vascular: Substitucion plastica de las arterias por las venas, o arterioplastia venosa, aplicado, como neuvo metodo, al traitamiento de los aneurismas. *Siglo Med.*, **53**, 561

89. Lexer, E. (1907). Die ideale Operation des arteriellen und des arteriellvenösen Aneurysma. *Arch. Klin. Chir.*, **83**, 459–77

90. Pringle, J.H. (1913). Two cases of vein-grafting for the maintenance of a direct arterial circulation. *Lancet*, **1**, 1795–6

91. Pringle, J.H. (1908). Notes on the arrest of hepatic hemorrhage due to trauma. *Ann. Surg.*, **48**, 541–9

92. Bernheim, B.M. (1916). The ideal operation for aneurisms of the extremity. Report of a case. *Bull. Johns Hopkins Hosp.*, **27**, 93–5

93. Leriche, R. and Kunlin, J. (1948). Possibilité de greffe veineuse de grande dimension (15 à 47 cm) dans les thrombose artérielles étendues. *Comptes rendu l'Acad. Sci.*, **227**, 939–40

94. Kunlin, J. (1949). Le traitement de l'artérite oblitérante par la greffe veineuse. *Arch. des Maladies du Coeur*, **42**, 371–2

95. Kunlin, J., Bitry-Boély, C., Volnié and Beaudry (1951). Le traitment de l'ischémie artérique par la greffe veineuse longue. *Revue de Chirurgie*, **70**, 206–35

96. Linton, R.L. and Darling, R.C. (1962). Autogenous saphenous vein bypass grafts in femoropopliteal obliterative arterial disease. *Surgery*, **51**, 62–73

97. Carrel, A. (1910). On the experimental surgery of the thoracic aorta and the heart. *Ann. Surg.*, **52**, 83–95

98. McAllister, F.F., Leighninger, D. and Beck, C. (1951). Revascularisation of the heart by vein graft from aorta to coronary sinus. *Ann. Surg.*, **133**, 153–65

99. Carrel, A. (1906). Transplantation de vaisseaux conservés au froit (en "cold storage") pendant plusieurs jours. *Comptes rendu Soc. Biol.*, **61**, 572–3

100. Levin, I. and Larkin, J.H. (1907–8). Transplantation of devitalized arterial segments. *Proc. Soc. Exp. Biol. Med.*, **5**, 109–11

101. Guthrie, C.C. (1919). End results of arterial restoration with devitalized tissue. *J. Am. Med. Assoc.*, **73**, 186

102. Guthrie, C.C. (1908). Transplantation of formaldehyde-fixed blood vessels. *Science*, **27**, 473

103. Klotz, O., Permar, H.H. and Guthrie, C.C. (1923). End results of arterial transplants. *Ann. Surg.*, **78**, 305–20

104. Yamanoüchi, H. (1911). Über die zirkularen Gefässnähte und Arterienvenenanastomosen, so wie über die Gefässtrans-plantationen. *Deutsche Ztschr. Chir.*, **112**, 1–118, 1 pl.

105. Gross, R.E., Bill, A.H., Jr and Pierce, C.E. III (1949). Methods of preservation and transplantation of arterial grafts: observation on arterial grafts in dogs. Report of transplantation of preserved arterial grafts in 9 human cases. *Surg. Gynecol. Obstet.*, **88**, 689

106. Dubost, C. *et al.* (1951). A propos du traitement des aneurysms de l'aorte; ablation de l'aneurysm; rétablissement de la continuité par greffe d'aorte conserve. *Mem. Acad. Chir.*, **77**, 381

107. Oudot, J. (1951). La greffe vasculaire dans les thromboses du carrefour aortique. *Presse Med.*, **59**, 234

108. Hufnagel, C.A. (1947). Permanent intubation of the thoracic aorta. *Arch. Surg.*, **54**, 382–9

109. Voorhees, A.B., Jaretzki, A. and Blakemore, A.H. (1952). The use of tubes constructed from Vinyon 'N' cloth in bridging arterial grafts. *Ann. Surg.*, **135**, 332–6

110. Voorhees, H. (1985). *Op. cit.*, p. 292

111. Levin, S.M. (1987). Reminiscences and ruminations: vascular surgery then and now. *Am. J. Surg.*, **154**, 158–62

112. Shumacher, H.B. (1980). A history of modern treatment of aortic aneurysms. *World J. Surg.*, **4**, 503–9

113. Clarke, C.P., Brandt, C.W.P., Cole, D.S. and Barratt-Boyes, B.G. (1967). Traumatic rupture of the aorta: diagnosis and treatment. *Br. J. Surg.*, **54**, 353

114. Gerbode, F., Braimbridge, M., Osborne, J.J., Hood, M. and French, S. (1957). Traumatic thoracic aneurysm: treatment by resection and grafting with the use of extracorporeal bypass. *Surgery*, **42**, 975

115. Passaro, E. Jr and Pace, W.G. (1959). Traumatic rupture of the aorta. *Surgery*, **46**, 787

116. Vasko, J.S., Raess, D.H., Williams, T.E. Jr, Kakos, G.S., Kilman, J.W. *et al.* (1977). Nonpenetrating trauma to the thoracic aorta. *Surgery*, **82**, 400

117. Gurin, D., Bulmer, J.W. and Derby, R. (1935). Dissecting aneurysm of the aorta: diagnosis and operative relief of acute arterial obstruction due to this cause. *NY State J. Med.*, **35**, 1200

118. Shaw, R.S. (1955). Acute dissecting aortic

aneurysm: treatment by fenestration of the internal wall of the aneurysm. *N. Engl. J. Med.*, **253**, 331

119. Paullin, J.E. and James, D.F. (1948). Dissecting aneurysm of aorta. *Postgrad. Med.*, **4**, 291

120. Johns, T.N.P. (1953). Dissecting aneurysm of the abdominal aorta: report of a case with repair of perforation. *Ann. Surg.*, **137**, 232

121. DeBakey, M.E., Cooley, D.A. and Creech, O. Jr (1955). Surgical considerations of dissecting aneurysm of the aorta. *Ann. Surg.*, **142**, 586

122. Spencer, F.C. and Blake, H. (1962). A report of the successful surgical treatment of aortic regurgitation from a dissecting aortic aneurysm in a patient with the Marfan syndrome. *J. Thorac. Cardiovasc. Surg.*, **44**, 238

123. Morris, G.C. Jr, Henly, W.S. and DeBakey, M.E. (1963). Correction of acute dissecting aneurysm of aorta with valvular insufficiency. *J. Am. Med. Assoc.*, **184**, 63

124. Lawrie, G.M. and Morris, G.C. (1978). Follow-up of dissecting aortic aneurysm. *J. Am. Med. Assoc.*, **239**, 724

125. DeBakey, M.E., Henly, W.S., Cooley, D.A., Morris, G.C. Jr, Crawford, E.S. and Beall, A.C. Jr (1964). Surgical management of dissecting aneurysm involving the ascending aorta. *J. Cardiovasc. Surg.*, **5**, 200

126. Osler, W. (1915). Remarks on arterio-venous aneurysm. *Lancet*, **1**, 949–55

127. Kirklin, J.W., Waugh, J.M., Grindlay, J.H., Openshaw, C.R. and Allen, E.V. (1953). Surgical treatment of arteriosclerotic aneurysms of the abdominal aorta. *AMA Arch. Surg.*, **67**, 632

128. DeBakey, M.E. and Cooley, D.A. (1953). Surgical treatment of aneurysm of abdominal aorta by resection and restoration of continuity with homograft. *Surg. Gynecol. Obstet.*, **97**, 157

129. Crawford, E.S., Snyder, D.M., Cho, G.C. and Roehm, J.O.F. Jr (1978). Progress in treatment of thoraco-abdominal and abdominal aortic aneurysms involving celiac, superior mesenteric, and renal arteries. *Ann. Surg.*, **188**, 404

130. Javid, H., Julian, O.C., Dye, W.S. and Hunter, J.A. (1962). Complications of abdominal aortic grafts. *Arch. Surg.*, **85**, 142

131. Creech, O. Jr (1966). Endoaneurysmorrhaphy and treatment of aortic aneurysm. *Ann. Surg.*, **164**, 935

132. Mortensen, J.D., Grindlay, J.H. and Kirklin, J.W. (1953). The arterial homograft bank. *Proc. Staff Meet. Mayo Clin.*, **28**, 713

133. Gross, R.E., Hurwitt, E.S., Bill, A.H. Jr and Peirce, E.C. (1948). Preliminary observations on the use of human arterial grafts in the treatment of certain cardiovascular defects. *N. Engl. J. Med.*, **239**, 578

134. Cooley, D.A. and DeBakey, M.E. (1952). Surgical considerations of intrathoracic aneurysms of the aorta and great vessels. *Ann. Surg.*, **135**, 660

135. Bahnson, H.T. (1953). Definitive treatment of saccular aneurysms of the aorta with excision of sac and aortic suture. *Surg. Gynecol. Obstet.*, **96**, 383

136. Johnson, J.B., Kirklin, J.W. and Brandenburg, R.O. (1953). The treatment of saccular aneurysms of the thoracic aorta. *Proc. Staff Meet. Mayo Clin.*, **28**, 723

137. Cooley, D.A. and DeBakey, M.E. (1956). Resection of entire ascending aorta in fusiform aneurysm using cardiac bypass. *J. Am. Med. Assoc.*, **162**, 1158

138. Hufnagel, C.A. and Rabil, P. (1955). Replacement of arterial segments utilizing orlon prostheses. *Arch. Surg.*, **70**, 105–10

139. Blakemore, A.H. and Voorhees, A.B. Jr (1954). The use of tubes constructed from Vinyon N cloth in bridging arterial defects – experimental and clinical. *Ann. Surg.*, **9**, 324

140. Deterling, R.A. Jr and Bhonslay, S.B. (1955). An evaluation of synthetic materials and fabrics suitable for blood vessel replacement. *Surgery*, **38**, 71

141. Borst, H.G., Schaudig, A. and Rudolph, W. (1964). Arteriovenous fistula of the aortic arch: repair during deep hypothermia and circulatory arrest. *J. Thorac. Cardiovasc. Surg.*, **48**, 443

142. Griepp, R.B., Stinson, E.B., Hollingsworth, J.F. and Buehler, D. (1975). Prosthetic replacement of the aortic arch. *J. Thorac. Cardiovasc. Surg.*, **70**, 1051

143. Bloodwell, R.D., Hallman, G.L. and Cooley, D.A. (1968). Total replacement of the aortic arch and the 'subclavian steal' phenomenon. *Ann. Thorac. Surg.*, **5**, 236

144. Crawford, E.S. and Saleh, S.A. (1981). Transverse aortic arch aneurysm: improved results of treatment employing new modifications of aortic reconstruction and hypothermic cerebral circulatory arrest. *Ann. Surg.*, **194**, 180

145. Hamby, W.B. (1952). *Intracranial Aneurysms*, p. 564. (Springfield, Illinois: Charles C. Thomas)

146. Gross, S.W. The history of carotid artery ligation. Read before the Johns Hopkins Hospital, April 7, 1967 at an International Symposium to honor Dr. A. Earl Walker

147. *Ibid.,* p. 221
148. Hamby, W.B. (1952). *Op. cit.*
149. Cooper, A. (1836). Account of the first successful operation performed on the common carotid artery for aneurysm in the year 1808 with the postmortem examination in the year 1821. *Guy's Hosp. Rep.*, **1**, 53
150. Gross, S.W. (1967). *Op. cit.*
151. *Ibid.*
152. Hamby, W.B. (1952). *Op. cit.*, p. 565
153. Matas, R. (1911). Testing the efficiency of the collateral system as a preliminary to the occlusion of the great surgical arteries. *Ann. Surg.*, **53**, 1
154. Gross, S.W. (1967). *Op. cit.*, p. 222
155. Gibbs, J.R. (1965). Torsion: a new technique for closure of the cervical carotid artery. *Br. J. Surg.*, **52**, 947
156. Thompson, J.E. (1986). History of carotid surgery. *Surg. Clin. N. Am.*, **66** (2), 225–31
157. Savory, W.S. (1856). Case of a young woman in whom the main arteries of both upper extremities and of the left side of the neck were throughout completely obliterated. *Med. Chir. Trans.*, **39**, 205–19
158. Broadbent, W.H. (1875). Absence of pulsation in both radial arteries, vessels being full of blood. *Trans. Clin. Soc.*, **8**, 165–8
159. Penzoldt, F. (1881). Uber Thrombose (autochtone oder embolische) der Carotis. *Dtsch. Arch. Klin. Med.*, **28**, 80–93
160. Chiari, H. (1905). Uber des verhalten des teilungswinkels der carotis communis bei der endarteriitis chronica deformans. *Verh. Dtsch. Ges. Pathol.*, **9**, 326–30
161. Hunt, J.R. (1914). The role of the carotid arteries, in the causation of vascular lesions of the brain, with remarks on certain special features of the symptomatology. *Am. J. Med. Sci.*, **147**, 704–13
162. Johnson, H.C. and Walker, A.E. (1951). Angiographic diagnosis of spontaneous thrombosis of the internal and common carotid arteries. *J. Neurosurg.*, **8**, 631–59
163. Fisher, M. (1951). Occlusion of the internal carotid artery. *AMA Arch. Neurol. Psychiatr.*, **65**, 346–77
164. Carrea, R.M.E., Molins, M. and Murphy, G. (1955). Surgical treatment of spontaneous thrombosis of the internal carotid artery in the neck, carotid-carotideal anastomosis; report of a case. *Acta Neurol. Lationam.*, **2**, 71–8
165. Wylie, E.J., Kerr, E. and Davies, O. (1951).

Experimental and clinical experiences with use of fascia lata applied as a graft about major arteries after thrombo-end-arterectomy and aneurysmorrhaphy. *Surg. Gynecol. Obstet.*, **93**, 257–72
166. Strully, K.J., Hurwitt, E.S. and Blankenberg, H.W. (1953). Thromboendarterectomy for thrombosis of the internal carotid artery in the neck. *J. Neurosurg.*, **10**, 474–82
167. DeBakey, M.E. (1975). Successful carotid endarterectomy for cerebrovascular insufficiency. Nineteen-year followup. *J. Am. Med. Assoc.*, **233**, 1083–5
168. Eastcott, H.H.G., Pickering, G.W. and Rob, C.G. (1954). Reconstruction of internal carotid artery in a patient with intermittent attacks of hemiplegia. *Lancet*, **2**, 994–6
169. Friedlander, W.J. (1972). About 3 old men: an inquiry into how cerebral arteriosclerosis has altered world politics. A neurologist's view. (Woodrow Wilson, Paul von Hindenburg, and Nikolai Lenin). *Stroke*, **3**, 467–73
170. Trendelenburg, F. (1907). Ueber die Operative Behandlung der Emboli der Lungenarterie. *Zentr. Chir.*, **44**, 1402
171. Willie Meyer discussion from G. Nystrom. (1930). Experiences with the Trendelenburg operation for pulmonary embolism. *Ann. Surg.*, **92**, 498
172. DaCosta, J.C. (1919). *Modern Surgery, General and Operative*, 8th edn., pp. 1027–8. (Philadelphia: W.B. Saunders Co.)
173. Meyer, W. (1913). The surgery of the pulmonary artery. *Ann. Surg.*, **58**, 191
174. *Ibid.*
175. *Ibid.*, pp. 193–4
176. Kirschner, M. (1924). *Arch. klin. Chir., Bd.*, 133
177. Meyer. *Surgery of Pulmonary Artery*, pp. 188–205
178. Letter from regular Berlin correspondent (1924). *J. Am. Med. Assoc.*, **83**, 136
179. Meyer, A.W. (1930). The operative treatment of embolism of the lungs. *Surg. Gynecol. Obstet.*, **50**, 891
180. Crafoord, C. (1929). Two cases of obstructive pulmonary embolism successfully operated upon. *Acta Chir. Scand.*, **64**, 172–86
181. Nystrom, G. (1930). Experiences with the Trendelenburg operation for pulmonary embolism, *Ann. Surg.*, **92**, 498–532
182. Steenburg, R. *et al.* (1958). A new look at pulmonary embolectomy. *Surg. Gynecol. Obstet.*, **107**, 214–20
183. Aristotle (1926). De partibus Animalium, Lib. III, Cap. 4 (Opera edidit Academia Regia

Borussica), 3, 328, quoted from Claude S. Beck, Wounds of the heart: the technique of suture. *Arch. Surg.*, **13**, 206

184. Fallopius (1600). Opera omnia tractatus de vulneribus in genere, Cap. 10 (Frankfort), p. 163, quoted from Beck: *Wounds of the Heart*, pp. 207–208

185. Fabricius ab Aquapendente (1666). Opera Chiurugica, Cap. 21 (Patavii), p. 104, quoted from Beck: *Wounds of the Heart*, p. 208

186. Beck: *Wounds of the Heart*, p. 205

187. Morgagni, J.B. (1829). De Sedibus et Causis Morborum (Lipsiae sumptibus Leopoldi Vossii), quoted from Beck: *Wounds of the Heart*, p. 209

188. Fischer, G. (1868). Die Wunden des Herzens und des Herzbeutels. *Arch. Klin. Chir.*, **9**, 571

189. Block (1882). Verhandlungen der Deutschen Gesellschaft für Chirurgie (Elften Congress, Berlin) part I, p. 108, quoted from Beck: *Wounds of the Heart*, p. 210

190. Del Vecchio, S. (1895). Sutura del Cuore. *Riforma Med.*, **11**, 38

191. Richardson, R.G. (1963). Billroth and cardiac surgery, *Lancet*, **1**, 1323

192. Nissen, R. (1963). Billroth and cardiac surgery. *Lancet*, **2**, 250

193. Harken, D. (1967). *Op. cit.*, p. 396

194. Absolon, K.B. (1983). Theodor Billroth and cardiac surgery. *J. Thorac. Cardiovasc. Surg.*, **86**, 451–52

195. McGoon, D.C. (1982). The John H. Gibbon, Jr. Lecture. *Bull. Am. Coll. Surg.*, p. 15

196. Borchart, E. (1920). Sammlung Lin. Vorträge. Neue Folge Chirurg., No. 113, 114, 806., in Ballance, C: Bradshaw Lecture on the Surgery of the Heart. *Lancet*, **1**, 1

197. Paget, S. (1896). *The Surgery of the Chest*, p.121. (Bristol: J. Wright and Co.)

198. Rehn, L. (1897). Ueber penetrirende Herzwunden und Herznah. *Arch. Klin. Chir.*, **55**, 315

199. Blatchford, J.W. (1985). Ludwig Rehn: the first successful cardiorraphy. *Ann. Thorac. Surg.*, **39**, 492–5

200. Farina (1896). Discussion. *Centralbl. Chir.*, **23**, 1224

201. Cappelen, A. (1896). Vulnia Cordis, Sutur af Hjertet, Norsk. Meg. Laegevidensk, 11, 285, Trans by Beck: *Wounds of the Heart*, p. 211

202. Rehn, L. (1907). Zur Chirurgie des Herzens und des Herzbeutels. *Arch. Klin. Chir.*, **83**, 723

203. Hill, L.L. (1902). A report of a case of successful suturing of the heart, and table of 37 other cases of suturing by different operators with various terminations, and the conclusions drawn. *Med. Rec.*, **62**, 846

204. Williams, D.H. (1897). Stab wound of the heart and pericardium – suture of the pericardium – patient alive three years afterwards. *Med. Rec.*, **31**, 437

205. Beck, C.S. (1926). Wounds of the heart. *Arch. Surg.*, **13**, 203–27

206. Elkin, D.C. (1936). Wounds of the heart. *J. Thorac. Surg.*, **3**, 390–603

207. Beck, C.S. and Griswold, R.A. (1930). Pericardiectomy in the treatment of the Pick syndrome. *Arch. Surg.*, **21**, 1064–113

208. Cox, D.M. (1928). Wounds of the heart. *Arch. Surg.*, **17**, 484–92

209. Griswold, R.A. and Drissen, E.M. (1936). Wounds of the heart. *Kentucky Med. J.*, **34**, 471–5

210. Mayer, J.M. (1936). The clinical management of injuries to the heart and pericardium. *Surg. Gynecol. Obstet.*, **62**, 852–64

211. Baderischer, V.A. (1940). Acute cardiac compression resulting from the restraining influence of the pericardium during acute dilatation of the heart. *Am. J. Surg.*, **50**, 367–70

212. Griswold, R.A. and Maguire, C.H. (1942). Penetrating wounds of the heart and pericardium. *Surg. Gynecol. Obstet.*, **74**, 406–18

213. Maguire, C.H. and Griswold, R.A. (1947). Further observations on penetrating wounds of the heart and pericardium. *Am. J. Surg.*, **74**, 721–31

214. Griswold, R.A. and Drye, J.C. (1954). Cardiac wounds. *Ann. Surg.*, **139**, 783–5

215. Martin, L.F., Mavroudis, C., Dyess, D.L., Gray, L.A. and Richardson, J.D. (1986). The first 70 years experience managing cardiac disruption due to penetrating and blunt injuries at the University of Louisville. *Am. Surg.*, **52**, 14–19

216. Borja, A.R., Lansing, A.M. and Ransdel, H.T. Jr (1970). Immediate operative treatment for stab wounds of the heart. *J. Thorac. Cardiovasc. Surg.*, **59**, 662–7

217. Elkin, D.C. and Campbell, R.E. (1951). Cardiac tamponade: treatment by aspiration. *Ann. Surg.*, **133**, 623–30

218. Ravitch, M.M. and Blalock, A. (1949). Aspiration of blood from pericardium in treatment of acute cardiac tamponade after injury. *Arch. Surg.*, **58**, 463–77

219. Ransdell, H.T. Jr and Glass, H. Jr (1960). Gunshot wound of the heart. *Am. J. Surg.*, **99**, 788–97

220. Richardson, J.D., Flint, L.M., Snow, N.J., Gray,

L.A. Jr and Trinkle, J.K. (1981). Management of transmediastinal gunshot wounds. *Surgery*, **90**, 671–6

221. Evans, J., Gray, L.A. Jr, Rayner, A. and Fulton, R.L. (1979). Principles for the management of penetrating cardiac wounds. *Ann. Surg.*, **189**, 777–84

222. Garrison, R.N., Richardson, J.D. and Fry, D.E. (1982). Diagnostic transdiaphragmatic pericardiotomy in thoracoabdominal trauma. *J. Trauma*, **22**, 147–9

223. Ravitch, M.M. (1981). *A Century of Surgery*, p. 188 (Philadelphia: JB Lippincott)

224. Kotte, J.H. and McGuire, J. (1951). Pericardial paracentesis. *Mod. Concepts Cardio-vasc. Dis.*, **20**, 102–3

225. Farrar, W.E. (1980). Parzival's pericardial puncture. *Ann. Int. Med.*, **92**, 640

226. von Eschenbach, W. (1961). *Parzival* (translated by Mustard, H.M. and Passage, C.E.), pp. 270–1. (New York: Random House (Vintage Books))

227. Jarcho, S. (1973). Thomas Jowett on Pericardiocentesis (1827). *Am. J. Cardiol.*, **31**, 273–6

228. Jowett, T. (1827). Case of dropsy of the pericardium in which the operation of tapping was performed. *Medico-Chirurgical Review*, **6**, 623–6

229. Weill, E. (1929). Traite des Maladies du Coeur chez les Enfants (Paris, 1895), p. 128, quoted from Edward D. Churchill: Decortication of the Heart (delorme) for Adhesive Pericarditis. *Arch. Surg.*, **19**, 1466

230. Delorme, E. (1898). *Gaz. d'Hôp.*, p. 1150, quoted from Churchill: Decortication of the Heart, p. 1466

231. Carl Beck in discussion of F.P. Norbury (1901). Some points in the treatment of pericarditis. *J. Am. Med. Assoc.*, **37**, 1585

232. Brauer, L. (1902). *München Med. Wchnschr.*, **49**, 1072, quoted from Churchill: Decortication of the Heart, p. 1467

233. Simon, R.M. (1912). A post-graduate lecture on cardiolysis. *Br. Med. J.*, **2**, 1649

234. Rehn, L. (1920). *Berl. klin. Wchnschr.*, p. 241, 1913; *Arch. klin. Chir.*, **102**, 1, 1914; *Med. Klin.*, **16**, 999

235. Schmieden, V. (1926). The technique of cardiolysis. *Surg. Gynecol. Obstet.*, **43**, 89

236. Churchill, E. (1929). *Decortication of the Heart*, p. 1457

237. Beck, C.S. and Griswold, R.A. (1930). Pericardiectomy in the treatment of the Pick syndrome. *Arch. Surg.*, **21**, 1064

238. Beck, C.S. and Moore, R.L. (1925). The significance of the pericardium in relation to surgery of the heart. *Arch. Surg.*, **11**, 550

239. Vesalius, A. (1543). *De humani corporis fabrica libri septum*, pp. 661–3. (Basel: Oporinus)

240. Bourne, W. (1936). Avertin anaesthesia for crippled children. *Can. Med. Assoc. J.*, **35**, 278

241. Trendelenburg, F. (1963). Beiträge zur den Operationen an den Luftwegen. 2. Tamponnade der Trachea. *Arch. Klin. Chir.*, **12**, 121, (1871), quoted from Thomas E. Keyes, The History of Surgical Anesthesia. (New York: Dover Publications)

242. Macewan, W. (1880). Introduction of tracheal tubes by the mouth instead of performing tracheotomy or laryngotomy. *Br. Med. J.*, **2**, 122

243. Maydl, K. (1893). Ueber de Intubation des Larynx als Mittel gegen das Einfliessenvon Blut in die Respirationsorgane bei Operationen. Wein. Med. Wchnscher., quoted from Keys, *History of Surgical Anesthesia*, **43**, 102

244. Eisenmenger, V. (1893). Tamponnade des Larynx nach Prof. Maydl, Wein. Med. Wchnschr., quoted from Keys, *History of Surgical Anesthesia*, **43**, 199

245. Tuffier and Hallion (1896). Operations Intrathoraciques avec respiration Artificielle par Insufflation. *Compt. Rend. Soc. Biol.*, **48**, 951

246. Matas, R. (1902). Artificial respiration by direct intralaryngeal intubation with a modified O'Dwyer tube and new graduated air-pump, in its application to medical and surgical practice. *Am. Med.*, **3**, 97

247. Fell, G. Fell Method: forced respiration: report of cases resulting in the saving of twenty-eight human lives: history and a plea for its general use in hospital and naval practice, section of general medicine. *1st Pan Am. Med. Congress*, p. 309

248. O'Dwyer, J. (1887). Fifty cases of croup in private practice treated by intubation of the larynx, with a description of the method and the dangers incident thereto. *Med. Rec.*, **32**, 557

249. Matas, R. (1899). On the management of acute traumatic pneumothorax. *Ann. Surg.*, **29**, 409

250. Parham, F.W. (1899). Thoracic resections for tumors growing from the bony wall of the chest. (Discussion by Rudolph Matas) T*rans. South. Surg. Gynecol. Assoc.*, **11**, 223

251. Quenu, E. and Lonquet, F. (1913). Notes sur quelques recherches experimentales concernant la chirurgie thoracique. *C.R. Soc. Biol.*, **48**, 1007, (1896), quoted from Keen, W.W. (ed.) *Surgery: its Principles and Practice*, chap. 149. (Philadelphia: W.B. Saunders)

252. Sauerbruch, F. (1904). Zur Pathologie des offenen Pneumothorax und die Grundlagen meines Verfahrens zu seiner Ausschaltung. *Mitt. Grenzgeb. Med. Chir.*, **13**, 399

253. Sauerbruch, F. (1904). Über die Ausschaltung der schädlichen Wirkung des Pneumothorax bei intrathorakalen Operationen. *Zentralbl. Chir.*, **31**, 146

254. Meyer, H.W. (1955). The history of the development of the negative differential pressure chamber for thoracic surgery. *J. Thorac. Surg.*, **30**, 114

255. Brauer, A. (1904). Mitt. Grenzgebieten, quoted from Keen (ed.), *Surgery*, chap. 149, p. 483

256. Brat and Schmieden (1908). Münch. Med. Woch., quoted from Keen (ed.), *Surgery*, chap. 149, no. 47

257. Tiegel, M. Beit. klin. Chir., quoted from Keen (ed.), *Surgery*, chap. 149, 64, 2

258. Barthélémy and Dufour (1907). L'Anesthésie dans la Chirurgie de la Face, quoted from Keys, History of Surgical Anesthesia. *Presse Med.*, **15**, 475

259. Meltzer, S.J. and Auer, J. (1911). Continuous respiration without respiratory movements. *J. Exp. Med.*, **11**, 662

260. Elsberg, C.A. (1910). The value of continuous intratracheal insufflation of air (Meltzer) in thoracic surgery. *Med. Rec.*, **77**, 493

261. Kirstein, A. (1895). Autokopie des Larynx und der Trachea. *Berliner Klin. Wchnschr.*, **32**, 476–8

262. Jackson, C. (1913). The technique of inserting of intratracheal insufflation tubes. *Surg. Gynecol. Obstet.*, **17**, 507

263. Rowbotham, E.S. and Magill, L. Anesthetics in the plastic surgery of the face and jaws. *Proc. R. Soc. Med.*, vol. 14, part I–II, p. 17

264. Johnson, S.L. (1970). *Op. cit.*, p. 56

265. Jackson, D.E. (1915). A new method for the production of general analgesia and anesthesia with a description of the apparatus used. *J. Lab. Clin. Med.*, **1**, 1

266. Waters, R.M. (1924). Clinical scope and utility of carbon dioxide filtration in inhalation anesthesia. *Curr. Res. Anesth. Analg.*, **3**, 20–2, 26

267. Waters, R.M. (1936). Carbon dioxide absorption from anaesthetic atmospheres. *Proc. R. Soc. Med.*, **30**, 11–12

268. Sword, B.C. (1930). The closed circle method of administration of gas anesthesia. *Curr. Res. Anesth. Analg.*, **9**, 198–202

269. Arens, J.F. (1985). Three decades of cardiac anesthesia. *Mount Sinai J. Med.*, **52**, 516–20

270. *Ibid.*, p. 516

271. *Ibid.*, p. 516

272. Libavius, A. (1954). Appendix Necessaria Syntagmatis Arcanorum Chymicorum (Frankfort, N. Hoffman, 1915), quoted from N.S.R. Maluf: History of Blood Transfusion. *J. Hist. Med.*, **9**, 59

273. Blundell, J. (1824). Researches physiological and pathological; instituted principally with a view to the improvement of medical and surgical practice, quoted from Maluf, *History of Blood Transfusion*. (London: E. Cox & Son)

274. Blundell, J. (1828). Successful case of transfusion, quoted from Maluf, History of Blood Transfusion, *Lancet*, **1**, 431

275. Ponfick, E. (1875). Experimentelle Beitrage zur Lehre von der Transfusion, quoted from Maluf, History of Blood Transfusion. *Virchow's Arch.*, **62**, 273

276. Landois, L. (1875). Die Transfusion des Blutes, quoted from Maluf, *History of Blood Transfusion*. (Leipzig: F.C.W. Vogel)

277. Landsteiner, K. (1901). Ueber Agglutinationserscheinungen normalen menschlichen Blutes. *Wien. Klin. Wschr.*, **14**, 1132

278. Funke, J. (1908). Test to determine the adaptability of the donor's blood to the receiver's blood in transfusion. *Ther. Gaz.*, **32**, 457

279. von Decastello, A. and Sturli, A. (1902). Ueber die Isoagglutinine im Serum gesunder and Kranker Menschen. *Münch. Med. Wschr.*, **49**, 1090

280. Gibbon, J.H. chap. 72, Surgical Technic, from Keen and DaCosta (eds.), *Surgery*, chap. 5, 5, 615

281. Ottenberg, R. (1911). Studies in isoagglutination. I. Transfusion and the question of intravascular agglutination, *J. Exp. Med.*, **13**, 425

282. Crile, G.W. (1907). The technique of direct transfusion of blood. *Ann. Surg.*, **46**, 329

283. Crile, G.W. (1909). Hemorrhage and transfusion, p. 313. (New York: D. Appleton & Co.)

284. Hewson, W. (1774). Experimental inquiries, part the first containing an inquiry into the properties of the blood. With remarks on some of its morbid appearances, quoted from Maluf, *History of Blood Transfusion*. (London: J. Johnson, 1st edn.)

285. Prévost, J.L. and Dumas, J.B.A. (1821). Examen du sang et de son action dans les divers phenomenes de la vie. Ann. Chim. (Phys.), quoted from Maluf, *History of Blood Transfusion*, Vol. 18

286. Arthus, M. and Pagés, C. (1890). Nouvelle

theorie chimique de la coagulation du sang, quoted from Maluf, History of Blood Transfusion. *Arch. Physiol. Norm. Path.*, **2**, 739

287. Lewisohn, R. (1958). The citrate method of blood transfusion in retrospect. *Surgery*, **43**, 325

288. DeBakey, M.E. and Cooley, D.A. (1955). Blood transfusion, the work of Crile and Hustin. *Bull. Soc. Int. Chir.*, **14**, 405

289. Hustin, A. (1914). Principe d'une nouvelle methode de transfusion muqueuse. *J. Med. Brux.*, **12**, 436

290. L'Agote (1915). Nueva procedimiento para la transfusion de sangre. *An. Inst. Model Clin. Med.*, **I**, nos. 1 and 3

291. Lewisohn, R. (1915). A new and greatly simplified method of blood transfusion. *Med. Rec., NY*, **87**, 141

292. Burton, Lee J. Transfusion of blood and its substitutes, from Keen (ed.) *Surgery*, chap. 12, **7**, 323

293. Weil, R. (1915). Sodium citrate in the transfusion of blood. *J. Am. Med. Assoc.*, **64**, 425

294. Rous, P. and Turner, J.R. (1916). The preservation of living red blood cells *in vitro*: I. Methods of preservation. *J. Exp. Med.*, **23**, 219

295. Rous, P. and Turner, J.R. (1916). The preservation of living red blood cells *in vitro*: II. The transfusion of kept cells. *J. Exp. Med.*, **23**, 239

296. Robertson, O.H. (1918). A method of citrate blood transfusion. *Br. Med. J.*, **1**, 477

297. Burton, Lee J. Transfusion of blood and its substitutes, from Keen (ed.) *Surgery*, chap. 12, **7**, 336–7

298. Shamov, V.N. (1937). The transfusion of stored cadaver blood. *Lancet*, **2**, 306

299. Yudin, S.S. (1936). Transfusion of cadaver blood. *J. Am. Med. Assoc.*, **106**, 997

300. Swan, H. and Schecter, D.C. (1962). The transfusion of blood from cadavers: a historical review. *Surgery*, **52**, 549–50

301. Yudin, S.S. (1937). La transfusion du sang de cadavre à l'homme, (Paris: Messon et Cie. 1933) quoted from S. Yudin: Transfusion of stored cadaver blood. *Lancet*, **2**, 361–6

302. Swan and Schecter. *Transfusion of Blood from Cadavers*, p. 546–7

303. Duran Jorda, F. (1939). The Barcelona blood-transfusion service. *Lancet*, **1**, 773–5

304. Saxton, R.S. (1937). The Madrid blood transfusion institute. *Lancet*, **2**, 606–7

305. Ficarra, B.J. (1942). The evolution of blood transfusion. *Ann. Med. Hist.*, **4**, 302–23

306. Fantus, B. (1937). The therapy of the Cook County Hospital. *J. Am. Med. Assoc.*, **109**, 128–31

307. Fantus, B. (1938). Cook County's blood bank. *Modern Hospital*, **50**, 57

308. Cotter, J. and MacNeal, W.J. (1938). Citrate solutions for preservation of fluid blood. *Proc. Soc. Exp. Biol. Med.*, **38**, 757–8

309. Loutit, J.F., Mollison, P.L. and Young, I.M. (1944). Citric acid-sodium citrate-glucose mixtures for blood storage. *Q. J. Exp. Physiol.*, **32**, 183–202

310. Decker, H.R. (1939). Foreign bodies in the heart and pericardium – should they be removed? *J. Thorac. Surg.*, **9**, 62–79

311. Harken, D.E. (1967). *Op. cit.*, ref.3, pp.393–401

312. Harken, D.E. Management of retained foreign bodies in the heart and great vessels, European theater of operations. From *Surgery in World War II*, vol. 2. *Thoracic Surgery*, pp. 353–95

313. Harken, D.E. (1946). A review of the activities of the thoracic center for the III and IV Hospital groups, 160th General Hospital, European theater of operations, June 10, 1944 to Jan. 1, 1945. *J. Thorac. Surg.*, **15**, 31

314. Harken, D.E. and Zoll, P.M. (1946). Foreign bodies in and in relation to the thoracic blood vessels and heart, III. Indications for the removal of intracardiac foreign bodies and the behavior of the heart during manipulation. *Am. Heart J.*, **32**, 1

315. Harken, D.E. and Williams, A.C. (1946). Foreign bodies in and in relation to the thoracic blood vessels and heart. II. Migratory foreign bodies within the blood vascular system. *Am. J. Surg.*, **72**, 80–90

316. Harken, D.E. (1946). Foreign bodies in and in relation to the thoracic blood vessels and heart. I. Techniques for approaching and removing foreign bodies from the chambers of the heart. *Surg. Gynecol. Obstet.*, **83**, 117–25

317. Johnson, S.L. (1970). *Op. cit.*, p. 25

318. *Ibid.*(1970) p. 26

319. Samways, D.W. (1898). Cardiac peristalsis: its nature and effects. *Lancet*, **1**, 927

320. Shumacher, H.B. (1968). Authority, research and publication. Reflections based upon some historical aspect of vascular surgery. *Ann. Surg.*, **168**, 169–82

321. Brunton, L. (1902). Possibility of treating mitral stenosis by surgical methods. *Lancet*, **1**, 352

322. Bourne, C. (1927). The surgical treatment of mitral stenosis. *St Bartholomew's Hosp. J.*, **35**, 22

323. (1902). Surgical operation for mitral stenosis. *Lancet*, **1**, 461

324. Brunton, L. (1902). Surgical operation for mitral stenosis. *Lancet*, **1**, 547

325. Samways, D.W. (1902). Letter to editors. *Lancet*, **1**, 548

326. Fisher, T. (1902). Letter to editors. *Lancet*, **1**, 547

327. Lane, W.A. (1902). Letter to editors. *Lancet*, **1**, 547

328. Shaw, L.E. (1902). Surgical operations for mitral stenosis. *Lancet*, **1**, 619

329. Tollemer, L. (1902). Traitement chirurgical du rétrécissement mitral (d'après Lauder Brunton). *Presse Méd.*, **1**, 233

330. Doyen, E. (1913). Chirurgie des malformations congenitales ou acquises du coeur. *Presse Med.*, **21**, (no. 86), 860

331. Cushing, H. and Branch, J.R.B. (1908). Experimental and clinical notes on chronic valvular lesions in the dog and their possible relation to a future surgery of the cardiac valves. *J. Med. Res.*, **17**, 471–86

332. Bernheim, B.M. (1909). Experimental surgery of the mitral valve. *Bull. Johns Hopkins Hosp.*, **20**, 107–10

333. Jeger, E. (1913). *Die Chirurgie der Blutgefässe und das Herzens*. (Berlin: A. Hirschwald)

334. Allen, D.S. and Graham, E.A. (1922). Intra-cardiac surgery: a new method. *J. Am. Med. Assoc.*, **79**, 1028–30

335. Allen, D.S. (1924). Intracardiac surgery. *Arch. Surg.*, **8**, 317–26

336. Meade, R.H. (1961). *A History of Thoracic Surgery*. (Springfield, Illinois: Charles C. Thomas)

337. Carrel, A. (1914). Experimental operations on the orifices of the heart. *Ann. Surg.*, **60**, 1

338. Tuffier, T. (1913). Etat actuel de la chirurgie intrathoracique XVIIth. *Internat. Congr. Med.*, London, sec. VII, pt. II, p. 247

339. Cutler, E.C. and Levine, S.A. (1923). Cardiotomy and valvulotomy for mitral stenosis. *Boston Med. Surg. J.*, **188**, 1023

340. Harken, D.W. (1967). *Op. cit.*, ref.3, p. 397

341. Souttar, H.S. (1925). Surgical treatment of mitral stenosis. *Br. Med. J.*, **2**, 603

342. Harken, D.W. (1967). *Op. cit.*, ref.3, p. 397

343. Cutler, E.C. and Beck, C.S. (1929). The present status of the surgical procedures in chronic valvular disease of the heart: final report of all surgical cases. *Arch. Surg.*, **18**, 403–16

344. Pribram, B.O.A. (1926). *Operative Behandlung der Mitralstenose*, 50. (Berlin: Tagung der deutschen Gesellschaft für Chirurgie)

345. Smithy, H.G., Pratt-Thomas, H.R. and Dryerle, H.P. (1948). Aortic valvulotomy. Experimental methods with early results. *Surg. Gynecol. Obstet.*, **86**, 513

346. Smithy, H.G., Boone, J.A. and Stallworth, J.M. (1950). Surgical treatment of constrictive valvular disease of the heart. *Surg. Gynecol. Obstet.*, **90**, 175–92

347. Bailey, C.P., Glover, R.P., O'Neill, T.J.E. and Redondo-Ramirez, H.P. (1950). Experiences with the experimental surgical relief of aortic stenosis. Preliminary report. *J. Thorac. Surg.*, **20**, 516

348. Mackenzie, J. and Orr, J. (1923). *Principles of Diagnosis and Treatment in Heart Affections*, 2nd edn. (London: Henry Frowde and Hodder and Stoughton)

349. Lewis, T. (1946). *Diseases of the Heart*, 4th edn., pp. 154 and 159. (London: Macmillan)

350. Murray, G., Wilkinson, F.R. and MacKenzie, R. (1938). Reconstruction of the valves of the heart. *Can. Med. Assoc. J.*, **38**, 317–19

351. Murray, G. (1950). The surgical treatment of mitral stenosis. *Can. Med. Assoc. J.*, **62**, 444–7

352. Murray, G. (1950). Treatment of mitral valve stenosis by resection and replacement of valve under direct vision. *Arch. Surg.*, **61**, 903–12

353. Bailey, C.P. (1949). The surgical treatment of mitral stenosis. *Dis. Chest.*, **15**, 377–97

354. Meade, R.H. (1961). Correspondence to Meade by Bailey. *Op. cit.*, p. 440

355. Bailey, C.P. Personal communication. In *Growth of Cardiac Surgery*, p. 27

356. Bailey, C.P., Glover, R.P. and O'Neill, T.J.E. (1950). The surgery of mitral stenosis. *J. Thorac. Surg.*, **19**, 16–45

357. Bailey, C.P. and Bolton, H.E. (1956). Criteria for and results of surgery for mitral stenosis. *NY J. Med.*, **56**, 825–39

358. Harken, D.E., Ellis, L.B., Ware, P.F. and Norman, L.R. (1948). The surgical treatment of mitral stenosis. I. Valvuloplasty. *N. Engl. J. Med.*, **239**, 804

359. Harken, D.E., Ellis, L.B. and Norman, L.R. (1950). The surgical treatment of mitral stenosis: progress in developing controlled valvuloplastic technique. *J. Thorac. Surg.*, **19**, 1–15

360. Ellis, L.B. and Harken, D.E. (1964). Closed valvuloplasty for mitral stenosis: a twelve year study of 1571 patients. *N. Engl. J. Med.*, **270**, 643

361. Harken, D.E., Ellis, L.B. and Norman, L.R. (1950). The surgical treatment of mitral stenosis. II. Progress in developing a controlled valvuloplastic technique. *J. Thorac. Surg.*, **19**, 1–15

362. Harken, D.E., Dexter, L., Ellis, L.B., Farrand, R.E. and Dickson, J.F. III (1951). The surgery of mitral stenosis. III. Finger-fracture valvuloplasty. *Ann. Surg.*, **134**, 722–41

363. Bailey, C.P., Bolton, H.E. and Redondo-Ramirez, H.P. (1952). Surgery of the mitral valve. *Surg. Clin. N. Am.*, pp. 1807–48

364. Baker, C., Brock, R.C. and Campbell, M. (1950). Valvulotomy for mitral stenosis: report of six successful cases. *Br. Med. J.*, **1**, 1283

365. Brock, R.C. (1948). Pulmonary valvulotomy for the relief of congenital pulmonary stenosis: report of three cases. *Br. Med. J.*, **1**, 1121

366. Sellors, T.H. (1948). Surgery of pulmonary stenosis: a case in which the pulmonary valve was successfully divided. *Lancet*, **1**, 988

367. Harken, D.E. (1980). Quoted in: Wertenbaker, L. *To Mend the Heart*, pp. 30–1. (New York: Viking Press)

368. Sweet, R.H. and Bland, E.F. (1949). The surgical relief of congestion in the pulmonary circulation in cases of severe mitral stenosis: preliminary report of 6 cases treated by means of anastomosis between pulmonary and systemic venous systems. *Ann. Surg.*, **130**, 384–97

369. (1948). A venous shunt for marked mitral stenosis: cases from the medical grand rounds, Massachusetts General Hospital. *Am. Pract.* **2**, 156–6

370. Dubost, C., Oteifa, G. and Blondeau, P. (1954). Le problème technique de la commissurotomie mitrale: résultats obtenus par la dilatation instrumentale de la sténose. *Mém. Acad. Chir.*, **80**, 321–9

371. Dubost, C., Blondeâu, P. and Pinwica, A. (1962). Instrumental dilatation using the transatrial approach in the treatment of mitral stenosis: a survey of 1,000 cases. *J. Thorac. Cardiovasc. Surg.*, **44**, 392–407

372. Edwards, F.R. (1964). Instrumental transatrial mitral valvotomy. *Dis. Chest*, **46**, 223–5

373. Logan, A. (1957). The transventricular route for mitral valvulotomy. *Kardiol. Pol.*, **1**, 49–50

374. Logan, A. and Turner, R. (1959). Surgical treatment of mitral stenosis with particular reference to the transventricular approach with a mechanical dilator. *Lancet*, **2**, 874–80

375. Tubbs, O.S. (1962). Transventricular mitral valvotomy. *Ned. Tidschr. Geneesk.*, **106**, 335

376. Romanos, A.N. and Derom, F.E. (1955). Scissors for posteromedial commissurotomy in mitral stenosis. *Lancet*, **2**, 1175

377. Bailey, C.P. and Hirose, T. (1958). Maximal reconstruction of the stenotic mitral valve by neostrophingic mobilization (rehinging of the septal leaflet). *J. Thorac. Surg.*, **35**, 559–83

378. Becker, O. (1872). Über die sichtbaren Erscheinungen der Blutbewegunginder menschlichen Netzhaut. *Arch. Opthalmol.*, **18**, 206

379. Klebs, E. (1976). Ueber operative Verletzingen der Herzklappen und deren Folgen. *Prager Med. Wochenschr.*, **1**, 29–36

380. Gross, R.E. and Hufnagel, C.A. (1945). Coarctation of the aorta: experimental studies regarding its surgical correction. *N. Engl. J. Med.*, **233**, 237

381. Glenn, W.W.L., Jaeger, C., Harned, H.S., Whittemore, R., Goodyer, A.V.N., Janzen, A. and Gentsch, T.O. (1955). The diverticulum approach to the chambers of the heart and great vessels. *Surgery*, **38**, 872

382. Carrel, A. (1910). On the experimental surgery of the thoracic aorta and the heart. *Ann. Surg.*, **52**, 83–95

383. Litvak, R.S. (1971). The growth of cardiac surgery: historical notes. *Cardiovasc. Clin.*, **3**, 5

384. *Ibid.*, p. 19

385. Tedeschi, C.G. and Nahas, H.C. (1955). The pericardial graft in mitral insufficiency (a morphological study of the aging graft). *Dis. Chest*, **28**, 599–609

386. Botwin, A.E. (1954). Pedunculated atrial flaps used for experimental cardiac surgery. *J. Thorac. Surg.*, **28**, 300–4

387. Chalnot, P., Benichoux, R., Chardot, C. and Fritsch, R. (1954). L'insuffisance mitrale expérimentale et sa correction par une prothèse matière plastique. *Arch. Mal. Coeur*, **47**, 315–21

388. Benichoux, R. and Chalnot, P. (1955). A method for the surgical correction of mitral insufficiency. *J. Thorac. Surg.*, **30**, 148–58

389. Carter, M.G., Gould, J.M. and Mann, B.F. Jr (1953). Surgical treatment of mitral insufficiency: an experimental study. *J. Thorac. Surg.*, **26**, 574–81

390. Johns, T.N.P. and Blalock, A. (1954). Mitral insufficiency: the experimental use of a mobile polyvinyl sponge prosthesis. *Ann. Surg.*, **140**, 335–41

391. DeWall, R.A., Warden, H.E., Lillehei, C.W. and Varco, R.L. (1956). A prosthesis for the palliation of mitral insufficiency. *Dis. Chest*, **30**, 133–40

392. Denton, G.R., Seymour, T. and Wiggers, H. (1953). A follow-up report on the development of a plastic prosthesis for the atrioventricular

valve. *Surg. Forum*, **4**, 83–7

393. Wible, J.H., Jacobson, L.F., Jordan, P. Jr and Johnston, C.G. (1956). Spring valve prosthesis for the control of valvular insufficiency. *Surg. Forum*, **7**, 230–2

394. Jordan, P. Jr and Wible, J. (1955). Spring valve for mitral insufficiency: preliminary report. *AMA Arch. Surg.*, **71**, 468–74

395. Ellison, R.G., Major, R.C., Pickering, R.W. and Hamilton, W.F. (1952). Further experiences with a technique of producing mitral stenosis of controlled degree. *Surg. Forum*, **3**, 305–11

396. McAllister, F.F. and Fitzpatrick, H.F. (1956). Constriction of the mitral annulus in the correction of certain types of mitral insufficiency and as an aid in by-passing the left ventricle. *Surgery*, **40**, 54–8

397. Kay, E.B. and Cross, F.S. (1955). Surgical treatment of mitral insufficiency: experimental observations. *J. Thorac. Surg.*, **29**, 618–20

398. Davila, J.C., Mattson, W.W. Jr, O'Neill, T.J.E. and Glover, R.P. (1954). A method for the surgical correction of mitral insufficiency. I. Preliminary considerations. *Surg. Gynecol. Obstet.*, **98**, 407–12

399. Davila, J.C., Glover, R.P., Trout, R.G., Mansure, F.S., Wood, N.E., Janton, O.H. and Iaia, B.D. (1955). Circumferential suture of the mitral ring: a method for the surgical correction of mitral insufficiency. *J. Thorac. Surg.*, **30**, 531–60

400. Borrie, J. (1954). Mitral regurgitation: circular suture tightening the A–V ring. *Proc. Univ. Otago M. School*, **32**, 24–6

401. Borrie, J. (1955). Mitral insufficiency: experimental circular suture around the atrioventricular ring. *J. Thorac. Surg.*, **30**, 687–97

402. Bailey, C.P., Jamison, W.L., Bakst, A.E., Bolton, H.E., Nichols, H.T. and Gemeinhardt, W. (1954). The surgical correction of mitral insufficiency by the use of pericardial grafts. *J. Thorac. Surg.*, **28**, 551–603

403. Johnson, A.S. (1956). A single surgical method for the correction of mitral regurgitation using the finger ring valve elevator. *J. Thorac. Surg.*, **32**, 557–61

404. Harken, D.E., Black, H., Ellis, L.B. and Dexter, I. (1954). The surgical correction of mitral insufficiency. *J. Thorac. Surg.*, **28**, 604–24

405. Davila, J.C., Glover, R.P., Voci, G., Jumbala, P., Trout, R.G. and Fritz, A.J. (1958). The clinical and physiologic criteria for surgical correction of mitral insufficiency. *J. Thorac. Surg.*, **35**, 206–29

406. Glover, R.P. and Davila, J.C. (1957). Surgical treatment of mitral insufficiency by total circumferential purse-string suture of the mitral ring. *Circulation*, **15**, 661–81

407. Glover, R.P. and Davila, J.C. (1957). The treatment of mitral insufficiency by the purse-string technique: initial clinical application. *J. Thorac. Surg.*, **33**, 75–101

408. Davila, J.C. and Glover, R.P. (1958). Circumferential suture of the mitral valve for the correction of regurgitation. *Am. J. Cardiol.*, **2**, 267–75

409. Harken, D.E., Black, H., Dexter, I. and Ellis, L.B. (1953). The surgical correction of mitral insufficiency. *Surg. Forum*, **4**, 4–7

410. Fay, T. and Henny, G.C. (1938). Correlation of foreign body segmental temperature and its relation to the location of carcinomatous metastasis. *Surg. Gynecol. Obstet.*, **66**, 512–24

411. Smith, L.W. and Fay, T. (1939). Temperature factors in cancer and embryonal cell growth. *J. Am. Med. Assoc.*, **113**, 653–60

412. Fay, T. (1940). Observations on prolonged human refrigeration. *NY State J. Med.*, **40**, 135–54

413. Smith, L.W. (1940). Refrigeration in cancer. *NY State J. Med.*, **40**, 1355–61

414. Bigelow, W.G., Lindsay, W.K. and Greenwood, W.F. (1950). Hypothermia; its possible role in cardiac surgery. An investigation of factors governing survival in dogs at low body temperatures. *Ann. Surg.*, **132**, 849–66

415. Bigelow, W.G., Lindsay, W.K., Harrison, R.C., Gordon, R.A. and Greenwood, W.F. (1950). Oxygen transport and utilization in dogs at low body temperatures. *Am. J. Physiol.*, **160**, 125–37

416. Bigelow, W.G., Callaghan, J.C. and Hopps, J.A. (1950). General hypothermia for experimental intracardiac surgery. *Ann. Surg.*, **132**, 531–9

417. Bigelow, W.G., Lindsay, W.K. and Greenwood, W.F. (1950). Hypothermia. *Ann. Surg.*, **132**, 849–66

418. Bigelow, W.G., Hopps, J.A. and Callaghan, J.A. (1952). Radiofrequency rewarming in resuscitation from severe hypothermia. *Can. J. Med. Sci.*, **30**, 185–93

419. Lewis, J.F. and Taufic, M. (1953). Closure of atrial septal defects with the aid of hypothermia; experimental accomplishments and the report of one successful case. *Surgery*, **33**, 52–9

420. Swan, H., Zeavin, I. and Blount, S.G. Jr (1953). Surgery of direct vision in the open heart during hypothermia. *J. Am. Med. Assoc.*, **153**, 1081–5

421. Swan, H. and Zeavin, I. (1954). Cessation of circulation in general hypothermia. III.

Technics of intracardiac surgery under direct vision. *Ann. Surg.*, **139**, 385–96

422. Cookson, B.A., Neptune, W.B. and Bailey, C.P. (1952). Hypothermia as a means of performing intracardiac surgery under direct vision. *Dis. Chest*, **22**, 245–60

423. Cookson, B.A., Neptune, W. and Bailey, C.P. (1952). Intracardiac surgery with hypothermia. *J. Int. Coll. Surg.*, **18**, 685–94

424. Boerema, I., Wildschut, W., Schmidt, W.J.H. and Broekhuysen, L. (1951). Experimental researches into hypothermia as an aid in the surgery of the heart. *Arch. Chir. Neerl.*, **3**, 25

425. Delorme, E.J. (1952). Experimental cooling of the blood-stream. *Lancet*, **2**, 914–15

426. Sellors, T.H. (1960). Atrial septal defects. *Minerva Cardioangiol. Eur.*, **8**, 172–83

427. Ross, D.N. (1954). Hypothermia. *Guy's Hosp. Rep.*, **103**, 97–138

428. Ross, D.N. (1954). Venous cooling: a new method of cooling the blood stream. *Lancet*, **1**, 1108–9

429. Brock, Sir R. and Ross, D.N. (1955). Hypothermia. *Guy's Hosp. Rep.*, **104**, 99–113

430. Horiuchi, T., Koyamada, K., Matano, I., Mohri, H., Komatsu, T., Honda, T., Abe, T., Ishitoya, T., Sagawa, Y., Matsuzawa, K., Matsumura, M., Tsuda, T., Ishizawa, E., Ishikawa, S., Suzuki, H. and Saito, Y. (1963). Radical operation for ventricular septal defect in infancy. *J. Thorac. Cardiovasc. Surg.*, **46**, 180

431. Hikasa, Y., Shirotani, H., Satomura, K., Muraoka, R., Abe, K., Tsushimi, K., Yokota, Y., Miki, S., Kawai, J., Mori, A., Okamoto, Y., Koie, H., Ban, T., Kanzaki, Y. and Yokata, M. (1967). Open heart surgery in infants with the aid of hypothermic anesthesia. *Archiv Japan Chirugie.*, **36**, 495

432. Eloesser, L. (1970). Milestones in chest surgery. *J. Thorac. Cardiovasc. Surg.*, **60**, 157

433. La Gallois, C.J. (1813). *Experiments on the Principle of Life.* (translated by Nancrede, N.C. and J.G.). (Philadelphia: M. Thomas)

434. Prévost, J.L. and Dumas, J.B. (1821). Examen du sang et de son action dans les divers phénomènes de la vie. *Ann. Chimie*, **18**, 280–96

435. Loebell, C.E. (1849). De conditionibus quibus secretiones in glandulis perficiuntur. *Diss Marburgi Cattorum: typ Elwerti*

436. Ludwig, C. and Schmidt, A. (1869). Das Verhalten der Gase, Welche mit dem Blut durch die reizbaren Säugethiermuskelz strömen. *Arb. Physiol. Annst. Leipz.*, **3**, 1–61

437. Bidder, E. (1862). *Beiträge zur Lehre von der Function der Nieren.* (Dorpat: E.J. Karow)

438. von Schröder, W. (1881–82). Uber die Bildungsstätte des Harnstoffs. *Arch. Exp. Pathol. Pharrankol, Leipzig*, **14–15**, 377

439. Jacobi, C. (1890). Apparat zur Durshblutung isolirter überlebender organe. *Arch. Path. Pharm.*, **26**, 388–400

440. Brodie, T.G. (1903). The perfusion of surviving organs. *J. Physiol.*, **29**, 255–75

441. Hooker, D.R. (1915). The perfusion of the mammalian medulla: the effect of calcium and of potassium on the respiratory and cardiac centers. *Am. J. Physiol.*, **38**, 200–8

442. Clark, L.C. Jr, Gollan, F. and Gupta, V.B. (1950). The oxygenation of blood by gas dispersion. *Science*, **III**, 85–7

443. von Frey, M. and Gruber, M. (1885). Ein respirations-apparat fur isolirte organe. *Arch. Physiol.*, **9**, 519–32

444. Richards, A.N. and Drinker, C.K. (1915). An apparatus for the perfusion of isolated organs. *J. Pharmacol. Exp. Ther.*, **7**, 467–83

445. Bayliss, L.E., Fee, A.R. and Ogden, E. (1928). A method of oxygenating blood. *J. Physiol.*, **66**, 443–8

446. Daly, I.D. and Thorpe, W.V. (1933). An isolated mammalian heart preparation capable of performing work for prolonged periods. *J. Physiol.*, **79**, 199–217

447. Björk, V.O. (1948). Brain perfusions in dogs with artificially oxygened blood. *Act. Chir. Scand.*, **96** (suppl. 137), 1–122

448. Cross, F.S. *et al.* (1956). Evaluation of a rotating disc type reservoir oxygenator. *Proc. Soc. Exp. Biol. Med.*, **93**, 210–14

449. Jongbloed, J. (1949). The mechanical heart-lung system. *Surg. Gynec. Obstet.*, **89**, 684–91

450. Jongbloed, J. (1951). Observations on dogs with mechanically sustained circulation and respiration. *J. Appl. Physiol.*, **3**, 642–8

451. Dale, H.H. and Schuster, E.H.J. (1928). A double perfusion-pump. *J. Physiol.*, **64**, 356–64

452. Carrel, A. and Lindbergh, C.A. (1935). The culture of whole organs. *Science*, **81**, 621–3

453. Gibbon, J.H. Jr (1937). Artificial maintenance of circulation during experimental occlusion of pulmonary artery. *Arch. Surg.*, **34**, 1105–31

454. Dogliotti, A.M. and Costantini, A. (1951). Primo caso di applicazione all' uomo di un apparecchio di circolazione sanguigna extracorporea. *Minerva Chir.*, **6**, 657–9

455. Sewell, W.H. Jr and Glenn, W.W.L. (1950).

Experimental cardiac surgery: I. Observation on the action of a pump designed to shunt the venous blood past the right heart directly into the pulmonary artery. *Surgery*, **28**, 474–94

456. Glenn, W.W. (1980). Some account of the early years of cardiac surgery. *Connecticut Med.*, **44**, 338–44

457. Clowes, G.H.A. Jr (1951). Experimental procedures for entry into the left heart to expose the mitral valve. *Ann. Surg.*, **134**, 957–68

458. Dodrill, F.D. *et al.* (1953). Pulmonary valvuloplasty under direct vision using the mechanical heart for a complete by-pass of the right heart in a patient with congenital pulmonary stenosis. *J. Thorac. Surg.*, **26**, 584–97

459. Lillehei, C.W. (1982). A personalized history of extracorporeal circulation. *Trans. Am. Soc. Art. Intern. Org.*, **28**, 5–16

460. Blum, L. and Megibow, S. (1950). Exclusion of the dog heart by parabiosis. *J. Mount Sinai Hosp. NY*, **17**, 38

461. Warden, H.E., Cohen, M., Read, R.C. and Lillehei, C.W. (1954). Controlled cross circulation for open intracardiac surgery. *J. Thorac. Surg.*, **28**, 331–43

462. Warden, H.E., Cohen, M., DeWall, R.A., Schultz, E.A., Buckley, J.J., Read, R.C. and Lillehei, C.W. (1954). Experimental closure of intraventricular septal defects and further physiologic studies on controlled cross circulation. *Surg. Forum*, **5**, 22–8

463. Lillehei, C.W., Cohen, M., Warden, H.E., Ziegler, N.R. and Varco, R.L. (1955). The result of direct vision closure of ventricular septal defects in 8 patients by means of controlled cross circulation. *Surg. Gynecol. Obstet.*, **101**, 447

464. Lillehei, C.W., Cohen, M., Warden, H.E., Read, R.C., Aust, J.B., DeWall, R.A. and Varco, R.L. (1955). Direct vision intracardiac surgical correction of the tetralogy of Fallot, pentalogy of Fallot, and pulmonary atresia defects, report of the first 10 cases. *Ann. Surg.*, **142**, 418

465. Lillehei, C.W., Cohen, M., Warden, H.E. and Varco, R.L. (1955). The direct-vision intracardiac correction of congenital anomalies by controlled cross circulation. *Surgery*, **38**, 11–29

466. Lillehei, C.W., Cohen, M., Warden, H.E., Read, R.C., DeWall, R.A., Aust, J.B. and Varco, R.L. (1955). Direct vision intracardiac surgery, Henry Ford Hospital. *International Symposium of Cardiovascular Surgery*, p. 371. (Philadelphia: W. B. Saunders)

467. Southworth, J.L. and Peirce, E.C. II (1952). Cross circulation for intracardiac surgery. *Arch. Surg.*, **64**, 58

468. Warden, H.E., Read, R.C., DeWall, R.A., Aust, J.B., Cohen, M., Ziegler, N.R., Varco, R.L. and Lillehei, C.W. (1955). Direct vision intracardiac surgery by means of a reservoir of 'arterialized venous' blood. *J. Thorac. Surg.*, **30**, 649–57

469. Sugarman, H.J., Wesolowski, S.A., Anzolo, J. and Welch, C.S. (1951). The use of an isolated homologous lung as a donor oxygenator. *Bull. N. Engl. Med. Center*, **13**, 107

470. Potts, W.J., Riker, W.L., DuBord, R. and Andrews, C.E. (1952). Maintenance of life by homologous lung and mechanical circulation. *Surgery*, **31**, 161

471. Mustard, W.T., Chute, A.L. and Simmons, E.H. (1952). Further observations on experimental extracorporeal circulation. *Surgery*, **32**, 803

472. Mustard, W.T., Chute, A.L., Keith, J.D., Sirak, A., Rowe, R.D. and Vlad, P. (1954). A surgical approach to transposition of the great vessels with extracorporeal circuit. *Surgery*, **36**–7

473. Campbell, G.S., Crisp, N.W. and Brown, E.B. Jr (1956). Total cardiac by-pass in humans utilizing a pump and heterologous lung oxygenator (dog lungs). *Surgery*, **40**, 364–71

474. *Ibid.*

475. Dennis, C., Spreng, D.S. Jr, Nelson, G.E., Karlson, K.E., Nelson, R.M., Thomas, J.V., Eder. W.P. and Varco, R.L. (1951). Development of a pump-oxygenator to replace the heart and lungs; an apparatus applicable to human patients and application to one case. *Ann. Surg.*, **134**, 709

476. Melrose, D.G. (1953). A mechanical heart-lung for use in man. *Br. Med. J.*, **ii**, 57–62

477. Melrose, D.G., Bassett, J.W., Beaconsfield, P., Graber, I.G. and Shackman, R. (1953). Experimental physiology of a heart-lung machine in parallel with normal circulation. *Br. Med. J.*, **ii**, 62–6

478. Aird, I., Melrose, D.G., Cleland, W.P. and Lynn, R.B. (1954). Assisted circulation by pump-oxygenator during operative dilation of the aortic valve in man. *Br. Med. J.*, **i**, 1284–7

479. Clark, L.C. Jr, Gollan, F. and Gupta, V.B. (1950). The oxygenation of blood by gas dispersion. *Science*, **111**, 85

480. Clark, L.C., Hooven, F. and Gollan, F. (1952). A large capacity, all-glass dispersion oxygenator and pump. *Rev. Sci. Instr.*, **23**, 748

481. Helmsworth, J.A., Clark, L.C. Jr, Kaplan, S., Sherman, R.T. and Largen, T. (1952). Artificial oxygenation and circulation during complete by-pass of the heart. *J. Thorac. Surg.*, **24**, 117

482. Helmsworth, J.A., Clark, L.C. Jr, Kaplan, S. and Sherman, R.T. (1953). An oxygenator-pump for use in total by-pass of heart and lungs. *J. Thorac. Surg.*, **26**, 617

483. Lillehei, C.W., DeWall, R.A., Read, R.C., Warden, H.E. and Varco, R.L. (1956). Direct vision intracardiac surgery in man using a simple disposable artificial oxygenator. *Dis. Chest*, **29**, 1

484. DeWall, R.A., Warden, H.E., Read, R.C., Gott, V.L., Ziegler, N.R., Varco, R.L. and Lillehei, C.W. (1956). A simple, expendable artificial oxygenator for open heart surgery. *Surg. Clin. North Am.*, **36**, 1025

485. Gott, V.L., DeWall, R.A., Paneth, M., Zuhdi, M.N., Weirich, W., Varco, R.L. and Lillehei, C.W. (1957). A self-contained disposable oxygenator of plastic sheet for intracardiac surgery. Experimental development and clinical application. *Thorax*, **12**, 1

486. Gott, V.L., Sellers, R.D., DeWall, R.A., Varco, R.L. and Lillehei, C.W. (1957). A disposable unitized plastic sheet oxygenator for open-heart surgery. *Dis. Chest*, **32**, 615

487. Hyman, E.S., Rosenberg, D., Hyman, A.L., Sayegh, S. and Kable, R. (1956). A simple artificial heart-lung: an approach to open heart surgery. Preliminary report. *J. Louisiana State Med. Soc.*, **108**, 134

488. Rygg, I.H. and Kyvsgaard, E. (1957). A disposable polyethylene oxygenator system applied to a heart-lung machine. *Acta Chir. Scand.*, **112**, 433

489. DeBakey, M. (1934). A simple continuous-flow blood transfusion instrument. *New Orleans Med. Sci. J.*, **87**, 386–9

490. Cooley, D.A. (1989). Recollections of early development and later trends in cardiac surgery. *J. Thorac. Cardiovasc. Surg.*, **98**, 817–22

491. Kolff, W.J., Effler, D.B., Groves, L.K. and Sones, F.M. Jr (1956). Disposable membrane oxygenator (heart lung machine) and its use in experimental surgery. *J. Thorac. Surg.*, **32**, 620

492. Clowes, G.H.A., Hopkins, A.L. and Neville, W.E. (1956). An artificial lung dependent upon diffusion of oxygen and carbon dioxide through plastic membranes. *J. Thorac. Surg.*, **32**, 630

493. Gentsch, T.O., Bopp, R.K., Siegel, J.H., Cev, M. and Glenn, W.W.L. (1960). Experimental and clinical use of a membrane oxygenator. *Surgery*, **47**, 301

494. Peirce, E.C. II (1962). The membrane lung: a critical study of a new multiple point support for Teflon film. *Surgery*, **52**, 777

495. Bramson, M.L., Osborn, J.J., Main, F.B., O'Brien, M.F., Wright, J.S. and Gerbode, F. (1965). A new disposable membrane oxygenator with integral heat exchange. *J. Thorac. Cardiovasc. Surg.*, **50**, 391

496. Lande, A.J., Parker, B., Subramanian, V., Carlson, R.G. and Lillehei, C.W. (1968). Methods for increasing the efficiency of a new dialyzer-membrane oxygenator. *Trans. Am. Soc. Artif. Intern. Organs*, **14**, 227

497. Lee, W.H. Jr, Krumhaar, D., Fonkalsrud, E.W., Schjeide, O.A. and Maloney, J.V. Jr (1961). Denaturation of plasma proteins as a cause of morbidity and death after intracardiac operations. *Surgery*, **50**, 29

498. Lee, W.H. Jr, Krumhaar, D., Derry, G., Sachs, D., Lawrence, S.H., Clowes, G.H.A. Jr and Maloney, J.V. Jr (1961). Comparison of the effects of membrane and nonmembrane oxygenators on the biochemical and biophysical characteristics of blood. *Surg. Forum*, **12**, 200

499. Gollan, F., Hoffman, J.E. and Jones, R.M. (1954). Maintenance of life of dogs below 10°C without hemoglobin. *Am. J. Physiol.*, **179**, 640

500. Neptune, W.B., Bougas, J.A. and Panico, F.G. (1960). Open-heart surgery without the need for donor-blood priming in the pump-oxygenator. *N. Engl. J. Med.*, **263**, 111

501. Gibbon, J.H. (1978). The development of the heart-lung apparatus. *Am. J. Surg.*, **135**, 608–19

502. Lillehei, C.W., Gott, V.L., DeWall, R.A. and Varco, R.L. (1957). Surgical correction of pure mitral insufficiency by annuloplasty under direct vision. *Lancet*, 446–9

503. Lillehei, C.W., Gott, V.L., DeWall, R.A. and Varco, R.L. (1958). The surgical treatment of stenotic or regurgitant lesions of the mitral and aortic valves by direct vision utilizing a pump-oxygenator. *J. Thorac. Surg.*, **35**, 154–90

504. Merendino, K.A. and Bruce, R.A. (1957). One hundred seventeen surgically treated cases of valvular rheumatic heart disease; with preliminary report of two cases of mitral regurgitation treated under direct vision with aid of a pump-oxygenator. *J. Am. Med. Assoc.*, **164**, 749–55

505. Nichols, H.T., Blanco, G., Uricchio, J.F. and Likoff, W. (1961). Open-heart surgery for mitral regurgitation and stenosis. *Arch. Surg.*, **82**, 128–36

506. Belcher, J.R. (1964). The surgical treatment of mitral regurgitation. *Br. Heart J.*, **26**, 513–23

507. Barratt-Boyes, B.G. (1963). Surgical correction of mitral incompetence resulting from bacterial endocarditis. *Br. Heart J.*, **25**, 415–20

508. Barnard, C.N. and Schrire, V. (1961). Surgery of mitral incompetence. *Postgrad. Med. J.*, **37**, 666–78

509. King, H., Su, C.S. and Jontz, J.G. (1960). Partial replacement of the mitral valve with synthetic fabric. *J. Thorac. Cardiovasc. Surg.*, **40**, 12–16

510. Johnson, F.E., Bascom, J.U., Peterson, T.A., Kiser, J.C., Telander, R.L., Bascom, J.F. and Farley, H.H. (1962). Prosthetic patch reconstruction of the aortic leaflet of the mitral valve in dogs. *Surg. Gynecol. Obstet.*, **114**, 426–30

511. Spencer, F.C. (1961). Discussion. In Merendino, K.A. *Prosthetic Valves for Cardiac Surgery*, pp. 224–6. (Springfield, Illinois: Charles C. Thomas)

512. Sauvage, L.R., Wood, S.J., Bill, A.H. Jr and Logan, G.A. (1962). Pericardial autografts in the mitral valve: a preliminary report. *J. Thorac. Cardiovasc. Surg.*, **44**, 67–72

513. Merendino, K.A., Thomas, G.I., Jesseph, J.E., Herron, P.W., Winterscheid, L,C. and Vetto, R.R. (1959). The open correction of rheumatic mitral regurgitation and/or stenosis; with special reference to regurgitation treated by posteromedial annuloplasty utilizing a pump-oxygenator. *Ann. Surg.*, **150**, 5–22

514. Frater, R.W.M. (1964). Anatomical rules for the plastic repair of a diseased mitral valve. *Thorax*, **19**, 458–64

515. Ellis, F.H. Jr, Frye, R.L. and McGoon, D.C. (1966). Results of reconstructive operations for mitral insufficiency due to ruptured chordae tendineae. *Surgery*, **59**, 165–72

516. McGoon, D.C. (1960). Repair of mitral insufficiency due to ruptured chordae tendineae. *J. Thorac. Cardiovasc. Surg.*, **39**, 357–62

517. Kay, J.H. and Egerton, W.S. (1963). The repair of mitral insufficiency associated with ruptured chordae tendineae. *Ann. Surg.*, **157**, 351–60

518. Kay, J.H., Tsuji, H.K. and Redington, J.V. (1965). The surgical treatment of mitral insufficiency associated with torn chordae tendineae. *Ann. Thorac. Surg.*, **1**, 269–75

519. Sanders, C.A., Scannell, J.G., Harthorne, J.W. and Austen, W.G. (1965). Severe mitral regurgitation secondary to ruptured chordae tendineae. *Circulation*, **31**, 506–16

520. Morris, J.D., Penner, D.A. and Brandt, R.L. (1964). Surgical correction of ruptured chordae tendineae. *J. Thorac. Cardiovasc. Surg.*, **48**, 772–80

521. Morris, J.D., Sloan, H., Wilson, W.S. and Brandt, R.L. (1962). An appraisal of clinical results in open mitral valvuloplasty. *J. Thorac. Cardiovasc. Surg.*, **43**, 17–32

522. Kay, J.H., Egerton, W.S. and Zubiate, P. (1961).The surgical treatment of mitral insufficiency and combined mitral stenosis and insufficiency with use of the heart-lung machine. *Surgery*, **50**, 67–73

523. Kay, J.H., Magidson, O. and Meihaus, J.E. (1962). The surgical treatment of mitral insufficiency and combined mitral stenosis and insufficiency using the heart-lung machine. *Am. J. Cardiol.*, **9**, 300–6

524. Wooler, G.H., Nixon, P.G.F., Grimshaw, V.A. and Watson, D.A. (1962). Experiences with the repair of the mitral valve in mitral incompetence. *Thorax*, **17**, 49–57

525. Carpentier, A. *et al.* (1980). Reconstructive surgery of mitral valve incompetence. *J. Thorac. Cardiovasc. Surg.*, **79**, 338

526. Gott, V.L., DeWall, R.A., Gonzales, J.L., Hodges, P.C., Varco, R.L. and Lillehei, C.W. (1957). The direct vision surgical correction of pure mitral insufficiency by use of annuloplasty or a valvular prosthesis. *Univ. Minnesota M. Bull.*, **29**, 69–79

527. Barnard, C.N., McKenzie, M.B. and Schrire, V. (1961). A surgical approach to mitral insufficiency. *Br. J. Surg.*, **48**, 655–62

528. McKenzie, M.B. (1960). The mitral valve: an experimental study with special reference to problems in the design and testing of a mobile prosthesis for the surgical correction of mitral insufficiency. *Thesis*, University of Capetown

529. Schimert, G., Sellers, R.D., Lee, C.B., Bilgutay, A.M. and Lillehei, C.W. (1961). Fabrication of mitral leaflets and aortic cusps from Silastic rubber-coated Teflon felt. In Merendino, K.A. *Prosthetic Valves for Cardiac Surgery*, pp. 368–84. (Springfield, Illinois: Charles C. Thomas)

530. Frater, R.W.M., Berghuis, J., Brown, A.L. Jr and Ellis, F.H. Jr (1963). Autogenous pericardium for posterior mitral leaflet replacement. *Surgery*, **54**, 260–8

531. Ellis, F.H. Jr (1961). Discussion. In Merendino, K.A. *Prosthetic Valves for Cardiac Surgery*, pp. 281–4. (Springfield, Illinois: Charles C. Thomas)

532. Ellis, F.H. Jr and Callahan, J.A. (1961). Clinical application of a flexible monocusp prosthesis: report of a case. *Proc. Staff Meet. Mayo Clin.*, **36**, 605–9

533. Ellis, F.H. Jr, McGoon, D.C., Brandenburg, R.O. and Kirklin, J.W. (1963). Clinical experience with total mitral valve replacement with prosthetic valves. *J. Thorac. Cardiovasc. Surg.*, **46**, 482–93

534. Young, W.P., Gott, V.L. and Rowe, G.G. (1965). Open-heart surgery for mitral valve disease, with special reference to a new prosthetic valve. *J. Thorac. Cardiovasc. Surg.*, **50**, 827–34

535. Braunwald, N.S., Cooper, T. and Morrow, A.G. (1961). Clinical and experimental replacement of the mitral valve: experience with the use of a flexible polyurethane prosthesis. In Merendino, K.A. *Prosthetic Valves for Cardiac Surgery*, pp. 307–19. (Springfield, Illinois: Charles C. Thomas)

536. Starr, A. and Edwards, M.L. (1961). Mitral replacement: clinical experience with a ball-valve prosthesis. *Ann. Surg.*, **154**, 726–40

537. Starr, A., Edwards, M.L. and Griswold, H. (1962). Mitral replacement: late results with a ball valve prosthesis. *Progr. Cardiovasc. Dis.*, **5**, 298–312

538. Starr, A. and Edwards, M.L. (1963). Mitral replacement: late results with a ball valve prosthesis. *J. Cardiovasc. Surg.*, **4**, 435–47

539. Swanson, J.S. and Starr, A. (1989). The ball valve experience over three decades. *Ann. Thorac. Surg.*, **48**, 551–2

540. Black, M.M., Drury, P.J. and Tindale, W.B. (1983). Twenty-five years of heart valve substitutes: a review. *J. R. Soc. Med.*, **76**, 667–80

541. Hufnagel, C.A. (1951). Aortic plastic valvular prosthesis. *Bull. Georgetown Univ. Med. Center.*, **4**, 128–30

542. Starr, A. (1961). Discussion. In Merendino, K.A. (ed.) *Prosthetic Valves for Cardiac Surgery*, p. 319. (Springfield, Illinois: Charles C. Thomas)

543. Herr, R., Starr, A., McCord, C.W. and Wood, J.A. (1965). Special problems following valve replacement: embolus, leak, infection, red cell damage. *Ann. Thorac. Surg.*, **1**, 403–10

544. Starr, A., Herr, R.H. and Wood, J.A. (1965). The present status of valve replacement. In *VII Congress of the International Cardiovascular Society*, Philadelphia, September 16–18, (Suppl. to J. Cardiovasc. Surg.), pp. 95–103

545. Morrow, A.G., Clark, W.D., Harrison, D.C. and Braunwald, E. (1964). Prosthetic replacement of the mitral valve: operative methods and the results of preoperative and postoperative hemo-dynamic assessments. *Circulation*, **29** (suppl. 1), 2–13

546. Cooley, D.A., Nelson, T.G., Beall, A.C. Jr and DeBakey, M.E. (1964). Prosthetic replacement of cardiac valves: results in 242 patients. *Dis. Chest*, **46**, 339–45

547. Beall, A.C. Jr, Bricker, D.L., Cooley, D.A. and DeBakey, M.E. (1965). Ball-valve prostheses. In surgical management of acquired valvular heart disease. *Arch. Surg.*, **90**, 720–31

548. Björk, V.O. (1964). The surgical treatment of mitral insuficiency: a comparison between annuloplastic procedures and total mitral valve replacement. *Thoraxchirurgie*, **12**, 291–5

549. Blondeau, P., d'Allaines, C., Pinwica, A., Cachera, J.P., Guilmet, D. and Dubost, C. (1965). Chirurgie de l'insuffisance mitrale. *Arch. Mal. Coeur*, **58**, 476–88

550. Windsor, H.M. and Shanahan, M. (1964). Mitral valve replacement. *Med. J. Aust.*, **2**, 613–18

551. Harken, D.E. I. (1965). A new caged-ball aortic and mitral valve and II. Monitoring and controlled respiration in critically ill patients. *J. Mt. Sinai Hosp. NY*, **32**, 93–106

552. Harken, D.E., Soroff, H.S., Taylor, W.J., Lefemine, A.A., Gupta, S.K. and Lunzer, S. (1960). Partial and complete prostheses in aortic insufficiency. *J. Thorac. Cardiovasc. Surg.*, **40**, 744

553. Smeloff, E.A., Cartwright, R.S., Cayler, G.G., Fong, W.Y. and Huntley, A.C. (1964). Clinical experience with a titanium double-caged full orifice ball valve. Read at the *VIII International Congress on Diseases of the Chest*, Mexico City

554. Magovern, G.J. and Cromie, H.W. (1963). Sutureless prosthetic heart valves. *J. Thorac. Cardiovasc. Surg.*, **46**, 726–36

555. Magovern, G.J., Kent, E.M., Cromie, H.W., Cushing, W.B. and Scott, S. (1964). Sutureless aortic and mitral prosthetic valves: clinical results and operative technique on sixty patients. *J. Thorac. Cardiovasc. Surg.*, **48**, 346–57

556. Magovern, G.J, Kent, E.M. and Cushing, W.B. (1966). Sutureless mitral valve replacement. *Ann. Thorac.Surg.*, **2**, 474–80

557. Barnard, C.N., Goosen, C.C., Holmgren, L.V. and Schrire, V. (1962). Prosthetic replacement of the mitral valve. *Lancet*, **2**, 1087–9

558. Hufnagel, C.A., Vilkgas, P.D. and Nahas, H. (1958). Experience with new types of aortic valvular prostheses. *Ann. Surg.*, **147**, 639

559. Schwartz, D.C. and Kaplan, S. (1966). The caged ball valve circa 1858. *Am. J. Cardiol.*, **18**, 942

560. Hammond, G.L., Laks, H. and Geha, A.S. (1980). Development of aortic valve prostheses. *Connecticut Med.*, **44**, 348–52

561. Emery, R.W., Anderson, R.W., Lindsay, W.G., Jorgenson, C.R. *et al.* (1979). *Surg. Forum*, **30**, 235–8

562. Ross, D.N. (1962). *Lancet*, **2**, 487

563. Wain, W.H., Greco, R., Ignegeri, A., Bodnar, E. and Ross, D.N. (1979). *International Journal of Artificial Organs*, **3**, 169–172, Woodroof, E.A. In Ionescu, M. I. (ed.) *Tissue Heart Valves*, p. 349. (London: Butterworths)

564. Ross, D.N. (1967). *Lancet*, **2**, 956

565. Senning, A. (1966). *Acta Chirurg. Scand. Suppl.*, **356B**, 17–20

566. Senning, A. (1971). *Thoraxchirurgie*, **19**, 304–8

567. Kaiser, G.A., Hancock, W.D., Lukban, S.B. and Litwak, R.S. (1969). *Surg. Forum*, **20**, 137–8

568. Edwards Laboratories Technical Bulletin (1976). *Carpentier-Edwards Bioprostheses.* (California: Edwards Laboratories)

569. Ionescu, M.I., Mary, D.A.S. and Abid, A. (1971). In Stalpaert, G. *et al.* (eds.) *Late Results of Valvular Replacements and Coronary Surgery*, p. 56. (Ghent: European Press)

570. Black, M.M., Drury, P.J. and Tindale, W.B. (1982). *Proceedings of the European Society for Artificial Organs*, **9**, 116–19

571. Carpentier, A. (1989). From valvular xenograft to valvular bioprosthesis: 1965–70. *Ann. Thorac. Surg.*, **48**, 573–4

572. Smeloff, E.A. (1989). Comparative study of heart valve design in the 1960s. *Ann. Thorac. Surg.*, **48**, 531–2

573. Siposs, G.G. (1989). Memoirs of an early heart-valve engineer. *Ann. Thorac. Surg.*, **48**, 56–7

574. Paton, B.C. and Vogel, J.H.K. (1985). Introduction: valve replacement: the first quarter century. *JACC*, **6**, 897–8

575. Brock, R. (1965). The development of heart surgery in children. *Arch. Dis. Child.*, **40**, 123

576. Munro, J.C. (1907). Ligation of the ductus arteriosus. *Ann. Surg.*, **46**, 335

577. Warren, R. (1984). Patent ductus arteriosus. *J. Am. Med. Assoc.*, **251**, 1203–7

578. Graybiel, A., Strieder, J.W. and Boyer, N.H. (1938). An attempt to obliterate the patent ductus arteriosus in a patient with subacute bacterial endarteritis. *Am. Heart J.*, **15**, 621

579. Jones, J.C., Dolley, F.S. and Bullock, L.T. (1940). The diagnosis and surgical therapy of patent ductus arteriosus. *J. Thorac. Surg.*, **9**, 413

580. Gross, R.E. and Hubbard, J.P. (1939). Surgical ligation of a patent ductus arteriosus. Report of first successful case. *J. Am. Med. Assoc.*, **112**, 729

581. Bourne, G., Keele, K.D., Tubbs, O.S. and Swain, R.H.A. (1941). Ligation and chemotherapy for infection of patent ductus arteriosus, with note on bacteriology. *Lancet*, **2**, 444–6

582. Tubbs, O.S. (1944). The effect of ligation on infection of the patent ductus arteriosus. *Br. J. Surg.*, **32**, 1–12

583. Crafoord, C. and Nylin, K.G.V. (1945). Congenital coarctation of the aorta and its surgical treatment. *J. Thorac. Surg.*, **14**, 347–61

584. Cleland, W.P. (1983). The evolution of cardiac surgery in the United Kingdom. *Thorax*, **38**, 887–96

585. Blalock, A. and Taussig, H.B. (1945). The surgical treatment of malformations of the heart in which there is pulmonary stenosis or pulmonary atresia. *J. Am. Med. Assoc.*, **128**, 189

586. Levy, S.E. and Blalock, A. (1939). Experimental observations on the effects of connecting by suture the left main pulmonary artery to the systemic circulation. *J. Thorac. Surg.*, **8**, 525

587. Taussig, H.B. (1965). On the evolution of our knowledge of congenital malformations of the heart. *Circulation*, **31**, 768–77

588. McNamara, D.G. (1984). The Blalock-Taussig operation and subsequent progress in surgical treatment of cardiovascular diseases. *J. Am. Med. Assoc.*, **251**, 2139–41

589. Baffes, T.G. (1987). Willis J. Potts: his contribution to cardiovascular surgery. *Ann. Thorac. Surg.*, **44**, 92–6

590. Potts, W.J., Smith, S. and Gibson, S. (1946). Anastomosis of the aorta to a pulmonary artery, certain types in congenital heart disease. *J. Am. Med. Assoc.*, **132**, 627

591. Glenn, W.W.L. (1958). Circulatory bypass of the right side of the heart. IV. Shunt between superior vena cava and distal right pulmonary artery – report of a clinical application. *N. Engl. J. Med.*, **259**, 117

592. Waterston, D.J. (1962). Treatment of Fallot's tetralogy in children under one year of age. *Rozhl. Chir.*, **41**, 181

593. Cooley, D.A. and Hallman, G.L. (1966). Intrapericardial aortic-right pulmonary arterial anastomosis. *Surg. Gynec. Obst.*, **122**, 1084

594. Gazzaniga, A.B., Lamberti, J.J., Siewers, R.D., Sperling, D.R., Dietrick, W.R., Arcilla, R.A. and Replogle, R.L. (1976). Arterial prosthesis of microporous expanded polytetrafluoroethylene for construction of aorta-pulmonary shunts. *J. Thorac. Cardiovasc. Surg.*, **72**, 357

595. Brock, R.C. (1948). Pulmonary valvotomy for the relief of congenital pulmonary stenosis.

Report of three cases. *Br. Med. J.*, **i**, 1121–6

596. Sellors, T.H. (1948). Surgery of pulmonary stenosis. *Lancet*, **1**, 988–9

597. Kirklin, J.W., Blackstone, E.H., Pacifico, A.D. *et al.* (1979). Routine primary repair vs two-stage repair of tetralogy of Fallot. *Circulation*, **60**, 373–85

598. De Laval, M.R., McKay, R., Jones, M. *et al.* (1981). Modified Blalock-Taussig shunt: use of subclavian artery orifice as flow regulator in prosthetic systemic pulmonary artery shunts. *J. Thorac. Cardiovasc. Surg.*, **81**, 112–19

599. Cohn, R. (1947). An experimental method for the closure of interauricular septal defects in dogs. *Am. Heart J.*, **33**, 453–7

600. Murray, G. (1948). Closure of defects in cardiac septa. *Ann. Surg.*, **128**, 843–53

601. Bailey, C.P., Downing, D.F., Geckeler, C.D., Likoff, W., Goldberg, H., Scott, J.C., Janton, O. and Redondo-Ramirez (1952). Congenital interatrial communications: clinical and surgical considerations with a description of a new surgical technic: atrio-septo-pexy. *Ann. Int. Med.*, **37**, 905–6

602. Dodrill, F.D. (1949). A method for exposure of the cardiac septa. *J. Thorac. Surg.*, **18**, 652–60

603. Marion, P. and Termet, H. (1950). Traitement chirurgical de la communication interauriculaire. *Lyon Chir.*, **45**, 583

604. Swan, H., Maresh, G., Johnson, M.E. and Warner, G. (1950). The experimental creation and closure of auricular septal defects. *J. Thorac. Surg.*, **20**, 542–51

605. Bailey, C.P., Bolton, H.E., Jamison, W.L. and Neptune, W.B. (1953). Atrio-septo-pexy for interatrial septal defects. *J. Thorac. Surg.*, **26**, 187

606. Hufnagel, C.A. and Gillespie, J.F. (1951). Closure of interauricular septal defects. *Bull. Georgetown Univ. Med. Center*, **4**, 137–9

607. Bailey, C.P., Downing, D.F., Geckeller, G.D., Likoff, W., Goldberg, H., Scott, J.C., Janton, O. and Redondo-Ramirez, H.P. (1952). Congenital interatrial communications: clinical and surgical considerations with a description of a new surgical technic: atrio-septo-pexy. *Ann. Intern. Med.*, **37**, 905

608. Gross, R.E., Pomeranz, A.A., Watkins, E. Jr and Goldsmith, E.I. (1952). Surgical closure of defects of the interauricular septum by use of an atrial well. *N. Engl. J. Med.*, **247**, 455

609. Watkins, E. Jr, Pomeranz, A.A., Goldsmith, E.I. and Gross, R.E. (1952). Experimental closure of atrial septal defects: techniques of an 'Atrial

Well' operation. *Surg. Forum*, **3**, 247–52

610. Gross, R.H., Pomeranz, A.A., Watkins, E. Jr and Goldsmith, E.I. (1952). Surgical closure of defects of the interauricular septum by use of an atrial well. *N. Engl. J. Med.*, **247**, 455–60

611. Gross, R.E., Watkins, E. Jr, Pomeranz, A.A. and Goldsmith, E.I. (1953). A method for surgical closure of interauricular septal defects. *Surg. Gynecol. Obstet.*, **96**, 1–23

612. Rashkind, W.J. and Miller, W.W. (1966). Creation of an atrial septal defect without thoracotomy: a palliative approach to complete transposition of the great arteries. *J. Am. Med. Assoc.*, **196**, 991–1

613. McNamara, D.G. (1983). Twenty-five years of progress in the medical treatment of pediatric and congenital heart disease. *JACC*, **1**, 164–273

614. McMillan, I.K.R., Johnson, A.M. and Machell, E.S. (1965). Total correction of tetralogy of Fallot in young children. *Br. Med. J.*, **i**, 348–50

615. Francois-Franck, C.A. (1899). Signification physiologique de la resection du sympathique dans la maladie de Basedow, l'eplepsie, l'idiote et la glaucome. *Bull. Acad. Natl. Med.*, (Paris) **4**, 565

616. Jonnesco, T. (1920). Angine de poitrine guerie par la resection du sympathetique cervico-thoracique. *Bull. Acad. Med.*, **84**, 93

617. Hudson, C.L., Moritz, A.R. and Wearn, J.T. (1932). The extracardiac anastomoses of the coronary arteries. *J. Exp. Med.*, **56**, 919

618. Moritz, A.R., Hudson, C.L. and Orgain, E.S. (1932). Augmentation of the extracardiac anastomoses of the coronary arteries through pericardial adhesions. *J. Exp. Med.*, **56**, 927

619. Beck, C.S. (1935). The development of a new blood supply to the heart by operation. *Ann. Surg.*, **102**, 801

620. O'Shaughnessy, L. (1936). An experimental method of providing a collateral circulation to the heart. *Br. J. Surg.*, **23**, 665

621. Obituary (1940). Laurence O'Shaughnessy. *Lancet*, **1**, 1100–01

622. Davies, D.T., Mansell, H.E. and O'Shaughnessy, L. (1938). Surgical treatment on angina pectoris and allied conditions. *Lancet*, **1**, 1

623. Vansant, J.R. and Muller, W.H. Jr (1960). Surgical procedures to revascularize the heart. A review of the Literature. *Am. J. Surg.*, **100**, 572–83

624. Beck, C.S. (1937). Coronary sclerosis and angina pectoris: treatment by Grafting a new blood supply upon the myocardium. *Surg. Gynecol. Obstet.*, **64**, 270

625. Wearn, J.T., Mettier, S.R., Klumpp, T.G. and Zschiesche, L.J. (1933). The nature of the vascular communications between the coronary arteries and the chambers of the heart. *Am. Heart J.*, **9**, 143–64

626. Gross, L. and Blum, L. (1935). Effects of coronary artery occlusion on dogs heart with total coronary sinus ligation. *Proc. Soc. Exp. Biol. Med.*, **32**, 1578–80

627. Beck, C.S. and Mako, A.E. (1941). Venous stasis in the coronary circulation; an experimental study. *Am. Heart J.*, **21**, 767–69

628. Beck, C.S., Stanton, E., Batiuchok, W. and Leiter, E. (1948). Revascularization of heart by graft of systemic artery with coronary sinus. *J. Am. Med. Assoc.*, **137**, 436–42

629. Beck, C.S. (1958). Coronary artery disease after twenty-five years. *J. Thorac. Cardiovasc. Surg.*, **36**, 329–51

630. Vineberg, A.M. (1946). Development of an anastomosis between the coronary vessels and a transplanted internal mammary artery. *Can. Med. Assoc. J.*, **55**, 117

631. McGoon, D.C. (1987). Prologue: from whence? *Cardiovascular Clinics*, **17**, 25

632. Vineberg, A.M. (1975). Medical news section. *J. Am. Med. Assoc.*, **234**, 693–4

633. Harken, D.E. (1968). Coronary artery disease: rest, repair or replacement. *J. Mt Sinai Hosp.*, **35**, 541–65

634. *Ibid.*

635. Smith, B.M., Hodes, R., Hall, H. *et al.* (1957). Auxiliary myocardial vascularization by prosthetic graft implantation. *Surg. Gynecol. Obstet.*, **104**, 263–8

636. Sabiston, D.C. Jr, Fauteaus, J.P. and Blalock, A. (1957). Experimental studies of the fate of arterial implants in the left ventricular myocardium. *Ann. Surg.*, **145**, 927–42

637. Olearchyk, A.S. (1988). Vasilii I. Kolesov: a pioneer of coronary revascularization by internal mammary-coronary artery grafting. *J. Thorac. Cardiovasc. Surg.*, **96**, 13–18

638. Kolesov, V.I. and Potashov, L.V. (1965). Operations on the coronary arteries. *Exp. Chir. Anaesth.*, **10**, 3–8

639. Kolesov, V.I. (1965). Contemporary problems in surgical treatment of coronary disease of the heart. Main lecture. (Leningrad: Meditsina Publishing Leningrad)

640. Kolesov, V.I. (1966). Coronary-thoracic anastomosis as a means of treating coronary heart disease. *Klin. Med.*, **7**, 7–12

641. Kolesov, V.I., (ed.) (1966). *Surgical Treatment of Coronary Disease of the Heart.* (Leningrad: Meditsina Publishing Leningrad)

642. Kolesov, V.I. (1967). The first experience in the treatment of angina pectoris by the establishment of coronary-systemic vascular anastomoses. *Kardiologiia*, **4**, 20–5

643. Kolesov, V.I. (1967). Mammary artery-coronary artery anastomosis as method of treatment for angina pectoris. *J. Thorac. Cardiovasc. Surg.*, **54**, 535–44

644. Kolesov, V.I. (1977). *The Surgery of Coronary Arteries of the Heart.* (Leningrad: Meditsina Publishing Leningrad)

645. Olearchyk, A.S. (1988). *Op. cit.*, p. 13

646. Kolesov, V.I., Kolesov, E.V. and Volodkovich, N.G. (1970). Mammary artery-coronary artery anastomosis as method of treatment for angina and myocardial infarction. *Khirurgiia*, **1**, 151–2

647. Kolesov, V.I., Kolesov, E.V. and Volodkovich, N.G. (1970). Treatment of acute and chronic coronary insufficiency by means of arterial shunting: cardiovascular research. *Abstracts of the Sixth World Congress on Cardiology, London*

648. Olearchyk, A.S. (1988). Coronary revascularization: past, present and future. *J. Ukr. Med. Assoc. N. Am.*, **35**, 3–29

649. Olearchyk, A.S. (1988). *Op. cit.*, p. 17

650. Effler, D.B. (1988). Vasilii I. Kolesov: pioneer in coronary revascularization. *J. Thorac. Cardiovasc. Surg.*, **96**, 183

651. Murray, G., Porcheron, R., Hilario, J. *et al.* (1954). Anastomosis of a systemic artery to the coronary. *Can. Med. J.*, **71**, 594

652. Bailey, C.P., May, A. and Lemon, W. (1957). Survival after coronary endarterectomy in man. *J. Am. Med. Assoc.*, **164**, 641–6

653. Longmire, W.P. Jr, Cannon, J.A. and Kattus, A.A. (1958). Direct-vision coronary endarterectomy for angina pectoris. *N. Engl. J. Med.*, **259**, 993–9

654. DeMarchi, G., Battezzati, M. and Tagliaferro, A. (1956). Influenze della legatura della arterie mammarie interne sulla insufficienza miocardica. *Minerva Medica*, **47**, 1184–95

655. Glover, R.P., Davila, J.C., Kyle, R.H. *et al.* (1957). Ligation of the internal mammary arteries as a means of increasing blood supply to the myocardium. *J. Thorac. Surg.*, **34**, 661–78

656. McGoon, D.C. (1987). *Op. cit.,* p. 6

657. Sauvage, L.R., Wood, S.J., Eyer, K.M. *et al.* (1963). Experimental coronary artery surgery. Preliminary observations of bypass venous grafts, longitudinal arteriotomies, and end-to-end

anastomoses. *J. Thorac. Cardiovasc. Surg.*, **46**, 826

658. Garrett, H.E., Dennis, E.W. and DeBakey, M.E. (1973). Aortocoronary bypass with saphenous vein graft. *J. Am. Med. Assoc.*, **223**, 792

659. Edwards, W.S. and Edwards, P.D. (1974). *Alexis Carrel, Visionary Surgeon.* (Springfield, Ill.: Charles C. Thomas)

660. Effler, D.B. (1978). Quoted by Comroe, J.H. Jr. In: *Retrospectroscope*, 2nd edn. (Menio Park, CA: Von Gehr)

661. Sabiston, D.C. Jr (1974). The coronary circulation. *Johns Hopkins Med. J.*, **134**, 314–29

662. Effler, D.B., Groves, L.K., Jones, F.M. Jr and Shirey, E.K. (1964). Endarterectomy in the treatment of coronary artery disease. *J. Thoracic Cardiovasc. Surg.*, **47**, 98–108

663. Effler, D.B., Goves, L.K., Suarez, E.L. and Favaloro, R.G. (1967). Direct coronary artery surgery with endarterectomy and patch-graft reconstruction. Clinical application and technical consideration. *J. Thorac. Cardiovasc. Surg.*, **53**, 101

664. Garrett, H.E., Dennis, E.W. and DeBakey, M.E. (1973). *Op. cit.*

665. Favaloro, R.G. (1968). Saphenous vein autograft replacement of severe segmental coronary artery occlusion. *Ann. Thorac. Surg.*, **5**, 334–9

666. Favoloro, R.G. (1983). The present era of myocardial revascularization – some historical landmarks. *Int. J. Cardiol.*, **4**, 331–44

667. Johnson, W.D., Flemma, R.J., Lepley, D. Jr and Ellison, E.H. (1969). Extended treatment of severe coronary artery disease: a total surgical approach. *Ann. Surg.*, **170**, 460–70

668. Bailey, C.P. and Hirose, T. (1968). Successful internal mammary – coronary arterial anastomosis using a minivascular suturing technique. *Int. Surg.*, **49**, 416–27

669. Green, G.E., Stertzer, S.H. and Reppent, E.H. (1968). Coronary arterial bypass grafts. *Ann. Thorac. Surg.*, **5**, 443–50

670. Green, G.E. (1972). Internal mammary – coronary artery anastomosis: three-year experience with 165 patients. *Ann. Thorac. Surg.*, **14**, 260–5

671. Edwards, W.S., Jones, W.B., Dear, H.D. and Kerr, A.R. (1970). Direct surgery for coronary artery disease: technique for left anterior descending coronary artery bypass. *J. Am. Med. Assoc.*, **211**, 1182–5

672. Loop, F.D., Spampinato, N., Cheanvechai, C. and Effler, D.B. (1973). The free internal mammary artery bypass graft. *Ann. Thorac. Surg.*, **15**, 53–6

673. Kay, E.B., Naraghipour, H., Beg, R.A., Demaney, M., Tambe, A. and Zimmerman, H.A. (1974). Long term follow up of internal mammary artery bypass. *Ann. Thorac. Surg.*, **18**, 269–75

674. Bernstein, B.B. (1986). The pursuit of the artificial heart. *Med. Heritage*, **2**, 80–100

675. Ross, R. (1923). *Memoirs.* (London: John Murray)

676. Chernin, E. (1988). *The Vivisector Vivisected, Perspectives in Biology and Medicine*, Spring, pp. 341–52

677. Akutsu, T. and Kolff, W.J. (1958). Permanent substitutes for valves and hearts. *Trans. Am. Soc. Artif. Intern. Organs*, **4**, 230

678. Kusserow, B.K. (1958). A permanently indwelling intracorporeal blood pump to substitute for cardiac function. *Trans. Am. Soc. Artif. Intern. Organs*, **4**, 227

679. Kolff, W.J. (1959). Mock circulation to test pumps designed for permanent replacement of damaged hearts. *Cleveland Clin. Q.*, **26**, 223

680. Hastings, F.W., Potter, W.H. and Molter, J.W. (1961). Artificial intracorporeal heart. *Trans. Am. Soc. Artif. Intern. Organs*, **7**, 323

681. Cooley, D.A., Liotta, D., Hallman, G.L., Bloodwell, R.D., Leachman, R.D. and Milam, J.D. (1969). Orthotopic cardiac prosthesis for two-staged cardiac replacement. *Am. J. Cardiol.*, **24**, 723

682. Hall, C.W. (1988). When did artificial heart implants begin? Letter to the editor. *J. Am. Med. Assoc.*, **259**, 1650

683. (1986). *New Options, New Dilemmas: an Inter-Professional Approach to Life or Death Decisions*, p.85. (Lexington, Mass: Lexington Books)

684. Cowart, V.S. (1988). When did artificial heart implants begin? Letter to the editor (in reply to Hall's letter). *J. Am. Med. Assoc.*, **259**, 1650

685. Dennis, C. (1969). In Gibbon, J.A., Sabiston, D.C. and Spencer, F.C. (eds.) *Assisted Circulation in Surgery of the Chest.* (Philadelphia: W.B. Saunders Co.)

686. Clauss, R.H., Birtwell, W.C., Albertal, G., Lunzer, S., Taylor, W.J., Fosberg, A.M. and Harken, D.E. (1961). Assisted circulation. I. The arterial counterpulsator. *J. Thorac. Cardiovasc. Surg.*, **41**, 447

687. Moulopoulos, S.C., Topaz, S. and Kolff, W.J. (1962). Diastolic balloon pumping (with carbon dioxide) in the aorta: mechanical assistance to the failing circulation. *Am. Heart J.*, **63**, 669

688. Schilt, W., Freed, P.W., Khalil, G. and

Kantrowitz, A. (1967). Temporary non-surgical intra-arterial cardiac assistance. *Trans. Am. Soc. Artif. Intern. Organs*, **13**, 322

689. Carrel, A. and Guthrie, C. (1905). The transplantation of veins and organs. *Am. Med.*, **10**, 1101

690. Carrel, A. (1907). The surgery of blood vessels. *Johns Hopkins. Hosp. Bull.*, **18**, 18

691. Mann, F.C., Priestley, J.T., Markowitz, J. and Yater, W.M. (1933). Transplantation of the intact mammalian heart. *Arch. Surg.*, **26**, 219

692. Demikhov, V.P. (1949). Homoplastic transplantation of the heart and lungs in warm-blooded animals (dogs). In *Problems of Thoracic Surgery*. (Medigiz)

693. Demikhov, V.P. (1950). Experimental homoplastic replacement of the heart and lungs. *Ibid.*, no. 5

694. Demikhov, V.P. (1950). A new and simpler variant of heart-lung preparation of a warm-blooded animal. *Ibid.*, no. 7

695. Demikhov, V.P. (1951). Experimental transplantation of the heart and lungs. Transactions of the AMN SSSR. *Problems of Clinical and Experimental Surgery*

696. Demikhov, V.P. (1952). Demonstration of the operation and of a dog with replaced heart and lungs at an extramural session of the AMN SSSR in Ryazan in 1950. Discussion. In *Nervous Regulation of the Circulation and Respiration*, p. 170. Transactions of the AMN SSSR

697. Demikhov, V.P. (1956). Transplantation of the heart and lungs and methods of preventing death during operation on the thoracic organs. *Transactions of the 26th All-Union Congress of Surgeons, Moscow*

698. Demikhov, V.P. (1959). Transplantation of the heart and lungs experimentally. *Trans. Acad. Med. Sci. USSR*, **12**, 18

699. Demikhov, V.P. (1962). *Experimental Transplantation of Vital Organs*. Authorized translation from the Russian by Basil Haigh. (New York: Consultants Bureau)

700. Sinitsyn, N.P. (1945). Homotransplantation of the frog's heart. *Usp. Sovrem. Biol.*, **19**, 2, 277

701. Demikhov, V.P. (1948). *Transplantation of the Heart as a New Method in Experimental Biology and Medicine*. Medigz

702. Demikhov, V.P. (1951). The ECG of the transplanted frog's heart. *Byull. Eksp. Biol. Med.*, **31** (2), 93

703. Goldberg, M., Berman, E.F. and Akman, L.C. (1958). Homologous transplantation of the canine heart. *J. Int. Coll. Surg.*, **30**, 575

704. Cass, M.H. and Brock, R.C. (1959). Heart excision and replacement. *Guy's Hosp. Rep.*, **180**, 285

705. Hardy, J.D., Chavez, C.M., Kurrus, R.D. *et al.* (1964). Heart transplantation in man: developmental studies and report of a case. *J. Am. Med. Assoc.*, **188**, 1132

706. Medawar, P.B. (1944). The behaviour and fate of skin autografts and skin homografts in rabbits. *J. Anat.*, **78**, 176

707. Medawar, P.B. (1961). Immunologic tolerance. *Nature (London)*, **189**, 14

708. Lower, R.R. and Shumway, N.E. (1960). Studies on orthotopic homotransplantation of the canine heart. *Surg. Forum*, **11**, 18

709. Barnard, C.N. (1967). The operation. *S. Afr. Med. J.*, **41**

710. Bernard, C. (1865). *Introduction à l'étude de la médicine expérimentale*. (Paris: Baillière)

711. Barnard, C. (1987). Reflections on the first heart transplant. *S. Afr. Med. J.*, **72**, 19–22

712. Shinebourne, E.A. (1984). Ethics of innovative cardiac surgery. *Br. Heart J.*, **52**, 597–601

713. DeVries, W.C., Anderson, J.L. and Joyce, L.D. (1984). Clinical use of the total artificial heart. *N. Engl. J. Med.*, **310**, 273–8

714. Dotter, C.T. and Judkins, M.P. (1964). Transluminal treatment of arteriosclerotic obstruction: description of a new technique and a preliminary report of its application. *Circulation*, **30**, 654

715. Dotter, C.T., Rosch, J. and Judkins, M.P. (1968). Transluminal dilatation of atherosclerotic stenosis. *Surg. Gynecol. Obstet.*, **127**, 794

716. Dotter, C.T. (1980). Transluminal angioplasty: a long view. *Radiology*, **135**, 561

717. Zeitler, E., Schoop. W. and Zahnow, W. (1971). The treatment of occlusive arterial disease by transluminal catheter angioplasty. *Radiology*, **99**, 19

718. Gruentzig, A. and Kumpe, D.A. (1979). Technique of percutaneous transluminal angioplasty with the Gruentzig balloon catheter. *Am. J. Radiol.*, **132**, 547

719. Gruentzig, A., Kuhlmann, U., Vetter, W., Luetof, U., Meier, B. and Siegenthaler, W. (1978). Treatment of renovascular hypertension with percutaneous transluminal dilatation of a renal-artery stenosis. *Lancet*, **1**, 801

720. Gruentzig, A.R., Senning, A. and Siegenthaler, W.E. (1979). Non-operative dilatation of coronary artery stenosis: percutaneous

transluminal coronary angioplasty. *N. Engl. J. Med.*, **301**, 61

721. Hurst, J.W. (1986). Andreas Roland Grüntzig: a free-spirited genius. *Cardiology*, **73**, 189–95

722. Kent, K.M., Bentivoglio, L.G., Block, P.C. *et al.* (1982). Percutaneous transluminal coronary angioplasty: report from the registry of the National Heart, Lung, and Blood Institute. *Am. J. Cardiol.*, **49**, 2011

723. Kent, K.M., Mullin, S.M. and Passamani, E.R. (eds.) (1984). Proceedings of the National Heart, Lung, and Blood Institute Workshop on the outcome of percutaneous transluminal angioplasty. *Am. J. Cardiol.*, **53**, IC

724. Barbash, G.I., Rabkin, M.T., Kane, N.M. and Baim, D.S. (1986). Coronary angioplasty under the prospective payment system: the need for a swift adjusted payment scheme. *J. Am. Coll. Cardiol.*, **8**, 784

725. Wohlgelernter, D., Cleman, M., Highman, H.A. and Zaret, B.L. (1986). Percutaneous transluminal coronary angioplasty of the culprit lesion for the management of unstable angina pectoris in patients with multivessel coronary artery disease. *Am. J. Cardiol.*, **58**, 460

726. DeFeyter, P.J., Serruys, P.W., Van den Brand, M., Balakumaran, K., Mochtar, B., Soward, A.L., Arnold, A.E.R. and Hugenholtz, P.G. (1985). Emergency coronary angioplasty in refractory unstable angina. *N. Engl. J. Med.*, **313**, 342

727. Braunwald, E. (1985). The aggressive treatment of acute myocardial infarction. *Circulation*, **71**, 1087

728. Meyer, J., Merx, W., Schmitz, H., Erbel, R., Kiesslich, T., Dorr, R., Lambertz, H., Bethge, C., Krebs, W., Bardos, P., Minale, C., Messmer, B.J. and Effert, S. (1982). Percutaneous transluminal coronary angioplasty immediately after intracoronary streptolysis of transmural myocardial infarction. *Circulation*, **66**, 905

729. Hartzler, G.O., Rutherford, B.D., McConahay, D.R., Johnson, W.L., McCallister, B.D., Gura, G.A., Conn, R.C. and Crockett, J.E. (1983). Percutaneous transluminal coronary angioplasty with and without thrombolytic therapy for treatment of acute myocardial infarction. *Am. Heart J.*, **106**, 965

730. Douglas, J.D., Gruentzig, A.R., King, S.B., Hollman, J., Ischinger, T., Meier, B., Craver, J.M., Jones, E.L., Waller, J.L., Bone, D.K. and Guyton, R. (1983). Percutaneous transluminal coronary angioplasty in patients with prior coronary bypass surgery. *J. Am. Coll. Cardiol.*, **2**, 745

731. Block, P.C., Cowley, M., Kaltenbach, M., Kent, K.M. and Simpson, J. (1984). Percutaneous angioplasty of stenoses of bypass grafts or of bypass graft anastomotic sites. *Am. J. Cardiol.*, **53**, 666

732. Waller, B.F., Rothbaum, D.A., Garfinkel, H.J., Ulbright, T.M., Linnemeir, T.J. and Berger, S.M. (1984). Morphologic observations after percutaneous transluminal balloon angioplasty of early and late aortocoronary saphenous vein bypass grafts. *J. Am. Coll. Cardiol.*, **4**, 784

733. Kan, J.S., White, R.I., Mitchell, S.E. and Gardner, T.J. (1982). Percutaneous balloon valvuloplasty: a new method for treating congenital pulmonary valve stenosis. *N. Engl. J. Med.*, **307**, 540

734. Kan, J.S., White, R.I., Mitchell, S.E., Anderson, J.H. and Gardner, T.J. (1984). Percutaneous transluminal balloon valvuloplasty for pulmonary valve stenosis. *Circulation*, **69**, 554

735. Walls, J.T., Lababidi, Z., Curtis, J.J. and Silver, D. (1984). Assessment of percutaneous balloon pulmonary and aortic valvuloplasty. *J. Thorac. Cardiovasc. Surg.*, **88**, 352

736. Lababidi, Z., Wu, J. and Walls, J.T. (1984). Percutaneous balloon aortic valvuloplasty: results in 23 patients. *Am. J. Cardiol.*, **53**, 194

737. Lock, J.E., Khalilullah, M., Shrivastava, S., Bahl, V. and Keane, J.I. (1985). Percutaneous catheter commissurotomy in rheumatic mitral stenosis. *N. Engl. J. Med.*, **313**, 1515

738. Zailbag, M.A., Kasab, S.A., Ribeiro, P.A. and Al Fagih, M.R. (1986). Percutaneous double-balloon mitral valvotomy for rheumatic mitral stenosis. *Lancet*, **1**, 6

739. McKay, R.G., Lock, J.E., Keane, J.F., Safian, R.D., Aroesty, J.M. and Grossman, W. (1986). Percutaneous mitral valvuloplasty in an adult patient with calcific rheumatic mitral stenosis. *J. Am. Coll. Cardiol.*, **7**, 1410

740. Block, P.C., Palacios, I.F., Jacobs, M.L. and Fallon, J.T. (1987). Mechanism of percutaneous mitral valvotomy. *Am. J. Cardiol.*, **59**, 178

741. McKay, R.G., Lock, J.E., Safian, R.D., Come, P.C., Diver, D.J. and Grossman, W. (1987). Balloon dilatation of mitral stenosis in adult patients: postmortem and percutaneous mitral valvuloplasty studies. *J. Am. Coll. Cardiol.*, **9**

742. Rahimtoola, S.H. (1987). Catheter balloon valvuloplasty of aortic and mitral valve stenosis in adults. *Circulation*, **75**, 895

743. Cribier, A., Savin, T., Berland, J., Rocha, P., Mechmeche, R., Saoudi, N., Behar, P. and Letac, B. (1987). Percutaneous transluminal balloon valvuloplasty of adult aortic stenosis: report of 92 cases. *J. Am. Coll. Cardiol.*, **9**, 381

744. McKay, R.G., Safian, R.D., Lock, J.E., Diver, D.J., Berman, A.D. and Grossman, W. (1987). Assessment of left ventricular and aortic valve function after aortic balloon valvuloplasty in adult patients with critical aortic stenosis. *Circulation*, **75**, 192

745. Rashkind, W.J. (1983). Transcatheter treatment of congenital heart disease. *Circulation*, **67**, 711

746. Park, S.C., Neches, W.H., Mullins, C.E., Girod, D.A., Olley, P.M., Falkowski, G., Garibjan, V.A., Mathews, R.A., Fricker, F.J., Beerman, I.B., Lenox, C.C. and Zuberbuhler, J.R. (1982). Blade arterial septostomy: collaborative study. *Circulation*, **66**, 258

747. Bommer, W.J., Lee, G., Riemenschneider, T.A., Ikeda, R.M. *et al.* (1983). Laser atrial septostomy. *Am. Heart J.*, **106**, 1152

748. Lock, J.E., Cockerham, J.T., Keane, J.F., Finley, J.P., Wakely, P.E. Jr and Fellows, K.E. (1987). Transcatheter umbrella closure of congenital heart defects. *Circulation*, **75**, 593

749. Abela, G.S., Normann, S.J., Cohen, D.M., Franzini, D., Feldman, R.L., Crea, F., French, A., Pepine, C.J. and Conti, C.R. (1985). Laser recanalization of occluded atherosclerotic arteries *in vivo* and *in vitro*. *Circulation*, **71**, 403

750. Eldar, M., Battler, A.A., Neufeld, H.N., Gaton, E., Arieli, R., Akselrod, S., Levite, A. and Katzir, A. (1984). Transluminal carbon dioxide-laser catheter angioplasty for dissolution of atherosclerotic plaques. *J. Am. Coll. Cardiol.*, **3**, 135

751. Isner, J.M., Donaldson, R.F., Deckelbaum, L.I., Clarke, R.H., Laliberte, S.M., Ucci, A.A., Salem, D.N. and Konstam, M.A. (1986). The excimer laser: gross, light microscopic and ultrastructural analysis of potential advantages for use in laser therapy of cardiovascular disease. *J. Am. Coll. Cardiol.*, **6**, 1102

752. Lee, G., Ikeda, R.M., Chan, M.C., Lee, M.H., Rink, J.L., Reis, R.L., Theis, J.H., Low, R., Bommer, W.J., Kung, A.H., Hanna, E.S. and Mason, D.T. (1985). Limitations, risks and complications of laser recanalization: a cautious approach warranted. *Am. J. Cardiol.*, **56**, 181

753. Choy, D.S.J., Stertzer, S.H., Myler, R.K., Marco, J. and Fournial, G. (1984). Human coronary laser recanalization. *Clin. Cardiol.*, **7**, 377

754. Ginsburg, R., Wexler, L., Mitchell, R.S., Profitt, D. (1985). Percutaneous transluminal laser angioplasty for treatment of peripheral vascular disease. Clinical experience with 16 patients. *Radiology*, **156**, 619

755. Simpson, J.B., Johnson, D.E., Tapliyal, H.V., Marks, D.S. and Braden, L.J. (1985). Transluminal atherectomy: a new approach to the treatment of atherosclerotic vascular disease. *Circulation*, **72**, (Suppl. III), 146

756. Leyser, L.J., Bundy, M.A., Abreo, F., Hanley, H.G., Fadely, D. and Walker, J.M. (1986). Evaluation of a coronary lysing system: results of a preclinical safety and efficacy study. *Cathet. Cardiovasc. Diagn.*, **12**, 246

757. Sigwart, U., Puel, J., Mirkovitch, V., Joffre, F. and Kappenberger, L. (1987). Intravascular stents to prevent occlusion and restenosis after transluminal angioplasty. *N. Engl. J. Med.*, **316**, 701

758. Sherry, S. (1989). The origin of thrombolytic therapy. *JACC*, **14**, 1085–92

759. Tillett, W.S. and Garner, R.L. (1933). The fibrinolytic activity of hemolytic streptococci. *J. Exp. Med.*, **58**, 485–502

760. Milstone, H. (1941). A factor in normal human blood which participates in streptococcal fibrinolysis. *J. Immunol.*, **42**, 109–16

761. Christensen, L.R. (1945). Streptococcal fibrinolysis: a proteolytic reaction due to a serum enzyme activated by streptococcal fibrinolysin. *J. Gen. Physiol.*, **28**, 363–83

762. Christensen, L.R. and MacLeod, C.M. (1945). A proteolytic enzyme of serum, characterization, activation and reaction with inhibitors. *J. Gen. Physiol.*, **28**, 559–83

763. Christensen, L.R. (1947). Protamine purification of streptokinase and effect of pH and temperature on reversible inactivation. *J. Gen. Physiol.*, **30**, 465–73

764. Johnson, A.J. and Tillett, W.S. (1952). Lysis in rabbits of intravascular blood clots by the streptococcal fibrinolytic system (streptokinase). *J. Exp. Med.*, **95**, 449–64

765. Kline, D.L. (1953). Purification and crystallization of plasminogen (profibrinolysin). *J. Biol. Chem.*, **204**, 949–55

766. Sherry, S., Lindermeyer, R.I., Fletcher, A.P. and Alkjaersig, N. (1959). Studies on enhanced fibrinolytic activity in man. *J. Clin. Invest.*, **38**, 810–22

767. Sherry, S. (1954). Fibrinolytic activity of streptokinase activated human plasmin. *J. Clin. Invest.*, **33**, 1054–63

768. Sherry, S., Titchener, A., Gottesman, L.,

Wasserman, P. and Troll, W. (1954). The enzymatic dissolution of experimental intravascular thrombi in the dog by trypsin, chymotrypsin and plasminogen activators. *J. Clin. Invest.*, **33**, 1303–13

769. Alkjaersig, N., Fletcher, A.O. and Sherry, S. (1959). The mechanism of clot dissolution by plasmin. *J. Clin. Invest.*, **38**, 1086–95

770. Fletcher, A.P., Alkjaersig, N., Smyrniotis, F.E. and Sherry, S. (1958). Treatment of patients suffering from early, myocardial infarction with massive and prolonged streptokinase therapy. *Trans. Assoc. Am. Physicians*, **71**, 287–96

771. Fletcher, A.P., Alkjaersig, N., Sherry, S., Genton, E., Hirsh, J. and Bachmann, F. (1965). Development of urokinase as a thrombolytic agent: maintenance of a sustained thrombolytic state in man by its intravenous infusion. *J. Lab. Clin. Med.*, **654**, 713–31

772. Macfarlane, R.G. and Pilling, J. (1946). Observations on fibrinolysis: plasminogen, plasmin, and antiplasmin content of human blood. *Lancet*, **2**, 562–5

773. DeWood, M.A., Spores, J., Notske, R., Mouser, L.T., Burroughs, R., Golden, M.S. and Lang, H.T. (1980). Prevalence of total coronary occlusion during the early hours of transmural myocardial infarction. *N. Engl. J. Med.*, **303**, 897

774. Buja, L.M. and Willerson, J.T. (1981). Clinicopathologic correlates of acute ischemic heart disease syndromes. *Am. J. Cardiol.*, **47**, 343

775. Willerson, J.T., Campbell, W.B., Winniford, M.D., Schmitz, I. *et al.* (1984). Conversion from chronic to acute coronary artery disease: specifications regarding mechanisms. *Am. J. Cardiol.*, **54**, 1349

776. Epstein, S.E. and Palmeri, S.T. (1984). Mechanisms contributing to progression of unstable angina and acute myocardial infarction: implications regarding therapy. *Am. J. Cardiol.*, **54**, 1245

777. Alpert, J.S. (1985). Coronary vasomotion, coronary thrombosis, myocardial infarction, and the camel's back. *J. Am. Col. Cardiol.*, **5**, 617

778. Feldman, R.L. (1987). Editorial. Coronary thrombosis, coronary spasm and coronary atherosclerosis and speculation on the link between unstable angina and acute myocardial infarction. *Am. J. Cardiol.*, **59**, 1187

779. Laffel, G.L. and Braunwald, E. (1984). Thrombolytic therapy. A new strategy for treatment of acute myocardial infarction. *N. Engl. J. Med.*, **311**, 710, 770

780. DeWood, M.A., Stifter, W.F., Simpson, C.S., Spores, J., Eugster, G.S., Judge, T.P and Hinnen, M.L. (1986). Coronary arteriographic findings soon after non-Q wave myocardial infarction. *N. Engl. J. Med.*, **315**, 417

781. Mandelkorn, J.B., Wolf, N.M., Singh, S., Shechter, J.A. *et al.* (1983). Intracoronary thrombus in nontransmural myocardial infarction and in unstable angina pectoris. *Am. J. Cardiol.*, **52**, 1

782. Rentrop, P., Blanke, H., Kostering, K. and Karsch, K.R. (1979). Acute myocardial infarction: intracoronary application of nitroglycerin and streptokinase in combination with transluminal recanalization. *Clin. Cardiol.*, **2**, 354–63

783. Gans, W., Buchbinder, N., Marcus, H., Mondkar, A., Madahi, J., Charuzi, Y., O'Connor, L., Shell, W., Fishbein, M.C., Kass, R., Miyamoto, A. and Swan, H.J.C. (1981). Intracoronary thrombolysis in evolving myocardial infarction. *Am. Heart J.*, **101**, 4

784. Markis, J.E., Malagold, M., Parker, J.A., Silverman, K.J., Barry, W.H., Als, A.V., Paulin, S., Grossman, W. and Braunwald, E. (1981). Myocardial salvage after intracoronary thrombolysis with streptokinase in acute myocardial infarction. *N. Engl. J. Med.*, **305**, 777

785. Schröder, R., Biamino, G., Enz-Rudiger, L. *et al.* (1983). Intravenous short-term infusion of streptokinase in acute myocardial infarction. *Circulation*, **63**, 536–48

786. Yusuf, S., Collins, R., Peto, R., Furberg, C., Stampfer, M.J., Goldhaber, S.Z. and Hennekens, C.H. (1985). Intravenous and intracoronary fibrinolytic therapy in acute myocardial infarction: overview of results on mortality, reinfarction, and side effects from 33 randomized control trials. *Eur. Heart J.*, **6**, 556

787. The TIMI Study Group (1985). The thrombolysis in myocardial infarction. TIMI trial. Phase I Findings. *N. Engl. J. Med.*, **312**, 932

30   Pharmacologic modalities

In primitive times, therapy was based on two principles: the law of similarity and the law of contagion. Cure was attempted through the law of similarity (*similia similibus curantur*) while the law of contagion was utilized in the formulation of the therapeutic agent itself. The magical ideas of primitive man followed the two laws. Mettler recounts how in following the law of similarity, parts of plants which resembled organs or portions of the body were considered to exert an influence over them. In applying the law of contagion, she cites as an example the use of moonstones in treating certain forms of insanity – the belief being that these were caused by the actions of the moon and since moonstones were also formed under the influence of the moon, they should exert a curative effect[1].

As communal life evolved and religious practices became established, pharmacotherapy began to emerge, rooted in mysticism, demonology and the belief that sickness was caused by an angry diety. In the Babylo-Assyrian era, incantations and water were the major elements of the *materia medica*. Balneology still continues as a favorite therapeutic tool in the spas of Europe though no longer on religious grounds. Besides water, the physician of the Babylo-Assyrian era also resorted to the use of botanicals. Medicaments derived from plants have been an important element of pharmacopeia throughout the ages, and continue to be so to this very day. Indeed in a book entitled *The Rivers Ran East*, the author (Clark) lists more than a hundred plants indigenous to the Brazilian Amazon that are sources of some very potent drugs.

The Babylo-Assyrian pharmacopeia (*Shammu*) was modest in number with the tablets of that era listing a little more than 300 drugs[2]. Jastrow describes a typical prescription for what appears to be an intraabdominal process[3]. 'If a man's inside is swollen and inflamed, and he is nauseated, then for his life … mix onion with cumin seed, let him drink it in wine without food and he will recover.

If ditto, take the green rind of the Il plant, mix with pig's fat, let him drink it with Du-Zab, unmixed wine and sweetened water, and he will recover'.

The Ebers papyrus mentions more than 700 drugs from which the Egyptian practitioner could choose. Among them were opium, olive oil, animal parts, precious stones, amulets, wormwood, and fresh dill juice. Herbs, however, played a prominent role in the Egyptian pharmacopeia.

Pharmakon is the Greek word for any drug, toxic or otherwise. It is the root word for all our nouns and adjectives relating to drugs. The Greek's pharmacopeia consisted mostly of herbal products and represented an adoption as well as an expanded form of Egyptian herbal polypharmacy. The herbal derivatives acted in most cases as the mediating agents since many of their therapeutic approaches were intimately intertwined with religious beliefs. The pagan polytheism of the ancient Greeks confused matters even more with invocations to several gods such as Apollo, Jupiter and Chiron, the centaur. The modern physician's 'Rx' symbol is derived from the ancient symbol for Jupiter whose name was invoked before prescribing the medicament itself.

The advent of the Asclepiads and the increasing numbers of adherents of Hippocrates gradually resulted in a simplification of this unwieldy polypharmacy. They tried for the most part practical corrective measures emphasizing diet, change in climate, purgatives and natural agents without recourse to precious stones, amulets, or alvine discharges to drive out the demons. An early expectorant as well as a diuretic was honey in vinegar. Hippocrates wrote that oxymel (honey in vinegar) '… promotes expectoration and freedom of breathing … It also promotes flatulent discharges from the bowels, and is diuretic, … and otherwise it diminishes the strength and makes the extremities cold; this is the only bad effect worth mentioning which I have known to arise from the oxymel'[4].

During this era, Theophrastus was the leading exponent of botanical remedies. He was a pupil of Aristotle, and utilized unsparingly Aristotle's entire botanical garden willed to him by the master himself. Theophrastus described about 500 drugs derived from plants. He described madder, which he called ereuthedanon, as having both diuretic and analgesic properties[5].

The Alexandrian period is noted for its emphasis on the use of poisons and their antidotes. Even royalty became involved in this nefarious aspect of *materia medica*. The most notorious was Mithridates, the sixth King of Pontus. Legend has it that he was so well versed in poisons that he even concocted a universal antidote. It is known to us as mithridatium, with obvious reference to him. It was made up of rue leaves, walnut, salt and figs. It had to be taken on a daily basis in order to be effective.

Mithridatium occupied an important role throughout a good part of Roman history. It was modified by Andromachus the Elder, archiater to Nero, by the addition of squill, viper's flesh, and opium[6]. This concoction was said to be Nero's first line of defense against being poisoned to death. Andromachus recommended it also as an effective agent in dropsy as well as in other conditions. The entire modified concoction came to be known as theriaca and under the eponym theriaca andromachi or under the alternate label of Venice treacle, it remained an important therapeutic agent as late as the mid-1700s[7]. The active ingredient in squill was not known at the time of Andromachus. In 1879, E. von Jamersted was the first to identify the active ingredient as being a glycoside; although, a century earlier, Francis Home of Edinburgh knew about the inhibitory cardiac action of squill[8]. Squill is also mentioned in Eber's papyrus and Pythagoras wrote a treatise on vinegar of squill, a mode of preparation which he introduced. Galen used it in epilepsy while Hippocrates employed it as an electuary in the treatment of empyema. Even Pliny had a use for it touting it as a very effective antihelminthic agent[9].

The Hindus and Chinese also relied on herbs and plants. The *Susruta*, a Hindu medical text, lists 760 herbs[10]. The father of Chinese *materia medica* is said to be Shen Nung (2735 BC). This emperor is credited with having written a 40 volume work entitled *Pun Tsao*, describing a large number of drugs, most of which were vegetable in origin. Among them were camphor and ephedrine-containing substances. They also used toad's eyelids which contain bufanin and bufotalin, both of which produce digitalis-like effects[11].

Going back to Rome, the 5th book of *De Medicina* by Celsus is devoted entirely to therapy. As far as the land and slave owners were concerned, this was probably the most useful portion of Celsus' *opus*. The book has 28 chapters and a considerable variety of therapeutic agents are described. They were culled from various sources. Very little mention is made of treating cardiac illness, as such; probably because the various manifestations of cardiac dysfunction were largely unknown at the time.

Dioscorides, a native of Anazarba, Cilica wrote the quintessential pharmacologic treatise of the period. It remained in vogue for almost 16 centuries[12].

Galen's entire pharmacopeia was based primarily on the humoral hypothesis of the Hippocratic era which by this time had become associated with the theory of the four elements. Buck quotes Galen as saying 'It is the business of pharmacology to combine drugs in such a manner − according to their elementary qualities of heat, cold, moisture and dryness − as shall render them effective in combating or overcoming the conditions which exist in the different diseases'[13]. Galen wrote some 30 books on the subject. Walsh emphasizes the careful detail with which Galen approached the use of drugs. 'In order to know drugs, inspect them not once or twice, but frequently, for though twins look alike to strangers, they are easily distinguished by friends'[14]. Galen had so little confidence in others that he had his own repository filled with a more than ample supply of drugs and herbs. In his travels he was always on the lookout for new additions to his *materia medica*. Galen's composition of the universal theriac contained 100 ingredients, among them being squill[15]. Galenicals were the mainstay of medicinals well into the 18th century; illustrative once more of Galen's firm entrenchment in medical practice.

The *materia medica* of the Byzantine era was characterized by adherence to superstitious faith in magical procedures coupled with complete immersion in galenical prescriptions. Paul of Aegina (Paulus Aeginata) stands out in this epoch with his rather heavy medical text consisting of 7 books, the last of which was devoted to *materia medica*[9]. He recommended drinking goat's blood with milk for the treatment of dropsy[16].

The Byzantines transmitted their medical knowledge to the Arabs with Dioscorides as the fountainhead of practically their entire medical lore. They introduced ambergris for the treatment of cramps, heart disease and brain disorders, and mace for cardiac diseases and indigestion[17].

Avicenna's text *al-Quanun-fi al-Tibb* (also known as the *Canon*) was already mentioned in Section 1. Figure 1 is a page from *Liber quintus Canonis* as translated by Gerardus Cremonensis. This manuscript dates back to the late 14th century.

The section devoted to *materia medica* lists 760 drugs, culled from Byzantine and Persian sources of Hindu agents. Avicenna's *Canon* exerted an important influence on western medicine even as late as the 17th century. It is still occasionally relied upon in Moslem countries[18]. The allusions to remedies for heart disease are repetitions of those found in Dioscorides. Figure 2 represents examples of prescriptions from Avicenna's *Liber Medicinalis*.

Avicenna's tract on cardiac drugs lists a total of 63. The tract itself consists of 17 sections. The 9th section analyzes the mode of action by virtue of which cardiac medicines produce exhilaration. Siddiqui and Aziz give as examples: 'wine acts by promoting growth and excellence of the soul, pearls or silk cocoons act by increasing the radiance and lustre of the soul, or myrobalans act by consolidating the soul, camphor and rose water by restoring the normal temperament of the heated soul by cooling it, burg-i-Gaozaban (leaves of *Onosma bracteatum*) by removing the vapours of black bile which were causing the turbidity of the soul'[19]. They also go on to say that 'some cardiac drugs exert their action by an unknown mode of action together with known ones. If these latter actions are partial they need correction; for correction such drugs are to be chosen as themselves possess cardiac properties'. Further critique of Avicenna's tract is as follows:

A careful study of the whole tract will give the readers insight into the mode of treatment of cardiac patients with drugs, diet and environmental adjustment. For example, Ibn Sina lays down the principles of the treatment according to the condition of the patient, thus: if a patient happens to have pure blood of normal consistency but having excess of heat, such a person will be choleric and this trait will interfere with the action of the cardiac drug. The drug to be prescribed must be of cold temperament and the patient must be kept in an environment which spares him from being exposed to circumstances which may excite anger; or, in case if the patient has pure but thin and cold blood he will have less capacity for anger or pleasure. Therefore he will require more potent cardiac drugs than the former case, while his diet should be so regulated as to restore the consistency and temperament of his blood to normal.

Throughout this medieval period, the western world continued to base its pharmacopeia on the Greco-Roman roots with Dioscorides remaining as the ultimate authority. Christian variations of pagan cults were also introduced as the magical components of superstitious practices. The pagan gods of the Aesculapian cult were replaced by the Christian saints. The church had such a powerful hold on current thought that very little progress was made towards establishing pharmacology as a scientific discipline. Self-medication was also practiced quite widely. The needs of the general populace were met in this way by compendia oriented towards the lay person. They were similar to our modern 'family physicians' and almanacs. Books of this sort remained in vogue even in the Renaissance, and perhaps, even more so because of the ease with which they could be printed as a result of Gutenberg's invention. Not all of them were printed, as the illustrations in Figures 3 and 4 indicate. Figure 3 is a page from a handwritten commonplace book by Giovanni Antonio Scandolisti. It is a *Tabulae de confortantibus* from Petrus Salernitanus (c. 1500). Figure 4 is an illustration of another page from the same commonplace book with notes on the practice of medicine, pulses, urines, etc.

Although the medieval commonplace manuscripts did not break new ground, they served a useful purpose in that they were able to hand down codified information from one generation to the next. The monks were particularly active in copying and translating manuscripts, many of them spending their entire lives in this work. Among the most noteworthy in the field of medicine was Aurelius Cassiodorus (480–575). While at the Benedictine monastery at Monte Cassino (badly damaged during World War II), he wrote of pharmacology in the following words[20]:

Learn to know the properties of herbs and the blending of drugs, but set all your hopes upon

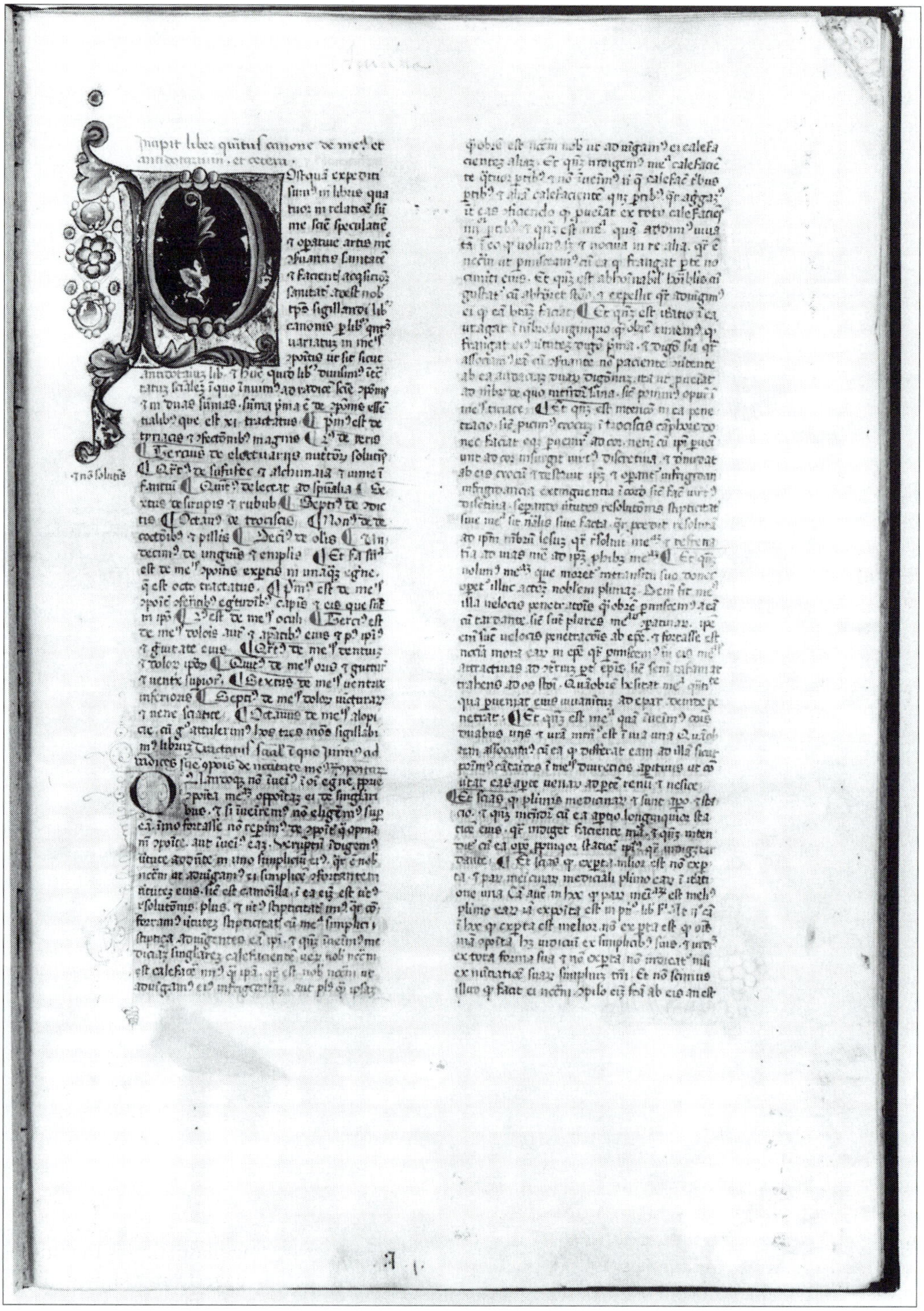

Figure 1 Reproduction of a page from 'Liber quintus Canonis' as translated by Gerardus Cremonensis. *Photo Source Wellcome Institute Library. Literary Source Avicenna, Liber quintus canonis, translated by Gerardus Cremonensis, s.l., n.d. (late 14th century). WIHM Western MS 104. fol 1. By courtesy of the Wellcome Trustees*

the Lord, who preserves life without end. If the language of the Greeks is unknown to you, you have the herb-book of Dioscorides, who has described and depicted the herbs of the field with astonishing accuracy. Afterwards read Hippocrates and Galen in Latin translation, i.e. the therapeutics of the latter, which he has dedicated to the philosopher Glaucon and the work of an unknown author, which, as would appear from investigation, is compiled from several writers. Study further the Medicine of Aurelius [Aurelianus] Caelius, the Hippocratic book upon herbs and healing methods, as well as a variety of other treatises upon the healing art which I have brought together in my library and have bequeathed to you.

The Salernitan school exerted its influence on pharmacology mainly during the 11th and 12th centuries. Two writers of importance emerged from this school. They were Nicolaus Salernitanus and Mathias Platearius. Again, no new ground was broken, their works being a reiteration of the traditional medications of Dioscorides.

Though geographically distant from southern Italy, Greece and the Moslem states, the practitioners of the British Isles were also influenced by their brethren in the Mediterranean area. Their *materia medica*, however, was corrupted with Druidic superstitions and a rather undisciplined attitude towards the efficacy and validity of their preparations. This is exemplified by the writings of Gilbert of England and John of Gaddesden; writings replete with the superstitions and worthless prescriptions of the day. The first published English herbal was printed by Richard Bankes of London. This work known to us as *Banckest Herbal*, contains characters from earlier Anglo-Saxon leech books and manuscript recipe books. Figure 5 is a reproduction of a page from a large collection of quaint medical and other receipts.

As the Renaissance began to dawn, alchemy began to insert itself as an integral part of the pharmacopeia. But it was not easy. It had to combat a resurgence of interest in botanical preparations because of the discovery and exportation of many new botanical specimens in the New World. Nicolas Monardes was a prime mover in introducing new Indian and American herbs and plants with medicinal properties. Even tobacco imported from America was touted as having marked

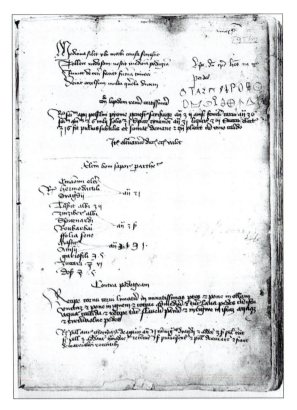

Figure 2 Examples of prescriptions from Avicenna's 'Liber Medicinalis'. *Photo Source Wellcome Institute Library. Literary source Avicenna, Liber Medicinalis, s. l. (German?), n.d. (c. 1430?) WIHM Western MS 105. By courtesy of the Wellcome Trustees*

healing powers. Jean Nicot, the French ambassador to Portugal, was able to get some tobacco plants and successfully cultivated them in his native country. The stimulant nicotine is named after Nicot.

Despite the existence of the printing press, many medical texts were still being published in the form of handwritten manuscripts. As mentioned in Section 1, isagogues were quite popular then. These were really introductions to more detailed studies. Figure 6 is a photograph of folio 1, labeled A from *Isagogica ad practicam medicinae*. It is from the late 16th century. The manuscript contains a list of diseases and their remedies in alphabetical order.

Another interesting illustration is the photograph in Figure 7. It is a page from Gasparo di Cagali's *Libro di recette medicinali*. The manuscript is written in the dialect of Verona. It contains a number of prescriptions and description of diseases for which they were written. The photograph is of the inside

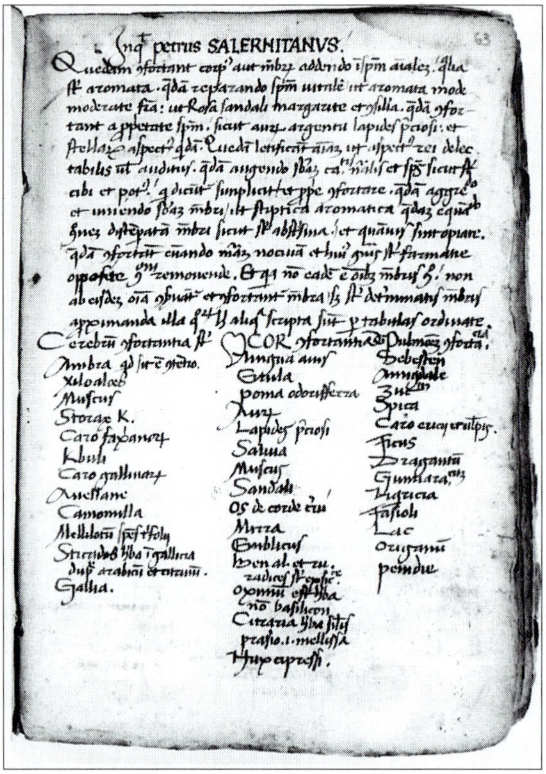

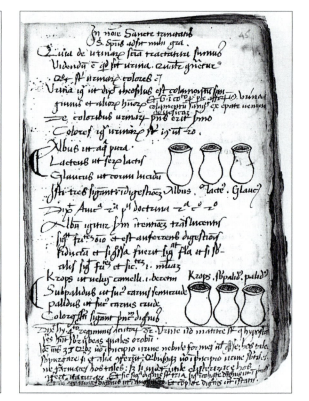

Figure 3 A page from a commonplace book by Giovanni Scandolisti. *Photo Source Wellcome Institute Library. Literary Source Giovanni Antonio Scandolisti, commonplace book, (14. Petrus Salernitanus, Tabulae de confortantibus) s.l., n.d. (c. 1500). WIHM Western MS 730, fol 63. By courtesy of the Wellcome Trustees*

Figure 4 Another page from Scandolisti's commonplace book with notes on the practice of medicine, pulses, urines, etc. *Photo Source Wellcome Institute Library. Literary Source Giovanni Antonio Scandolisti, commonplace book, (3. Notes on the practice of medicine, pulses, urines,etc.) s.l., n.d. (c. 1500) WHIM Western MS 730, fol 45. By courtesy of the Wellcome Trustees*

of the front cover. It shows a pen drawn coat of arms of the writer and notes of his personal affairs beginning with 'Questo libero sie di M gasparro barbiro e ciroicho che fu fiolo di m antonio ceroicho da Legnago di chagalii habito in la contra di S. Zen … e questo libero fu scritto adi agosto 1529'. The birth of a daughter on 14 November 1527 is also mentioned.

While Europe was being inundated with New World botanicals, the alchemists continued to plod away in their search for the philosopher's stone and elixir of life. Paracelsus acted as the catalyst in espousing chemical remedies[21]. He introduced 'Lilium Paracelsi' as a constituent of a theriacal elixir. It contained tin, copper and iron alloys of antimony. A protracted controversy ensued over the alleged benefits and toxicity of antimony. The controversy lasted for more than a century

when it was resolved temporarily by a French royal decree in 1566 prohibiting its use. The most vociferous opponent of antimony in France was the satirist, Guy Patin. His pharmacopeia was simple, limited to syrup of roses or senna and blood-letting. He thought so little of theriaca and its antimony ingredient that his words dripped with disdain.

The reputation of theriaca is without effect and without foundation, it comes only from the apothecaries who do all they can to persuade people to use compositions and would take from them if they could the knowledge and use of simple remedies which are most useful. If I were bitten by a venomous animal I would not trust in theriaca, nor in any cardiac, external or internal of the shops. I would scarify the wound deeply,

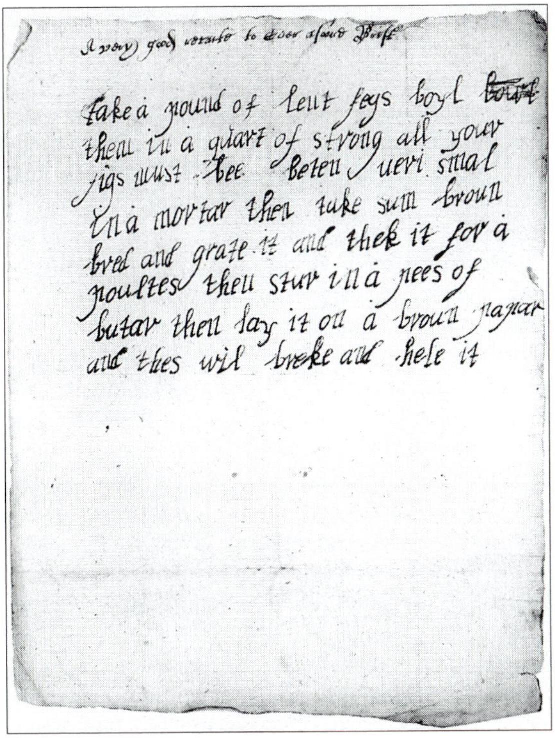
take a pound of lent figs boyl them in a quart of strong all your figs must bee beten veri smal in a mortar then take sum broun bred and grate it and thek it for a poultes then stur in a pees of butar then lay it on a broun papar and thes wil breke and hele it

Figure 5 A page from a large collection of quaint medical and other receipts. *Photo Source The Wellcome Institute Library. Literary Source Manuscript: WMS 400. By courtesy of the Wellcome Trustees*

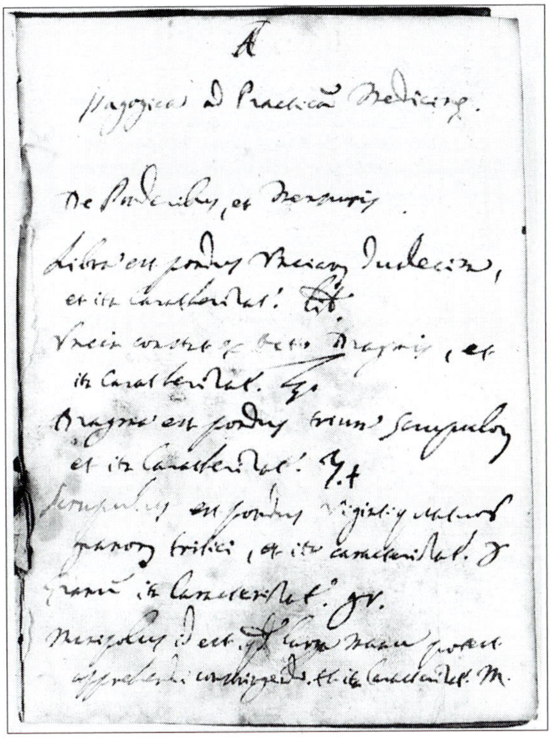
A

Isagogica ad Practicam Medicinae.

Figure 6 Photograph of folio 1, labeled A, of 'Isagogica ad practicam medicinae'. *Photo Source The Wellcome Institute Library. Literary Source Manuscript, WMS 371. By courtesy of the Wellcome Trustees*

> and apply to it powerful attractives and only have myself bled for the pain, fever or plethora. But by good fortune there are scarcely any venomous animals in France. In recompense we have Italian favorites, partisans, many charlatans, and much antimony.[22]

Nothwithstanding Patin's vituperative remarks, antimony was reinstated as a legitimate remedy by still another royal decree, a century after it was prohibited. King Louis XIV bestowed his royal approval on it because he was 'miraculously cured of typhoid fever with the antimony preparation'.

Theodore Turquet de Mayerne of Geneva was responsible for introducing some order in the preparation and dispensing of drugs in England during the early part of the 17th century. He apparently had the power to do so because of his position as royal physician to James I and Charles I. His initial step in unraveling the confusion was to separate the grocer's guild from that of the apothecaries. In tune with this a new set of standards had to be in place by which medications could be properly prepared. The *Pharmacopoeia Londonensis*, a reference book that de Mayerne helped to sponsor, lent itself quite nicely to this purpose. The book was nothing else but a copy of the 6th edition of the *Augsburg Pharmacopoeia*, and although originally without merit, it acquired real significance after undergoing several revisions and editions[23].

The 18th century saw the chemists and herbalists establishing a more cooperative relationship. This is not surprising since many advances being made in chemistry were utilizing crude botanical specimens as their source of purer agents. It was to take many years, however, before the chemists would be able to synthesize pure chemical agents without the need of a herb or plant.

If nothing else, this survey until now should have served, at least, to emphasize that up until the 19th century, medical therapy of heart disease was

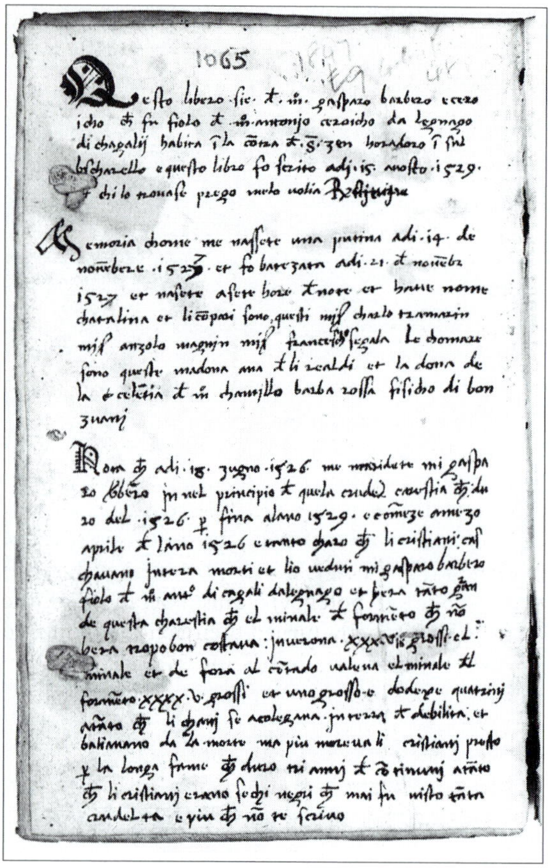

Figure 7 Photograph of the inside of the front cover of 'Libro di recette medicinali' by Gasparo di Cagali, Verona, 1529. *Photo Source The Wellcome Institute Library. Literary Source Manuscript: WMS 174. By courtesy of the Wellcome Trustees*

virtually non-existent. What few agents were available were crude in composition, unpredictable in action and laden with untoward effects. Blood letting was a popular therapeutic modality and held in esteem primarily because of the teachings of Corvisart, Bouillaud and other luminaries of the time. Hydragogue cathartics including saline were used in the treatment of dropsy. Squill, a survivor from the days of ancient Egypt and still an ingredient of the ubiquitous theriacal elixir, was used without rhyme or reason. Even digitalis leaf was used but without sufficient knowledge of its pharmacological actions nor for the right reason despite Withering's monumental monograph on the subject.

A clear picture of the *materia medica* in heart disease can be had by referring to Hope's *Diseases of the Heart* published in 1839[24]. Mercury competed with antimony as the anchor sheet of treatment. It came in the form of the 'blue pill' or calomel. Hyoscyamus and digitalis were given for nervousness and acute endocarditis. Dropsy was the umbrella term for fluid retention regardless of cause, and it was treated with a host of agents that had diuretic properties such as squill again, juniper, tartrates, acetates, decoction of broom, spirits of nitrous ether, potassium nitrate, and cantharides. The list is not complete but noteworthy because of its emphasize on chemical agents rather than botanical preparations. Digitalis leaf was used frequently in dropsy under the belief that it was a diuretic agent rather than a cardiotonic drug. Digitalis was also used for palpitation but under the mistaken notion that this disorder was due to a nervous state rather than an underlying arrhythmia. No specific drugs were used for cardiac hypertrophy or cardiac dilatation, the latter being a synonymn for heart failure. Blood letting was still 'de rigeur' for cardiac hypertrophy, at least during the first half of the 19th century. Inadvertently, this practice, by decreasing blood volume, could have benefited somewhat those in whom the cardiac hypertrophy was a consequence of hypertension. This physiologic factor in maintaining blood pressure was, of course, not known to the practitioners of the time. When valvular disease was present, mercury and antiphlogistics were given during the early phase when there was no evidence of heart failure. When heart failure supervened, purges, diuretics and diaphoretics were resorted to.

The therapeutic objectives in aortic aneurysm were a slow heart and a reduction in myocardial contractility. Digitalis was mistakenly given as a negative inotropic agent simultaneously with diuretics and purgatives. Albertina and Valsalva advocated vigorous blood letting. Hope still adhered to their advice but tempered it by reducing the amount of blood withdrawn and the frequency of its removal. Leeches were used as an adjunct to phlebotomy.

This constituted virtually the entire spectrum of cardiac medical management with blood-letting as the most important protagonist of the scenario. No wonder they had such disastrous results. There was good cause for the therapeutic nihilism that prevailed during the first half of the 19th century. An anonymous verse of the era rather clearly underscores the disdain with which cardiac therapy was regarded by the cognoscenti of the times. 'The King employs three doctors daily, Willis, Heberden and Baillie. All exceeding clever men, Baillie, Willis, Heberden. Uncertain which most sure to kill is Baillie, Heberden, or Willis'[25].

The 19th century saw the evolution of anti-anginal treatment undergo several stages with various drugs being tried on an empirical basis or on the mistaken concepts of the underlying pathophysiology. The prevailing notion prior to Herrick and Heberden was that heart disease need not be present. The stomach was thought to be the culprit in many cases, and therapy was directed towards relief of acidity, gas or residual undigested gastric contents. Acidity was combated with soda or prepared chalk. Antispasmodic agents were also given, in the belief that the gastro-intestinal tract was the seat of the difficulty. This could be given in the form of a belladonna plaster. Tincture or extract of opium was also used, mostly because of its sedative action. Blood-letting or application of leeches over the precordium were reserved for those experiencing a great deal of pain. Counter-irritants were also applied to the precordium until blistering occurred. This too was reserved only for protracted pain.

It is easy to see with this litany of agents how the pathophysiologic basis of angina completely eluded the early 19th century clinician. Laénnec himself was of the belief that angina pectoris was neuralgic in origin. He used two strongly magnetized steel plates, one over the precordium, and the other over the left scapular area. This mode of therapy appeared to have favorable results only in the hands of Laénnec. Hope wrote that 'It should be remarked that they who witnessed the application of the magnet by Laénnec, did not, in general, form so favourable an opinion of its utility as that author himself'[26].

The usage of a nitrogenous group of chemicals for the palliative relief of angina pectoris began with the discovery of nitroglycerin. Since the history of the medical applications of nitroglycerin is so intimately intertwined with that of the early days of homeopathy, a few words about this almost defunct branch of medical therapy are most appropriate at this time.

Samuel Hahnemann of Meissen (1769–1843) was responsible for introducing homeopathy. Though it proved to be a useless system of therapeutics, it was much simpler than allopathy and had an intriguing appeal as an alternative to the therapeutic nihilism

that greeted the allopathic remedies of the day. Hahnemann was a well-meaning physician and in no way could he be accused of fraud or quackery. He was simply lost in the confusion of his convictions. He presented his theory of therapeutics in a landmark paper entitled *Organon der rationellen Heilkunde*[27]. T. Sollman, a well-known pharmacologist of the 20th century, wrote an excellent critique of homeopathy in his *Manual of Pharmacology* published in 1932[28].

Hahnemann believed that disease depends upon a perversion of the purely spiritual vital powers and is entirely immaterial in its nature. Logically, a thing spiritual could not be combated by material remedies, and hence, Hahnemann turned to a spiritual power which he believed to be bound up in plants and liberated by dilution. The activity would therefore increase with the dilution, and be the greater, the smaller the dose (doctrine of potency). This liberation of the principles exactly turned their action around, so that the action of his dilutions was, he stated, exactly the opposite of that of the concentrated drug, and could be used for the relief of such symptoms as the latter produced: *Similia similibus curantur*. This was the first tenet of Hahnemann. The second was that the nature of the disease being unsizeable, it was not subject to treatment, but that only its symptoms could be treated. Hence, homeopathy, in so far as it follows the principles of its founder, has no place for the medical sciences, such as physiology, anatomy, pathology, or chemistry. Any one with an indexed book of symptoms and their remedies would be able to practice it without an elaborate study or preparation.

In marked contrast to the above is the third dictum: that the medicinal treatment must be supported by dietetic and hygienic measures.

The claims of homeopathy as a rational system hinge on the proof of the similia similibus theory and the doctrine of potentiation by dilution. Most of its advocates seem to deny altogether the relevance of scientific testimony, and to base themselves purely on the slippery ground of empirical experience. Others, while they neglect the great body of scientific experience which disproves their theory, avail themselves of the few experimental facts, which, through a variety of sophistications, can be twisted into a specious support. Hahnemann himself seems to have started from the observation that large doses of drugs produce the opposite effects from moderate doses. The correctness of this principle may be granted, for many cases. But it is a very unwarranted feat of logic to assume that infinitesimal doses must again cause effects opposite to those of moderate doses!

Schonbein's discovery of the powerful explosive, 'gun cotton' was the stimulus of an intensive search for another explosive among a nitrogenous group of chemicals[29]. This search resulted in the synthesis of nitroglycerin in 1846 by Sobrero, an Italian chemist. He combined nitric and sulphuric acids with glycerol[30,31]. It was just at this time that homeopathy was enjoying an increasing popularity as an alternative therapeutic approach to that of allopathic medicine.

Constantin Hering, a homeopathic physician, native of Germany who later lived in Philadelphia, was the first among the homeopaths to see the therapeutic possibilities of nitroglycerin. Although initially an agnostic of homeopathy, once converted he became its most ardent proselytizer and was very instrumental in encouraging the growth of homeopathy in America, his adopted country. Hering began to experiment with nitroglycerin in the late 1840s. He and a group of homeopathic colleagues conducted the initial observations on themselves. This approach was nothing new among homeopaths. Hahnemann, himself, routinely used self-experimentation when evaluating the therapeutic value of various agents[32]. They were called provings and the term was applied to observations in clinical trials of patients as well as on themselves.

The acronym 'glonoine' was bestowed upon nitroglycerin by Hering. On the basis of a year of provings he concluded,

This new substance has caused headache with all who tasted it: thus … it will cure such headaches and other complaints in the sick as are similar to the symptoms produced by it on the healthy.

He also observed,

The kind of headache, being in the highest degree a throbbing one, lead me to the examination of the pulse, and in all cases the pulse was altered. I urged that the pulse should be felt, and so made the important discovery, the glonoine, even in very small quantities, exercised a more decided influence upon the activity of the heart than any

other remedy had done before. The pulse was accelerated in almost every prover, and so soon after taking it, that the acceleration is sometimes already felt by the finger when the globules can scarcely have melted on the tongue.

Every patient was a 'prover' of the clinical effects of the drug. Hering's glonoine was an alcoholic solution of nitroglycerin embedded in a sugar pellet[33]. The pellets were placed on the tongue. They dissolved rapidly resulting in an equally rapid absorption of the nitroglycerin.

Fye recounts how the results of 4 years of proving were published in a German journal of homeopathy in 1851 but remained unknown to Americans until 1874 when Hering republished them with additional observations[34]. Besides the headache and rapid forceful pounding of the heart, Hering described in addition, the onset of anginoid symptoms. Despite the various forms of chest discomfort that occurred, Hering never thought to implement the basic dictum of homeopathy *similia similibus curantur* for the relief of angina pectoris. Fye is of the opinion that this may have been due to the perception among physicians of the late 19th century, allopaths as well as homeopaths, that angina pectoris was a rare disorder and therefore not easily brought to mind in evaluating chest distress of any kind[35]. Thus, glonoine became a standard homeopathic remedy for a number of conditions but never for angina pectoris.

Alfred Field, a British subject, was the first among allopathic physicians to study in depth the clinical effects of nitroglycerin. He thought it was a gastrointestinal antispasmodic and used it for the first time on a 69 year old woman who had frequent episodes of 'intense pain in the epigastrium, extending up to the top of the chest, and then down the innerside of the left arm'[35]. Field published his paper in 1858. It came to the attention of several other British physicians who added observations of their own to those of Field[36,37].

In 1864, the German physician, J. Albers, published the first truly scientific evaluation of nitroglycerin. It was a physiologic and therapeutic study emphasizing its effects on the heart and circulation[38]. In 1876, Allan Hamilton presented his animal and self-experimental observations on the neurologic actions of nitroglycerin. He thought it would be quite useful in treating spasm of the cerebral vessels[39,40].

T. L. Brunton presented a short but quite formidable list of antianginal agents in his textbook of pharmacology, therapeutics and materia medica published in 1885. He had apparently developed an impressive clinical experience in the symptomatic relief of angina. Included among his list were amyl nitrite, aconite, arsenic, phosphorous, strychnia, and turpentine. Brunton was responsible for introducing in 1867 the inhalation of amyl nitrite for the anginal episode[41]. His reasoning for adopting this agent was wrong, as he thought that the vasodilation relieved pain by reducing systemic pressure. At any rate, it worked and remained in use even as late as the 1950s. Brunton did not recommend nitroglycerin as an antianginal agent simply because of the headache it precipitated. He had tried it on himself and felt that the headache outweighed its benefits. This apparently did not bother William Murrell who introduced it again in 1879. In fact, Murrell was the first allopathic physician to advocate the use of nitroglycerin in angina pectoris. His review on the subject appeared in *The Lancet*[42,43]. Thirty-five patients were studied, all of whom described the same throbbing headache, tachycardia and forceful heart beat that he experienced when he first tried the drug on himself. Murrell, in later studies, documented the changes in pulse with the recently invented sphygmograph (see Section 5). He noticed the similarity in action between nitroglycerin and amyl nitrite, which led him to comment: 'From a consideration of the physiological action of the drug and more especially from the similarity existing between its general action and that of nitrite of amyl, I concluded that it would probably prove of service in the treatment of angina pectoris, and I am happy to say that this anticipation has been realized[42].

Within a year of Murrell's paper, a British chemist, William Martindale, prepared nitroglycerin in tablet form in a dose of 1/100 of a grain. The apothecary system of posology was in use then. The current metric system did not appear until the latter part of the 20th century. Martindale's tablet dissolved rapidly when placed in the mouth accounting for its rapid absorption and immediate relief of symptoms. He vouched for its safety by saying that it was stable, non-volatile, and that it could not be detonated when taken in this manner[44]. Parke-Davis was the first American pharmaceutical house to prepare and market nitroglycerin in tablet form[45,46].

In 1883, Mathew Hay published a paper describing his experiments on the pharmacology of nitroglycerin[47]. He was able to delineate to some extent the chemical nature and physiological action of this agent. Hay was a demonstrator of practical materia medica at the University of Edinburgh. His observations with other antianginal remedies, however, led him to favor nitrite of sodium rather than nitroglycerin or even the amyl nitrite that Brunton preferred. Figure 8 is a reproduction of the opening paragraphs of his handwritten manuscript on the value of some nitric, nitrous and nitro- compounds in angina pectoris.

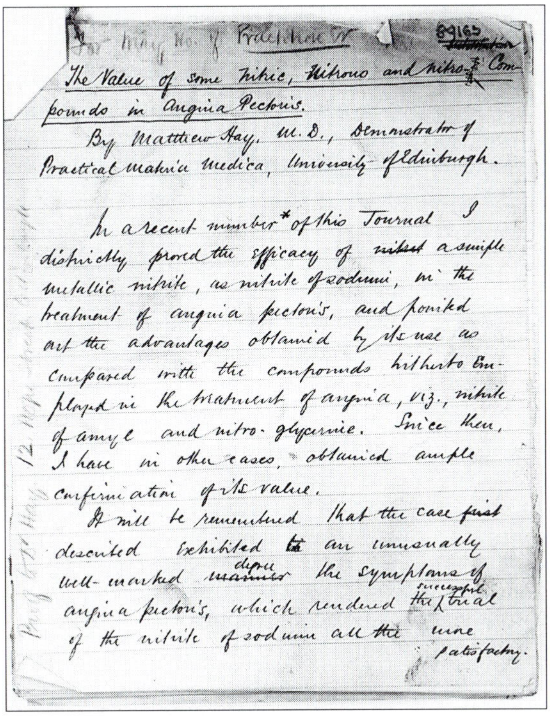
The Value of some Nitric, Nitrous and Nitro- Compounds in Angina Pectoris.
By Matthew Hay, M. D., Demonstrator of Practical Materia Medica, University of Edinburgh.

In a recent number* of this Journal I distinctly proved the efficacy of a simple metallic nitrite, as nitrite of sodium, in the treatment of angina pectoris, and pointed out the advantages obtained by its use as compared with the compounds hitherto employed in the treatment of angina, viz., nitrite of amyl and nitro-glycerine. Since then, I have in other cases, obtained ample confirmation of its value.

It will be remembered that the case first described exhibited an unusually well-marked degree the symptoms of angina pectoris, which rendered the successful trial of the nitrite of sodium all the more satisfactory.

Figure 8 Mathew Hay: 'The value of some nitric, nitrous and nitro-compounds in angina pectoris', Edinburgh, 1883. *Photo Source The Wellcome Institute Library. Literary Source Manuscript: WMS 2794. By courtesy of the Wellcome Trustees*

Despite the headache, which is of short duration only, nitroglycerin sublingually has continued to remain in constant use since its introduction by Murrell as an allopathic agent. It has proven its value time and again. Practically every patient today with coronary artery disease carries a small bottle of nitroglycerin tablets for emergency use as the need arises. Experimental techniques of the 20th century, especially angiography, made it possible to prove the vasodilating properties of nitrates and nitroglycerin as well as their hemo-dynamic effects on preload and afterload.

The longer acting nitrates did not appear until the 1940s. By this time several large pharmaceutical houses turned their attention towards the development of drugs capable of sustained vasodilatation of the coronary arteries. The true pathophysiologic basis of angina pectoris was now well-recognized and relief of ischemia appeared to be the logical route in the medical management of the anginal syndrome. A number of nitrate-based vasodilating agents were introduced beginning with pentaer-ythritol tetranitrate by Parke-Davis. Other companies introduced the isosorbide dinitrates and still others manufactured nitroglycerin in the long-acting form. An interesting and quite successful approach was the formulation of nitroglycerin as a paste, ointment or patch for delivery through the skin.

The 20th century saw a veritable avalanche of pharmaceutical agents in the management of cardiac disturbances. Antianginal nitrates were but a small part of this huge outpouring, as the 20th century unfolded. In the succeeding paragraphs and in other sections of this text, we shall see how other antianginal agents were introduced along with inotropic, diuretic, antiarrhythmic and antihypertensive pharmaceuticals. All these new drugs were a result of the marked changes that have occurred in the preparation and distribution of cardiac and other remedies during this century, the most striking difference being the removal of their preparation from the apothecary or practitioner with their ubiquitous mortar and pestle to the huge pharmaceutical establishments with their sophisticated equipment. Most importantly, a truly scientific atmosphere was now in place for the development of physiologically effective drugs. Research and development are the hallmark of the pharmaceutical industry in this fiercely competitive field. The populace has benefited from all this; there is no doubt about this. But, all is not so 'rosy,' as a pervasive and unrelenting hucksterism continues to mar the scientific achievements of the pharmaceutical firms. One glaring example is that each new discovery brings with it second and third generation congeners with claims of enhanced efficacy and minimal adverse effects. That such is not the case is all too well known, and one of the pitfalls of this hucksterism.

The apothecary today is no longer in existence. He has been replaced by the pharmacist with a university degree, who, though functioning for the most part as a distributor of factory-prepared drugs, is, nevertheless, learned enough to act as the watch-dog of the physician's prescription.

The apothecary of yesteryear was in essence a shopkeeper with a small area set aside where he compounded pills, ointments, suppositories and infusions. For many years he did not have to be nor was he a learned man. For centuries he did not possess a degree or diploma. His training consisted of an apprenticeship, upon completion of which, he would be able to open his own shop. His equipment for many years was largely a herb garden, but he also had cupboards stocked with remedies from foreign lands. Figure 9 is an outdoor scene of a pharmacy during the last decade of the 16th century showing the collecting of plants and the compounding of drugs. Figure 10 is another woodcut, also of a scene during the 16th century.

The apothecary did not enjoy any significant degree of social esteem. He was neither a part of the gentry nor of the learned professions. The surgeon of the medieval age and throughout the Renaissance was only a step higher than the apothecary in the social hierarchy. Surgeons were originally barbers and the guilds or schools of barber-surgeons were still extant in the 18th century. Figure 11 depicts the interior of a barber-surgeon's establishment in 1652. Two patients are being treated and blood-letting pans are seen hanging from the ceiling.

As mentioned before, blood-letting was so common that it prompted the illustration in Figure 12. The artist was George Woodward and in a satirical vein it shows a doctor in purgatory approached by many demons who start to purge and bleed him. Are the demons representative of his former patients?

Although surgeons were not on the same social footing as physicians, the barber-surgeons' guilds were, nevertheless, a force with considerable clout, zealously defending their rights and privileges. A copy of the original charter of the barber-surgeons' guild of London is illustrated in Figure 13. This copy was made for Charles John Shoppee in 1858 with the frontispiece depicted in Figure 14 and the coat of arms reproduced in Figure 15.

The guild was the precursor of the Royal College of Surgeons of England. It was not until the end of the 18th and the beginning of the 19th centuries that surgery became firmly established as part of the medical curriculum.

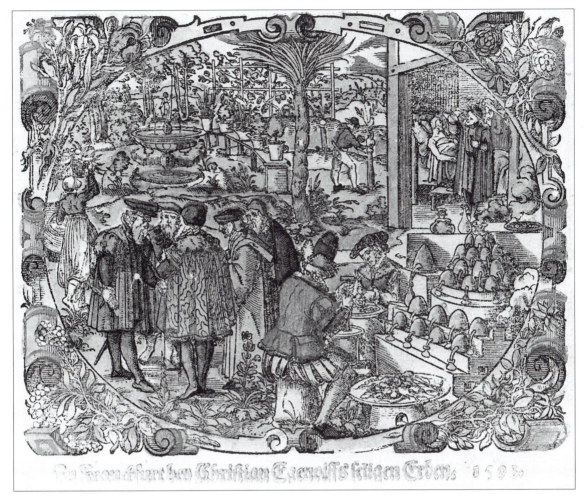

Figure 9 A woodcut of an outdoor scene in the late 16th century showing the collecting of plants and the compounding of drugs. *Photo Source National Library of Medicine. Literary Source Lenitzer, A. (1593). Kreuterbuch. Frankfurt. Courtesy of National Library of Medicine*

In contrast to both the apothecary and barber-surgeons, the physician occupied an entirely higher position in the social pecking order. Although he usually served an apprenticeship, he also earned a university degree. He was, in essence, a man of education. England during the 18th century paid special homage to such men bestowing upon them titles, favors and opportunities for advancement.

It was against this background that William Withering entered the rank of notables in cardiology with his account of the foxglove and some of its medical uses. Although he, himself, was unaware of the true actions of digitalis, his monograph was the first of a series of papers dealing with positive inotropic agents. Although more than two centuries have elapsed since Withering's landmark monograph, digitalis continues to remain one of the most widely used drugs in cardiologic practice.

William Withering was born in Wellington, Shropshire, England in 1741 and died in 1799. He was the only son of the local apothecary. The father was prosperous enough to send young William to the University of Edinburgh from whence he received his doctorate in medicine at the age of 25. Before entering the university, William was trained as an apothecary familiar with herbal medicinal preparations.

He established a quiet country practice at Stafford but after just a few years, he moved to Birmingham where he soon enjoyed one of the

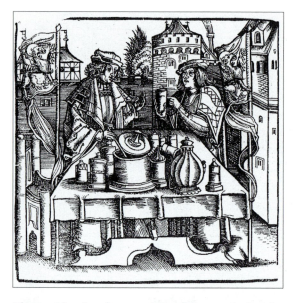

Figure 10 Another woodcut of a scene during the 16th century showing a pharmacy with two men behind a table compounding remedies. *Photo Source National Library of Medicine. Literary Source Brunschwig, H. (1537). Das neu distilier Buch…Stassburg. Courtesy of National Library of Medicine*

largest provincial practices of the day. As a member of Birmingham's Lunar Society, Withering became part of a circle that included some of the leading scientists of England. Withering always maintained a strong interest in scientific matters and despite the demands of a busy practice he pursued especially his botanical investigations. Early in his career he began a systematic collection of the flora indigenous to the Stafford area. In due time, he eventually added to his herbarium plants from all parts of Great Britain. At the age of 35, and only 10 years after receiving his MD, Withering published a classification of Great Britain's botanical specimens. It was entitled *A Botanical Arrangement of All The Vegetables Naturally Growing in Great Britain*. It was in this book that Withering first set down the therapeutic potentialities of *Digitalis purpurea*. The book underwent several editions during his lifetime, the last one just three years before his death. It definitely established him as a botanist of repute. He was held in such high esteem that the French botanist L'Héretier de Brutelle named a genus of plants (of the Salamaceae family) *Witheringia*.

Withering's other interests included chemistry and meteorology. He was the first to demonstrate

that naturally occurring barium carbonate is a compound distinct from other barium salts. Withering's name was again commemorated when the mineralogist, Abraham Werner, referred to barium carbonate as 'witherite'.

Withering's interest in the weather may have been fueled by his chronic pulmonary illness which was probably tuberculosis, and which is known to be affected by climatic changes. As far as cardiology is concerned, Withering's masterpiece was his monograph entitled *An Account of the Foxglove And Some of its Medical Uses: with Practical Remarks on Dropsy, And Other Diseases*. It was published in 1785. Figure 16 is a reproduction of the frontispiece of this great classic on digitalis[48,49].

Withering described in detail his experience with the drug in a series of 163 patients over a span of 9 years. Several important elements were underscored in his treatise. They were his discovery that the active ingredient of the foxglove plant was digitalis; the use of a standardized preparation for proper evaluation of a dose-response relationship; and his description of the effects of the drug including toxic manifestations[50].

Withering's botanical knowledge was of such magnitude that he was able to identify the foxglove plant as the essential ingredient in a secret prescription dispensed by a locally known rural herbalist. She was an old woman in Shropshire who had acquired a reputation for being able to effect cures when the regular practitioners failed. She was known by the sobriquet 'Old Mother Hutton'[51]. In his monograph, Withering describes how he first became aware of the diuretic properties of digitalis. 'In the year 1775, my opinion was asked concerning a family recipe for the cure of the dropsy, I was told that it had long been kept a secret by an old woman in Shropshire (by some named as 'Old Mother Hutton') who had sometimes made cures after the more regular practitioners had failed. I was informed also that the effects produced were violent vomiting and purging; for the diuretic effects seemed to have been overlooked. This medicine was composed of twenty or more different herbs; but it was not very difficult for one conversant in these subjects to perceive that the active herb could be no other than the Foxglove'. Figure 17 is a photograph of *Digitalis purpurea*, the foxglove plant.

Although Withering did comment on 'the power of the drug' over 'the motion of the heart',

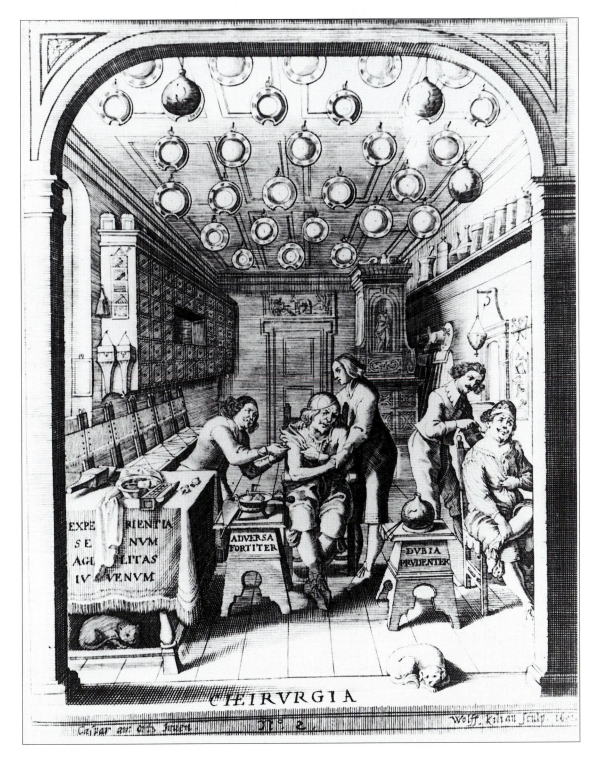

Figure 11 Engraving by W. Kilian (c.1652) showing interior of barber-surgeon's establishment with two patients being treated and blood-letting pans hanging from the ceiling. *Photo Source National Library of Medicine. Literary Source Photo Archives. Courtesy of National Library of Medicine*

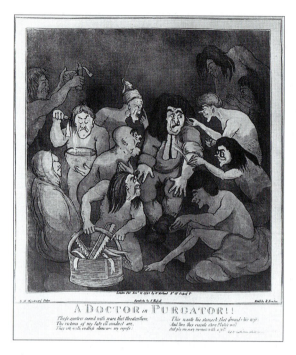

Figure 12 A doctor is approached by many demons (patients?) in purgatory, who start to bleed, purge and treat him. *Photo Source National Library of Medicine. Literary Source Etching and aquatint. London, W. Holland, Nov. 11, 1792. Courtesy of National Library of Medicine*

In the name of god amen. In the tenthe
dai of may. the zeer of oure lord athou-
sand. cccc. and. xxv. in the zeer of kyng
herry the. vi. the. iiij. By the good ad-
vijs of the worschipful men of the craft
or science of cirurgie in the citee of london. and at the comounalte of the same
craft a composicioun or an ordinance
in this matere is maad. and assentid stabli
to stonde euer here aftir. ¶ ffirst that
zeerli the seid craft come togidere on the
dai of Seint Cosme and Damian afore noon.
and chese hem .iiij. maistris for the zeer as
oold custum was. to rule and gouerne
wel and truli the seid craft. And that
tho maistris haue the tresour and co-
moun godis of the same craft or felo-
schip i gouernaunce the said zeer and
ther to be bounden therfore att the valu

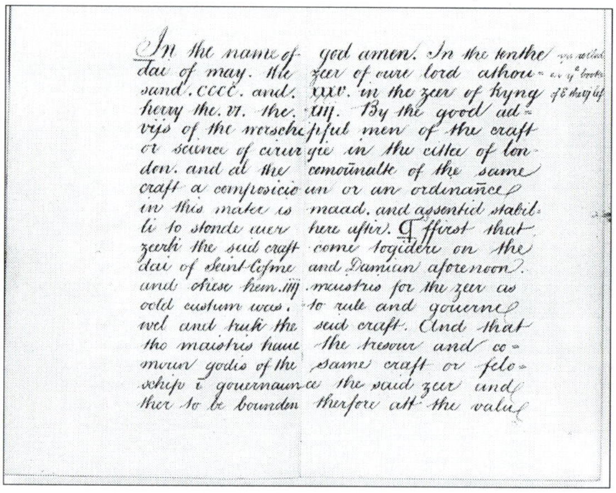

Figure 13 Copy of the original charter of the barber-surgeons of London, 1858. *Photo Source The Wellcome Institute Library. Literary Source WIHM Western MS 1054. The charter. By courtesy of the Wellcome Trustees*

he had absolutely no idea what the mechanism was. Withering used the drug primarily in dropsy mistakenly attributing the favorable effects to a diuretic action rather than a cardiotonic one. In fact, only subsequent research by others identified digitalis as a cardiac glycoside. Though not called by that name and with their mechanism of action completely unknown, cardiac glycosides date their use back to antiquity, long before Withering's time.

Probably the oldest known cardiac glycoside-containing plant is squill. Mention of this plant is to be found in the Ebers Papyrus and in *De Universa Medicina*, the encyclopedic materia medica of Dioscorides. Neither the actual chemical composition nor its action on the heart was known at the time. It was used as an ingredient in the preparation of the theriacal drugs.

The use of digitalis came at a much later date. The name is derived from the latin designation for the foxglove plant, *Digitalis purpurea* when L. Fuchs originally described it in 1542[52]. The plant was known in Germany as fingerhut which means thimble. The Latin word for thimble is 'digitalibum'. The original English name for the plant was 'folksglove' with the glove part of the name alluding to its shape, that of the finger of the glove. Folksglove later evolved into foxglove.

In his *De Historia Stirpium Commentarii*, Fuchs ascribed to the plant both purgative and emetic properties. He also thought it would be useful in dropsy, and he recommended that it be given in the form of a decoction or infusion[53]. The foxglove became a popular remedy in English folk medicine. The English herbalists used the plant frequently throughout the 16th and 17th centuries. Both Gerarde and Parkinson mention it in their herbals[50]. There were many indications for its use but never once was there any mention of a heart disorder being one of them. Welsh physicians of the 13th century had used the herbal preparation as an external medicament and it was still being used in the 17th century as a remedy for skin diseases. It was also used in epilepsy and scrofula, the king's evil[53]. Dodoens described its use in 1554 as an expectorant prepared by boiling the leaves in wine[53].

The plant was used more widely in England than anywhere else. The *London Pharmacopoeia* listed it for the first time in 1661, but when the medical reform movement reached its height in the 1740s, it was deleted from the list of acceptable remedies. The lack of the drugs efficacy in relieving or curing the diverse maladies for which it was used, as well as its alarming toxicity accounted for its removal from the *London Pharmacopoeia*.

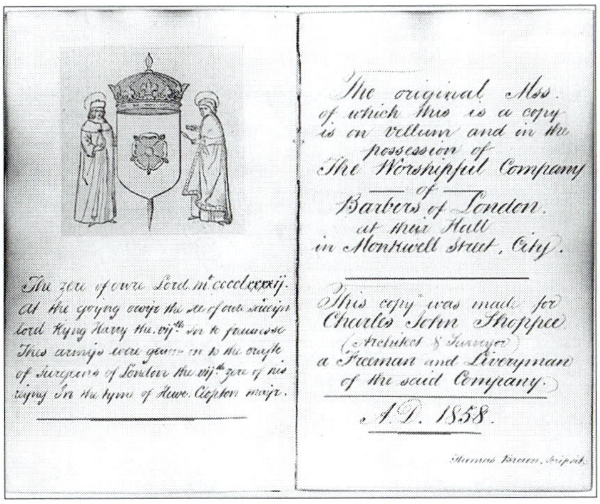

Figure 14 Copy of title-page and end of charter of the barber-surgeons of London. *Photo Source The Wellcome Institute Library. Literary Source Manuscript: WMS 1054. By courtesy of the Wellcome Trustees*

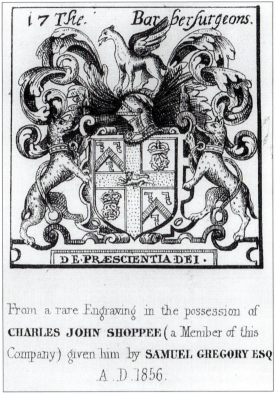

Figure 15 Coat of arms of the barber-surgeons' guild. *Photo Source The Wellcome Institute Library. Literary Source Manuscript: WMS 1054. By courtesy of the Wellcome Trustees*

When Withering introduced the foxglove as a successful remedy in the relief of dropsy he was quite shrewd in its posology, managing in this manner to decrease the frequency of toxic reactions. This he learned through experience since in his earlier days with the drug he too was plagued with its toxicity. Withering finally arrived at a dose of one grain twice a day – mixed with opium to control nausea and vomiting. The drug was given in the form of either an infusion of leaves or the dried leaf itself. Only four years after Withering's monograph was published, digitalis became part of Edinburgh's *Infirmary Pharmacopeia*. Jonathan Stokes was primarily responsible for alerting the Edinburgh physicians to this medicament[50].

Lack of specific knowledge regarding the pharmacological spectrum of digitalis compounded by ignorance on the part of practitioners regarding titration of dosage were impediments to the acceptance of the drug as a valuable therapeutic agent. Somberg recounts the abuses suffered by digitalis in the hands of several generations of physicians following the publication of Withering's monograph[50]. There was, however, some recognition of its effects on the cardiovascular system, the very same year that Withering died. In 1799, John Ferriar described the cardiac effects in his *An essay on the medical properties of Digitalis purpurea or foxglove*[54]. He wrote that the 'extractions from the leaf furnish us a means of regulating the pulse to

our wish and supporting it in a given state of velocity as long as we may judge it proper'. The positive inotropic effect of digitalis was recognized by another contemporary, Thoma Beddoes. Jacobs quotes him as saying that 'digitalis increases the organic action of the contractile fibers'[53].

Kreysig in 1814 was the first to postulate a central nervous system effect with digitalis. He ascribed the slowing of the pulse to a narcotic action on the brain, considering this a side effect with the principal action of the drug still concerning itself specifically with the heart[50].

Bouillaud in 1835 described cases in which digitalis controlled a rapid intermittent irregular pulse[55]. It was because of this quieting effect on the heartbeat that Bouillaud called digitalis the 'opium of the heart'[56].

The entire 19th century was punctuated by clinical and animal studies on the foxglove. Gradually there began to emerge from these

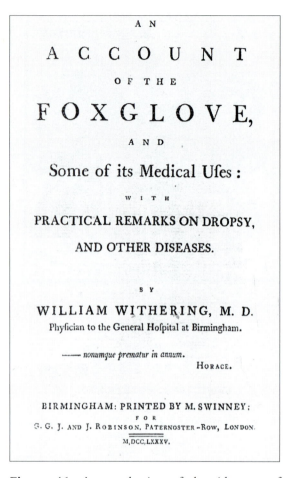

AN

ACCOUNT

OF THE

FOXGLOVE,

AND

Some of its Medical Ufes :

WITH

PRACTICAL REMARKS ON DROPSY,

AND OTHER DISEASES.

BY

WILLIAM WITHERING, M. D.

Phyfician to the General Hofpital at Birmingham.

———— nonumque prematur in annum.

HORACE.

BIRMINGHAM: PRINTED BY M. SWINNEY;

FOR

G. G. J. AND J. ROBINSON, PATERNOSTER-ROW, LONDON.

M,DCC,LXXXV.

Figure 16 A reproduction of the title-page of Withering's monograph on digitalis. *Photo Source National Library of Medicine. Literary Source Photo Archives. Courtesy of National Library of Medicine*

studies, the wide spectrum of pharmacologic activity that digitalis possessed. Consonant with these studies an intensive and prolonged search was carried on to isolate the active principles of the plant. Many of these studies continued into the first half of the 20th century.

Some of the first animal experiments were conducted in the mid-19th century. Vulpian in France and Fothergill of England were quite active in the field[49-59]. Fothergill poisoned a heart with aconite and watched its contractility rebound with digitalis. He called this the 'action par excellence of digitalis'.

Frank's experiments in 1895 indicated that digitalis increased cardiac output only in the compromised heart and had no effect on output in the normal frog heart[60-62]. This was confirmed by

Bijlsma and Roessingh in 1922[63]. Further proof became available when Anitschkow and Trendelenburg conducted a definitive experiment in 1928 wherein they showed that strophanthin had little effect on the normal heart but markedly reduced right atrial pressure and increased cardiac output in the failing heart[64]. After Krayer refined their experimental method, it became a standard technique for determining the positive inotropic effect of a variety of agents[65].

Many other studies during the early 20th century supported the concept that digitalis had a positive inotropic action. In 1927, Wiggers and Stimson used optical recording techniques to delineate various hemodynamic parameters after administration of digitalis and strophanthin in the normal dog[66]. They showed that these drugs increased the gradient of pressure development and left ventricular systolic pressure. This was a very important study and so was that conducted by Gold and Cattell in 1940[57]. The latter demonstrated beyond a doubt that digitalis had a positive inotropic action on cardiac muscle. They used the right ventricular papillary muscle of the cat to delineate the mechanism whereby digitalis abolished heart failure.

The earliest studies of the 20th century in man were carried out by Mackenzie and Sir Thomas Lewis. They were interested mainly in the effect on cardiac rhythm. Mackenzie suggested that the primary action of digitalis was to slow the ventricular rate[67,68]. Sir Thomas Lewis also noted the bradycardia induced by digitalis, like Mackenzie, especially in the presence of atrial fibrillation. This eventually came to be one of the prime indications for digitalis, which had a notably beneficial effect in chronic atrial fibrillation[69,70].

In 1928, Cohn and Stewart used a moving X-ray film that recorded decreases in cardiac shadow in dogs during both systole and diastole indicative of improved contractility[71-73]. In 1932, these two men confirmed that clinical trials in man induced the same effects on cardiac output whether the heart was normal or failing[74]. Other investigators in the US, France and Germany also noticed improvement in cardiac function in humans even in the presence of normal ryhthm.

Mason and Braunwald, and also Smith and Haber, summarized in 1968 and 1973 respectively the currently held view on digitalis[75,76]. It is that digitalis has a positive inotropic effect in patients with heart failure and normal sinus rhythm. This is its primary action. Its chronotropic effect is exerted through the vagus nerve and by a direct depressant action on atrioventricular conduction. However, both its inotropic and chronotropic effects can be modified by the action of digitalis on autonomic reflexes, blood vessels and conduction.

The search for the active principles of the foxglove began in the early decades of the 19th century and continued into the 20th century. The initial extraction studies were based on the mistaken belief that the active ingredients were alkaloid in nature rather than glycosides.

In 1824, Leroyer of Geneva extracted from the plant an alkali from which Prevost later obtained a fine crystalline material which he labeled 'digitaline' thinking that it was an alkaloid[52]. Subsequent experiments proved that it was not an alkaloid despite its biological activity. In 1840, Donovan attributed the biological activity of digitaline to a resin that it contained[77].

The continued search for the active principle was fostered by La Société de Pharmacie de Paris. In 1835, the society offered a prize of 500 francs. This was doubled to 1000 francs in 1840, and one year later the prize was won by E. Homolle and Theodore A. Quevenne when they extracted from the plant a biologically active material in crystalline form[78,79]. In 1935, an American chemist, Robert Elderfield, thought that the awardees had probably isolated an impure form of digitoxin, though these men called it digitaline[80].

The name digitaline (without the e when it was definitely known not be be an alkaloid) subsequently created a great deal of confusion because it was applied to several quite different products. The first step in this confusion occurred in 1869, when a French pharmacist, Claude Adolphe Nativelle, isolated from the foxglove a crystalline material which he called 'digitaline crystalisée'[81]. Six years later, Johann Schmiedeberg extracted a well-defined crystalline substance that was cardioactive and which he named 'digitoxin'[77]. Some subsequent workers expressed the opinion that Nativelle's digitalin was really digitoxin[82]. Schmiedeberg also added to the confusion when he investigated a commercial product prepared from the seeds of the foxglove and marketed under the name 'digitalin'. He extracted a fraction from this commercial product which he termed 'digitalin'.

Both Schmiedeberg's digitoxin and the digitalin from the seeds underwent extensive chemical

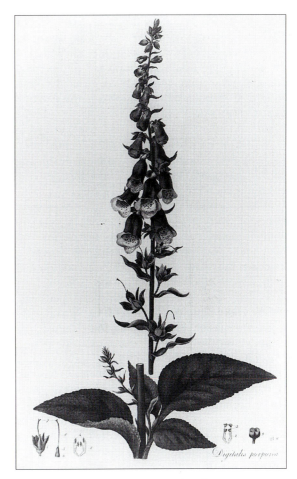

Figure 17 *Digitalis purpurea*, the foxglove plant. *Photo Source National Library of Medicine. Literary Source Photo Archives. Courtesy of National Library of Medicine*

analyses by several chemists working independently of each other. They were finally classified as glycosides and recognized as the active ingredients of *Digitalis purpurea*. Cloetta proved in 1920 that digitoxin was the most potent cardiac glycoside then available[83]. It was known commercially as digitaline nativelle. I, myself, prescribed it in the 1950s under this name.

Windaus completed the analytical investigation in 1928[84,85]. Windaus and his co-workers were also active in the investigation of digitalin from the seeds of the foxglove plant[85]. Cloetta and Kraft extracted still another glycoside from the leaves of the plant. They called it gitoxin[85]. *Digitalis lanata*, a plant related to foxglove, yielded an entirely new glycoside and a current favorite called digoxin[86].

It was extracted by Sidney Smith in 1930. Arthur Stoll and his co-workers also set their sights on *Digitalis lanata*. They were able to extract from it the natural precursors of digitoxin, gitoxin and digoxin. The three precursors were called digilanid A, B & C. Stoll called the digilanids the genuine digitalis glycosides[52].

In 1951, the Ciba Foundation tried to create order out of the chaotic morass in nomenclature. They proposed the root name 'cardanolide' for the digitalis-like compounds and 'bufanolide' for the glycosides found in squill[87].

Withering's admonition expressed in his monograph is worth repeating: 'After all, in spite of opinion, prejudice, or error, time will fix the real value upon this discovery, and determine whether I have imposed upon myself and others, or contributed to the benefit of science and mankind'[88].

As the foregoing words have indicated, the toxicity of digitalis has been a particularly worrisome thorn in clinical practice. Indeed for many years, the foxglove was listed among the poisonous plants. The therapeutic–toxic ratio is one of the smallest in clinical remedies. One of Withering's greatest contribution in his monograph was his admonition regarding overdose. His graphic description of a well-meaning but ill-informed wife in preparing an infusion of digitalis leaves for her husband should never be forgotten. 'This good woman knew the medicine of her country, but not the dose of it, for the husband narrowly escaped with his life'[88]. This was his comment when he described how the wife almost caused her husband's death when she boiled a large handful of digitalis leaves in a half pint of water and gave the concoction to her husband for his asthma.

Over the past two hundred years there have been repeated reports and warnings concerning its toxicity. Its poisonous effects have caused it to play a homicidal role in fiction. Mary Webb, Dorothy Sayers and Agatha Christie impugned the foxglove in this manner. Gwilt and Gwilt in listing the elements of Agatha Christie's poisonous pharmacopeia mention the use of digitalis six times[89]. Dame Agatha's familiarity with the poisonous potentiality of digitalis is exemplified especially in the short story entitled *The Herb of Death*. Parson reviewed in detail the case of Dr Coutis de Pommerais of Paris who was a notorious murderer and killed two of his former patients with lethal doses of digitalis. His trial took place in the late 19th century[90].

Burchell's paper on digitalis poisoning is a goldmine of anecdotal information on the subject and should be read in its entirety[91]. I was particularly impressed with his recounting of a scam that was uncovered during the 1930s involving many doctors and lawyers wherein the electrocardiographic changes of digitalis were used to buttress fraudulent claims of heart disease. This led to the suicide of a notable New York physician, who, though innocent, was unwittingly part of the scam. Ironically he had been the leading co-author of a paper entitled *A dangerous preparation of digitalis*, published not too long before his involvement became known[92]. Burchell quotes a letter by Dr Kossmann written just before Dr Wyckoff committed suicide. It is as follows:

When all of the dirty business came to a head in 1937 I was a clinical assistant visiting physician at Bellevue ... Wyckoff was a strict disciplinarian with himself and with others. One evening, I believe in February or March, 1937, I was called by Wyckoff to come to his private patient office. I think on East 37th Street. When I arrived he handed me two electrocardiograms and asked me what I thought of them. Each showed abnormalities of the T wave. I gave my standard correlative interpretation of them, namely, that 'they displayed abnormalities of the T wave ascribable to myocardial disease, digitalis or both. The light in the waiting room, now devoid of patients, was dim but I thought I perceived a further tightening of his usually tightly compressed lips. He thanked me, turned to enter his consulting room, and left me to find my way out, a brusqueness I had come to expect from him. I thought no more of the episode ... until after the holiday week-end of 1937. On returning by train, I was shocked to read ... that John Wyckoff had been found in coma in the anatomy laboratory of the Medical School. This straight-laced, rigidly honest, puritanically ethical man just could not cope with the disgrace that might be heaped upon him by colleagues and the public who would never believe that he had been duped by dishonest and avaricious doctors and lawyers...

There are several substances derived from amines which also exhibit positive inotropic properties like digitalis but differ from it in that they cause an increase in heart rate. They are classified as catecholamines and include the well-known epinephrine and norepinephrine as well as dopamine, dobutamine, amrinone and milrinone.

Foremost among them in terms of longevity is epinephrine, also known as adrenaline. It was in 1894 and 1895, that G. Oliver and E. Schäfer extracted from the adrenal glands, a substance that had very interesting physiological properties[93]. They found that when a large amount of this adrenal extract was given intravenously to rabbits it resulted in their death. On the other hand when a small amount was given it caused an immediate and marked rise in blood pressure. Subsequent experiments indicated that the rise in blood pressure was due to increased peripheral resistance through a generalized constriction of the arterioles. They did not know what the active principle was but were rather certain that it came from the medullary portion of the adrenal gland[94].

Their discovery stirred up a great deal of interest among physiologists, and those who had a chemical bent set out to isolate the active principle. Within two years, John Jacob Abel, who was the first professor of pharmacology in the western hemisphere, presented a paper before the Association of American Physicians wherein he described his method of isolating the active principle and which he named epinephrine. In rapid succession he published two other papers all of which established him as being the first to isolate this important hormone[94–97].

On November 5, 1900, Jokichi Takamine applied for a US patent on an extract of the adrenal gland which he called 'adrenalin'[94]. Six months later he was granted the right to use the word 'adrenalin' as a trademark[98]. Later Takamine assigned the license to produce it to Parke, Davis & Co. Takamine was an entrepreneur who labored in secret while attempting to isolate adrenalin. Later, when fully protected by the patent laws, he did his utmost to publicize the product in conjunction with Parke, Davis & Co. by publications and presentations before learned societies[99–103]. In all of these activities he extolled the therapeutic versatility of adrenalin claiming that it was useful in deafness, heart disease, Addison's disease and exophthalmic goiter.

Takamine went on to make a fortune while Abel remained an academician searching for ways to purify his epinephrine and simultaneously engaging in controversy on the matter with other investigators including, of course, Takamine. Abel persistently

asserted that Takamine's adrenalin was not pure, and, in this, he was right because subsequent studies proved that it contained a good deal of norepinephrine. The controversy died down when Abel turned his attention to other projects.

In 1905 Eliot's paper on the action of adrenalin appeared in the *Journal of Physiology*[104]. He outlined in detail the positive inotropic and chronotropic effects of adrenaline; excellent attributes but marred by its propensity to induce arrhythmias. It was this particular adverse reaction that caused a new search for other inotropic agents in the catecholamine family.

Goldberg described the cardiovascular and renal action of dopamine with its potential clinical applications in 1972[105]. Tuttle in 1975 described the ability of another catecholamine 'dobutamine' to selectively increase cardiac contractility[106]. Still others were synthesized but failed to make the grade in clinical practice.

Most recently two new products were introduced as effective inotropes. These are amrinone and milrinone. They both have a positive inotropic action with vasodilative properties and minimal effects on heart rate[107,108]. As with the others, these new agents carry a high price by their side reactions with the trade-off definitely not in their favor. The ideal inotropic agent still eludes us.

The history of Ca^{++} antagonists is interminably entwined with the efforts of one man, A. Fleckenstein. The identification and development began and continued in his laboratory in the Physiological Institute at the University of Freiburg. In his paper on the history of calcium antagonists he divided its evolution into three periods[109]. The first period consists of the primary events which gave birth to the concept of calcium antagonism. Extensive studies on the mechanism and sites of action constitute the second period while the third concerns itself with the acceptance of the principles and the development of congeners.

Two pharmaceutical companies (Knoll and Hoechst) were responsible for getting Dr Fleckenstein involved. In his own words this is what Fleckenstein had to say about it:

The discovery of Ca^{++} antagonism occurred by chance. It happened in November 1963, that I was asked by two German pharmaceutical companies (Knoll and Hoechst) to have a look on two newly synthesized coronary vasodilators with unexplained cardiodepressant side effects. One of these compounds was prenylamine. The other compound had not yet a name, but was later called Isoptin, Iproveratril, or by the generic name verapamil. To our surprise, it rapidly became evident that both compounds mimicked the cardiac effects of simple Ca^{++} withdrawal. As I reported in 1964, both substances, like Ca^{++} deficiency, inhibited cardiac excitation–contraction coupling in that they diminished contractile force without a major change in the action potential (Fleckenstein, 1964). Moreover, both substances decreased Ca^{++} dependent high-energy phosphate utilization in the beating ventricles and lowered extra oxygen consumption strictly in parallel with the depression of contractile activity. However, all of these inhibitory effects of the two drugs could be neutralized promptly with the help of additional Ca^{++}, β-adrenergic catecholamines, or cardiac glycosides that is to say, by measures which were suitable to increase or restore the Ca^{++} supply to the contractile system. These observations led us to suppose that the common action of verapamil and prenylamine might consist of an interference with the mediator function of Ca^{++} in excitation–contraction coupling of heart muscle. In fact, the explanatory assumption of a β–receptor-blocking activity of both drugs, initially put forward by the two drug companies, had definitely been disproved by us in 1967. Hence, as an alternative, the concept of Ca^{++} antagonism as a new pharmacodynamic principle arose.[109]

In 1968, the chief chemist of the Knoll company, Dr Ferdinand Dengel, brought Fleckenstein a methoxy derivative of verapamil which was labeled D600. It proved to be much stronger than verapamil. D600 stood for the fact that it was the 600th compound synthesized by Dengel. It was later named gallopamil. A year later another friend visited Fleckenstein. He was Professor Kroneberg, a senior pharmacologist at the Bayer Co. He had with him two bottles labeled 'Bay a 1040' and 'Bay a 7168', both coronary vasodilators but with marked negative inotropic action. Kroneberg was seeking clarification of this dual action. Fleckenstein obliged, and in due time he was able to show that these two agents had a mechanism of action in common with verapamil, prenylamine

and D600. He decided to call this entire new family of vasodilators, 'calcium-antagonists'. The actual name of the Bayer drugs was a carefully kept secret, and it was only after Fleckenstein issued his reports did it become known that Bay a 1040 was nifedipine and Bay a 7168 was nilupidine.

Fleckenstein continued his research with this class of compounds in collaboration with Kohlhardt. Over a period of years they established that these drugs selectively inhibited the slow transsarcolemmal inward Ca^{++} current in the myocardial fibers, and for this reason the drugs came to be known as calcium channel blocking agents even though Fleckenstein preferred his original designation of Ca^{++} antagonist. This was the second period of Fleckenstein's historical outline. Notice too that we are dealing with agents that are purely chemical in origin and synthetically made through the manipulation of chemical structures. Herbs, botanical plants and the apothecary are no longer to be found. The giant pharmaceutical firms of the 20th century have established their pre-eminence in their search for physiologically active agents.

All smooth muscle cells are dependent upon the inward flux of Ca^{++} ions for contraction with the coronary smooth muscle exhibiting the greatest sensitivity to the spasmolytic action of Ca^{++} antagonists. Peripheral arterioles also are affected by inhibition of the inward migration of Ca^{++} ions. This important physiological fact was brought out by Grün and Fleckenstein in 1972[110–112]. Moreover, Fleckenstein's basic research served to establish a new principle in cardiac pathophysiology. This was that when the myocardium is overloaded with uninhibited Ca^{++} ion penetration, necrosis of the myocardial fibers occurs, and that this process could be prevented with Ca^{++} antagonists[113,114]. A number of workers subsequently showed that even hypoxic and ischemic hearts could be protected against Ca^{++} induced damage with Ca^{++} antagonists such as verapamil[115,116], or diltiazem[117,118].

Clinical trials conducted in the early 1960s documented the anticipated beneficial effects of the calcium antagonists in coronary artery disease. Germany was the first to use these drugs as antianginal agents but it took several more years before the Food and Drug Administration (FDA) would allow their use in the USA as coronary vasodilators.

Bender in 1966 was the first to demonstrate the antiarrhythmic effects of verapamil[119]. Shamroth confirmed this in 1972, and over the next several years verapamil was found to be quite effective in the treatment of supraventricular tachycardias[120]. Not all Ca^{++} antagonists have this therapeutic effect. Electrophysiologic studies begun in 1970 showed that some of the Ca^{++} antagonists already on the market had a depressant effect on SA node automaticity and atrioventricular conduction. Contributors to an understanding of this mode of action were Zipes and Fischer in 1974 and Wit and Cranefield, also in 1974[121,122].

As a result of all this a dualistic concept of cardiac excitation emerged. Ca^{++} antagonists would inhibit the slow Ca^{++} channel dependence of impulse generation in the SA node and conduction of impulse to the AV node whereas they had no effect on the Na^{+} dependent excitatory events in the atrial myocardium, His bundle, Purkinje fibers and ventricular myocardium. The Japanese led by Taira and Narimatsu documented this with their cross-circulated AV node experiments on dogs between the years 1972 and 1975[123–125].

Since 1970, the beginning of Fleckenstein's third period, there has been a phenomenal increase in the use of calcium channel blocking agents. They have repeatedly demonstrated their ability to counteract anginal episodes, decrease blood pressure by virtue of their arterial dilating properties, protect the degeneration of the myocardium from Ca^{++} overload, control certain arrhythmias, and most recently, demonstrate an antiatherogenic effect. These are formidable properties for a class of drugs that did not even exist before the 1960s. The Germans were not the only ones responsible for their development. Diltiazem, for example, originated in Japan and its clinical profile was delineated by Nakajima and associates in 1975[126].

The family of Ca^{++} antagonists has grown rapidly since Fleckenstein's original efforts, and it continues to do so thanks to the research efforts of the major pharmaceutical houses. Moreover, the various drugs being developed most recently have a specific physiological orientation. One group selectively suppresses the slow Ca^{++} current but does not inhibit the effects of Mg^{++}. Examples of this group are diltiazem and the nifedipine derivatives. Another group, examples of which are terodiline and carroverine, affects both the electrogenic Ca^{++} and Mg^{++} activity.

Beta blockers were introduced to cardiology in the 1960s. Since then they have assumed an important role in the pharmacological management of hypertension, ischemic heart disease and certain arrhythmias.

It was Ahlquist who first postulated the hypothesis that catecholamine activity was mediated through alpha and beta adrenergic receptors[127]. This was in 1948. The seemingly contradictory actions of the various catecholamines could be explained only with this hypothesis. For example, it was found that epinephrine can both excite and inhibit smooth muscle. Ahlquist theorized that if epinephrine attached itself to certain receptors located in the target smooth muscle which he labeled alpha, constriction would occur. On the other hand, stimulation of the beta receptors would result in relaxation. This stimulated interest in searching for agents that could block these receptors and thus neutralize catecholamine effects. When agents capable of doing this were identified, it not only proved a boon in medical management but also served to confirm Ahlquist's concepts.

In 1958, Powell and Slater synthesized an agent with beta-blocking ability[128]. It was dichloroisoproterenol. Unfortunately, this compound was also a partial agonist which made it unsuitable for clinical application in view of the potential adverse effects it could precipitate. The synthesis of this drug, however, laid the groundwork for other workers in their search for a compound without any agonistic catecholamine action. The first such product was introduced by Sir James Black and associates in the late 1950s. The drug was called pronethalol. It, too, could not be used clinically because it produced thymic tumors in mice. The search continued for safer compounds. Success was achieved in 1962 when Black and Stephenson described their observations with propranolol[129,130]. They found that propranolol was a competitive beta-adrenergic antagonist devoid of any agonist activity, and any clinically significant adverse effects. It was marketed under the trade name of Inderal and in a very short time it became the prototype for numerous congeners.

By this time Ahlquist's simple classification had mushroomed with subdivisions of the alpha receptors into many subsets and with a similar division of the beta receptors. In particular beta-1 receptors were seen localized to the myocardium while the beta-2 type were found in the smooth muscle of other sites such as the bronchi. In 1989 Emorine isolated a human gene that encodes still another beta-adrenergic receptor. He called it beta-3.

It is about ten times more sensitive than epine-phrine and is relatively resistant to blockade by such antagonists as propranolol[131].

Pharmaceutical houses competed with each other in producing beta blockers that had more affinity for beta-1 rather than beta-2 receptors when the prime indication was cardiac dysfunction. Numerous antiadrenergic compounds flooded the market, each with varying properties. Some blocked alpha-adrenergic receptors. Others had differences in lipid solubility allegedly to minimize central nervous system reactions. Some had intrinsic sympathomimetic activity. Again, marketing claims of superiority, efficiency and minimal side reactions were counterproductive and degraded somewhat the fruitful research efforts of the pharmaceutical industry. This is a sad commentary but no different from the boastful claims by the physicians of yesteryear with their secret formulations.

The development of true diuretics is a phenomenon of the 20th century and represents a triumph of the synthetic chemist. The empiricism that governed the use and selection of botanically derived agents was no longer necessary. The advances of the chemist, however, did require the elucidation of essential knowledge regarding glomerular filtration and tubular reabsorption of salt and water. This knowledge was worked out by A. N. Richards in the 1930s. In his Croonian lecture presented before the Royal Society of Medicine, he outlined in detail the processes of urine formation utilizing the micropuncture technique in the frog kidney[132]. Richards had already established the Merck institute at the request of George Merck, the founder of the Merck pharmaceutical firm. The merger of Merck with Sharp and Dohme, another large pharmaceutical house, did not come about until 1951. This prestigious firm was very instrumental in furthering the development of sulfonamide-derived oral diuretics.

Richards' observations in the frog were also seen in the mammalian kidney. These were reported by Walker and associates in 1941 utilizing the same micropuncture technique[133]. Included in this team was Jean Oliver, who eventually acquired an outstanding reputation as a renal physiologist.

The earliest synthetic diuretics of the early 20th century were the organomercurial agents[134]. These were widely used in the 1940s, especially as adjunct therapy in congestive heart failure. The addition of ammonium chloride tablets was supposed to enhance the diuretic effect of Mercupurine and Mercuhydrin, the trade-name of these organo-mercurials in the USA, but this was more theoretical than factual since repeated scout films of the abdomen constantly revealed unabsorbed ammonium chloride tablets in the intestinal tract. The organomercurials were thought to exert their diuretic action by blocking sulfhydryl-catalyzed dehydrogenases thereby making available hydrogen ions for the exchange reabsorption of sodium ions. Although quite effective as diuretics, these compounds could be given only parenterally, a major drawback for those in need of chronic therapy.

In 1940, Mann and Keilin demonstrated that sulfanilamide was a specific inhibitor of carbonic anhydrase[135]. Five years later Pitts and Alexander clarified the role of carbonic anhydrase in acidifying the urine at the renal tubular level[136]. This was followed by Krebs' report in 1948 confirming that sulfonamides in general possessed the property of inhibiting carbonic anhydrase[137]. These reports led Schwartz to investigate the effects of sulfanilamide on salt and water excretion in congestive heart failure[138]. In 1949 he proposed that sulfanilamide might be a weak natriuretic–diuretic agent.

At the same time, certain pharmaceutical firms were directing their research chemists to synthesize sulfonamide congeners for the inhibition of carbonic anhydrase. In 1950, two Lederle Laboratory researchers, Roblin and Clapp, reported their results with several such inhibitors[139]. Diamox (acetazolamide) was among them, and as a result of Maren's report in 1952[140], it became quite popular as an oral diuretic agent. However, its diuretic effect was nowhere near as potent as the organo-mercurials.

Another pathway of diuresis was now entertained. It was based on the simple notion that if the tubular reabsorption of sodium ions was prevented, the intrinsic osmotic property of this ion would result in the elimination of a good deal of urine. The goal then was to find a congener of the sulfonamides that was a saluretic agent. Diamox was not in this category.

The chemists at Sharp and Dohme became quite active in looking for such an agent. Karl Beyer headed this group[141]. At a symposium of the International Physiology Congress in 1953, Beyer presented a new carbonic anhydrase inhibitor derived from the sulfonamide family that had in addition a saluretic action. It was p-carboxyben-zenesulfonamide (CBS)[142]. It never did achieve any degree of acceptance, probably because of the popularity of Diamox. At any rate, Beyer and his colleagues continued their search for a clinically useful saluretic and in 1958 they were able to publish their initial reports on chlorothiazide[143,144]. This was the first orally active saluretic sulfonamide. In a very short time, the thiazides became an important component of diuretic therapy. Chlorothiazide was marketed as Diuril and hydrochlorothiazide as Hydrodiuril.

The so-called loop diuretics came into being during the 1960s[145–147]. They are actually chloruretic agents. These were initially furosemide and then ethacrynic acid. More recently bumetanide was introduced by Duchin and Davies working independently of each other[148,149]. The loop diuretics were eagerly accepted by the clinician not only because they could be given orally as well as parenterally but also because they possessed potent diuretic capability. However, these new compounds also proved to have a marked kaliuretic effect, a clinically significant defect in that hypopotassemia is now known to predispose to cardiac arrhythmias. In an effort to get around this, amiloride and triamterene were introduced in the 1960s[150,151]. These increased the excretion of sodium by inhibiting its reabsorption in exchange for potassium in the distal portion of the renal tubule: in essence they work as aldosterone antagonists[152,153].

Aldosterone antogonism was another interesting pathway of diuresis that had been previously explored in the 1950s. The physiological role of aldosterone came to light in 1954 through the efforts of Simpson and co-workers[154]. This adrenal cortical hormone causes the retention of sodium and the excretion of potassium. Obviously, an antagonist to this mechanism would appear to be a suitable pathway for the elimination of sodium with its attendant diuresis. The first agent with aldosterone antagonistic properties was spironolactone. It was described by Kagawa and his associates at the Searle Laboratories in 1959[155].

The treatment of hypertension did not begin until the sphygmomanometer was developed. It was only then that hypertension was recognized as a disease entity with ultimately fatal complications, and measures were instituted in an attempt to combat its relentless progress.

Unwittingly the phlebotomists of old may have saved the life of many an individual through blood letting. This simple method of reducing blood volume would most certainly have had a temporary salutory effect on those with elevated blood pressure.

Before 1950 the list of remedies for controlling high blood pressure was astounding besides being useless and often too toxic. They ran the gamut of botanical extracts to rice diets, sodium restriction, nephrectomy and so on. The list is too long to enumerate. Smithwick's sympathectomy appeared to be the only valid approach but this required surgical intervention.

The evolution of antihypertensive therapy since 1950 is also a tribute to modern pharmacology. As in diuretic therapy, advances were made as a direct result of enlightenment on the physiologic mechanisms for the regulation of blood pressure. In a matter of just a few decades the ineffectual therapy of the past was transformed into one with notable physiological efficacy. In particular, the 1980s saw a steam-rolling effect in the multiple approaches towards the pharmacological management of essential hypertension. The final beneficial effects, if any, on the target organs, are still not known but all indications point to a favorable outcome. This is not to imply that the drugs currently used are ideal, but, at least, they appear to be oriented in the right direction. The incidence of side effects is still a major problem and excessive interference with normal homeostatic mechanisms is still a factor that has not been resolved.

Smithwick introduced sympathectomy as a means of permanently blocking the alpha-adrenergic constricting mechanism on the peripheral arterioles. Ganglionic blocking drugs with the same effect were introduced in 1950 as a chemical alternative to the surgical procedure. Several workers were involved in proposing this approach. They were Paton and Zaimis in 1949[156], Smirk[157] and Turner[158] in 1950, Freis in 1951[159] and Schroeder in 1953[160]. Hexamethonium was the initial ganglionic blocking agent. What a relief this drug brought to the practitioner. I, myself, was impressed because prior to its introduction, all I could offer was salt restriction and elixir of phenobarbital.

Shortly after hexamethonium appeared, Smirk introduced as a more efficacious agent, pentolinum[161]. These drugs were quite effective in lowering blood pressure but they often caused alarming side reactions. Despite this, ganglionic-blocking agents were considered for some time the main drug to be used in controlling the blood pressure. Since many of the side reactions of the ganglionic blockers were dose dependent, it was felt that concomitant administration of other agents would allow smaller doses of the ganglionic blockers and thus minimize side effects. It was at about this time that reserpine and hydralazine were introduced and incorporated into the antihypertensive regimen as adjunctive therapy. This so-called 'background' therapy with these two agents was fostered by Vakil (1949)[162], Freis (1954)[163], Taylor, Dustan, Corcoran and Page (1952)[164] and Wilkins (1954)[165]. All of these authors were the leading investigators of hypertension during that era. It should be noted that reserpine was a botanical byproduct of the Indian plant, *Rauwolfia serpentina*, while hydralazine was a synthetic chemical.

A veritable wagonload of drugs was developed by various pharmaceutical houses fiercely competing with each other in what was and continues to be perceived as a highly lucrative market. There was no shortage of clinical investigators throughout the world willing and eager to try each new compound as it was introduced. To enumerate them would have no truly historical value. They all shared the common characteristic of peripheral arteriolar dilatation with or without reduction in cardiac output and/or blood volume. Reductions in cardiac output were accomplished through the negative inotropic and chronotropic effects of beta blockers. This approach, in itself, produced a whole cadre of agents, some short-acting, and others with extended pharmacologic activity. Reduction in blood volume was accomplished primarily through the action of the thiazide diuretics. Peripheral arteriolar dilatation has been effected through centrally acting agents, calcium antagonists and the new angiotensin converting enzyme inhibitors.

Although they have all proven to be, in general, quite effective, the associated penalty, in terms of side effects, has often been quite frustrating. Properly used, these drugs have no doubt prolonged life by postponing the inevitable effects of persistent hypertension on the heart, brain and kidneys. At the same time, their usage has demanded on the part of the practitioner an inexhaustable amount of patience and therapeutic maneuverability in the titration of dose and the avoidance of annoying or, at times, severe side effects.

Throughout all this, it should be quite obvious by now that the main thrust has been a reduction in blood pressure through the sympathetic pathways. This treatment, unfortunately, is purely a symptomatic approach though based on sound physiological principles. The root cause of essential hypertension has yet to be deciphered. It could be a metabolic defect related to the function of smooth muscle, kidney or brain. It is only when the root cause is uncovered can we then truthfully say a cure for this common ailment is in the offing.

Historically the early attempts in the treatment of thromboembolic disorders focused on prevention of thrombus formation, and once formed, prevention of extension or embolization of the clot. The earliest antithrombotic agents were heparin for intravenous administration and the oral anticoagulants belonging to the coumarin group of drugs. More recently antiplatelet agents have been introduced and most recently an immunologic approach against platelet aggregation appears to hold much promise.

The use of anticoagulants in medicine is not new. Leeches with their ability to draw blood freely and without clotting were a valid alternative to blood-letting by venesection for more than a thousand years. Haycraft confirmed this anticoagulating ability of leeches in 1884 with his own observations on the matter[166]. First of all he noted that a leech bite caused blood to flow freely without clotting. In addition, he found that the blood of the common leech, *Hirudo medicinales*, an annelid worm, did not clot even after being ejected by the animal. The active anticoagulant principle in this blood was isolated by Jacoby in 1904[167]. He extracted it from the same type of leech and gave it the logical name of 'hirudin'. This active principle became a useful tool in animal experimentation when clotting was to be avoided. John Jacob Abel, the noted pharmacologist, was responsible for suggesting the use of hirudin in this manner[168]. He demonstrated that hirudin could be used to prevent the blood of a dog from clotting without ill effects while he was conducting his experiments that led to the development of 'plasmapheresis', a word he coined[168]. It was never used clinically. The crystalline form was extracted in 1929 and again in 1957.

Leeches are still used today in Europe and particularly in Russia. As Vigran recounts, the local druggist in these parts keeps them in glass jars filled with water overlying a sandy bottom. He also recounts how in certain parts of Europe 'it is still not uncommon to find a score of leeches applied over the enlarged liver of a patient suffering from congestive heart failure'[169]. I remember as a young boy growing up on the lower East Side of New York City how well stocked our local barbershops were with leeches for use by the newly arrived immigrants from Italy. Application of leeches and cupping were considered the first line of therapy for pneumonia in this preantibiotic era.

Heparin was discovered in the early 1900s. Two men were involved in its discovery. They were William Howell and Jay McLean. There is some controversy regarding the role each played in its discovery and development.

Howell is recognized as an outstanding authority on blood coagulation[170-173]. Howell was fortunate in being able to pursue his premedical studies at Johns Hopkins University. Although relatively new, the school had already created an image of fostering original research that bore no comparison with other American Universities. As a candidate for the Ph.D, Howell was working in Newell Martin's department of biology. The master assigned Howell the task of investigating the difference in coagulability between arterial and venous blood. He spent no more than two months on this project before he put it aside to work instead on finding the origin of the fibrin formed in the coagulation of blood. In his autobiographical notes, this is what Howell had to say about this period in his career. 'After working at it for a month or two without any assistance I came to the conclusion that there was nothing in the problem, and made a formal call upon Martin … to ask his permission to substitute another problem that had been suggested by my reading. He agreed, and I worked at my experiments very happily for the rest of the year; with only an occasional short visit from him to enquire how things were going. But when I took the finished dissertation to him he expressed himself as pleased with the results, and thereafter admitted me to a sort of inner circle'. Howell's thesis, *The Origin of the Fibrin Formed in the Coagulation of the Blood*, was published in December 1884[174].

Upon receiving his doctorate Howell remained with Martin as his chief assistant while carrying on a heavily laden teaching schedule. He soon left Johns Hopkins for a faculty position at the University of Michigan. He stayed only long enough to obtain a medical degree while attempting to engage in further research. He had left Johns Hopkins because of the excessive teaching demands that deprived him of much research time, but it was no better at Michigan. By this time, Howell's interest in research was such that he foresook clinical medicine for a career in physiology. After a year's stint at Harvard, Howell returned to his *alma mater* as professor of physiology in the newly established medical school. Howell was now well recognized as a physiologist, a reputation augmented and solidified by his recently published textbook on physiology. As head of his own department he could now allocate whatever time was needed in the pursuit of his interests in blood coagulation. In particular he focused on proving that the normal mammalian blood contained physiological inhibitors of coagulation. He demonstrated the presence of such a substance in 1911 and called it antithrombin[175].

Howell's investigations laid the groundwork for the isolation of heparin in 1916 by Jay McLean, a medical student from California, who was at that time working in Howell's laboratory. Howell had given McLean the problem of determining what was the significance and role of the clotting substance. It was during the course of this work that McLean discovered the anticoagulant. Acting against his mentor's wishes, the young student rushed into print the results of his research efforts[176]. He called it cephalin. The substance was quite impure and very toxic. It was left to Howell to prepare a more purified form.

McLean was a rather determined young man who was very anxious to establish himself as the leading individual in isolating heparin and to indicate that Howell had a subordinate role in this endeavor. This desire to protect his 'rights' as the discoverer of heparin may have been the reason for McLean's precipitous publication of his findings. He expressed his concern to Charles Best of Toronto in 1940. Best revealed this in his paper on heparin in 1959[177]. That same year McLean also recounted the circumstances surrounding his discovery of heparin in a paper published in *Circulation*[178].

Within two years after McLean's discovery Howell was already totally immersed in this new finding. In 1918, he described the anticoagulant in more detail and labeled it now heparin rather than antiprothrombin which he had initially suggested[179]. A detailed description of its physiologic and chemical behavior was presented by Howell in 1928[180]. By this time heparin's ability to prevent intravascular clotting was amply demonstrated in numerous animal experiments. Best's interest in heparin led him to be the first to administer it in humans in 1935[181]. Three years later Irving Wright turned his attention to it when he himself fell victim to a severe bout of thrombophlebitis causing him to inquire about an effective anticoagulant. That very same year Wright called upon Best and Murray to treat a patient under his care with refractory thrombophlebitis. These Canadians did their best but could not effectuate a complete cure because their supply of heparin ran out and could not be replenished in time[182].

The prophylactic value of heparin in postsurgical thrombosis was fully shown by Crafoord in 1937[183]. I have already mentioned the invaluable role that heparin played in the evolution of modern cardiovascular surgery. Recently there has been a resurgence of interest in assessing the role of heparin as an anticoagulant following thrombolytic therapy.

Heparin's major limitation has always been the inability to give it orally. It is for this reason that the coumarin derivatives became heparin's alternative in the diverse clinical indications that required prolonged or chronic therapy with anticoagulants.

The story begins in the early 1920s in that region of North America wherein North Dakota and Alberta are located. Cattle were being decimated by a peculiar disorder characterized by hemorrhage. Two veterinarians by the name of Schofield and Roderick were able to implicate sweet clover as the cause of the epidemic[184]. The disturbance came to be known as sweet clover disease. Nothing else was known about it and the matter rested there until 1933 when Karl Link was confronted by a distraught farmer with a dead calf covered with hematomas. The farmer was desperate and sought Link's help in trying to find out why sweet clover wreaked such havoc in cattle. There was a raging blizzard that night in Wisconsin, a farmer with a dead calf and with the instrument of its death, the sweet clover that the farmer used to feed the cattle since there was no other hay available because of the severe weather[185].

Link took up the challenge. Little did he realize that seven years would roll by before he could find the cause for the bleeding diathesis in those cattle unfortunate enough to eat sweet clover. This he did when in 1940 he identified the causal agent as dicoumarol. He was also able to synthesize this agent and over the course of the next two years his laboratory at the Agricultural Experimental Station was able to synthesize more than 100 related hydroxycoumarins. These were logged by number in accordance with their basic chemical structure. Those with the numbers 40 through 65 were studied in more detail because of their perceived potentialities as anticoagulants. Out of this group, two were found as being much more potent when administered to the rat or dog. He selected no. 42 as being ideal for killing rats and gave it the name warfarin. It is still sold today as a rodenticide under the same generic name. Warfarin is an acronym with 'warf' derived from the first letters of the Wisconsin Alumnae Research Foundation (that funded his research) and the 'arin' from coumarin[186]. Warfarin became available for clinical use upon the recommendation of S. M. Gordon of the Endo Laboratories, who, in turn, was pressured to do so by his friend, Karl Link. Endo marketed it under the trade name coumadin. Prior to that clinicians were using dicoumarol but soon found that coumadin was a better product.

Oral anticoagulation with dicoumarol had been started in a limited fashion in 1941 by the Mayo Clinic and O. O. Meyer at the University of Wisconsin[186]. The concept of oral anticoagulation in the treatment of coronary thrombosis seemed a logical step, and with an oral anticoagulant now available, along with vitamin K as a satisfactory antidote, clinical investigations were begun with this in mind. Multicenter trials were set up throughout the United States under the energetic leadership of Irving Wright in 1948[187]. This study generated so much enthusiasm that for almost two decades it was considered foolhardy for a physician to refrain from this therapeutic approach in myocardial infarction. Subsequent clinical studies doused the fire of its earlier acceptance until finally it was no longer considered proper as a routine measure[188-191]. The major point was that none of the clinical trials came up with irrefutable proof that treatment of myocardial infarction with anticoagulants lowered mortality. But this is not hard to understand since death from myocardial infarction has a multifactorial basis such as arrhythmias, congestive heart failure, cardiogenic shock, rupture of the myocardium and so on. One study did show that mortality due to thromboembolic complications was definitely lowered and within these parameters anticoagulant therapy was probably beneficial in this subset of patients[192].

The advent of thrombolytic therapy in the emergency management of acute myocardial infarction and unstable angina has created a resurgence of interest in anticoagulation as adjunctive therapy following successful thrombolysis. The pendulum now has swung back to anticoagulation but with a more selective focus in mind, namely, to prevent further formation of thrombus in the affected coronary artery.

During the past decade, antiplatelet agents have become part of the anticlotting armamentarium. This is especially so in coronary artery disease since it is now firmly established that arterial thrombosis is predominantly precipitated by the clumping of platelets. These agents include aspirin, dipyridamole and sulfinpyrazone. Dipyridamole is a vasodilator that is often used in conjunction with Coumadin to prevent the formation of clots on prosthetic valves. It has also become a component of the aspirin regimen in the alleged prevention of coronary artery thrombosis. The role of sulfinpyrazone at this writing is still controversial[193].

Aspirin has been found to be so effective that it was recently recognized as an antiplatelet agent by the National Heart, Lung, and Blood Institute Consensus Conference on antithrombotic therapy[194]. Aspirin has an interesting background, and it seems as though every day a new therapeutic door is opened with this commonplace drug.

Prior to 1876, the treatment of rheumatic fever was hopelessly shackled by the blood-letting practice so firmly entrenched in western medicine. Hope's book again is the repository for this therapeutic modality. He wrote: 'After one full bleeding, or even two, in robust subjects, but without any bleeding in the feeble and delicate, I give, every night calomel, and opium, according to the age and the severity of symptoms'[195]. The poor unfortunates were also given daily infusions of senna or magnesium sulphate, and, at times, wine of colchicum and powdered ipecac.

In 1876, J. J. Maclagen introduced salicylates in the treatment of rheumatic fever. He was apparently an advocate of botanically derived agents. This is how he came to select salicylates for rheumatic fever:

On reflection it seemed to me that the plants whose haunts best corresponded to this description, were those belonging to the various forms of willow. Among these therefore, I determined to search for a remedy for rheumatism.

The bark of many species of willow contains a bitter principle called salicin. This principle was exactly what I wanted. To it, therefore I determined to have recourse.

I began to use salicin in the treatment of rheumatism in November, 1874. A short experience sufficed to show that my expectations were likely to be more than realized ... But no one ever claimed for these remedies the power to rob acute rheumatism of all its dangers.[196]

How wise he was in realizing that salicylates gave relief but did not protect against the cardiac aftermath. 'Rheumatic fever licks the joints but bites the heart' was a clinical aphorism that has remained with me ever since my days in medical school.

Maclagen's observations on the use of salicin were unique in that the drug was used by him only for the treatment of rheumatic fever. However, its antipyretic powers were also being recognized; so much so, that the chemists became involved in finding congeners of salicin. Dressar's efforts resulted in the synthesis of acetylsalicylic acid in 1899[197]. Little did he realize what a monumental achievement this was to be. For many years aspirin (as it came to be known) was the standard salicylate remedy in acute rheumatic fever. The mid-20th century saw its use extended to the role of an anti-clotting agent, and currently there seems to be no doubt how beneficial aspirin is in this regard. Dressar coined the word 'aspirin' by combining 'a' with 'spir'. Spir was extracted from 'spiraeic acid', a term no longer used for salicylic acid. The 'a' came from 'acetyl' as in acetylsalicylic acid.

The list of antiarrhythmic drugs at the disposal of cardiologists has had an accordian-like pattern for the past several decades. The variability in the length of this list serves to emphasize that the ideal agent has yet to be found. Each newly introduced drug has carried with it its own peculiar side effects, often causing its demise.

Prior to 1950 the only useful antiarrhythmic drug available was quinidine. It has the distinction of being the only one with a botanical root. It is related to quinine which in turn has its origin in the cinchona bark. Quinidine like digitalis is a survivor. Despite its many adverse reactions it is still a widely used antiarrhythmic.

Two drugs appeared in 1950 that successfully competed with quinidine for the cardiologists' attention. They were procainamide and lidocaine. Both were local anesthetics. The 1960s saw the introduction of disopyramide, beta blockers, calcium antagonists and blockers of the late potassium outward current. As more knowledge accumulated about the sarcolemmal channels, drugs appeared that interfered with the fast sodium channel. In addition replacements were sought for the potentially toxic quinidine and lidocaine. The most important group that emerged from these efforts was that class of drugs characterized by their blocking effect on the fast inward sodium current. Some were effective against atrial arrhythmias while others were effective only in those arrhythmias arising from the ventricles. They included aprundine, disopyramide, lorcainide, tocainide, and mexiletine.

Over the course of time evidence was uncovered to support the belief that disturbances of the potassium gradient enhanced the probability of cardiac arrhythmias and that this was accompanied by a modified sensitivity to certain cardioactive drugs[198]. During the same period Hondeghem and Katzung[199] and independently Hille[200] formulated a 'modulated-receptor' hypothesis that interpreted the blocking of sodium channels in terms of association–dissociation of a blocking substance with a channel receptor. In 1982, Sanchez-Chapula and associates delineated in more detail the effects of lidocaine and benzocaine on cardiac sodium current[201].

The antiarrhythmic effect of calcium antagonists became increasingly evident ever since Fleckenstein first described their mode of action. This was repeatedly confirmed by Bigger[202], Kass[203] and Nawrath[204]. Kass and his coworkers also showed that the calcium antagonists blocked to a variable extent the late outward potassium current. This observation provided the explanation for the prolonged duration of the action potential rather than the reverse as one would expect if only inward calcium movement were blocked.

The focus on channel activity produced a number of antiarrhythmic agents. This eventually brought about a classification based on which ionic channel was blocked. In an attempt to improve drug selectivity, compounds were developed that blocked ionic channels in a way that depended on the state of the channel, that is, if the channel were in a resting, active or inactivated state.

The pharmacological management of arteriosclerosis had to wait for clarification of the role of cholesterol in its pathogenesis. This did not occur as we have seen until the 20th century (see Section 2). The development of cholesterol lowering agents did not start until the midportion of the century. The initial preparations acted only in the gut preventing the absorption of ingested cholesterol through the binding action of resins. An attempt was made during the 1960s to lower blood cholesterol levels by blocking its synthesis in the body. Although the concept was good the preparation (MER 29) blocked the synthesis at its penultimate precursor level with disastrous consequences. In the 1980s lovastatin was introduced as a CoA reductase inhibitor. This drug gained wide acceptance simply because it is very effective in blocking the hepatic synthesis of cholesterol at its earliest stage without too many adverse effects. In the 1990s reports began to appear that regression of atherosclerosis could be brought about by lowering serum cholesterol. Blankenhorn played a leading role in describing this beneficial turn of events with angiographic documentation of regression.

REFERENCES

1. Mettler, C.C. (1947). *History of Medicine* p. 173
2. Jastrow, M. (1917). Babylonian–Assyrian medicine. *Ann. M. Hist.*, **1**, 244
3. *Ibid.*, p. 238
4. Adams, F. (1849). *The Genuine Works of Hippocrates*, 2 vols., **2**, 725. (London)
5. Hort, A. (1916). *Theophrastus: Enquiry into Plants*, 2 vols. (London)
6. Mettler, C. *Op. cit.*, p.178.
7. Allbutt, C. (1901). Greek medicine in Rome. *Lancet*, **2**, 1332
8. von Jamersted, E. (1879). Ueber das Scillain. *Arch. Exp. Path. Pharmakol.*, **11**, 22–38
9. Adams, F. (1844–47). *The Seven Books of Paulus Aeginata*, vol. 3, p. 515. (London)
10. Frazer, J.G. (1926). *The Magic Art*, vol. 2. p. 33. (London)
11. Mettler, C. *Op. cit.*, pp. 177–8
12. Gunther, R.T. (1934). *The Greek Herbal of Dioscorides.* (Oxford)
13. Buck, A. (1917). *Growth of Medicine*, p. 317. (New Haven: Yale Univ. Press)
14. Walsh, J. (1927). Galen visits the Dead Sea and the copper mines of Cyprus. *Bull. Geogr. Soc. Phila.*, **25**, 99
15. Walsh, J. (1930). Galen's second sojourn in Italy and his treatment of the family of Marcus

Aurelius. *M. Life*, **37**, 490

16. Adams, F. (1844–47). *Op. cit.*, **3**, 1–2

17. Adams, F. (1844–7). *Op. cit.*, **2**, 238

18. Hitti, P. (1939). *History of the Arabs*, p. 368. (New York)

19. Siddiqui, H.H. and Aziz, M.A. (1963). A note on Ibn Sina's tract on cardiac drugs. *Planta Medica*, Jabrgong 11, Heft 4

20. Neuburger, M. (1910). *History of Medicine*, **2**, 8. (London)

21. Buck, A. (1917). *Op. cit.*, p. 404

22. Packard, F.R. (1922). Guy Patin and the medical profession in Paris in the seventeenth century. *Ann. M. Hist.*, **4**, 136–65, 215–40, 375–85, see p. 228

23. Mettler, C. *Op. cit.*, p. 206.

24. Hope, J. (1839). *A Treatise on the Diseases of the Heart and Great Vessels*. (London: John Churchill)

25. East, T. (1958). *The Story of Heart Disease*, p. 102. (London: William Dawson and Sons)

26. Hope, J. (1839). *Op. cit.*, pp. 501–2

27. Wheeler, C.E. (1913). *Organon of the Rational Art of Healing*, (translation of Hahnemann's paper published in Dresden in 1810). (London)

28. Sollman, T. (1932). *A Manual of Pharmacology*, p. 99. (Philladelphia)

29. Krantz, J.C. (1975). Historical background. In Needleman, P. (ed.) *Organic Nitrates*, p. 1. (New York: Springer-Verlag)

30. Hering, C. (1875). Glonoin or nitro glycerin. [Americanische Arzpneiprüfungen, translated with additions.] History as proved and applied by C. Hering, Philadelphia, 1847–1851. *N. Eng. Med. Gaz.*, **9**, 255, 337, 385, 433, 481, 529, **10**, 1

31. Munch, J.C. and Petter, H.H. (1965). Story of glyceryl trinitrate, development of glonoin. *J. Am. Pharmacol. Assoc.*, n.s. **5**, 493

32. Haehl, R. (1927). *Samuel Hahnemann, his Life and Work*. (London: Homoeopathic Publishing Co.)

33. Hering, C. (1849). Glonoine, a new medicine for headache. *Am. J. Homeopathy*, **4**, 3

34. Fye, W.B. (1986). Nitroglycerin: a homeopathic remedy. *Circulation*, **2**, 21–9

35. Field, A.G. (1858). On the toxical and medicinal properties of nitrate of oxyde of glycyl. *Med. Times Gazette*, **16**, 291

36. Fuller, H.W. (1858). Nitro-glycerine-glonoin. *Med. Times Gazette*, **1**, 356

37. Harley, G. (1858). Nitro-glycerin-glonoin. *Med. Times Gazette*, **1**, 356

38. Albers, J.F.H. (1864). Die physiologische und therapeutische Wirkung des Nitroglycerins.

Dtsch. Klin No., **42**, 405

39. Neuberger, M. (1981). *The Historical Development of Experimental Brain and Spinal Cord Physiology before Flourens*, translated by Clark E. Baltimore. (Johns Hopkins University Press)

40. Minor, A.J. and Hamilton, A.H. (1876). Tri-nitro-glycerine. Its physiological effects and therapeutical indications. *Am. Psychol. J.*, **3**, 103

41. Brunton, T.L. (1885). *A Textbook of Pharmacology, Therapeutics and Materia Medica*. (Philadelphia: Lea Brothers and Co.)

42. Murrell, W. (1879). Nitro-glycerine as a remedy for angina pectoris. *Lancet*, **1**, 80, 113, 151, 225

43. Smith, E. and Hart, F.D. (1971). William Murrell, physician and practical therapist. *Br. Med. J.*, **3**, 632

44. Martindale, W. (1880). Nitroglycerin in pharmacy. *Practitioner*, **24**, 35

45. Murrell, W. (1882). *Nitro-glycerine as a Remedy in Angina Pectoris*. (London: H.K. Lewis)

46. Murrell, W. (1885). Nitro-glycerine tablets. *Lancet*, **2**, 546

47. Hay, M. (1883). The chemical nature and physiological action of nitro-glycerin. *Practitioner*, **30**, 422

48. Peck, T.W. and Wilkinson, K.D. (1950). *William Withering of Birmingham, M.D., FRS., John Wright & Son, Ltd. (Bristol)*. (London: Simpkin Marshall)

49. Gillespie, C.C. (1976). (Editor in Chief) *Dictionary of Scientific Biography*, vol. XIV, pp. 463–4. (New York: Charles Scribner's Sons)

50. Somberg, J., Greenfield, P. and Tepper, D. (1985). Digitalis: historical development in clinical medicine. *J. Clin. Pharm.*, **25**, 484–9

51. Willius, F.A. and Dry, T.J. (1948). *A History of the Heart and the Circulation*, p. 10, 310. (Saunders)

52. Paterson, G.R. and Locock, M.J. (1967). The history of cardiac glycosides. *Applied Therapeutics*, January, pp. 60–5

53. Jacobs, M. (1936). A history of digitalis therapy. *Ann. Med. Hist.*, **8**, 492–9

54. Ferriar, J. (1799). *An Essay on the Medical Properties of Digitalis purpurea or Foxglove*. (Manchester, England: Sowler and Russell)

55. Bouillaud, J. (1835). *Traite Clinique des Maladies du Coeur*. (Paris)

56. McMichael, J. (1972). The history of ideas on digitalis action. In Marks, B. and Weissler, A. (eds.) *Basic and Clinical Pharmacology of Digitalis*, pp. 5–14. (Springfield, Ill.: Charles C. Thomas)

57. Gold, H. and Cattell, M. (1940). Mechanism of digitalis action abolishing heart failure. *Arch.*

Intern. Med., **65**, 263–78

58. Vulpian, M. (1855). *Gazette Med.*, **10**, 59

59. Aranson, J.K. (1984). Digitalis. In Parnham, M.J. and Bruinvels, J. (eds.) *Discoveries in Pharmacology*, vol. 2, pp. 163, 184. (Amsterdam: Elsevier Science Publishers)

60. Frank, O. (1959). Zur Dynamick des Herzmuskels. *Z. Biol.*, **32**, 370–409, 1895; (see also translation by Chapman, C.B. and Wasserman, E.): *Am Heart J.*, **58**, 282–467

61. Straub, W. (1924). Die Digitalis Gruppe. *Heffters Handbuch der experimentellen Pharmakologie*, vol. II 2, pp. 1335–452. (Berlin: Springer Verlag)

62. Lendle, L. (1935). Digitaliskorper und verwandte herzwirksame Glykoside (Digitaloide). Heffters Handbuch der experimentellen Pharmakologie. *Erganzungswerk*, vol. I. p. 193. (Berlin: Springer Verlag)

63. Bijlsma, U.G. and Roessingh (1922). Die Dynamik des Saugertierherzens unter dem Einfluss Von Stoffen der Digitalisgruppe. *Naunyn Schmiedebergs Arch Pharmacol.*, **94**, 235

64. Anitschkow, S.W. and Trendelenburg, P. (1928). Die Wirkung des Strophanthin auf das suffiziente und unsuffiziente Warmbluterherz. *Dtsch. Med. Wochenschr.*, **2**, 1672

65. Krayer, O. (1931). Versche am insuffizienten Herzen. *Naunyn Schmiedebergs Arch. Pharmacol.*, **162**, 1–28

66. Wiggers, C.J. and Stimson, B. (1927). Studies on the cardiodynamic of drugs. III, The mechanism of cardiac stimulation by digitalis and strophanthin. *J. Pharmacol. Exp. Ther.*, **30**, 251

67. Mackenzie, J. (1905). New methods of studying affections of the heart. *Br. Med. J.*, **1**, 587

68. Mackenzie, J. (1919). Digitalis. *Heart* (London), **2**, 273

69. Lewis, T. (1920). *The Mechanism and Graphic Registration of the Heart Beat*, pp. 308–9. (New York: Paul Hoeber)

70. Lewis, T. (1919). On cardinal principles in cardiological practice. *Br. Med. J.*, **2**, 621

71. Cohn, A.E. and Stewart, H.J. (1928). The relation between cardiac size and cardiac output per minute following the administration of digitalis in normal dogs. *J. Clin. Invest.*, **6**, 53

72. Cohn, A.E. and Stewart, H.J. (1928). The relation between cardiac size and cardiac output per minute following the administration of digitalis in dogs in which the heart is enlarged. *J. Clin. Invest.*, **6**, 79

73. Stewart, H.J. and Cohn, A.E. (1932). Studies on the effect of the action of digitalis on the output of blood from the heart. II, The effect on the output of the hearts of dogs subject to artificial auricular fibrillation. *J. Clin. Invest.*, **11**, 897

74. Stewart, H.J. and Cohn, A.E. (1932). Studies on the effect of the action of digitalis on the output of blood from the heart. III. Part 1, The effect on the output in normal human hearts; and Part 2, The effect on the output of hearts in heart failure with congestion in human beings. *J. Clin. Invest.*, **11**, 917

75. Mason, D.T. and Braunwald, E. (1968). Digitalis, new facts about an old drug. *Am. J. Cardiol.*, **22**, 151

76. Smith, W. and Haber, F. (1973). Digitalis. *N. Engl. J. Med.*, **289**, 945, 1063

77. Donovan, M. (1840). On the injurious effects of the pharmaceutical treatment of *Digitalis purpurea*, in forming its tincture, with a proposal for a more efficacious formula. *Dublin Journal of Medical Science*, May, 1839; through *Am. J. Pharm.*, **11**, 204

78. Homolle, E. Memoire sur la digitale pourpree, *J. Pharm. Chim.*, 3rd series, **7**, 57 (1845). Homolle, M., *Am. J. Pharm.*, **17**, 97–105, (1846)

79. Homolle, E. and Quévenne, T.A. (1935). *Arch. Physiol. Therap. Hygien.*, (Bouchardat) 1 (1854); through Elderfield, R.C., *Chem. Rev.*, **17**, 185

80. Elderfield, R.C. (1935). *Chem. Rev.*, **17**, 185,

81. Nativelle, C.A. (1869). *J. Pharm. Chim.*, 4th. series, **9**, 255

82. Movitt, E.R. (1946). *Digitalis and other Cardiotonic Drugs*, p. 112. (Oxford Press)

83. Cloetta, M. (1920). *Arch. Exp. Pathol. Pharmakol.*, **88**, 113

84. Windaus, A. and Stein, G. (1928). *Ber.*, **6**, 2436

85. Stoll, A. (1937). *The Cardiac Glycosides.* (London: Pharmaceutical Press)

86. Smith, S.J. (1930). *Chem. Soc.*, p. 508

87. Cahn, R.S. *et al.* (1951). *Chem. Ind.*, SN 1

88. Withering, W. (1785). *An Account of the Foxglove and Some of It's Medical Uses: Practical Remarks on Dropsy and Other Diseases.* (Birmingham, UK: M. Sweney)

89. Gwilt, P.R. and Gwilt, J.R. (1978). Dame Agatha's poisonous pharmacopoeia. *Pharm. J.*, **221**, 572–3

90. Parson, J. (1971). Le Médicin Criminel Coutis de la Pommerais. *Histoire de la Medicine*, **21**, 33–45

91. Burchell, H.B. (1983). Digitalis poisoning: historical and forensic aspects. *J. Am. Coll. Cardiol.*, **2**, 506–16

92. Wyckoff, J. and Gold, H. (1930). A dangerous

preparation of digitalis. *J. Am. Med. Assoc.*, **94**, 627

93. Oliver, G. and Shäfer, E.A. (1895). On the physiological action of extract of the suprarenal capsules. *J. Physiol.*, London, **16**, i–iv, 1894; **17**, ix–xiv, 1895; **18**, 230–79

94. Davenport, H.W. (1982). Epinephrin(e), *The Physiologist*, **25**

95. Abel, J.J. and Crawford, A.C. (1897). On the blood-pressure-raising constituent of the suprarenal capsule. *Johns Hopkins Hosp. Bull.*, **8**, 151–7

96. Abel, J.J. (1898). Further observations on the chemical nature of the active principle of the suprarenal capsule. *Johns Hopkins Hosp. Bull.*, **9**, 215–18

97. Abel, J.J. (1899). Ueber den blutdruck-erregendes Bestandtheil des Nebenniere, das Epinephrin. *Hoppe-Seylers Z. Physiol. Chem.*, **28**, 318–62

98. United States Trade Mark **86**, 269; 16 Apr. 1901

99. Takamine, J. (1902). The blood-pressure-raising principle of the suprarenal gland. *J. Am. Med. Assoc.*, **38**, 153–5

100. English Patent 1467; 22 Jan. 1901

101. Takamine, J. (1901). The blood-pressure-raising principle of the suprarenal glands: a preliminary report. *Ther. Gaz. Detroit*, **16**, 221–4

102. Takamine, J. (1902). Adrenalin; the active principle of the suprarenal gland. *Scott. Med. Surg. J.*, **10**, 131–8

103. Takamine, J. (1901). Adrenalin; the active principle of the suprarenal gland. *Am. J. Pharm.*, **73**, 523–31, 1901. Houghton, E.M. The pharmacological assay of preparations of the suprarenal gland. *Am. J. Pharm.*, **73**, 531–5

104. Elliot, R. (1905). The action of adrenalin. *J. Physiol.* (London), **32**, 401

105. Goldberg, L.I. (1972). Cardiovascular and renal action of dopamine. Potential clinical application. *Pharmacol. Rev.*, **24**, 1

106. Tuttle, R.R. and Mills, J. (1975). Dobutamine: development of a new catecholamine to selectively increase cardiac contractility. *Circ. Res.*, **36**, 185

107. Alousi, A.A,, Farah, A.E., Lesher, G.Y. and Opalka, C.J. (1979). Cardiotonic activity of amrinone, Win 40680 [5-amino-3,4' bipyridine-6-(1H)-one]. *Circ. Res.*, **45**, 666

108. Alousi, A.A., Stankus, G.P., Stuart, J.C. and Walton, L.H. (1983). Characterization of the cardiotonic effects of milrinone, a new and potent cardiac bipyridine on isolated tissue from several animal species. *J. Cardiovasc. Pharmacol.*, **5**, 804

109. Fleckenstein, A. (1983). History of calcium antagonists. *Circ. Res.*, Suppl. I, Calcium Channel-blocking Drugs, vol. **52**, no. 2

110. Fleckenstein, A. and Grün, G. (1969). Reversible Blockierung der elektromech-anischen Koppelungsprozesse in der glatten Muskulatur des Rattenuterus mittels organischer Ca++ -Antagonisten (1proveratril, D600, Prenylamin). *Pfluegers Arch.*, **307**, R26

111. Grün, G. and Fleckenstein, A. (1972). Die elektromechanische Entkoppelung der glatten Gefaàmuskulature als Grundprinzip der Coronar-dilatation durch 4-(2'-Nitrophenyl)-2,6-dimethyl-1,4-dihydropyridin-3,5-dicarbonsaure-dimethylester (Bay a 1040, Nifedipin). *Arznei-mittelforsch*, **22**, 334–44

112. Grün, G., Fleckenstein, A. and Byon, Y.K. (1971). Hemmung der Motilität isolierter Uterus-Streifen aus gravidem und nicht gravidem menschlichen Myometrium durch Ca++ -Antagonisten und Sympathomimetica. *Arzneimit-telforsch*, **21**, 1585–90

113. Fleckenstein, A. (1968). Myokardstoffwechsel und Nekrose. In Heilmeyer, I. and Holtmeier, H.J. (eds.) *VI Symposium der Deutsch. Ges. für fortschritte auf dem Gebiet der Inneren Medizin über Herzinfarkt und Schock*, November 8, 1969, in Freiburg, pp. 94–109. (Stuttgart: Georg Thieme Verlag)

114. Fleckenstein, A. (1970/71). Specific inhibitors and promoters of calcium action in the excitation-contraction coupling of heart muscle and their role in the production or prevention of myocardial lesions. In Harris, P. (ed.) *Calcium and the Heart, Proceedings of the Meeting of the European Section of the International Study Group for Research in Cardiac Metabolism*, London, September 6, 1970. I. Opie., pp. 135–88. (New York: Academic Press)

115. Nayler, W.G., Grau, A. and Slade, A. (1976). A protective effect of verapamil on hypoxic heart muscle. *Cardiovasc. Res.*, **10**, 650–62

116. Henry, P.D., Shuchleib, R., Borda, L.J., Roberts, R., Williamson, J.R. and Sobel, B.C. (1978). Effects of nifedipine on myocardial perfusion and ischemic injury in dogs. *Circ. Res.*, **43**, 372–80

117. Bing, R.J., Weishaar, R., Rackl, A. and Pawlik, G. (1979). Antianginal drugs and cardiac metabolism. In Bing, R.J. (ed.) *New Drug Therapy with a Calcium Antagonist, Diltiazem,*

Hakone Symposium, 1978, pp. 27–37. (Amsterdam-Princeton: Excerpta Medica)

118. Nagao, T., Matlib, M.A., Franklin, D., Millard, R.W. and Schwartz, A. (1980). Effects of diltiazem, a calcium antagonist, on regional myocardial function and mitochondria after brief coronary occlusion. *J. Mol. Cell. Cardiol.*, **12**, 29–43

119. Bender, F., Kojima, N., Reploh, H. and Oelmann, G. (1966). Behandlung tachykarder Rhythmusstörungen des Herzens durch Beta-Rezeptorenblockade des Atrioventrikular-gewebes. *Med. Welt.*, **17**, 1120–3

120. Schamroth, I,. Krikler, D. and Garrett, C. (1972). Immediate effects of intravenous vera-pamil in cardiac arrhythmias. *Br. Med. J.*, **I**, 660–2

121. Zipes, C.P. and Fischer, J.C. (1974). Effects of agents which inhibit the slow channel on sinus node automaticity and atrioventricular conduction in the dog. *Circ. Res.*, **34**, 184–92

122. Wit, A.L. and Cranefield, P.F. (1974). Effect of verapamil on the sinoatrial and atrioventricular nodes of the rabbit and the mechanism by which it arrests reentrant atrioventricular nodal tachycardia. *Circ. Res.*, **35**, 413–25

123. Narimatsu, A. and Taira, N. (1976). Effects on atrioventricular conduction of calcium antagon-istic coronary vasodilators, local anaesthetics and quinidine injected into the posterior and the anterior septal artery of the atrioventricular node preparation of the dog. *Naunyn Schmiedebergs Arch. Pharmacol.*, **294**, 169–77

124. Taira, N. and Narimatsu, A. (1975). Effects of nifedipine, a potent calcium-antagonistic coro-nary vasodilator, on atrioventricular conduction and blood flow in the isolated atrioventricular node preparation of the dog. *Naunyn Schmiedebergs Arch Pharmacol.*, **290**, 107–12

125. Taira, N., Motomura, S., Narimatsu, A., Satoh, K. and Yanagisawa, T. (1980). The effect of calcium-antagonists on atrioventricular con-duction. In Fleckenstein, A. and Roskamm, H. (eds.) *Calcium-Antagonismus*, pp. 42–3. (Berlin-Heidelberg-New York: Springer Verlag)

126. Nakajima, H., Hoshiyama, M., Yamashita, K. and Kiyomoto, A. (1975). Effect of diltiazem on electrical and mechanical activity of isolated cardiac ventricular muscle of guinea-pig. *Jpn. J. Pharmacol.*, **25**, 383–92

127. Ahlquist, R.P. (1948). A study of the adreno-tropic receptors. *Am. J. Physiol.*, **153**, 586–600

128. Powell, C.E. and Slater, I.H. (1958). Blocking of inhibitory adrenergic receptors by a dichloro analog of isoproterenol. *J. Pharmacol. Exp. Ther.*, **122**, 480–8

129. Black, J.W. and Stephenson, J.S. (1962). Pharmacology of a new beta-adrenergic receptor blocking compound. *Lancet*, **2**, 311–14

130. Black, J.W. and Prichard, B.N.C. (1973). Activation and blockade of β-adrenoceptors in common cardiac disorders. *Br. Med. Bull.*, **29**, 163–7

131. Emorine, L.J., Marullo, S., Briend-Sutren, M.M., Patey, G., Tate, K., Delavier-Klutchko, C. and Strosberg, D. (1989). Molecular characterization of the human β3-adrenergic receptor. *Science*, **245**, 1118–21

132. Richards, A.N. (1938). The Croonian lectures. Processes of urine formation. *Proc. R. Soc., London (Biol.)*, **126**, 398

133. Walker, A.M., Bott, P.A., Oliver, J. and MacDowell, M.C. (1941). The collection and analysis of fluid from single nephrons of the mammalian kidney. *Am. J. Physiol.*, **134**, 580

134. Saxl, P. and Heilig, R. (1920). Ueber die diuretische Wirkung von Novasurol und anderen Quecksilberinjektionen. *Wien. Klin. Wochenschr.*, **33**, 943

135. Mann, T. and Keilin, D. (1940). Sulfanilamide as a specific inhibitor of carbonic anhydrase. *Nature (London)*, **146**, 164

136. Pitts, R.F. and Alexander, R.S. (1945). The nature of the renal tubular mechanism for acidifying the urine. *Am. J. Physiol.*, **144**, 239

137. Krebs, H.A. (1948). Inhibition of carbonic anhydrase by sulfonamides. *Biochem. J.*, **43**, 525

138. Schwartz, W.B. (1949). The effect of sulfanil-amide on salt and water excretion in congestive heart failure. *N. Engl. J. Med.*, **240**, 173

139. Roblin, R.O. Jr and Clapp, J.W. (1950). The preparation of heterocyclic sulfonamides. *J. Am. Chem. Soc.*, **72**, 4890

140. Maren, T.H. (1952). Pharmacological and renal effects of Diamox (6063), a new carbonic anhydrase inhibitor. *Trans. N. Y. Acad. Sci.*, **15**, 53

141. Beyer, K.H. Jr (1977). Diuretics in perspective. *J. Clin. Pharm.*, 618–24

142. Beyer, K.H. (1954). Factors basic to the development of useful inhibitors of renal transport mechanisms. *Arch. Int. Pharmacodyn.*, **98**, 97

143. Beyer, K.H., Baer, J.E., Russo, H.F. and Noll, R. (1958). Electrolyte excretion as influenced by chlorothiazide. *Science*, **127**, 146

144. Beyer, K.H. (1958). Chlorothiazide and other diuretic agents. *Ann. N. Y. Acad. Sci.*, **71**, 321

145. Beyer, K.H. and Baer, J.E. (1960). Newer diuretics. *Fortschr. Arzneimittelforsch.*, **2**, 9

146. Beyer, K.H., Baer, J.E., Michaelson, J.K. and Russo, H.F. (1965). Renotropic characteristics of ethacrynic acid: a phenoxyacetic saluretic–diuretic agent. *J. Pharmacol.*, **147**, 1

147. Hook, J.B. and Williamson, H.E. (1965). Effect of furosemide on renal medullary sodium gradient. *Proc. Soc. Exp. Biol. Med.*, **118**, 372

148. Duchin, K. and Hutcheon, D. (1974). Renal pharmacology of bumetanide. A new sulfamoyl-metanilic acid diuretic. *J. Clin. Pharmacol.*, **14**, 396

149. Davies, D.L., Lant, A.F., Millard, N.R., Smith, A.J., Ward, J.W. and Wilson, G.M. (1974). Renal action, therapeutic use and pharmacokinetics of the diuretic bumetanide. *Clin. Pharmacol. Ther.*, **15**, 141

150. Baer, J.E., Jones, C.B., Spitzer, S.A. and Russo, H.F. (1967). The potassium-sparing and natriuretic activity of N-amidino-3, 5-diamino – 6 chloro -pyraziinecarboxamide hydrochloride dihydrate (amiloride hydrochloride). *J. Pharmacol.*, **157**, 472

151. Wiebelhaus, V.D., Weinstock, J., Brennan, F.T., Sosnowski, G. and Larsen, T.J. (1961). A potent, non-steroidal orally active antagonist of aldosterone. *Fed. Proc.*, **20**, 409

152. Barratt, L.J. (1975). Effects of amiloride on the transepithelial potential difference of the distal tubule of the rat kidney. *Clin. Exp. Pharmacol. Physiol.*, **2**, 88

153. Crabbe, J. (1968). A hypothesis concerning the mode of action of amiloride and triamterene. *Arch. Int. Pharmacodyn.*, **173**, 474

154. Simpson, S.A., Tait, J.F., Wettstein, A., Neher, R., von Euw, J., Schlindler, O. and Reichstein, T. (1954). Die Konstitution des Aldosterons: Ueber Bestandteile der Nebennierenrinde und verwandte Stoffe. *Helv. Chim. Acta.*, **37**, 1200

155. Kagawa, C.M., Sturtevant, F.M. and Van Arman, C.G. (1959). Pharmacology of a new steroid that blocks salt activity of aldosterone and desoxycorticosterone. *J. Pharmacol.*, **126**, 123

156. Paton, W.D.M. and Zaimis, E.M. (1949). The pharmacological actions of polymethylene bistrimethyl-ammonium salts. *Br. J. Pharmacol. Chemother.*, **4**, 381–400

157. Smirk, F.H. (1950). Methonium compounds in hypertension. *Lancet*, **2**, 477

158. Turner, R. (1950). Medical sympathectomy in hypertension. A clinical study of methonium compounds. *Lancet*, **2**, 353–8

159. Freis, E.D. (1951). Methonium compounds in hypertension. *Lancet*, **1**, 909

160. Schroeder, H.A. (1953). *Hypertensive Diseases: Causes and Control.* (London: Henry Kimpton)

161. Smirk, F.H. (1953). Action of a new methonium compound in arterial hypertension. *Lancet*, **1**, 457–64

162. Vakil, R.J. (1949). A clinical trial of rauwolfia serpentina in essential hypertension. *Br. Heart J.*, **11**, 350–5

163. Freis, E.D. (1954). Mental depression in hypertensive patients treated for long periods with large doses of reserpine. *N. Engl. J. Med.*, **251**, 1006–8

164. Taylor, R.D., Dustan, H.P., Corcoran, A.C. and Page, I.H. (1952). Evaluation of 1-hydrazinophthalazine (apresoline) in treatment of hypertensive disease. *Arch. Intern. Med.*, **90**, 734–49

165. Wilkins, R.W. (1954). Rauwolfia in the treatment of essential hypertension. *Am. J. Med.*, **17**, 703–11

166. Haycraft, J.B. (1884). On the action of secretion obtained from the medical leech on the coagulation of blood. *Proc. R. Soc. London*, **36**, 478

167. Jacoby, C. (1904). Über Hirudin. *Deutsche Med. Wochenschr.*, **30**, 1786

168. Parascandola, J. (1982). John J. Abel and the early development of pharmacology at the Johns Hopkins University. *Bull. Hist. Med.*, **56**, 512

169. Vigran, I.M. (1974). History of anticoagulants. *Heart and Lung*, **3**, 812–16

170. Erlanger, J. (1950). Biographical memoir of William Henry Howell 1860–1945. *Natl. Acad. Sci. Biog. Memoirs*, **26**, 153

171. The celebration of the sixtieth anniversary of Dr. William H. Howell's graduation from the Johns Hopkins University. *Bull. Johns Hopkins Hosp.*, **68**, 291

172. (1961). An anniversary tribute to the memory of the late William Henry Howell. *Bull. Johns Hopkins Hosp.*, **109**, 1

173. Harvey, A.M. (1975). Fountainhead of American physiology; H. Newell Martin and his pupil, William Henry Howell. *Johns Hopkins Med. J.*, **136**, 38

174. Howell, W.H. (1884). The origin of the fibrin formed in the coagulation of blood. *Stud. Biol. Lab. Johns Hopkins Univ.*, **3**, 63

175. Howell, W.H. (1911). The role of antithrombin and thromboplastin (thromboplastic substance) in the coagulation of blood. *Am. J. Physiol.*, **29**, 187

176. McLean, J. (1916). The thromboplastic action of cephalin. *Am. J. Physiol.*, **41**, 250

177. Best, C.H. (1959). Preparation of heparin and its use in the first clinical cases. *Circulation*, **19**, 79

178. McLean, J. (1959). The discovery of heparin. *Circulation*, **19**, 75

179. Howell, W.H. and Holt, E. (1918). Two new factors in blood coagulation: heparin and pro-antithrombin. *Am. J. Physiol.*, **47**, 328

180. Howell, W.H. and Holt, E. (1928). The purification of heparin and its chemical and physiological reactions. *Bull. Johns Hopkins Hosp.*, **47**, 199

181. Best, C.H. (1959). *Op. cit.*

182. Wright, I.S. (1959). Experience with anticoagulants. *Circulation*, **19**, 110

183. Crafoord, C. (1965). The development of cardiovascular surgery. *J. Cardiovasc. Surg.*, (Torino) (Suppl.), **1**

184. Link, K.P. (1959). The discovery of dicoumarol and its sequels. *Circulation*, **19**, 97

185. Hunter, R.B. (1961). Review of the action of oral anticoagulants on the coagulation mechanism. *Symposium on Anticoagulant Therapy, Report of the Proceedings*. (London: Harvey & Blythe, Ltd)

186. Butt, H.R., Allen, E.V. and Bollman, J.L. (1941). Preparation from spoiled sweet clover (3,31-methylene-bis-4-hydroxycoumarin) which prolongs the coagulation and prothrombin time of blood: preliminary report of experimental and clinical studies. *Proc. Staff Meet. Mayo Clin.*, **16**, 388

187. Wright, I.S., Marple, C.D. and Beck, D.F. (1948). Report of the committee for evaluation of anticoagulants in the treatment of coronary thrombosis with myocardial infarction. *Am. Heart J.*, **38**, 801–15

188. Report of the Working Party on Anticoagulant Therapy in Coronary Thrombosis to the Medical Research Council (1969). Assessment of short-term anticoagulant administration after cardiac infarction. *Br. Med. J.*, **1**, 335–42

189. Cooperative Study (1969). Long-term anticoagulant therapy after myocardial infarction: final report of the Veteran Administration cooperative study. *J. Am. Med. Assoc.*, **207**, 2263

190. International Anticoagulant Review Group (1970). A collaborative analysis of long term anticoagulant administration following acute myocardial infarction. *Lancet*, **1**, 203

191. Meuwissen, O.J.A.T., Vervoorn, A.C., Cohen, O. *et al.* (1969). Double-blind trial of long-term anticoagulant treatment after myocardial infarction. *Acta Med. Scand.*, **186**, 361

192. Results of a Cooperative Clinical Trial (1973). Anticoagulants in acute myocardial infarction. *J. Am. Med. Assoc.*, **225**, 724

193. Anturane Reinfarction Trial Policy Committee (1982). The Anturane Reinfarction Trial: reevaluation of outcome. *N. Engl. J. Med.*, **306**, 1005–8

194. Hirsh, J., Fuster, V. and Salzman, E. (1986). Antiplatelet agents: the relationship among dose, side effects, and antithrombotic effectiveness. *Chest.*, **89** (Suppl.), 4S–10S

195. Hope, J. (1839). *Op cit.*, p. 179

196. Maclagan, T.J. (1886). *Rheumatism, Its Nature, Its Pathology and Its Successful Treatment*, p. 156. (London)

197. Feil, H. (1959). History of the treatment of heart disease in the nineteenth century. Read at *The Symposium of the Heart, American Association for the History of Medicine*, 32nd annual meeting, Cleveland, Ohio

198. Dryfus, L.S., de Azevedo, I.M. and Watanabe, Y. (1974). Electrolyte and antiarrhythmic drug interaction. *Am. Heart J.*, **88**, 995–1007

199. Hondeghem, L.M. and Katzung, B.G. (1977). Time and voltage-dependent interactions of antiarrhythmic drugs with cardiac sodium channels. *Biochem. Biophys. Acta*, **472**, 373–98

200. Hille, B. Local anesthetics: hydrophilic and hydrophobic pathways for drug–receptor reaction. *J. Gen. Physiol.*, **69**, 497–515

201. Sanchez-Chapula, Tsuda, T.Y., Josephson, I. and Brown, A.M. (1982). Effects of lidocaine and benzocaine on cardiac sodium current. *Biophys. J.*, **37**, 238a (Abstr.)

202. Bigger, J.T. and Mandel, W.J. (1970). Effect of lidocaine on the electrophysiological properties of ventricular muscle and Purkinje fibers. *J. Clin. Invest.*, **49**, 63–77

203. Kass, R.S. and Tsien, R.W. (1975). Multiple effects of calcium antagonists on plateau currents in cardiac Purkinje fibers. *J. Gen. Physiol.*, **66**, 169–92

204. Nawrath, H., Tenfick, R.E., McDonald, T.F. and Trautwein, W. (1977). On the mechanism underlying the action of D600 on slow inward current and tension in mammalian myocardium. *Circ. Res.*, **40**, 408–14

Index

Klein, O.   560–561
Kleist, Ewald von   241
Klotz, Oscar   109, 116
Kluge, T.   43
knives in mitral valve surgery   634, 636
Knoll, Philipp   348
Kobylinski, O.   403
Koch, E.   325
Koelliker, Rudolph Albert von   36
Kolesov, Vasillii I.   661
Kolff, W.J.   666
Köllicker, A.   520, 532, 534
Kolte, Harold   568
Kon, Y.   118
Kopp, W.   411
Korotkoff (Nicolai Sergeyevich)   497–499
    sounds   497–499, 512
Koster, G.   268
Kouwenhoven, William   365–366, 367
Krause, S.   130
Krayer, O.   716
Kreb's cycle   230, 233
Krehl, L.   77
Kreysig, Friedrich Ludwig   65, 715
Krogh, August   208
Kronecker, Hugo   249
Kümmell, Hermann   601
Kussmaul, Adolph   452
kymograph (kymography)   556
    Ludwig's manometer and   207–208, 218, 496, 501–502,
    504

La Gallois, Julian Cesar   641
Labbé, M.   305
Ladon, A.   268
Laénnec, René Theophile-Hyacinthe   75, 84, 85, 89, 94,
    148, 162, 454, 463, 466, 468–472, 473, 480–482
Laffont, M.   267
Lambert–Hallowell operation   600
Lamont, Austin   622
Lancisi, Maria   56–57, 87, 98–100
Landis, E.M.   326
Landois, Leonard   623
Landouzy–Déjérine dystrophy   134
Landsteiner, Karl   623
Lane, Sir Arbuthnot   628
Langley, John Newport   269, 269–270
Laragh, John   329–330
Larry, M.J.   406
Larson, E.W.   96
laryngoscopy   621
Lau, E.   515
Lauterbur, P.C.   592
Lavoisier, Antoine Laurent   206, 207, 557
law of heart, Starling's   225–228
Lazari, Julio   340
leads
    ECG   530
    pacemaker   376

Leared, Arthur   474
Leary, Timothy   119
Leatham, Aubrey   507, 509–512
Lebowitz, E.   586
Leckrome, Michael   375
leeches   724–725
Leeuwenhoek, Antoni van   41, 43
Lenard, Philipp   533
Lenègre, Jean   336, 563
lens, apochromatic, string galvanometers and   519
lentigenes, multiple (in LEOPARD syndrome)   406, 407
LEOPARD syndrome   406–407
Lerich, René   605
Levin, Sheldon M.   607–608
Levine, Samuel   535, 629, 630, 631
Levy, Alfred Goodman   335, 365
Levy, S.E.   325
Lewinski, L.   321–322
Lewis, John   639
Lewis, Sir Thomas   256, 269, 299, 340, 342, 347, 349,
    350, 351–352, 353, 353–354, 354, 364–365, 502, 505,
    531–533, 632, 716
Lexer, Erich   605
Leyden, Ernst Victor von   298, 320–321
Leyden jar/flask   241, 242, 243, 245
Li, T.W.   119
Libavius, Andreas   622–623
Libman, Emanuel   66, 299
lidocaine   727, 728
Lidwill, Mark C.   370–372
Liebreich, Richard   324
ligament, Botallo's   23
ligation
    with aneurysms   599
    carotid artery   611
    ductus arteriosus   654–655
    internal mammary artery   662
Liljestrand, G.   209, 211
Lillehei, C. Walton   642, 643–644, 645, 648
Lillehei–Kaster valve   652
limb–girdle muscular dystrophy   134
Lincoln, Abraham
    aortic insufficiency   455, 456
    Marfan's syndrome   413, 455
Lindbergh, Charles   602, 642
Lindenthal, O.T.   565
linear array transducers in echocardiography   578
Ling, G.   258, 260
Ling–Gerard electrode   258, 260
Link, Karl   726
lipid (fat)
    dietary, atherosclerosis and   117–121
    elevated levels
        genetic factors causing   428–430
        pharmacotherapy   728
lipiodol   566
lipoma, cardiac   129
lipoprotein, low-density (LDL)   427
    atherosclerosis and   117, 120, 121